D1619537

SPINE and SPINAL CORD TUMORS

Advanced Management and Operative Techniques

Spine and Spinal Cord Tumors

Advanced Management and Operative Techniques

EDITED BY

Christopher P. Ames, MD

Professor of Neurosurgery; Director of Spine Tumor Surgery,
Department of Neurological Surgery,
University of California San Francisco, San Francisco, California

Stefano Boriani, MD

Director, Department of Oncologic and Degenerative Spine Surgery,
Rizzoli Orthopedic Institute, Bologna, Italy

Rahul Jandial, MD, PhD

Assistant Professor, Division of Neurosurgery,
City of Hope Comprehensive Cancer Center,
Los Angeles, California

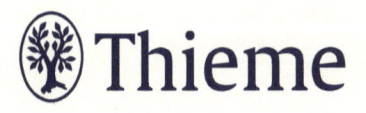

Thieme

Director, Editorial Services: Mary Jo Casey
International Production Director: Andreas Schabert
International Marketing Director: Fiona Henderson
International Sales Director: Louisa Turrell
Director of Sales, North America: Mike Roseman
Senior Vice President and Chief Operating Officer: Sarah Vanderbilt
President: Brian D. Scanlan

**Library of Congress Cataloging-in-Publication Data
is available from the publisher upon request.**

© 2014 Thieme Medical Publishers, Inc.
Thieme Publishers New York
333 Seventh Avenue, New York, NY 10001 USA
+1 800 782 3488, customerservice@thieme.com

Thieme Publishers Stuttgart
Rüdigerstrasse 14, 70469 Stuttgart, Germany
+49 [0]711 8931 421, customerservice@thieme.de

Thieme Publishers Delhi
A-12, Second Floor, Sector-2, Noida-201301
Uttar Pradesh, India
+91 120 45 566 00, customerservice@thieme.in

Thieme Publishers Rio, Thieme Publicações Ltda.
Edifício Rodolpho de Paoli, 25º andar
Av. Nilo Peçanha, 50 – Sala 2508
Rio de Janeiro 20020-906, Brasil
+55 21 3172 2297

Cover design by Thieme Publishers, Inc.

Printed in Germany by CPI Books   5 4 3 2

ISBN 978-1-62623-646-2
Also available as an e-book:
eISBN 978-1-62623-903-6

Important note: Medicine is an ever-changing science undergoing continual development. Research and clinical experience are continually expanding our knowledge, in particular our knowledge of proper treatment and drug therapy. Insofar as this book mentions any dosage or application, readers may rest assured that the authors, editors, and publishers have made every effort to ensure that such references are in accordance with **the state of knowledge at the time of production of the book.**

Nevertheless, this does not involve, imply, or express any guarantee or responsibility on the part of the publishers in respect to any dosage instructions and forms of applications stated in the book. **Every user is requested to examine carefully** the manufacturers' leaflets accompanying each drug and to check, if necessary in consultation with a physician or specialist, whether the dosage schedules mentioned therein or the contraindications stated by the manufacturers differ from the statements made in the present book. Such examination is particularly important with drugs that are either rarely used or have been newly released on the market. Every dosage schedule or every form of application used is entirely at the user's own risk and responsibility. The authors and publishers request every user to report to the publishers any discrepancies or inaccuracies noticed. If errors in this work are found after publication, errata will be posted at www.thieme.com on the product description page.

Some of the product names, patents, and registered designs referred to in this book are in fact registered trademarks or proprietary names even though specific reference to this fact is not always made in the text. Therefore, the appearance of a name without designation as proprietary is not to be construed as a representation by the publisher that it is in the public domain.

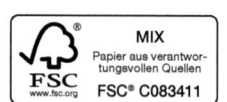

This book, including all parts thereof, is legally protected by copyright. Any use, exploitation, or commercialization outside the narrow limits set by copyright legislation without the publisher's consent is illegal and liable to prosecution. This applies in particular to photostat reproduction, copying, mimeographing or duplication of any kind, translating, preparation of microfilms, and electronic data processing and storage.

*I dedicate this work to my children, Peaarson, Sebastian, and Scarlett.
It is my hope that they find careers that they love,
because that is the key to true success.
I also dedicate this work to my spinal tumor patients,
who have shown me so many times the real meaning of courage
and who have taught me so much about life.*

C.P.A.

To Lori, my love and my best friend.

S.B.

*To my mother, Sushma Jandial,
for always reminding me that you are who you choose to be.*

R.J.

Contributors

Frank L. Acosta, Jr., MD
Associate Professor, Department of Neurosurgery, University of Southern California, Los Angeles, California

Luca Amendola, MD
Doctor, Department of Orthopedics and Traumatology–Spine Surgery, Maggiore Hospital, Bologna, Italy

Christopher P. Ames, MD
Professor of Neurosurgery; Director of Spine Tumor Surgery, Department of Neurological Surgery, University of California San Francisco, San Francisco, California

Henry E. Aryan, MD, FACS, FAANS
Associate Professor of Clinical Neurosurgery, Department of Neurological Surgery, University of California San Francisco, San Francisco, California

Kurtis Ian Auguste, MD
Associate Physician, Department of Neurological Surgery, University of California San Francisco, San Francisco; Staff Neurosurgeon, Department of Neurological Surgery, Children's Hospital and Research Center Oakland, Oakland, California

Ali A. Baaj, MD
Assistant Professor of Surgery; Director of Spinal Neurosurgery, Department of Surgery, University of Arizona Medical Center, Tucson, Arizona

Stefano Bandiera, MD
Department of Oncologic and Degenerative Spine Surgery, Rizzoli Orthopedic Institute, Bologna, Italy

Nicholas M. Barbaro, MD
Betsey Barton Professor and Chair, Department of Neurological Surgery, Indiana University, Indianapolis, Indiana

S. Samuel Bederman, MD, PhD, FRCSC
Assistant Clinical Professor, Department of Orthopaedic Surgery, University of California Irvine, Orange, California

Jacqueline Benjamin, MD
Assistant Professor of Pathology; Associate Director of Neuropathology, Department of Pathology, University of Southern California, Los Angeles, California

Sara G. Bennett, MS, CCC-SLP
Speech Language Pathologist, Department of Rehabilitative Services, University of California San Francisco Medical Center, San Francisco, California

Mark H. Bilsky, MD
Attending Surgeon, Department of Neurosurgery, Memorial Sloan-Kettering Cancer Center; Professor, Department of Neurosurgery, Weill Medical College of Cornell University, New York, New York

Frank S. Bishop, MD
Director, Spine Health, Department of Neurological Surgery, Neuroscience and Spine Institute, Kalispell Regional Healthcare, Kalispell, Montana

Stefano Boriani, MD
Director, Department of Oncologic and Degenerative Spine Surgery, Rizzoli Orthopedic Institute, Bologna, Italy

Damien Bresson, MD
Department of Neurosurgery, Hôpital Lariboisière, Paris, France

Michaël Bruneau, MD, PhD
Associate Professor, Department of Neurosurgery, Hôpital Erasme, Brussels, Belgium

Shane Burch, MD, MSc, FRCSC
Associate Professor in Residence, Department of Orthopaedic Surgery, University of California San Francisco, San Francisco, California

David S. Chang, MD, FACS
Assistant Clinical Professor, Department of Surgery, University of California San Francisco, San Francisco, California

Bihong T. Chen, MD, PhD
Clinical Associate Professor, Department of Diagnostic Radiology, City of Hope National Medical Center, Duarte, California

Mike Y. Chen, MD, PhD
Assistant Professor; Section Head—Malignant Brain Tumor Program, Division of Neurosurgery, City of Hope National Medical Center, Duarte, California

Cynthia T. Chin, MD
Associate Professor of Clinical Radiology, Department of Radiology, University of California San Francisco, San Francisco, California

Dean Chou, MD
Associate Professor of Neurosurgery, Department of Neurosurgery, University of California San Francisco, San Francisco, California

Neil R. Crawford, PhD
Associate Professor, Department of Spinal Biomechanics, Barrow Neurological Institute, Phoenix, Arizona

Julie Damiano, MS, OTR/L
Occupational Therapist, Department of Rehabilitation, University of California San Francisco, San Francisco, California

Wali E. Danish, BA, MS
Medical Student, Georgetown University School of Medicine, Washington, DC

Satoru Demura, MD
Assistant Professor, Department of Orthopaedic Surgery, Kanazawa University, Kanazawa, Japan

Vedat Deviren, MD
Professor Clinical Orthopaedics, Department of Orthopaedic Surgery, University of California San Francisco, San Francisco, California

Doniel Drazin, MD, MA
Department of Neurosurgery, Cedars-Sinai Medical Center, Los Angeles, California

Jan M. Eckermann, MD
Chief, Division of Neurosurgery, Department of Surgery, Kern County Medical Center, Bakersfield, California

Ivan Homer El-Sayed, MD, FACS
Associate Professor; Director of Minimally Invasive Skull Base Surgery Center, Department of Otolaryngology–Head and Neck Surgery, University of California San Francisco, San Francisco, California

J. Bradley Elder, MD
Assistant Professor, Department of Neurological Surgery, The Ohio State University Medical Center, Columbus, Ohio

Daniel K. Fahim, MD
Director, Spine Tumor Program, Department of Neurosurgery, Oakland University William Beaumont School of Medicine, Royal Oak, Michigan

Azadeh Farin, MD
Staff Neurosurgeon, Department of Neurosurgery, Los Angeles Medical Center, Los Angeles, California

Charles G. Fisher, MD, MHSc, FRCSC
Associate Professor, Department of Orthopaedic Surgery, University of British Columbia, Vancouver, British Columbia, Canada

Yoshiyasu Fujimaki, MD
Assistant Professor, Department of Orthopaedic Surgery, Kanazawa University, Kanazawa, Japan

Julio Garcia-Aguilar, MD, PhD
Chief Attending, Colorectal Service; Stuart H.Q. Quan Chair in Colorectal Surgery, Department of Surgery, Memorial Sloan-Kettering Cancer Center, New York, New York

Alessandro Gasbarrini, MD
Department of Oncologic and Degenerative Spine Surgery, Rizzoli Orthopedic Institute, Bologna, Italy

Bernard George, MD
Professor and Staff Surgeon, Department of Neurosurgery, Hôpital Lariboisière, Paris, France

Peter C. Gerszten, MD, MPH, FACS
Peter E. Sheptak Professor, Departments of Neurological Surgery and Radiation Oncology, University of Pittsburgh Medical Center, Pittsburgh, Pennsylvania

Michael E. Glover, PT, NCS
Physical Therapist; Clinical Specialist, Department of Rehabilitative Services, University of California San Francisco Medical Center, San Francisco, California

Ziya L. Gokaslan, MD, FACS
Donlin M. Long Professor; Professor of Neurosurgery, Oncology and Orthopaedic Surgery; Director, Neurosurgical Spine Program; Vice Chair, Department of Neurosurgery, Johns Hopkins University School of Medicine, Baltimore, Maryland

Sally Greenberg, MBBS
Medical Oncologist, Department of Oncology, Western Hospital, Melbourne, Victoria, Australia

Nalin Gupta, MD, PhD
Professor, Department of Neurological Surgery and Pediatrics, University of California San Francisco; Chief, Division of Pediatric Neurosurgery, UCSF Benioff Children's Hospital, San Francisco, California

Yoon Ha, MD, PhD
Associate Professor of Neurosurgery, Department of Neurosurgery, College of Medicine, Yonsei University, Seoul, Korea

Van Halbach, MD
Clinical Professor of Radiology, Neurological Surgery, Neurology and Anesthesia, University of California San Francisco Medical Center, San Francisco, California

Andrea L. Harzstark, MD
Assistant Professor of Medicine, Department of Medicine, University of California San Francisco, San Francisco, California

Joyce Ho, MD
Surgical Fellow, Division of General and Oncologic Surgery, City of Hope National Medical Center, Duarte, California

William Y. Hoffman, MD
Professor and Chief, Division of Plastic and Reconstructive Surgery; Steven J. Mathes Endowed Chair in Plastic Surgery, Department of Surgery, University of California San Francisco, San Francisco, California

Thierry M. Jahan, MD
Professor of Clinical Medicine, Department of Medicine, Division of Hematology/Oncology, University of California San Francisco, San Francisco, California

Rahul Jandial, MD, PhD
Assistant Professor, Division of Neurosurgery, City of Hope Comprehensive Cancer Center, Los Angeles, California

Andrew Jea, MD, FAANS, FACS, FAAP
Associate Professor, Department of Neurosurgery, Baylor College of Medicine, Texas Children's Hospital, Houston, Texas

Eric B. Jelin, MD
Chief Resident, Department of Surgery, University of California San Francisco, San Francisco, California

Brian J. Jian, MD, PhD
Department of Neurosurgery, Kaiser Permanente, Sacramento, California

Walter D. Johnson, MD, FACS
Department of Neurosurgery and Radiation Medicine, Loma Linda University, Loma Linda, California

David Josephson, MD
Tower Urology Institute of Minimally Invasive Surgery, Cedars-Sinai Medical Center, Los Angeles, California

Norio Kawahara, MD
Professor, Department of Orthopaedic Surgery, Kanazawa Medical University, Kanazawa, Japan

Sassan Keshavarzi, MD
Division of Neurosurgery, University of California San Diego, San Diego, California

Brendan D. Killory, MD
Director of Epilepsy and Functional Neurosurgery, Department of Neurosurgery, Hartford Hospital, Hartford, Connecticut

Keung Nyun Kim, MD, PhD
Professor of Neurosurgery, Department of Neurosurgery, College of Medicine, Yonsei University, Seoul, Korea

Tyler R. Koski, MD
Associate Professor, Department of Neurological Surgery, Northwestern University, Chicago, Illinois

Ted H. Leem, MD, MS
Assistant Professor, Chief, Denver VAMC Otolaryngology, Department of Otolaryngology–Head and Neck Surgery, University of Colorado School of Medicine, Aurora, Colorado

Dzenan Lulic, MD
Department of Neurosurgery, University of South Florida, Tampa, Florida

Quang D. Ma, DO
Department of Neurosurgery, Arrowhead Regional Medical Center, Colton, California

Rex A.W. Marco, MD
Professor, Department of Orthopaedic Surgery, University of Texas Medical School at Houston, Houston, Texas

Jamal McClendon, Jr., MD
Chief Resident, Department of Neurological Surgery, Northwestern University, Feinberg School of Medicine; Northwestern Memorial Hospital, Chicago, Illinois

Matthew Mei, MD
Fellow, Department of Hematology/Oncology, City of Hope National Medical Center, Duarte, California

Jennifer Moore, MS, CCC-SLP
Speech Language Pathologist, Department of Rehabilitative Services, University of California San Francisco Medical Center, San Francisco, California

Lee Jae Morse, MD
Orthopaedic Resident, Department of Orthopaedic Surgery, University of California San Francisco, San Francisco, California

Hideki Murakami, MD
Associate Professor, Department of Orthopaedic Surgery, Kanazawa University, Kanazawa, Japan

Rebecca L. Mustille, MPT
Physical Therapist, Department of Inpatient Rehab Services, University of California San Francisco Medical Center, San Francisco, California

Peter Nakaji, MD
Professor of Neurosurgery, Division of Neurosurgery, Barrow Neurological Institute, Phoenix, Arizona

Agne Naujokas, DO
Dermatopathology Fellow, Department of Pathology, University of California San Francisco, San Francisco, California

Richard J. O'Donnell, MD
Professor of Clinical Orthopaedic Surgery, Department of Orthopaedic Surgery, Helen Diller Family Comprehensive Cancer Center, University of California San Francisco, San Francisco, California

Susan Onami, BA
Department of Medical Oncology and Experimental Therapeutics, City of Hope Comprehensive Cancer Center, Duarte, California

Stephen L. Ondra, MD
Professor of Neurological Surgery, Department of Neurological Surgery, Northwestern University, Feinberg School of Medicine; Senior Vice President and Chief Medical Officer, Health Care Service Corporation, Chicago, Illinois

A. Orlando Ortiz, MD, MBA, FACR
Chairman, Department of Radiology, Winthrop–University Hospital, Mineola; Professor of Clinical Radiology, Stony Brook University School of Medicine, Stony Brook, New York

Sumanta Kumar Pal, MD
Assistant Professor, Division of Genitourinary Malignancies, Department of Medical Oncology and Experimental Therapeutics, City of Hope Comprehensive Cancer Center, Los Angeles, California

Andrew T. Parsa, MD, PhD
Michael J. Marchese Professor and Chair, Department of Neurological Surgery, Northwestern University, Feinberg School of Medicine, Chicago, Illinois

Murat Pekmezci, MD
Assistant Clinical Professor, Department of Orthopedic Surgery, University of California San Francisco, San Francisco, California

Julie A. Ressler, MD
Clinical Associate Professor, Department of Diagnostic Radiology, City of Hope National Medical Center, Duarte, California

Laurence D. Rhines, MD
Professor; Director Spine Program, Department of Neurosurgery, University of Texas MD Anderson Cancer Center, Houston, Texas

Lary A. Robinson, MD
Professor of Surgery (Thoracic), Department of Interdisciplinary Oncology, University of South Florida College of Medicine; Senior Member, Division of Thoracic Oncology, Moffitt Medical Group, Moffitt Cancer Center, Tampa, Florida

Hope S. Rugo, MD
Professor of Medicine, Department of Medicine, University of California San Francisco Medical Center, San Francisco, California

Justin K. Scheer, BS
Medical Student, University of California San Diego, La Jolla, California

Meic H. Schmidt, MD, MBA
Associate Professor, Department of Neurosurgery, University of Utah, Salt Lake City, Utah

Joseph H. Schwab, MD, MS
Instructor, Department of Orthopaedic Surgery, Massachusetts General Hospital, Boston, Massachusetts

Daniel M. Sciubba, MD
Assistant Professor of Neurosurgery, Oncology, and Orthopaedic Surgery; Director of Spine Research, Department of Neurosurgery, Johns Hopkins University School of Medicine, Baltimore, Maryland

Dr. med Matthias Setzer
Neurosurgical Clinic, J.W. Goethe Universität Frankfurt, Frankfurt, Germany

Luigi Simonetti, MD
Director, Department of Emergency Interventional Radiology and Neuroradiology, Maggiore Hospital, Bologna, Italy

Jerry D. Slater, MD
Professor and Chair, Department of Radiation Medicine, Loma Linda University, Loma Linda, California

George Somlo, MD, FACP
Professor, Department of Medical Oncology and Hematology and Hematopoietic Cell Transplantation, City of Hope National Medical Center, Duarte, California

Robert F. Spetzler, MD
Professor, Department of Neurosurgery, University of Arizona College of Medicine, Tucson; Director and J.N. Harber Chairman of Neurological Surgery, Department of Neurological Surgery, Barrow Neurological Institute, Phoenix, Arizona

John Street, MD, PhD, FRCSI, FRCS(Tr&Orth)
Assistant Professor, Department of Orthopedics, University of British Columbia; Spine Surgeon, Combined Neurosurgical and Orthopedic Spine Program, Vancouver General Hospital, Vancouver, Canada

Peter P. Sun, MD
Clinical Associate Professor, Department of Neurosurgery, University of California San Francisco, San Francisco; Director, Department of Pediatric Neurosurgery, Children's Hospital Research Center–Oakland, Oakland, California

Matthew C. Tate, MD, PhD
Resident, Department of Neurological Surgery, University of California San Francisco, San Francisco, California

James K. Tatum, MD
Interventional Neuroradiologist, Department of Neuroscience, Sierra Providence Health Network, El Paso, Texas

Nicholas Theodore, MD, FAANS, FACS
Professor of Neurological Surgery; Chief, Spine Section; Director, Neurotrauma Program, Division of Neurological Surgery, Barrow Neurological Institute, Phoenix, Arizona

Pierre Reynald Theodore, MD
Associate Professor, Department of Cardiothoracic Surgery, University of California San Francisco, San Francisco, California

Tarik Tihan, MD, PhD
Professor of Pathology, Department of Pathology, University of California San Francisco, San Francisco, California

Katsuro Tomita, MD
President, Kanazawa University Hospital, Kanazawa, Japan

Przemyslaw Twardowski, MD
Clinical Professor of Medical Oncology, Department of Medical Oncology, City of Hope Cancer Center, Duarte, California

Frank D. Vrionis, MD, MPH, PhD
Professor of Neurosurgery, Orthopaedics and Oncology, College of Medicine, University of South Florida; Chief of Neurosurgery, Department of Neurooncology, H. Lee Moffitt Cancer Center, Tampa, Florida

Jean-Paul Wolinsky, MD
Associate Professor of Neurosurgery and Oncology, Department of Neurosurgery, Johns Hopkins University School of Medicine, Baltimore, Maryland

Rebecca Wu, MD
Radiology Resident, Department of Radiology, Winthrop–University Hospital, Mineola, New York

Rosanna Wustrack, MD
Assistant Professor, Department of Orthopedic Surgery, University of California San Francisco, San Francisco, California

Yoshiya Yamada, MD, FRCPC
Associate Radiation Oncologist, Department of Radiation Oncology, Memorial Sloan-Kettering Cancer Center, New York, New York

Do Heum Yoon, MD, PhD
Professor of Neurosurgery, Department of Neurosurgery, College of Medicine, Yonsei University, Seoul, Korea

Chi-Shing Zee, MD
Professor of Radiology, Department of Radiology, University of Southern California, Los Angeles, California

Foreword

Spinal oncology is an evolving field, and operative techniques as well as clinical acumen are constantly improving. Advances in medical and radiation oncology and earlier detection of disease are extending patient life expectancy. The role of the spine surgeon is expanding, and simple decompressions are often no longer satisfactory. Today curative wide resections and durable, complex reconstructions are technically feasible. Although spine tumor surgeons must be comfortable with these advanced approaches, we must also exercise restraint in the treatment of a patient in whom the odds of cure are near zero, and the goals of surgery are mostly palliative. Thus a firm understanding of the pathology underlying disease processes, prognosis, and outcomes are paramount in the surgeon's decision-making process.

Spine and Spinal Cord Tumors: Advanced Management and Operative Techniques, edited by Drs. Ames, Boriani, and Jandial, is a valuable addition to the field of spinal oncology. The reader will find chapters dedicated to specific disease processes that have traditionally been grouped in a single umbrella chapter. This approach assists the reader to a deeper understanding of why, for example, one may need to treat two patients with spinal epidural metastasis very differently. Medicine is moving toward a multimodality, team-based approach to provide individualized plans of care for each patient, and this is the overarching theme of this book.

Dr. Ames, following his residency at UCSD and fellowship at the Barrow Neurologic Institute, is the director of the spine tumor and deformity section at UCSF. Dr. Jandial, also a product of UCSD, is now at City of Hope in Los Angeles. Dr. Boriani is currently the director of the Department of Oncologic and Degenerative Spine Surgery at the Rizzoli Orthopedic Institute in Italy. All three are very well known and are truly world leaders in the field. Their publication record and contributions to the field have been extraordinary, and their efforts in assembling this text have been tireless.

This is not merely a book on techniques; each topic is thoroughly discussed, from detailed coverage of each pathologic condition to treatment options, indications, decision-making, operative intervention, and outcomes. Valuable cases are included, as are Tips From the Masters and Bailout Techniques. The figures and tables are carefully chosen to complement the discussion. The audience for this text is quite broad; it has invaluable insights for medical students, residents, practitioners, and basic scientists alike. This is indispensable reading for anyone wishing to advance his or her understanding of spinal oncology.

Ali Kemal Ozturk, MD
Instructor of Neurosurgery,
Department of Neurosurgery,
Johns Hopkins University School of Medicine,
Baltimore, Maryland

Ziya L. Gokaslan, MD, FACS
Donlin M. Long Professor;
Professor of Neurosurgery,
Oncology and Orthopaedic Surgery;
Director, Neurosurgical Spine Program;
Vice Chair, Department of Neurosurgery,
Johns Hopkins University School of Medicine,
Baltimore, Maryland

Preface

As the field of spine tumor treatment has rapidly evolved over the past decade, multidisciplinary approaches have increasingly been used in planning treatment and treatment alternatives as part of the shared patient and physician decision-making process. Spinal oncology has come into its own as a specialty, with full integration of medical oncology, radiation oncology, radiosurgery, and spinal surgery.

Advancements in surgical technique and postgraduate training have led to increased application of en bloc resection for primary tumors, as well as wider access to this type of treatment at regional centers of excellence across the world. Treatment of metastatic tumors has evolved from transcavitary approaches to transpedicular corpectomy to "separation surgery" as an adjunct to radiosurgery. In parallel, medical oncology has made tremendous advances in many sites of primary diseases, such as the breast, lung, and prostate, that frequently metastasize to the spine.

This book represents an attempt to bring the advancements in medical oncology, radiation oncology, surgical techniques, and combined therapy together in one comprehensive resource to guide clinicians in improving the care of spine tumor patients. Accordingly, the organization of this textbook offers chapters that are presented as part of a didactic flow that can provide the dedicated reader with a complete knowledge base—or chapters can be read individually for focused learning and refinement of existing skills.

Logically arranged into four sections, this book begins with a section on Fundamentals that contains introductory topics on anatomy, radiation, and rehabilitation. A chapter on "Plastic Surgery for Primary Reconstruction" provides guidance for treating spine wounds with flaps and free tissue transfer. The second section focuses on Oncology and presents chapters on the biology and medical management of both primary and metastatic tumors as well as tumors arising from the spinal roots and cord. With the anatomic and medical background established, the text transitions to the third and most robust section, Operative Techniques. The chapters in this section provide exhaustive coverage of an advanced surgical repertoire that brings together international experts to define the leading edge of operative techniques for tumors of the spine and spinal cord. Within each chapter, Tips From the Masters and Bailout Techniques provide additional insights. The book concludes with a final section on Complications and

Outcomes, with key chapters on the common complications encountered in spine tumor surgery and outcome reporting. In addition, videos of key operative procedures are demonstrated on the accompanying DVD to provide a visual reference for challenging techniques.

Our contributors and Section Editors, Drs. Mark Bilsky, Frank Vrionis, Vedat Deviren, Yoshiya Yamada, and Rex Marco, are the leading experts in the fields of oncology, radiosurgery, and spine surgery. Many of them are pioneers and innovators who have graciously given of their time, despite busy clinical practices. We sincerely appreciate their dedication as they met tight deadlines and made certain that their contributions reflect the current state of the art. Without their incredibly hard work, this text would not have been possible.

We hope that this book will provide valuable guidance for surgeons, both experienced and new to practice, who are engaged in treating spine and spinal cord tumors, and that it will provide a source of new information, stimulate thought, foster innovation, and forge new solutions to ongoing problems and challenges.

Christopher P. Ames
Stefano Boriani
Rahul Jandial

Acknowledgments

We would like to extend a special thank you to the dedicated team at Quality Medical Publishing for supporting this project's concept from its inception, for fostering its direction, and for the creation of this textbook.

We would also like to thank Carlo Piovani for his invaluable assistance with collecting data, storing images, and anatomic and surgical drawings.

Contents

Foreword xv

Preface xvii

Section I

Fundamentals

1. Spine and Spinal Cord Anatomy for Tumor Surgery 3
   Rahul Jandial, Rebecca Wu, Bihong T. Chen, A. Orlando Ortiz

2. Spine Biomechanics and Balance of Tumor Reconstruction 39
   Ali A. Baaj, Nicholas Theodore, Neil R. Crawford

3. Scoring System for Metastatic Tumors: Palliative or Aggressive Resection and Reconstruction 53
   Satoru Demura, Katsuro Tomita, Norio Kawahara, Hideki Murakami

4. Imaging of Spinal Cord Tumors 63
   Cynthia T. Chin

5. Heavy-Particle Radiation 87
   Jan M. Eckermann, Jerry D. Slater, Walter D. Johnson

6. Spine Stereotactic Radiosurgery 99
   J. Bradley Elder, Yoshiya Yamada, Peter C. Gerszten, Mark H. Bilsky

7 Plastic Surgery for Primary Reconstruction 113
David S. Chang, William Y. Hoffman

8 Physical and Occupational Therapy 127
Julie Damiano, Michael E. Glover, Rebecca L. Mustille

9 Speech and Swallow Management 161
Sara G. Bennett, Jennifer Moore

Section II

Oncology

10 Chordoma 175
Jamal McClendon, Jr., Christopher P. Ames, Frank L. Acosta, Jr.

11 Chondrosarcoma of the Spine 201
Daniel M. Sciubba, Jean-Paul Wolinsky, Ziya L. Gokaslan

12 Giant Cell Tumors 213
Rosanna Wustrack, Shane Burch

13 Aneurysmal Bone Cysts 225
Joseph H. Schwab, Luigi Simonetti, Alessandro Gasbarrini, Stefano Bandiera, Luca Amendola, Stefano Boriani

14 Hemangiomas 237
Jamal McClendon, Jr., Stephen L. Ondra, Frank L. Acosta, Jr.

15 Osteoid Osteomas and Osteoblastomas 251
Shane Burch

16 Osteosarcoma 259
Lee Jae Morse, Vedat Deviren

17 Soft Tissue Sarcomas and Malignant Peripheral Nerve Sheath Tumors 275
Azadeh Farin, Jacqueline Benjamin, Christopher P. Ames

18 Systemic Treatment of Advanced Lung Cancer   301
    Thierry M. Jahan

19 Renal Cell Carcinoma   313
    Matthew Mei, Andrea L. Harzstark

20 Breast Cancer   325
    Sally Greenberg, Hope S. Rugo

21 Prostate Cancer   353
    Sumanta Kumar Pal, Susan Onami, David Josephson, Przemyslaw Twardowski

22 Plasmacytoma and Multiple Myeloma   371
    Quang D. Ma, George Somlo, Mike Y. Chen

23 Intradural Extramedullary Tumors   379
    Agne Naujokas, Tarik Tihan

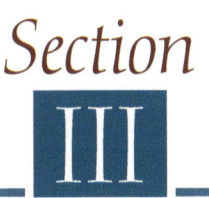

Section III

Operative Techniques

24 Approaches to Percutaneous Image-Guided Spine Biopsy   411
    Bihong T. Chen, Mike Y. Chen, Julie A. Ressler, Chi-Shing Zee

25 Embolization and Test Occlusion   435
    James K. Tatum, Van Halbach

26 Intramedullary Spinal Cord Tumors   457
    Yoon Ha, Keung Nyun Kim, Do Heum Yoon, Brian J. Jian, Andrew T. Parsa, Christopher P. Ames

27 Surgical Management of Nerve Sheath Tumors   473
    Matthew C. Tate, Nicholas M. Barbaro, Pierre Reynald Theodore, Christopher P. Ames

28 T-Saw Laminoplasty   487
    Yoshiyasu Fujimaki, Hideki Murakami, Norio Kawahara, Katsuro Tomita

29 Paramedian Transpedicular Approach for Ventral Intradural Extramedullary Tumors of the Cervical and Cervicothoracic Spine   497
Frank L. Acosta, Jr., Christopher P. Ames

30 Combined Far-Lateral Approaches and Reconstruction for Tumors of the Craniocervical Junction   511
Brendan D. Killory, Peter Nakaji, Robert F. Spetzler

31 Transoral and Transglossal Approach or Transmandibular Circumglossal Approach to the Cervical Spine   529
Ted H. Leem, Ivan Homer El-Sayed

32 Vertebral Artery Sacrifice and Mobilization   551
Bernard George, Michaël Bruneau, Damien Bresson

33 Pancoast Tumors   565
Matthias Setzer, Lary A. Robinson, Frank D. Vrionis

34 Advanced Thoracic Approaches to the Spine   591
Eric B. Jelin, Pierre Reynald Theodore

35 Thoracoscopic Resection and Reconstruction   607
Frank S. Bishop, Meic H. Schmidt

36 Sagittal Osteotomy for En Bloc Resection of Lateralized Tumors of the Lumbar Spine   629
S. Samuel Bederman, Christopher P. Ames, Vedat Deviren

37 Combined Lateral/Posterior Approach for Large Anterior/Lateral Lesions   647
Daniel K. Fahim, Laurence D. Rhines

38 Approaches and Techniques for C2 Tumors: Transpedicular Corpectomy and Spondylectomy   679
Justin K. Scheer, Azadeh Farin, Frank D. Vrionis, Christopher P. Ames

39 En Bloc Resection of Primary Tumors of the Cervical Spine   705
Frank L. Acosta, Jr., Doniel Drazin, Christopher P. Ames

40 En Bloc Spondylectomy: Single-Stage Thoracic Spine   719
Hideki Murakami, Katsuro Tomita, Norio Kawahara, Satoru Demura

41 En Bloc Spondylectomy: Two-Stage Thoracic/Lumbar Spine 735
Dean Chou, Wali E. Danish

42 Transpedicular Approach for Anterior Decompression and Reconstruction 745
Sassan Keshavarzi, Dzenan Lulic, Henry E. Aryan

43 Hemipelvectomy and Hemicorporectomy: Hindquarter Amputation 759
Richard J. O'Donnell, Shane Burch

44 Reconstruction of the Sacroiliac Joint and Pelvis 777
Murat Pekmezci, Christopher P. Ames, Vedat Deviren

45 Sacral Resection 791
Joyce Ho, Julio Garcia-Aguilar

46 Distal Sacrectomy 815
Dean Chou, Wali E. Danish

47 Proximal Sacrectomy and Pelvic Reconstruction 825
Jamal McClendon, Jr., Tyler R. Koski, Stephen L. Ondra, Frank L. Acosta, Jr.

48 Pediatric Spine and Spinal Cord Tumors 845
Andrew Jea, Nalin Gupta, Peter P. Sun, Kurtis Ian Auguste

Section IV

Complications and Outcomes

49 Complications in Spine Tumor Surgery 879
Jean-Paul Wolinsky, Daniel M. Sciubba

50 Outcomes Reporting in Tumor Surgery 889
John Street, Charles G. Fisher

Index 903

Video Contents

Foramen Magnum Meningioma
Schahrazed Bouazza, Sebastien Froelich, Bernard George

Chordoma of the Cranio-Cervical Junction
Damien Bresson, Schahrazed Bouazza, Bernard George

Four-Level En Bloc Cervical Chordoma
Christopher P. Ames

Neurinoma
Damien Bresson, Sebastien Froelich, Bernard George

C5-6 Foramen Decompression
Schahrazed Bouazza, Bernard George

Vertebral Artery Loop at C5-6
Muneyoshi Yasuda, Bernard George

270-Degree En Bloc Thoracic Chondrosarcoma
Christopher P. Ames

Single-Stage Thoracic En Bloc With the Tomita Saw System
Christopher P. Ames

Lumbar En Bloc Resection
Christopher P. Ames

Double-Approach Vertebrectomy
Stefano Boriani, Alessandro Gasbarrini, Riccardo Ghermandi

En Bloc Total Sacrectomy and Reconstruction
Christopher P. Ames

Section I

Fundamentals

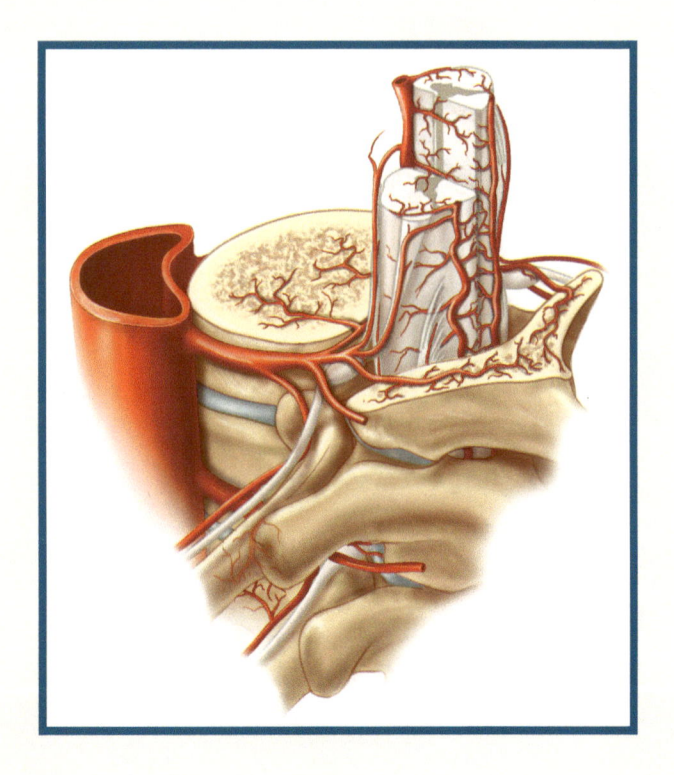

Chapter 1

Spine and Spinal Cord Anatomy for Tumor Surgery

Rahul Jandial, Rebecca Wu, Bihong T. Chen,
A. Orlando Ortiz

*U*nderstanding the anatomy and imaging characteristics of the spine can greatly facilitate surgery, radiation, and/or other interventional spine treatments. Various imaging modalities, such as CT, MRI, and conventional radiography, have become an essential part of preoperative planning and postsurgical management of spine tumors. In this chapter the radiologic anatomy of the spinal axis is reviewed according to anatomic segments from the cervical spine through the lumbosacral spine.

CERVICAL SPINE

The cervical spine is the most superior segment of the spine and is composed of seven cervical vertebrae (Fig. 1-1, *A* through *C*). The upper cervical spine includes C1 and C2, which demonstrate a unique appearance. C1, or the atlas, contains no vertebral body but is formed by a complete ring consisting of anterior and posterior arches (Fig. 1-1, *D* through *G*). In addition, paired lateral masses and transverse processes arise from the lateral aspects of this osseous ring. The superior aspect of the lateral masses articulates with each occipital condyle to form the atlantooccipital joint. The inferior aspect of each lateral mass articulates with the superior aspect of the axis, or C2, at the atlantoaxial joint. C2 has a body and an odontoid process, or dens, that articulates with the anterior arch of C1 (see Fig. 1-1, *A* through *C*). C3 through C7 can be grouped together, as all of these vertebrae are composed of a body, bilateral pedicles, laminae, and articulating facets (both superior and inferior) (see Fig. 1-1, *D* through *G*).[1,2]

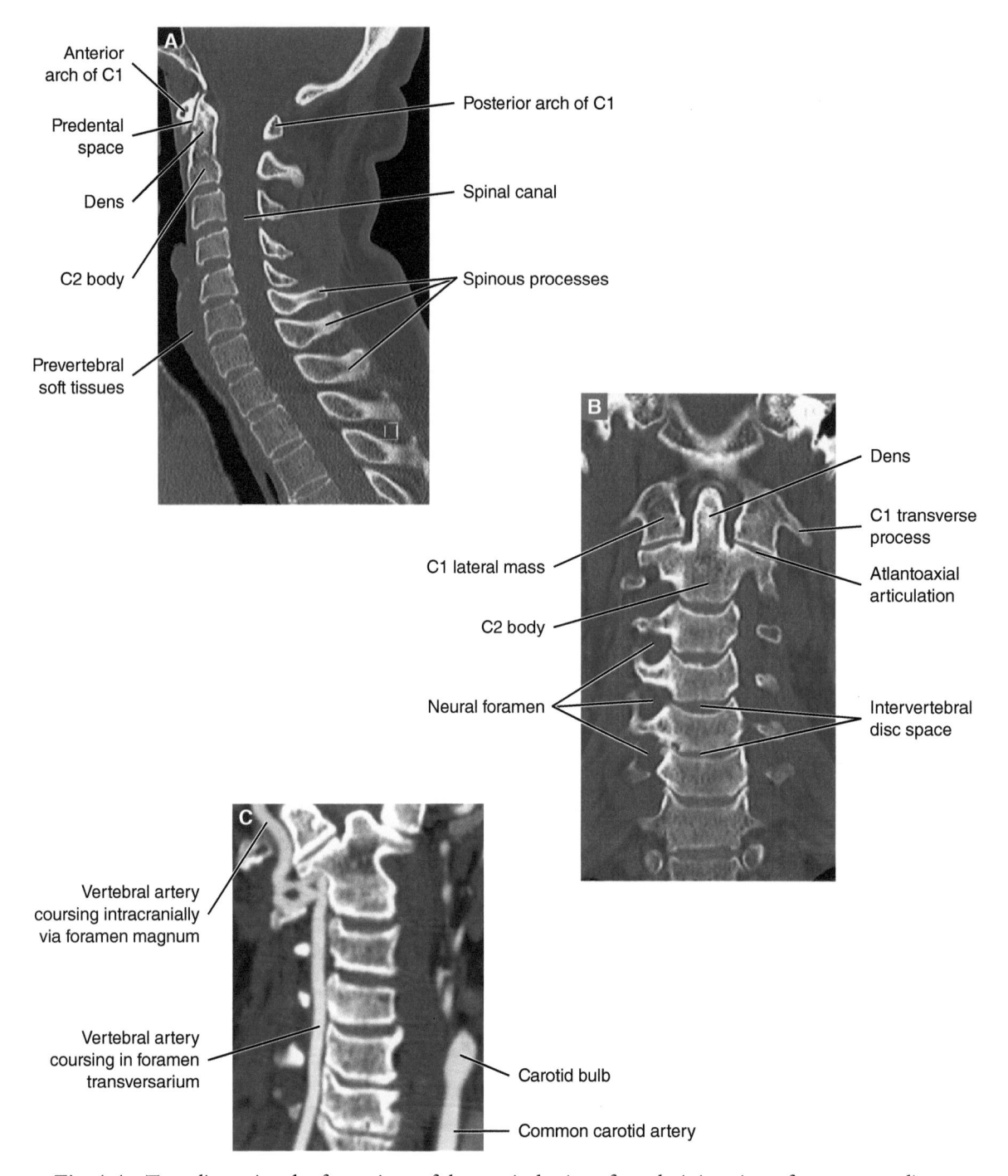

Fig. 1-1 Two-dimensional reformations of the cervical spine after administration of contrast medium with bone window algorithm in the **A,** sagittal and **B** and **C,** coronal planes.

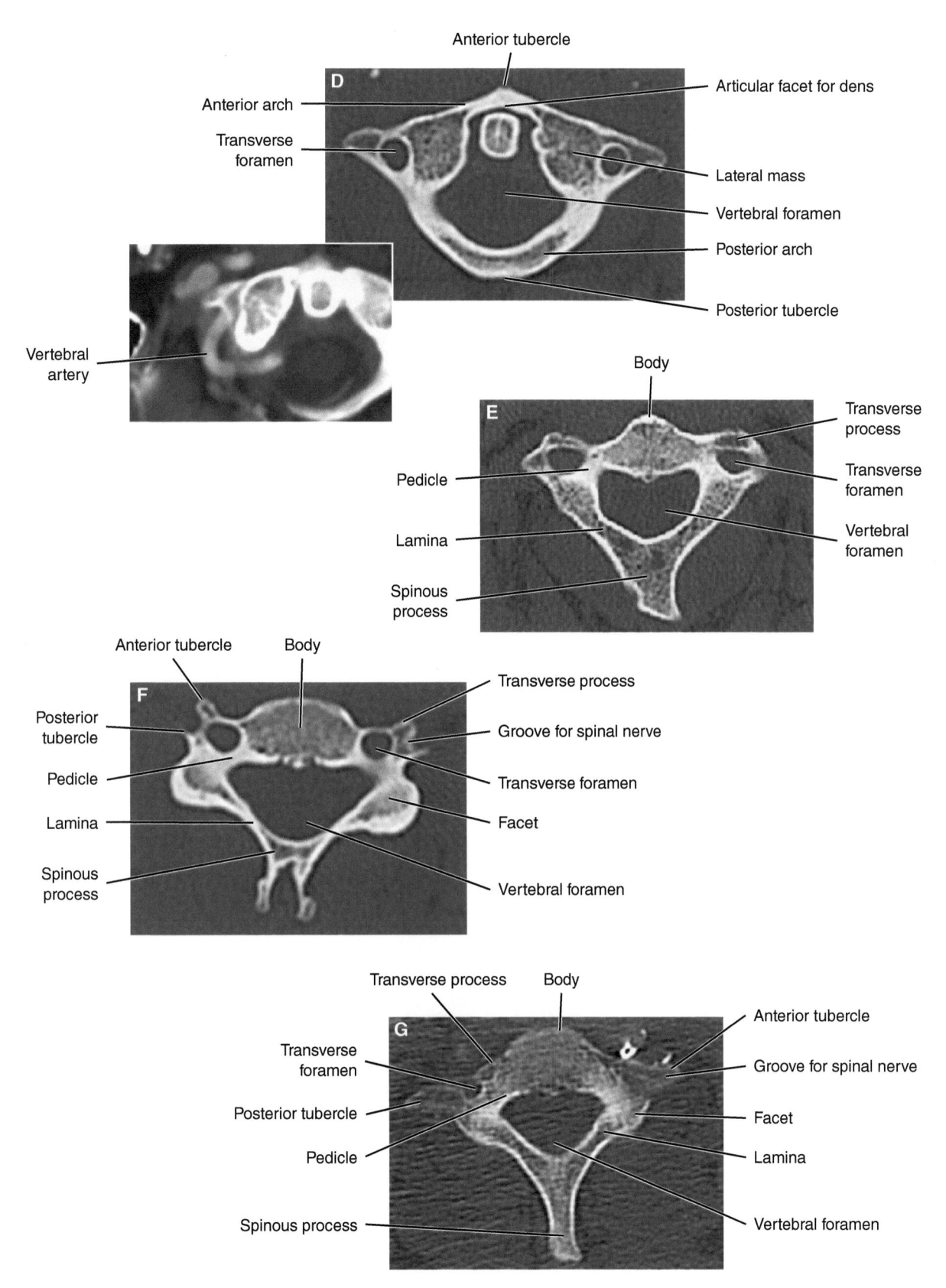

Fig. 1-1, cont'd **D,** Axial CT images (bone window algorithm) of the cervical spine at C1, with and without intravenous contrast agent as well as at **E,** C2, **F,** C4, and **G,** C7 levels.

The C1-2 articulation between the dens and the atlas is stabilized by the transverse ligament, which is located posterior to the dens. The alar ligament connects the tip of the dens to the occipital condyles. The anterior and posterior atlantooccipital membranes extend from the upper aspect of C1 to the anterior and posterior aspects of the foramen magnum, respectively. Further stabilization of the cervical spine is provided by the anterior and posterior longitudinal ligaments, which attach to the basiocciput at their most superior extent and will be discussed later in this chapter (Fig. 1-2). The cervical intervertebral discs are comprised of an annulus fibrosus and a central nucleus pulposus, and they are smaller than the discs in the thoracic and lumbar spine.[1]

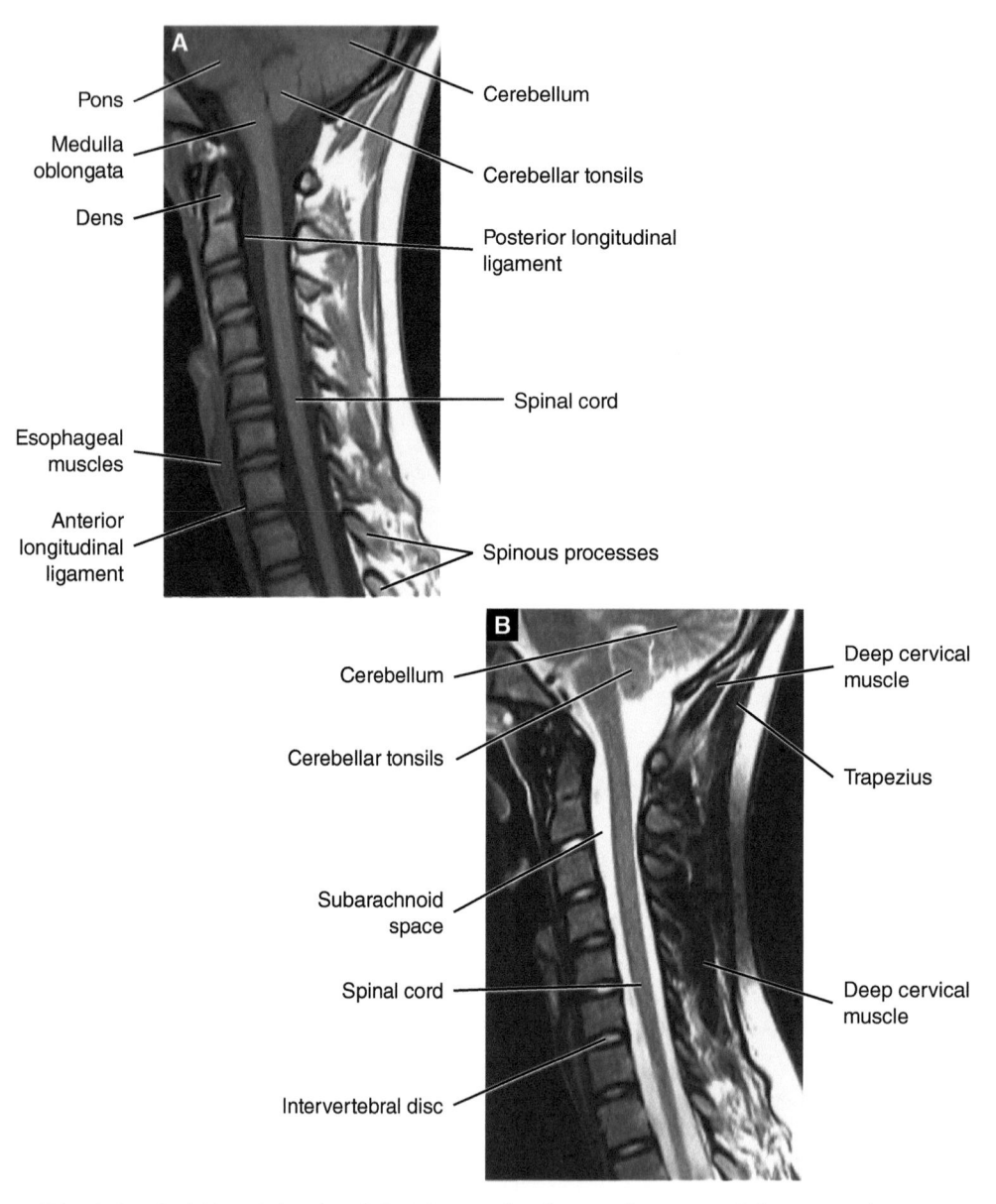

Fig. 1-2 **A,** T1-weighted and **B,** T2-weighted sagittal images of the cervical spine.

The cervical spinal cord lies within the vertebral canal and is covered by the meninges, including the pia, arachnoid, and dura from the innermost layer to the periphery. Eight paired spinal nerves exit the lower part of the neural foramina in the cervical spine. The neural foramina are oriented anterolaterally in contrast to the thoracic and lumbar regions. Cervical cord segments usually lie one numbered-spine level higher than their corresponding vertebrae (e.g., the C6 cord segment lies adjacent to the C5 vertebra). The first cervical nerves course above C1, the second cervical nerves course above C2, and the C3 nerves traverse the C2-3 neural foramina (Fig. 1-3). This pattern continues to C7-T1 where the C8 nerves emerge from their respective foramina.

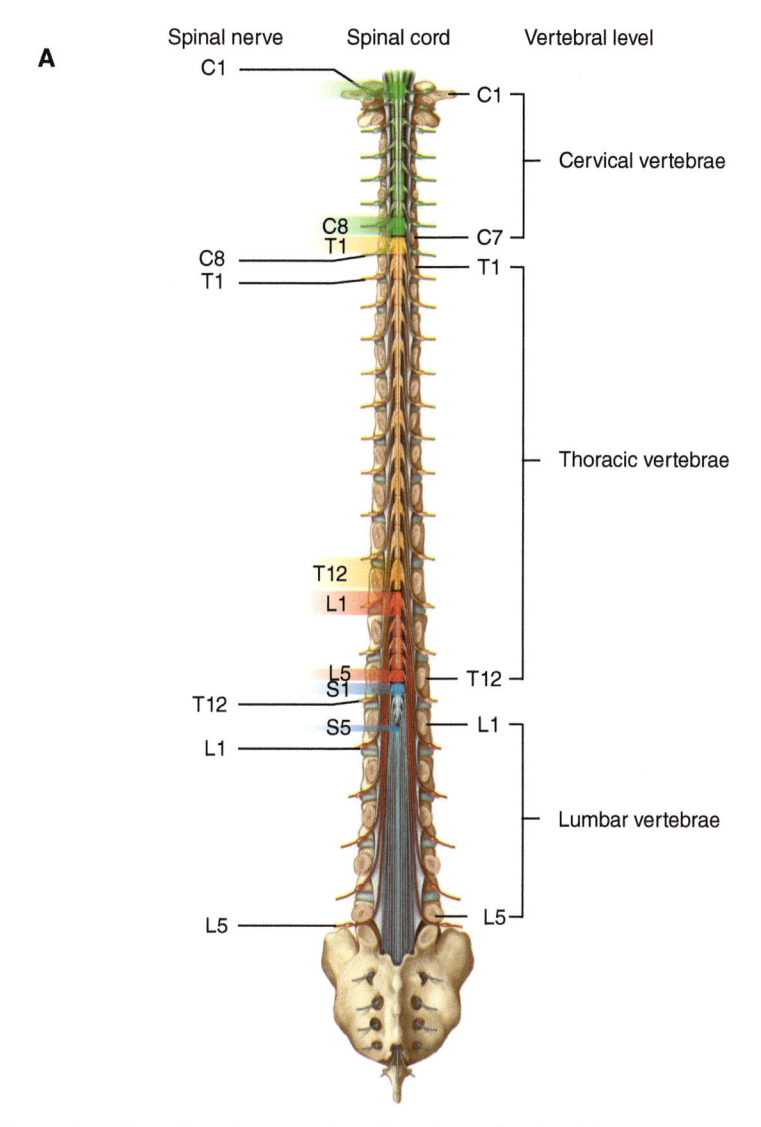

Fig. 1-3 **A,** Posterior view showing spinal cord and vertebral column. Each spinal nerve bears the name and numeral of the vertebrae superior to it, with the exception of the cervical region. C1 exits superior to vertebra C1, and C8 exits between vertebrae C7 and T1.

Continued

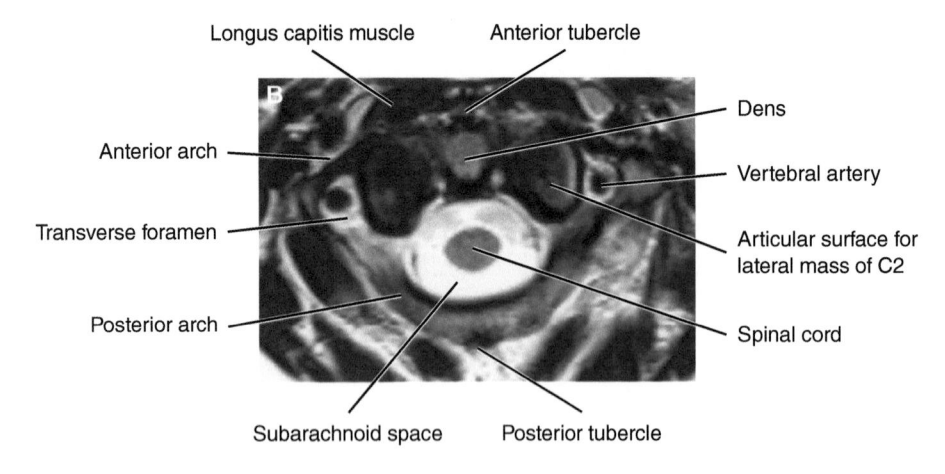

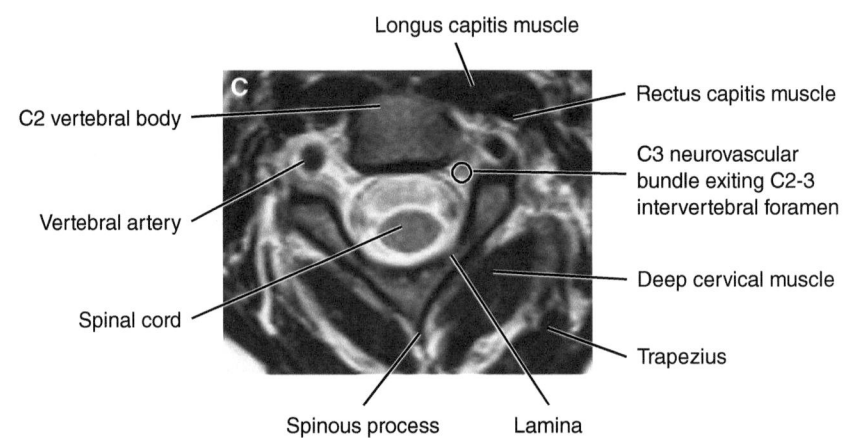

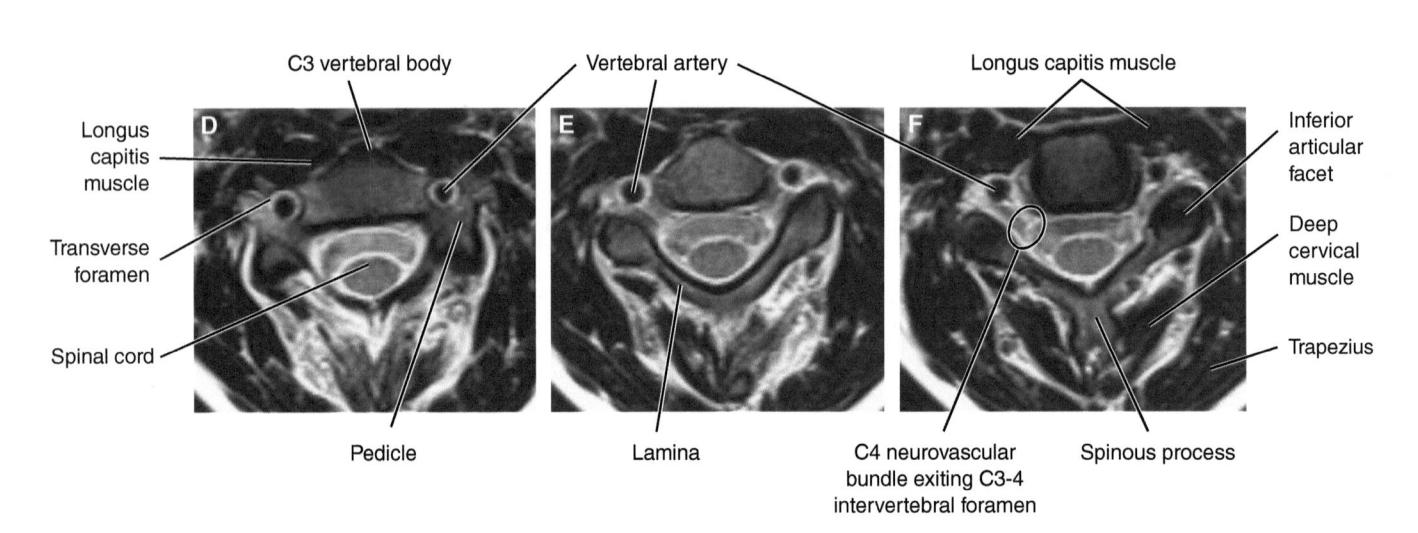

Fig. 1-3, cont'd **B,** T2-weighted axial MR images of the cervical spine at C1 as well as at **C,** C2, and **D-F,** C3.

THORACIC SPINE

The thoracic spine is composed of 12 vertebrae with less variation in morphology compared to the cervical spine (Fig. 1-4, *A* through *D*). There is considerable variation in size, with each vertebral body increasing in size by a factor of approximately two as the thoracic spine is traversed in a caudal direction.[3] Also, the dorsal aspect of the vertebral body is slightly higher than the ventral aspect, a feature that contributes to the normal gentle kyphosis of the thoracic spine (see Fig. 1-4, *A* and *B*).

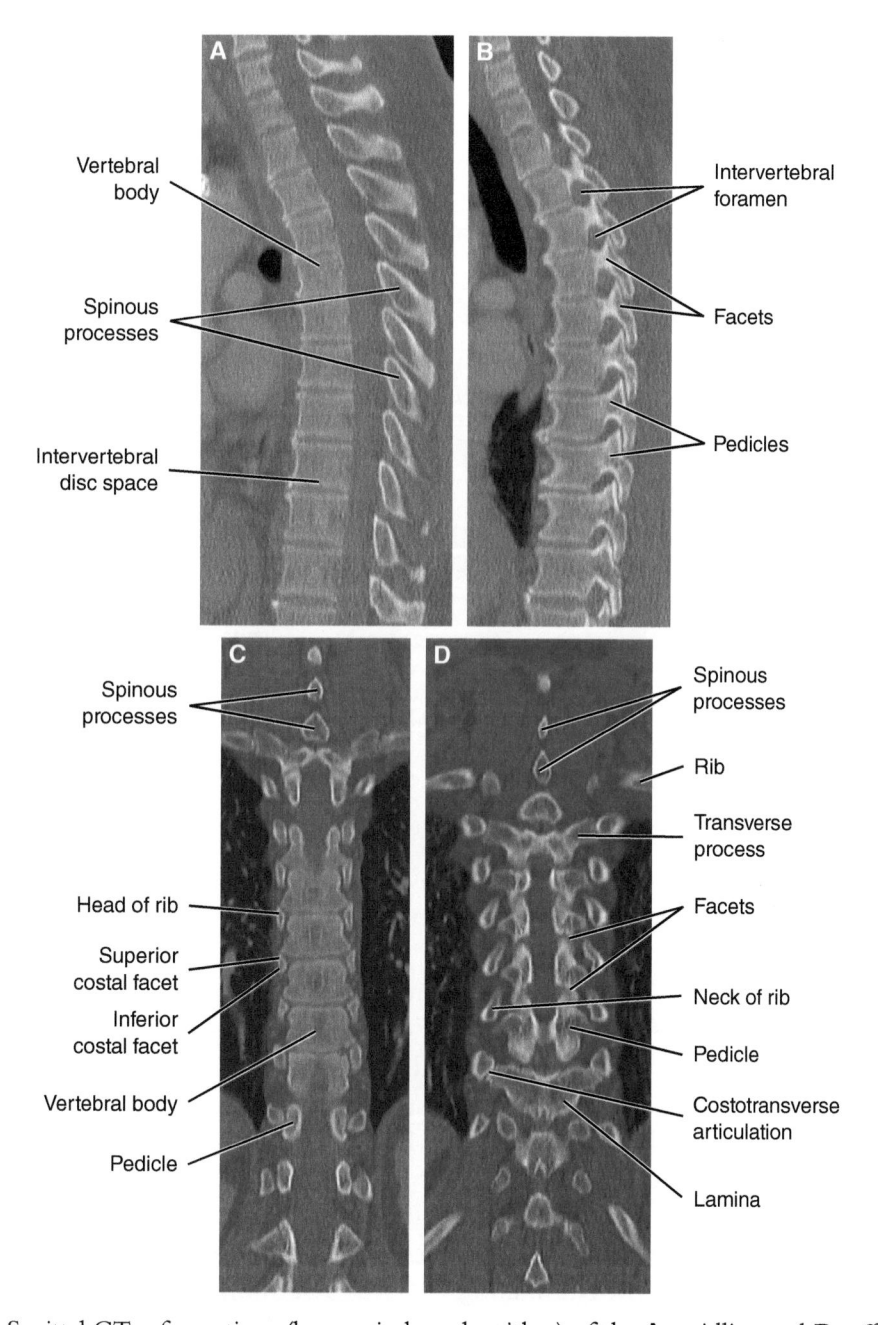

Fig. 1-4 Sagittal CT reformations (bone window algorithm) of the **A,** midline and **B,** off-midline thoracic spine. Coronal CT reformations (bone window algorithm) of the thoracic spine at the **C,** vertebral body and **D,** posterior element level.

Continued

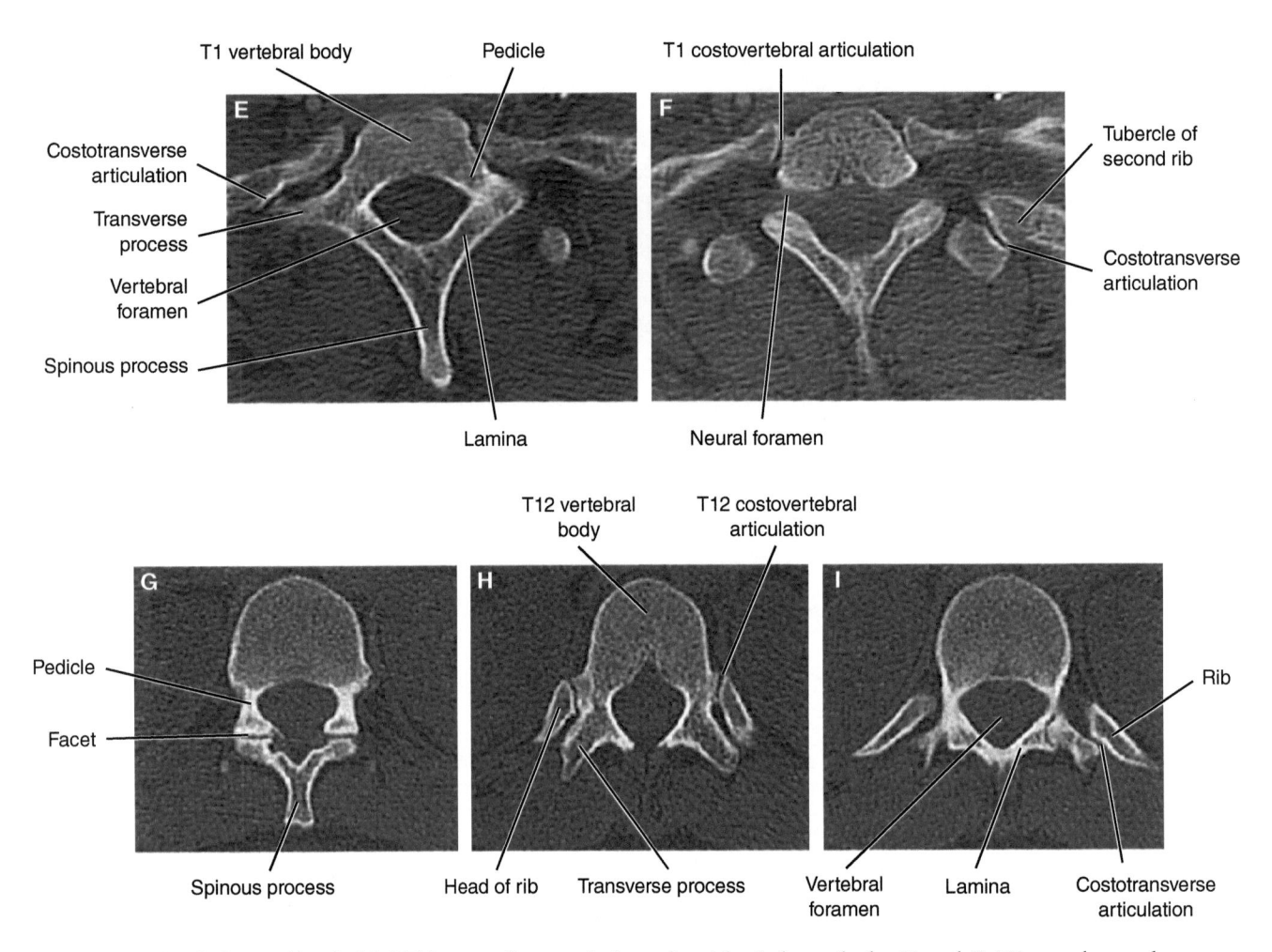

Fig. 1-4, cont'd Axial CT images (bone window algorithm) through the **E** and **F,** T1 vertebra and **G-I,** T12.

When viewed in cross-section, the ventral aspect of the vertebral body is convex anterior and the dorsal aspect is concave posterior (Fig. 1-4, *E* through *I*).

All 12 thoracic vertebrae support ribs, forming a unit that protects critical intrathoracic structures such as the heart and thoracic aorta. Each thoracic vertebral body has costal facets at the dorsolateral aspect to which the ribs articulate. In the midthoracic spine the heads of the ribs articulate with the vertebral bodies in a configuration that spans the intervertebral disc space (see Fig. 1-4, *C* and *D*). The articular surfaces on the vertebral bodies are essentially demifacets, with one component at the inferior margin of a body and the other at the superior margin of the body below it. The first thoracic vertebra is unique because it possesses a complete facet on each side of its body for the head of the first rib in addition to a lower demifacet for the head of the second rib. The lowest two thoracic vertebral bodies, T11 and T12, only display one costal facet on either side to support their respective ribs.

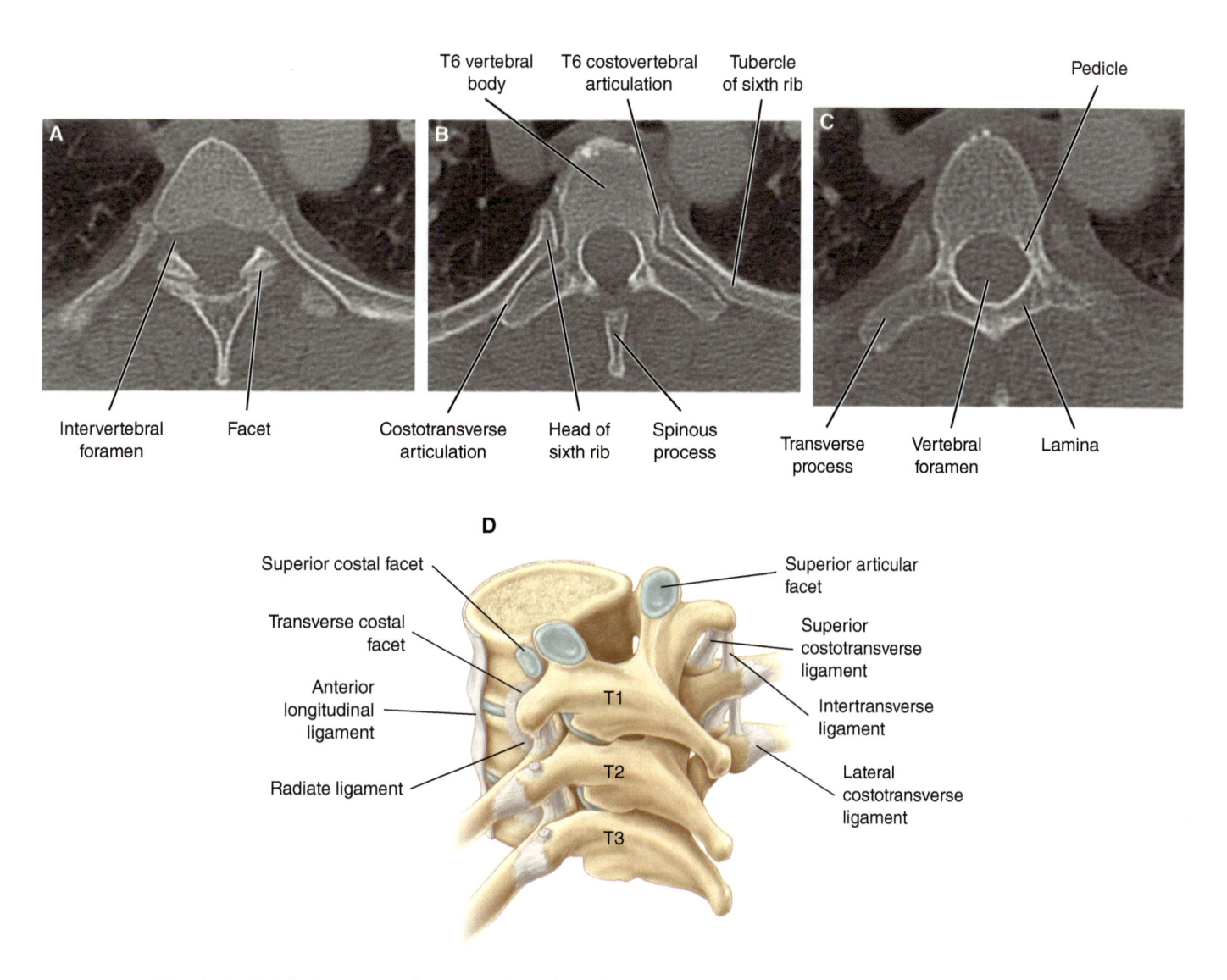

Fig. 1-5 Axial CT images (bone window algorithm) through the **A-C,** T6 vertebra. **D,** Posterolateral view of thoracic vertebrae showing facets and ligaments.

The tubercles of the ribs also articulate with the thoracic vertebrae. At the lateral aspect of the transverse processes, a concave facet exists along the ventral aspect to which the tubercles articulate (Fig. 1-5, *A* through *C*). The transverse processes of T11 and T12 are smaller than their more superior counterparts and are unable to buttress the ribs, hence the term *floating ribs.* At each level a group of ligaments reinforce the costovertebral and costotransverse articulations. The radiate ligament spans the intervertebral disc space and secures the head of the rib to the vertebral bodies. The superior and lateral costotransverse ligaments connect the superior and posterior aspects of the neck to the transverse process above at the level of the rib, respectively. The transverse processes on each side are connected to the transverse processes above and below by the intertransverse ligament (Fig. 1-5, *D*).

Posterolateral to the costovertebral articulation is the pedicle, a three-dimensional structure filled with cancellous bone that arises from the superior aspect of the vertebral body (see Fig. 1-4, *E* through *I*).[4] The size and orientation of the pedicles depend largely on the level of the thoracic spine being examined. In terms of size, the pedicle height and width typically decrease from T1 to T4 and increase from T4 to T12, with the smallest pedicles occurring at T3-6.[4] The T1 and T2 pedicles exhibit an oblique orientation, in part reflecting the transition in morphology of the vertebrae between the cervical and thoracic spine. In the more caudal thoracic spine the pedicles are oriented in an anteroposterior direction (see Fig. 1-4, *E* through *I*). This change in orientation is important to keep in mind when introducing transpedicular hardware (i.e., screws) to avoid malpositioning. It is important to note that the medial wall of the pedicle is significantly thicker than the lateral wall,[5] which is a possible explanation for why pedicle fractures related to screws are more commonly seen laterally.

The spinous processes of the thoracic vertebrae are longer than those in the cervical and lumbar spine (see Fig. 1-4, *A* and *B*). The acuity with which the spinous process projects from the posterior arch depends on the level of the thoracic spine. The spinous processes of T1 through T4 project posteriorly at an angle of approximately 40 degrees from the horizontal. In comparison, the T5 through T8 spinous processes project posteriorly at a more acute angle of approximately 60 degrees from the horizontal. In this segment of the thoracic spine, there is complete overlap of the spinous process with the one just inferior to it. The interspinous ligament reinforces the connection between each spinous process.

There are 12 pairs of thoracic nerve roots. The position of the nerve roots in the neurovascular bundle as they exit the neural foramen is different from that seen in the cervical spine. Unlike in the cervical spine, the neurovascular bundle in the thoracic spine exits the neural foramen inferior to the same numbered pedicle (Fig. 1-6, *A* and *B*).

For example, the T1 nerve root is found beneath the T1 pedicle (Fig. 1-6, *C* through *F*), and the T12 nerve root is found beneath the T12 pedicle (Fig. 1-6, *G* through *J*). The nerve roots course superiorly within the bundle and are in close proximity to the roof of the neural foramen.

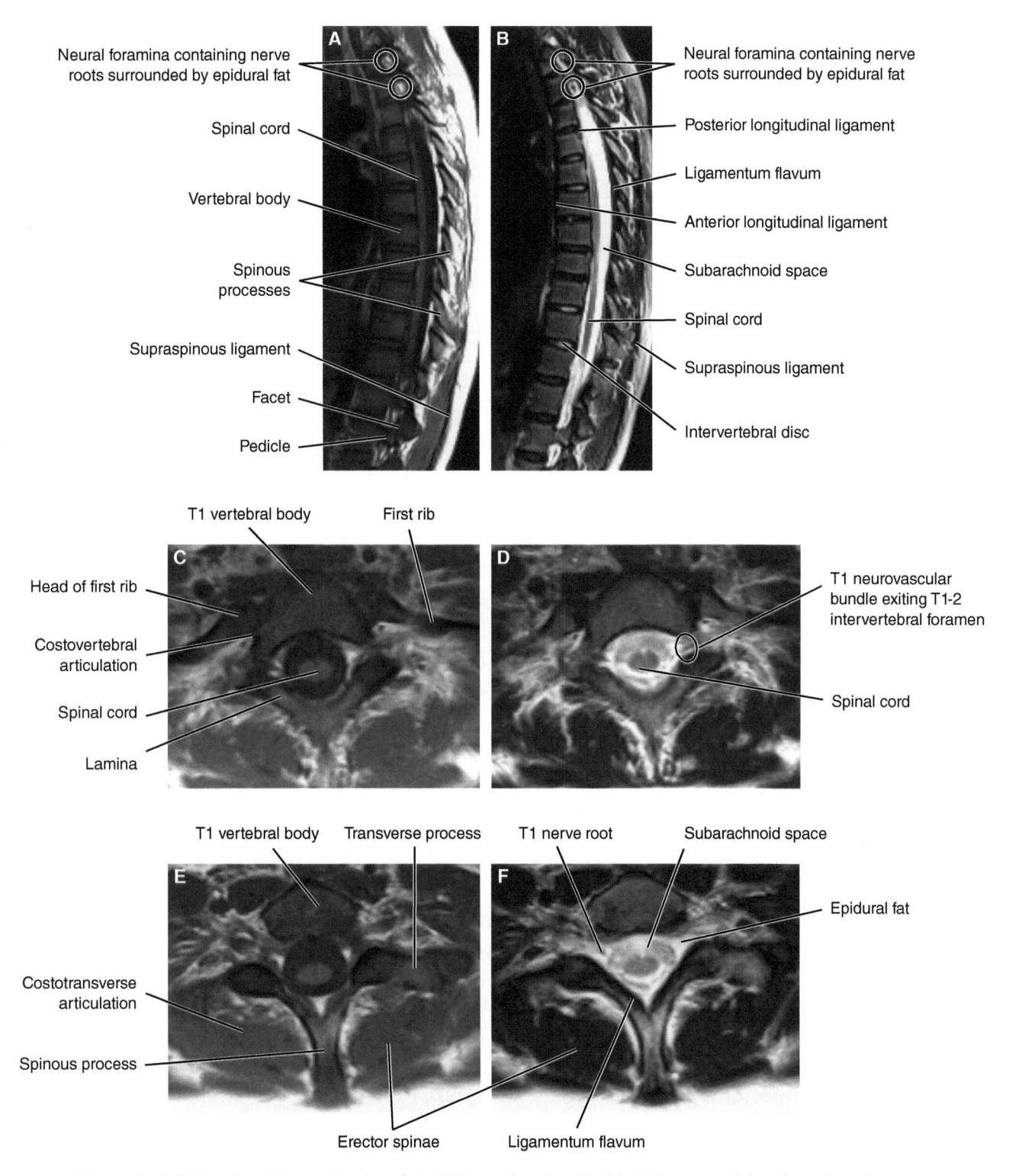

Fig. 1-6 Midline **A,** T1-weighted and **B,** T2-weighted sagittal MR images of the thoracic spine. **C** and **D,** T1-weighted and **E** and **F,** T2-weighted axial MR images at the level of the T1 vertebra.

Continued

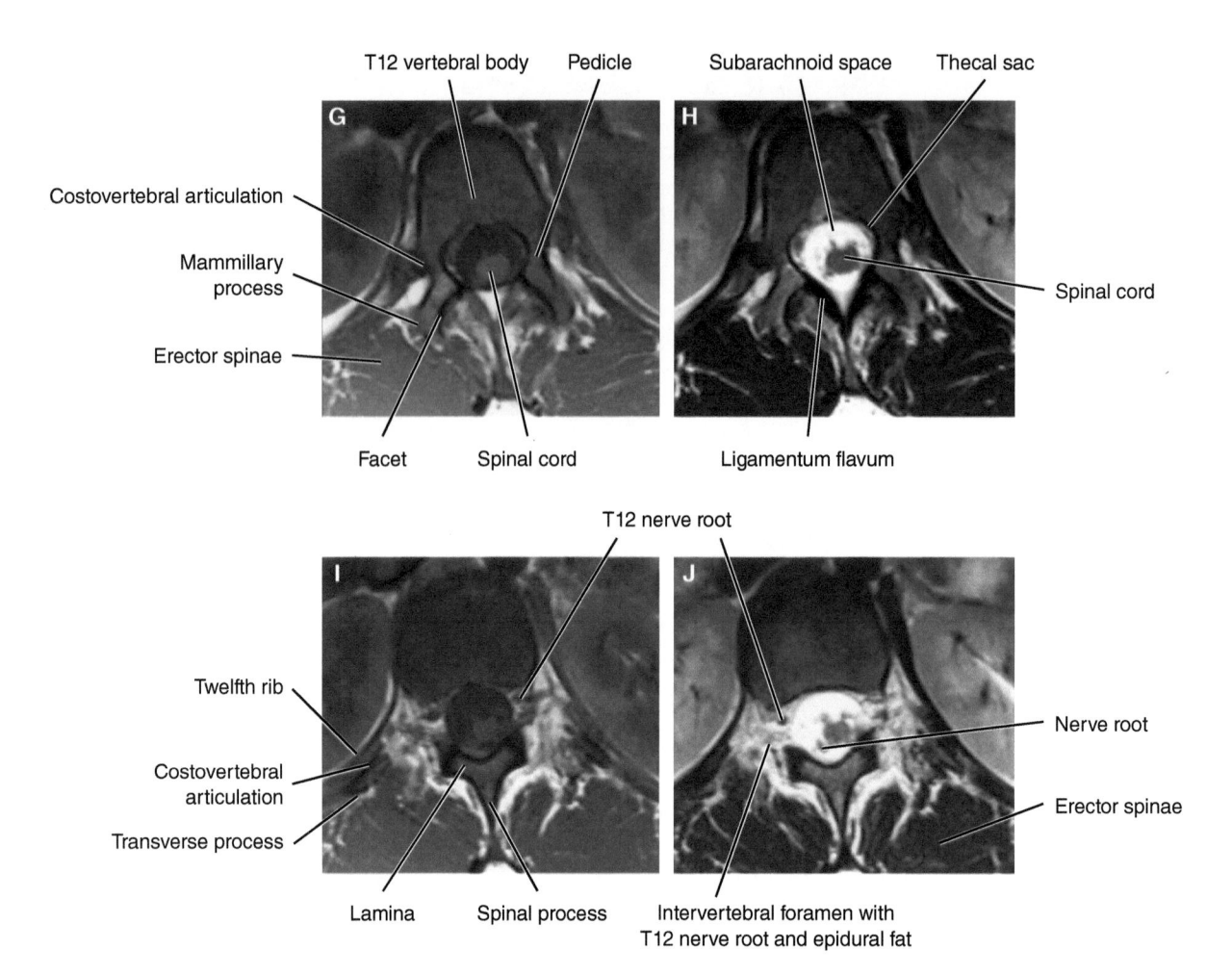

Fig. 1-6, cont'd **G** and **I**, T1-weighted and **H** and **J**, T2-weighted axial MR images at the level of the T12 vertebra.

LUMBAR SPINE

The most caudal section of the presacral column is the lumbar spine. The lumbar vertebrae are easily distinguished from the other presacral vertebral bodies by their lack of transverse foramina, as seen in the cervical spine, and costal articulations, as seen in the thoracic spine.[6] The lumbar vertebral bodies are the largest in the spine, and they are slightly thicker anteriorly than posteriorly in concordance with the normal lumbar lordosis (Fig. 1-7, *A* and *B*). They are also greater in transverse dimension than in anteroposterior dimension (Fig. 1-7, *C* through *G*). The other vertebral elements are proportionately larger than their more cranial counterparts within the spinal axis (Fig. 1-7, *H* through *J*).

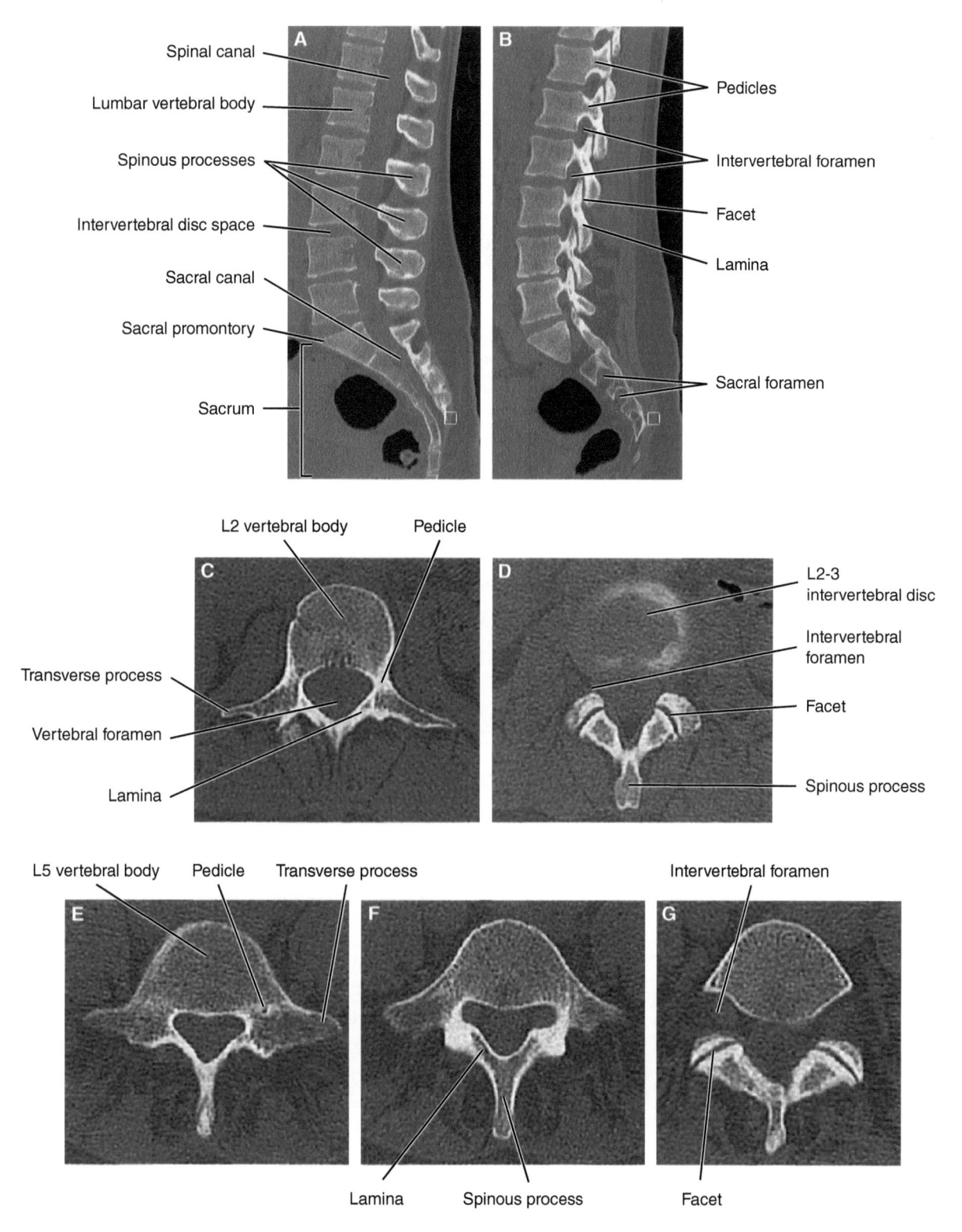

Fig. 1-7 Sagittal CT reformations (bone window algorithm) of the **A,** midline and **B,** off-midline lumbar spine. Axial CT images (bone window algorithm) through **C** and **D,** the L2 vertebra and **E-G,** the L5 vertebra.

Continued

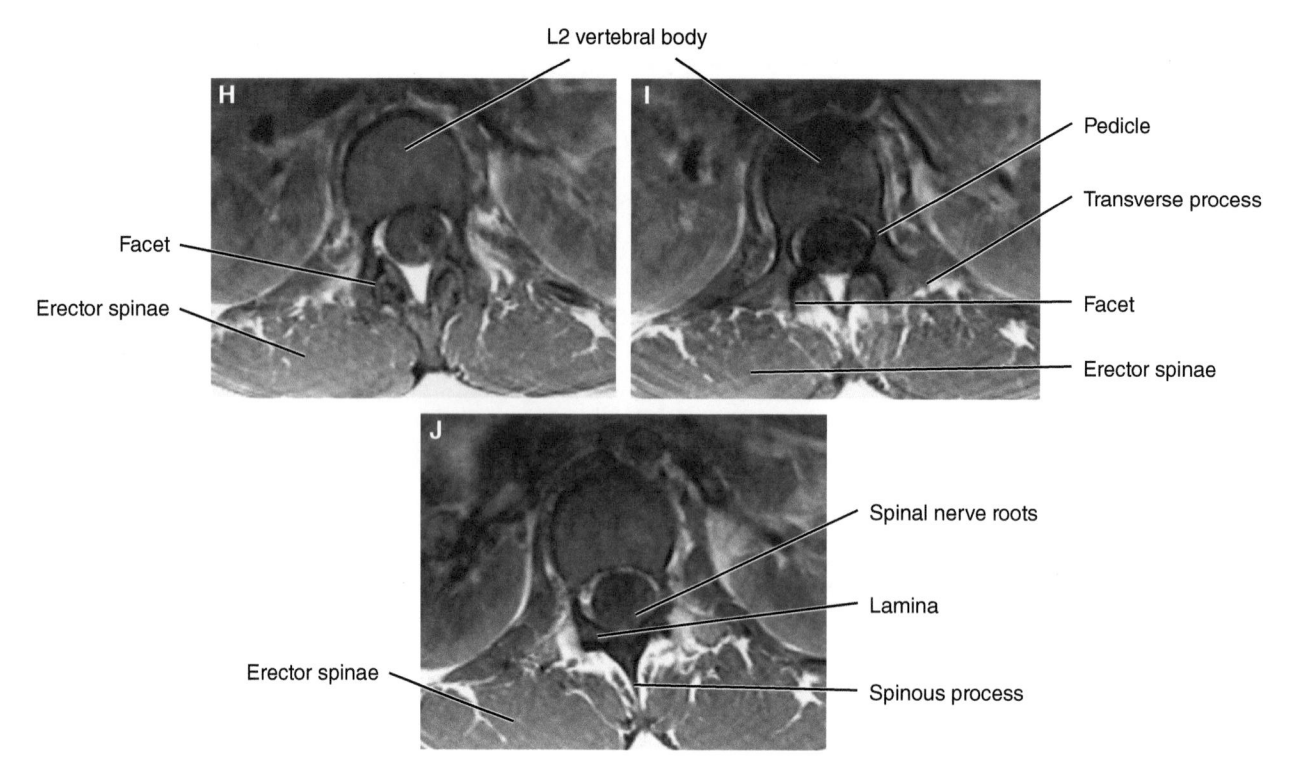

Fig. 1-7, cont'd **H-J,** T1-weighted axial MR images at the level of the L1 vertebra.

The pedicles in the lumbar spine are thicker and arise from the superolateral aspect of each lumbar vertebral body to form the lateral margins of a triangle-shaped spinal canal (see Fig. 1-7, *A* through *G*).[4] The laminae complete the triangular shape posteriorly. The pedicle orientation varies from L1 to L5, with those of L1 oriented in an anteroposterior direction similar to the lower thoracic spine. The angle of the pedicles increases in obliquity toward the lower lumbar spine and is greatest at L5 (see Fig. 1-7, *C* through *G*).[3]

The lumbar vertebrae can also be distinguished from those in the other segments by their articulations. The superior articular facets arise from the junction of the pedicles and laminae, with surfaces that are slightly concave (see Fig. 1-7, *A* and *B*), in contrast to the convex surfaces seen in the thoracic spine. The superior facets are oriented dorsomedially so that the inferior processes projecting down from the laminae above

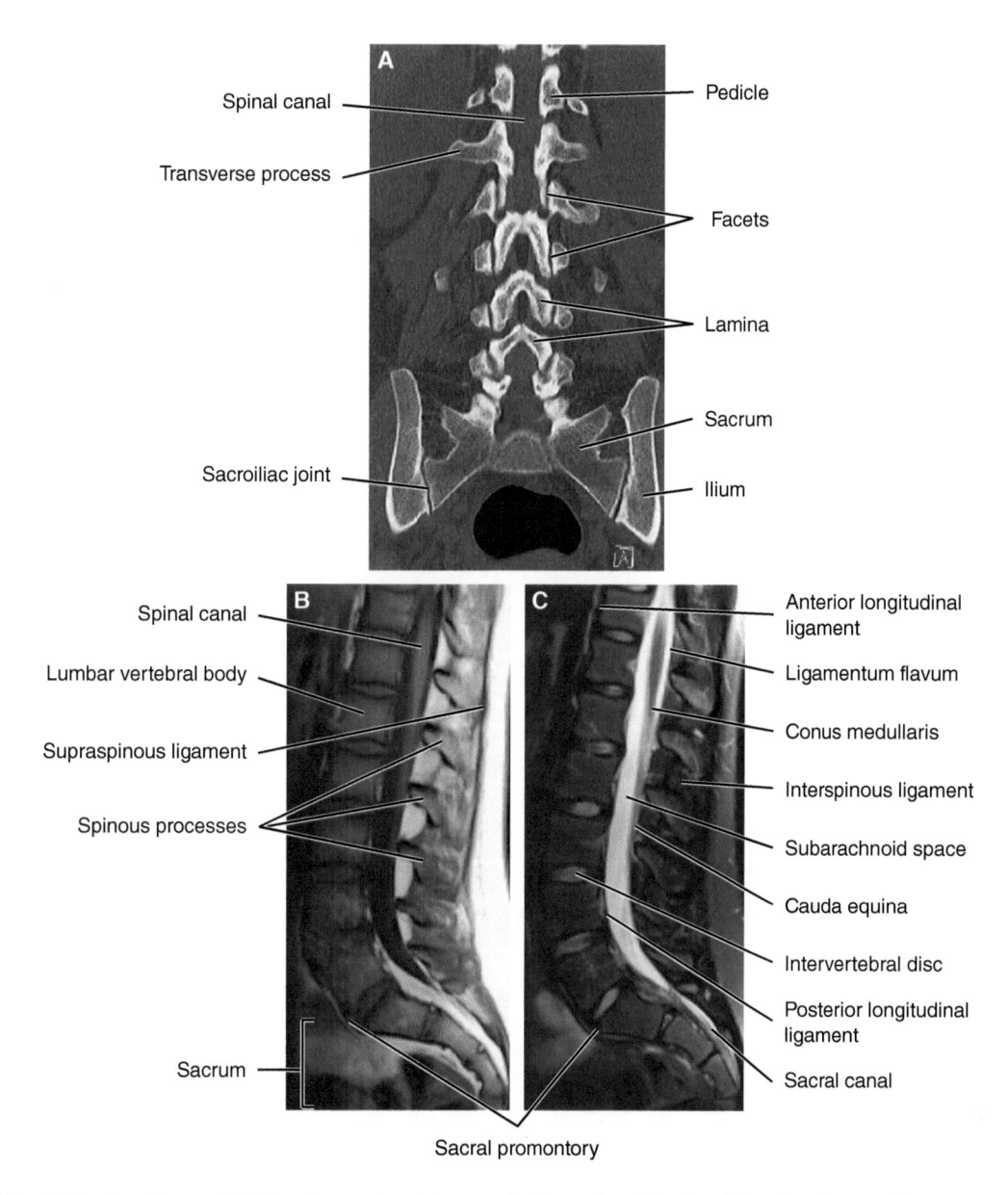

Fig. 1-8 **A,** Coronal CT reformation (bone window algorithm) of the lumbosacral spine at the posterior element level. Midline **B,** T1-weighted and **C,** T2-weighted sagittal magnetic resonance images of the lumbar spine.

larticulate in a manner that restricts both rotation and flexion in this segment of the spine (Fig. 1-8, *A*) (see also Fig. 1-7, *C* through *J*).[6] The L5 transverse process on either side is connected to the iliac crest by the iliolumbar ligament. As in the thoracic spine, the spinous processes in the lumbar spine are reinforced by the interspinous and supraspinous ligaments (Fig. 1-8, *B* and *C*).

Five paired lumbar nerve roots are typically found in the lumbar spine. These nerve roots course anteriorly and laterally through the neural foramina. Each lumbar nerve root exits the spinal canal through the neural foramen inferior to the corresponding pedicle of its respective spinal segment. For example, the L1 nerve root emerges from the spinal canal inferior to the L1 pedicle, and the L2 nerve root emerges inferior to the L2 pedicle (Fig. 1-9).

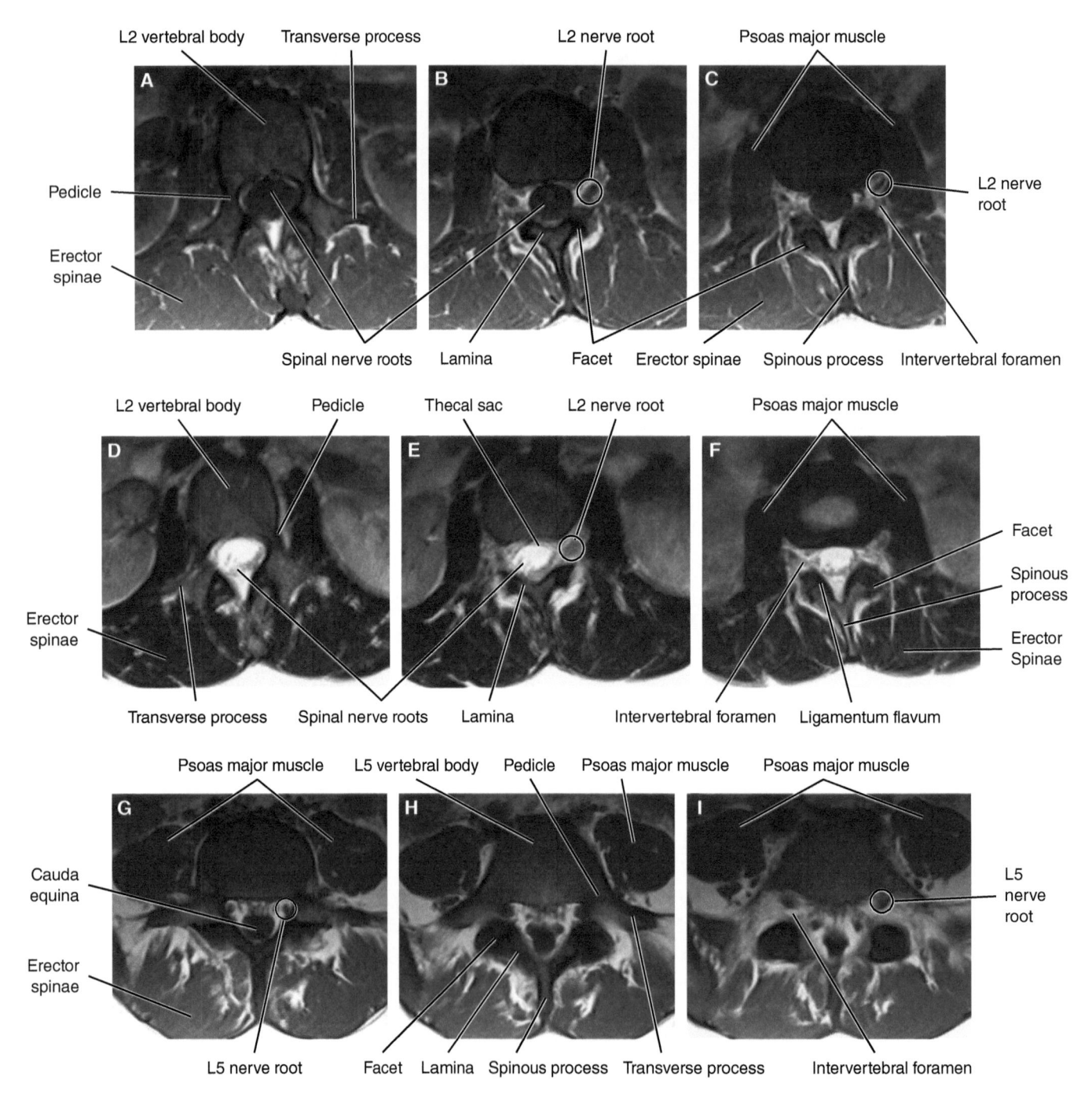

Fig. 1-9 **A-C,** T1-weighted axial MR images at the level of the L2 vertebra. **D-F,** T2-weighted axial MR images at the level of the L2 vertebra. **G-I,** T1-weighted axial MR images at the level of the L5 vertebra.

SACRUM

The sacrum is located at the caudal end of the spinal axis and articulates with the lumbar spine at the intervertebral disc, often L5-S1 (see Figs. 1-7, *A* and *B*, and 1-8, *B* and *C*). The sacrum projects posteriorly at this articulation, forming the lumbosacral angle. Caudally the sacrum articulates with the coccyx at the sacrococcygeal joint. The anterior anatomic relations of the sacrum include the presacral space, which is comprised of fat, and the rectum. Posteriorly the sacrum is covered by the medial aspect of the gluteal musculature, the caudal aspect of the posterior paraspinal musculature, and the subcutaneous fat and skin. The lateral relations of the sacrum include the sacroiliac joints and the iliac bones (Fig. 1-10).

The sacrum consists of five sacral segments. Unlike other regions of the spinal axis, the sacral vertebrae are fused anteriorly and posteriorly.[7] This produces a large complex triangular or somewhat pyramidal configuration to the sacrum. The sacral segments get progressively smaller in a cranial to caudal direction. The first sacral vertebra, S1, is the largest and its anterior-superior aspect forms the sacral promontory (see Figs. 1-7, *A* and *B*; 1-8, *B* and *C*; and 1-10). The lateral masses of the sacrum are fused to form the sacral ala (see Fig. 1-10). The sacral ala, a wing-shaped structure, is prominent at S1 and progressively decreases in size along with the more caudal sacral vertebra. The lateral aspects of the sacral ala articulate with the iliac bones at the sacroiliac joints. The sacral ala are marrow-containing structures and, given their overall greater volume compared with other vertebral structures, are not an uncommon site for osseous me-

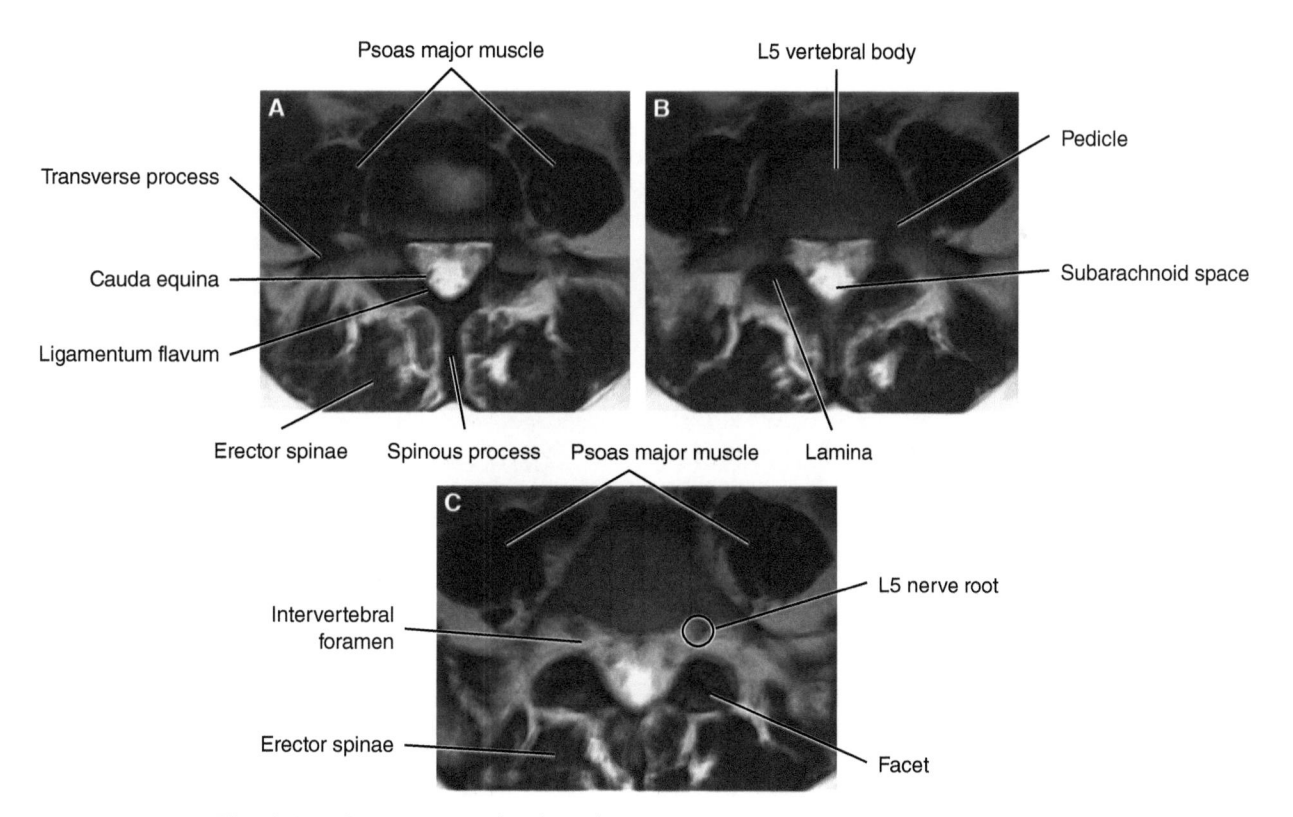

Fig. 1-10 **A-C,** T2 weighted axial MR images at the level of the L5 vertebra.

tastases. The trabecular density within the sacral ala is decreased relative to the adjacent osseous structures.[8] These regions of diminished trabeculae or alar voids are the sites that are affected by stress and insufficiency fractures. In certain cases the striking imaging appearance of these fractures may mimic the presence of neoplastic processes in these locations. The cortical thickness of the sacrum is relatively uniform throughout.

The posterior elements of the sacrum are fused so that they form a circumferential enclosure of the sacral spinal canal (see Fig. 1-10).[9] Rudimentary spinous processes are present. These spinous processes are fused and comprise the median sacral crest. The posterior contour of the sacrum is convex and the inner surface is concave. At the fifth sacral segment, or S5, an opening is present at the posterior aspect of the sacrum. This aperture, or sacral hiatus, is the terminal point of the spinal canal. The sacral hiatus is bordered posteriorly and laterally by the sacral cornu, which is covered by the sacral ligaments. The sacral canal is the caudal continuation of the lumbar spinal canal (Fig. 1-11). It contains the meninges, the sacral and coccygeal nerve roots, and the filum terminale. The extradural contents of the sacral canal from S5 to approximately S3 consist of epidural fat and veins. The dural sac terminates at S2 to S3. Given that this is the most dependent location of the cerebrospinal fluid–containing dural sac, this anatomic location is not an infrequent site of drop metastases. Unlike the other levels of the spine, an anterior and posterior foramen is present at each sacral level, allowing for passage of the respective sacral nerve roots (S1 to S4). The ventral rami exit anteriorly and the dorsal rami exit through the posterior foramen. There are four pairs of sacral foramina that demonstrate an oblique orientation within the sacrum so that the posterior foramen is medial relative to the anterior foramen.

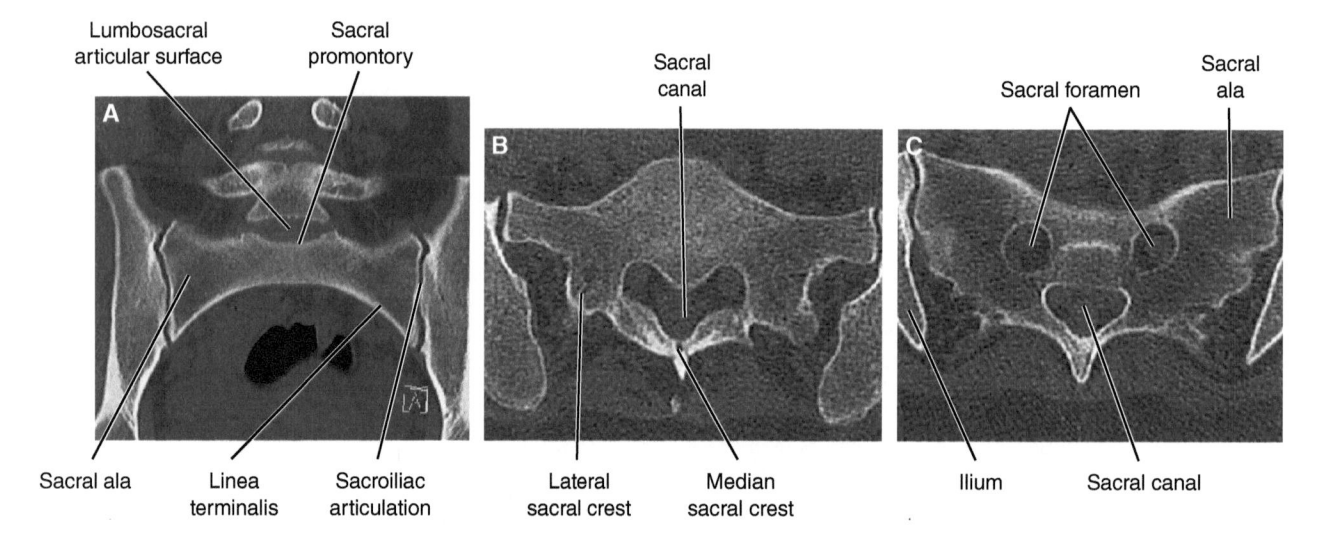

Fig. 1-11 **A,** Coronal CT reformation. **B** and **C,** Axial CT images in bone window algorithm of the sacrum.

The lumbosacral plexus is formed by the ventral rami of the L4, L5, and S1 through S4 nerves.[10] It consists of a large superior band and a small inferior band that join to form the sciatic nerve at the level of the greater sciatic foramen. The superior band consists of the lumbosacral trunk (L4, L5, and S1), and the inferior band is comprised of S2, S3, and S4. The lumbosacral trunk is located medial to the psoas muscle and sacroiliac joint and anterior to the sacral ala. Caudally the sacral plexus is found posterior to the iliac artery and vein and anterior to the piriformis muscle. The sacral sympathetic plexus is located at the L5-S1 level between the common iliac vessels (Fig. 1-11, *D*). The ganglion impar is the union of the distal sympathetic chains; it is located anterior to the sacrococcygeal junction posterior to the rectum.

The sacroiliac joints are located between the sacral alae and the iliac bones (see Fig. 1-11). The sacral side of the sacroiliac joint is lined by a layer of hyaline cartilage with a thickness of 3 to 5 mm. A 1 mm thick layer of fibrocartilage lines the iliac side of the sacroiliac joint.[11] The sacroiliac joints are complex and consist of synovial and fibrous compartments. The synovial portion of the joint is the lower one third to one half of the joint. The remaining fibrous joint compartment is formed by the interosseous portion of the sacroiliac ligaments. This interosseous ligament is surrounded anteriorly by the ventral sacroiliac ligament and posteriorly by the dorsal sacroiliac ligament. The ventral and dorsal sacroiliac ligaments also surround the synovial component of the sacroiliac joint. Two additional sacral ligaments, the sacrotuberous and sacrospinous ligaments, contribute to further stabilization of the sacrum. The sacrotuberous ligament connects the sacrum to the ischial tuberosity, the posterior iliac spine, and the coccyx, whereas the sacrospinous ligament connects the caudal aspect of the sacrum to the ischial spine and coccyx.

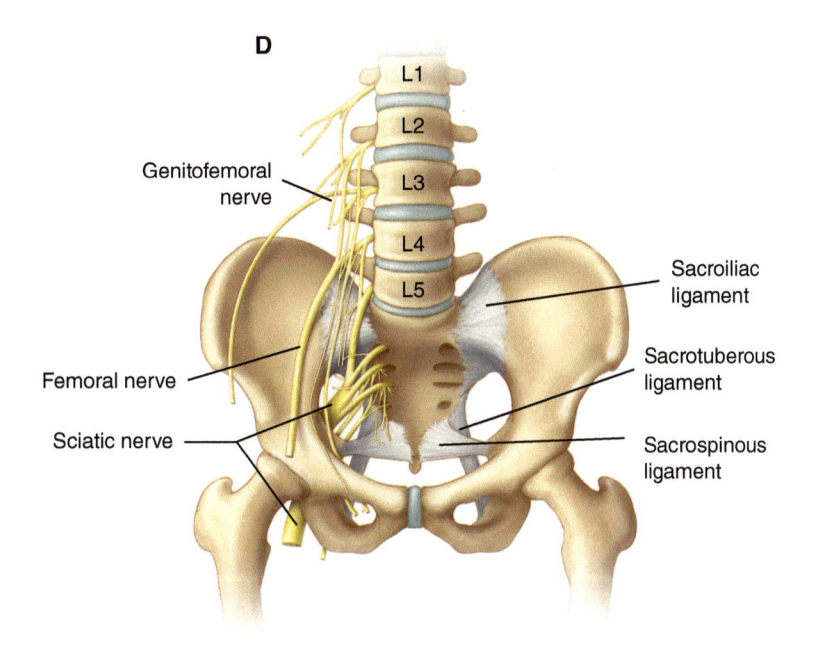

Fig. 1-11, cont'd **D,** Anterior view showing pelvic ligaments and the major nerves of the lumbosacral plexus.

The sacrum functions as a weight-bearing structure for the spinal axis. The sacrum's wedge-shaped configuration acts as a keystone within the pelvic ring and is involved in bidirectional load transfer not only from above but also from the lower extremities through the pelvic girdle.[12] The sacrum contributes to the posterior stability of the pelvis, particularly during standing, walking, and running. It also serves to protect the contents of the pelvic cavity.

TRANSITIONAL VERTEBRA

The most common pattern of vertebral segments consists of seven cervical vertebrae, 12 thoracic vertebrae, and five lumbar vertebrae for a total of 24 vertebral segments. In some individuals an anomalous pattern of total segments may be encountered in which there are 23 to 25 total vertebral segments. The most consistent finding, however, is the presence of seven cervical vertebrae. The vertebral count in the thoracic spine may result in 11, 12, or 13 rib-bearing vertebral segments. Similarly, four, five, or six lumbar vertebral segments may be encountered in the lumbar spine. A transitional vertebra is a hybrid structure that retains features of the spinal segment above and below it. These can occur at the thoracolumbar junction or the lumbosacral junction,[13] although transitional vertebrae are most frequently identified at the lumbosacral junction. Furthermore, a complete S1-S2 disc is associated with lumbosacral transitional vertebrae. In a series of 147 subjects, transitional vertebrae were seen in 15% of the subjects at the lumbosacral junction, and 4.1% of the subjects had transitional segments in the thoracolumbar junction.[13]

It is imperative that the possible presence of a transitional vertebra and an anomalous number of total vertebrae be routinely considered when evaluating results of spine imaging examinations. Potential treatment implications exist in these patients not only with respect to treatment planning and correct level identification, but also with their clinical presentation. For example, patients with lumbosacral transitional vertebrae have dermatomal variations. Appropriate communication and review of all pertinent studies between the radiologist and the clinician is recommended to identify the presence of a transitional vertebra and to clarify the number and level of a specific lesion along the spinal axis.

UNCOVERTEBRAL AND FACET JOINTS

The facet joints are paired apophyseal joints between the posterior elements of two adjacent vertebrae with a steep oblique orientation to the sagittal plane (see Figs. 1-4, *A* through *D* and 1-7, *A* and *B*). Facet joints are synovial joints that are subjected to the stresses of normal motion. Degenerative facet arthropathy is not uncommon in middle-aged to elderly adults and can often mimic posterior element lesions on skeletal scintigraphy. Facet joints are found between C2-3 caudally to the L5-S1 level.

In addition, within the cervical spine, additional articulations are found between the cervical vertebrae from C2 to T1. They are referred to as the uncovertebral joints. The lateral edges of the superior surface of each cervical vertebral body curve upward to form the uncinate processes, creating somewhat of a shallow concavity into which the vertebra above settles (see Fig. 1-1, *A* through *C*). The inferior surface of the vertebral body above is shaped in a complementary broad-based convexity. This synovial-lined articulation between these two surfaces forms the uncovertebral joint characteristic of the cervical spine.

The facet joints in the thoracic and lumbar spine demonstrate a different morphology. In the thoracic and lumbar spine each vertebra contributes two articular processes, one on each side, to form a curved facet joint with the vertebra just inferior to it (see Figs. 1-4, *E* through *I*; 1-5, *A* through *C*; and 1-7, *C* through *G*). The joint contains a synovial lining and is reinforced by a fibrous capsule. The median branch of the dorsal ramus of the ipsilateral spinal nerve innervates each facet joint as well as the joint immediately beneath it.[4] In the thoracic spine the superior articular facets project from the junction of the lamina and pedicle on either side. The joint surfaces are ovoid and slightly convex with a subtle superolateral orientation (see Figs. 1-4, *A* through *D*; 1-7, *A* and *B*; and 1-8, *A*). The paired interior articular facets are formed by the inferior edges of the laminae with a shape and orientation that are complementary to those of the paired superior articular facets. In the lumbar spine the origins of the paired superior articular facets are similar to those in the thoracic spine. The difference lies in their shape and orientation. The articular facets are concave in shape, and they are oriented dorsomedially so that their surfaces almost face each other (see Fig. 1-7, *C* through *G*). As in the thoracic spine, the paired inferior articular facets of the lumbar spine arise from the laminae with a shape and orientation complementary to the superior articular facet projected from the vertebrae below. The articulation between the superior and inferior facets in the lumbar spine occurs in a mortise-and-tenon fashion, which restricts both rotation and flexion in this spinal segment.

INTERVERTEBRAL DISCS

The intervertebral discs are supportive structures of the spinal axis that, in combination with facet joints, allow for complex motion between two adjacent vertebrae. The discs are located between vertebral bodies in the cervical, thoracic, and lumbar spine with a couple exceptions: an intervertebral disc is not present at the C1-2 articulation, and an S1-2 intervertebral disc may be seen within the upper sacrum, which should not be confused with the L5-S1 intervertebral disc space. Aside from these aforementioned exceptions and the rare occurrence of congenitally fused or "block" vertebra, an intervertebral disc is located between two vertebral bodies.

The disc forms an amphiarthrosis between the superior and inferior vertebral end plates and is comprised of a hyaline cartilage plate, a more peripheral annulus fibrosus and a central nucleus pulposus. The cartilage plate lines the vertebral endplate and is surrounded by the ring epiphysis of the vertebral body endplate. Because of its location, the hyaline endplate possesses a shock-absorbing feature.

The annulus fibrosus is made up of a layered matrix of laminated fibrocartilaginous fibers. One layer is oriented in a specific direction, with the adjacent layer oriented at 50 to 70 degrees. The inner fibers of the annulus fibrosus attach to the cartilaginous endplate. Most of the outer fibers of the annulus fibrosus attach to the ring epiphysis and to the anterior and posterior longitudinal ligaments. A few of the outer annulus fibrosus fibers, or Sharpey's fibers, attach directly to the cortex of the vertebral body. The annulus fibrosus, therefore, assists in stabilizing the spinal axis by interacting with the nucleus pulposus to transmit axial and nonaxial forces associated with spinal motion and weight transfer. The nucleus pulposus consists of a complex gelatinous matrix that is rich in proteoglycans and in normal spinal columns also possesses abundant water content. In the lumbar spine the nucleus pulposus is located slightly posterior to the central vertical axis of the vertebral body.

SPINE LIGAMENTS

Two major ligaments help to stabilize the spine and ensure that its individual elements are in proper alignment while, at the same time, affording the flexibility required by the spine to accomplish everyday movements. These structures are the anterior longitudinal ligament (ALL) and the posterior longitudinal ligament (PLL) (see Figs. 1-2; 1-6, A and B; and 1-8, B and C). The ALL is a band of ligamentous fibers that courses along the anterior surface of the spine from the skull base to the sacrum. This strong band of fibers reinforces the spine and provides added stability to its individual elements. The ALL attaches to the atlas and axis in the upper cervical spine, where it is the narrowest with a cordlike appearance. Moving inferiorly down the spine, the ALL increases in width until it blends completely into the presacral fibers. The composition of the ALL includes three different layers: deep, intermediate, and superficial. The deep layer spans only one intervertebral disc space and is covered by the intermediate layer, which spans two to three vertebrae. Finally, the superficial layer unites four to five vertebrae at a time. The periosteum along the anterior surface of each vertebra is formed where the ALL adheres to the bony surface, although, for the most part, the ALL is adherent to the anterior surface of the spine. There are points at which the ALL is more loosely attached and can be elevated from the spine, such as at the midsection of the intervertebral disc where it attaches to the annulus fibrosus.[6]

The posterior counterpart to the ALL is the PLL, which courses along the posterior surface of the vertebrae and intervertebral discs within the vertebral canal. Similar to the ALL, the PLL extends from the base of the skull to the sacrum. Unlike the ALL, which is adherent to the spine, the PLL exhibits a segmental denticulate configuration

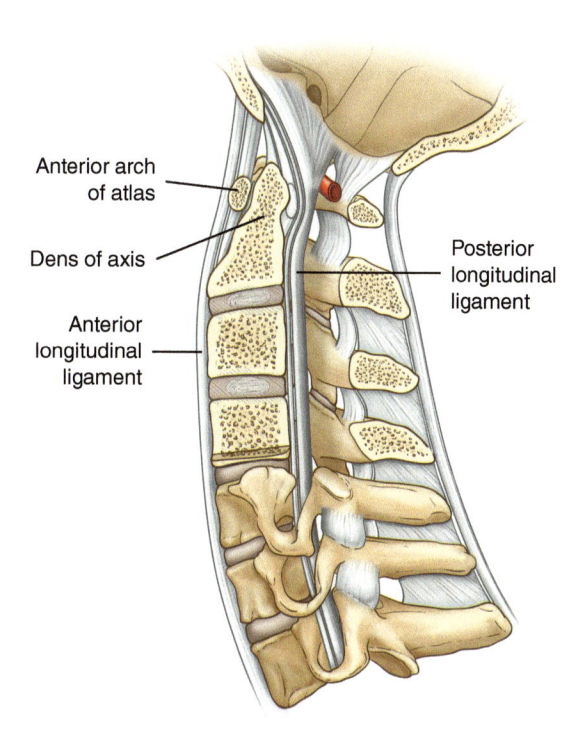

Fig. 1-12 Cross section of cervical vertebrae showing the anterior longitudinal ligament and the posterior longitudinal ligament.

in which a thick band of connective tissue arches across the concave dorsal aspect of the vertebral body to allow vascular elements to enter and exit the medullary sinuses deep to the fibers (Fig. 1-12). This configuration is most commonly seen in the lower thoracic and lumbar spine. Whereas the ALL comprises three fibrous layers, the PLL is composed of only two layers: deep fibers that span two vertebral elements and longer superficial fibers that bridge several vertebrae.

PARASPINAL MUSCLES

Spine tumors may involve any or all elements of the spine (e.g., vertebrae, spinal cord, nerve roots, and blood vessels) and may demonstrate intracanalicular or extracanalicular extension. Although neoplastic extension into the spinal canal is a major concern in terms of potential involvement of the neural elements, extracanalicular extension into the paraspinal muscles may be just as problematic. In some cases the extent of paraspinal involvement may be so pronounced that it causes compression of the paraspinal and iliopsoas muscles. The proximity of the tumor capsule to these soft tissue structures may present a challenge for surgical resection. Although it is a rare occurrence, the possibility of primary tumors arising from the paraspinal soft tissues themselves must also be entertained and factored into the management algorithm. As such, knowledge of the paraspinal muscle anatomy is important for appropriate surgical planning.

The paraspinal muscles are the deep muscles of the back with direct attachments to the spine from the skull base to the sacrum (Fig. 1-13). The primary function of these muscles is to provide additional stability and support to the vertebral column while enabling simple or complex motions of the spine. The paraspinal muscles are divided into anterior and posterior groups on the basis of their location relative to the vertebral column. These muscles can also be divided based on their location within the segmental spine (e.g., cervical, thoracic, or lumbar). The size and complexity of each segmental muscle group are dependent on the type of motion permitted at that particular level of the spine.

The cervical paraspinal muscles are the most complex, given the variety of movements permitted at the craniocervical junction, and they are discussed separately from the rest of the spine (see Figs. 1-2 and 1-3). The paraspinal muscles in this region extend from the base of the skull to the thoracic inlet and are divided into anterior and posterior groups, with the posterior group being the major component. The muscles within this group are located in the posterior cervical space and are further subdivided into superficial, intermediate, and deep layers (Table 1-1).

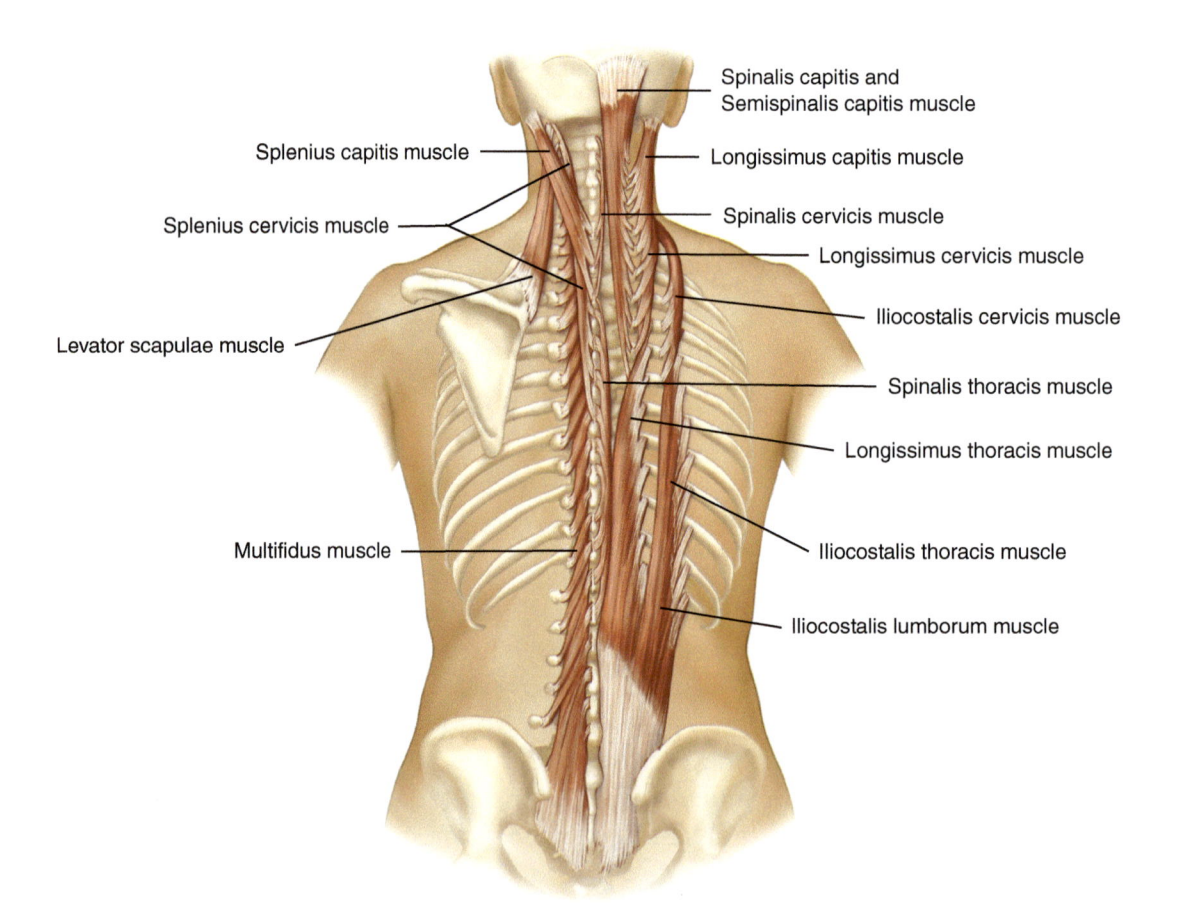

Fig. 1-13 Posterior view of the deep back muscles.

Table 1-1 Superficial, Intermediate, and Deep Cervical Paravertebral Muscles

Layer	Muscle	Origin	Insertion
Superficial	Trapezius	Medial third of the superior nuchal line External occipital protuberance Ligamentum nuchae C7 and T1-12 spinous processes	Lateral third of the clavicle Medial margin of the acromion Scapular spine
Intermediate	Levator scapulae	C1 and C2 transverse processes Posterior tubercles of C3 and C4 transverse processes	Superior angle and upper medial border of the scapula
	Splenius capitis	Lower half of the ligamentum nuchae C7-T3 spinous processes	Mastoid process of the temporal bone Lateral aspect of the superior nuchal line
	Splenius cervicis	T3-6 spinous processes	Posterior tubercles of C1 through C3 or C4 transverse processes
	Semispinalis cervicis	T1 through T5 or T6 transverse processes	C2-5 spinous processes
	Semispinalis capitis	Tips of C7 through T6 or T7 transverse processes	Between the superior and inferior nuchal lines of the occipital bone
	Longissimus cervicis	Tips of T1 through T4 or T5 transverse processes	Posterior tubercles of C2-6 transverse processes
	Longissimus capitis	T1 through T4 or T5 transverse processes Articular processes of lower 3 or 4 cervical vertebrae	Posterior margin of mastoid process of the temporal bone
Deep	Iliocostalis cervicis	Angles of ribs 3-6	Posterior tubercles of C4-6 transverse processes
	Spinalis capitis	Spinous processes of lower cervical and upper thoracic vertebrae	Between superior and inferior nuchal lines of occipital bone
	Spinalis cervicis	C7-T2 spinous processes Ligamentum nuchae	C2-4 spinous processes
	Multifidus	Articular processes of lower 4 cervical vertebrae	Spinous processes of higher vertebrae (each muscle spans 2-4 vertebrae)
	Rotatores cervicis	Articular processes of cervical vertebrae	Base of spinous processes of cervical vertebrae immediately superior
	Interspinales	Superior surface of spinous processes	Inferior surface of spinous processes immediately superior
	Intertransversarii	Superior surface of transverse processes	Inferior surface of transverse processes immediately superior

The anterior cervical muscles are located in the prevertebral space and have attachments at the skull base and the upper thoracic spine (Table 1-2).

The deep muscles of the thoracolumbar spine also consist of anterior and posterior groups (see Figs. 1-6, *C* through *J;* and 1-7 through 1-9). The posterior lumbar paraspinal muscles include the paired erector spinae, multifidus, interspinalis, and intertransversarii muscles (Table 1-3).

The erector spinae is a superficial muscle that is further subdivided into the iliocostalis, longissimus, and spinalis muscles. As a group the paired erector spinae muscles originate from the iliac crests to insert onto the inferior margins of the six or seven most caudal ribs.

The paired psoas and quadratus lumborum constitute the anterior thoracolumbar muscles. Similar to the erector spinae muscles, the quadratus lumborum muscles also originate from the iliac crests with insertions on the lowest ribs and transverse processes of L1-4.

Table 1-2 Cervical Prevertebral Muscles

Muscle		Origin	Insertion
Longus colli	Superior oblique	Anterior tubercles of C3-5 transverse processes	Tubercle of the anterior arch of C1
	Inferior oblique	Anterior surface of T1 through T2 or T3 vertebral bodies	Anterior tubercles of C5-6 transverse processes
	Vertical	Anterolateral surface of C5-T3 vertebral bodies	Anterior surfaces of C2-4 vertebral bodies
Longus capitis		C3-6 transverse processes via tendinous slips	Inferior surface of basilar occipital bone
Rectus capitis anterior		Anterior surface of lateral masses of C2 C2 transverse processes	Inferior surface of basilar occipital bone
Rectus capitis lateralis		Superior surface of C1 transverse processes	Inferior surface of jugular process of occipital bone

Table 1-3 **Posterior Thoracic and Lumbar Paravertebral Muscles**

Muscle			Origin	Insertion
Erector spinae	Iliocostalis	Lumborum	Iliac crest Common tendon Erector spinae	Ribs 6-12
		Thoracis	Ribs 6-12	Ribs 1-6 C7 transverse process
		Cervicis	Ribs 3-6	C4-6 transverse processes
	Longissimus	Thoracis	Transverse processes of lumbar vertebrae	Ribs 3-12 T1-12 transverse processes
		Cervicis	T1-5 transverse processes	C2-6 transverse processes
		Capitis	T1-5 transverse articular processes	Mastoid process of temporal bone
	Spinalis	Thoracis	T11-L2 spinous processes	T1-8 spinous processes (variable)
		Cervicis	C7 spinous process T1-2 vertebrae Ligamentum nuchae	C2-4 spinous processes
		Capitis	Lower cervical/upper thoracic spinous processes	Semispinalis capitis muscle
Multifidus			Lumbar mammillary processes Thoracic transverse processes Lower 4 cervical articular processes	Lumbar spinous processes
Rotatores		Lumborum	Lumbar mammillary processes	Spinous process immediately above
		Thoracis	Thoracic transverse processes	Spinous process immediately above
		Cervicis	Cervical articular processes	Spinous process above C7

VASCULAR SUPPLY—VERTEBRAL COLUMN

Each vertebra is supplied by nutrient vessels derived from paired segmental arteries arising from the posterior surface of the aorta.[6] These arteries course along the anterolateral surface of the vertebral bodies and give rise to dorsal and lateral branches (Fig. 1-14). In the thoracic spine the lateral branch continues on to become the intercostal artery, and in the lumbar spine the lateral branch continues as the lumbar artery. The dorsal branch divides into the posterior central, prelaminar, and intermediate neural branches, which provide the major blood supply to the bone and contents of the vertebral canal (i.e., neural elements, meninges, and epidural tissues). Two additional nutrient vessels, the anterior central and postlaminar branches, are derived from arteries external to the vertebral column. The paired segmental arteries that course to the right form ipsilateral anastomoses over the anterior aspect of the spine are called *prevertebral anastomoses*. Those that course to the left of the aorta communicate with each other through paravertebral anastomoses.

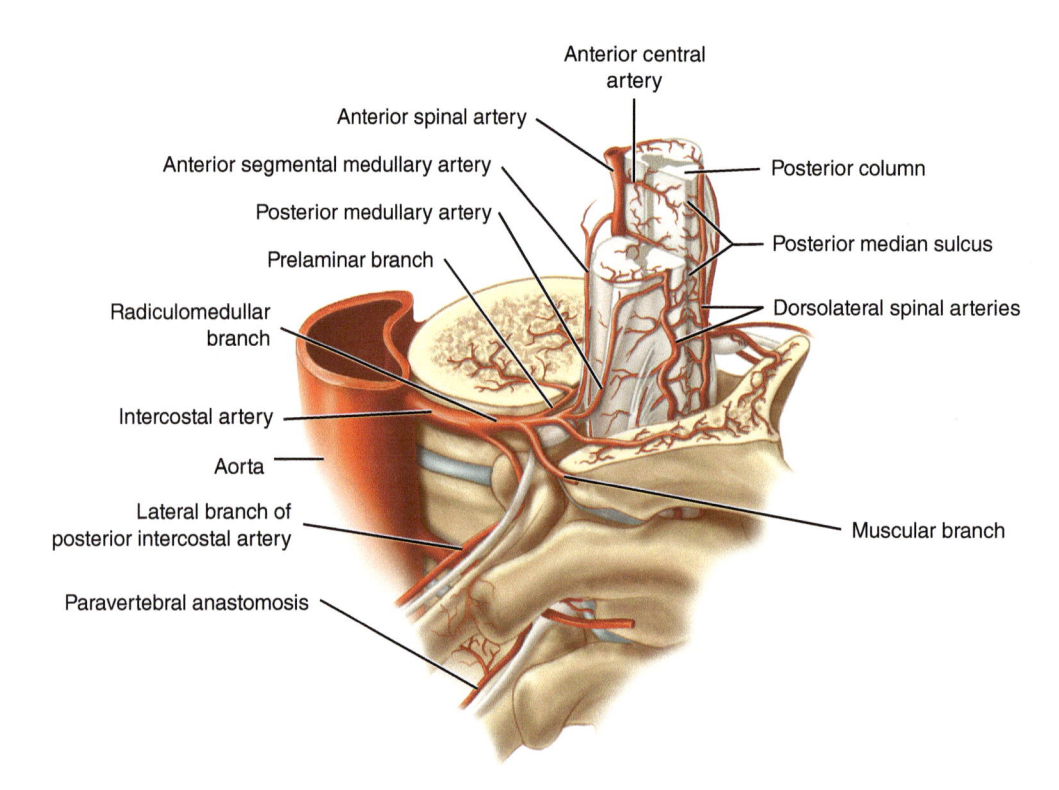

Fig. 1-14 Posterolateral view showing blood supply to the spinal cord and vertebrae.

The venous drainage of the vertebral column is valveless, and the direction of flow varies on the basis of intraabdominal and intrathoracic pressures.[6] The spinal venous system is divided into external and internal venous plexuses with distributions approximating that of the arterial supply. The external and internal venous plexuses can further be divided into an anterior and posterior network of veins. The anterior external venous plexus is smaller and receives draining veins from the anterior and lateral portions of the vertebral body. The more extensive posterior external venous plexus is a paired network that exists on either side of the vertebral column with anastomoses across the spinous processes along the entire length of the spine. The internal venous system drains into the external plexus through tributaries that pass through the intervertebral foramina.

The internal venous plexus is an extensive network of veins in the epidural space that is intimately associated with the epidural fat. These epidural sinuses are also divided into anterior and posterior segments, referred to as the anterior and posterior internal vertebral (epidural) venous plexuses, respectively. The anterior internal vertebral plexus lies medial to the pedicles on either side and converge medially into the larger basivertebral vein. Venous channels perforating the vertebral body proper serve as a connection between the basivertebral vein and the anterior external venous plexus. Although these tributaries serve as a connection between the epidural sinuses and the external venous plexus, the major external connection is through the veins that pass through the intervertebral foramen, appropriately called the *intervertebral veins*. The potential for bidirectional flow within the epidural sinuses presents a hematogenous route for metastasis between pelvic malignancies and the central nervous system.

VASCULAR SUPPLY—SPINAL CORD

The segmental arteries from the aorta give rise to radiculomedullary branches in addition to the previously mentioned lateral branches. The radiculomedullary arteries supply the exiting nerve roots and also provide variable supply to the spinal cord. Three longitudinal vessels receive blood from the segmental spinal arteries through medullary feeder arteries and distribute the oxygen- and nutrient-rich blood to the spinal cord. They are composed of a single unpaired anterior spinal artery (ASA) and two smaller paired dorsolateral spinal arteries (DSAs). The ASA lies in the ventral median fissure and supplies 75% of the cord substance and all of the gray matter.[6] It is formed by two branches derived from the vertebral arteries just proximal to their formation of the basilar artery with additional supply from the spinal segmental arteries through medullary feeder vessels. The number of feeder arteries varies for each spinal segment, although the typical distribution of anterior medullar arteries is three in the cervical region, one or two in the thoracic region, and one large vessel in the lumbosacral region (artery of Adamkiewicz). The paired DSAs provide less nutritional support for the spinal cord, as reflected by their diminished caliber. They arise from the posterior inferior cerebellar arteries, as well as from scattered radiculomedullary branches in the thoracic spine, and receive more medullary feeder vessels than the ASA.

Table 1-4 Distribution of the Vertebral Artery in the Foramen Transversarium

Vertebral Artery Segment	Distribution in Foramen Transversarium
V1	Subclavian artery to the C6 foramen transversarium
V2	C6 to C1
V3	Atlas to foramen magnum
V4	Extends intradurally from the foramen magnum to meet with the contralateral vertebral artery to form the basilar artery

Data from Peng CW, Chou BT, Bendo JA, et al. Vertebral artery injury in cervical spine surgery: anatomical considerations, management, and preventive measures. Spine J 9:70-76, 2009.

In the cervical spine the vertebral arteries travel in the foramina transversaria between C1 and C6 (see Fig. 1-1). The left vertebral artery is usually larger and dominant in patients with vertebral artery asymmetry, and it is the main blood supply to the posterior circulation of the brain. The most cephalad anterior spinal artery branch arises at the junction of the two vertebral arteries. This provides the vascular supply to most of the cervical spinal cord. The vertebral artery is divided into four segments, V1 through V4, in the surgical literature[15] (Table 1-4).

The vertebral artery is most vulnerable at several points where it is not surrounded by an osseous channel: anteriorly at C7, laterally at C3 to C7, and posteriorly at C1 and C2. There are various anatomic anomalies of the vertebral artery that operators should be aware of.[14,15] The artery can course beneath the C1 posterior arch without passing through the transverse foramen. Some patients have a high-riding C2 transverse foramen on at least one side. Rheumatoid arthritis has a known predilection for pannus formation at the atlantoaxial joint resulting in subluxation and an abnormally located transverse foramen. Detailed imaging studies of the cervical spine with recognition of arterial anomalies and pathologic conditions can help the surgeon minimize possible vertebral artery injury during high cervical spine instrumentation.

In the thoracic and lumbar spine, the anterior spinal artery derives contributions from several segments. The largest of these is the artery of the lumbar enlargement, also referred to as the artery of Adamkiewicz (Fig. 1-15). This artery tends to arise from a lower thoracic intercostal artery branch on the left side between T9 and T12 in approximately 75% of cases. However, it may arise lower or higher along the spinal axis or on the right side. Smaller contributions to the anterior spinal artery supply may also be observed from other thoracic intercostal radiculomedullary branches. A border zone of the arterial vascular supply may be encountered at the level of the cervicothoracic junction.

Similar to the venous drainage of the vertebral column, the veins draining the spinal cord are also divided into an anterior and a posterior system. The anterior portion of the spinal cord is drained by the anterior sulcal vein, which empties into the anterior

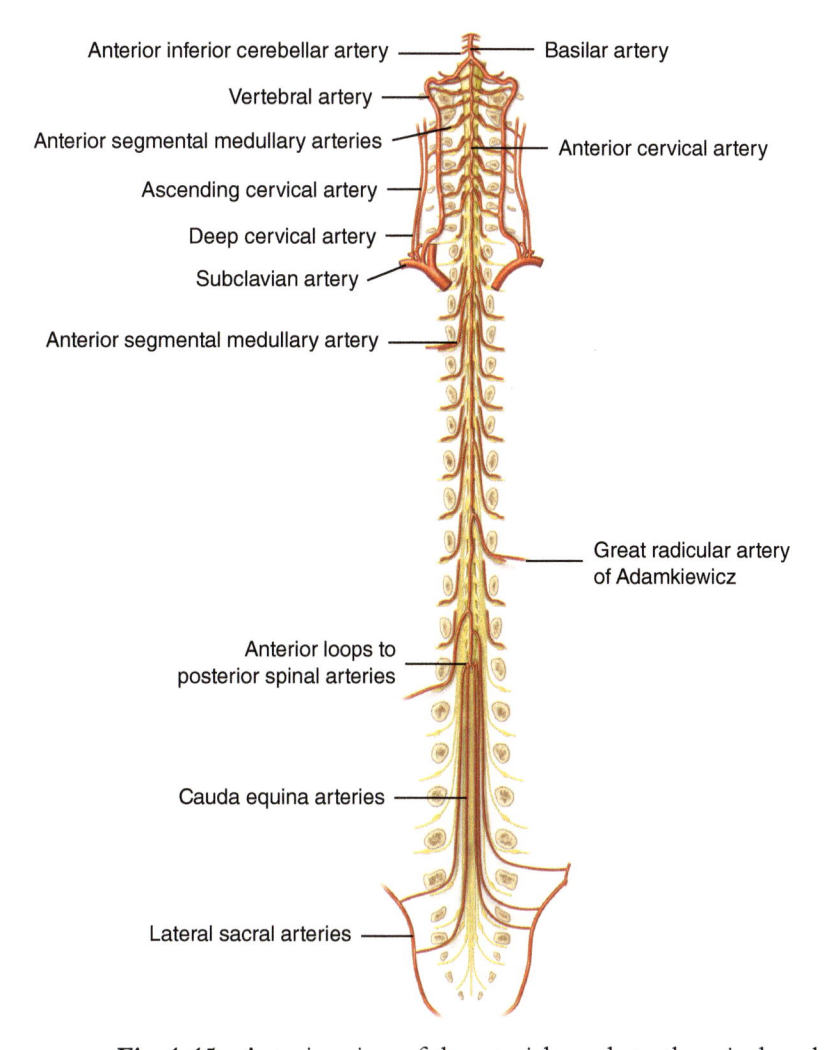

Fig. 1-15 Anterior view of the arterial supply to the spinal cord.

spinal vein followed by the anterior segmental medullary vein. The anterior spinal vein runs parallel to the ASA. Posteriorly the spinal cord is drained by the posterior sulcal vein, posterior spinal vein, and posterior segmental medullary vein. Both the anterior and posterior segmental medullary veins communicate with the extravertebral venous system through the intervertebral vein, which exits at each level through the neural foramen as part of the neurovascular bundle.

OTHER CRITICAL STRUCTURES

In addition to the paraspinal muscles, knowledge of the regional anatomy at each level of the spine is crucial to surgical planning. Critical structures to avoid in the cervical region include the great vessels (e.g., common and internal carotid arteries, vertebral arteries, internal jugular veins, and so forth) (see Fig. 1-1), nerves or nerve roots (e.g., brachial plexus, vagus, phrenic, recurrent laryngeal, and so forth) (see Fig. 1-3), and trachea, esophagus, and thyroid and parathyroid glands.[16] Major structures to avoid from the thoracic inlet to the lower thoracic spine include the aortic arch, superior vena cava, intercostal vessels and nerves, sympathetic chains, tracheobronchial tree, and lungs. Resection of anterior paraspinal tumors in the lumbar spine could potentially require mobilization of the aortic branch vessels, femoral nerves, and adjacent organs (e.g., pancreas, liver, spleen, kidneys, and so forth). Finally, critical structures to avoid at the sacral level are the iliac vessels, sacral nerve roots, and pelvic organs.

Major nerve plexuses are also found along the length of the spine, and their locations should be noted during surgical planning (Fig. 1-16). The sympathetic trunk is a paired nervous structure that flanks the vertebral column on either side and courses subpleurally in close apposition to the heads of the ribs. Dilatations corresponding to ganglia are seen along the length of the sympathetic trunk at most intercostal spaces. The stellate ganglion, or cervicothoracic ganglion, is a paired structure formed by fusion of the inferior cervical and first thoracic sympathetic ganglia. This paired ganglion is larger than its more inferior counterparts and is located at the C7 level anterior to the transverse process and head of the first rib. The stellate ganglion varies in size and shape, with as much as 25% of the general population exhibiting a significant right-to-left asymmetry in terms of morphology.[17] The primary sympathetic innervation of the head, neck, and upper extremities is provided via pathways through the stellate ganglion. The cervical sympathetic chain and its ganglia are formed by the coalescence of strands that arise from the cephalad aspect of the stellate ganglion and lies anterior to the longus colli muscle. In addition, the vertebral artery travels between the individual strands that form the cervical sympathetic chain and, in some cases, may be encased by the nerve fibers. During the preoperative planning process, it is important to note the close relationship of these structures to avoid potential harm to the nerves or vessels.

The celiac plexus constitutes the largest visceral nerve plexus in the abdomen; it supplies the sympathetic, parasympathetic, and visceral sensory afferent fibers to the upper abdominal viscera. This complex neural structure consists of a network of retroperitoneal nerve fibers that course along the anterolateral aspect of the aorta just caudal to the origin of the celiac artery.[18] The preganglionic sympathetic efferent nerve fibers, derived from the greater splanchnic (T5 through T9), lesser splanchnic (T10 and T11), and least splanchnic (T12) nerves, are the main components of the celiac plexus.[19] This nerve plexus also includes the celiac, superior mesenteric, and aorticorenal ganglia. The celiac trunk also contains parasympathetic efferent nerve fibers, which are derived from the posterior trunk of the vagus nerve. The afferent nerve fibers from the upper abdominal viscera travel to and terminate in the spinal cord through the celiac plexus.

The celiac plexus and splanchnic nerves are separated by the diaphragmatic crura, with the celiac plexus in the antecrural space and the splanchnic nerves in the retrocrural space. Although there is some variability in the position of the celiac ganglia with respect to the spine, approximately 94% are located at the T12 or L1 level.[18,19] Given this variability, the celiac artery is considered to be a more reliable landmark for localization of the celiac plexus because its relationship to the artery is more consistent. It is also important to note that the celiac ganglion on the left is positioned slightly inferior to the one on the right. Localization of this major nerve plexus and its ganglia before surgery is essential to avoid injuring this critical structure.

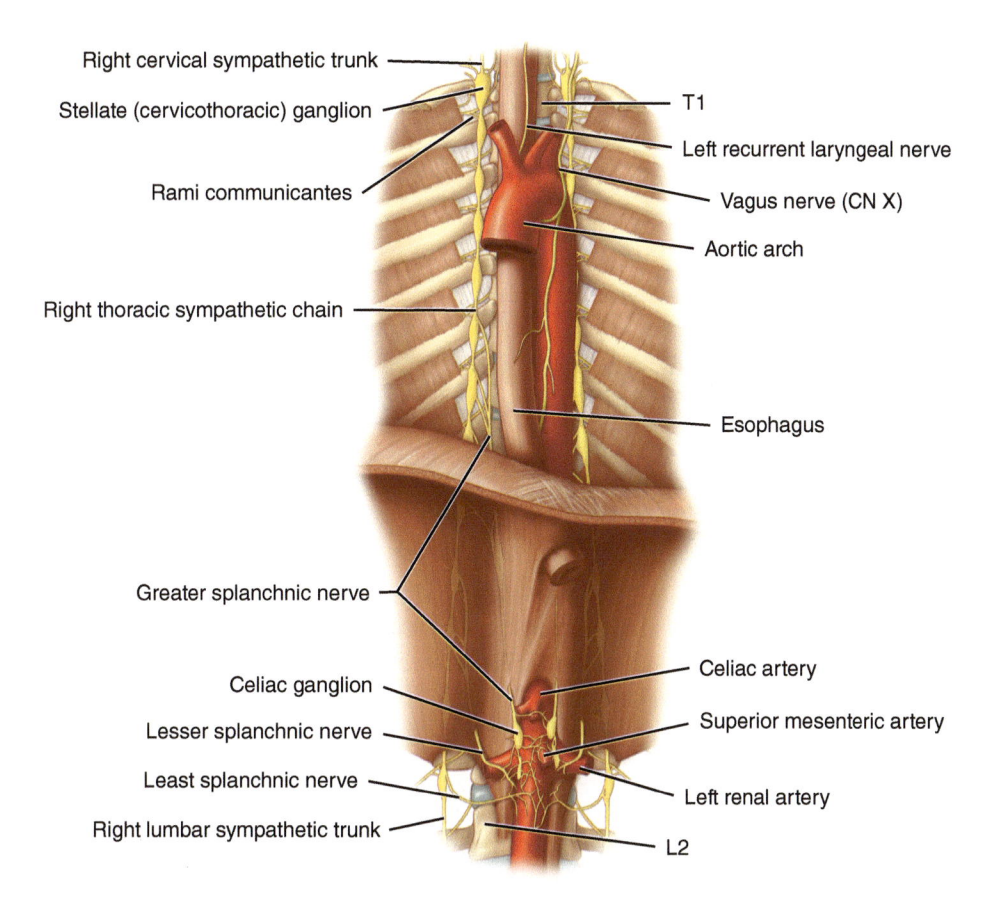

Fig. 1-16 Anterior view of autonomic nerves, including the stellate ganglion (cervicothoracic ganglion) and the celiac ganglion.

IMAGING MODALITIES FOR THE SPINE

Several imaging modalities are used in the evaluation of the spinal axis. MRI is the preferred imaging modality for evaluating musculoskeletal and neurologic diseases of the spine. MRI provides superior soft tissue detail, which improves the detection of processes that may involve the vertebral bodies, intervertebral discs, neural foramina, ligaments, spinal cord, nerve roots, and/or caudal portion of the posterior fossa structures. The imaging characteristics of cerebrospinal fluid and fat on the various MRI sequences aid in identification of the spinal cord, thecal sac, nerve roots, and vessels of the spine as well as potential abnormalities that may affect these structures. Cerebrospinal fluid exhibits low signal intensity on T1-weighted images and high signal intensity on T2-weighted images. Fat demonstrates the opposite with high signal intensity on T1-weighted images and relatively lower signal intensity on T2-weighted images. For example, the normal appearance of bone marrow varies based on the degree of fatty replacement. The spinal cord itself demonstrates an intermediate signal on T1-weighted images and a very low in signal on T2-weighted images because of the densely packed myelinated fibers and inherent low water content. The option of contrast-enhanced MRI can help further identify and characterize inflammatory or neoplastic processes in the spine. Postcontrast sequences are typically fat suppressed to differentiate high signal from contrast enhancement versus high signal from fat on the T1-weighted sequences.

Morphologic abnormalities of vertebral endplates are best appreciated on sagittal and coronal fat-suppressed sequences.[20] In some cases subtle endplate abnormalities may be the only clue to disc degeneration and a possible explanation for the patient's pain. To appreciate abnormalities, it is important to first be familiar with what is considered normal. The cartilaginous endplate normally appears hypointense to isointense on T1-weighted images and hypointense on T2-weighted images relative to the normal intervertebral disc.

Although there are many advantages to using MRI, this particular imaging modality is not without its disadvantages. Because of the long scanning time, motion artifacts are a frequent occurrence, particularly in patients who have back pain. In some instances, motion degradation may be so pronounced that it renders the images uninterpretable. Even with patient cooperation, motion artifacts may still arise from pulsatile flow within blood vessels, cerebrospinal fluid pulsation, or normal respiratory motion. Techniques are available to reduce these potential sources of artifacts, but they are at the expense of increased scanning time. Magnetic susceptibility artifacts from spinal hardware may also pose a problem in patients who have had prior surgery.

Additional imaging techniques, such as CT, CT myelography, nuclear medicine bone scans, and positron emission tomography (PET), are available to supplement MRI or serve as an alternative imaging modality for patients who are unable to undergo MRI evaluation. CT is superior to MRI in depicting the osseous elements of the spine, as well as any sclerotic or lytic processes that may affect the spine. Paraspinal soft tissues are also fairly well demonstrated on CT. As with MRI, a variety of artifacts are inherent to CT as an imaging modality. Beam-hardening artifact from low-energy photons or the presence of spinal hardware can present a challenge to image interpretation. However, despite the challenges, when these imaging techniques are employed, presurgical evaluation of the spine is a less daunting task.

IMAGING AND ANATOMIC LOCALIZATION OF SPINE TUMORS

Tumors that arise from or extend or spread to the spine may be localized within one or more spinal structures. To facilitate a radiographic differential diagnosis, a compartmental approach is used to place or localize the lesion or lesions to one or more spinal compartments. These compartments are based on two key anatomic landmarks: the dura mater and the spinal cord proper. Lesions located outside of the dura are referred to as being located within the extradural compartment and are often found within the spinal column, the vertebrae and/or intervertebral discs, or the adjacent paraspinal soft tissue structures. They include entities such as metastases, multiple myeloma, and, less commonly, primary bone tumors of the spine. These lesions can extend into the spinal canal either directly or through the neural foramina. Lesions located within the dura but outside of the spinal cord are referred to as *intradural* and *extramedullary*. These lesions are often related to the spinal covering, or meninges, or the exiting nerve roots (i.e., meningiomas, schwannomas, and neurofibromas). Lesions located within the spinal cord are described as being located within the intramedullary compartment. Spinal cord astrocytomas and ependymomas comprise most of these lesions.

Most neoplasms of the spine are located within the extradural compartment. Osseous tumors often display a predilection for specific sites in the skeleton. Benign osseous tumors and tumor-like lesions that favor the spine include aneurysmal bone cysts, osteoblastomas, Langerhans cell histiocytosis, and hemangiomas.[21] Malignant lesions with a predilection for the spine include chordoma, multiple myeloma, and osseous metastases. The distribution of tumors or tumorlike lesions within a vertebra has some value in predicting whether the lesion is benign or malignant. Malignant lesions occur predominantly in the anterior part of the vertebra, whereas benign lesions typically affect the posterior elements. Primary myeloma of the spine in its early stages may spare the pedicles. This is in contrast to metastatic disease, which usually affects the pedicles. The most common malignant spine tumors are metastatic disease, myeloma, and lymphoma, whereas the most common benign spine tumors are hemangiomas.[22] In the case of a solitary spine lesion, a primary tumor must be considered.

Patients presenting with spinal lesions are often evaluated by means of conventional radiography, CT, and MRI. The radiologic appearance of these tumors can help narrow the differential diagnosis and guide treatment, whether conservative or surgical. Correlation with patient age and clinical history contributes to the diagnostic evaluation. Tumors of the spine are uncommon in patients less than 30 years of age and, if present, are often benign.[23] The exceptions are Ewing's sarcoma and osteosarcoma.[23] In contrast, patients older than 30 years presenting with spinal lesions often have tumors that are malignant, with the exception of hemangiomas and bone islands.[22,24,25]

Although conventional radiography plays a lesser role in the evaluation of spinal lesions, this imaging modality is still complementary to CT and MRI evaluation. Spinal radiographs, which are often obtained on an urgent or emergent basis in patients with severe back pain, may show subtle signs of pedicle destruction, a unilateral missing pedicle on the frontal radiographic projection, pathologic vertebral compression deformities, or abnormal paraspinal soft tissue density. In addition, weight-bearing full-spine radiographs may play a role in surgical planning. CT with multiplanar reformats is the preferred imaging modality for the evaluation of osseous integrity and the degree of tumor involvement. Magnetic resonance, on the other hand, is used primarily for evaluation of the epidural space and neural elements, and the administration of gadolinium helps delineate vascular structures and tumor enhancement patterns. Tumors that are intimately associated with the spinal vessels may require CT or MR angiography to define the relationship between the tumor and adjacent blood vessels.[22] Spinal catheter angiography may be indicated for the evaluation of a suspected hypervascular spinal mass, such as an aggressive hemangioma of the vertebral body or a renal metastasis. The distribution of metastatic disease in the vertebra follows the distribution of hematopoietic marrow. For example the sacrum, which is rich in hematopoietic marrow in adults, is a common site of both metastatic disease and hematologic malignancies.

References (With Key References in Boldface)

1. Netter FH. Cervical vertebrae. In Dalley AF II, ed. Atlas of Human Anatomy. East Hanover, NJ: Novartis Medical Education, 1998 (Plates 9-16).
2. Lustrin ES, Karakas SP, Ortiz AO, et al. Pediatric cervical spine: normal anatomy, variants, and trauma. Radiographics 23:539-560, 2003.
3. **Mathis JM, Shaibani A, Wakhloo AK. Spine anatomy. In Mathis JM, Golovac S, eds. Image-Guided Spine Interventions. New York: Springer, 2011, pp 8-32.**
4. **Ortiz O, Deramond H. Spine anatomy. In Imaging of the Spine. Philadelphia: Saunders/Elsevier, 2011, pp 7-23.**
5. Kothe R, O'Holleran JD, Liu W, et al. Internal architecture of the thoracic pedicle. An anatomic study. Spine 21:264-270, 1996.
6. **Parke WW. Applied anatomy of the spine. In Rothman-Simeone, ed. The Spine. Philadelphia: Saunders/Elsevier, 2011 pp 35-87.**
7. Diel J, Ortiz O, Losada RA, et al. The sacrum: pathologic spectrum, multi-modality imaging, and subspecialty approach. Radiographics 21:83-104, 2001.
8. Peretz AM, Hipp JA, Heggenes MH. The internal bony architecture of the sacrum. Spine 23:971-974, 1998.
9. Whelan MA, Gold RP. CT of the sacrum: 1. Normal anatomy. AJR Am J Roentgenol 139:1183-1190, 1982.
10. Blake LC, Robertson WD, Hayes CE. Sacral plexus: optimal imaging planes for MR assessment. Radiology 199:767-772, 1996.
11. Resnick D. Anatomy of individual joints. In Resnick D, ed. Diagnosis of Bone and Joint Disorders, 3rd ed. Philadelphia: WB Saunders, 1995, pp 716-719.
12. White AA, Panjabi MM. Clinical Biomechanics of the Spine, 2nd ed. Philadelphia: Lippincott-Raven, 1990, pp 362-363.
13. Carrino JA, Campbell PD, Lin DC, et al. Effect of spinal segment variants on numbering vertebral levels at lumbar MR imaging. Radiology 259:196-202, 2011.
14. Peng CW, Chou BT, Bendo JA, et al. Vertebral artery injury in cervical spine surgery: anatomical considerations, management, and preventive measures. Spine J 9:70-76, 2009.
15. Goldberg AL, Kershah SM. Advances in imaging of vertebral and spinal cord injury. J Spinal Cord Med 33:105-116, 2010.
16. Spitzer AL, Ceraldi CM, Wang TN, et al. Anatomic classification system for surgical management of paraspinal tumors. Arch Surg 139:262-269, 2004.
17. Hogan QH, Erickson SJ. MR imaging of the stellate ganglion: normal appearance. Am J Roentgenol 158:655-659, 1992.
18. **Kambadakone A, Thabet A, Gervais DA, et al. CT-guided celiac plexus neurolysis: a review of anatomy, indications, technique, and tips for successful treatment. Radiographics 31:1599-1621, 2011.**
19. Zhang XM, Zhao QH, Zeng NL, et al. The celiac ganglia: anatomic study using MRI in cadavers. Am J Roentgenol 186:1520-1523, 2006.
20. Naidich TP, Castillo M, Cha S, et al. Imaging of the Spine. Philadelphia: Saunders/Elsevier, 2011.
21. Greenspan A. Tumors and tumor-like lesions. In Orthopedic Imaging: A Practical Approach. Philadelphia: Lippincott Williams & Wilkins, 2011, pp 545-786.
22. Rodallec MH, Feydy A, Larousserie F, et al. Diagnostic imaging of solitary tumors of the spine: what to do and say. Radiographics 28:1019-1041, 2008.
23. Greenspan A. Radiologic evaluation of tumors and tumor-like lesions. In Orthopedic Imaging: A Practical Approach, 5th ed. Philadelphia: Lippincott Williams & Wilkins, 2004, pp 547-588.
24. Banna M. Clinical Radiology of the Spine and the Spinal Cord. Rockville, MD: Aspen System, 1985.
25. Ortiz AO, Lefkowitz D. Imaging of spinal tumors. In Castillo M, ed. Spinal Imaging: State of the Art. Philadelphia: Hanley & Belfus, 2001, pp 145-167.

Chapter 2

Spine Biomechanics and Balance of Tumor Reconstruction

Ali A. Baaj, Nicholas Theodore, Neil R. Crawford

A number of primary and secondary neoplasms affect the vertebral column. These tumors range from benign osteoid osteomas to the more malignant osteosarcomas and metastatic tumors. The decision to intervene surgically is multifactorial, based on the histopathologic findings and natural history of the primary disease, the patient's age, comorbid conditions, neurologic function, and the structural integrity of the involved vertebral column segment or segments. When warranted, the goals of oncologic surgical intervention are to decompress the neural elements; resect the lesion en bloc, if possible and if necessary; restore spinal alignment; and stabilize the vertebral column.

Given the aggressive nature of most spinal column tumors, with the goal of en bloc resection for some, complex reconstruction is often necessary. An understanding of the strengths and weaknesses of various fixation techniques is required to ensure a favorable surgical outcome and preservation of neurologic function. In this chapter we first discuss the basic principles of spinal biomechanics relevant to tumor reconstruction. We then highlight the properties of various complex fixation techniques in spinal oncology surgery.

KEY BIOMECHANICAL PRINCIPLES

One key biomechanical consideration with regard to tumor reconstruction is stress shielding. In surgery for trauma or degeneration, this consideration is typically less important, because the cross-section of hardware tends to be much smaller than the cross-section of the remaining bone. However, wide tumor resections often require a wide span of reconstruction. According to Wolff's law, bone under compression will grow and bone shielded from loading will resorb. At surgery, options to encourage a good environment for bone growth and prevent stress shielding, including the selection of biomaterials and locations of fixation points, are important considerations.

The expansive nature of tumor reconstruction often leads to lengthy constructs and thereby long moment arms. A moment is the product of force and distance. In the context of spine reconstruction, forces are applied by the muscles to the spine, and the distance under consideration is the distance across the hardware construct. Understanding how moment arms are introduced and counteracted by different portions of instrumentation can prevent subsequent failures.

Another concept closely linked to stress shielding and moment arms is sagittal balance. Whether the spine's favored upright posture is balanced well so the center of gravity is equally distributed over the anterior and posterior portions of the spine can be greatly affected by surgery. Fusing the spine in poor sagittal balance can exaggerate stress shielding, increase moment arms, lead to muscle spasms as the body tries to compensate (rebalance), and accelerate spinal decompensation.

OCCIPITOCERVICAL JUNCTION

The occipitocervical (OC) junction of the spine is a complex region formed by the base of the occiput, C1 and C2, and the associated neurovascular and ligamentous components (Fig. 2-1). The primary motions at this level are flexion and extension (O-C1) and axial rotation (C1-2). Fixation therefore markedly restricts the corresponding range of motion (ROM), depending on which motion segments are fused. Fixation of O-C1 or O-C2 is sometimes necessary after resection of aggressive foramen mag-

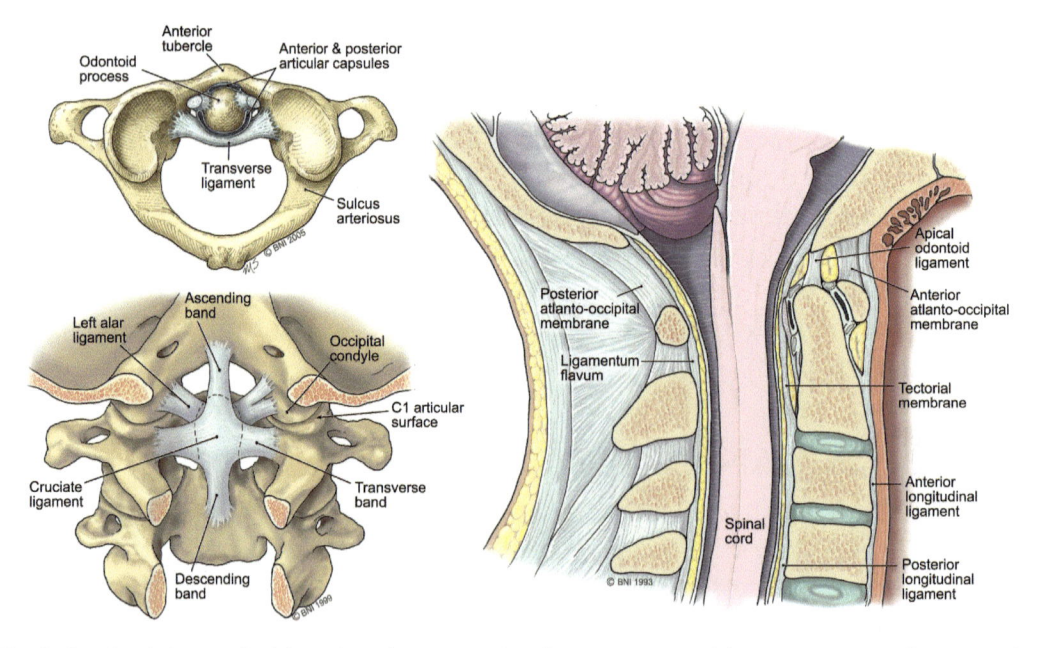

Fig. 2-1 Occipitocervical junction demonstrating ligamentous and bony structures that contribute to stability. (Courtesy of Barrow Neurological Institute.)

num or atlantoaxial primary osseous and metastatic tumors, especially if the principal articulating joints have been compromised.

Stabilization techniques at the OC junction primarily involve fixation of any of the following structures: the occipital bone, occipital keel, and occipital condyle; the C1 lateral mass and posterior arch; and the C2 pars interarticularis, pedicle, or lamina. Fixation strategies, similar to those used in other parts of the spinal column, include using a combination of screws, hooks, wires, plates, and rods. In general, OC constructs have short moment arms and less stress shielding, because a limited amount of bone is resected and hardware is limited to the posterior region. Sagittal balance, however, can easily be disturbed because of the difficulty of fixating the OC junction in "perfect" sagittal alignment, because the alignment desired at surgery is difficult to assess from fluoroscopy and head position (Fig. 2-2). A global analysis of the patient's sagittal balance can be an important consideration during a spine reconstruction of the OC

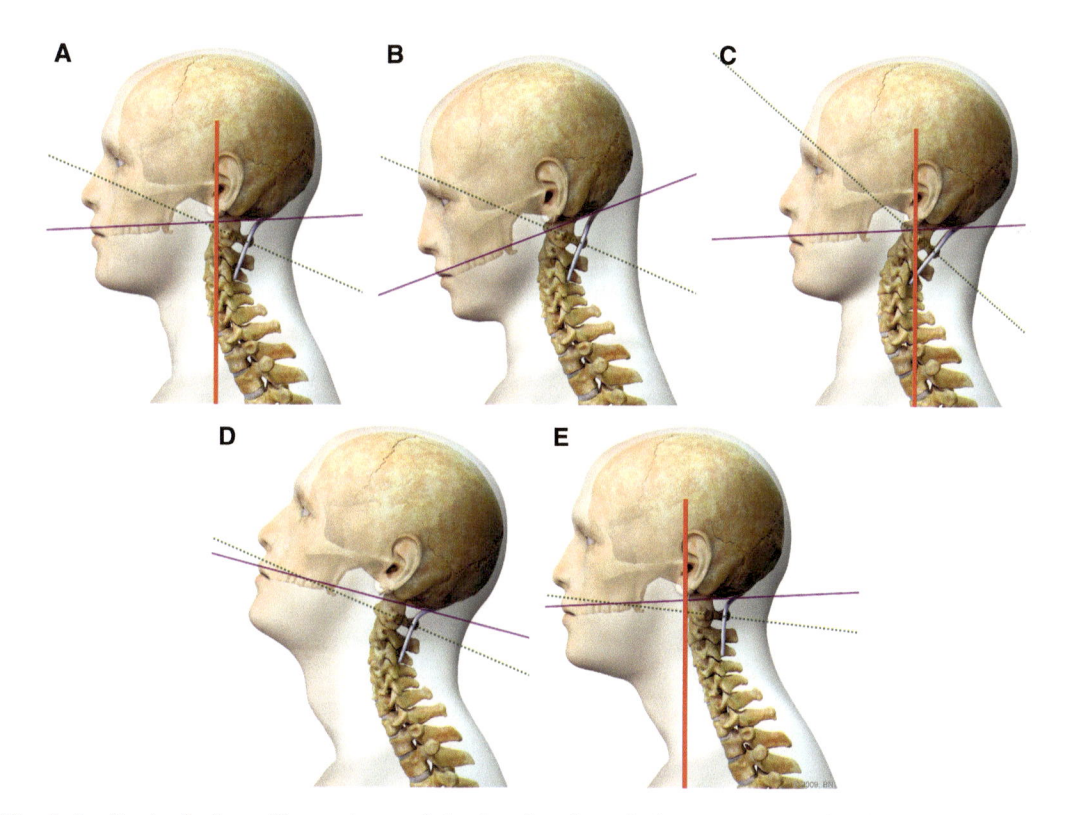

Fig. 2-2 Sagittal plane illustrations of the head and neck demonstrating the theoretical effect of occipitocervical fusion on sagittal balance and posture. It may be difficult for the surgeon to estimate intraoperatively the correct neutral sagittal angle, particularly at the occipitoatlantal (O-C1) joint. **A,** If O-C1 is positioned and fused in the correct neutral alignment within an O-C3 construct *(indicated by the angle between the solid violet and dotted green lines)*, then overall sagittal balance *(indicated by the red vertical line)* is good postoperatively. **B,** If O-C1 is fused in a kyphotic (flexed) alignment intraoperatively, then the patient compensates through exaggerated lordosis (extension) at caudal levels postoperatively, resulting in **C,** a final head position with sagittal balance shifted posteriorly. **D,** If O-C1 is fused in a lordotic alignment intraoperatively the patient compensates by kyphosing caudal levels postoperatively, resulting in **E,** a final head position with sagittal balance shifted anteriorly. (Courtesy of Barrow Neurological Institute.)

junction after tumor resection; therefore preoperative fluoroscopy is recommended to ensure that the patient is fixated in the desired OC alignment. This is particularly important for constructs that cross both the occipitocervical and cervicothoracic junctions.

Multiple studies have attempted to determine which OC construct provides the greatest biomechanical stability. Oda et al[1] evaluated the biomechanics of five different OC constructs with the use of an unstable C2 dens fracture model:
1. Occipital and sublaminar wiring with rectangular rod
2. Two occipital screws and C2 lamina claw hooks/rod
3. Two occipital screws, two foramen magnum screws, and C1-2 transarticular screws/rod
4. Two occipital screws and C1-2 transarticular screws/Y-plate
5. Six occipital screws and C2 pedicle screws/rod

C1-2 transarticular screws or C2 pedicle screws offered the greatest stiffness compared with sublaminar wiring or lamina hooks.

A recent study in our laboratory compared the stability provided by three occipitoatlantal fixation techniques (O-C1 transarticular screws, occipital keel screws rigidly interconnected with C-1 lateral mass screws, and suboccipital/sublaminar wired contoured rod).[2] Application of O-C1 transarticular screws with a wired graft reduced the mean ROM to 3% of normal. During extension and lateral bending, occipital keel-C1 lateral mass screws (also with graft) offered less stability than transarticular screws ($p < 0.02$), reducing ROM to 17% of normal (Fig. 2-3). The wired contoured rod reduced ROM to 31% of normal, providing significantly less stability than either screw fixation technique. Fatigue increased ROM in constructs fitted with transarticular screws, keel screws/lateral mass screw constructs, and contoured wired rods, by a mean of 19%, 5%, and 26%, respectively. In all constructs, adding a structural graft significantly improved stability, but the extent depended on the loading direction. We concluded that O-C1 transarticular screws and occipital keel–C1 lateral mass screws are approximately equivalent in performance for occipitoatlantal stabilization. A posteriorly wired contoured rod is less likely to provide a favorable fusion environment because it offers less stability and has a greater likelihood of loosening with fatigue. However, wired contoured rod constructs spanning at least O-C2 have proved to be quite biomechanically robust in clinical experience.[3]

In a recent cadaveric biomechanics study, Dmitriev et al[4] evaluated the biomechanics of intralaminar, pars, and pedicle screw fixation at C2. In terms of stiffness, C2 intralaminar fixation was comparable to pedicle screws, but only with an intact atlantoaxial ligament complex. When the dens is fractured or resected, however, pedicle and pars screw fixation offers greater stiffness.

Substantial biomechanical data demonstrate the superiority of using the occipital keel, C1 lateral mass, and C2 pars or pedicle for the most rigid immediate fixation at the

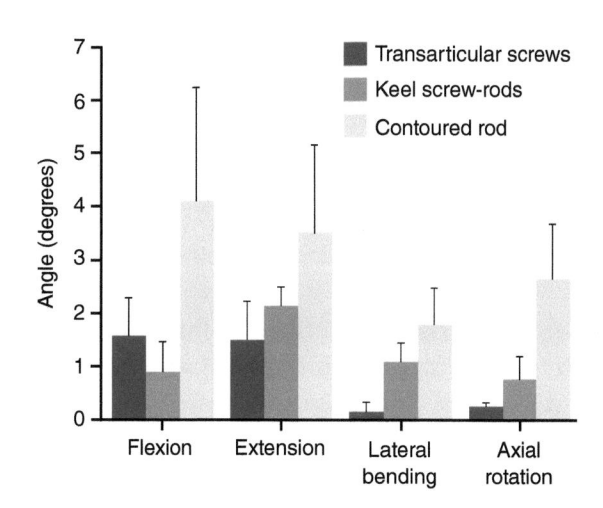

Fig. 2-3 Bar graph comparing mean ROM at O-C1 for three fusion constructs studied by Bambakidis et al[2]: bilateral O-C1 transarticular screws, occipital keel screws interconnected through rods to C1 lateral mass screws, and horseshoe-shaped contoured rod attached to the skull base suboccipitally and C1 sublaminarly with the use of crimped, braided titanium cable. Error bars show standard deviations. (Courtesy of Barrow Neurological Institute.)

OC junction. Given the involvement of the posterior elements, the use of intralaminar and sublaminar devices is often precluded in spine tumor surgery. In all cases the construct should be augmented by a structural autograft (iliac crest or rib) or allograft (cadaveric fibula). Unless bony resection is extensive, stress shielding should not occur. However, some sagittal imbalance may occur, depending on the method of fixation and the ability to identify normal curvature.

SUBAXIAL CERVICAL SPINE

Key features of the subaxial cervical spine (C3-7) include its lordotic curvature and coronally oriented facets. The vertebral bodies account for the weight-bearing capability in the flexed position, but the facets are loaded during extension. In the subaxial cervical spine, as in the thoracolumbar region, fixation should be directed at the region of the resected segment. That is, if a corpectomy is performed, the anterior column should be reconstructed with a cage or strut graft and plating. When the posterior elements are resected, fixation should be performed posteriorly. When an extensive multilevel resection is performed, circumferential fixation affords the most biomechanically advantageous construct. However, significant resection and circumferential reconstruction in the subaxial spine induce stress shielding, create long moment arms, and may cause sagittal imbalance. Long-segment, unidirectional fixation, with either posterior or anterior multilevel reconstruction, is more likely to cause sagittal imbalance than other types of constructs. It is typically easier in the subaxial cervical spine than in the upper cervical spine to identify (on radiographs) and match the normal curvature of the neck to avoid sagittal imbalance.

Panjabi et al[5] investigated the failure of the screw-vertebra interfaces in one- and three-level corpectomy models. In both models the motion at the lower ends was greater than at the upper ends. Fatigue increased three-level model ranges of motion at the lower end by 171% during flexion, 164% during extension, 153% during lateral bending, and 115% during axial rotation. Similar increases were observed in neutral zones. Panjabi et al[5] concluded that screw loosening in such lower constructs may explain the clinically observed failures at the caudal end of long anterior cervical plate constructs.

Singh et al[6] evaluated the stability of anterior, posterior, and anterior/posterior constructs with and without instrumentation after a two-level cervical corpectomy. The combined anterior/posterior instrumentation reconstruction model and the posterior-only instrumentation model were significantly more rigid than the anterior-only instrumentation model ($p < 0.05$). There was no statistically significant difference between the combined anterior plate/posterior instrumentation model and the posterior instrumentation–only model.

An in vitro study from our laboratory[7] compared stability after a three-column injury stabilized by posterior, anterior, or combined anterior/posterior fixation. Posterior, anterior, and combined instrumentation each significantly improved stability ($p < 0.05$). Combined fixation provided significantly better stability than either anterior or posterior instrumentation alone (Fig. 2-4). Circumferential fixation will likely balance moment arms and bring the axis of rotation to a more neutral position. It should be noted that the clinical relevance of the stability of one construct over another becomes less important if the spine ultimately fuses in a favorably balanced position.

Another study from our laboratory[8] further highlighted the importance of circumferential fixation in unstable corpectomy and spondylectomy models. Pure moments were applied to destabilized specimens (C5 corpectomy and spondylectomy) before and after anterior, posterior, or combined fixation. Results demonstrated the superiority of circumferential fixation in providing immediate stiffness to both models. Circumferential fixation (anterior graft/plating with C4-6 lateral mass screws) exhibited greater stiffness after corpectomy than after spondylectomy during lateral bending and axial rotation. Extended posterior fixation (C3-7) exhibited greater stiffness after corpectomy than after spondylectomy during extension and axial rotation (Fig. 2-5).

Although resection of posterior elements at a single level is unlikely to cause destabilization, wide resections that involve facet joints posteriorly or vertebral bodies anteriorly require fixation. Ample evidence from biomechanical studies demonstrates the superiority of circumferential fixation, especially with multilevel corpectomies. However, because of loss of bony support, multilevel corpectomies require extensive anterior reconstruction that will likely result in stress shielding and excessive moment arms. These moment arms should be balanced with circumferential fixation, and stress shielding should be countered by ensuring that grafts or cages are under compression. These goals are achieved by sizing hardware to ensure a large area for bony ingrowth and by using a fusion substrate to encourage rapid bone growth.

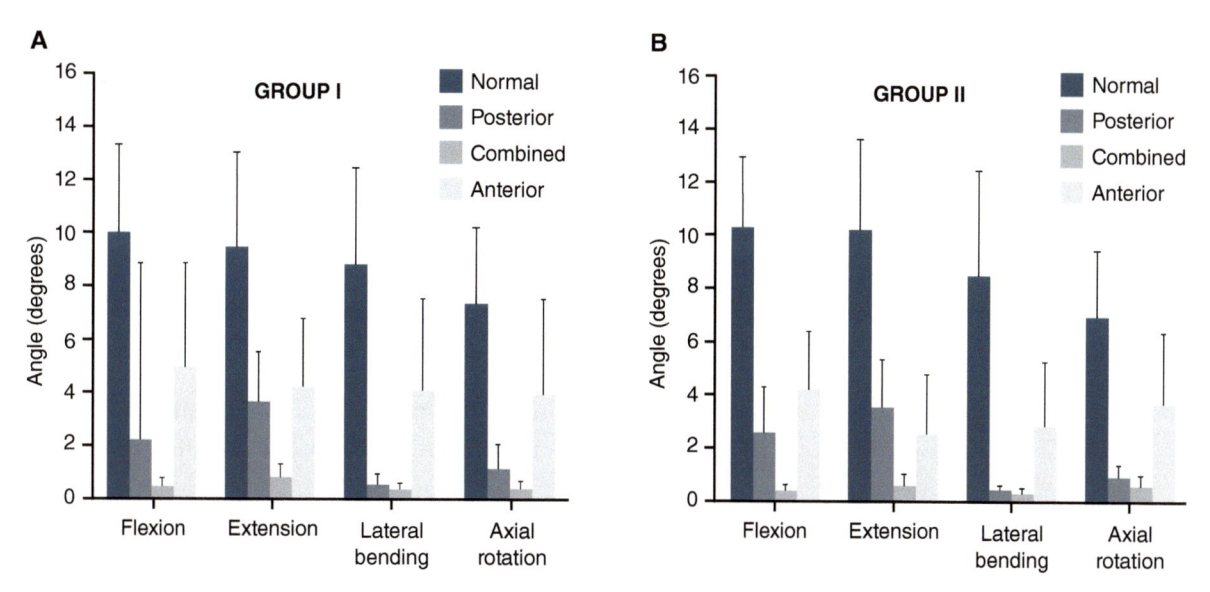

Fig. 2-4 **A,** Bar graphs showing the mean ROM across C5-7 in two 2-level posterior screw-rod constructs: group I (lateral mass screws at C5 and C6 and pedicle screws at C7) and **B,** group II (pedicle screws at C5, C6, and C7) studied by Bozkus et al.[7] Error bars show standard deviation. (Courtesy of Barrow Neurological Institute.)

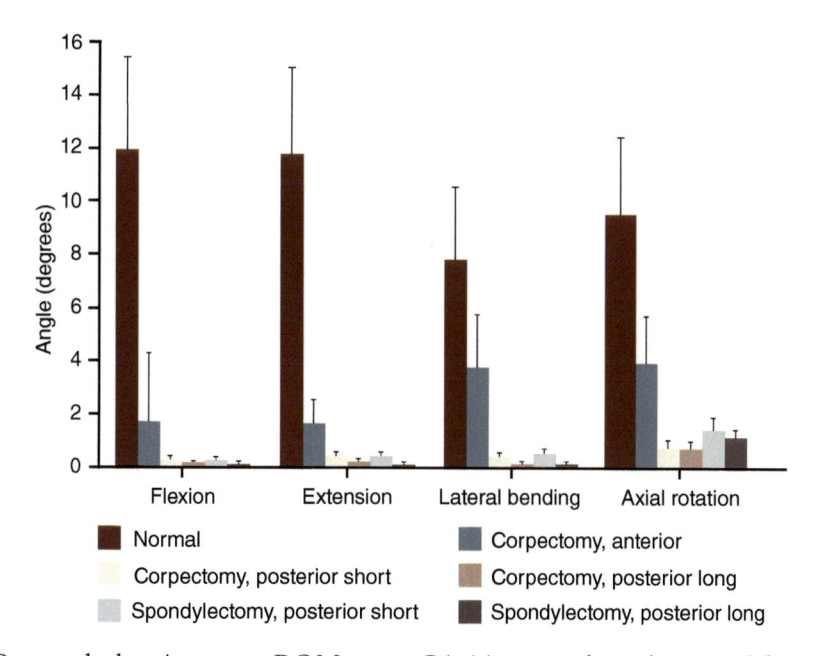

Fig. 2-5 Bar graph showing mean ROM across C4-6 in normal condition and five reconstructed conditions studied by Dogan et al[8]: corpectomy stabilized with two-level anterior plate, corpectomy stabilized with two-level posterior screws-rods, corpectomy stabilized with four-level posterior screws-rods, spondylectomy stabilized with two-level posterior screws-rods, and spondylectomy stabilized with four-level posterior screws-rods. Error bars show standard deviation. (Courtesy of Barrow Neurological Institute.)

CERVICOTHORACIC JUNCTION

In terms of reconstruction, the cervicothoracic junction (CTJ) is a challenging region of the spine. It is a transitional point between the mobile lordotic cervical spine and the relatively rigid kyphotic thoracic region. The size of the vertebral bodies increases along the CTJ, and the facets begin to lose their coronal orientation. In a clinical retrospective review of patients undergoing surgery at the CTJ, Steinmetz et al[9] found that laminectomy at the CTJ was strongly associated with failure. Failure was defined as construct failure, deformity (progression or de novo), or instability.

In an in vitro cadaveric study, Prybis et al[10] evaluated the effectiveness of different CTJ constructs. They studied four different constructs after destabilization:
1. C7-T1 two-column distractive flexion injury with posterior instrumentation
2. C7-T1 three-column injury (anterior disc additionally disrupted) with posterior instrumentation
3. C7-T1 three-column injury with anterior interbody cage/plate and posterior instrumentation
4. C7-T1 three-column injury plus C7 corpectomy with anterior cage/plate and posterior instrumentation

Posterior instrumentation consisted of screws and rods that spanned C5-T1, C5-T2, or C5-T3. The results showed that for a three-column injury, posterior fixation alone was insufficient to provide appropriate stiffness in flexion. For two-column injuries, there were no statistically significant differences in stability ($p > 0.05$), although flexibility tended to decrease as the number of fixated thoracic levels increased.

In another in vitro study, we evaluated different constructs across the CTJ in a trauma model.[11] Flexion, extension, lateral bending, and axial rotation were studied in cadaveric specimens during application of nondestructive pure moments in the following sequence of conditions: (1) intact, (2) after destabilization (simulated three-column injury involving two segments with wedge fracture), (3) with posterior instrumentation from C6-T1 or T2, and (4) with corpectomy/graft and anterior instrumentation alone or combined anterior/posterior instrumentation. Our results demonstrated an 89% decrease in ROM during lateral bending ($p = 0.01$) and a 64% decrease in ROM during axial rotation ($p = 0.04$) with the use of posterior instrumentation compared to anterior instrumentation (Fig. 2-6). Circumferential instrumentation, however, outperformed both anterior and posterior instrumentation alone. Most biomechanical measurements of stability improved when posterior instrumentation was extended from T1 to T2. When feasible, therefore, circumferential fixation across the CTJ is preferable.

Given that the CTJ is a transitional point in the spine between natural lordosis and kyphosis, extensive resection will alter overall sagittal balance in unpredictable ways. Methods for minimizing alterations to natural curvature should be considered when devising reconstruction and fixation strategies.

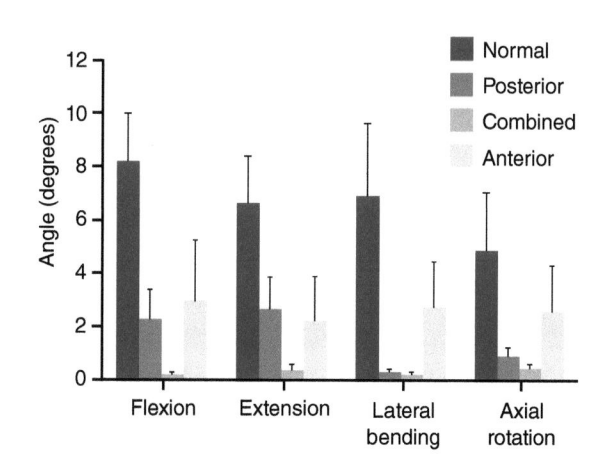

Fig. 2-6 Bar graph showing mean angular ROM with posterior instrumentation (C6 lateral mass screws, no screws in C7-T1 pedicle screws), anterior plate from C6-T1, and combined anterior and posterior instrumentation, as studied by Ames et al.[11] (Courtesy of Barrow Neurological Institute.)

THORACOLUMBAR SPINE

The thoracic spine is the most frequently involved segment in metastatic spine disease.[12] Tumors in these segments of the spine typically involve either the anterior or combined anterior/posterior elements of the spine. A common presentation is a pathologic compression fracture of the vertebral body. Given that the vertebral body and the intervertebral disc comprise the load-bearing portion of the spine, it is especially important that this feature be considered when planning reconstruction. Depending on the extent of the disease, surgical stabilization methods include vertebral body augmentation, anterior reconstruction alone, and circumferential fixation. Anterior reconstruction improves load sharing and restores lordosis and sagittal balance.

In the rigid thoracic spine, the rib cage acts as a "fourth column" of support. In the region of true ribs, the ribs also serve the useful purpose of maintaining sagittal alignment during surgical resection and reconstruction of the thoracic spinal column. Unless there is extensive resection of multiple thoracic levels and associated rib attachments, a significant disturbance in sagittal balance is unlikely. Similarly, stress shielding is unlikely to be an issue unless wide tumor resection, including removal of rib sections, leads to a need to place circumferential hardware. If extended posterior instrumentation is needed, it may be necessary to offset the long moment arm that has been introduced by augmenting the construct with an anterolateral device.

In an in vitro cadaveric study, Oda et al[13] evaluated the stability of anterior, posterior, and circumferential fixation after L2 spondylectomy. After implantation of an anterior titanium mesh as a strut graft, the testing sequences were as follows: (1) anterior instrumentation at L1-3 with multisegmental posterior instrumentation at T12-L4, (2) anterior instrumentation at L1-3 with short posterior instrumentation at L1-3,

(3) anterior instrumentation at L1-3, (4) multilevel posterior instrumentation at T12-L4, and (5) short posterior instrumentation at L1-3. During all loading modes, circumferential instrumentation techniques were significantly stiffer than the intact spine ($p < 0.05$). Even short circumferential fixation provided more stability than multilevel posterior instrumentation ($p < 0.05$).

A cadaveric study from our laboratory[14] examined the biomechanical properties of various anterior fixation techniques in the thoracolumbar spine. Both one- and two-level thoracic corpectomy models were tested. An interbody mesh cage was placed in the corpectomy site, and three types of anterior fixation devices were used: a single-screw plate, a two-screw plate, and a dual-rod system (Fig. 2-7). Testing demonstrated equivalent stabilization among all three techniques for both one- and two-level corpectomies. Depending on the extent of surgical resection, augmenting any of these anterior fixation techniques with posterior fixation may reduce the moment arm, increase stiffness, and ensure that the construct is locked into the appropriate sagittal alignment. Clinically, however, it should be noted that the additional surgery required for circumferential stabilization is not always advisable and in some cases may carry unnecessary risks.

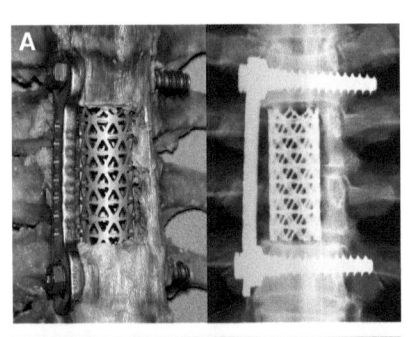

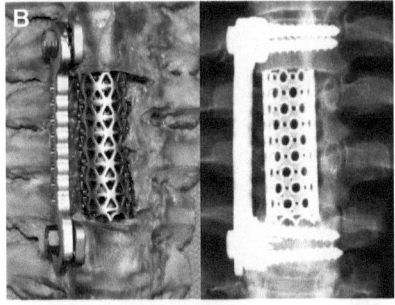

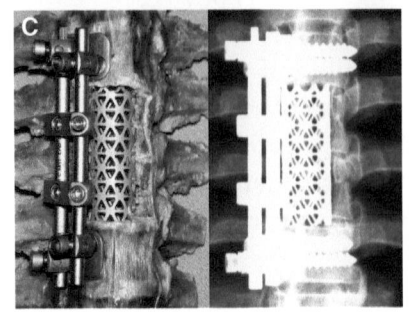

Fig. 2-7 Postoperative photographs juxtaposed with radiographs of fully instrumented conditions studied by Chou et al.[14] One- and two-level corpectomies with supplementary hardware were studied sequentially; only two-level corpectomy conditions are shown. **A,** Specimen with titanium mesh reconstruction cage and plate/bolt hardware; bolts are inserted first and the plate is then locked to the head of the bolt with a nut. **B,** Specimen with mesh cage and plate/screw hardware; two screws hold staples in place, and the plate is then locked to the staples with a nut. **C,** Specimen with mesh cage and dual-rod hardware; screws are placed through staples and rods and then connected directly to the screw heads. Two cross-links reinforce the construct. (From Chou D, Larios AE, Chamberlain RH, et al. A biomechanical comparison of three anterior thoracolumbar implants after corpectomy: are two screws better than one? J Neurosurg Spine 4:213-218, 2006.)

LUMBOSACRAL-PELVIC REGION

The two most important points to consider in the lumbar region are that the vertebral bodies provide most of the weight-bearing load and that the pedicles provide the strongest means of segmental fixation. These facts have implications when planning and performing a wide resection and reconstruction.

The biomechanical implications of incorporating the sacrum into a fixation construct, as in partial or total sacrectomy, or of extending fixation caudally to support the lower lumbar region, must be understood. The first key point involves the ability or need to maintain or restore overall sagittal balance. Maintaining sagittal balance decreases the incidence of pathologic compensatory kinematics, back pain, and construct failure.[15] A second key point involves the lumbosacral pivot point, which is located at the dorsal aspect of the L5-S1 annulus fibrosus (Fig. 2-8). To achieve maximal flexion resistance, fixation should extend caudally and ventrally to this point when feasible.[16]

Fixation of the lower lumbar vertebrae to the sacroiliac region typically involves using the S1 pedicles. In terms of placing S1 pedicle screws, the anterior midline has the highest bone mineral density and thus offers the greatest resistance to pullout. When feasible, therefore, S1 screws should be bicortical and aimed toward the sacral promontory.[17]

When extensive resection and caudal extension of fixation constructs are considered, as when tumor invades the lower lumbar region and sacrum, it should be noted that iliac screw fixation provides the greatest stiffness. O'Brien[18] identified three zones in the sacroiliac region. Zone 1 is composed of the S1 body and top of the ala, zone 2 is the inferior part of the ala, S2 through the coccyx, and zone 3 includes both ilia. O'Brien[18] demonstrated that stiffness increases as more zones are incorporated into the fixation construct. Furthermore, several studies have demonstrated the utility of iliac screw fixation in augmenting and protecting sacral alar and lower lumbar screw constructs.[16,19,20]

Fig. 2-8 Midsagittal perspective of the lumbosacral pivot point where sagittal rotation occurs. This point is the most critical for spinal sagittal balance; therefore positioning of instrumentation relative to this point and length of moment arms created relative to this point should be considered when selecting surgical hardware. (Courtesy of Barrow Neurological Institute.)

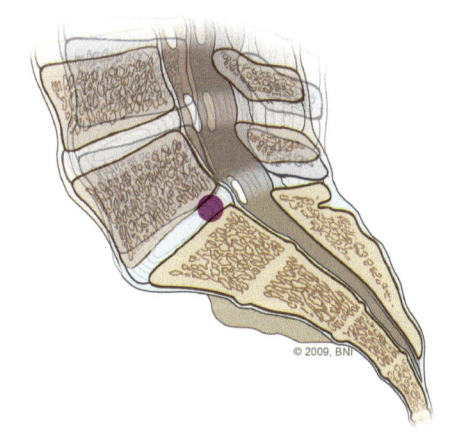

Wide resection at the lumbosacral transition point may lead to significant sagittal imbalance, which is even more deleterious than imbalance at the CTJ or the thoracolumbar junction, because the orientation of the entire spine above the lumbosacral junction is affected. Current technology, including lordotic implants and expandable cages, should allow balance to be restored even after extensive bony removal. Stress shielding is an issue when entire corpectomies or even spondylectomies are performed. Inducing mechanical compression across the interbody device may help induce good bone formation before stress shielding leads to resorption. Extending the fixation caudally, rostrally, or both with devices of transitional stiffness may help relieve high-stress points caused by moment arms across fusion constructs. When clinically needed and technically feasible, circumferential fixation, with multiple fixation points, increases stiffness.

CONCLUSION

Vertebral column tumors pose a challenge for spine surgeons. In cases of metastatic tumors, it should always be remembered that the pathology is a systemic disease that is often present at multiple levels of the spine. The kinematics of the spinal column are drastically altered because of the frequent need for wide en bloc resection. Derangements in sagittal balance, moment arms, and stress shielding are common. The biomechanical principle of multiple fixation points is particularly pertinent when reconstruction is needed because of a wide resection, osteopenia, instability, and decreased likelihood of fusion. When clinically appropriate and technically feasible, circumferential reconstruction, which provides the most immediate stability, is recommended. With posterior fixation alone, extended segmental fixation is likely needed to produce a favorable moment arm, lock in good sagittal balance, and prevent construct failure. Aiming for maximal biomechanical stability is prudent in the clinical setting of spine tumor surgery, because adjuvant chemotherapy and radiation create a hostile environment for fusion and the durability of the repair relies more on the hardware.

TIPS FROM THE MASTERS

- Ensuring spinal stability after resection of spine tumors can be challenging, especially with increased emphasis on wide resection margins and with the resulting longer term patient survival. Most biomechanical studies have focused purely on ROM and not fatigue testing of reconstructions for oncologic disease.
- Radiation and recurrent tumor can further compromise fusion rates and adjacent-level fixation.
- Additional points of fixation and 360-degree fusion surgery should be strongly considered, especially when projected survival is thought to be significant and the fusion substrate is likely to be poor.

References (With Key References in Boldface)

1. Oda I, Abumi K, Sell LC, et al. Biomechanical evaluation of five different occipito-atlanto-axial fixation techniques. Spine (Phila Pa 1976) 24:2377-2382, 1999.
2. **Bambakidis NC, Feiz-Erfan I, Horn EM, et al. Biomechanical comparison of occipitoatlantal screw fixation techniques. J Neurosurg Spine 8:143-152, 2008.**
3. Horn EM, Feiz-Erfan I, Lekovic GP, et al. Survivors of occipitoatlantal dislocation injuries: imaging and clinical correlates. J Neurosurg Spine 6:113-120, 2007.
4. Dmitriev AE, Lehman R Jr, Helgeson MD, et al. Acute and long-term stability of atlantoaxial fixation methods: a biomechanical comparison of pars, pedicle, and intralaminar fixation in an intact and odontoid fracture model. Spine (Phila Pa 1976) 34:365-370, 2009.
5. **Panjabi MM, Isomi T, Wang JL. Loosening at the screw-vertebra junction in multilevel anterior cervical plate constructs. Spine (Phila Pa 1976) 24:2383-2388, 1999.**
6. Singh K, Vaccaro AR, Kim J, et al. Biomechanical comparison of cervical spine reconstructive techniques after a multilevel corpectomy of the cervical spine. Spine (Phila Pa 1976) 28:2352-2358, 2003.
7. **Bozkus H, Ames CP, Chamberlain RH, et al. Biomechanical analysis of rigid stabilization techniques for three-column injury in the lower cervical spine. Spine (Phila Pa 1976) 30:915-922, 2005.**
8. Dogan S, Baek S, Sonntag VK, et al. Biomechanical consequences of cervical spondylectomy versus corpectomy. Neurosurgery 63:303-308, 2008.
9. Steinmetz MP, Miller J, Warbel A, et al. Regional instability following cervicothoracic junction surgery. J Neurosurg Spine 4:278-284, 2006.
10. Prybis BG, Tortolani PJ, Hu N, et al. A comparative biomechanical analysis of spinal instability and instrumentation of the cervicothoracic junction: an in vitro human cadaveric model. J Spinal Disord Tech 20:233-238, 2007.
11. **Ames CP, Bozkus MH, Chamberlain RH, et al. Biomechanics of stabilization after cervicothoracic compression-flexion injury. Spine (Phila Pa 1976) 30:1505-1512, 2005.**
12. Gokaslan ZL, York JE, Walsh GL, et al. Transthoracic vertebrectomy for metastatic spinal tumors. J Neurosurg 89:599-609, 1998.
13. Oda I, Cunningham BW, Abumi K, et al. The stability of reconstruction methods after thoracolumbar total spondylectomy. An in vitro investigation. Spine (Phila Pa 1976) 24:1634-1638, 1999.
14. **Chou D, Larios AE, Chamberlain RH, et al. A biomechanical comparison of three anterior thoracolumbar implants after corpectomy: are two screws better than one? J Neurosurg Spine 4:213-218, 2006.**
15. Benzel EC. Lumbosacral pelvic constructs. In Benzel EC, ed. Biomechanics of Spine Stabilization. Rolling Meadows, IL: American Association of Neurologic Surgeons, 2001, pp 297-298.
16. McCord DH, Cunningham BW, Shono Y, et al. Biomechanical analysis of lumbosacral fixation. Spine (Phila Pa 1976) 17:S235-S243, 1992.
17. **Lehman RA Jr, Kuklo TR, Belmont PJ Jr, et al. Advantage of pedicle screw fixation directed into the apex of the sacral promontory over bicortical fixation: a biomechanical analysis. Spine (Phila Pa 1976) 27:806-811, 2002.**
18. O'Brien MF. Sacropelvic fixation in spinal deformity. In DeWald RL, ed. Spinal Deformities: The Comprehensive Text. New York: Thieme, 2003, pp 601-614.
19. Lebwohl NH, Cunningham BW, Dmitriev A, et al. Biomechanical comparison of lumbosacral fixation techniques in a calf spine model. Spine (Phila Pa 1976) 27:2312-2320, 2002.
20. Alegre GM, Gupta MC, Bay BK, et al. S1 screw bending moment with posterior spinal instrumentation across the lumbosacral junction after unilateral iliac crest harvest. Spine (Phila Pa 1976) 26:1950-1955, 2001.

Chapter 3

Scoring System for Metastatic Tumors: Palliative or Aggressive Resection and Reconstruction

Satoru Demura, Katsuro Tomita, Norio Kawahara, Hideki Murakami

Metastatic tumors of the spine are an increasingly prevalent pathology encountered by oncologists and spine surgeons in caring for patients with cancer. As a result of improved systemic therapies for the most common solid organ malignancies, this increase in spinal metastases poses a significant threat to the functional independence and quality of life of these patients. In light of this increase in spinal metastases, algorithms and strategies for multidisciplinary management of this disease entity have evolved and will be discussed in this chapter.

Indications for surgical management of spinal metastases are based on signs of neurologic deficits, the presence of intractable pain, spinal cord compression, and spinal instability. Harrington[1] devised a five-category classification scheme for metastatic spine tumors that is based on the degree of bone destruction and neurologic compromise, with nonsurgical therapy recommended for classes I, II, and III and surgical intervention for classes IV and V (Box 3-1).

Box 3-1 **Classification of Metastatic Spine Tumors**

Class I	No significant neurologic involvement
Class II	Involvement of bone without collapse or instability
Class III	Major neurologic impairment (sensory or motor) without significant involvement of bone
Class IV	Vertebral collapse with pain resulting from mechanical causes or instability but with no significant neurologic compromise
Class V	Vertebral collapse or instability combined with major neurologic impairment

SCORING SYSTEMS

Tokuhashi et al[2] originally proposed a prognostic scoring system for the preoperative evaluation of patients with metastatic spine tumors. Recently they revised their scoring system and evaluated treatment outcomes by means of their prognostic scoring system.[3,4] This scoring system is based on the following six variables:

1. General medical condition
2. Number of extraspinal metastases
3. Number of vertebral metastases
4. Visceral metastases
5. Primary tumor type
6. Presence of neurologic deficits

Each parameter is evaluated and assigned a score ranging from 0 to 2 or 0 to 5 points, with a maximum total score of 15. Excisional surgery would be indicated for patients with a total score of 12 or higher, whereas palliative resection would be appropriate for patients with a score of 9 to 11. In patients with a total score of 8 or less, conservative or palliative radiation treatment is indicated (Fig. 3-1 and Table 3-1).

Predicted prognosis	Total score	Treatment
>6 months	0-8	Conservative treatment
≤6 months	9-11	Palliative surgery • Single lesion • No metastases to the major internal organs
≤1 year	12-15	Excisional surgery

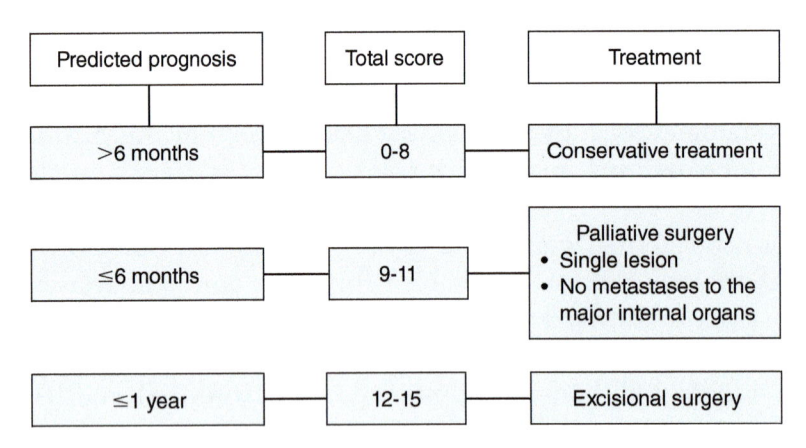

Fig. 3-1 Strategy for treatment of spinal metastases. (Adapted from Tokuhashi Y, Matsuzaki H, Oda H, et al. A revised scoring system for preoperative evaluation of metastatic spine tumor prognosis. Spine (Phila Pa 1976) 30:2186-2191, 2005.)

Table 3-1 Revised Evaluation System for Prognosis of Metastatic Spine Tumors*

Characteristic	Score
General Conditions	
Poor (PS 10% to 40%)	0
Moderate (PS 50% to 70%)	1
Good (PS 80% to 100%)	2
Number of Extraspinal Bone Metastases Foci	
≥3	0
1-2	1
0	2
Number of Metastases in the Vertebral Body	
≥3	0
2	1
1	2
Metastases to the Major Internal Organs	
Unremovable	0
Removable	1
No metastases	2
Primary Site of Cancer	
Lung, osteosarcoma, stomach, bladder, esophagus, pancreas	0
Liver, gallbladder, unidentified	1
Others	2
Kidney, uterus	3
Rectum	4
Thyroid, breast, prostate, carcinoid tumor	5
Palsy	
Complete (Frankel A, *B*)	0
Incomplete (Frankel C, *D*)	1
None (Frankel E)	2

From Tokuhashi Y, Matsuzaki H, Oda H, et al. A revised scoring system for preoperative evaluation of metastatic spine tumor prognosis. Spine (Phila Pa 1976) 30:2186-2191, 2005.
*Criteria of predicted prognosis: Total score (TS) 0-8 = >6 months; TS 9-11 = ≤6 months; TS 12-15 = ≤1 year
PS, Performance status.

Cappuccio et al[5] and Gasbarrini et al[6] proposed a flow chart to be used as a guide for the treatment of spinal metastases (Fig. 3-2). This approach considers the following variables: anesthetic assessment (ASA), presence of spinal compression with a neurologic deficit, possibility of recovery, risk of pathologic fracture, sensitivity to adjuvant therapy, number of vertebral metastases, and therapeutic possibilities for osseous and/or visceral metastases. In a retrospective review, these investigators reported improved quality of life for patients who adhered to the proposed treatment algorithms.

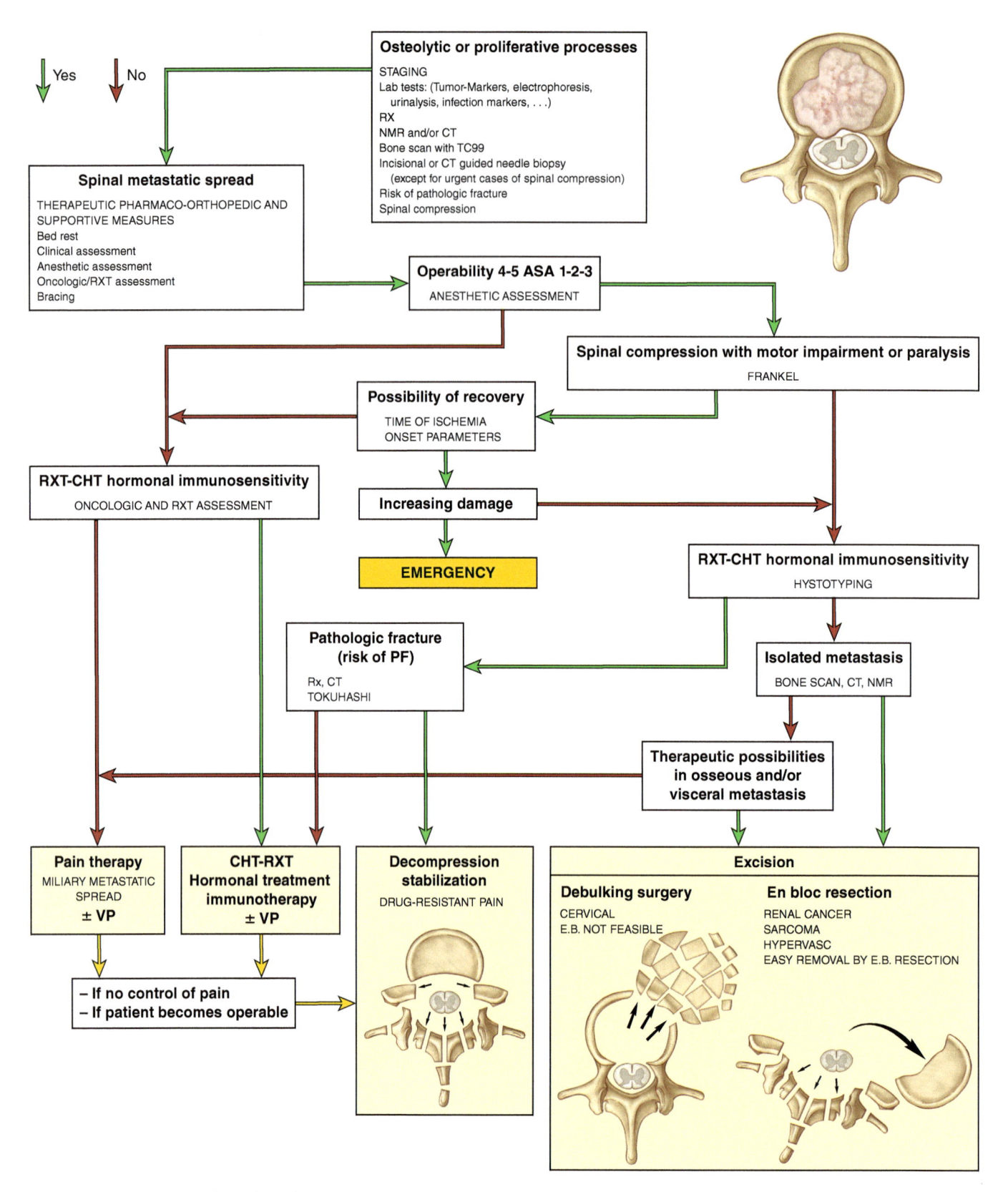

Fig. 3-2 Flow chart for the treatment of spinal metastases. (Adapted from Cappuccio M, Gasbarrini A, Van Urk P, et al. Spinal metastasis: a retrospective study validating the treatment algorithm. Eur Rev Med Pharmacol Sci 12:155-160, 2008.)

SURGICAL DECISION-MAKING

We have proposed a surgical strategy for spinal metastases that can be used both to decide whether surgical intervention is needed and to determine the type of surgical procedure. Building on previous efforts, we employed the three most important prognostic factors: grade of malignancy of the primary tumor, visceral metastases to vital organs, and bone metastases (spine inclusive) (Fig. 3-3).[7-9]

When considering surgery for patients with spinal metastases, our prerequisite is a minimum score of 3 or less according to the Eastern Cooperative Oncology Group performance status[10] or 30% or more on the Karnofsky performance scale,[11] which are the same requirements for administrating chemotherapy. Our scoring system consists of three prognostic factors that are regarded as the most influential factors for life expectancy, and these scores are assigned on the basis of each hazard ratio:
1. Pathologic ≒ clinical grade of malignancy (low grade ≒ slow growth: 1 point; intermediate grade ≒ moderate growth: 2 points; high grade ≒ rapid growth: 4 points)
2. Metastases to vital organs (no metastasis: 0 points; controllable: 2 points; uncontrollable: 4 points)
3. Bone metastases (isolated: 1 point; multiple: 2 points)

These three factors are added together to yield a total prognostic score between 2 and 10 points. We discovered that neurologic deficits cannot be considered a direct influential factor for life expectancy; thus it is not counted. The aim of treatment for each patient is set according to this prognostic score and the patient's life expectancy.[12]

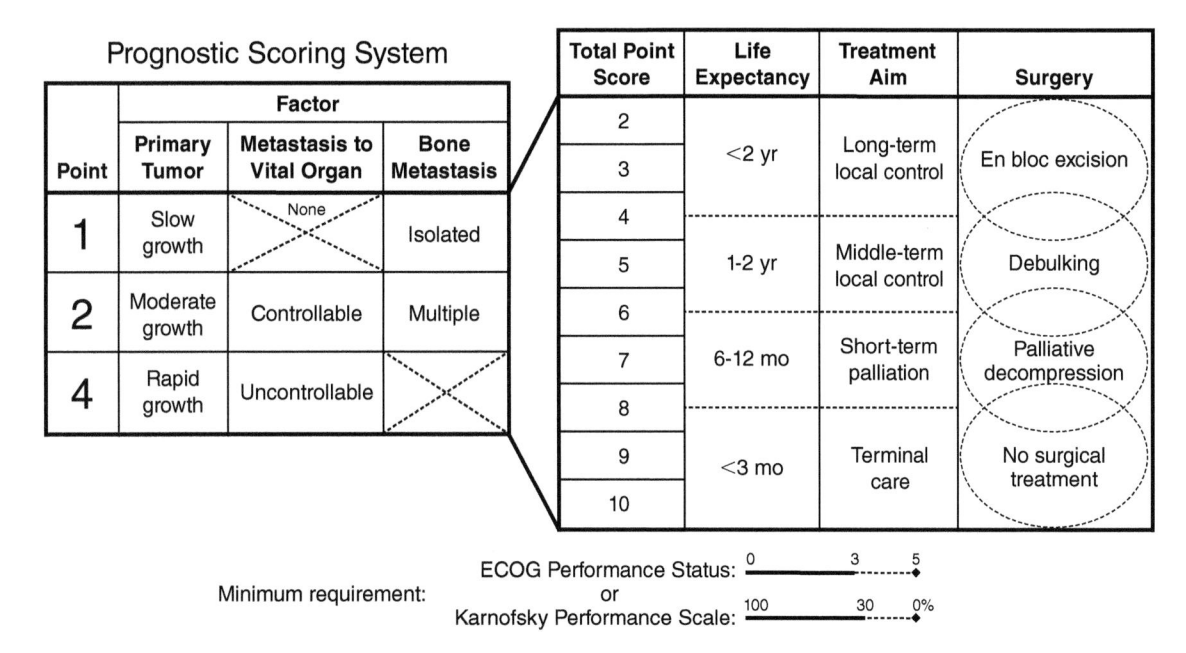

Fig. 3-3 Surgical strategy for spinal metastases. (From Tomita K, Kawahara N, Murakami H, et al. Total en bloc spondylectomy for spinal tumors: improvement of the technique and its associated basic background. J Orthop Sci 11:3-12, 2006.)

We have also devised a surgical classification of spine tumors[12,13] that is based on both the pattern of local vertebral tumor progression and the type of surgery used to excise it. Metastatic tumors frequently grow or settle in the middle posterior part of the vertebral body from where they can easily extend to the posterior arch through the pedicles; these are known as intracompartmental lesions, or type 1, 2, and 3 lesions. These tumors generally grow outside of the compartment (extracompartmentally) into the spinal canal (type 4) or extend outside of the vertebra (type 5) and finally reach the adjacent vertebra or vertebrae (type 6). Multiple lesions in the spinal column (type 7) are referred to as skip lesions (Fig. 3-4).

A wide surgical margin, or at least a marginal margin, can be achieved around the affected vertebra when the lesion is intracompartmental (type 1, 2, or 3), particularly when the vertebra is cut at the healthy part of the pedicle or lamina. For type 4, or for tumors invading the paravertebral areas (type 5 or 6), a marginal margin may only be possible if the lesion is well encapsulated with a fibrous reactive membrane.[14,15]

After deciding on the surgical strategy for each patient, along with the treatment aims, the extent of the spinal metastases is stratified according to the surgical classification of spine tumors. The most technically appropriate and feasible surgical procedure (e.g., en bloc excision, debulking, palliative decompression, or no surgical treatment) is deter-

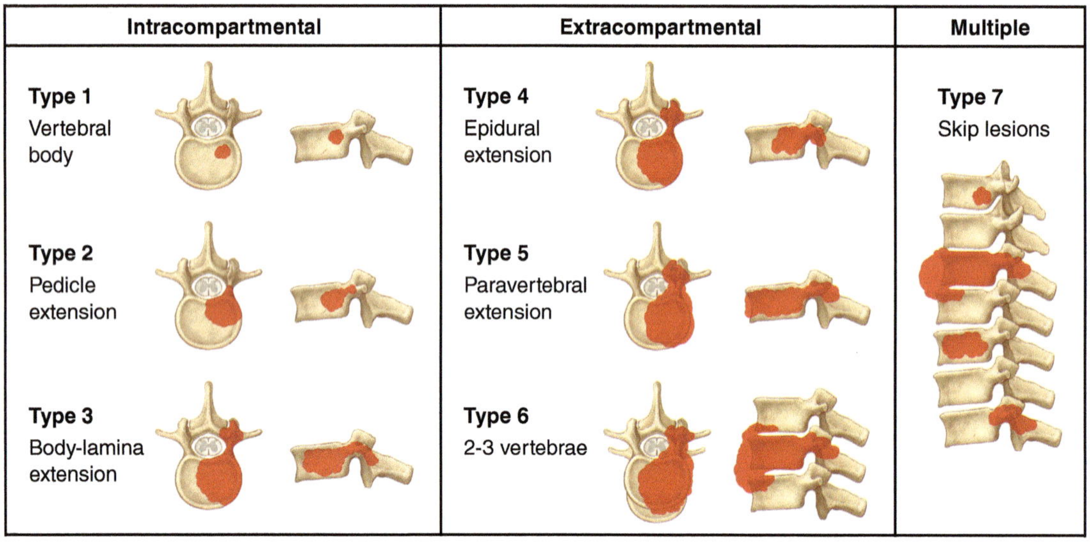

Fig. 3-4 Surgical classification of spinal tumors. (Adapted from Tomita K, Kawahara N, Kobayashi T, et al. Surgical strategy for spinal metastases. Spine 26:298-306, 2001.)

mined for each patient based on the surgical strategy for spinal metastases and surgical classification of spine tumors. Treatment options should be offered after discussion with the spine surgeon, medical oncologist, radiation oncologist, and the patient.

OUTCOMES

From 1993 to 2008, a total of 185 patients with spinal metastases were surgically treated and followed until death or for at least 1 year at Kanazawa University Hospital. Among the 185 patients with metastatic tumors, the primary organ was the kidney in 42, the breast in 28, the lung in 24, the thyroid gland in 17, the colon in 14, the liver in 11, and the prostate in 7; in 9 patients the primary organ was unknown, and 33 patients had some other type of carcinoma. The mean length of survival after surgery was 23 months (range 1 to 131 months). Patients' 50% survival rates and length of survival were associated with prognostic scores as follows: 2 to 4 points, 42.3 months; 4 to 6 points, 17 months; 6 to 8 points, 11 months; and those with a score of 8 to 10 points survived only 3 months (Fig. 3-5).

Total en bloc spondylectomy (TES) was performed in 93 of 185 patients with spinal metastases. Aggressive piecemeal excision or debulking surgery was the primary procedure in 44 patients, and palliative surgery, such as posterior decompression and stabilization, was performed in 48 patients with spinal metastases.

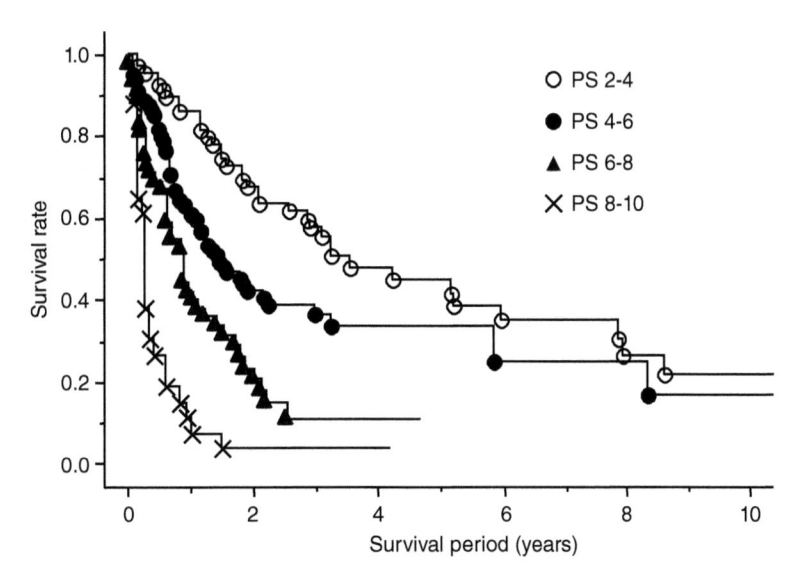

Fig. 3-5 Survival curves (Kaplan-Meier method) for patients with prognostic scores (PS) of 2 to 4, 4 to 6, 6 to 8, and 8 to 10.

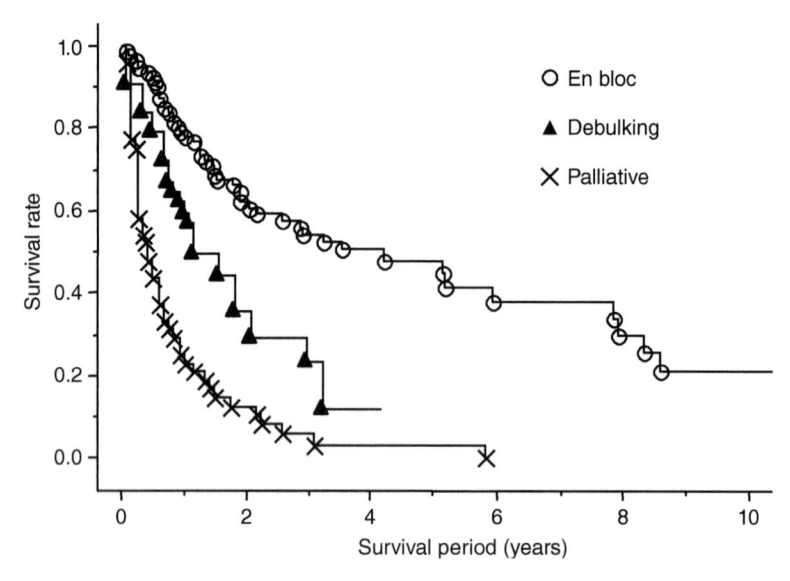

Fig. 3-6 Survival curves (Kaplan-Meier method) for patients with en bloc excision, debulking surgery, and palliative surgery.

Among 93 patients who underwent TES, 2-year survival was 62.0% and 5-year survival was 47.6%. Forty-four patients who underwent aggressive piecemeal excision or debulking surgery had a 1-year survival rate of 62.0% and 2-year survival of 35.2%. Among 48 patients who underwent palliative surgery, 6-month survival was 47.9% and 1-year survival was 25.0% (Fig. 3-6). Overall survival based on Kaplan-Meier curves showed a significant difference among the groups ($p < 0.001$).

Eighty-eight of 93 patients (95.7%) who underwent TES showed no tumor recurrence at the time of death or last follow-up. Five of 93 patients (5.3%) had a local recurrence, and the mean length of time between the operation and the recurrence was 23 months. All five patients had a local recurrence from residual tumor tissue. In three patients the tumor extended farther than expected into the adjacent level, and in another patient the recurrence was from the dural area. One patient had an inadequate spinal osteotomy, which was followed by curettage of the remainder of the tumor.

CONCLUSION

As the biological landscape continues to improve and generate novel cancer therapies, patients with systemic malignancies will develop more spinal metastases. Although treatment of these metastases is mostly palliative, and management should include the contributions of a multidisciplinary team, improvements in spinal instrumentation and techniques is allowing for improvements in quality of life and a reduction in local recurrence rates that were not possible in the past. We expect this evolution to increasingly favor an aggressive approach for selected spinal metastases in appropriate patients.

TIPS FROM THE MASTERS

- It is often very difficult to obtain accurate predictions of life expectancy from medical oncologists. Scoring systems can help guide spine surgeons who are trying to decide which type of surgery, if any, to offer their often-debilitated patients.
- With tremendous evolution in technique, much of it driven by the senior author of this chapter (K.T.), surgeons have many options for treating metastatic disease, ranging from piecemeal resection and decompression to en bloc resection for isolated metastases. The choice of surgery should be guided by intimate knowledge of the underlying biology of the primary tumor, current staging and its likely future responsiveness to adjuvant therapy, as well as the patient's medical status and the surgeon's best judgment.

References (With Key References in Boldface)

1. **Harrington KD. Metastatic disease of the spine. J Bone Joint Surg Am 68:1110-1115, 1986.**
2. Tokuhashi Y, Matsuzaki H, Toriyama S, et al. Scoring system for the preoperative evaluation of metastatic spine tumor prognosis. Spine (Phila Pa 1976) 15:1110-1113, 1990.
3. Tokuhashi Y, Ajiro Y, Umezawa N. Outcome of treatment for spinal metastases using scoring system for preoperative evaluation of prognosis. Spine (Phila Pa 1976) 34:69-73, 2009.
4. **Tokuhashi Y, Matsuzaki H, Oda H, et al. A revised scoring system for preoperative evaluation of metastatic spine tumor prognosis. Spine (Phila Pa 1976) 30:2186-2191, 2005.**
5. **Cappuccio M, Gasbarrini A, Van Urk P, et al. Spinal metastasis: a retrospective study validating the treatment algorithm. Eur Rev Med Pharmacol Sci 12:155-160, 2008.**
6. Gasbarrini A, Cappuccio M, Mirabile L, et al. Spinal metastases: treatment evaluation algorithm. Eur Rev Med Pharmacol Sci 8:265-274, 2004.
7. **Tomita K, Kawahara N, Kobayashi T, et al. Surgical strategy for spinal metastases. Spine (Phila Pa 1976) 26:298-306, 2001.**
8. **Tomita K, Kawahara N, Murakami H, et al. Total en bloc spondylectomy for spinal tumors: improvement of the technique and its associated basic background. J Orthop Sci 11:3-12, 2006.**
9. Bauer H, Tomita K, Kawahara N, et al. Surgical strategy for spinal metastases. Spine 27:1124-1126, 2002.
10. Oken MM, Creech RH, Tormey DC, et al. Toxicity and response criteria of the Eastern Cooperative Oncology Group. Am J Clin Oncol 5:649-655, 1982.
11. Karnofsky DA, Abelmann WH, Craver LF, et al. The use of nitrogen mustards in the palliative treatment of carcinoma with particular reference to bronchogenic carcinoma. Cancer 1:634-669, 1948.
12. Tomita K, Kawahara N, Baba H, et al. Total en bloc spondylectomy for solitary spinal metastasis. Int Orthop 18:291-298, 1994.
13. Tomita K, Kawahara N, Baba H, et al. Total en bloc spondylectomy. A new surgical technique for primary malignant vertebral tumors. Spine (Phila Pa 1976) 22:324-333, 1997.
14. **Enneking WF, Spanier SS, Goodman MA. A system for the surgical staging of musculoskeletal sarcoma. Clin Orthop Relat Res 153:106-120, 1980.**
15. Fujita T, Ueda Y, Kawahara N, et al. Local spread of metastatic vertebral tumors. A histologic study. Spine (Phila Pa 1976) 22:1905-1912, 1997.

Chapter 4

Imaging of Spinal Cord Tumors

Cynthia T. Chin

Spine tumors account for 15% of all central nervous system (CNS) tumors. Intramedullary neoplasms account for 5% to 10% in adults and 35% in children. Ninety to 95% of spinal cord tumors are glial tumors. Ependymomas, astrocytomas, and gangliogliomas are the more common intramedullary tumors followed by hemangioblastomas and metastases. Ependymomas are the most common glial tumors in adults, whereas astrocytomas are the most common intramedullary tumors in children.

Intramedullary tumors have a varied radiologic appearance, including many overlapping imaging characteristics that can make it challenging to differentiate the lesions. Imaging modalities may aid in both diagnosis and, when necessary, guidance for interventional procedures. In addition, imaging studies aid in monitoring results during and after treatment.

Techniques available for imaging of spinal cord tumors range from noninvasive (magnetic resonance imaging [MRI], computed tomography [CT], radiography, and nuclear medical imaging) to invasive (CT myelography and catheter angiography) procedures.

MAGNETIC RESONANCE IMAGING

MRI is the modality of choice for viewing the spinal cord. MRI identifies associated abnormalities, such as cysts, syringohydromyelia, hemorrhage, and edema, and also serves as a guide for surgical resection.

MRI studies should include unenhanced T1- and T2-weighted images in the sagittal and axial planes and contrast-enhanced T1-weighted images in the sagittal and axial planes. T1-weighted sequences are used in routine imaging of the spine; they are sensitive for the presence of infiltrative processes, such as neoplasms, as well as edema and reactive degenerative changes, particularly in the marrow.[1] Fast spin-echo (FSE) T2-weighted sequences are used to evaluate the spinal cord, the nerve roots, the caliber of the spinal canal, and vertebral marrow edema. FSE sequences are advantageous compared with conventional spin-echo T2 sequences, because they have a shorter acquisition time, which decreases artifact from patient motion, and they also are less sensitive to cerebrospinal fluid pulsation artifact.[2] In addition, FSE imaging and short-T1 inversion-recovery (STIR) sequences are less distorted by metallic artifact and are, therefore, useful in postoperative imaging of the spine.

In the vast majority of spinal cord neoplasms, including even low-grade forms, views are enhanced after administration of contrast material, to at least some degree. Enhanced areas probably represent more active portions of the tumors and may indicate potential sites for biopsy if resection is not feasible. Contrast-enhanced images are especially valuable for determining the solid portion of an intramedullary neoplasm and for identifying associated cysts and other features that often modify the differential diagnosis.[3]

Postoperative imaging of patients who have undergone spinal instrumentation is often limited by metallic magnetic susceptibility artifacts. Titanium alloys produce fewer artifacts relative to stainless steel.[4] Imaging of postoperative patients may be challenging and, for purposes of suppressing the signal from fat while avoiding severe metal-related artifacts, the STIR pulse sequence is preferable. Use of lower magnetic field strength is also desirable. If a high–field strength magnet is used, the imaging parameters chosen (e.g., small field of view, high-resolution image matrix, thin sections, increased echo train length, and higher gradient strength for small voxel sizes) may help reduce metal-related artifacts.[5,6]

The recently developed *i*terative *d*ecomposition of water and fat with *e*cho *a*symmetry and *l*east-squares estimation (IDEAL) technique can be used to achieve very high signal-to-noise efficiency and is insensitive to magnetic field inhomogeneity.[7]

MYELOGRAPHY

Myelography is useful in patients for whom MRI is contraindicated (i.e., those with metallic foreign bodies or cardiac pacemakers). It is an invasive study and generally should be used as a secondary imaging modality to answer questions not addressed by MRI or CT scans. It is essentially an exploration of the subarachnoid space. Myelography can reveal an intramedullary mass as a complete or partial block to the flow of intrathecal contrast material. When extensive hardware from spine fusion is obscuring the details of the spinal canal on MRI, myelography may be a helpful imaging technique. However, it can rarely help define the characteristics of spinal cord lesions.

INTRAMEDULLARY NEOPLASMS

The following three MRI features are important in evaluating spinal cord tumors: the presence of cord expansion, enhancement, and associated cysts, both tumoral and nontumoral. Most intramedullary spinal neoplasms are enhanced after intravenous administration of gadolinium-based contrast material.[8] Contrast-enhanced images in at least two different planes are crucial for differential diagnosis and surgical planning. However, the absence of enhancement does not preclude the possibility of intramedullary neoplasms in the presence of cord expansion.

Cysts located at the poles of the solid portion of the tumor may represent reactive dilatation of the central canal (syringomyelia). Approximately 60% of all intramedullary spine tumors demonstrate these polar or satellite cysts. These cysts are nontumoral and nonenhancing, and they are thought to develop from fluid produced by the tumor into the central canal. These polar cysts will either decompress on removal of the solid tumor portion or they can be aspirated at resection. They are not septated and do not show echogenicity within their walls on intraoperative ultrasonography. In contrast, tumoral cysts are located within the tumor itself and show peripheral enhancement. Identification of the location of the solid enhancing portion of the tumor (including enhancing tumoral cysts) is crucial for surgical planning.[9,10]

EPENDYMOMAS

Prevalence

Ependymomas constitute approximately 60% of intramedullary tumors in adult patients and 30% of all CNS ependymomas. Cord ependymomas are most common in the cervical cord. These tumors are typically solitary, but they can be multiple in association with other tumors (e.g., meningiomas and schwannomas) in patients with neurofibromatosis type II. These tumors may also occur as secondary metastases from a primary intracranial ependymoma.[11]

Ependymomas are slow-growing tumors that arise from the ependymal lining of the central canal or ependymal rests along the conus medullaris and cauda equina. Myxopapillary ependymomas of the filum terminale are a histologic variant that accounts for 80% of ependymomas in the conus.

Subependymomas are another variant of ependymomas and are rare within the cord. Their benign course and lack of symptoms account for incidental detection at autopsies.

Pathology

Ependymomas are classified according to the World Health Organization (WHO) grading system as follows: ependymoma (WHO grade II), myxopapillary ependymoma (WHO grade I), subependymoma (WHO grade I), and anaplastic ependymoma (WHO grade III). Most ependymomas displace rather than infiltrate adjacent neural tissue and result in symmetrical cord expansion. These tumors are well marginated and often demonstrate small feeding vessels. Histologic examination typically reveals uniform hyperchromatic nuclei. The presence of perivascular pseudorosettes establishes the diagnosis of ependymoma. Cystic degeneration and hemorrhage are common.

Imaging

Patients with ependymomas may demonstrate scoliosis, canal widening, vertebral body scalloping, pedicle erosion, or laminar thinning on conventional radiography. Conventional myelography may demonstrate complete or partial blockage of the flow of contrast material.[12]

Characteristic imaging features of ependymomas include their central cord location (because of the ependymal progenitor) and their tendency to be well circumscribed. Ependymomas are typically isointense to hypointense on T1 imaging and hyperintense on T2 imaging. Polar caps, a feature of ependymomas, are cysts that arise from the rostral or caudal extreme of the tumor. These cysts can also contain blood products as a sequela of hemorrhage within this vascular tumor. Ependymomas can also demonstrate intratumoral cysts, which, unlike polar caps, will be enhanced (Fig. 4-1).

Hemorrhage is common and results in T2 susceptibility artifact. In addition, ependymomas may show dystrophic calcification. These calcifications are easily identifiable on CT imaging but may not be discernible on MRI because both calcification and hemorrhage cause T2 susceptibility artifact.[13,14]

Syringohydromyelia may be present, and syringomyelia fluid content may be consistent with an exudate, resulting from a disruption of the blood-brain barrier.[15] The vast

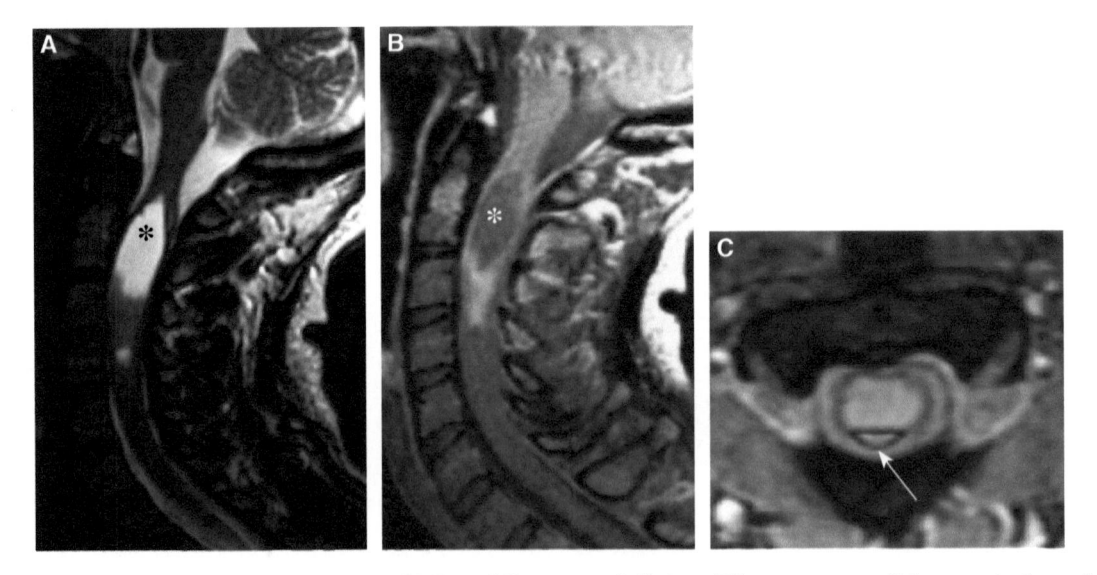

Fig. 4-1 Ependymoma. **A,** Sagittal T2 and **B,** postgadolinium T1 sequences of the cervical cord demonstrate an enhancing ependymoma with associated hemorrhage and **C,** hematocrit level on the axial gradient echo sequence *(arrow)*. The tumor is centrally located within the cord with an enhancing tumoral cyst *(asterisk)*.

majority of spinal cord ependymomas show enhancement after intravenous administration of gadolinium-based contrast material.

Given its central intramedullary location, compression or disruption of medullary spinal tracts may be found on diffusion tensor imaging.[16]

Myxopapillary Ependymoma

Prevalence
This ependymoma variant makes up approximately 13% of spinal ependymomas, is seen at an earlier age, and is more common in male patients. These tumors have a distinct predilection for the conus medullaris or filum terminale; they arise from the ependymal glia of the filum and are, therefore, the most common neoplasms in this region.

Pathology
Myxopapillary ependymomas often appear as encapsulated soft lobular masses. These tumors typically produce mucin. The mucin and papillary zones are mixed with cellular regions made of rosettes and pseudorosettes.

Imaging
Myxopapillary tumors, unlike the common cellular type, may be hyperintense both on T1 and T2 imaging because of their highly proteinaceous/mucinous contents and/or hemorrhaging. Siderosis may also be seen, as is the case with highly vascular tumors. These tumors typically show enhancement. The location of these tumors at the conus medullaris is suggestive of the diagnosis[17,18] (Fig. 4-2).

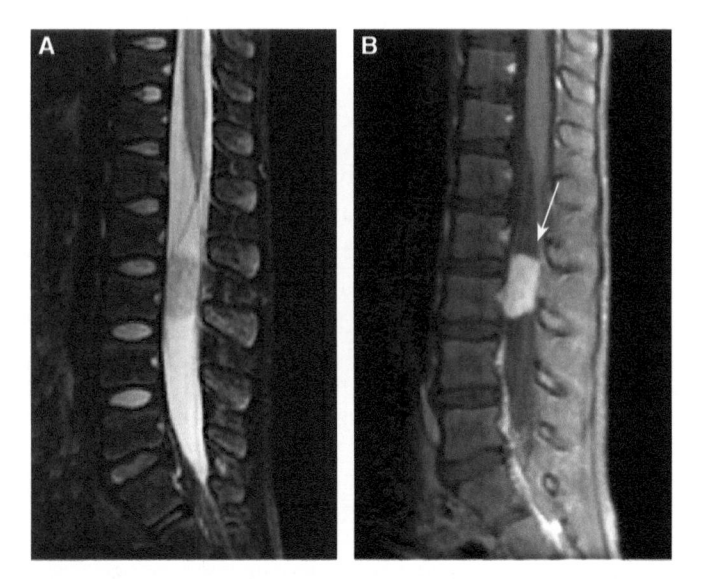

Fig. 4-2 Grade 1 myxopapillary ependymoma. **A,** Sagittal T2 and **B,** postgadolinium T1 sequences of the lumbar spine in a 10-year-old girl with 2 years of low back pain radiating to both legs demonstrate an intradural extramedullary well-defined centrally located enhancing mass associated with the filum *(arrow)*.

Subependymoma

Prevalence
Subependymomas are thought to arise from pluripotential cells of the subependymal plate. The cells of origin, tanycytes, bridge the pial and ependymal layers (from the Greek word *tanyos,* "to stretch"). Spinal cord subependymomas have been reported predominantly in male patients, with a mean age at presentation of 42 years. These tumors may recur after surgical resection.

Pathology
Spinal cord subependymomas are typically avascular gray-yellow masses with no evidence of cysts. Histologic examination shows that ependymal cells are distributed among the predominant fibrillary astrocytes.

Imaging
Subependymomas are well defined and eccentrically located. They demonstrate variable enhancement and associated edema. On MRI they appear with fusiform dilatation of the spinal cord with well-defined borders. MRI findings are not sufficiently unique to allow differentiation between ependymomas and subependymomas.[19-22]

ASTROCYTOMAS

Prevalence
Astrocytomas originate from astrocytic glial cells and represent approximately 30% of intramedullary tumors, but they are the most common intramedullary tumor in the pediatric population. The incidence is approximately 2.5 per 100,000 per year; these tumors are more common in males and present at a mean age of 29 years, which is relatively younger than the mean age for ependymomas. These tumors most often occur in the thoracic spine and usually within the upper spinal cord. In children the entire cord may be involved.

Pathology
The histologic subtypes of low-grade (WHO grade I and II) spinal cord astrocytomas include pilocytic astrocytoma and diffuse astrocytoma, respectively. The high-grade (WHO grade III and IV) subtypes include anaplastic astrocytoma and glioblastoma multiforme, respectively. Up to 90% of spinal astrocytomas are WHO grade 1 pilocytic astrocytomas or fibrillary astrocytomas (grade II). The tumors are characterized by ill-defined diffuse fusiform cord enlargement. Neoplastic astrocytes infiltrate along a scaffolding of normal astrocytes, oligodendrocytes, and axons of surrounding neural tissue. Histologic examination reveals enlarged irregularly shaped hyperchromatic nuclei.

Pilocytic astrocytomas demonstrate varying proportions of bipolar cells with Rosenthal fibers. Low-grade diffuse astrocytomas show tumor cells of uniform morphology within a dense fibrillary matrix. Glioblastomas are highly cellular pleomorphic tumors with necroses and hypercellular pseudopalisading border zones and vascular proliferations.[23]

Imaging

On MRI pilocytic astrocytomas are usually well delineated; they often show cystic formation and have variable enhancement. Diffuse astrocytomas have poorly defined margins and appear hyperintense on T2-weighted images. Differentiation of tumor borders from adjacent edema may be difficult. Enhancement alone cannot differentiate between low-grade and high-grade gliomas. Associated cysts are commonly observed especially with the pilocytic tumors. Hemorrhage is uncommon relative to ependymomas. As astrocytomas arise from the cord parenchyma, they are generally T1 hypointense and T2 hyperintense, with enhancement of the central nodular component; tumoral cysts will show peripheral enhancement typically located eccentrically within the cord. Cross-sectional localization of tumor on axial T2-weighted images is important for surgical planning. Unlike ependymomas, which usually are found centered in the cord, astrocytomas are eccentric in location and ill-defined and irregular. Exophytic tumor growth has also been described with astrocytomas. The surrounding reactive cysts and edema that arise will not enhance[24,25] (Figs. 4-3 and 4-4).

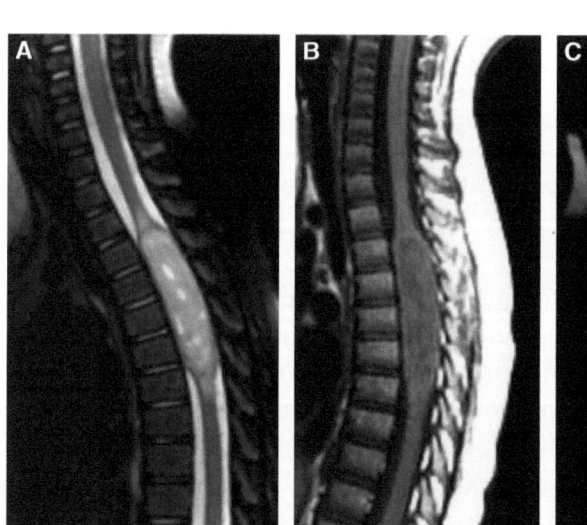

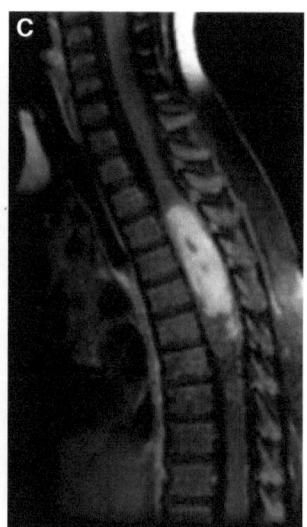

Fig. 4-3 Juvenile pilocytic astrocytoma. **A,** Sagittal T2, **B,** T1, and **C,** postgadolinium T1 sequences demonstrate a well-defined enhancing thoracic cord mass with focal expansion and tumoral cysts in a 3-year-old girl with 5 months of back pain waking her from sleep.

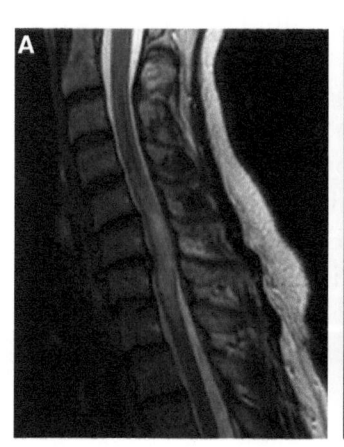

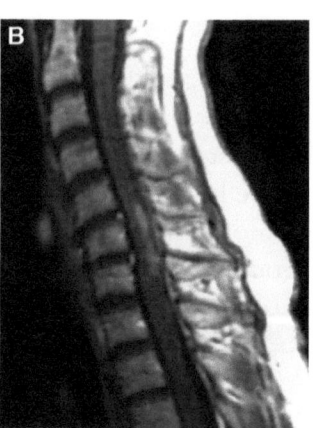

Fig. 4-4 Grade II astrocytoma. **A,** Sagittal T2 and **B,** postgadolinium T1 sequences of the cervical cord in a 43-year-old woman with a 3-month history of neck pain and radicular symptoms demonstrate cord expansion with an ill-defined enhancing increased T2 signal.

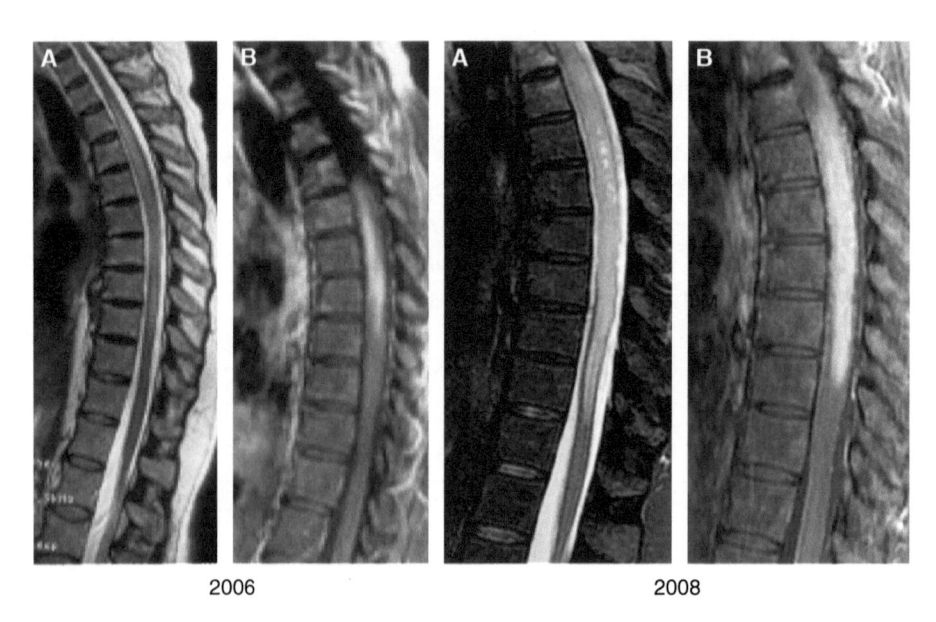

Fig. 4-5 Glioblastoma. **A,** Sagittal T2 and **B,** postgadolinium T1 sequences of the thoracic spine demonstrate progression of spinal cord glioblastoma over a 2-year period. Note interval increase in ill-defined cord expansion, abnormal T2 signal, and enhancement.

Primary spinal cord glioblastoma multiforme is rare and demonstrates intense peripheral enhancement and edema. In 60% of patients there is associated leptomeningeal spread[26] (Fig. 4-5).

It is difficult to differentiate ependymomas from astrocytomas by means of MRI alone. Spinal cord ependymomas are the most common type in adults, and cord astrocytomas are most common in children. Together they constitute up to 70% of all intramedullary neoplasms. A central location within the spinal cord, presence of a cleavage plane, intense homogeneous enhancement, and the presence of hemosiderin are imaging features that favor an ependymoma. Intramedullary astrocytomas are usually eccentrically located within the cord; they are ill-defined and have patchy enhancement after administration of intravenous contrast material. Even with these characteristics, it may not be possible to differentiate these two entities on the basis of imaging features alone.[9]

Although MRI allows earlier detection of spinal cord tumors, histologic grading on the basis of MRI is often inaccurate. Diffusion tensor imaging is an advanced MRI technique that can show motor and sensory fiber tracts and their relationship to spinal cord tumors. This technique, when available, may be helpful in differentiating between resectable and nonresectable tumors based on preoperative imaging. Ependymomas and hemangioblastomas are typically noninfiltrative lesions with a distinct tumor–spinal cord plane. They are considered resectable, whereas fibrillary astrocytomas, because of their infiltrative characteristic, are considered nonresectable.[16]

Gangliogliomas

Prevalence

Gangliogliomas are a rare subset of astrocytomas; they account for 0.4% to 6.25% of all primary CNS tumors and approximately 1.1% of all spine neoplasms. They are more common in children, and they are most common in the cervical spinal cord. Less commonly, gangliogliomas may involve the conus medullaris or the entire spinal cord. They are typically located eccentric within the cord and demonstrate tumoral cysts more frequently (more than 40%) than spinal astrocytomas (20%) and ependymomas (3%).

Pathology

Gangliogliomas represent a mixture of mature but neoplastic neuronal elements (neurons or ganglion cells) and glial elements (primarily neoplastic astrocytes) at histologic examination. Because the proportions of cells may vary from one tumor to another, various synonyms have been used to describe these lesions, including ganglioglioneuroma, ganglionic neuroma, neuroastrocytoma, neuroganglioma, ganglionic glioma, neuroma gangliocellulare, and neuroglioma.

These tumors are classified histologically on the basis of the relative differentiation of the neuronal component and the presence of glial elements. Gangliocytomas (WHO grade I) are composed of mature neuronal components without glial components; gangliogliomas (WHO grade I/II) contain additional neoplastic astrocytic elements; anaplastic gangliogliomas (WHO III) are extremely rare.

Although the potential for malignancy is low, spinal cord gangliogliomas have a recurrence rate of 27%, which is approximately three to four times that of cerebral gangliogliomas.

Imaging

As a result of the histologic mixture, these tumors are generally slow growing, and they have an insidious onset. The chronicity may result in scalloping and deformity of the spine and may cause scoliosis. Osseous changes, including scoliosis and remodeling, are much more common in spinal gangliogliomas compared with other types of tumors.

The MRI characteristics are similar to those of astrocytomas, with a mixed T1, hyperintense T2 signal that is often associated with a tumoral cyst. The mixed signal intensity may be caused by the dual cellular population (i.e., neuronal and glial elements). Additional findings that can aid in the diagnosis are lack of significant associated cord edema and absence of a hemosiderin cap, because surrounding edema is less commonly seen in spinal gangliogliomas than in cord ependymomas or astrocytomas.

Most spinal gangliogliomas show at least some degree of enhancement after the administration of contrast material. Patchy enhancement is the most common pattern,

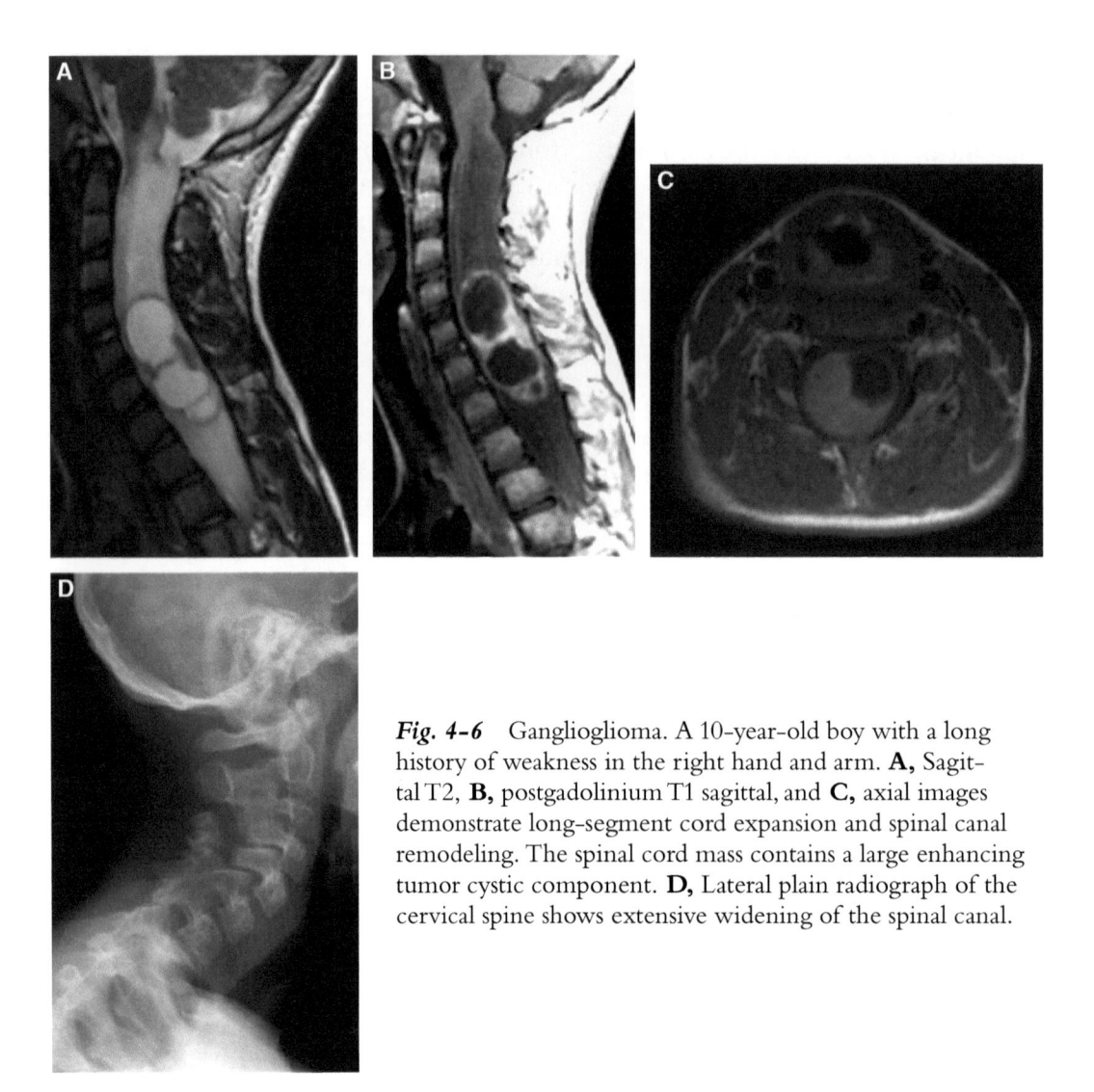

Fig. 4-6 Ganglioglioma. A 10-year-old boy with a long history of weakness in the right hand and arm. **A,** Sagittal T2, **B,** postgadolinium T1 sagittal, and **C,** axial images demonstrate long-segment cord expansion and spinal canal remodeling. The spinal cord mass contains a large enhancing tumor cystic component. **D,** Lateral plain radiograph of the cervical spine shows extensive widening of the spinal canal.

but enhancement of the pial surface is also common. Approximately 15% of these lesions show no enhancement[27-29] (Fig. 4-6).

HEMANGIOBLASTOMAS

Prevalence
Hemangioblastomas constitute 1.0% to 7.2% of all spinal cord neoplasms and show no gender predilection. These meningothelial-related tumors have an unknown cell of origin and are predominantly intramedullary (75%), but they may involve the intradural space or may even be extradural. Extramedullary hemangioblastomas are commonly attached to the pia mater of the dorsal cord or nerve roots. These slow-growing lesions involve the thoracic cord most commonly (50% of patients), followed closely by the cervical cord (40%). Most cord hemangioblastomas (70% to 80%) are solitary and occur in patients younger than 40 years, usually with impaired proprioception given their preferential location near or in the dorsal column.

Multiple lesions may be an indication of von Hippel–Lindau syndrome (VHL). VHL is an autosomal dominant disorder resulting in tumors in various organ systems. Associated tumors include retinal hemangioblastomas, pheochromocytomas, renal cell carcinomas, renal cysts, pancreatic cystadenomas, and pancreatic neuroendocrine tumors. Nearly 70% of patients with VHL will develop hemangioblastomas of the CNS as part of the syndrome during their lifetimes.

A tumor suppressor gene located on chromosome 3p25-26 is responsible for the disease when it is inactivated. Genetic testing for VHL mutations should be considered in patients with hemangioblastomas. One third of patients have VHL, with retinal or cerebellar findings usually preceding spinal cord manifestations.

Rarely, spinal hemangioblastomas may be a source of subarachnoid hemorrhage or hematomyelia. Patients may present with acute subarachnoid or intramedullary hemorrhage because of the high vascularity of these tumors.

Pathology
Hemangioblastomas are highly vascular, discrete, nodular, red-to-orange masses that are often found along the walls of large cysts and abutting the leptomeninges with prominent dilated and tortuous vessels on the posterior cord surface. An associated syrinx is common. Occasionally these tumors may exophytically extend from the spinal cord. The tumors consist of large and vacuolated stromal cells that lie in a matrix of abundant vascular cells forming thin-walled vessels. The stromal cells express S100 and neuron-specific enolase. The cell of origin remains unknown.

Imaging
Hemangioblastomas classically appears as a cystic mass with an intensely enhancing mural nodule. Diffuse cord expansion is common, which may be attributable to venous congestion and edema. Tortuous flow voids representing feeding arteries are invariably present and are helpful in the differential diagnosis. The tumors have variable signal intensity on T1-weighted images and are hyperintense on T2-weighted images. Up to 25% of hemangioblastomas may appear to be solid.

Magnetic resonance angiographic sequences are an important noninvasive method for preoperative evaluation demonstrating feeding vessels. Diagnostic angiography can also be performed preoperatively to demonstrate the highly vascular mass with prolonged blush and prominent draining veins and to perform preoperative embolization. Screening MRI of the brain and spine is recommended for patients with a positive family history of VHL syndrome. The presence of a well-defined mass and homogeneous signal intensity facilitates the differentiation of these lesions from spinal arteriovenous fistulas, which may otherwise mimic a spinal cord hemangioblastoma at imaging.

Hemangioblastomas of the spine are relatively uncommon, accounting for less than 5% of spinal cord tumors. One third of spinal hemangioblastomas are associated with VHL syndrome, and the ratio of intracranial hemangioblastomas to VHL lesions is approximately the same. The lesions are fairly evenly distributed throughout the cord with the bulk arising in the thoracic spine (50%) and the cervical spine (40%). Hemangioblastomas are peripherally located in the cord and always come in contact with the subpial surface.

A notable characteristic of these tumors is the intense enhancement. The lesions are highly vascular and result in extensive spinal cord edema and potential syrinx that is disproportionate to the size of the tumor. These lesions may mimic vascular malformations because there are often associated larger veins and arteries overlying the lesion. The extensive edema is similar to that seen in dural arteriovenous fistulas of the spine. Clinically hemangioblastomas with minimal edema may be occult; symptoms are proportional to the edema and surrounding cord changes rather than a direct reflection of tumor size. After resection, the marked edema will typically resolve.

Although hemangioblastomas avidly enhance, they can resemble intramedullary cysts, which will not enhance. These tumors are typically hyperintense on T2-weighted images and variable on T1-weighted images because of their high protein content.

Catheter angiography may aid in the diagnosis when the clinical picture is difficult to discern from that of other vascular lesions[30-32] (Figs. 4-7 and 4-8).

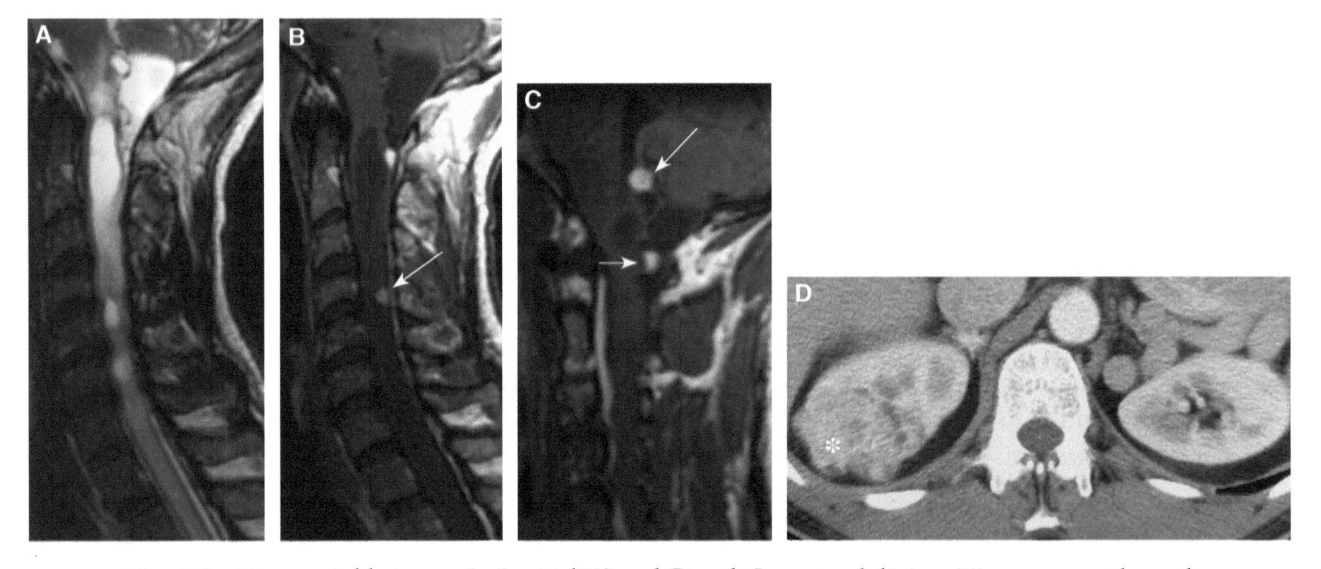

Fig. 4-7 Hemangioblastoma. **A,** Sagittal T2 and **B** and **C,** postgadolinium T1 sequences through the cervical spine in a 39-year-old patient with VHL demonstrate extensive cord edema, cysts, and multiple enhancing pial nodules *(arrows)*. This patient also has renal cell carcinoma, which is demonstrated on axial contrast-enhanced CT scan through the kidneys and shows an enhancing mass in **D,** the right kidney *(asterisk)*.

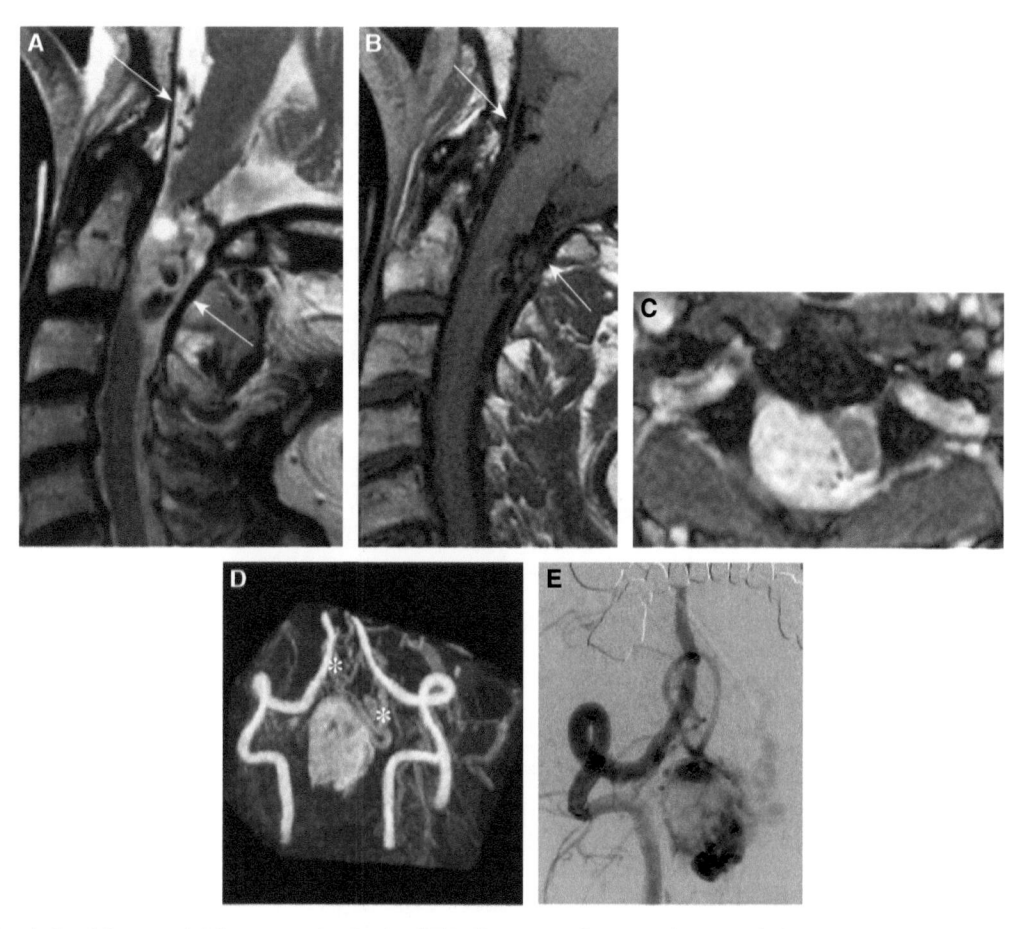

Fig. 4-8 Hemangioblastoma. **A,** Sagittal T2, **B,** T1, and **C,** axial postgadolinium T1 images through the cervical spine demonstrate a heterogeneous enhancing exophytic mass with prominent flow voids, which is compatible with a highly vascular tumor *(arrows)*. **D,** Anteroposterior view from a magnetic resonance angiogram demonstrates prominent arterial feeders from the vertebral arteries to this vascular tumor *(asterisks)* correlating with **E,** conventional angiography, which was performed for preoperative embolization.

LYMPHOMA

Prevalence
Lymphoma confined to the spinal cord is rare, comprising only 3.3% of CNS lymphoma, and is predominantly solitary (98%). The cervical cord is the most commonly affected site, followed by the thoracic cord and the lumbar region. There is a slight female predominance, and mean age at presentation is 47 years. Patients with primary intramedullary spinal lymphoma may have a better prognosis than those with primary intracranial CNS lymphoma.

Pathology
Histologic examination demonstrates a homogeneous collection of lymphocytes. Immunohistochemical stains may identify the dominant B-cell lymphocytes. A T-cell lineage is an unusual feature in CNS lymphoma. Human T-cell lymphotropic virus type I may be a precursor to T-cell spinal cord lymphoma.

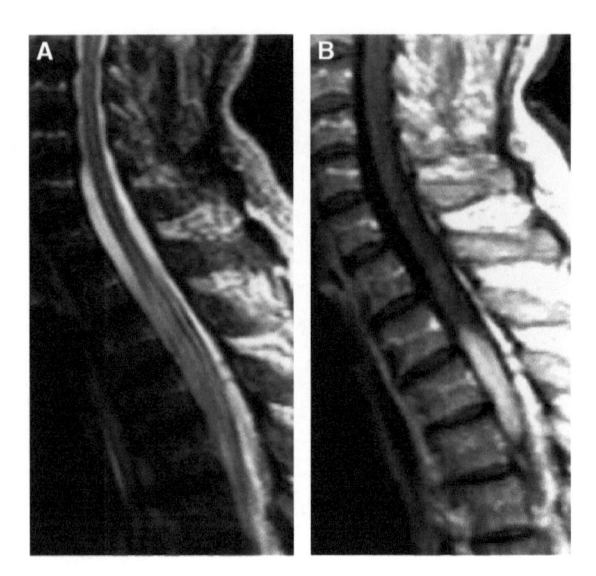

Fig. 4-9 Lymphoma. **A,** Sagittal T2 and **B,** postgadolinium T1 images demonstrate an intermediate T2 signal homogeneously enhancing intramedullary mass within the thoracic cord.

Imaging
More often than not, lymphoma within the spinal cord is metastatic, although the primary lymphoma is unknown. Although intracranial lymphoma typically demonstrates low signal intensity on T2-weighted images, spinal cord lymphomas may show high signal intensity on T2-weighted images. These tumors may be isointense or show a variable signal relative to the spinal cord on unenhanced T1-weighted images, and they are homogeneously enhanced after administration of contrast material. Unlike primary cord tumors, lymphomas may not expand the cord[33-35] (Fig. 4-9).

Metastasis
Prevalence
Although osseous metastases are the most commonly occuring bone tumors of the spine, metastasis directly to the parenchymal cord is rare. The rate of intramedullary metastasis at autopsy is reported to be less than 2% in the literature. These tumors can arise from primary intracranial CNS neoplasms through cerebrospinal fluid seeding and hematogenous spread of systemic carcinomas. Extension along the Batson venous plexus from retroperitoneal tumors or extension along the perineural lymphatic ducts is also a possibility. Most metastases occur in the cervical cord and are solitary.

The most common primary sources for cord metastases are lung carcinoma (40% to 85%), breast carcinoma (11%), melanoma (5%), renal cell carcinoma (4%), colorectal carcinoma (3%), and lymphoma (3%); 5% of the primary sites are unknown.

Although primary intramedullary neoplasms of the spine may demonstrate symptoms over a long period of time, patients with spinal cord metastasis (75%) may have symptoms for less than 1 month before diagnosis. These patients with spinal cord metastasis tend to have a poor prognosis, with two thirds of them dying within 6 months. Radiation and corticosteroid therapy are the treatments of choice for these metastases.

Pathology
Spinal cord tumor metastases often resemble their tissues of origin and are therefore all histologically different. These lesions frequently appear as circumscribed, rounded, gray-white or tan masses and often show central necrosis or hemorrhage.

Imaging
Cord metastases typically are isointense on T1-weighted images. If there is associated hemorrhaging, these lesions may be T1 hyperintense and show susceptibility artifact associated with hemosiderin deposition. Melanoma lesions may also be intrinsically T1 bright because of the melanotic composition, regardless of hemorrhagic conversion. Metastatic lesions are T2 hyperintense, reflecting edema or tumor infiltration, and typically enhance. Spinal cord edema is often disproportionately increased for the size of the lesion. Lesions typically produce mild cord expansion over several segments[36-39] (Fig. 4-10).

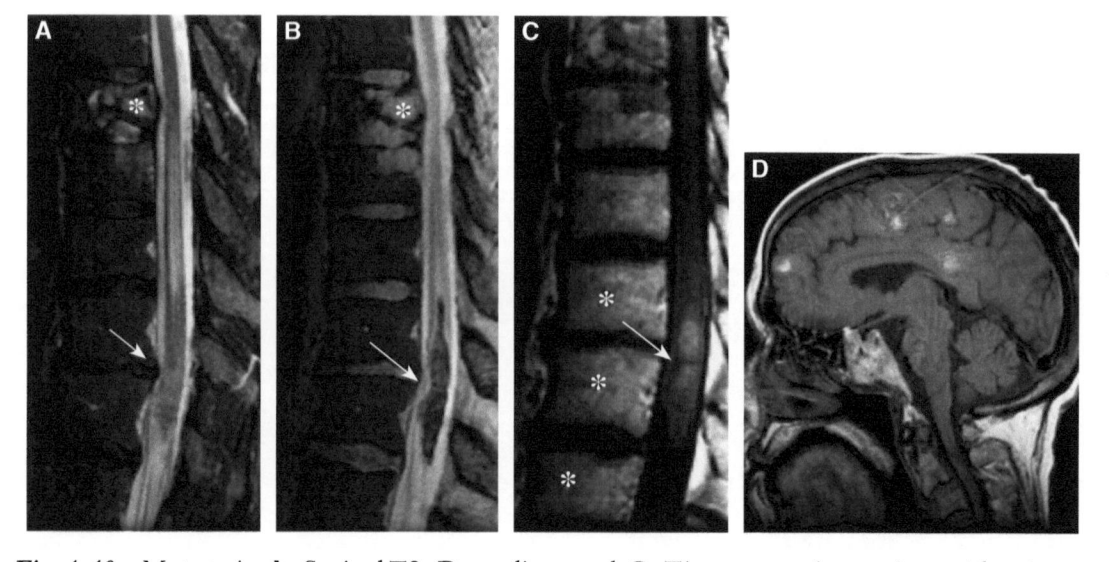

Fig. 4-10 Metastasis. **A,** Sagittal T2, **B,** gradient, and **C,** T1 sequences in a patient with primary breast carcinoma demonstrates a focal hemorrhagic mass within the conus *(arrows)* with associated extensive edema. There is evidence of osseous metastatic disease within collapsed vertebrae *(asterisks)*. The source for the intramedullary conus metastasis is likely through subarachnoid seeding given the multiple hemorrhagic intracranial metastases in this patient seen on **D,** the sagittal T1 sequence through the brain.

INTRAMEDULLARY TUMORS: DISTINGUISHING NEOPLASTIC FROM NON-NEOPLASTIC LESIONS

Notwithstanding its unsurpassed sensitivity, MRI has limited specificity and cannot differentiate the wide variety of possible etiologies of intramedullary lesions. Non-neoplastic etiologic factors, such as demyelinating disease, sarcoidosis, and dural arteriovenous fistulas, can mimic spinal cord tumors. Distinguishing neoplastic from non-neoplastic causes is crucial for the surgeon. Once the non-neoplastic cause is confirmed, appropriate (and usually nonsurgical) therapy can be instituted. In a series of 212 patients suspected of having intramedullary disease, nine (4%) had non-neoplastic lesions. None of the nine patients had evidence of spinal cord expansion on imaging studies.[40,41]

MULTIPLE SCLEROSIS

Most focal plaques are less than two vertebral body lengths in size; they occupy less than half of the cross-sectional diameter of the cord and are characteristically located peripherally. Lesions within the cord are twice as likely to involve the cervical cord compared with the lower cord levels. When an isolated cord lesion is demonstrated, MRI of the head is helpful in detecting additional lesions and supporting a diagnosis of primary demyelinating disease. However, approximately 10% to 15% of patients with spinal cord lesions have no intracranial disease.

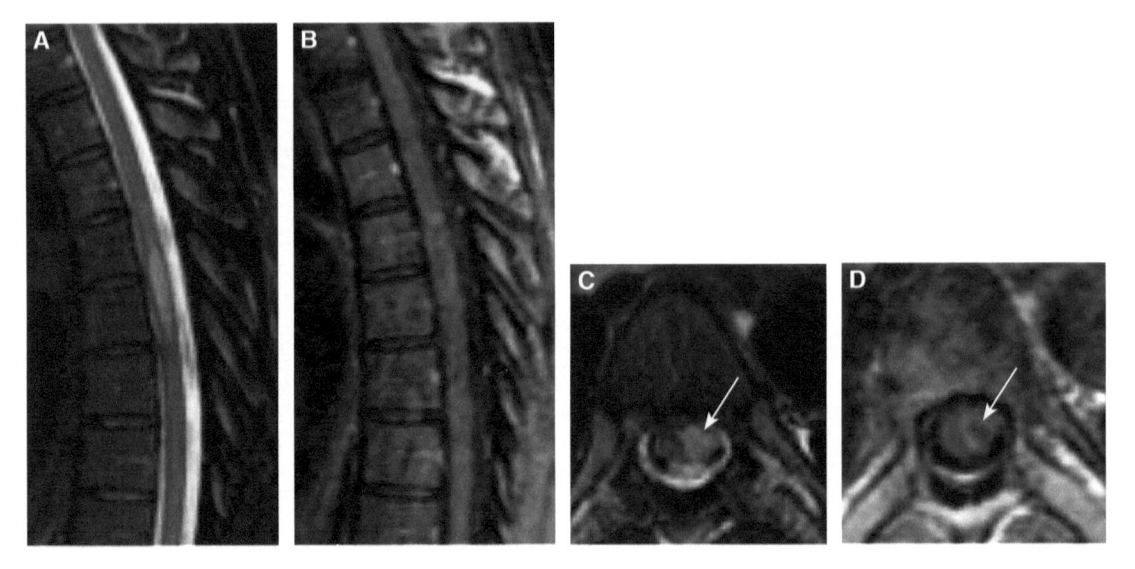

Fig. 4-11 Multiple sclerosis. **A,** Sagittal T2 and **B,** postgadolinium T1 sequences through the thoracic cord demonstrate a focal intramedullary lesion without significant expansion. **C,** Axial T2 sequence demonstrates the peripheral location of the lesion within the left hemicord. Note evidence of incomplete marginal enhancement of the lesion on the **D,** axial postgadolinium image, which is compatible with a primary demyelinating process *(arrows)*.

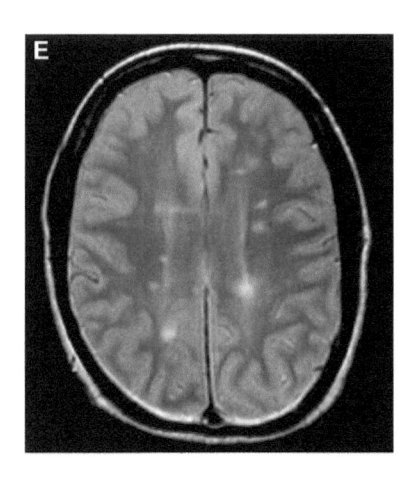

Fig. 4-11, cont'd Multiple sclerosis. **E,** Axial T2 sequence through the brain reveals multiple deep periventricular and callosal white matter foci compatible with MS.

The lesions appear as foci of increased signal intensity on T2-weighted images and possible low signal intensity on T1-weighted sequences. There may be associated cord expansion during the acute phase of the disease and cord atrophy in the late stages. In one series, more than half of all cord plaques longer than two vertebral segments were accompanied by cord atrophy or swelling. Cord swelling occurred only in patients with relapsing-remitting multiple sclerosis (MS) and in patients with Devic's syndrome.[42] Diffuse cord abnormalities have been shown to correlate with primary or secondary subtypes of progressive clinical MS.

The presence of enhancement appears to correlate with active disease. In very old plaques there is evidence of Wallerian degeneration, and iron deposition has been demonstrated at the edge of plaques, which may account for some of the foci of low signal intensity seen on the T2-weighted sequences. There is a lack of precise correlation between clinical and MRI evidence of spinal cord activity because newly detected plaques are not necessarily associated with new clinical signs[43,44] (Fig. 4-11).

ACUTE TRANSVERSE MYELOPATHY

The MRI appearance of this acute inflammatory monophasic process is quite variable. Although the size of the regions of abnormal cord hyperintensity on T2-weighted images can vary, these regions tend to extend for three or more spinal segments and, unlike MS plaques, they generally involve more than two thirds of the cross-sectional area of the spinal cord on transverse images.

MRI studies of the head are useful because approximately one third of these patients will demonstrate the intracranial lesions typical of MS. These patients have a high probability of developing clinical MS. It has been shown that in patients with small, ovoid enhancing spinal cord lesions without cord swelling, there is a high likelihood that they will develop clinically definitive MS. Those patients who demonstrated long segments of cord swelling with inhomogeneous gadolinium enhancement did not go on to develop MS.[45-47]

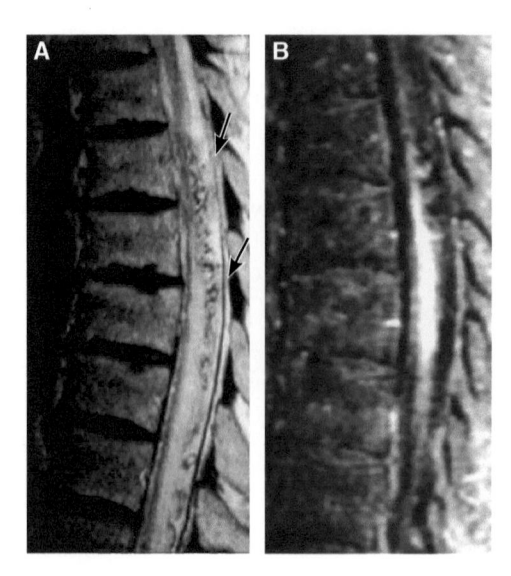

Fig. 4-12 Dural arteriovenous fistula. **A,** Sagittal T2 and **B,** postgadolinium sequences through the thoracic cord demonstrate diffuse increased T2 signal compatible with associated venous congestion and enhancement within the cord. Prominent flow voids are identified along the dorsal margin of the cord, which is highly suggestive of a dural arteriovenous fistula *(arrows)*.

SUBACUTE NECROTIZING MYELOPATHY

Most cases of this rare progressive myelopathy, which occurs frequently in elderly patients, are thought to be related to a spinal dural arteriovenous fistula (AVF). In an analysis of patients with suspected spinal dural AVFs who underwent spinal angiography, myelography, and MRI, 100% of patients who were diagnosed with spinal dural AVFs by means of spinal angiography demonstrated vessels on supine myelography and abnormal T2 hyperintense signals within the cord on MRI. Gadolinium enhancement was seen in 88%. Mass effect and flow voids were seen in less than half of the patients. Among patients with normal spinal angiograms, vessels were demonstrated on supine myelography in 92%. However, very few (17%) demonstrated an abnormal cord signal on T2-weighted images[48-51] (Fig. 4-12).

ACQUIRED IMMUNE DEFICIENCY SYNDROME

Vacuolar myelopathy is a spongy degeneration of the spinal cord that involves predominantly the posterior and lateral columns; it is the most common spinal cord disease in patients with acquired immune deficiency syndrome (AIDS). On MRI there may be atrophy and symmetrical abnormal hyperintense signals on T2-weighted sequences within the dorsal columns over several spine segments. There is no cord swelling, and characteristically there is no enhancement.[52,53]

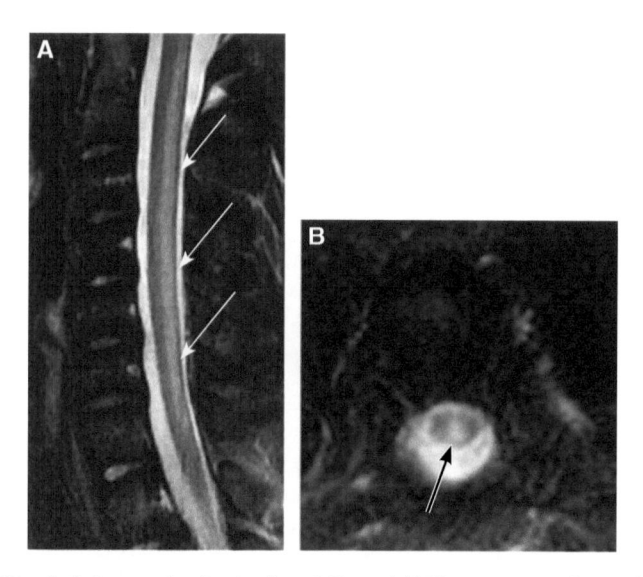

Fig. 4-13 Vitamin B_{12} deficiency. **A,** Sagittal and **B,** axial T2 sequences through the cervical cord in a patient with vitamin B_{12} deficiency demonstrate abnormal increased T2 signal diffusely throughout the entire cervical cord in a typical distribution within the dorsal columns without cord expansion or enhancement *(arrows)*.

SUBACUTE COMBINED DEGENERATION

Subacute combined degeneration (SCD) is a complication of vitamin B_{12} deficiency. MRI shows an abnormal increased signal within the dorsal columns on T2-weighted sequences. There is a corresponding improvement in these radiologic findings along with improved clinical function after vitamin B_{12} supplementation.

Nitrous oxide toxicity can also result in a pathophysiologic process and radiologic images identical to those of SCD because of the inactivation of cobalamin[54] (Fig. 4-13).

RADIATION MYELOPATHY

The incidence of radiation myelopathy correlates with the total dosage of radiation, dose per fraction, and length of spinal cord irradiated. A 50% incidence of radiation myelopathy can be expected if the cord has received between 68 and 73 Gy and only 5% when the cord receives between 57 and 61 Gy. The time course for development of radiation myelopathy demonstrates two peaks: the first at 12 to 14 months and the second at 24 to 28 months.

MRI findings are variable with no correlation between MRI appearance and the latency period. Less than 8 months after the onset of symptoms, low T1- and high T2-weighted signal intensity may be seen within a long segment of the spinal cord, possibly with cord swelling and focal enhancement. Images obtained 3 years after the onset of symptoms reveal cord atrophy[55,56] (Fig. 4-14).

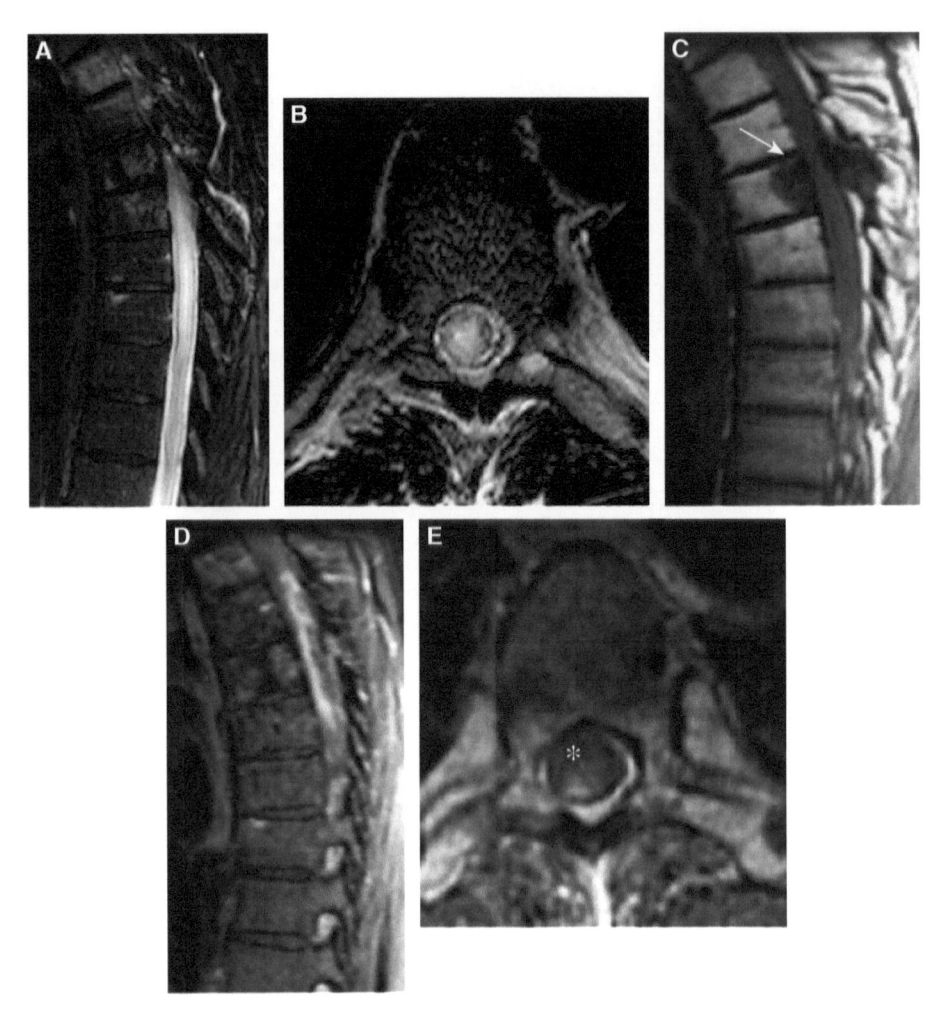

Fig. 4-14 Radiation myelitis. **A,** Sagittal and **B,** axial T2 sequences demonstrate long-segment abnormal increased signal within the thoracic spinal cord involving the entire transverse dimension compatible with edema. **C,** Sagittal T1 sequence through the thoracic spine demonstrates the osseous metastatic lesion that was previously irradiated *(arrow)*. Radiation myelitis. **D,** Sagittal and **E,** axial postgadolinium T1 sequences demonstrate irregular enhancement within the cord at the irradiated level *(asterisk)*.

CONCLUSION

Intramedullary neoplasms of the spine have limited distinguishing radiographic features. MRI results often permit a likely diagnosis. Features favoring an ependymoma include a central location, a well-circumscribed mass, the presence of hemorrhage, a location in the conus medullaris or filum terminale; and focal, intense, homogeneous enhancement. Astrocytoma is favored when the mass is eccentric, ill-defined, and enhances in a patchy, irregular fashion. Myxopapillary ependymomas are the most common neoplasms of the conus medullaris or filum terminale. Gangliogliomas characteristically involve eight or more vertebral segments and have mixed signal intensity on T1-weighted images, a finding unique among spinal cord tumors. Hemangioblastomas are highly vascular lesions and may have prominent flow voids near the mass. Less common intraspinal neoplasms include metastases and lymphoma.

Neoplastic spinal cord lesions must be differentiated from non-neoplastic conditions that can mimic intramedullary tumors, such as demyelination, inflammatory and vascular lesions, metabolic disease, infection, and radiation.

TIPS FROM THE MASTERS

- The presence of hemorrhage or hemosiderin in a well-defined centrally located intramedullary mass favors ependymoma.
- In addition to vascular malformations, prominent vessels may be detected in ependymomas and hemangioblastomas.
- Primary demyelinating disease is a common mimic of intramedullary tumors. An MRI of the head can be helpful in evaluating additional central nervous system involvement.

References (With Key References in Boldface)

1. Smoker WR, Godersky JC, Knutzon RK, et al. The role of MR imaging in evaluating metastatic spinal disease. AJR Am J Roentgenol 149:1241-1248, 1987.
2. Gillams AR, Soto JA, Carter AP. Fast spin echo vs conventional spin echo in cervical spine imaging. Eur Radiol 7:1211-1214, 1997.
3. Sze G. New applications of MR contrast agents in neuroradiology. Neuroradiology 32:421-438, 1990.
4. **Stradiotti P, Curti A, Castellazzi G, et al. Metal-related artifacts in instrumented spine. Techniques for reducing artifacts in CT and MRI: state of the art. Eur Spine J 18(Suppl 1):102-108, 2009.**
5. Georgy BA, Hesselink JR. MR imaging of the spine: recent advances in pulse sequences and special techniques. AJR Am J Roentgenol 162:923-934, 1994.
6. Valk J. Gd-DTPA in MR of spinal lesions. AJR Am J Roentgenol 150:1163-1168, 1988.
7. **Cha JG, Jin W, Lee MH, et al. Reducing metallic artifacts in postoperative spinal imaging: usefulness of IDEAL contrast-enhanced T1- and T2-weighted MR imaging—phantom and clinical studies. Radiology 259:885-893, 2011.**
8. Parizel PM, Baleriaux D, Rodesch G, et al. Gd-DTPA-enhanced MR imaging of spinal tumors. AJR Am J Roentgenol 152:1087-1096, 1989.
9. **Koeller KK, Rosenblum RS, Morrison AL. Neoplasms of the spinal cord and filum terminale: radiologic-pathologic correlation. Radiographics 20:1721-1749, 2000.**
10. **Waldron JS, Cha S. Radiographic features of intramedullary spinal cord tumors. Neurosurg Clin North Am 17:13-19, 2006.**
11. Plotkin SR, O'Donnell CC, Curry WT, et al. Spinal ependymomas in neurofibromatosis Type 2: a retrospective analysis of 55 patients. J Neurosurg Spine 14:543-547, 2011.
12. Ferrante L, Mastronardi L, Celli P, et al. Intramedullary spinal cord ependymomas—a study of 45 cases with long-term follow-up. Acta Neurochir (Wien) 119:74-79, 1992.
13. Kahan H, Sklar EM, Post MJ, et al. MR characteristics of histopathologic subtypes of spinal ependymoma. AJNR Am J Neuroradiol 17:143-150, 1996.
14. Heuer GG, Stiefel MF, Bailey RL, et al. Acute paraparesis from hemorrhagic spinal ependymoma: diagnostic dilemma and surgical management. Report of two cases and review of the literature. J Neurosurg Spine 7:652-655, 2007.

15. Lohle PN, Wurzer HA, Hoogland PH, et al. The pathogenesis of syringomyelia in spinal cord ependymoma. Clin Neurol Neurosurg 96:323-326, 1994.
16. **Setzer M, Murtagh RD, Murtagh FR, et al. Diffusion tensor imaging tractography in patients with intramedullary tumors: comparison with intraoperative findings and value for prediction of tumor resectability. J Neurosurg Spine 13:371-380, 2010.**
17. Wippold FJ II, Smirniotopoulos JG, Moran CJ, et al. MR imaging of myxopapillary ependymoma: findings and value to determine extent of tumor and its relation to intraspinal structures. AJR Am J Roentgenol 165:1263-1267, 1995.
18. Kumar V, Solanki RS. Myxopapillary ependymoma of the filum terminale. Pediatr Radiol 39:415, 2009.
19. Hoeffel C, Boukobza M, Polivka M, et al. MR manifestations of subependymomas. AJNR Am J Neuroradiol 16:2121-2129, 1995.
20. Scheithauer BW. Symptomatic subependymoma. Report of 21 cases with review of the literature. J Neurosurg 49:689-696, 1978.
21. Shimada S, Ishizawa K, Horiguchi H, et al. Subependymoma of the spinal cord and review of the literature. Pathol Int 53:169-173, 2003.
22. Zenmyo M, Ishido Y, Terahara M, et al. Intramedullary subependymoma of the cervical spinal cord: a case report with immunohistochemical study. Int J Neurosci 120:676-679, 2010.
23. Henson JW. Spinal cord gliomas. Curr Opin Neurol 14:679-682, 2001.
24. Schittenhelm J, Ebner FH, Tatagiba M, et al. Holocord pilocytic astrocytoma—case report and review of the literature. Clin Neurol Neurosurg 111:203-207, 2009.
25. **Seo HS, Kim JH, Lee DH, et al. Nonenhancing intramedullary astrocytomas and other MR imaging features: a retrospective study and systematic review. AJNR Am J Neuroradiol 31:498-503, 2010.**
26. Ng C, Fairhall J, Rathmalgoda C, et al. Spinal cord glioblastoma multiforme induced by radiation after treatment for Hodgkin disease. Case report. J Neurosurg Spine 6:364-367, 2007.
27. Patel U, Pinto RS, Miller DC, et al. MR of spinal cord ganglioglioma. AJNR Am J Neuroradiol 19:879-887, 1998.
28. Lonergan GJ, Schwab CM, Suarez ES, et al. Neuroblastoma, ganglioneuroblastoma, and ganglioneuroma: radiologic-pathologic correlation. Radiographics 22:911-934, 2002.
29. Satyarthee GD, Mehta VS, Vaishya S. Ganglioglioma of the spinal cord: report of two cases and review of literature. J Clin Neurosci 11:199-203, 2004.
30. Silbergeld J, Cohen WA, Maravilla KR, et al. Supratentorial and spinal cord hemangioblastomas: gadolinium enhanced MR appearance with pathologic correlation. J Comput Assist Tomogr 13:1048-1051, 1989.
31. Miller DJ, McCutcheon IE. Hemangioblastomas and other uncommon intramedullary tumors. J Neurooncol 47:253-270, 2000.
32. Baker KB, Moran CJ, Wippold FJ II, et al. MR imaging of spinal hemangioblastoma. AJR Am J Roentgenol 174:377-382, 2000.
33. Schild SE, Wharen RE Jr, Menke DM, et al. Primary lymphoma of the spinal cord. Mayo Clinic Proc 70:256-260, 1995.
34. Caruso PA, Patel MR, Joseph J, et al. Primary intramedullary lymphoma of the spinal cord mimicking cervical spondylotic myelopathy. AJR Am J Roentgenol 171:526-527, 1998.
35. Flanagan EP, O'Neill BP, Porter AB, et al. Primary intramedullary spinal cord lymphoma. Neurology 77:784-791, 2011.
36. Findlay JM, Bernstein M, Vanderlinden RG, et al. Microsurgical resection of solitary intramedullary spinal cord metastases. Neurosurgery 21:911-915, 1987.
37. Post MJ, Quencer RM, Green BA, et al. Intramedullary spinal cord metastases, mainly of non-neurogenic origin. AJR Am J Roentgenol 148:1015-1022, 1987.
38. Lim V, Sobel DF, Zyroff J. Spinal cord pial metastases: MR imaging with gadopentetate dimeglumine. AJR Am J Roentgenol 155:1077-1084, 1990.
39. Pellegrini D, Quezel MA, Bruetman JE. Intramedullary spinal cord metastasis. Arch Neurol 66:1422, 2009.

40. Lee M, Epstein FJ, Rezai AR, et al. Nonneoplastic intramedullary spinal cord lesions mimicking tumors. Neurosurgery 43:788-794; discussion 794-795, 1998.
41. **Do-Dai DD, Brooks MK, Goldkamp A, et al. Magnetic resonance imaging of intramedullary spinal cord lesions: a pictorial review. Curr Probl Diagn Radiol 39:160-185, 2010.**
42. Wiebe S, Lee DH, Karlik SJ, et al. Serial cranial and spinal cord magnetic resonance imaging in multiple sclerosis. Ann Neurol 32:643-650, 1992.
43. Trop I, Bourgouin PM, Lapierre Y, et al. Multiple sclerosis of the spinal cord: diagnosis and follow-up with contrast-enhanced MR and correlation with clinical activity. AJNR Am J Neuroradiol 19:1025-1033, 1998.
44. Hickman SJ, Miller DH. Imaging of the spine in multiple sclerosis. Neuroimaging Clin N Am 10:689-704, 2000, viii.
45. Choi KH, Lee KS, Chung SO, et al. Idiopathic transverse myelitis: MR characteristics. AJNR Am J Neuroradiol 17:1151-1160, 1996.
46. Campi A, Filippi M, Comi G, et al. Acute transverse myelopathy: spinal and cranial MR study with clinical follow-up. AJNR Am J Neuroradiol 16:115-123, 1995.
47. **Goh C, Phal PM, Desmond PM. Neuroimaging in acute transverse myelitis. Neuroimaging Clin North Am 21:951-973, 2011.**
48. Gilbertson JR, Miller GM, Goldman MS, et al. Spinal dural arteriovenous fistulas: MR and myelographic findings. AJNR Am J Neuroradiol 16:2049-2057, 1995.
49. Rodesch G, Lasjaunias P. Spinal cord arteriovenous shunts: from imaging to management. Eur J Radiol 46:221-232, 2003.
50. Krings T, Lasjaunias PL, Hans FJ, et al. Imaging in spinal vascular disease. Neuroimaging Clin North Am 17:57-72, 2007.
51. Sharma AK, Westesson PL. Preoperative evaluation of spinal vascular malformation by MR angiography: how reliable is the technique: case report and review of literature. Clin Neurol Neurosurg 110:521-524, 2008.
52. Chong J, Di Rocco A, Tagliati M, et al. MR findings in AIDS-associated myelopathy. AJNR Am J Neuroradiol 20:1412-1416, 1999.
53. Thurnher MM, Post MJ, Jinkins JR. MRI of infections and neoplasms of the spine and spinal cord in 55 patients with AIDS. Neuroradiology 42:551-556, 2000.
54. Ravina B, Loevner LA, Bank W. MR findings in subacute combined degeneration of the spinal cord: a case of reversible cervical myelopathy. AJR Am J Roentgenol 174:863-865, 2000.
55. Marcus RB Jr, Million RR. The incidence of myelitis after irradiation of the cervical spinal cord. Int J Radiat Oncol Biol Phys 19:3-8, 1990.
56. Bou-Haidar P, Peduto AJ, Karunaratne N. Differential diagnosis of T2 hyperintense spinal cord lesions: part B. J Med Imaging Radiat Oncol 53:152-159, 2009.

Chapter 5

Heavy-Particle Radiation

Jan M. Eckermann, Jerry D. Slater,
Walter D. Johnson

*I*onizing radiation applied to biological tissue exerts its function primarily through the Compton effect, described as the change in wavelength of an incoming x-ray or gamma ray after its interaction with biological matter.[1] This phenomenon was discovered by American physicist Arthur Holly Compton, for which he received the Nobel Prize in physics in 1929. The direction of the ray is also altered after tissue interaction, which has been referred to as *Compton scattering* (Fig. 5-1).

These ionizing rays exert their biological effect by removing orbital electrons from intracellular molecules and thus produce large amounts of reactive free radicals, resulting in irreversible and lethal tissue damage.[2] Apoptosis and terminal growth inhibition (metabolic cell death) are implicated in radiation-induced cell destruction and contrasted with that associated with dividing cells, which is called *mitosis-linked cell*

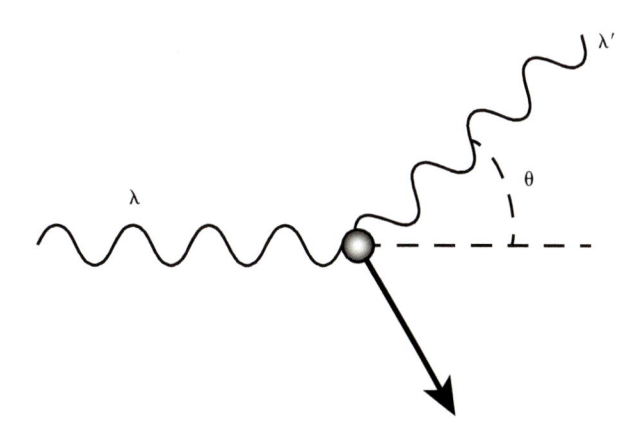

Fig. 5-1 Compton effect and scattering. The wavelength λ of the ionizing source is changed to λ' after interaction with matter. The direction is changed by the angle θ.

death. Radiation exerts its desired target cell death by destruction of the nuclear DNA, primarily by breaking the double helix and preventing transcription and translation from occurring, ultimately resulting in cell death.[3] The higher replication rate of tumor cells compared with nontumor cells makes them more vulnerable to this damage.

CURRENT SOURCES OF RADIATION TREATMENT

Current sources of radiation treatment can be divided into photons and hadrons (heavy particles) (Fig. 5-2). The hadron group includes helium, protons, and other heavy ions, such as carbon, and is generated through cyclotrons or synchrotrons.[4]

Gamma Knife units (GKUs), which use gamma rays, and linear accelerators (linacs), which use electrons, both rely heavily on the creation of reactive oxygen free radical species, which in turn cause irreversible DNA damage.[5] Heavy particles, on the other hand, accomplish most of their destruction by direct particle interaction with the cell's DNA. This is an important distinction because many tumors harbor hypoxic areas that allow for some radioresistance.[6] However, this problem does not present itself when heavy particles are deployed.

GKUs use a ^{60}Co source with multiple beams (201) centered at the isocenter.[7] Linacs produce x-rays through *bremsstrahlung.* Bremsstrahlung, literally translated from the German *bremsen,* "to brake," and *Strahlung,* "radiation," is electromagnetic radiation produced by the acceleration of a charged particle, such as an electron, on another charged particle.[8]

One of the greatest concerns and limitations in radiosurgery and radiation oncology is the undesired effect of ionizing radiation on the surrounding healthy tissue.[9] This creates an especially formidable challenge in the treatment of spine tumors because of the immediate proximity of healthy, radiosensitive tissue, specifically the spinal cord and brainstem.[10] Careful planning will sufficiently separate the dose-response curves of each tissue to maximize tumor dose and curtail the dose delivered to normal tissue. This is possible only by precisely configuring dose delivery portals to minimize dose and target volume of normal tissue.

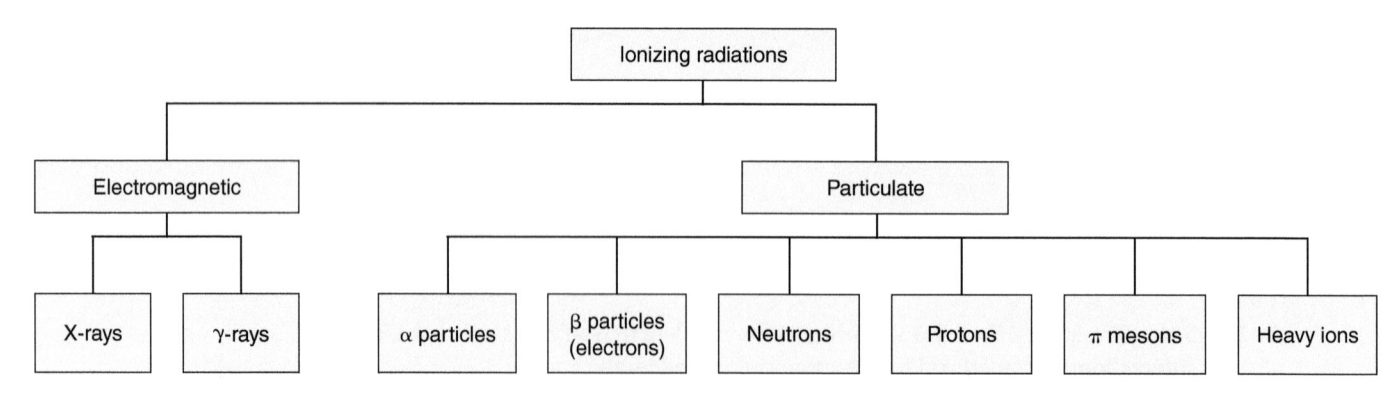

Fig. 5-2 Different forms of ionizing radiation. The major subdivisions are electromagnetic (photons) and particulate (hadrons).

Models, formulas, and calculations have been described in detail to predict cell death, specific tissue radiosensitivity, adequate dosage, and healthy tissue damage.[11] The most commonly used mathematical model to describe the relationship between cell survival and radiation dosage is the linear-quadratic model. This model finds the best-fit curve and slope of variables, such as radiation sensitivity of cells, an effect-threshold dose, and the repair capacity of cells.[12] The proportion of cell death to dose increases linearly as a result of destruction of double-strand DNA, and the proportion grows quadratically as a result of single-strand DNA destruction. The most important factor in the relationship between surviving cells and radiation dose is the intrinsic cellular radiosensitivity, which describes the dose necessary to achieve a 37% cell survival fraction.

Protons are positively charged particles resulting from the ionization of hydrogen atoms. Once released, the proton is accelerated through a cyclotron or synchrotron to a desired energy and then extracted as a linear beam. As the protons travel through tissue planes, only very small portions of energy are lost as a consequence of interaction with electrons and nuclear collisions, consequently exhibiting a much lower entrance dose compared with photons.[13] However, when the proton stops within the target volume, large amounts of energy are deposited within this volume, resulting in a rapid rise in energy absorbed, the high point of which is known as the *Bragg peak*.[14,15] The width of the Bragg peak is only a few millimeters for a single beam, but this energy can be modulated to create a spread-out Bragg peak, allowing this target volume to receive a precisely placed, relatively high dose of radiation energy. Fig. 5-3 compares the differences in tissue energy transfer of GKU, linacs, and protons.

Of significance is the steep and practically immediate drop-off in proton-delivered energy distal to the target as compared with the exponential decay of photonic radiation. This can dramatically limit the radiation exposure to neighboring tissues,

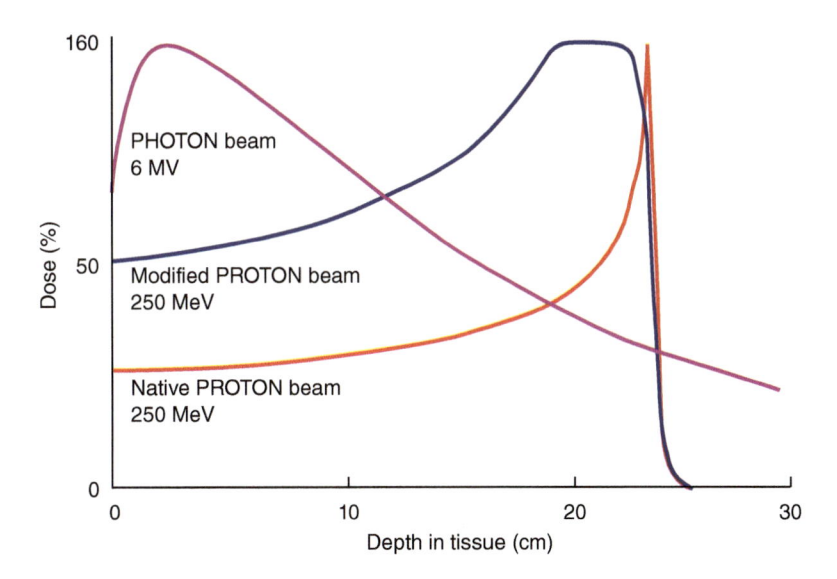

Fig. 5-3 Comparison of dose deposition of proton beam versus photons. Note the Bragg peak and spread-out Bragg peak, as well as the decreased entrance dose of protons compared with photon beams.

making it a particularly attractive choice for radiation of lesions adjacent to the spinal cord, brainstem, or other highly radiosensitive tissue.

ADVANTAGES OF HEAVY-PARTICLE RADIATION

Heavy-particle radiation has several advantages. Primarily it has greater controllability because of the higher charge and mass of the particles. This allows control in not only targeting tumor volume but also in targeting the tumor margins, thus minimizing damage to adjacent tissue. Although other types of radiation require multiple beams to produce a highly focal dose distribution, the Bragg peak phenomenon allows this to be done with only two to six beams.

As seen in Fig. 5-3, the x-ray dose climbs rapidly at a fairly shallow tissue depth, falls off exponentially within the target area, and then continues into adjacent normal tissue distal to the target, mostly uncontrolled. Conversely, the modulated proton beam delivers a much lower dose to tissue proximal to the target, a higher dose to the target, and then abruptly decays with virtually no dose delivered distal to the target.[16]

A third advantage is the ionization density (referred to as linear energy transfer, or LET) produced by the particle, each type of particle having a different LET. High LET causes tissue damage in normal tissues, whereas lower LET provides sufficiently for normal tissue recovery and repair after radiation injury. Because malignant cells are less capable of repair caused by ionization damage, the low LET characteristic of protons makes them ideal for minimizing risk to adjacent tissue.

The fourth relative advantage is that proton beams may be used for applications in any target within the body with precision and effectiveness.

Heavy particles were first generated and used medically at Lawrence Berkley Laboratory in 1949.[17] Several centers in Europe began using protons to treat cancer throughout the 1950s. In 1963 the Harvard cyclotron was being built and used for cancer therapy. At that time all cyclotrons were built as part of the various physics departments and research laboratories. Loma Linda University Medical Center built the world's first hospital-based proton accelerator and treatment center, treating its first patient in 1991.[18,19] Massachusetts General Hospital began with a proton accelerator and treatment facility at Massachusetts Institute of Technology[20] but recently opened a hospital-based center. Currently eight hospital-based proton accelerator treatment centers are available for treatment of patients in the United States. Over the past several decades, more than 40,000 patients have been treated with proton beam therapy worldwide.

The Gesellschaft fur Schwerionenforschung, the leading investigative group on heavy-particle radiation in Germany, and the Heavy Ion Medical Accelerator group in Japan are the first and largest facilities to use and study carbon ion (C-ion) beams as a heavy particle for radiation therapy.[21,22] The C-ion beams provide unique advantageous biological and physical properties in radiation therapy for malignant tumors. C-ion beams have a high relative biological effectiveness resulting from the high LET. In terms of their physical characteristics, C-ion beams exhibit a spread-out Bragg peak and make for a better dose distribution of the target volume by specified beam modulations. C-ion properties appear to be very similar to protons. However, much more experience is currently reported with proton beam therapy.

INDICATIONS AND CONTRAINDICATIONS

Benign tumors with a gross total resection more than likely do not need radiation but will require close, long-term radiologic follow-up examinations. All subtotal resections of benign spine tumors warrant an evaluation for radiation therapy as do any anaplastic or frankly malignant tumors. Metastatic lesions may receive radiation therapy as the primary and only treatment or, on occasion, before surgical resection.[23]

One contraindication for spine irradiation is prior radiation therapy, particularly if the target and dose distribution curves are unknown. If expected survival is shorter than the time to anticipated effect of radiation, radiation is most likely not indicated, although it may play a role in palliative pain reduction.

PREOPERATIVE EVALUATION

Complete history and thorough physical examination play an integral part in establishing a successful physician-patient relationship and formulating a treatment plan. Patient history and physical examination can be narrowed to the specific problem because patients are almost always referred by other health care professionals (i.e., spine surgeons and neurologists). However, careful attention must be paid to a history of prior radiation, previous resections and spinal stability, wound healing, nutrition, and the patient's overall medical condition.

High-quality and thorough neuroimaging is critical. CT scans and MRIs with and without contrast enhancement must be up to date and in a system that is supported by the local digital system and the radiation-administering software. Furthermore, positron emission tomography (PET) and/or full-body CT scans are warranted to rule out a potential primary malignancy with a prognosis that is worse than the natural history of the spine lesion being addressed. Identifying the location of the lesion in terms of intramedullary or extramedullary and intradural or extradural may narrow the differential diagnosis list and may provide clues regarding the originating tissue (primary versus metastatic).

It is also very important to study the bony anatomy at the location of the lesion and to determine the integrity of the spinal column. The first-order decision will be whether surgical intervention is required before radiation and, if so, what approach would be optimal. If the lesion requires significant bone removal, stabilization with arthrodesis and instrumentation needs to be done. When evaluating images, careful attention is paid to the relationship between the targeted lesion and the surrounding tissues, especially the spinal cord, such as the margin between the cord and tumor. In addition, the patient's functional status will dictate how important this margin is. For example, a patient with fixed neurologic deficits resulting from the tumor (such as paraplegia) will not be substantially altered by maximal irradiation to the cord at that level. The next step is to calculate the volume of the target lesion, define the isocenter or isocenters, and calculate the appropriate dosage. Furthermore, fractionation of the dose will be considered, depending on the proximity and radiosensitivity of adjacent healthy tissue.

CLINICAL DECISION-MAKING

Once the diagnosis of spine tumor has been established, it is important to take a multidisciplinary approach to define a customized, patient-focused treatment plan. Careful physical examination and documentation cannot be overemphasized. A thorough metastatic workup is standard for patients with spine tumors. Then, with the multidisciplinary team, which would involve radiation and medical oncologists as well as surgeons, the benefits of radiation, chemotherapy, and surgery are discussed. This will include several key questions, including the following: Is surgical resection indicated, or is just a biopsy sufficient for tissue diagnosis? What is the timing of surgery in relation to both chemotherapy and radiation? What are the ultimate goals and likely success of the proposed treatment? Furthermore, existing instrumentation should be discussed as a potential factor in negatively influencing applied radiation and may warrant a nontraditional choice of path for the radiation beam to circumvent the obstruction.

TECHNIQUE

Treatment planning begins with high-quality neuroimaging, generally CT, but may include MRI and PET. These images are then used to generate a three-dimensional image of the target and thus determine the sophisticated shaping of dose distribution. Appropriate beam-shaping devices are used.

Patient positioning and stabilization are of primary importance during treatment planning and delivery. Patients are immobilized most commonly by means of either a face mask or some type of body molding, which ensures identical patient positioning during each treatment session. These are designed for patient comfort and, for the most part, are fairly well tolerated during treatment. Once immobilization is completed, radiation therapy simulation is initiated. First, a virtual simulation using the three-dimensional imaging techniques is done to plan the approach, then the complete treatment is planned with regard to gross tumor volume. The tumor volume is delineated based on imaging studies, clinical target volume, and the visualized tumor, plus adjacent areas at risk. Planning target volume, which is a slightly enlarged clinical target volume, includes margin of error for patient motion, setup errors, and linear accelerator alignment errors. These target volumes, optimal dosing, and beam direction require input from radiation therapists, medical physicists, and dosimetrists. Once planning is optimized, normally in approximately 14 days, treatment can begin.

OUTCOMES WITH EVALUATION OF RESULTS

We have successfully treated a wide variety of spine tumors at the Loma Linda University Proton Beam Center. Pathologic diagnoses include chordomas, chondrosarcomas, sarcomas, malignant schwannomas, and myxopapillary ependymomas. The most immediate and most common complication is delayed wound healing. This is managed with aggressive wound care and, at times, hyperbaric oxygen therapy. Spinal cord edema and occasional radiation necrosis may be more delayed complications with limited treatment options other than oral steroids. Because of the favorable characteristics of heavy particles, radiation necrosis is less frequent compared with conventional radiation therapy.

SIGNATURE CASES

A 71-year-old man had a recurrence of a C4 chordoma 1 year after a previous resection with instrumentation (Fig. 5-4, *A* and *B*). He underwent an en bloc C4 corpectomy with instrumentation followed by proton beam therapy. MRI at 2 years' follow-up showed good tumor control Fig. 5-4, *C* and *D*).

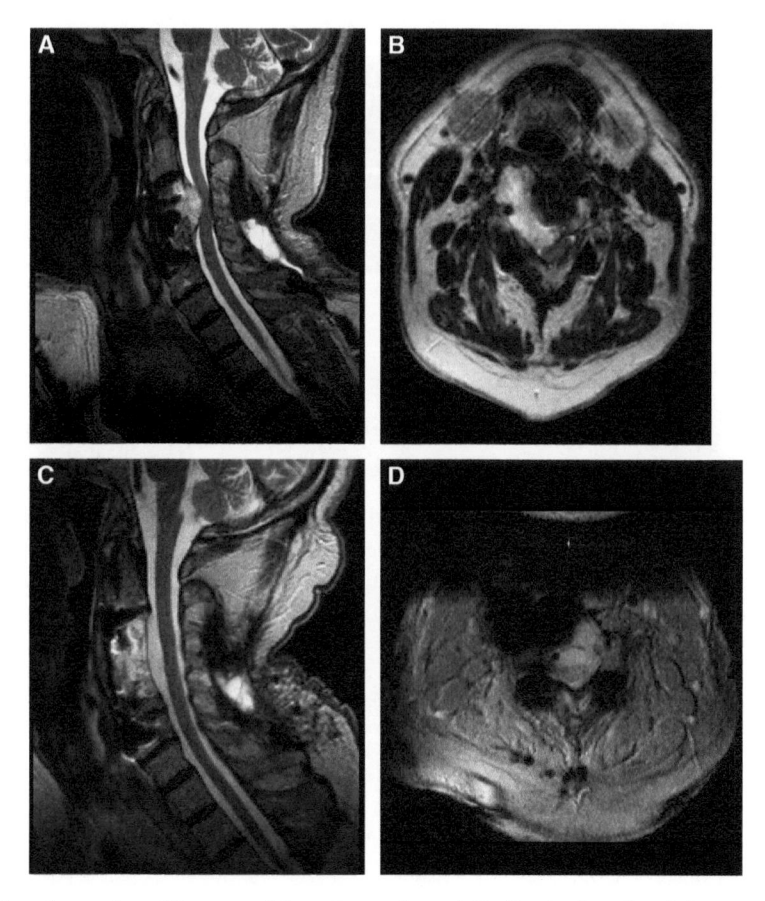

Fig. 5-4 C4 chordoma in a 71-year-old patient. **A** and **B,** Sagittal and axial, preoperative non–contrast-enhanced, T2-weighted MRI images of the cervical spine. **C** and **D,** Postoperative and postradiation T2-weighted MRI images demonstrating good tumor control at 2 years' follow-up. This patient required instrumentation for stabilization.

A 61-year-old man presented with an L1 plasma cell myeloma (Fig. 5-5, *A* and *B*). He underwent a transpedicular tumor resection and corpectomy with posterior instrumentation. MRI at 6 months' follow-up demonstrated good tumor control (Fig. 5-5, *C* and *D*). Although there is no evidence that proton beam therapy is superior to other types of radiation therapy, it was selected by the patient's radiation oncologist for postoperative treatment.

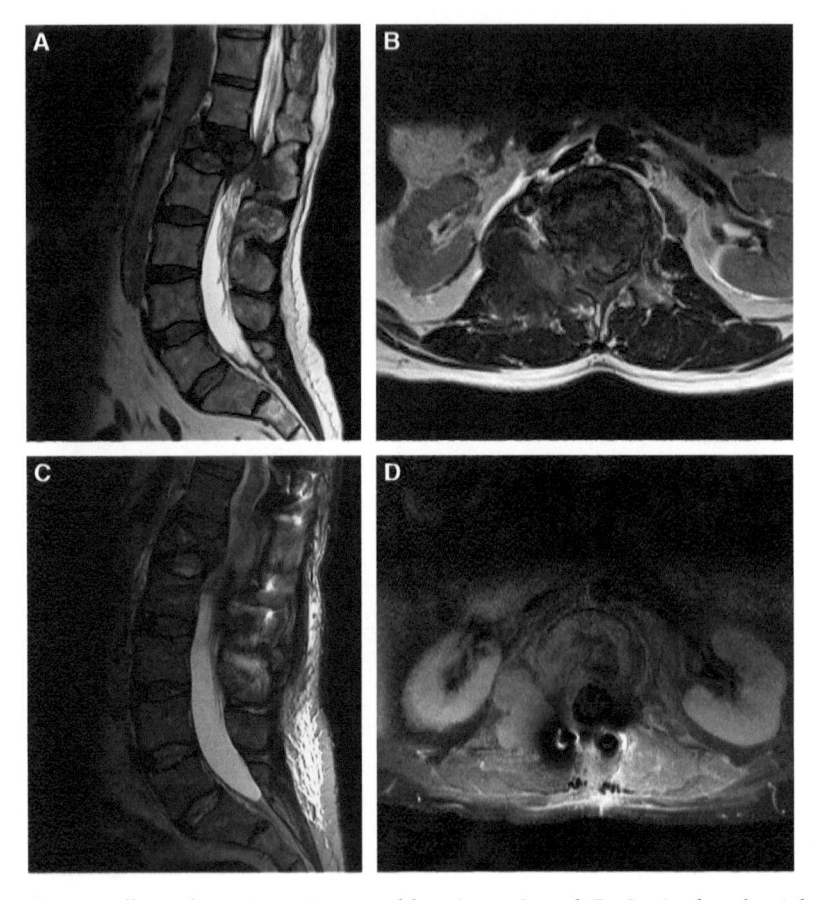

Fig. 5-5 L1 plasma cell myeloma in a 61-year-old patient. **A** and **B,** Sagittal and axial, preoperative non–contrast-enhanced, T2-weighted MRIs of the lumbar spine. **C** and **D,** Postoperative and postradiation T2-weighted MRIs demonstrating good tumor control at 6 months' follow-up. This patient required instrumentation for stabilization.

A 39-year-old man presented with a recurrent sacral schwannoma with malignant features (Fig. 5-6, *A* and *B*). He underwent resection without instrumentation, and MRI at 2 years' follow-up showed good tumor control (Fig. 5-6, *C* and *D*).

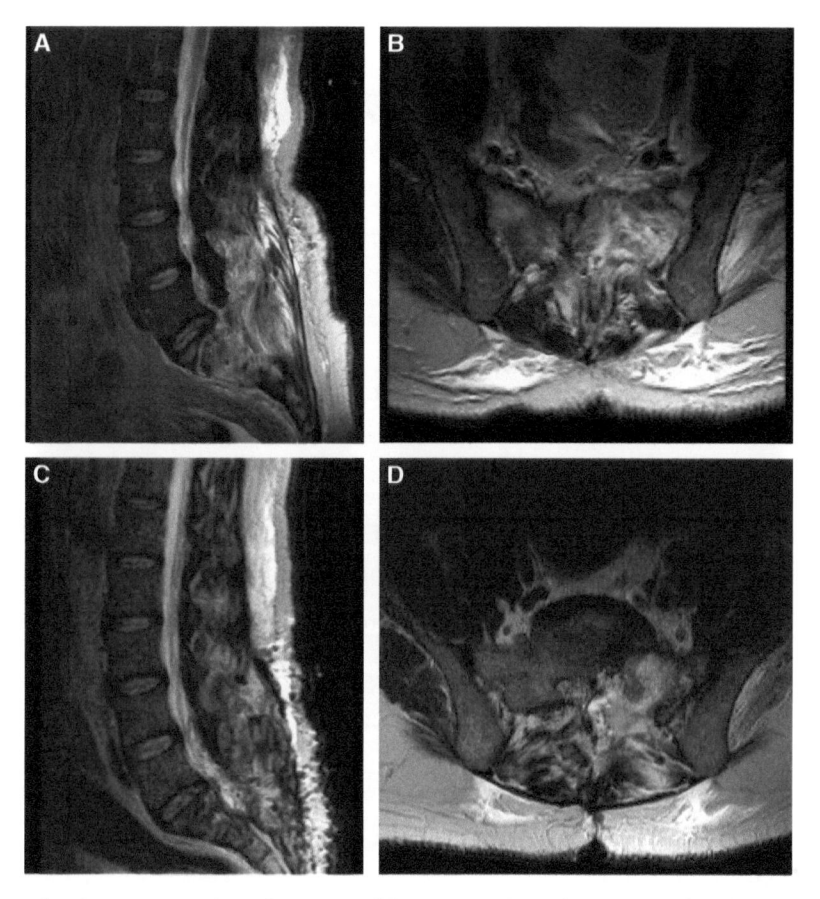

Fig. 5-6 Sacral schwannoma in a 39-year-old patient. **A** and **B,** Sagittal and axial, preoperative non–contrast-enhanced, T2-weighted MRIs of the lumbosacral spine. **C** and **D,** Postoperative and postradiation T2-weighted MRIs demonstrating good tumor control at 2 years' follow-up.

CONCLUSION

Current heavy-particle radiation techniques are well suited for the treatment of spine tumors. Careful planning and a multidisciplinary team approach that includes spine surgeons, radiation and medical oncologists, medical physicists, and radiation dosimetrists are critical in the development of an optimal treatment strategy for patients with spine tumors. Heavy-particle radiation has some particular advantages over conventional radiation techniques because of the well-defined range and accuracy of the particles and the steep drop-off immediate distal to the target, which has the potential of protecting adjacent normal tissues, especially when high doses of radiation are required.

TIPS FROM THE MASTERS

Heavy-particle radiation offers the following advantages:
- Delivery of high-dose radiation while sparing closely adjacent spinal cord
- Excellent tumor control
- High controllability with minimal dosage proximal or distal to target

References (With Key References in Boldface)

1. Sahoo S, Gribakin GF, Shabbir Naz G, et al. Compton scatter profiles for warm dense matter. Phys Rev E Stat Nonlin Soft Matter Phys 77:2-4, 2008.
2. Yamada H, Kobayashi K, Hieda K. Effects of the K-shell X-ray absorption of phosphorus on the scission of the pentadeoxythymidylic acid. Int J Radiat Biol 63:151-159, 1993.
3. Bernhard WA, Mroczka N, Barnes J. Combination is the dominant free radical process initiated in DNA by ionizing radiation: an overview based on solid-state EPR studies. Int J Radiat Biol 66:491-497, 1994.
4. Coutrakon GB. Accelerators for heavy-charged-particles radiation therapy. Technol Cancer Res Treat 6(4 Suppl):49-54, 2007.
5. Zhao W, Diz DI, Robbins ME. Oxidative damage pathways in relation to normal tissue injury. Br J Radiol 80:23-31, 2007.
6. Gerszten PC, Ryu S. Spine Radiosurgery. New York: Thieme, 2008.
7. Leksell L. Cerebral radiosurgery. I. Gammathalamotomy in two cases of intractable pain. Acta Chir Scand 134:585-595, 1968.
8. Hettinger G, Starfelt N. Bremsstrahlung spectra from roentgen tubes. Acta Radiol 50:381-394, 1958.
9. Cerqueira EM, Meireles JR, Lopes MA, et al. Genotoxic effects of x-rays on keratinized mucosa cells during panoramic dental radiography. Dentomaxillofac Radiol 37:398-403, 2008.
10. Bayrakli F, Dincer A, Sav A, et al. Late brain stem radionecrosis seventeen years after fractionated radiotherapy. Turk Neurosurg 19:182-185, 2009.
11. Elsasser T, Brons S, Psonka K, et al. Biophysical modeling of fragment length distributions of DNA plasmids after X and heavy-ion irradiation analyzed by atomic force microscopy. Radiat Res 169:649-659, 2008.
12. Chun LS, Regine WF, eds. Principles and Practice of Stereotactic Radiosurgery. New York: Springer, 2008.
13. **Slater JM. Selecting the optimum particle for radiation therapy. Technol Cancer Res Treat 6:35-39, 2007.**

14. Kjellberg RN, Nguyen NC, Kliman B. [The Bragg Peak proton beam in stereotaxic neurosurgery] Neurochirugie 18:235-265, 1972.
15. Chong CY, Linfoot JA, Lawrence JH. High-energy heavy particles in medicine. Radiol Clin North Am 7:319-343, 1969.
16. **Bush DA, McAllister CJ, Loredo LN, et al. Fractionated proton beam therapy for acoustic neuroma. Neurosurgery 50:273-275, 2002.**
17. **Skarsgard LD. Radiobiology with heavy charged particles: a historical review. Phys Med 14(Suppl 1):1-19, 1998.**
18. Slater JM, Miller DW, Archambeau DO. Development of a hospital-based proton beam treatment center. Int J Radiat Oncol Biol Phys 14:761-775, 1988.
19. Nelson GA, Green LM, Gridley DS, et al. Research activities at the Loma Linda University and Proton Treatment Facility—an overview. Phys Med 17:30-32, 2001.
20. Sisterson JM, Cascio E, Koehler AM, et al. Proton beam therapy: reliability of the synchrocyclotron at the Harvard Cyclotron Laboratory. Phys Med Biol 36:285-290, 1991.
21. Haettner E, Iwase H, Schardt D. Experimental fragmentation studies with 12C therapy beams. Radiat Prot Dosimetry 122:485-487, 2006.
22. Inaniwa T, Furukawa T, Matsufuji N, et al. Clinical ion beams: semi-analytical calculation of their quality. Phys Med Biol 52:7261-7279, 2007.
23. Gerszten PC, Welch WC. Cyberknife radiosurgery for metastatic spine tumors. Neurosurg Clin N Am 15:491-501, 2004.

Chapter 6

Spine Stereotactic Radiosurgery

J. Bradley Elder, Yoshiya Yamada,
Peter C. Gerszten, Mark H. Bilsky

More than 180,000 new cases of spinal metastases are diagnosed in North America each year, with 20,000 clinical cases of spinal cord compression.[1-3] The incidence and prevalence of spine tumors are expected to rise in the future with improvements in systemic therapy. Thus these tumors represent a growing source of morbidity among patients with cancer. The goals of treatment are pain relief, improved or maintained neurologic status, local tumor control, spinal stability and, ultimately, improved quality of life. The principal decisions must take into account that treatment for spinal metastases is palliative not curative, and most patients will present with or develop widespread systemic visceral and bone disease. Many patients also have significant comorbid conditions that may preclude aggressive surgical treatment. With few exceptions, such as multiple myeloma, lymphoma, and carcinomas of the breast and prostate gland, chemotherapy and hormones play a limited role in the treatment of metastatic spine tumors. The principal treatment modalities for solid tumor spinal metastases are radiation therapy and surgery. Because of the inherent morbidity of surgery, radiation therapy has been considered the mainstay of treatment for spinal metastases. However, surgery continues to play a role in the treatment of metastatic disease for high-grade epidural spinal cord resulting from solid tumor malignancies and gross spinal instability.

For most metastatic tumors, radiation offers the best chance of durable long-term local tumor control or cure when delivered either as definitive therapy or as a postsurgical adjuvant treatment. Despite the less-invasive nature of radiation compared with surgery, conventional external beam radiation therapy (cEBRT) has not always afforded effective palliation. The role of radiation is well established for metastatic spine tumors.[2-8] However, the effectiveness of cEBRT (such as 30 Gy in 3 Gy/fraction) is limited by spinal cord tolerance, which is defined as 50 Gy in 1.8 to 2.0 Gy per fraction for a 5 to 10 cm length of spinal cord.[4] This cEBRT dose is subtherapeutic for most metastatic spine tumors, particularly solid tumors.[4a]

Stereotactic radiosurgery (SRS) is defined as high-dose conformal photon therapy delivered as a single fraction or hypofractionated regimen (2 to 5 fractions). SRS enables the delivery of a potentially cytotoxic dose that can spare normal tissue in areas such as the spinal cord, bowel, kidney, and esophagus. Technological advances in imaging, computerized inverse treatment planning, tumor localization, and sophisticated image-guided delivery systems allow radiation doses that provide effective palliation with limited morbidity.

SRS is being used with increasing frequency to treat primary malignant and benign spine tumors.[5-7] However, the discussion in this chapter will be limited to metastatic spine tumors, which represent the largest experience to date. The integration of SRS into the decision frameworks for metastatic spine tumors is predicated on redefining the concept of radiation responsiveness. Tumors that are radioresistant to cEBRT, such as renal cell carcinoma and melanoma, have shown marked responses to SRS. Improved control rates are observed with the use of SRS both as definitive therapy and as postoperative adjuvant therapy. The improved local control rates with SRS may reduce the need for aggressive or en bloc resection of metastatic spine tumors.

PRINCIPLES OF STEREOTACTIC RADIOSURGERY

Spinal radiosurgery procedures are divided into the following four components:
1. Target identification
2. Treatment planning
3. Patient immobilization and isocenter verification
4. Dose delivery

Numerous systems have been developed to evaluate each of these components, including the following: Trilogy (Varian Medical Systems, Palo Alto, CA), Synergy (Electa, Stockholm, Sweden), Novalis (Varian Medical Systems, Palo Alto, CA, and Brainlab, Westchester, IL), and CyberKnife (Accuray, Sunnyvale, CA). Each has advantages and disadvantages that need to be carefully weighed before choosing a system. Treatment planning and delivery are coordinated in a multidisciplinary fashion among spine surgeons, radiation oncologists, and radiation physicists, and all of these specialists need to be comfortable with each step of the process.

Target Identification

Regardless of the system, one of the most important steps in treatment planning is target identification. Unlike cEBRT, in which the tumor and normal surrounding structures essentially receive the same radiation dose, SRS targets the tumor while sparing normal tissue. The International Commission on Radiation Units and Measurements (ICRU) defines target volumes that play a significant role in SRS planning.[8]

The gross tumor volume (GTV) is contoured to the radiologically identified tumor based on CT or MRI scans. The clinical target volume (CTV) includes the GTV and the adjacent anatomic areas with a high likelihood of tumor involvement or microscopic disease. For instance, the CTV for a small GTV in the vertebral body is often contoured to include the entire vertebral body because of the high risk of marginal recurrence. The CTV is then expanded to define the planning target volume (PTV), which is typically a 3 mm expansion of the CTV, taking care to avoid transgression of the spinal cord contour. The PTV accounts for uncertainties of setup and delivery inherent in the system. Organs at risk are then contoured, including the spinal cord, esophagus, great vessels, bowel, and kidney. Treatment planning is currently based on CT images, although targets may be better visualized on MRI scans. For this reason, many systems have the capacity to fuse MRI and CT images for target delineation. At Memorial Sloan-Kettering Cancer Center, myelography/CT is routinely used to identify the spinal cord for planning purposes, particularly in the postoperative setting in which metallic implants have been placed.

TREATMENT PLANNING

Once treatment volumes have been identified, treatment doses and beam delivery are determined based on inverse treatment planning. This planning takes into account the therapeutic dose to the tumor, as well as the constraints of normal tissue tolerance. The prescribed tumoral dose is predicated on the tumor histology, spinal cord volume, and previous radiation exposure to normal tissue, especially the spinal cord. No large experience with spinal radiosurgery has resulted in guidelines for the optimal doses and dose constraints. Common dosage regimens range from 14 to 24 Gy in a single fraction or hypofractionated regimens, such as 5 Gy in 6 fractions or 9 Gy in 3 fractions.[9-14]

IMAGE-GUIDED TECHNIQUES

All treatment systems have effectively developed different methods of target localization, immobilization, and beam delivery. Patient setup and isocenter verification are essential for precision beam delivery that is well in excess of normal tissue tolerance. Patient immobilization, which is essentially target immobilization, is managed with a variety of stereotactic body frames and immobilization cradles. Once the patient is positioned on the table, most systems employ cone beam CT to ensure a three-dimensional matched registration to the digitally reconstructed radiographs used for simulation treatment planning. Positioning errors are noted in all three planes and corrections are made. The CyberKnife has solved the problem by using a different paradigm. This system takes repeat two-dimensional localization images throughout the procedure, and the linear accelerator mounted on a robotic arm makes automated corrections.

Photon beams are created by a linear accelerator. The proper beam angles and directions are selected to provide the best tumoral coverage while avoiding normal tissues. The high-dose delivery to the target with sparing of normal tissue is created by the intersection of noncoplanar beams at the isocenter. The dose and shape of the beams are modified by mini-multileaf collimators that optimize treatment delivery. This beam delivery is defined as intensity-modulated radiation therapy (IMRT). The use of three-dimensional near real-time image verification with cone beam CT and IMRT beam delivery is called image-guided intensity-modulated radiation therapy (IGRT). IGRT can be used to deliver SRS as a single fraction (for example, 14 to 24 Gy), hypofractionated (24 Gy in 3 fractions), or conventional fraction radiation (30 Gy in 10 fractions). Most commonly at Memorial Sloan-Kettering Cancer Center, single-fraction radiation is used to treat metastatic tumors as initial therapy. Hypofractionated radiation is used primarily to reirradiate tumors that were previously treated unsuccessfully with cEBRT, although it can also be used as initial treatment, especially for tumors causing spinal cord compression. High-dose conventional fraction radiation is rarely used to treat metastatic tumors; it is instead used to treat primary spine tumors. The dose schedule is determined from the sarcoma or chordoma experience using proton beam therapy.[6] However, high-dose single-fraction radiation may also be effective in treating primary bone tumors.[5]

RADIATION AS INITIAL TREATMENT
CONVENTIONAL EXTERNAL-BEAM RADIATION THERAPY

The variable radioresponsiveness of spinal metastases was initially reported in a series by Greenberg et al[15] that compared outcomes after a combination of surgery and cEBRT with results of cEBRT alone. The surgical approach was principally laminectomy without instrumentation, which makes the operative technique somewhat antiquated. The evolution of anterior transcavitary or posterolateral approaches with instrumentation has resulted in markedly improved surgical outcomes. Although the surgical data may no longer be relevant, Greenberg et al[15] demonstrated marked differences in radiation response rates based on tumor histology. Patients with breast carcinoma and hematologic malignancies showed improved outcomes compared to patients with relatively radioresistant tumors, such as renal and lung carcinoma.

Maranzano and Latini[16] also demonstrated the histology-dependent responses based on radiosensitivity. This prospective study evaluated two different fractionation schedules: 30 Gy in 10 fractions compared with three 5 Gy doses plus five 3 Gy doses delivered in a split course. Of 275 patients, 20 were excluded for gross spinal instability. No differences were demonstrated in fractionation schedules. Of the 209 evaluable patients, 98% maintained ambulation, whereas only 60% recovered the ability to ambulate. Of those who regained ambulation, 70% had tumors that were considered to have responded favorably or were radiosensitive to cEBRT; these tumors included hematologic malignancies (such as lymphoma or multiple myeloma), seminoma, and carcinoma of the breast and prostate. Tumors that responded unfavorably or were relatively radioresistant included hepatocellular, bladder, renal cell, non–small cell lung, and colon carcinoma. For example, breast carcinoma demonstrated an 80% response rate compared to hepatocellular carcinoma with a 20% response rate. Furthermore, the durability of the response was 10 to 16 months for relatively radiosensitive tumors, compared with 1 to 3 months for relatively radioresistant tumors. A number of other studies have demonstrated this variable response based on tumor histology.[17-20]

Patchell et al[21] presented a prospective randomized trial comparing surgery and cEBRT to cEBRT alone for high-grade spinal cord compression that demonstrated the overall lack of radiosensitivity for solid tumor malignancies. Hematologic malignancies were excluded because of their exquisite radiosensitivity, although other relatively radiosensitive solid tumors malignancies, such as breast carcinoma, were included. Surgery showed significant advantages in terms of overall maintenance and recovery of ambulation, continence, narcotic requirements, and even survival. While helping to establish surgery as the optimal treatment for patients with solid tumors harboring high-grade epidural spinal cord compression, the poor responses to cEBRT were compelling. Patients undergoing cEBRT alone had a 57% rate of overall ambulation, but the durability was only 13 days. Three of 16 nonambulatory patients (19%) recovered ambulation.[21] However, the study design was an intention-to-treat analysis. All three patients who recovered ambulation crossed over to the surgical arm. The study design did include patients with instability, which potentially confounds the outcome.[27]

The application of SRS to spine tumors has improved the ability to deliver a cytotoxic dose to the tumor and spare normal tissue. Essentially, tumors that are relatively radioresistant to cEBRT are rendered relatively radiosensitive with the use of SRS. This response appears to be histology independent. Renal cell carcinoma has traditionally been considered markedly radiation resistant to cEBRT. The potential of improving radiation sensitivity with coadministration of antiangiogenic agents is being explored. Gerszten et al[22] reported 60 cases of renal cell carcinoma treated with single-fraction SRS. Most of them (48 of 60) had progressed through prior cEBRT. Doses ranged from 14 to 21 Gy with the mean maximum tumoral dose of 20 Gy. The median follow-up was 37 months. Axial pain improved in 34 of 38 patients (89%) who presented with pain, and tumor control was achieved in seven of eight patients who presented with tumor progression. Only 6 of 60 patients (10%) required surgery for progressive neurologic symptoms. Despite the high number of reirradiated patients in this study who were undergoing single-fraction radiation for salvage, no radiation myelopathy or other toxicity was seen in the follow-up period.

Gerszten et al[23] also reported on 500 tumors, all with differing histologic findings (breast, lung, melanoma), that were treated with SRS at all levels of the spine. The maximum intratumoral dose ranged from 12.5 to 25 Gy (mean 20 Gy). Pain control and radiographic tumor control were achieved in 86% and 90% of cases, respectively. Radiographic tumor control differed based on primary pathology reports, with breast and lung carcinoma showing 100% radiographic tumor control compared with renal cell carcinoma (87%) and melanoma (75%).

Yamada et al[24] reported 101 cases treated with single-fraction SRS predominantly to relatively radioresistant histologic findings, with the exception of six patients with breast cancer. None of the patients had prior radiation therapy or surgery of the treated area. The treatment paradigm was a dose escalation from 18 to 24 Gy, with the maximum spinal cord dose maintained at less than 14 Gy to a single voxel on the spinal cord. At a median follow-up of 16 months, the overall radiographic control rate was 90%. Seven failures occurred at a median time of 9 months. A statistically significant dose-response difference was demonstrated at 24 Gy compared with less than 24 Gy—95% versus 80%, respectively. Yamada et al[24] reanalyzed the data in 248 patients receiving single-fraction radiation, and this dose-response difference was maintained at the 5-year follow-up. Only grade 1 and 2 skin and esophageal toxicity were noted in this study. None of the patients demonstrated myelopathy or functional radiculopathy.

Chang et al[25] reported on 63 patients with 74 spine tumors who were treated with hypofractionated SRS (27 Gy in 3 fractions). The median follow-up was 21 months. The actuarial tumor-free progression was 84%. The principal risk of failure was both adjacent-segment progression and tumor in the epidural space. No myelopathy or functional radiculopathy was observed. These investigators concluded that the liberalization of spinal cord doses may prevent epidural tumor progression.

POSTOPERATIVE ADJUVANT THERAPY

Most patients with spinal instability benefit from open surgery or a percutaneous procedure that uses vertebral body cement augmentation or pedicle screws, alone or in combination. However, the ongoing debate in the SRS community concerns the treatment of high-grade epidural spinal cord compression. Currently most patients with high-grade spinal cord compression resulting from relatively radioresistant metastatic solid tumors or gross spinal instability benefit from surgery.[21,26,27] Spinal instability is usually treated with an open operation or a percutaneous procedure that uses vertebral body cement augmentation or pedicle screws, alone or in combination. Tumors that are sensitive to cEBRT can often be treated effectively with low-dose SRS in the setting of spinal cord compression.[28,29] Tumors that are relatively radioresistant to cEBRT probably require SRS doses that are well above levels tolerated by the spinal cord to achieve local tumor control.[30] However, reducing the tumoral dose at the margin of the thecal sac so that it remains within the limits of spinal cord tolerance probably increases the likelihood of delivering a subtherapeutic dose to the tumor, which may increase the likelihood of local recurrence, resulting in progressive compression and the development of myelopathy. In addition, even with an effective dose of radiation, the soft tissue tumor may take weeks or months to resolve, resulting in ongoing compression.

Surgery is very effective for spinal cord decompression, neurologic salvage, and stabilizing the spine, but it is not effective in providing durable tumor control. Radiation therapy is essential for achieving postoperative local tumor control.

The poor local control rates achieved with cEBRT prompted exploration of SRS as a postoperative adjuvant treatment.

Moulding et al[31] reviewed the histologic findings of 21 patients who underwent posterolateral decompression and instrumentation for radioresistant tumors. Notably, the

GTV was delineated on the basis of the preoperative tumor volume rather than the postoperative residual tumor. The spinal cord and thecal sac contour were established by means of CT myelography, which provides excellent anatomic detail in the presence of spinal implants. The GTV received 24 Gy in 16 patients and 18 to 21 Gy in five patients. Overall, the local control rate was 81%, with an estimated 1-year failure rate of 9.5%. Local control was significantly better in the cohort receiving 24 Gy compared with the group receiving less than 24 Gy, 94% versus 60%, respectively. The ability to achieve local tumor control probably reduces the need for aggressive resection, particularly in large paraspinal masses. Local tumor control appears equivalent to that seen with the use of SRS in the up-front setting.

COMPLICATIONS

The most feared complication of SRS is spinal cord or functional nerve root injury, but normal tissue tolerance should be considered for the skin, great vessels, esophagus, bowel, and kidneys. Spinal cord constraints are variably reported in the literature as either a percentage of the spinal cord or a maximum dose to a single voxel on the spinal cord (cord D_{max}). Ryu et al[32] defined spinal cord tolerance as a maximum of 10 Gy to 10% of the spinal cord.

Yamada et al[24] reported safely treating to a cord D_{max} of 14 Gy. Gibbs et al[33] reported spinal cord data for 1075 patients undergoing CyberKnife radiosurgery for benign and malignant spine tumors who developed delayed myelopathy. Six patients were identified at a median of 6.4 months (range 2 to 9 months) who had delayed myelopathy resulting from SRS. Three tumors were metastatic in the middle to upper thoracic spine, and the remaining three were benign cervical lesions. Three tumors had previously been irradiated. No specific dosimetric factors were identified, but three patients received spinal cord equivalent doses greater than 8 Gy.

In our own experience, brachial plexus and nerve roots are contoured but receive full-dose irradiation. No toxicity has been noted, and often functional nerve root recovery can be seen. No significant toxicity has been reported in other organs other than grade 1 or 2 skin and esophageal toxicity.[14]

Most studies have focused on neurologic toxicity, but Rose et al[34] reviewed the records of 62 patients undergoing single-fraction SRS for solid tumor malignancies at 71 sites. They determined a 39% risk of delayed fracture of the vertebral body in this population. Multivariate regression analysis showed significant risk factors were lytic tumors, which had a 6.8 times risk compared with sclerotic or mixed lytic-sclerotic tumors, and thoracolumbar or lumbar tumor locations had a risk that was 4.6 times that of other levels of the spine. In addition, patients with more than 40% lytic destruction of the vertebral body had an 85% probability risk of progressive fracture. This has led investigators to explore the role of prophylactic percutaneous cement augmentation in at-risk patients.

SIGNATURE CASES
STEREOTACTIC RADIOSURGERY ALONE

A 69-year-old woman had pain in the low back and right hip. MRI of the spine showed a tumor at L2-3 suggestive of metastatic disease. Additional studies included a CT scan of the chest, which showed a right middle lobe mass measuring 7.4 cm. The patient had no mechanical radiculopathy or neurologic deficits in her legs and was ambulating well. Total spine MRI showed no other spine disease. The patient underwent a needle biopsy, which confirmed the suspected histologic diagnosis of adenocarcinoma of the lung. She then underwent image-guided radiation therapy, 24 Gy in a single fraction. One month after SRS, the patient's back pain had improved significantly. She had no side effects from the radiation, and 6 months after SRS she remained ambulatory (Fig. 6-1).

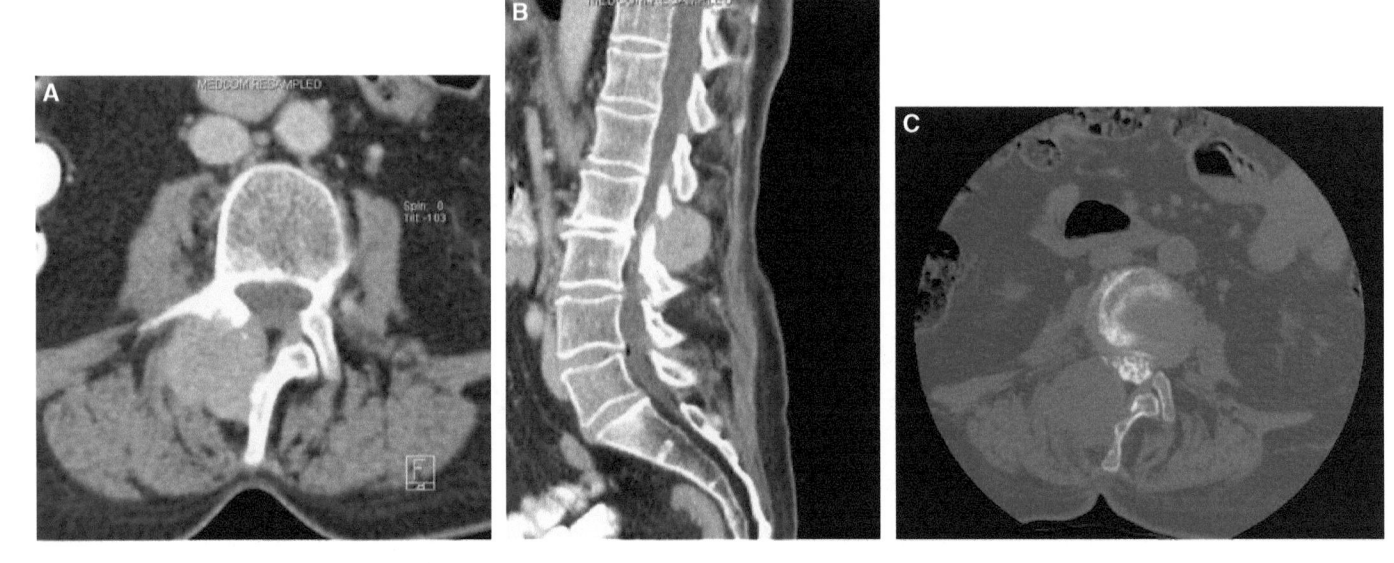

Fig. 6-1 **A,** Axial and **B,** sagittal CT reconstruction demonstrating tumor centered within and destroying the right lamina of L2. **C,** CT myelogram shows no compression of the thecal sac.

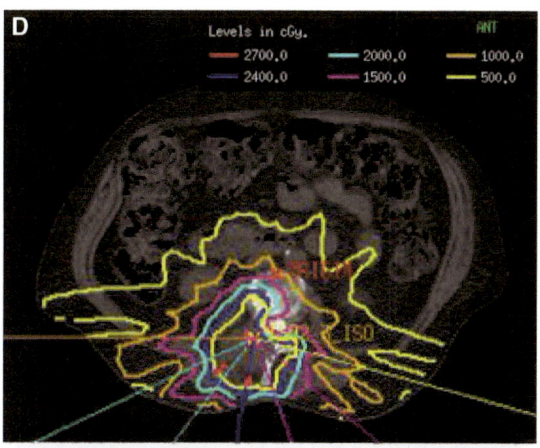

Fig. 6-1, cont'd **D,** Axial, **E,** coronal, and **F,** sagittal CT reconstructions show **G,** SRS planning and treatment volumes, which are also numerically depicted. Note the PTV (*dark blue* on the CT images) showing the 24 Gy isodose line.

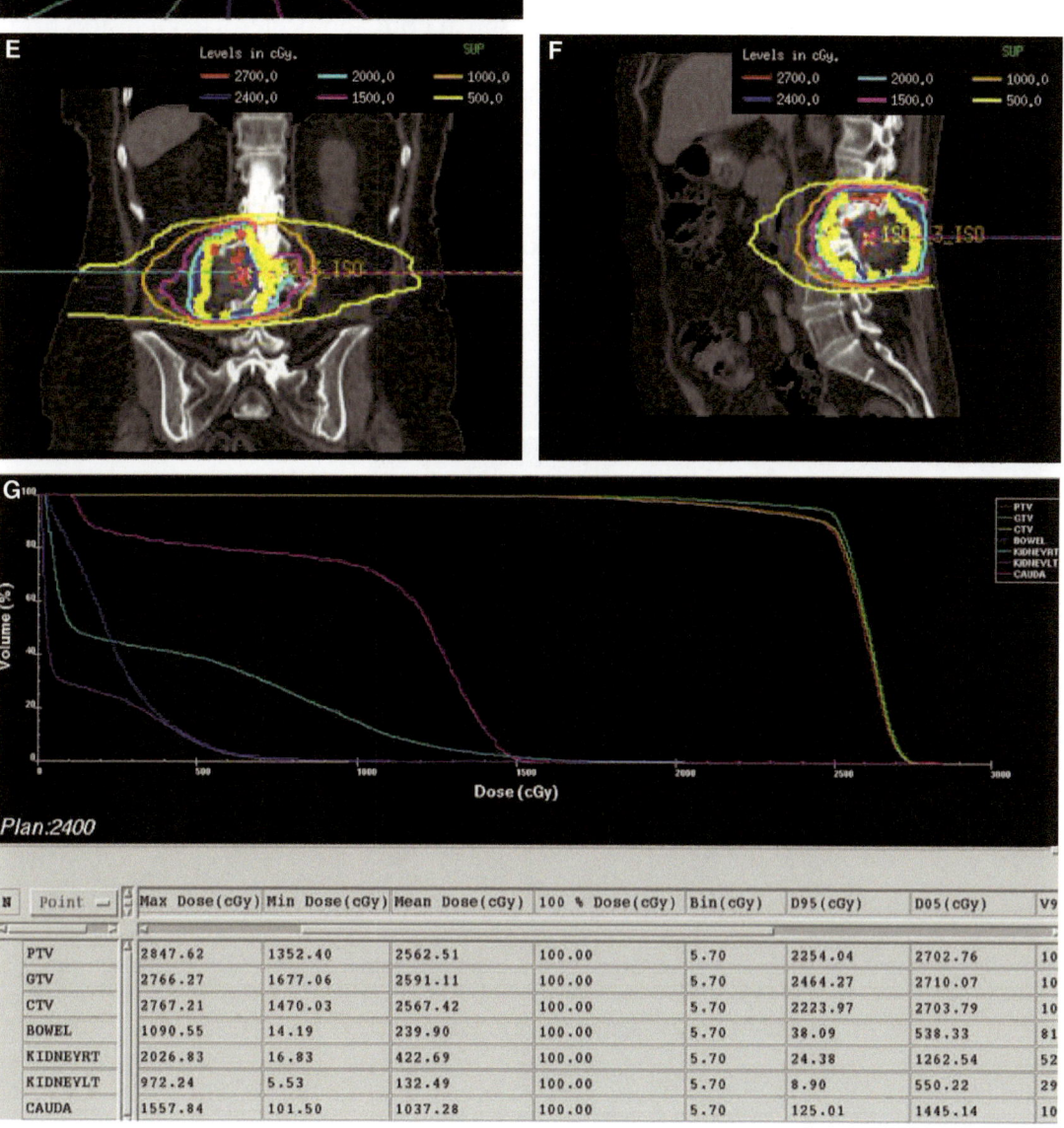

Point	Max Dose(cGy)	Min Dose(cGy)	Mean Dose(cGy)	100 % Dose(cGy)	Bin(cGy)	D95(cGy)	D05(cGy)
PTV	2847.62	1352.40	2562.51	100.00	5.70	2254.04	2702.76
GTV	2766.27	1677.06	2591.11	100.00	5.70	2464.27	2710.07
CTV	2767.21	1470.03	2567.42	100.00	5.70	2223.97	2703.79
BOWEL	1090.55	14.19	239.90	100.00	5.70	38.09	538.33
KIDNEYRT	2026.83	16.83	422.69	100.00	5.70	24.38	1262.54
KIDNEYLT	972.24	5.53	132.49	100.00	5.70	8.90	550.22
CAUDA	1557.84	101.50	1037.28	100.00	5.70	125.01	1445.14

Surgery and Postoperative Adjuvant Stereotactic Radiosurgery

A 64-year-old man was referred to the spine clinic because of a 2-week history of upper back pain located between the scapulae, bilateral lower extremity paresthesia, and progressive difficulty ambulating. The patient had full strength in all four extremities but had decreased pinprick sensation and light touch sensation below the nipple level. He had hyperreflexia of the right lower leg (knee and ankle) with a positive Babinski sign. Left lower extremity reflexes were normal. The patient had a history of chondrosarcoma of the right foot that had been resected 10 years previously; he had had no evidence of disease for 10 years until the current symptoms appeared. MRI of the spine revealed a lesion at T3 causing severe spinal cord compression. The patient underwent surgery for decompression of the spinal cord and posterolateral fusion from T1 to T5. Histologic findings showed the tumor to be a chondrosarcoma. CT myelography after surgery demonstrated decompression of the thecal sac with reconstitution of the cerebrospinal fluid space around the spinal cord. The patient underwent SRS (24 Gy in 1 fraction) 4 weeks after surgery. One month after SRS, the patient's pain had improved dramatically. He regained his ability to ambulate, although he had to use a cane because of persistent sensory deficits in his right leg (Fig. 6-2).

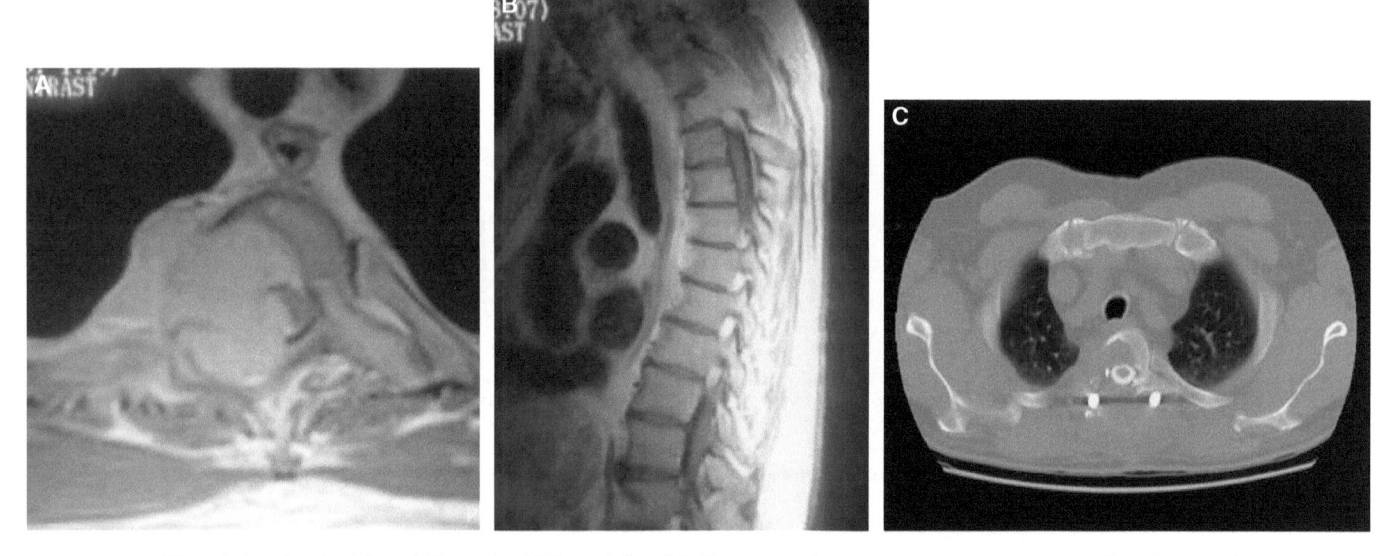

Fig. 6-2 **A,** Axial and **B,** sagittal T1-weighted MRI scans demonstrate tumor centered within and destroying the right pedicle of T3, causing severe spinal cord compression and deformation. **C,** CT myelography performed after surgery shows decompression of the thecal sac and complete reconstitution of the cerebrospinal fluid space around the spinal cord.

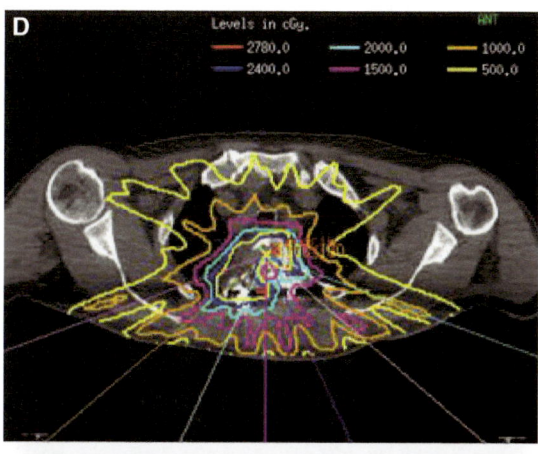

Fig. 6-2, cont'd **D,** Axial, **E,** coronal, and **F,** sagittal CT reconstructions show **G,** SRS planning and treatment volumes, which are also numerically depicted. Note the PTV (*dark blue* on the CT images) showing the 24 Gy isodose line.

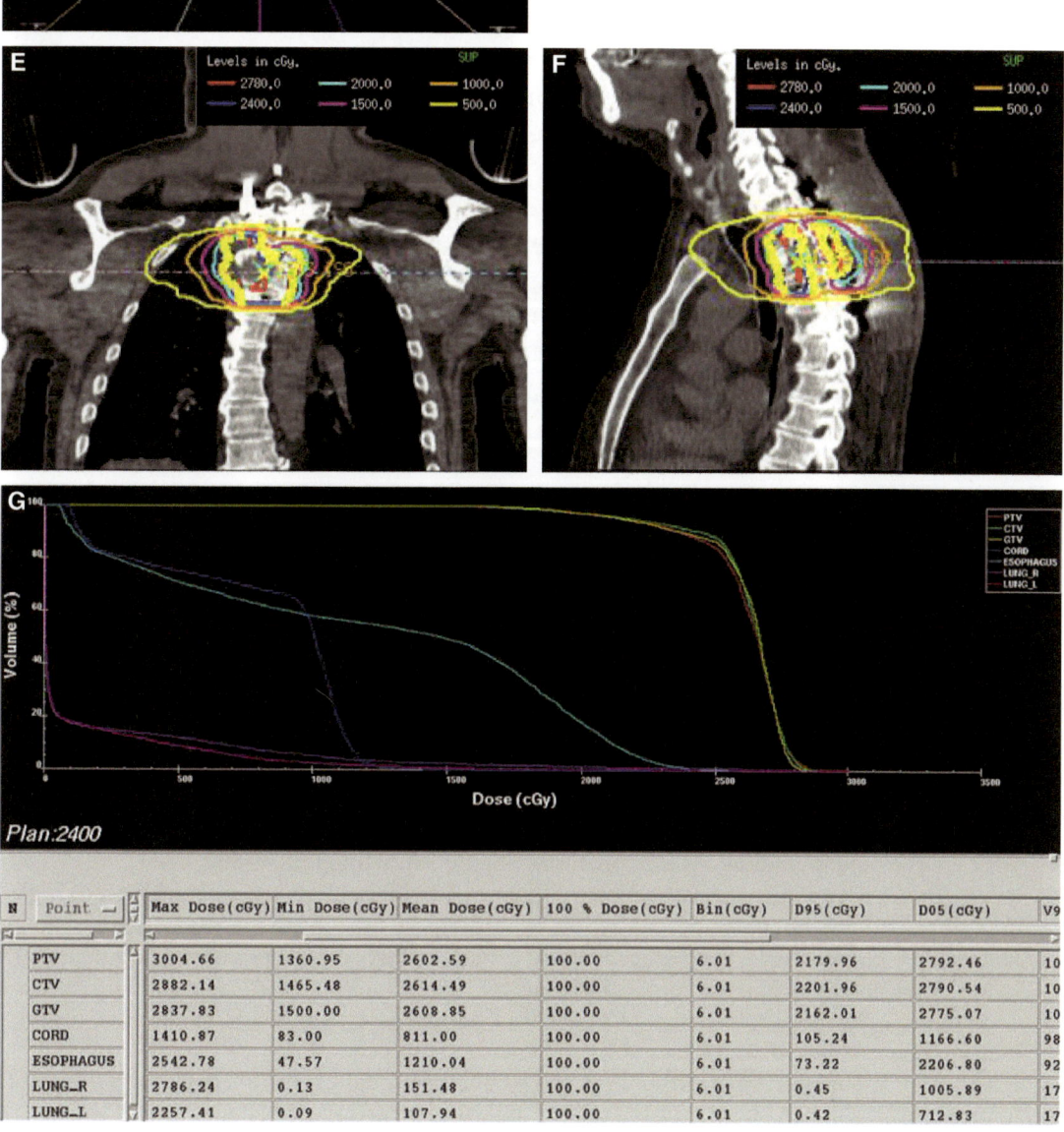

N	Point	Max Dose(cGy)	Min Dose(cGy)	Mean Dose(cGy)	100 % Dose(cGy)	Bin(cGy)	D95(cGy)	D05(cGy)	V9
	PTV	3004.66	1360.95	2602.59	100.00	6.01	2179.96	2792.46	10
	CTV	2882.14	1465.48	2614.49	100.00	6.01	2201.96	2790.54	10
	GTV	2837.83	1500.00	2608.85	100.00	6.01	2162.01	2775.07	10
	CORD	1410.87	83.00	811.00	100.00	6.01	105.24	1166.60	98
	ESOPHAGUS	2542.78	47.57	1210.04	100.00	6.01	73.22	2206.80	92
	LUNG_R	2786.24	0.13	151.48	100.00	6.01	0.45	1005.89	17
	LUNG_L	2257.41	0.09	107.94	100.00	6.01	0.42	712.83	17

CONCLUSION

The utility and power of SRS are still being explored for the treatment of metastatic spine disease, both as initial treatment and as postoperative adjuvant therapy. Preliminary evidence suggests that local control rates with SRS are better than those achieved with cEBRT. Toxicity profiles of normal tissue tolerance are being established. Tumoral responses seem to be independent of histologic findings. Clinical trials are now underway to establish safety profiles and outcomes for the use of SRS in the treatment of metastatic spine tumors.

TIPS FROM THE MASTERS

- SRS delivered as a high-dose single fraction (for example, 24 Gy) or hypofractionated radiation (8 to 10 Gy times 3) provides excellent durable tumor control for metastatic tumors considered to be relatively resistant to conventional external beam radiation, such as renal cell carcinoma and melanoma.
- Tumor control rates greater than 90% are seen when SRS is delivered either as the definitive therapy or as postoperative adjuvant radiation therapy.
- Radiation-dose constraints on normal tissues such as the spinal cord, kidney, and bowel are essential for the safe delivery of tumoricidal doses of radiation.
- Delayed vertebral body fractures may be a sequelae of SRS.

References (With Key References in Boldface)

1. Black P. Spinal metastasis: current status and recommended guidelines for management. Neurosurgery 5:726-746, 1979.
2. Gokaslan ZL, York JE, Walsh GL, et al. Transthoracic vertebrectomy for metastatic spinal tumors. J Neurosurg 89:599-609, 1998.
3. Yamada Y, Lovelock DM, Bilsky MH. A review of image-guided intensity-modulated radiotherapy for spinal tumors. Neurosurgery 61:226-235; discussion 235, 2007.
4. Emami B, Lyman J, Brown A, et al. Tolerance of normal tissue to therapeutic irradiation. Int J Radiat Oncol Biol Phys 21:109-122, 1991.
4a. Gerszten PC, Mendel E, Yamada Y. Radiotherapy and radiosurgery for metastatic spine disease: what are the options, indications, and outcomes? Spine 34(22 Suppl):S78-S92, 2009.
5. Wu AJ, Bilsky MH, Edgar MA, et al. Near-complete pathological response of chordoma to high-dose single-fraction radiotherapy: case report. Neurosurgery 64:E389-E390, 2009.
6. DeLaney TF, Liebsch NJ, Pedlow FX, et al. Phase II study of high-dose photon/proton radiotherapy in the management of spine sarcomas. Int J Radiat Oncol Biol Phys 74:732-739, 2009.
7. Gerszten PC, Burton SA, Ozhasoglu C, et al. Radiosurgery for benign intradural spinal tumors. Neurosurgery 62:887-896, 2008.
8. ICRU Report 50: Prescribing, Recording, and Reporting Photon Beam Therapy. Bethesda, MD: International Commission on Radiation Units and Measurements, 1993, pp 1-72.
9. Bilsky MH, Yamada Y, Yenice KM, et al. Intensity-modulated stereotactic radiotherapy of paraspinal tumors: a preliminary report. Neurosurgery 54:823-830; discussion 830-831, 2004.
10. Chang EL, Shiu AS, Lii M-F, et al. Phase I clinical evaluation of near-simultaneous computed tomographic image-guided stereotactic body radiotherapy for spinal metastases. Int J Radiat Oncol Biol Phys 59:1288-1294, 2004.

11. Klish MD, Watson GA, Shrieve DC. Radiation and intensity-modulated radiotherapy for metastatic spine tumors. Neurosurg Clin North Am 15:481-490, 2004.
12. Rock JP, Ryu S, Yin F-F. Novalis radiosurgery for metastatic spine tumors. Neurosurg Clin North Am 15:503-509, 2004.
13. Ryu S, Yin FF, Rock J, et al. Image-guided and intensity-modulated radiosurgery for patients with spinal metastasis. Cancer 97:2013-2018, 2003.
14. Yamada Y, Lovelock DM, Yenice KM, et al. Multifractionated image-guided and stereotactic intensity-modulated radiotherapy of paraspinal tumors: a preliminary report. Int J Radiat Oncol Biol Phys 62:53-61, 2005.
15. Greenberg HS, Kim JH, Posner JB. Epidural spinal cord compression from metastatic tumor: results with a new treatment protocol. Ann Neurol 8:361-366, 1980.
16. Maranzano E, Latini P. Effectiveness of radiation therapy without surgery in metastatic spinal cord compression: final results from a prospective trial. Int J Radiat Oncol Biol Phys 32:959-967, 1995.
17. Maranzano E, Bellavita R, Rossi R, et al. Short-course versus split-course radiotherapy in metastatic spinal cord compression: results of a phase III, randomized, multicenter trial. J Clin Oncol 23:3358-3365, 2005.
18. Katagiri H, Takahashi M, Inagaki J, et al. Clinical results of nonsurgical treatment for spinal metastases. Int Radiat Oncol Biol Phys 42:1127-1132, 1998.
19. Rades D, Karstens JH, Hoskin PJ, et al. Escalation of radiation dose beyond 30 Gy in 10 fractions for metastatic spinal cord compression. Int J Radiat Oncol Biol Phys 67:525-531, 2007.
20. Rades D, Fehlauer F, Schulte R, et al. Prognostic factors for local control and survival after radiotherapy of metastatic spinal cord compression. J Clin Oncol 24:3388-3393, 2006.
21. Patchell RA, Tibbs PA, Regine WF, et al. Direct decompressive surgical resection in the treatment of spinal cord compression caused by metastatic cancer: a randomised trial. Lancet 366:643-648, 2005.
22. Gerszten PC, Burton SA, Ozhasoglu C, et al. Stereotactic radiosurgery for spinal metastases from renal cell carcinoma. J Neurosurg Spine 3:288-295, 2005.
23. Gerszten PC, Burton SA, Ozhasoglu C, et al. Radiosurgery for spinal metastases: clinical experience in 500 cases from a single institution. Spine 32:193-199, 2007.
24. Yamada Y, Bilsky MH, Lovelock DM, et al. High-dose, single-fraction image-guided intensity-modulated radiotherapy for metastatic spinal lesions. Int J Radiat Oncol Biol Phys 71:484-490, 2008.
25. Chang EL, Shiu AS, Mendel E, et al. Phase I/II study of stereotactic body radiotherapy for spinal metastasis and its pattern of failure. J Neurosurg Spine 7:151-160, 2007.
26. **Bilsky MH, Laufer I, Burch S. Shifting paradigms in the treatment of metastatic spine disease. Spine 34:S101-S107, 2009.**
27. **Bilsky M, Smith M. Surgical approach to epidural spinal cord compression. Hematol Oncol Clin North Am 20:1307-1317, 2006.**
28. Gagnon GJ, Henderson FC, Gehan EA, et al. Cyberknife radiosurgery for breast cancer spine metastases: a matched-pair analysis. Cancer 110:1796-1802, 2007.
29. Klekamp J, Samii H. Surgical results for spinal metastases. Acta Neurochir (Wien) 140:957-967, 1998.
30. Rock JP, Ryu S, Shukairy MS, et al. Postoperative radiosurgery for malignant spinal tumors. Neurosurgery 58:891-898, discussion 891-898, 2006.
31. **Moulding HD, Elder JB, Lis E, et al. Local disease control after decompressive surgery and adjuvant high-dose single-fraction radiosurgery for spine metastases. J Neurosurg Spine 13:87-93, 2010.**
32. Ryu S, Jin JY, Jin R, et al. Partial volume tolerance of the spinal cord and complications of single-dose radiosurgery. Cancer 109:628-636, 2007.
33. **Gibbs IC, Patil C, Gerszten PC, et al. Delayed radiation-induced myelopathy after spinal radiosurgery. Neurosurgery 64:A67-A72, 2009.**
34. Rose PS, Laufer I, Boland PJ, et al. Risk of fracture after single fraction image-guided intensity-modulated radiation therapy to spinal metastases. J Clin Oncol 27:5075-5079, 2009.

Chapter 7

Plastic Surgery for Primary Reconstruction

David S. Chang, William Y. Hoffman

Wounds of the spine are among the most challenging to treat. The relative lack of adjacent tissue and the frequent presence of instrumentation make primary closure difficult and skin grafting not an option. Flaps are the primary mode of reconstruction. Muscle, skin and muscle (musculocutaneous), and skin and fascia (fasciocutaneous) flaps all provide well-vascularized tissue for soft tissue coverage. The availability of these flaps depends on the location of the wound, when available. Muscle flaps have the advantage of filling dead space. Drains are used liberally in both the subfascial space beneath flaps and within the subcutaneous space created by elevation of flaps.

The back can be divided into three anatomic regions: upper, middle, and lower (see Fig. 7-1). Most wounds related to spinal column reconstruction are in the midline. The upper third extends between the base of the neck and the midscapula, the middle third from the midscapula to the waistline, and the lower third from the waist to the sacrococcygeal region. The location of the wound relative to its anatomic region will determine the reconstructive options available. For the spine surgeon, consultation with a plastic surgeon who is well versed in flaps is recommended.

INDICATIONS AND CONTRAINDICATIONS

There are no absolute contraindications to reconstructive surgery. Patients who are candidates for tumor extirpation or spinal instrumentation, by default, are also candidates for reconstructive surgery. However, in cases of infected instrumentation, flap closure is not a substitute for appropriate management, which may require prolonged treatment with antibiotics or even removal of instrumentation.

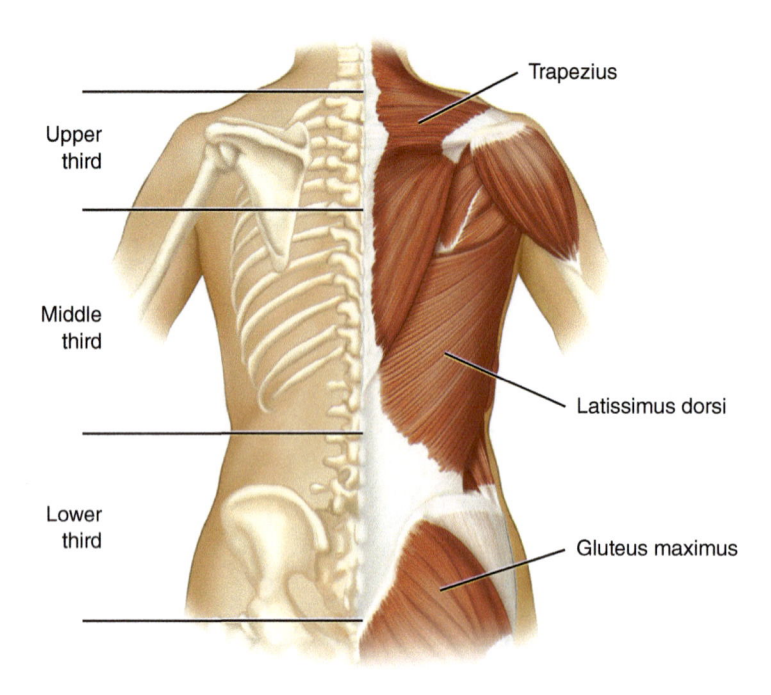

Fig. 7-1 The back with upper, middle, and lower thirds outlined.

PREOPERATIVE EVALUATION

Preoperative evaluation consists of obtaining a complete history, paying particular attention to comorbid conditions, nutritional status, and underlying pathology. Previous operations and scars should be noted on examination, because they can alter the operative plan. Assessing the surrounding skin and underlying musculature is also critical. A history of radiation therapy may render local tissues unusable as an option for reconstruction. The presence of infection may necessitate a staged approach to closure after debridement of devitalized tissue and treatment with antibiotics.

Physical examination, computed tomography, and magnetic resonance imaging will help localize the tumor. Determining the extent of the resection is critical to decide which anatomic region will need to be reconstructed and, ultimately, what choices are available for the reconstruction.

CLINICAL DECISION-MAKING

The first step in clinical decision-making is to determine whether wound coverage can be achieved in one stage. Primary wounds of the spine should be covered at the time of the primary spine procedure, whether it is tumor extirpation or spinal instrumentation. In secondary cases that may involve infection or tissue necrosis, final wound coverage should be staged after debridement of devitalized tissue and grossly contaminated tissue. Under these circumstances, temporary wound coverage and staged debridement may be necessary to convert a contaminated wound into a clean wound. Salvage of instrumentation with muscle flaps may be possible in these cases.

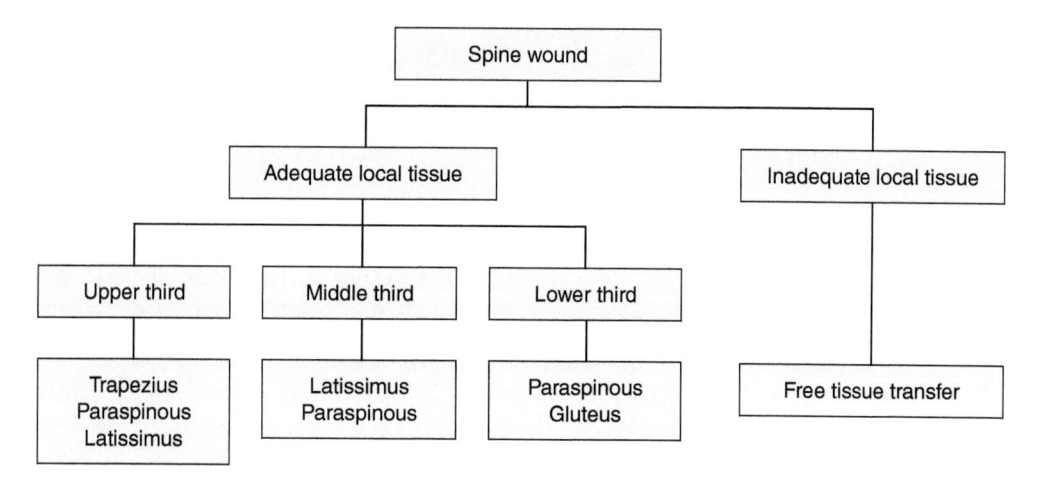

Fig. 7-2 Decision-making algorithm for reconstructing spine wounds.

Flap selection will depend on the size and location of the defect (Fig. 7-2). Muscle flaps can help to obliterate dead space, in addition to providing well-vascularized tissue to cover a wound. When skin is also deficient, a musculocutaneous flap with a skin island may be necessary. Upper-third defects are best reconstructed with trapezius (cephalic half) or latissimus dorsi (caudal half) muscle flaps.[1-5] Other options include fasciocutaneous flaps based on perforating vessels or a random flap with a length-to-width ratio of less than 2:1. Middle-third defects are effectively covered with latissimus dorsi flaps.[1,6] The transverse back flap is a large fasciocutaneous flap that can also be used in middle-third skin defects.[7] Lower-third defects can be covered with paraspinous and gluteus maximus muscle flaps.[8-14] Occasionally, omentum or rectus abdominis flaps can be brought through the peritoneal cavity to the spine.[13,15,16] Free tissue transfer is the final option when no local options are available.[13] Because of the relative lack of donor vessels in the back, long vein grafts are frequently necessary.

TECHNIQUES
GENERAL
Most spine wounds encountered by plastic surgeons are located in the lower third. The first choice for closure of these wounds is a paraspinous muscle flap, which is discussed herein. All wounds are closed over closed-suction drains (for example, 19 Fr Blake drains or 10 mm flat Jackson-Pratt drains). All wounds are closed primarily in layers, including deep sutures in Scarpa's fascia, buried deep dermal sutures, and nylon skin sutures. Vertical or horizontal mattress skin sutures are used to provide better eversion of tissue at the skin level. We use absorbable monofilament for all buried sutures.

UPPER THIRD
The upper third can be further divided into cephalic and caudal portions. The cephalic half is best suited to coverage with the trapezius muscle, whereas the lower half is better treated with the latissimus dorsi muscle.

Cephalic Portion

The trapezius muscle originates on the external occipital protuberance, the medial third of the superior nuchal line, the ligamentum nuchae, the spinous process of the seventh cervical vertebra, and all 12 thoracic vertebrae. Its insertion is the lateral third of the clavicle, the spine of the scapula, and the acromion (Fig. 7-3, *A*). A flap based on the dominant pedicle, the transverse cervical artery and vein (Fig. 7-3, *B*), can be raised and rotated to cover the cephalic portion of the upper third (Fig. 7-3, *C* and *D*) and, in fact, this flap will reach onto the occipital skull. For flap elevation, the fibers of the muscle are identified through the existing wound. The skin over the muscle is elevated, taking care to dissect in a plane directly on top of the muscle. The muscle is then separated from the chest wall. The middle and inferior portions of the muscle are elevated up to the superior border of the scapula. The pedicle is seen on the deep

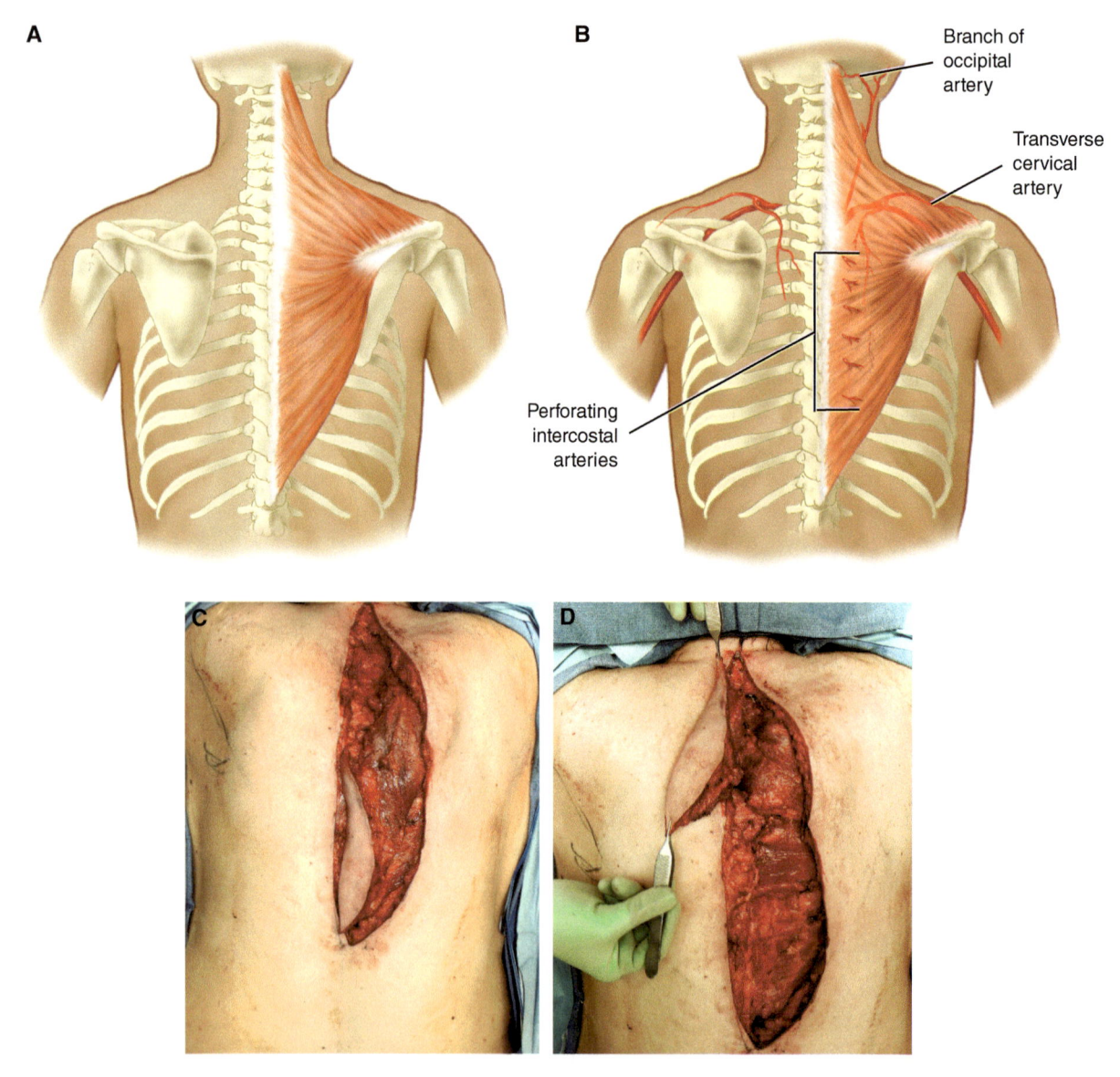

Fig. 7-3 **A,** Trapezius flap in situ. **B,** Blood supply of the trapezius flap. **C,** Trapezius flap elevated with skin paddle. **D,** Trapezius flap rotated to cover upper thoracic spine.

surface of the muscle just cephalad to the rhomboid minor muscle. If a skin island is used, muscle fibers are identified around the margins of the skin island. The skin island is vertically oriented and centered between the posterior midline medially, the vertebral border of the scapula laterally, the midportion of the scapula cephalically, and the posterior superior iliac crest caudally. The superior portion of the muscle is preserved to avoid shoulder droop.

Caudal Portion

The caudal half of the upper third of the spine is effectively covered by the latissimus dorsi (Fig. 7-4, *A*), which can be raised with or without a skin island. Raised on the dominant pedicle, the thoracodorsal artery and vein (Fig. 7-4, *B*), the latissimus will reach up to the midscapular level. The muscle originates on the lower six thoracic vertebrae, the sacral vertebrae, and the posterior iliac crest. The muscle fibers converge to insert on the intertubercular groove of the humerus. Its superior fibers are deep to the trapezius, but most of the muscle lies superficial to the other muscles of the trunk. The entire muscle can be elevated on its vascular pedicle with division of the origin and insertion. Ideally the landmarks are marked with the patient sitting or standing upright. The borders of the muscle are the tip of the scapula superiorly, the midline vertebrae medially, and the posterior iliac crest inferiorly. The lateral border extends from the axilla to the posterior iliac crest. Flap elevation for a latissimus muscle flap begins at the margins of the skin incision. The skin is undermined directly on top of the muscle, which is then separated from the chest wall. If the insertion is divided, a separate counterincision may be necessary in the posterior axilla. A skin island centered obliquely over the proximal two thirds of the muscle will reliably reach the midline (Fig. 7-4, *C*). The donor site is closed primarily.

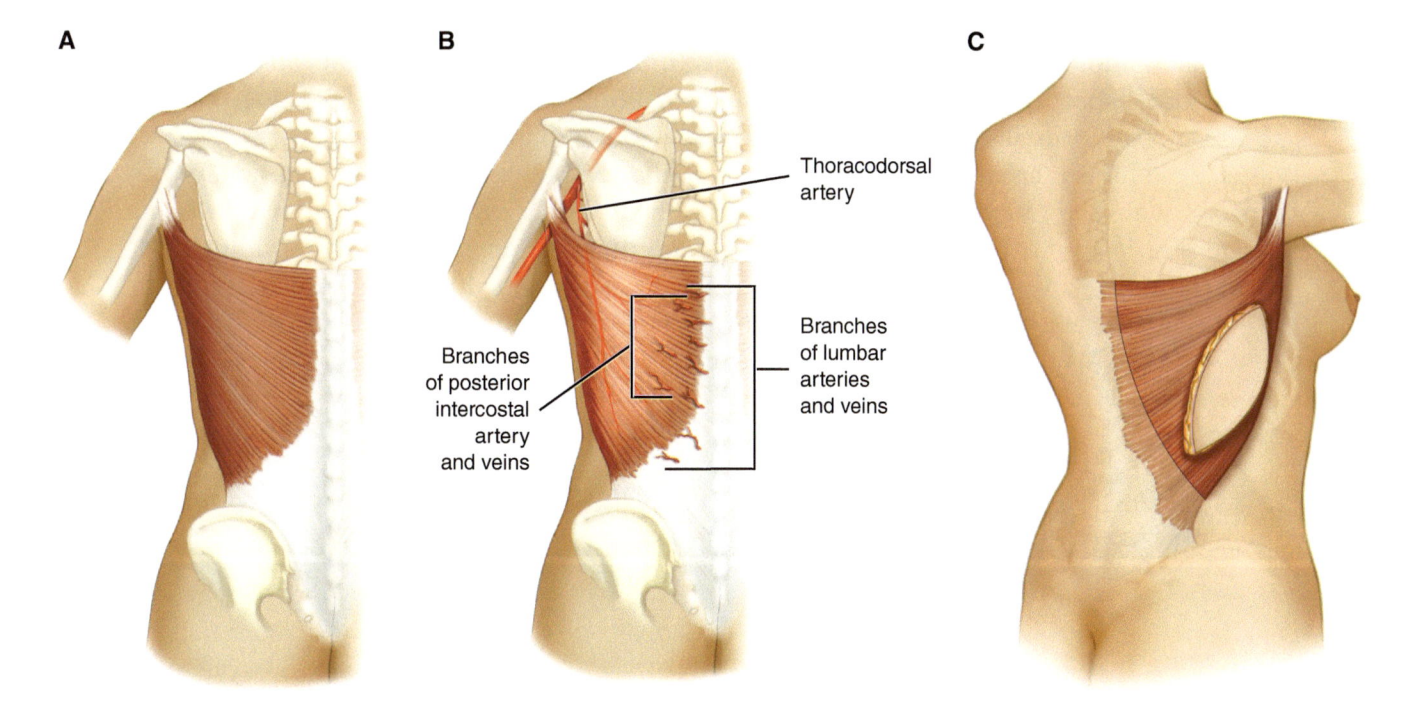

Fig. 7-4 **A,** Latissimus flap in situ. **B,** Blood supply of latissimus flap. **C,** Latissimus with skin island.

The latissimus dorsi is an expendable muscle in patients with intact bilateral shoulder girdle muscles. Because most of the muscle is off of the midline, the latissimus dorsi is especially helpful in radiation wounds, because it can bring healthy nonirradiated tissue to close the defect. In patients with contralateral absence or paralysis of the latissimus dorsi, use of the only functioning latissimus dorsi muscle is not advised. In patients with paraplegia, the latissimus dorsi muscle may be more important functionally for wheelchair use and transfers, and an effort should be made to find another option for reconstruction.

Middle Third

The latissimus dorsi is also suitable for covering defects of the middle third of the back. For smaller defects the muscle can be advanced bilaterally by undermining the muscle from the chest wall and suturing it together in the midline (Fig. 7-5, *A*). In addition to a standard flap raised on the major pedicle, as described for the upper third, the muscle can also be raised as a reverse flap based off of its minor blood supply medially from the lumbar artery and veins.[4] It is important to establish that these vessels are still intact after spine surgery. The flap can be raised segmentally, leaving a portion of the origin and insertion intact to function normally (Fig. 7-5, *B*). The muscle is turned over on itself, similar to a page in a book. Flap elevation without a skin island begins through a separate oblique skin incision. If a skin island is used, the muscle is identified through the skin incision for the skin island. The surrounding skin is elevated to define the muscle, which is then segmentally divided. Undermining of the muscle must remain at least 4 to 6 cm from the midline to avoid injuring the segmental blood supply. The flap is based on one or two of these vessels and is rotated 90 to 180 degrees into the defect.

Lower Third

The paraspinous muscles are a paired group of muscles that run deep to the latissimus dorsi and trapezius muscles along the length of the spine. The muscles include the longissimus, iliocostalis, and spinalis. Blood supply to the muscles comes from the intercostal and lumbar arteries. Skin flaps are elevated directly over muscle fascia. Relaxing incisions are then made in the fascia approximately 5 to 7 cm lateral to the wound edge (Fig. 7-6, *A*). The paraspinous muscles are then advanced toward the midline and sutured in a vest-over-pants fashion with the use of 0 or 1 mattress sutures (Fig. 7-6, *B*). Clinical examples of flaps covering wounds are shown in Fig. 7-7.

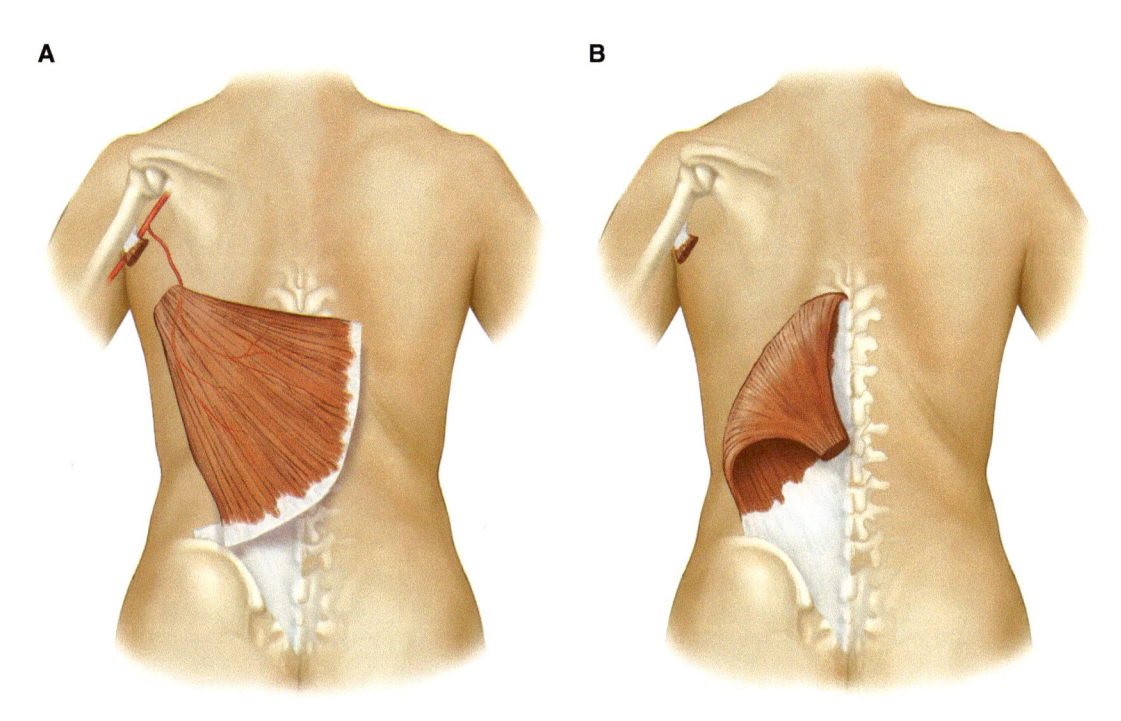

Fig. 7-5 **A,** Latissimus dorsi flap as an advancement flap. **B,** Latissimus flap as a reverse flap.

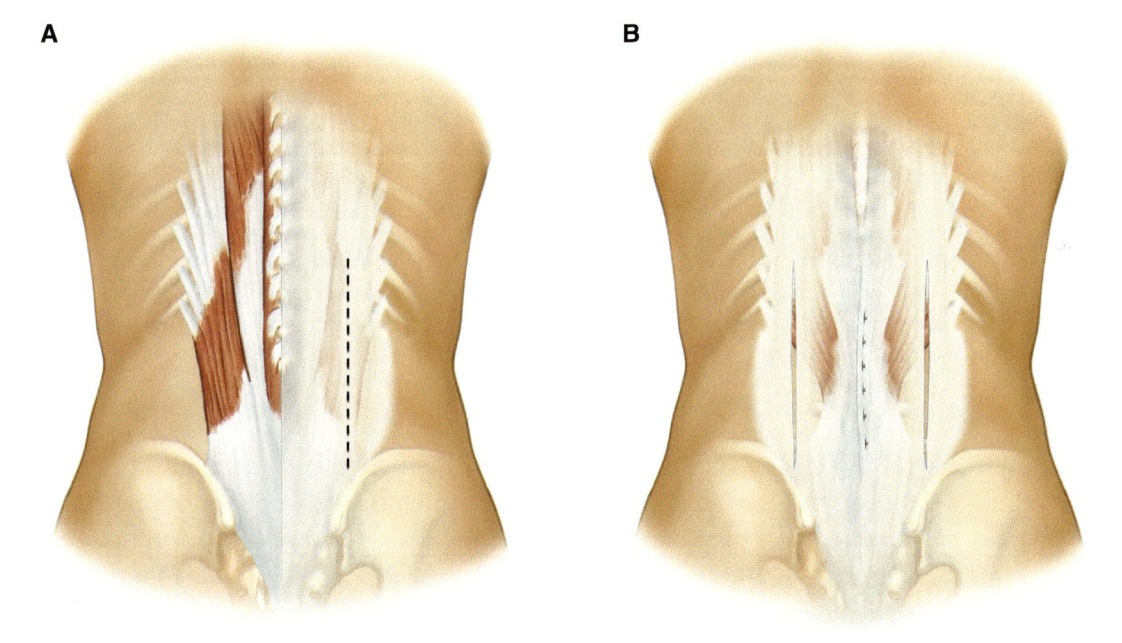

Fig. 7-6 **A,** Paraspinous muscle flap in situ. Relaxing incisions in fascia of paraspinous muscles. **B,** The muscles are sutured in the midline.

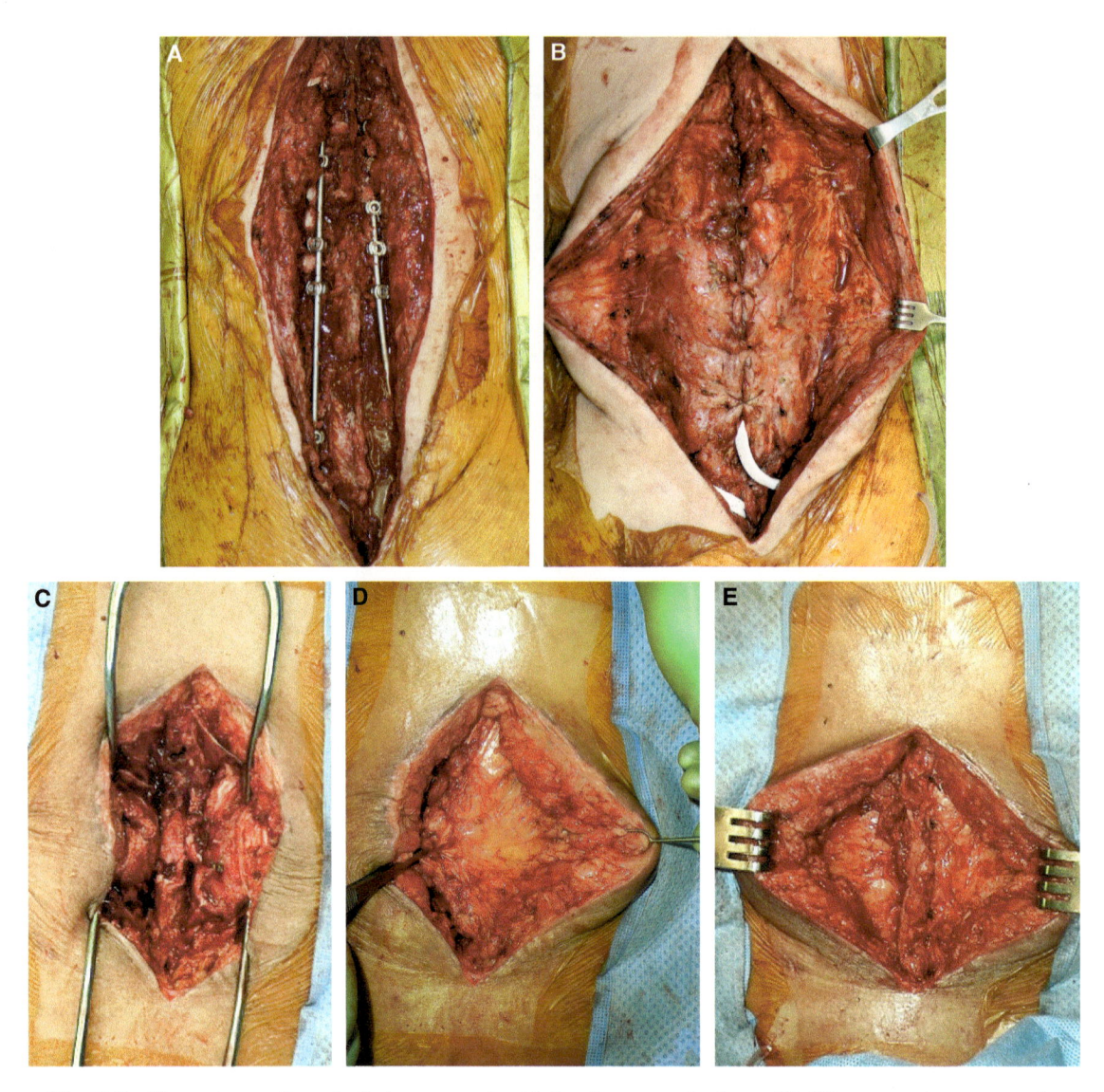

Fig. 7-7 Paraspinous flap. **A,** Spine wound with hardware at the base. **B,** The paraspinous muscles are advanced and sutured in the midline to cover the hardware. **C,** Spine wound infection after debridement. **D,** The paraspinous muscle flap is advanced past the midline. **E,** The paraspinous muscles are sutured in the midline to cover the defect.

The gluteus maximus flap is a versatile flap that can be raised in different ways to cover lower-third wounds in the lumbosacral region. In ambulatory patients, preservation of the inferior or superior half of the muscle is necessary to preserve function, specifically terminal extension of the hip, which is critical for ascending stairs. The muscle can be raised on either the superior gluteal or inferior gluteal vessels as a segmental turnover flap to fill defects of the sacrum (Fig. 7-8, *A*). It can also be advanced as a V-Y musculocutaneous flap (Fig. 7-8, *B* through *D*) or rotated as a gluteal island flap (Fig. 7-8, *E* through *G*). If skin is not needed, the flap can be deepithelialized and buried in the defect.

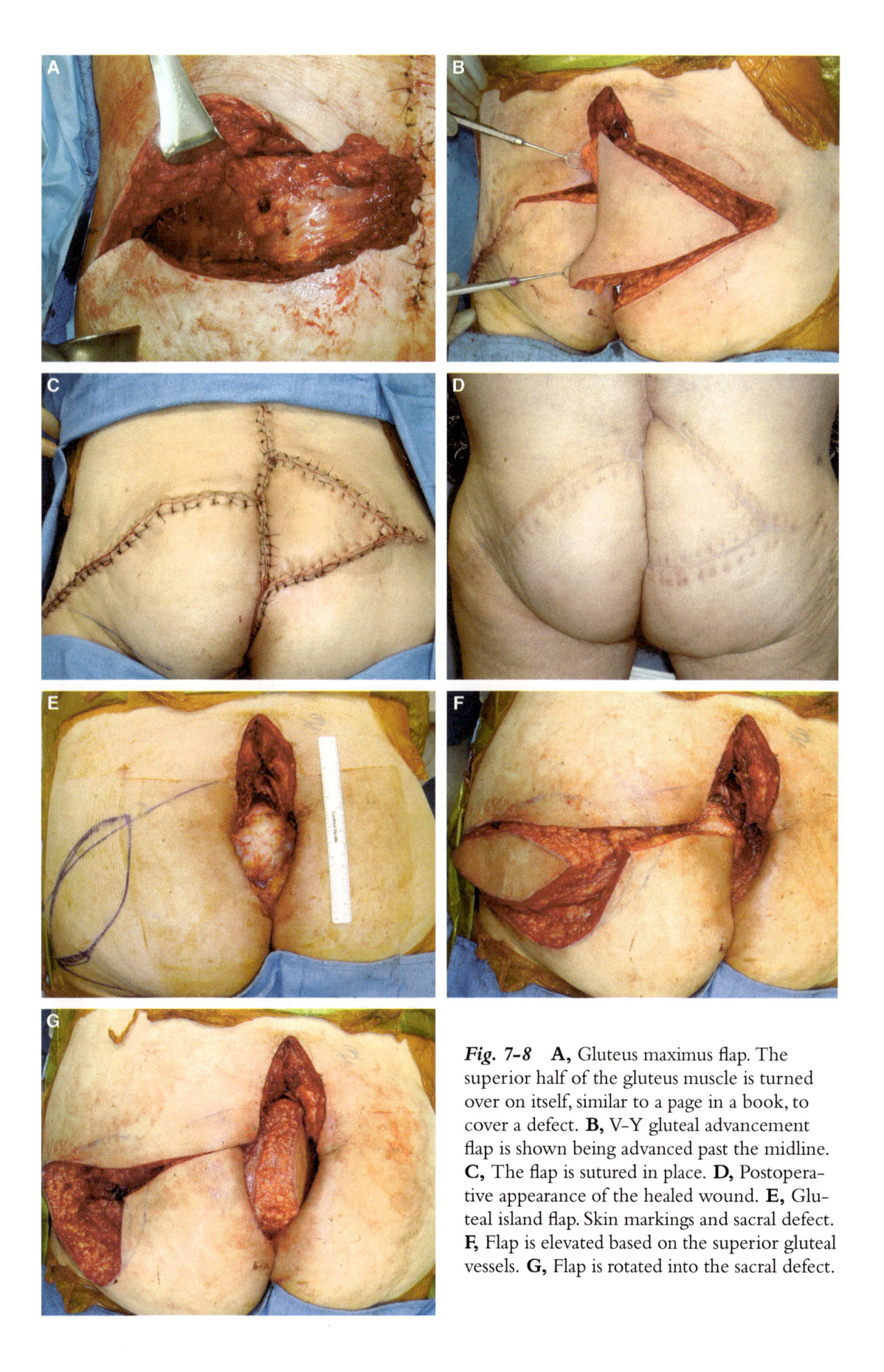

Fig. 7-8 **A,** Gluteus maximus flap. The superior half of the gluteus muscle is turned over on itself, similar to a page in a book, to cover a defect. **B,** V-Y gluteal advancement flap is shown being advanced past the midline. **C,** The flap is sutured in place. **D,** Postoperative appearance of the healed wound. **E,** Gluteal island flap. Skin markings and sacral defect. **F,** Flap is elevated based on the superior gluteal vessels. **G,** Flap is rotated into the sacral defect.

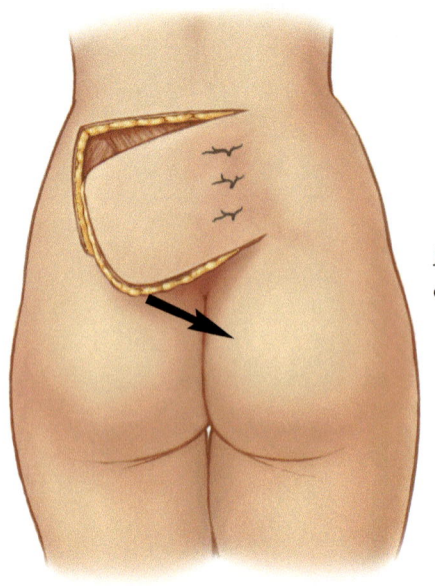

Fig. 7-9 Transverse back flap. Flap can rotate to cover sacral wounds.

The transverse back flap is a fasciocutaneous flap that consists of the skin overlying the lumbar trunk between the posterior costal margin and the sacrum. It has a segmental blood supply from perforating arteries of the lumbar and intercostal arteries. The point of rotation is the lateral edge of the paraspinous muscles, and the lateral extent of the flap should not extend past the posterior axillary line. The flap rotates 90 degrees to cover sacral defects (Fig. 7-9). Skin grafts are used for the resulting donor site. Patients should remain prone during the early postoperative period to avoid compression of the flap pedicle. Previous posterior midline incisions at the level of the flap base are a contraindication to this type of flap. This flap is only recommended for small sacral wounds, when all other options have been exhausted.

The greater omentum is an intraabdominal organ that contains mostly fat and blood vessels. The omental flap is usually raised on the right gastroepiploic vessels and passed transabdominally to fill spine wounds.[15] Some advantages of the omental flap are its structural laxity and its capacity to absorb cerebrospinal fluid and exudates.[17] However, elevating this flap requires a laparotomy incision, and transposing and insetting the flap can be challenging because of the presence of intraabdominal organs, which must be mobilized.

Rectus abdominis flaps can be elevated with a vertically oriented skin island based on the inferior epigastric vessels and its medial and lateral row of perforating vessels (Fig. 7-10). This flap provides both bulk in the form of muscle and skin to fill sacrectomy defects.[16] The flap is elevated during the anterior portion of the spine procedure. The inferior insertion on the pubis is left intact to prevent excessive tension on the vascular pedicle. The flap is then left in the peritoneal cavity until the posterior portion of the procedure, which may be carried out with the patient under the same anesthesia or 24 to 48 hours later. The flap is retrieved from the posterior approach and brought through to fill the posterior sacral defect.

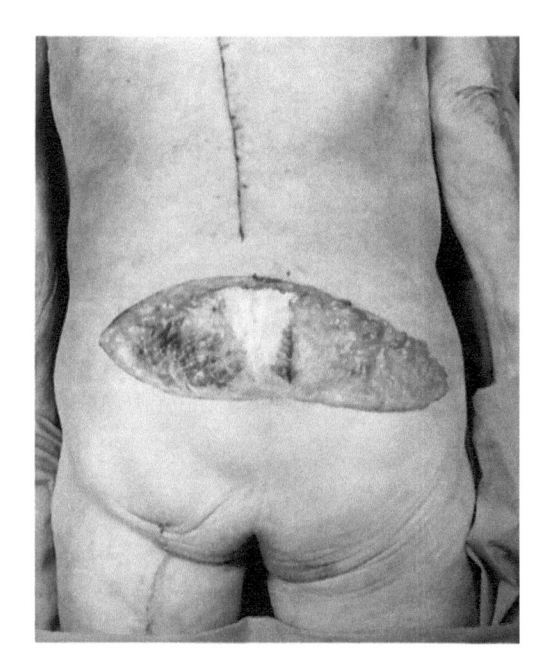

Fig. 7-10 A transverse back flap has been elevated across the midline.

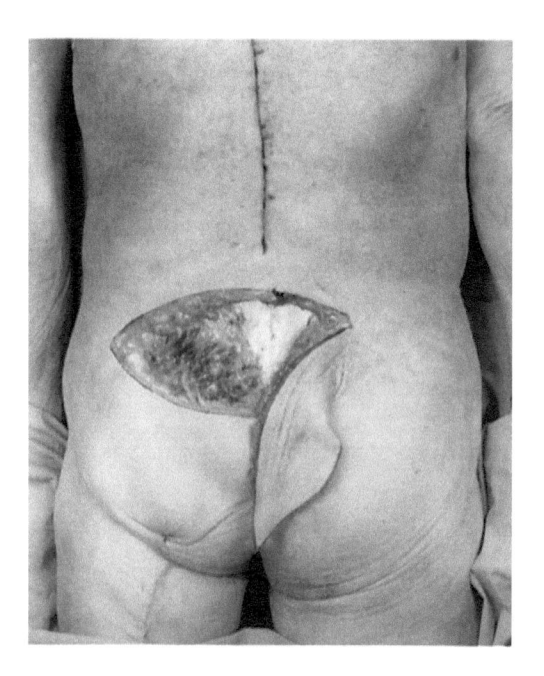

Fig. 7-11 Transverse back flap rotated to cover sacrum.

FREE FLAPS

Free tissue transfer (free flap) is an option for wound coverage when pedicled flaps are not available. This technique involves the autologous transplantation of tissue from another part of the body to the back, by means of microvascular techniques, to reestablish inflow and outflow to the flap. The advantages of free tissue transfer are the versatility (the size of the flap can be selected depending on the size of the wound) and the ability to bring well-vascularized tissue to the wound. These flaps are technically more demanding than pedicled flaps and may require repositioning the patient from supine to prone, depending on the location of the flap harvest and the donor vessel. Furthermore, vein grafting to lengthen the arterial and venous pedicles may be necessary.[18] The most commonly used free flap to the back is the latissimus dorsi flap, which was described previously. The muscle can be raised on its pedicle and transposed to any part of the back. To accomplish this, the pedicle is first transected. An arteriovenous loop is then created between the thoracodorsal vein and artery with the use of reversed saphenous vein. This loop is then divided to create two vein grafts, which are then anastomosed to the latissimus dorsi pedicle, essentially lengthening the pedicle to allow the muscle to reach the wound (Fig. 7-11). The microvascular portion of the procedure can be performed with the latissimus dorsi still perfused by its secondary pedicles (posterior perforating branches), minimizing ischemia time to the muscle.

Complex spinal reconstruction may occasionally require more than soft tissue reconstruction. Tumor extirpation or debridement of vertebral osteomyelitis can necessitate bony reconstruction. The vascularized fibula flap is versatile and can provide both structural support with bone, and soft tissue when harvested with a skin paddle.[19] It has been described for reconstruction of bony defects throughout the body. In the spine, it has been described for cervical arthrodesis,[20] fusion following debridement of osteomyelitis,[21] and reconstruction of large bone defects from tumor resection.[22,23,24] Compared with a nonvascularized bone graft (e.g., the iliac crest), a vascularized graft does not undergo resorption and results in more rapid healing. Time to bony union can take up to 4 months. Vascularized grafts are also more resistant to infection and can provide healthy tissue to previously radiated beds.

The vascular pedicle to the fibula flap is the peroneal artery and vein. The flap is harvested under tourniquet control, and a skin paddle can be included with the flap measuring up to 8 times 20 cm. It is important to leave 8 cm of fibula distally and 6 cm proximally to avoid ankle or knee instability.[25] The graft can be osteotomized and folded on itself to create a double barrel and be placed posteriorly or anteriorly in the spine with hardware fixation. Disadvantages of the fibula flap include the requirement of microsurgical expertise, adequate recipient vessels, and additional operative time. In the cervical spine, the external carotid artery and internal jugular vein provide the recipient vessels. In the thoracic spine, a segmental intercostal artery or vein may be used for the recipient vessels. Recipient vessels for the lumbar spine and sacrum are the common iliac artery and vein. Vein grafts may occasionally be necessary.

OTHER OPTIONS

Local skin flaps based on a random blood supply from the subdermal plexus can be used for small superficial wounds that are not amenable to other flaps. These flaps are typically used in a 2:1 length-to-width ratio, which can be increased to 3:1 when raised as bipedicled flaps. These flaps are frequently limited by the arc of rotation and should be reserved for cases in which no other flap options are available.

POSTOPERATIVE CARE

Patients are mobilized according to post–spine surgery protocols and are typically out of bed on postoperative day 1 or 2. Patients are kept in a lateral decubitus position for 2 weeks. Drains are left in place until the output is less than 30 cc per day for 2 consecutive days. Patients with drains that communicate with instrumentation are placed on prophylactic antibiotics until the drains are removed. Sutures are left in place for at least 2 weeks.

Complications include dehiscence and wound infection. Any wound dehiscence should be evaluated to determine the depth of the wound. Wounds that are superficial will often heal secondarily with local wound care. Negative-pressure dressings can help control exudate and minimize dressing changes. If the wound communicates with the deep space, the patient should be managed more aggressively with operative washout and reclosure over drains. Similarly, infections that are superficial to the muscle fascia are often self-limiting and are managed with debridement and antibiotics. Infections that are deep to fascia and communicate with hardware should be managed more aggressively. These infections require operative debridement of devitalized tissue and washout of hardware followed by muscle flap closure over drains. Hultman et al[9] reported an 80% hardware salvage rate with this approach. Cerebrospinal fluid leaks are managed with lumbar drains. As is often the case, spinal instrumentation cannot be removed, and long-term suppressive antibiotic therapy is indicated.

CONCLUSION

Spine wounds can present a challenge to spine and reconstructive surgeons. Successful coverage will depend on the location of the wound and the availability of local tissues. Basic principles of management include thorough evaluation of the problem, careful planning, debridement of devitalized tissue, and coverage with flaps. Muscle flaps can help eliminate dead space and bring well-vascularized tissue to the wound. Free tissue transfer is a salvage procedure when no other options are available.

TIPS FROM THE MASTERS

- Determine whether there is adequate local tissue for wound coverage.
- The location of the wound will dictate flap options.
- Paraspinous muscle flaps will be first line for most lower midline wounds.
- For upper middle or lower third wounds, consider the trapezius, latissimus or gluteus muscle flaps, respectively.

References (With Key References in Boldface)

1. Mathes SJ, Nahai F. Latissimus dorsi flap. In Reconstructive Surgery: Principles, Anatomy, and Technique. New York: Churchill Livingstone, 1997, pp 565-615.
2. Mathes SJ, Nahai F. Trapezius flap. In Reconstructive Surgery: Principles, Anatomy, and Technique. New York: Churchill Livingstone, 1997, pp 651-677.
3. **Disa JJ, Smith AW, Bilsky MH. Management of radiated reoperative wounds of the cervicothoracic spine: the role of the trapezius turnover flap. Ann Plast Surg 47:394-397, 2001.**
4. Meiners T, Flieger R, Jungclaus M. Use of the reverse latissimus muscle flap for closure of complex back wounds in patients with spinal cord injury. Spine (Phila Pa 1976) 28:1893-1898, 2003.
5. Mathes SJ, Stevenson TR. Reconstruction of posterior neck and skull with vertical trapezius musculocutaneous flap. Am J Surg 156:248-251, 1988.
6. **Casas LA, Lewis VL Jr. A reliable approach to the closure of large acquired midline defects of the back. Plast Reconstr Surg 84:632-641, 1989.**
7. Mathes SJ, Nahai F. Transverse back flap. In Reconstructive Surgery: Principles, Anatomy, and Technique. New York: Churchill Livingstone, 1997, pp 643-650.
8. Manstein ME, Manstein CH, Manstein G. Paraspinous muscle flaps. Ann Plast Surg 40:458-462, 1998.

9. **Hultman CS, Jones GE, Losken A, et al. Salvage of infected spinal hardware with paraspinous muscle flaps: anatomic considerations with clinical correlation. Ann Plast Surg 57:521-528, 2006.**
10. Saint-Cyr M, Nikolis A, Moumdjian R, et al. Paraspinous muscle flaps for the treatment and prevention of cerebrospinal fluid fistulas in neurosurgery. Spine (Phila Pa 1976) 28:E86-E92, 2003.
11. Wendt JR, Gardner VO, White JI. Treatment of complex postoperative lumbosacral wounds in nonparalyzed patients. Plast Reconstr Surg 101:1248-1253; discussion 1254, 1998.
12. Koh PK, Tan BK, Hong SW, et al. The gluteus maximus muscle flap for reconstruction of sacral chordoma defects. Ann Plast Surg 53:44-49, 2004.
13. **Miles WK, Chang DW, Kroll SS, et al. Reconstruction of large sacral defects following total sacrectomy. Plast Reconstr Surg 105:2387-2394, 2000.**
14. Mathes SJ, Nahai F. Gluteus maximus–gluteal thigh flap. In Reconstructive Surgery: Principles, Anatomy, and Technique. New York: Churchill Livingstone, 1997, pp 501-535.
15. Ladin D, Rees R, Wilkins E, et al. The use of omental transposition in the treatment of recurrent sarcoma of the back. Ann Plast Surg 31:556-559, 1993.
16. **Glatt BS, Disa JJ, Mehrara BJ, et al. Reconstruction of extensive partial or total sacrectomy defects with a transabdominal vertical rectus abdominis myocutaneous flap. Ann Plast Surg 56:526-530; discussion 530-531, 2006.**
17. O'Shaughnessy BA, Dumanian GA, Liu JC, et al. Pedicled omental flaps as an adjunct in the closure of complex spinal wounds. Spine (Phila Pa 1976) 32:3074-3080, 2007.
18. Few JW, Marcus JR, Lee MJ, et al. Treatment of hostile midline back wounds: an extreme approach. Plast Reconstr Surg 105:2448-2451, 2000.
19. Ackerman DB, Rose PS, Moran SL, et al. The results of vascularized-free fibular grafts in complex spinal reconstruction. J Spinal Disord Tech 24:170-176, 2011.
20. Lee MJ, Ondra SL, Mindea SA, et al. Indications and rationale for use of vascularized fibula bone flaps in cervical spine arthrodeses. Plast Reconstr Surg 116:1-7, 2005.
21. Erdmann D, Mead RA, Lins RE, et al. Use of the microvascular free fibula transfer as a salvage reconstruction for failed anterior spine surgery due to chronic osteomyelitis. Plast Reconstr Surg 117:2438-2445, 2006.
22. Chang DW, Fortin AJ, Oates BD, et al. Reconstruction of the pelvic ring with vascularized double-strut fibular flap following internal hemipelvectomy. Plast Reconstr Surg 121:1993-2000, 2008.
23. Sakuraba M, Kimata Y, Iida H, et al. Pelvic ring reconstruction with the double-barreled vascularized fibular free flap. 116:1340-1345, 2005.
24. Choudry UH, Moran SL, Karacor Z. Functional reconstruction of the pelvic ring with simultaneous bilateral free fibular flaps following total sacral resection. Ann Plast Surg 57:673-676, 2006.
25. Mathes SJ, Nahai F. Reconstructive Surgery: Principles, Anatomy, & Technique. New York: Churchill Livingstone/Quality Medical Publishing, 1997.

Chapter 8

Physical and Occupational Therapy

Julie Damiano, Michael E. Glover,
Rebecca L. Mustille

Rehabilitation is a vital component of surgical management of patients with spine tumors. Many of these patients initially present with neurologic deficits or other related symptoms that interfere with or diminish their quality of life. In fact, one study showed that as many as 95% of patients with metastatic spinal cord compression had back pain so severe that it limited participation in daily activities.[1] One medical dictionary defines rehabilitation as "the processes of treatment and education that leads the disabled individual to attainment of maximum function, a sense of well-being, and a personally satisfying level of independence."[2] Early involvement by a rehabilitation team, which includes physical therapists, occupational therapists, and speech therapists, is critical. Therapists in these disciplines are skilled at identifying factors that limit functional independence and helping patients to overcome these limitations. The goals of treatment include prevention of deficits, restoration of function, and minimization of disabilities.[3] Rehabilitation has been shown to minimize disabilities and maximize a person's functional level after spine surgery. In one study, patients who underwent rehabilitation not only lived longer but also had a better quality of life for the remainder of their lives.[4] The value of rehabilitation is solidified by the finding that the benefits of rehabilitation, with regard to pain, depression, and self-perceived quality of life, persist for the remainder of patients' lives. Through rehabilitation, patients gain functional independence and improvement in overall strength to become ready to be discharged home.[4]

Many factors contribute to the success of rehabilitation, including patient age, degree of initial neurologic injuries, comorbidity, prognosis, motivation, and social support. Patients with limited support face extra challenges; thus facilitating maximum independence to allow these patients to return to their homes, as opposed to a facility, is essential during rehabilitation. Inclusion of the rehabilitation team in discussions surrounding a patient's prognosis is paramount in determining an appropriate course of treatment. For those who have undergone palliative surgery, the rehabilitative goals may be to prevent complications, such as pressure ulcers and painful loss of range of motion (ROM), or to help patients return to their homes or families in a safe and comfortable way. For patients pursuing aggressive treatment to facilitate a longer lifespan, rehabilitation becomes much more wide ranging and will encompass all areas of self-care, mobility, work, and leisure. Regardless of the specific goals or limiting complications, rehabilitation can provide patients with a directed purpose in difficult recoveries after spine surgery.

Together with various members of the medical team, physical, occupational, and speech therapists play a valuable role in determining a safe discharge plan for patients after surgery. Frequently patients require continued rehabilitation that is provided at multiple venues outside of the hospital, including inpatient rehabilitation and skilled nursing facilities, the patient's home, and outpatient clinics. A comprehensive discussion of rehabilitation would ideally include a subsection for each level of care, as well as information about all team members (recreational therapists, case managers, social workers, psychologists, and so forth). However, this chapter will focus on the acute care setting. The subsequent information will be divided into physical therapy and occupational therapy to examine the specific contributions each discipline provides to patients after surgery. By outlining physical evaluation and examination, creation of a comprehensive treatment plan, specific interventions used, and a review of available adaptive equipment, this chapter will help surgeons to appreciate the contributions that rehabilitation can offer to their patients after surgery.

PHYSICAL THERAPY

Physical therapists are health care professionals who maintain, restore, and improve movement, activity, and health, enabling individuals of all ages to have optimal functioning and quality of life.[5] Physical therapists serve as movement specialists who identify ROM, strength, and functional movement ability and limitations.[6] Physical therapists also help prevent conditions associated with loss of mobility through fitness and wellness programs to achieve a healthy lifestyle. In the acute postsurgical setting, physical therapists facilitate an increase in function by focusing on ambulation and exercise programs that assist in preventing many of the potential side effects that can occur with immobility. The process of identifying abilities and impairments begins with an initial assessment. From the initial assessment, physical therapists, patients, and their families or caregivers can establish a patient-centered plan of care to achieve desired outcomes. Physical therapists develop care plans by incorporating treatment techniques that promote optimal health and fitness, reduce pain, restore and improve movement, maintain cardiopulmonary function, and limit disabilities from injury, surgery, or disease. Physical therapy is a vital part of the interdisciplinary team approach for patients in an acute hospital care setting. Goals include restoration or maintenance of sensory and motor abilities to prevent, reverse, or minimize functional limitations and/or disabilities.[5] The underlying goal of physical therapy is to improve quality of life for patients and their caregivers while preserving the highest and safest level of functional mobility.

PHYSICAL THERAPY EVALUATION
DIAGNOSIS

It is essential that the physical therapist perform a detailed and comprehensive review of the patient's medical chart to gain an accurate understanding of the diagnosis on admission according to the International Classification of Disease. For the physical therapist to establish treatment and goals, a rehabilitation diagnosis is imperative to establish physical and functional deficits. The skilled physical therapist will extrapolate a working diagnosis before beginning the evaluation to narrow the focus of the evaluation and expedite patient care.

PREVIOUS MEDICAL AND SURGICAL HISTORY

The medical history should include all medical diagnoses, along with the surgical history, to obtain a holistic view of patient-centered intervention. A thorough review of the past medical history will assist the therapist in obtaining information on all pertinent comorbid conditions. The therapist should assess all systems of the body, including neurologic, orthopedic, endocrine, cardiovascular, lymphatic, integumentary, and sensory systems.

SUBJECTIVE INFORMATION
SOCIAL HISTORY

As part of the patient interview process, it is imperative that the therapist gain an understanding of the mobility expectations required before the patient can be safely discharged. As part of a comprehensive social history, the physical therapist must assess the home setup in terms of the physical, environmental, and social support to which the patient will be returning after being discharged from the hospital. The therapist should assess physical barriers limiting the patient's entry in the home, including the number of stairs, surface grade, and topography. Once inside the home, it is necessary to assess the functional expectations for mobilization in daily activity. The physical therapist should assess the layout of the patient's bedroom and bathroom. As part of the assessment process, it is imperative that the following questions be asked:

1. Is the patient's primary or available bedroom on the ground floor, or are stairs necessary? Does the patient have the option to use a handrail? If a first-floor bedroom is not available, is modification of the home setup feasible?
2. Is the patient's primary bathroom on the ground floor, or does the patient have to ascend a flight of stairs to reach it? Is a first-floor bathroom modification of the home setup feasible?
3. Does the bathroom have a shower over a tub bath or a walk-in shower? Are there grab bars available for assistance? Is a shower bench or chair available?
4. Does the patient have a standard toilet? Does the patient have an elevated toilet seat or elevated commode? Are there grab bars available for assistance?

The physical therapist can initiate a functional treatment plan on the basis of these functional demands. All of the preceding questions are imperative to gain an understanding of the functional demands and necessary goals of discharge for the patient and the caregiver.

Along with the physical and environmental demands on the patient, it is important to fully understand the level of family and caregiver support. It is imperative that the following questions be asked:

1. Does the patient live alone?
2. Does the patient have in-home support of family, caregivers, and/or home health aides?
3. If so, how much support does the patient have? Is the available caregiver physically able to assist at the patient's current functional status?

Previous Level of Function/Durable Medical Equipment Owned

A baseline level of functional ability must be established to effectively establish therapeutic goals and develop an appropriate plan of care. The patient and the caregiver must offer a clear picture of previous functional ability. It is appropriate to establish realistic and obtainable goals for rehabilitation to help the patient return to the previous level of function. To create an understanding of function, the following questions must be asked:

1. Before this surgery, was the patient able to ambulate household distances? Did the patient require the use of an assistive device? What kind of assistive device did the patient use? What level of assistance/supervision did the patient require?
2. Before this surgery, was the patient able to ambulate community distances? Was the patient able to ambulate through a store? Did the patient require the use of an assistive device? What kind of assistive device did the patient use?
3. Does the patient have any other durable medical equipment or home modifications?

4. How far was the patient able to ambulate before requiring a rest break, and what was the limiting factor?
5. Had the patient ever fallen? How frequent were the falls? Was the patient aware of any patterns to the falls (time of day, surface characteristics, level of fatigue or distraction)?
6. Before this surgery, was the patient able to perform activities of daily living (ADLs), including bathing, dressing, and grooming? Did the patient require assistance or any assistive devices?
7. Before this surgery, was the patient able to perform instrumental ADLs, including cooking, cleaning, and bookkeeping? Did the patient require assistance or any adaptive equipment or assistive devices?
8. What are the patient's hobbies, interests, and activities that offer enjoyment?

The answers to many of these questions are important to take into consideration when establishing a plan of care. Obtaining a full understanding of a patient's medical equipment needs will assist in appropriate ordering for a safe discharge. Collaborating in a patient-centered treatment plan with a list of patient-driven goals will promote effective outcomes. Patient ownership of treatment and personal investment of participation are highly correlated with satisfaction with the treatment plan.[7] Incorporating the patient's interests and obtainable, functional goals will increase compliance and the chance for a successful return to the previous level of function.

PAIN

Pain may be a limiting factor in therapeutic interventions. Pain is a debilitating side effect of spine surgery and can create difficulties within all areas of daily life. Patients suffering from pain may have difficulty performing ADLs, ambulating, concentrating, and finding enjoyment in daily life. Neuropathy is a particular type of pain that is caused by damaged or dysfunctional nerve fibers and may be seen in patients after spine surgery. It is often recommended by rehabilitation practitioners, and found to be beneficial by both rehabilitation practitioners and patients, to premedicate patients for pain before they participate in any activities. Interdisciplinary communication with the nursing staff is vital to maximize rehabilitation potential.

OBJECTIVE MEASURES
RANGE OF MOTION

Physical therapists are specialists in musculoskeletal function and movement. One of the principal roles of the physical therapist is to assess both passive and active movement and function in all extremities, the trunk, and the spine. Movement may be assessed with active function and physical mobility. When appropriate, it is the role of the physical therapist to assess functional limitations and measure deficits. Joint kinesiology and goniometric tools establish an objective baseline for evaluation. It is outside the scope of this chapter to further discuss complete goniometric measurements.

STRENGTH

Another principal role of the physical therapist is to assess muscle strength and active movement in all extremities, the trunk, and the spine. Physical therapists use a standardized manual muscle testing measurement scale (Box 8-1). Major muscle groups to measure standard manual muscle grades are the key to establishing spinal cord involvement and functional impairments. Box 8-2 reviews major muscle groups and proximal nerve root distributions.

When spinal cord function is impaired as a result of tumor invasion, establishment of a baseline objective measurement for all major muscle groups and spine levels is imperative (see Box 8-2). The American Spinal Injury Association (ASIA) has developed a standard neurologic classification of spinal cord injuries, which is often referred to as the ASIA scale.[7] It is recommended that the ASIA scale be employed during the initial evaluation and at each subsequent reevaluation to track changes related to motor and sensory levels of impairment.

Box 8-1 Manual Muscle Testing

5/5	*Normal:*	Full active ROM against maximum resistance
4+/5	*Good plus:*	Full active ROM against moderate/maximum resistance
4/5	*Good:*	Full active ROM against moderate resistance
4−/5	*Good minus:*	Full active ROM against minimum/moderate resistance
3+/5	*Fair plus:*	Full active ROM against minimum resistance
3/5	*Fair:*	Full active ROM against gravity
3−/5	*Fair minus:*	Unable to perform active ROM against gravity, although >50%
2+/5	*Poor plus:*	Active ROM is initiated against gravity, although <50%
2/5	*Poor:*	Full active ROM, gravity eliminated
2−/5	*Poor minus:*	Unable to perform full active ROM, gravity eliminated
1/5	*Trace:*	Active muscle facilitation
0/5	*Zero:*	No active facilitation noted

Box 8-2 Key Muscle Level: Motor Function

C5: Elbow flexors	T1: Finger abductors	L2: Hip flexors	L5: Great toe extensors
C6: Wrist extensors		L3: Knee extensors	S1: Ankle-plantar flexion
C7: Elbow extensors		L4: Ankle dorsiflexors	
C8: Wrist flexors			

SKIN INTEGRITY

Skin integrity is a vital component of a patient's health and recovery. A proactive approach to maintaining skin integrity is to educate patients, their families, and caregivers before skin complications occur. A visual assessment of the skin is appropriate to evaluate postoperative incisions, pressure ulcerations, skin breakdown, and shearing abrasions resulting from movement and transfers. If any of these skin complications are noted, it will assist in interdisciplinary dialog among patients, families, caregivers, and nursing staff to teach appropriate bed and wheelchair positioning, bed mobility, and transfer techniques.

SENSORY IMPAIRMENT

The spinal cord carries multiple tracts offering peripheral somatosensory feedback. When spinal cord function is impaired, it is imperative to establish baseline objective measurements of light touch, deep pressure, pinprick, vibration, and thermoregulation. The ASIA has developed a standard neurologic classification of spinal cord injury that is often referred to as the ASIA scale.[7]

PROPRIOCEPTION

The dorsal column of the spinal cord is the primary location for all proprioceptive afferent tracts. Proprioception is assessed in many forms, including static kinesthetic joint position sense, dynamic posturing, and active facilitation. It is within the scope of the physical therapist's role to accurately assess all facets of proprioception. Joint kinesthetics can be assessed by passively facilitating joint movement and asking the patient to blindly offer joint position sense. Static kinesthetics may also be identified by passively positioning the patient's upper or lower extremity and asking the patient to mirror the position sense on the contralateral limb.

Lesions of the dorsal column may also appear with dynamic posturing and active facilitation deficits. These deficits are common in intramedullary tumor resections. Patients may have functional deficits resulting from impaired awareness of self in space. Loss of proprioceptive input may alter a patient's motor planning with activity and ultimately will jeopardize the patient's safety.

COORDINATION

Standard objective measurements of coordination are appropriate for each patient assessment to ensure functional gains and postoperative recovery. Activities tested are rapid alternating movement for determination of gross motor function in the upper and lower extremities. An alternative activity for assessment of upper extremities includes the finger-nose-finger test. The patient is offered a target object to tap with the index finger. Once the target is successfully reached, the patient is cued to touch his or her own nose and return to touch the original object. The therapist is evaluating the patient's purposeful movement, pursuit of tracking, and accuracy in reaching the target. Lower extremity assessment includes sliding the heel on the opposite shin. The patient is cued to take the right heel and slide it from the left medial malleolus to the left knee along the tibial tuberosity. The patient is cued to perform the same task with the opposite lower extremity. The therapist is evaluating the patient's purposeful movement and smooth pursuit of tracking.

SPASTICITY

Spasticity is a motor disorder characterized by a velocity-dependent increase in tonic stretch reflexes (muscle tone) with exaggerated tendon jerks, resulting from hyperexcitability of the stretch reflex, as one component of upper motor neuron syndrome. Spastic musculature may be beneficial or detrimental postoperatively. Potential side effects may include limitations to ROM, pain, interference with ADLs, effects on posture and positioning, skin breakdown, and disorders affecting movement and functional mobility. When spasticity is identified, it is appropriate to objectively grade the hypertonia. One standard scale that is used is the Modified Ashworth Scale, which employs the following grading system:

- 0 = No increase in muscle tone
- 1 = Slight increase in muscle tone, manifested by a catch and release or by minimal resistance at the end ROM, when the part is moved in flexion or extension/abduction or adduction, and so forth
- 1+ = Slight increase in muscle tone, manifested by a catch, followed by minimal resistance throughout the remainder (less than half) of the ROM
- 2 = More marked increase in muscle tone through most of the ROM, but the affected part is easily moved
- 3 = Considerable increase in muscle tone, but passive movement is difficult
- 4 = Affected part is rigid in flexion or extension

Upper motor neuron lesions may be present with spine tumors that occur with lesions involving the spinal cord and peripheral nerves proximal to alpha motor neurons. The presence of clonus may interfere with functional activity progression. The awareness of onset, exacerbation, and resolution of clonus will assist the physical therapist in planning treatment sessions and progression appropriately.

Clonus Test

The therapist offers a quick stretch of the gastrocnemius by advancing the foot into dorsiflexion. A positive result presents with a subsequent beat or repeated pulsation of dorsiflexion and plantar flexion.

Babinski Test

The therapist applies a stroking movement on the lateral aspect of the patient's plantar aspect of the foot and moves medially across the metatarsal heads. A positive result is an extension of the great toe and flare of the lateral four digits.

FUNCTIONAL MOBILITY

Once the objective and neurologic measurements are identified, the physical therapist incorporates all findings to define functional mobility. The postoperative patient is assessed in functional progression of bed mobility, transfers, balance, and gait. The functional assist level is offered by the level of care provided by the therapist for the patient to achieve the desired goal of treatment. Standard language used by the medical team to grade the patient's level of independence includes the following:

1. *Independent*: The patient performs the task without assist or verbal cues.
2. *Modified independent*: The patient performs the task without assistance or verbal cues but requires an assistive device, an altered physical environment (e.g., elevated height of a chair or bed), or adaptive equipment to safely perform the task.
3. *Standby assist, supervision*: The patient completes the task without physical assistance but requires verbal cues or setup of the physical environment for safety.
4. *Contact guard assist*: The patient completes the task with intermittent physical assistance for safety only and may require verbal cues or setup of the physical environment.
5. *Minimal assistance*: The patient completes more than 75% to 100% of the task, but the therapist offers physical assistance for the patient to safely perform the task.
6. *Moderate assistance*: The patient completes more than 50% to 74% of the task, but the therapist offers physical assistance for the patient to safely perform the task.
7. *Maximum assistance*: The patient completes more than 25% to 49% of the task, but the therapist offers physical assistance for the patient to safely perform the task.
8. *Dependent assistance*: The patient can perform up to 24% of the task, but the therapist offers physical assistance for the patient to safely perform the task.

The physical therapist performs a gross functional mobility assessment of bed mobility, transfers, and gait. It is important to obtain a baseline functional progression of ability and to evaluate postoperative function. In the context of this chapter, ability will be addressed from basic to advanced progression, starting with the patient in the supine position.

Rolling

Bed mobility is addressed with the patient in the supine position to test the ability to roll to left side-lying and right side-lying. The physical therapist must educate the patient on the importance of the log-rolling technique to limit rotation of the spine. The patient may require the assistance of the bed rails to pull to side-lying if allowed by the surgeon. Use of side rails is usually permitted for patients with instrumentation in the cervical and lumbar spine but is often prohibited for patients with instrumentation in the thoracic spine.

Supine to Sit Edge of Bed

Once the patient has achieved full side-lying posture, the patient is instructed to push upright to a sitting position with bilateral upper extremities.

Sitting Balance

Static Sitting Balance   Balance is assessed with and without the use of single and bilateral upper extremities; this is documented as appropriate.

Dynamic Sitting Balance   This is an assessment of sitting balance when the patient is reaching outside of the base of support and performing functional ADLs. It is appropriate to assess balance with and without the use of single and bilateral upper extremities; this is documented as appropriate.

Common language used by physical and occupational therapists to quantify balance typically rates balance as *good*, *fair*, or *poor*. Standardized assessments for balance that have been researched as valid and reliable are the Berg Balance Scale, the Tinetti Balance Assessment Tool, and the Timed Up and Go Test.

Sit to Stand

This includes functional progression from the sitting surface to a complete standing position. It is important to note the surface and height from which the patient is standing and the functional use of upper extremities.

Static Standing Balance

It is appropriate to assess balance with and without the use of single and/or bilateral upper extremities; this is documented as appropriate.

Dynamic Standing Balance

This is an assessment of standing balance when the patient is reaching outside of the base of support and performing functional ADLs. It is appropriate to assess balance with and without the use of single and/or bilateral upper extremities or an assistive device; this is documented as appropriate.

Chair Transfer

This is an assessment of the patient's mobility from the static surface to a chair. Use of upper extremities assistance, external assistance, or an assistive device must be noted.

Gait

This is an assessment of functional ambulation of distance, endurance, use of assistive devices, and external assistance. A primary role of the physical therapist is to analyze gait deviations and educate patients to facilitate appropriate gait patterns.

Stairs

The physical therapist will assess the functional ascending and descending of stairs, number of stairs, endurance, use of the railing, as well as the assistive device or external assistance required to perform safely. A primary role of the physical therapist is to analyze gait deviations and educate patients accordingly.

PHYSICAL THERAPY: POSTOPERATIVE MANAGEMENT

Once evaluation of the patient is complete, the role of the physical therapist is to establish a postoperative treatment plan. This patient-centered plan of care should reflect the functional goals of the patient and the interdisciplinary team to maximize independence. Research in rehabilitative science is geared to stimulate neuroplasticity in the brain and spinal cord, including neuronal outgrowth, synaptogenesis, and neurogenesis.[8]

Supine positioning in bed after surgical intervention is responsible for many complications, including skin breakdown, physical deconditioning, lung congestion and the potential for infection, equilibrium disturbances, thromboembolic disorders, and decline in cognitive status. Early mobilization and progression to sitting on the edge of the bed are imperative for functional progression. For postoperative patients, absence of regular physical activity will result in a functional decline of balance and muscle strength.[8] Education and reinforcement of the log-rolling technique to maintain a static spine are important to maintain postoperative precautions. The patient should be educated to roll to the side of the bed, keeping the pelvis and shoulders in alignment. Once in the full side-lying position, the patient is instructed to push upward with bilateral upper extremities to obtain a static midline sitting position.

Once the patient is sitting at the edge of the bed, the physical therapist will evaluate static sitting balance, along with the patient's ability to find, and awareness of, the body-centered midline. Education concerning midline awareness and the functional base of support will offer the patient insight into the center of gravity. The patient may require the use of both arms to increase the base of support to maintain static and dynamic sitting balance. Offering appropriate physical perturbations, the physical therapist can assess the return to established midline. Postoperatively patients may have vestibular and proprioceptive impairments as associated body awareness deficits. The use of a mirror may offer visual input and knowledge of performance to establish midline and sensory integration.[9] The use of upper extremities in reaching to recover or block loss of balance reassures the therapist that the patient has appropriate righting reactions. Righting reactions indicate positive rehabilitative outcomes to reach functional goals.[8]

As midline awareness is discovered and dynamic balance is within safe functional limits, therapeutic exercises for core strengthening are indicated in the sitting position. Seated pelvic tilts (contraindicated with lumbar and lumbosacral fusions), alternating raising and lowering of the upper and lower extremities, and reaching outside the base of support all encourage antagonist contraction to stabilize the core muscle groups. The dynamic progression of sitting balance also demonstrates the patient's functional balance, with unilateral or no upper extremity support. Reaching outside the base of support for an activity of daily living or a therapeutic exercise with established core and midline awareness encourages progression to standing by ensuring core trunk strength and functional righting reactions. In the seated position, gravity-eliminating therapeutic exercises offer a further challenge to sitting balance and core-strengthening exercises. It is important to emphasize the closed-chain therapeutic intervention to incorporate multiple muscle groups while offering joint approximation and sensory input. A handout of progressing therapeutic exercises may offer increased awareness and compliance with the established program.

Ambulation is typically one of the patient's primary postoperative goals. It is a primary skill set of the physical therapist to promote the safest and most energy-efficient gait pattern. Once the patient has safely and successfully achieved edge-of-bed static and dynamic sitting balance, pregait activity should be initiated. Transferring from sitting at the edge of the bed to standing incorporates a multisystem integration of motor and sensory planning. The patient must facilitate bilateral lower extremities and equal distribution of weight-bearing. If the patient is unable to achieve standing balance, he or she can brace the arms on a bedrail or the armrest of a chair, or use a cane or walker. The physical therapist must offer tactile cues to ensure equal weight-bearing distribution between bilateral lower extremities to initiate active muscle facilitation, joint approximation, and sensory input.[10] Physical and occupational therapists offer the patient this tactile input to promote accurate muscle facilitation with all standing progression when performing ADLs.

Standing exercises are equally important for safe functional balance and gait progression. Educating patients on standing active ROM offers unilateral strengthening and contralateral balance exercises. Repeated sit-to-stand and minisquat exercises offer closed-chain exercises that encourage antagonist muscle facilitation, joint approximation, and sensory input. Alternating the base of support initiates a therapeutic balance program; the therapist can facilitate this by encouraging a narrow base of support with feet together, tandem stance, and single-leg stance.

Locomotor training, as defined by Behrman et al,[11] is a physiologically based approach to retraining after a focal spine injury that capitalizes on the intrinsic mechanisms of the spinal cord to generate stepping in response to specific afferent input associated with the task of walking. Bilateral and equal weight-bearing offers maximum loading of the lower extremities. The goal of the physical therapist is to provide the appropriate sensory input to generate stepping activity while minimizing compensatory strategies. Overground walking speed at premorbid mobility has been found to be effective for maximizing rehabilitative recovery. Those trained at premorbid gait speed have been found to have improved functional results.[10] Behrman et al[11] describes the three essential elements of ambulation as *stepping, balance,* and *adaptability*. Stepping is the most intrinsic and primitive level of reciprocal movement. The intrinsic stepping patterns have been linked to sensory signals and spinal interneurons, often referred as central pattern generators.[10,11] Rhythmic patterns of stepping initiate a functional gait progression. Sherrington[12] was the first to propose that full hip extension is important to initiate the flexor burst into the swing phase of the gait cycle.[11] For a safe ambulation progression, patients must be able to right the trunk over the lower extremity stepping pattern. Balance requires a multisystem integration of equilibrium during propulsive movement, including visual, sensory, and vestibular systems. If any component is compromised, the body may learn to compensate for the system in a deficient system in order to safely adapt. Adaptability is the integration of motor, sensory, and behavioral goals within the external and environmental constraints. These three components uniquely overlap to promote the greatest functional recovery and direct the plan of care and rehabilitative treatment strategies. The most ideal motor learning scenario occurs when patient-centered performance is matched with the environment and motor and sensory integration.[10]

When independent ambulation is not obtained or is considered unsafe for a patient's reentry into the household or community, it is appropriate to offer a gait assistive device for the patient to achieve modified independence. It is standard practice to offer the patient the least cumbersome and restrictive device possible for safe ambulation. The physical therapist will educate the patient to minimize compensatory strategies that divert loading to the paretic or weak lower extremity. Research endorses minimizing, or even eliminating, the use of assistive devices with therapeutic intervention. This paradigm shift shows that weight-bearing through the upper extremities and onto the assistive device will force a flexed trunk, with hip flexion restricting hip extension and diminishing appropriate lower extremity loading, ground reaction forces with gait pattern.[11]

OCCUPATIONAL THERAPY

Occupational therapy aims to provide patients with the skills needed to regain their independence with regard to daily occupations. These occupations, or ADLs, range from self-care to work and leisure and encompass everything that is done on a day-to-day basis that allows a person to participate in and enjoy life. Patients with spine tumors often experience a major disruption in most areas of their lives, and these changes can have a profound effect on their psychological well-being. Beyond needing assistance with everyday tasks, many patients are forced to relinquish roles within the family and community, lose the ability to partake in social activities they once enjoyed, and ultimately experience isolation and depression. Routines become disrupted and self-worth diminishes because many people feel they have become a burden and are no longer able to make valuable contributions to their families or society. These psychosocial changes can be as difficult to navigate as the physical changes. Occupational therapy becomes vital as it is "founded on an understanding that engaging in occupation structures everyday life and contributes to health and well-being."[13] Participating in simple tasks allows patients with spine tumors to regain some control as they face their many challenges.

Occupational therapy is a holistic approach that recognizes the importance of treating all areas affecting the ADLs, including motor, sensory, cognitive, perceptual, and psychosocial components encompassing cultural, social, personal, and spiritual aspects of life.[14] Occupational therapists are uniquely trained to recognize required activity demands, including objects used and their properties, space demands, social demands,

Table 8-1 Donning Pants

Activity	Physical Requirements	Modifications
Retrieve article of clothing	Ambulate or wheel self to closet or drawer Reach to get item Grasp item and pull out Intact cognition and vision (address as needed)	Keep clothing at waist level Keep clothing at bedside Use long-handled reacher
Loop pants over each foot	Maintain balance sitting or standing Hold pants Bend forward or flex hips above 90 degrees (contraindicated for various surgical levels) Lift leg For some, manage over ankle-foot orthotic	Sit in a chair that supports upright position Prop with one arm in seated position Lie down and perform at bed level Use seated cross-legged technique Use arms or leg lifter to position legs Use reacher or dressing stick to thread over feet
Pull up pants	Maintain balance Grasp pants Pull over hips	Prop against a wall Use reacher or dressing stick Sit and shift weight side-to-side Perform at bed level
Fasten	Fine motor coordination to manage buttons or tie	Use pants with elastic or snaps Use button hook Have caregiver assist at any of the above steps

sequencing and timing, required actions, required body functions, and required body structures.[13] The ability to perform detailed activity analysis enables occupational therapists to break down daily tasks into several components to help identify barriers limiting independence and recommend modifications that will enable patients to experience success. These adaptations vary according to need and can include placing a patient in a certain posture through physical support, education concerning a new technique, use of adaptive equipment, modifying the environment, and caregiver training to assist patients in maximizing their independence in terms of occupational performance. Table 8-1 details the steps necessary to perform the simple task of putting on a pair of pants and the suggestions an occupational therapist may make to a patient experiencing limited success.

A more complex task, such as riding on public transportation, which involves navigating the station, purchasing a ticket, boarding the train, taking a seat, holding on for support, exiting the train, and navigating a new station, requires an expanded knowledge of activity analysis to facilitate patient participation. Determining the limiting steps and modifying the activity to facilitate success are the hallmarks of occupational therapy. Modifications may need to be implemented at each stage to allow independence, and by breaking down activities to a step-by-step process, occupational therapists can provide their patients with the skills they need to improve functional outcomes.

Occupational therapists use many strategies to encourage patients to participate in daily occupations while adjusting to the demands of the tasks. Therapeutic use of self is a core tenet of occupational therapy and involves drawing on personal experiences or personality traits to engage patients to participate in tasks.[15] This tool is especially useful when working with patients and families who are dealing with end-of-life issues, because it highlights the therapist's ability to appreciate the patient's perspective and, ideally, assist in overcoming some of the difficult emotions. Keeping patients motivated with positive encouragement is essential, particularly in patients with terminal illnesses, and can have a significant effect on functional outcome after spine surgery.

OCCUPATIONAL THERAPY EVALUATION
OCCUPATIONAL PROFILE

Establishing a baseline of previous functional ability is required to effectively establish therapeutic goals and an appropriate plan of care. Understanding the roles, routines, habits, and priorities of the patient, as well as the context in which occupational performance is conducted, is a vital component of the occupational therapy evaluation.[16] Patients are asked to describe their abilities before surgery, including participation in ADLs, instrumental ADLs, such as cooking and cleaning, sexual activity, sleep patterns, functional mobility, employment status, assistive devices used, and recreational or leisure activities enjoyed. Patients are also asked to provide information regarding the home environment, any adaptive devices or equipment available at discharge, and the amount of assistance that would be available once they are discharged home. This information should include the layout and physical requirements necessary to enter or navigate throughout the home, including the patient's bedroom and bathroom, and any environmental modifications that have already been made (i.e., installing a ramp or grab bars). Along with the physical and environmental demands on the patient, it is important to fully understand the level of support the patient will have at home, whether live-in help or help from an external source. Support may be in the form of family, friends, hired caregivers, or home health aides and can range from grocery shopping to assisting with bathing and dressing. This information is vital in that it helps to define the direction of therapy.

OCCUPATIONAL PERFORMANCE

ADLs are assessed to determine whether patients can perform basic activities related to self-care before discharge. These basics include the following:
1. *Self-feeding*: Patients are evaluated to determine whether they can access food (i.e., open tops or sugar packets), set up the environment (i.e., cut food or place butter on toast), manipulate utensils, and bring food or drink to the mouth.
2. *Grooming and hygiene*: To determine a level of independence in this category, patients are given a variety of tasks, such as combing hair, brushing teeth, shaving, or applying makeup.
3. *Upper body bathing and dressing*: Patients are assessed to determine whether they can retrieve, don, arrange, and fasten an article of clothing, including a brace, if applicable, as well as access all areas for self-bathing.

4. *Lower body bathing and dressing*: Patients are assessed to determine whether they can retrieve, don, arrange, and fasten an article of clothing, including a brace, if applicable, as well as access all areas for self-bathing. Patients are also asked to don socks and shoes and to manage fasteners.
5. *Toileting*: Therapists determine whether patients can independently perform perineal care, as well as maintain balance and manage clothing during the activity.

Given the time limitations, functional observation of occupational performance is the most time-efficient method used for acute care. If warranted, occupational therapists may also perform standardized tests that offer a detailed, objective look at a patient's ability to engage in ADLs. Tests such as the Assessment of Motor and Process Skills (AMPS) and the Kohlman Evaluation of Living Skills (KELS) can be valuable tools for determining a safe discharge plan and setting goals.

ACTIVITY DEMANDS

Occupational therapists take particular note of not only the type and amount of effort exerted during various activities, but also the tools used, the effect of the current environment, the time required, and the effects on other systems, including neuromuscular, cardiovascular, and respiratory systems, and the patient's mood related to the performance.[13] The Model of Human Occupation, a framework used by many occupational therapists, emphasizes that to understand human occupation, it is also necessary to understand the physical and social environment in which it takes place. Assessing all of these components allows occupational therapists to determine the exact areas limiting success and create a plan of care that will allow their patients to return to the highest level of function possible. This initial evaluation helps to identify the barriers limiting performance of ADLs and serves as a framework on which to build a plan that promotes success. Depending on the patient's level, the evaluation may need to be completed over the course of many visits to gain a complete picture of the patient's functional level. For example, some patients are in too much pain to tolerate sitting on the edge of the bed, whereas others, once they are up, may become ill and need to return to bed.

OCCUPATIONAL THERAPY: POSTOPERATIVE MANAGEMENT

Once patients have completed the evaluation, the occupational therapist will detail a specific strategy to assist patients in achieving their goals. When designing a treatment plan, occupational therapists take many factors into account, including the patient's age, ability to tolerate activity, comorbid conditions, prognosis, social support, and discharge plans, as well as the patient's wishes. It is also important to determine patients' adaptive performance skills—that is, how resourceful they are in compensating for functional deficits and learning new modified strategies. In the case of metastatic lesions, knowledge of the prognosis is paramount in helping patients to set realistic, attainable goals. Patients and/or their family members may have unrealistic expectations about what patients will be able to achieve, so setting clear goals and outlining reasonable outcomes is an important role of the rehabilitation team.[17] Often this is the first time a person becomes aware of the impact of his or her condition, and open, direct communication allows adjustment to current and future situations. For those facing a shortened lifespan, spending a month in a rehabilitation facility might not be the best option when that time may be better spent with family. The person with limited support faces extra challenges, so facilitating maximum independence to allow a return to home versus a facility is critical. Great care is taken to ensure that the patient's goals are being addressed and not necessarily what a typical program would dictate when selecting an appropriate course of treatment. For example, a patient may have no interest in self-bathing or dressing but would rather focus on ways to return to computer use or dining out in a favorite restaurant. This type of client-centered rehabilitation encourages patients to spend time in meaningful pursuits and encourages patients to become actively involved in their recovery.[18]

Treatment at an acute care hospital is subject to the patient's medical stability. It is imperative to monitor patients' vital signs, because many of them have orthostasis or decreased oxygen saturation with activity. At the onset of intervention, some patients are unable to tolerate even sitting at the edge of the bed, so treatments may be spent on education or answering the many questions patients and their families often have as they contemplate the uncertainty of the future. Family training is a large component of rehabilitation, because often family support is increasingly needed for the patient to be successful with daily tasks.

Functional mobility is addressed by both occupational and physical therapists because accessing a patient's environment is relevant to all members of the rehabilitation team. Typically postsurgical patients demonstrate difficulties with all aspects of self-care, ranging from self-feeding and showering to shopping and cooking. The specific limitations usually correspond to the location of the tumor and the level of surgical intervention.

Many activities need to be avoided, such as driving, mowing the lawn, or playing golf; however, countless other activities can be performed in altered ways. To facilitate a safe return to the home, most patients are provided with recommendations to alter the environment to ensure the home is free from barriers or possible dangers. Some of these recommendations include removing throw rugs and clutter, avoiding low chairs or those with wheels, checking doorway widths for wheelchair access and, for elderly patients, use of a lifeline in the event they need assistance and are unable to access a phone. General modifications for safety in the bathroom that are helpful to all patients recovering from spine surgery include the following: use of a commode with adjustable legs or a raised toilet seat to replace a standard low toilet, use of a shower chair or tub bench, applying a nonslip surface to the floor of the shower or tub, and use of long-handled sponges, "soap-on-a-rope" (attached to the chair), or wall-mounted soaps and shampoos. Falls in the bathroom are quite common, so specific measures should be taken to decrease this risk. In addition to these general tips, there are numerous activities that require modification, depending on the level of surgery. To examine these, the levels will be separated into the following categories: cervical, thoracic/lumbar, and sacral.

CERVICAL SURGERY

There are a vast number of daily activities that involve motion at the neck. For 6 to 8 weeks after surgery, most patients are required to wear a brace 24-hours a day and to avoid all neck movements, shoulder flexion above 90 degrees, and lifting, pushing, or pulling more than 10 pounds. To maintain compliance with 24-hour bracing, the patient will be given a cervical collar for daily use and for bathing (Fig. 8-1). This necessitates adaptations in daily functioning, whether they involve learning how to perform tasks in a modified way, using specific equipment, or avoiding activities for a period of time. Occupational therapists are uniquely trained in the area of self-care and can educate patients on alternative ways of performing tasks to achieve independence. Table 8-2 is an example of the step-by-step analysis. The role of occupational therapist is to assist with the patient's improvement and participation in functional activities after cervical surgery.

Patients are taught to don and doff a neck brace while standing in front of a mirror to minimize the risk of unintentional neck movements. Examples of less obvious tasks involving neck movements that are often mentioned to patients include getting in and out of a car, turning to look when one's name is called and looking down when eating, climbing stairs, going to sit on a chair or flush the toilet, pronounced sneezing, and head position when sitting at a computer. To maximize safety and avoid neck flexion and falls, patients may also be taught to use textured tape to denote thresholds in the home and to place a bell on the collar of small animals. Hand or finger splints can be

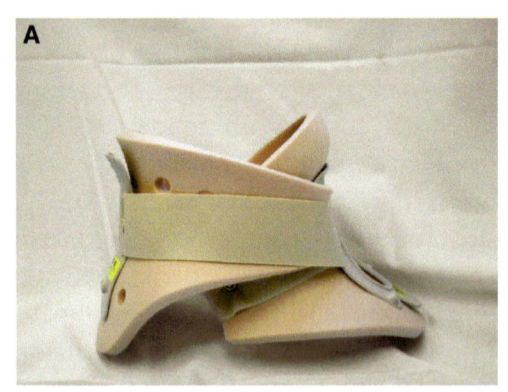

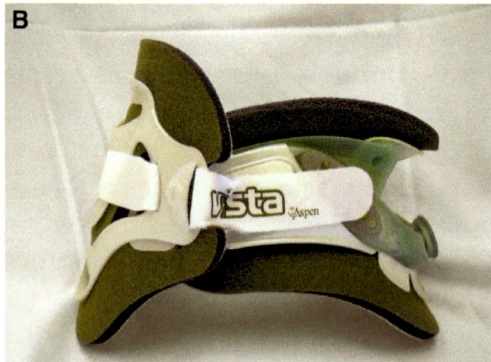

Fig. 8-1 **A,** Philadelphia collar. **B,** Aspen cervical collar.

Table 8-2 Sample Activity for Cervical Precautions

Activity	Physical Requirements	Modifications
Self-feeding	Neck flexion to locate food Neck extension to drink liquid Fine motor coordination	Keep food at arm's reach to avoid looking down Use straws Use curved utensils or those with built-up handles
Shaving	Neck extension, lateral flexion	Use electric razor Use wall-mounted mirror Move skin with fingers to make it taut instead of moving neck
Brushing teeth	Neck flexion	Rinse with a cup or spittoon
Shampooing/combing hair	Neck extension	Use detachable, long-handled showerhead
Donning shirt	Raising arms above 90 degrees	Pull garment over head first; then thread arms Use wide, V-neck, or button-down shirt
Urinating (men)	Neck flexion	Use urinal Sit to urinate Use angled mirror
Talking on the phone	Lateral flexion	Keep elbow elevated at side to prevent head drifting laterally Use earpiece and microphone Use speaker phone

used in patients who have cervical level complications to enable increased occupational performance. Patients who have had cervical operations can also face issues with eating and swallowing that are addressed by both occupational therapists and speech-language pathologists. Occupational therapists typically work on physical capability, bringing the patient's hand to the mouth, manipulating a utensil, and containing spillage, whereas speech-language pathologists usually address the mechanics of the swallow itself. In some facilities, however, occupational therapists who have undergone advanced training also address these issues.

THORACIC AND LUMBAR SURGERY

As with cervical precautions, countless activities are affected during the first 6 to 8 weeks after thoracic or lumbar surgery. The surgeon may indicate that the patient is to be externally braced for postoperative management. The patient is educated regarding self-donning techniques for such braces. Two primary braces are prescribed: a lumbosacral corset and a thoracolumbosacral orthosis, often referred to as a *TLSO* (Fig. 8-2). The precautions associated with this level of surgery include avoiding trunk flexion, extension, and lateral flexion or rotation; limiting all lifting, pushing, or pulling

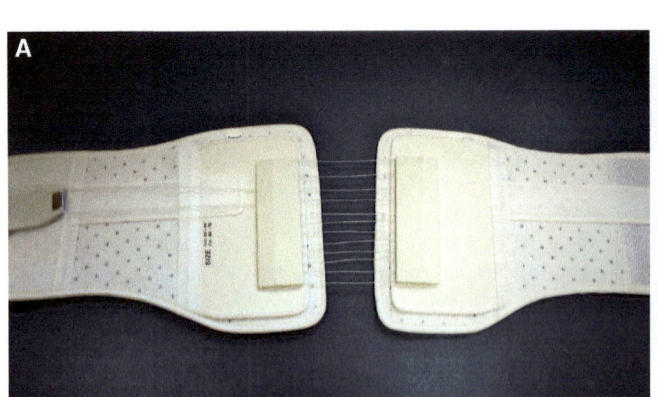

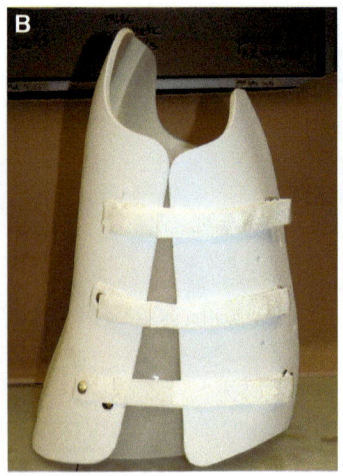

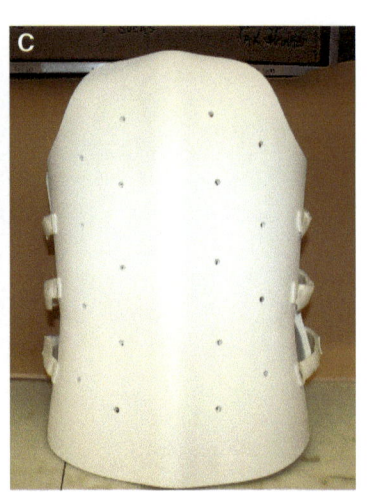

Fig. 8-2 **A,** Cybertech brace. **B,** Lateral view and **C,** posterior view of thoracolumbosacral orthosis.

to less than 5 to 10 pounds, and avoiding sitting for longer than 40 minutes at a time. These precautions have a much greater impact on ADLs involving the lower body, as well as functional mobility. Many people lack the flexibility to put their pants, socks, and shoes on without bending. One strategy is to use the seated cross-legged technique, where the patient sits and brings one foot up over the opposite knee to don the article of clothing while maintaining an upright posture. If the patient is unable to use this maneuver, either the family can assist or the patient can use adaptive equipment to address this need (Fig. 8-3). A reacher is a device that uses a pincer mechanism attached to a long handle to thread pants over the feet and pull them up until the clothing is within arm's reach without the need to bend forward. A reacher can also be used to retrieve lightweight items from the floor or manipulate the environment to facilitate independence while following precautions. Another option for pants is a dressing stick, which entails the use of a long stick with curved ends to manage clothing. For donning socks, patients are commonly provided with a sock aid after surgery. This device works by slipping a sock over a formed surface and then, by holding two long straps, the patient is able to slide the foot in and pull on the straps to remove the device while leaving the sock on the foot. To address shoes and shoelaces, patients can be given a long-handled shoehorn, as well as elastic shoelaces, to prevent the need for tying. Patients who are unable to lift their legs to the edge of the bed are given a leg lifter. To improve safety and allow adherence to thoracic and lumbar spine precautions, occupational therapists usually provide a quick review of daily activities that involve bending, twisting, and lifting and offer techniques that will alter the activity demands to allow success. Some common tasks include getting in and out of a car, going from

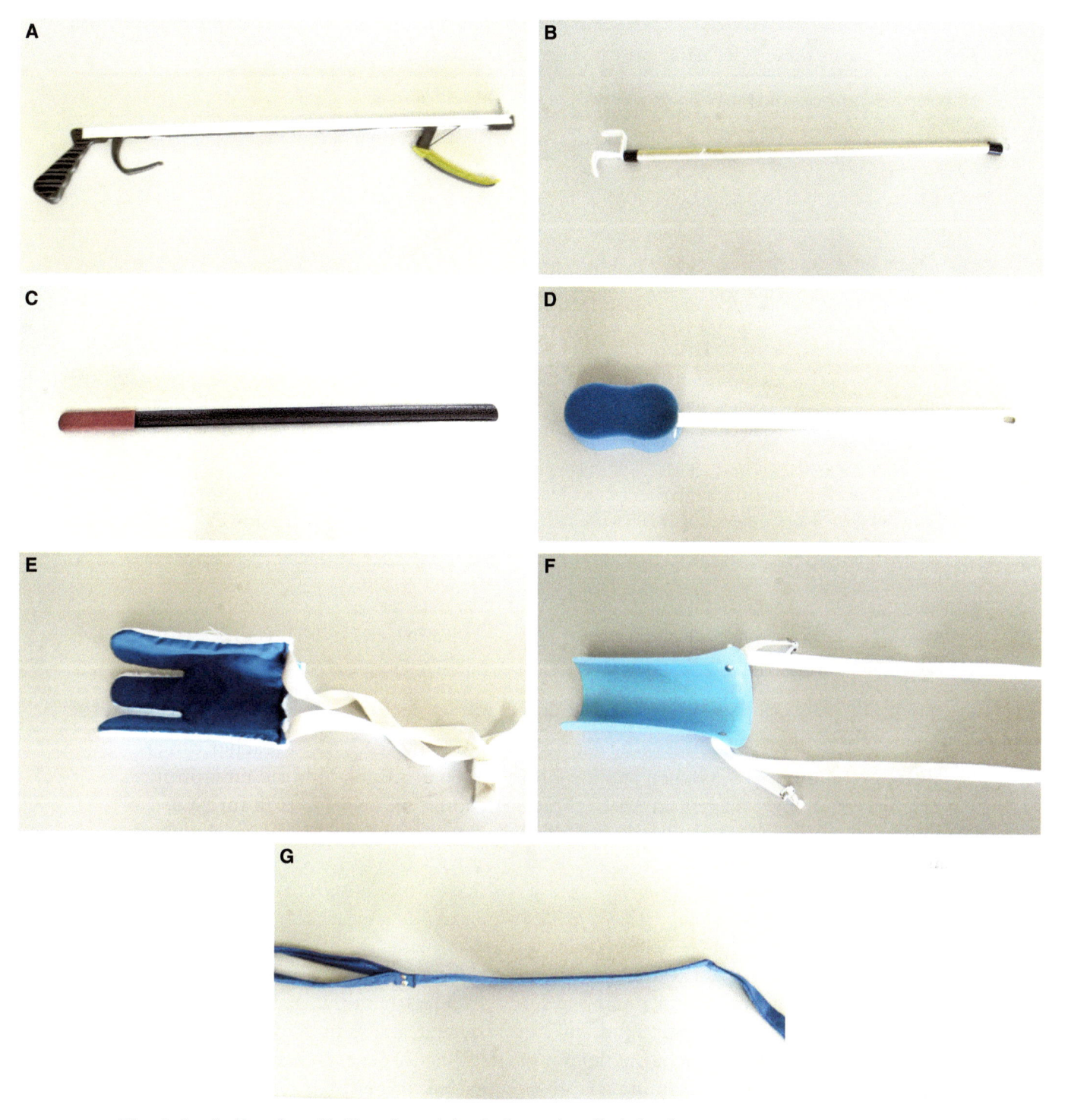

Fig. 8-3 **A,** Reacher. **B,** Dressing stick. **C,** Long-handled shoehorn. **D,** Long-handled sponge. **E,** Soft sock aid. **F,** Hard sock aid. **G,** Leg lifter.

Table 8-3 Sample Activity Analysis for Thoracic/Lumbar Precautions

Activity	Physical Requirements	Modifications
Brushing teeth	Thoracic/lumbar flexion	Rinse with a cup or spittoon Bend at the hips
Lower body dressing	Thoracic/lumbar flexion	Use seated cross-legged technique Use adaptive equipment (see Figs. 8-1, *A*; 8-2, *A* and *C*; 8-3, *A* and *B*)
Lower body bathing	Thoracic/lumbar flexion	Use long-handled sponge Sit on shower chair or tub bench and bring legs up Place soapy washcloth on floor and use reacher to retrieve before exiting shower
Toileting	Thoracic/lumbar flexion Thoracic/lumbar rotation (for some)	Use long-handled toilet aid Stand and bend knees as needed Reach behind back, taking care not to twist Use bidet
Reaching items below waist	Thoracic/lumbar flexion	Bend knees Use reacher Ask for assistance
Reaching object outside of arm's reach	Thoracic/lumbar flexion Thoracic/lumbar rotation	Take a step closer Turn feet and face object Use reacher

sitting to standing and standing to sitting positions, performing light meal preparation, reaching for items on a bottom shelf, cleaning, feeding animals, and picking up pets or children (see Table 8-3 for details and sample activities and modifications that might increase success).

SACRAL SURGERY

Sacral precautions include avoiding trunk flexion, extension, lateral flexion or rotation, limiting all lifting, pushing, or pulling to less than 5 to 10 pounds, avoiding sitting for longer than 40 minutes at a time, and no hip flexion greater than 90 degrees. Coupled with no bending, avoidance of hip flexion greater than 90 degrees mandates that either the family assist or the patient use adaptive equipment to perform all ADLs involving the lower body. These patients also are only able to sit on surfaces high enough to prevent this excessive flexion, including a raised toilet seat. Table 8-4 highlights some common modifications provided during a typical occupational therapy session.

Table 8-4 Sample Activity Analysis for Sacral Precautions

Activity	Physical Requirements	Modifications
Lower body dressing	Thoracic/lumbar flexion	Perform sitting Use adaptive equipment
Lower body bathing	Thoracic/lumbar flexion	Use long-handled sponge Sit on shower chair or tub bench Place soapy washcloth on floor and use reacher to retrieve before exiting shower
Toileting	Thoracic/lumbar flexion Thoracic/lumbar rotation (for some)	Use toilet aid Stand and bend knees as needed Reach behind back, taking care not to twist Use bidet
Reaching items below waist	Thoracic/lumbar flexion	Bend knees Use reacher Ask for assistance
Reaching object outside of arm's reach	Thoracic/lumbar flexion Thoracic/lumbar rotation	Take a step closer Turn feet and face object Use reacher

POTENTIAL POSTOPERATIVE COMPLICATIONS

NEUROLOGIC COMPLICATIONS

Upper motor neuron lesions may be present with tumors involving the spinal cord and peripheral nerves proximal to alpha motor neurons. It is common for the medical team to assess patients for signs of these lesions. The presentation of a lesion will assist in establishing impairments and in measuring prognostic, postoperative recovery. The rehabilitation team works in tandem with the medical team to track the progression and waning of upper motor lesions to establish functional gains in active motor control and functional rehabilitation potential.

Motor Function

After surgery, patients may regain lost motor function. The role of occupational therapists and physical therapists is to facilitate this recovery through strengthening exercises and education on proper joint alignment for functional use. During treatment sessions, therapists place their patients in positions or postures that will compensate for the loss and facilitate functional movements.

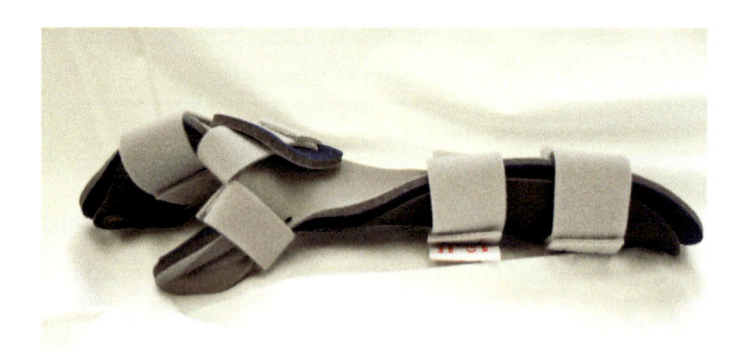

Fig. 8-4 Resting hand splint.

Postoperative patients may lose motor control distal to the level of surgical intervention. This loss of function may be unilateral or bilateral in presentation. The spinal level of impairment may be different on each side of the body. It may become necessary to offer these patients adaptive equipment or bracing to safely accommodate the desired activity.

Upper Extremity Bracing
A variety of upper extremity orthotics are available after injury. The most effective and applicable devices are those that offer the greatest joint approximation while allowing functional weight-bearing and use of the affected/impaired extremity. If the extremity has no active facilitation, joint integrity is imperative to maintain. The glenohumeral joint must not be permitted to subluxate, and appropriate positioning to eliminate impairment is warranted. Finally, placing a resting hand splint to the distal upper extremity bracing the forearm and wrist will maintain the arches of the hand (Fig. 8-4). The intent of all orthotic bracing is to maximize the functional position of the extremity in an attempt to regain functional recovery.

Lower Extremity Bracing
A variety of orthotic devices are available to control paretic lower extremity function. Often the orthosis is intended to maximize functional independence, but the device may also limit functional progression. The orthosis is named by the most proximal joint and distal contribution. For example, any device that controls movement of the knee, ankle, and foot is simply referred to as a knee-ankle-foot orthosis (KAFO). An ankle-foot orthosis (AFO) is the most commonly prescribed orthotic device (Fig. 8-5). The AFO offers ankle control, stability for joint protection in ambulation, and potentially facilitates mobility. On the contrary, the AFO may alter limb mechanics of gait, diminish ground reaction forces and afferent input, and inhibit responses to sensory input. Ultimately, the use of an AFO depends on the clinical judgment of the physical therapist as it pertains to patient function and safety.

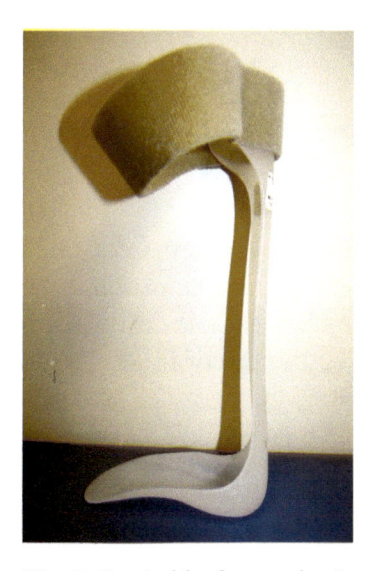

Fig. 8-5 Ankle-foot orthosis.

Sensory Considerations

Postoperative patients may lose sensation distal to the level of surgical intervention. Because of the anatomy of the spinal tracts, light touch and deep pressure lie on separate tracts from pain and temperature. The distinct assessment and separation of these tracts on examination will assist in assessing functional recovery and teaching of compensatory strategies. Patients who lack sensations for light touch and deep pressure may have characteristics similar to those of patients with proprioceptive deficits. These patients may appear to ambulate or perform ADLs with dysmetric and ataxic movements. Compensatory strategies may be necessary to educate these patients with regard to their safety. For patients who lack pain and temperature sensation, the therapist will need to educate them in terms of safely accommodating for their deficits. Such strategies include assessing the temperature of bath water with the nonaffected extremity before placing the affected extremity in the water to avoid burning the skin. Those patients who lack pain awareness must be educated to regularly assess the skin for breakdown and potential noxious stimuli in the environment that may cause a potential lesion.

Proprioception

Similar to the reflex loop, proprioceptive deficits may be present after surgical intervention. Golgi tendon organs are located at the junction of the tendon and the skeletal muscle and contribute to a feedback loop that identifies physical awareness in space. A feedback control system exists between the gamma motor neuron, the 1b afferent fibers, and the intrafusal muscle fibers.[19] A disruption of this system creates a lack of awareness of the upper or lower extremities in movement. A patient will often present with ataxic or dysmetric movements that appear uncoordinated, inaccurate, or clumsy. If a patient has proprioceptive deficits, the rehabilitation team will educate the patient with regard to awareness of the extremity in space. Strategies to promote awareness include visual attention to the task and extremity approximation, target practice that includes space and cadence sequencing, and distal extremity weighting that offers rhythmic damper of tremor.[8,20]

Coordination

Coordination deficits are common in patients with neurologic impairment and may involve impaired sequencing and timing that can interfere with successful performance of ADLs and mobility. Exercises can be demonstrated that address dexterity and control, along with modifications to the environment, to facilitate success.

Reflexes

Postsurgical intervention may disrupt signals relayed to the upper motor neurons within the spinal cord. A feedback control system between the alpha motor neuron, 1a afferent fibers, and the muscle spindle may be impaired and cause hyporeflexia or hyperreflexia.[19] Hyporeflexia or hyperreflexia may cause impairments in ADLs, functional transfers, and gait progression. These symptoms typically wax and wane depending on surgical recovery, disease progression, medication cycle, level of fatigue, or active muscular facilitation. It is important that patients become cognizant of any fluctuation in reflexes to ensure functional safety. When reflexive deficits arise, patients must realize it may be unsafe to perform ADLs, functional transfers, and gait progression. The rehabilitation team must educate these patients on signs and symptoms of hyporeflexia or hyperreflexia to ensure safe functional activity for them.

Tone

Spasticity is a motor disorder that is characterized by a velocity-dependent increase in tonic stretch reflexes (muscle tone) with exaggerated tendon jerks, resulting from hyperexcitability of the stretch reflex, as one component of upper motor neuron syndrome. Spastic musculature may be beneficial or detrimental postoperatively. Potential side effects may include limits to range of motion, pain, interference with ADLs, effects on posture and positioning, skin breakdown, and disorders with movement and functional mobility. When movement disorders are identified, it is the role of the interdisciplinary team, including the physician, pharmacist, nurse, rehabilitation team, patient, and family/caregivers, to establish appropriate interventions and a treatment plan. When hypotonicity or hypertonicity is present, it is the goal of the rehabilitation team to identify appropriate intervention to maximize ROM and minimize muscle contractures. ROM programs, whether passive movements performed by the caregiver or active therapeutic exercises, are essential to maintain viable muscle tensile mobility. In extreme cases the rehabilitation team may recommend splinting joints in resting positions to prevent pain and skin breakdown and maximize functional activity. Ultimately, the rehabilitation therapists work in concert with the nursing and medical teams to promote functional active ROM.

Continence Disorders

Loss of bladder and bowel control accompanies sacral level injuries and is a problem that affects a significant number of patients undergoing spine surgery. In one study 56% of patients preoperatively demonstrated continence dysfunction.[21] This signifies the pervasiveness of these disorders, which can be especially devastating because feelings of shame and embarrassment often interfere with social interactions. Symptoms can range from frequent urges and mild leaks to full loss of control. Occupational and physical therapists commonly educate patients on exercises that strengthen core muscle groups, including the pelvic floor (Kegel exercises), abdominal wall, and lumbar musculature. If the problem centers around frequent urges, use of timed voiding can be helpful. Patients who are unable to completely empty their bladders are at increased risk for urinary tract infections and therefore may benefit from keeping a voiding diary or voiding on a timed schedule. A timed voiding schedule for bowel control is standard practice in rehabilitation. It is recommended that a regular voiding schedule be established. Patients who are unable to establish a regular bowel program are at increased risk for medical complications. One complication is constipation, which can lead to further medical complications, such as fecal impaction, hemorrhoids, and small bowel obstruction. An additional complication is frequency of loose stools, which can lead to impaired skin integrity, public embarrassment, and possible dehydration. Some basic adaptations that can assist patients in addressing mild urinary and fecal incontinence include use of incontinence pads, adult diapers, or less restrictive clothing, as well as strategies for eliminating odors. If mobility is a constraint, placing a commode or urinal within reach can add to success. When in public, locating the nearest restroom or sitting close to one can help ease the anxiety that often accompanies incontinence. In severe cases patients will be required to self-catheterize or rely on family members who have been trained to assist with this task. For fecal incontinence, education on diet, suppositories, laxatives, and medication may help to regulate the bowels.

Sexual Dysfunction

Sexual dysfunction is caused by a combination of sensory and motor complications resulting from the interrelationship between the sympathetic and parasympathetic nervous systems, with a compromising tumor or spinal impairment. Although both men and women can have impaired function, these impairments will have significantly different psychological and social effects, depending on individual life roles, expectations, and goals. It is necessary to address each person at the time of the initial injury. In some cases, life roles, expectations, and goals may change, and the projection or speculation of future life goals may be appropriate to address. It may be outside the scope of the rehabilitation team to address these goals, and referral to a rehabilitation psychologist or social worker may be indicated.

Male Response

When bowel and bladder function is compromised, sexual dysfunction is often impaired. Erectile dysfunction is often greater in upper motor neuron and incomplete lesions. This is important to consider in the scope of this chapter, with regard to spine tumors and level or invasiveness of disease. Ejaculatory dysfunction is greater in lower motor neuron and incomplete lesions. Unfortunately, because of the conflicting erectile and ejaculation injury location, procreation may be difficult through sexual intercourse. It is indicated that the rehabilitation team educate men in the early disease progression to acquire seminal fluid and sperm samples when children and procreation are life goals.

Female Response

There is little research on postinjury responses in women. It has been speculated that the reason for this is that fertility is rarely affected. Recent studies have shown that women respond similarly to men, with regard to sexual injury, with diminished engorgement of the labia and clitoris.[22] Conception and pregnancy remain possible after spinal injury in women. Childbirth and uterine contractions will be present because of hormone control, but the mother may not be able to offer active facilitation of the abdominal wall to forcefully deliver the child, and a cesarean-type surgical intervention may be necessary for a safe birth. The rehabilitation team may offer female patients suggestions for appropriate lubrication for comfort, skin integrity, and partner pleasure. Postpartum education of pelvic floor and abdominal musculature integrity may be indicated to promote functional posture and sitting balance.

Integument

After surgical intervention for a spine tumor, patients may have decreased ability to mobilize in bed, leading to increased pressure and skin breakdown at bony prominences. The rehabilitation team and nursing staff must collaborate with these patients to ensure changes in position every 1 to 2 hours when the patient is in bed. Postoperative spine precautions state that the patient should reposition every 40 minutes to avoid ischemia at the surgical site. Physical therapists and occupational therapists educate patients and their families about pressure relief when a patient is in bed or sitting and adaptive seating for patients in wheelchairs. Specialized boots that relieve pressure from the heels can also be used to assist in prevention of skin breakdown (Fig. 8-6).

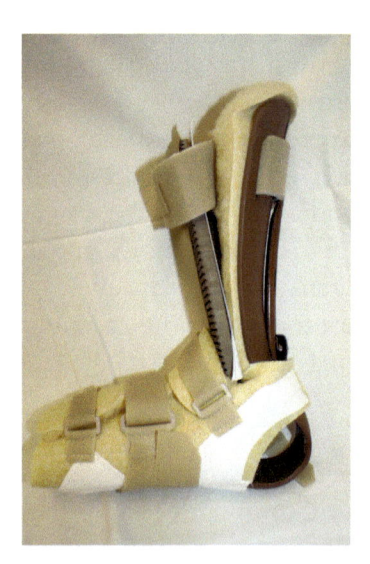

Fig. 8-6 Multipodus boot.

Deep Venous Thrombosis

According to the "Surgeon General's Call to Action to Prevent Deep Vein Thrombosis and Pulmonary Embolism," more than 350,000 individuals are affected by deep venous thrombosis (DVT) and/or pulmonary embolisms each year. DVT is a postsurgical complication that can have a negative impact on functional mobility and activity. Signs and symptoms of DVT include pain, shiny skin, decreased palpable pulse, edema, redness, and purple skin. Part of the role of the rehabilitative team in the inpatient setting is to identify listed signs and symptoms and notify appropriate hospital staff. The rehabilitative team plays an integral role in limiting the risk of DVT through active movement. Active movement is the body's natural way of circulating blood and preventing venous stasis. Physical and occupational therapists will educate patients about therapeutic activity. In immobile patients, or in patients with limited mobility, placement of a sequential compressive device is recommended. For patients with a diagnosis of DVT, most surgeons will order pharmaceutical management and may ask for the rehabilitation team to postpone therapy until the international normalized ratio, prothrombin time, and partial thromboplastin time are within a therapeutic range. A complication such as DVT may decrease functional progression with therapy, cause pain that limits patient activity, and place patients at increased risk for additional complications, including pulmonary embolism.

Orthostasis

One potential side effect of early mobilization is orthostatic hypotension. Orthostatic hypotension is a rapid decrease in systolic blood pressure when transitioning to a sitting or standing position. Signs and symptoms often include dizziness, light-headedness, blurred vision, numbness, tingling, and vasovagal syncope. The primary cause is blood pooling in the skeletal muscles of the lower extremities and the abdominal cavity. Education concerning lower extremity muscle facilitation of ankle pumps and deep breathing initiates the venous return of blood supply. Secondary causes in postsurgical patients may be the result of blood loss, postsurgical anesthesia, and multiple medications. If active muscle facilitation and deep breathing do not counter the orthostatic hypotension, the patient should be returned to a supine or semireclined position to avoid episodes of syncope and risk of injury. Ultimately, it remains the goal of the rehabilitation team to improve patient mobility. Many noninvasive therapeutic interventions are possible to manage blood pressure. Physical and occupational therapists may recommend compression stockings or therapeutic Ace bandages to promote circulation and abdominal binding to reduce blood pooling and venous stasis. In patients with severe orthostasis, a gradual increase in upright posturing with the aid of a hospital bed or tilt table is indicated to further improve the patient. Ultimately, upright positioning of the postoperative patient is indicated to achieve the greatest functional gains.

Psychological Factors

Many patients also exhibit psychosocial symptoms, such as depression, anxiety, and confusion, as they try to adjust to changes in their functional abilities, including maintaining familial and community connections, as well as possible end-of-life issues.[16,23] These emotions must be addressed early in the recovery process because, if left unchecked, they can progress to social isolation and further diminish a patient's quality of life. The National Comprehensive Cancer Network recognizes that life-threatening illness affects all aspects of life. Advanced training in the area of daily life qualifies occupational and physical therapists to assist patients in managing the wide-ranging effects of disease and overcoming or adjusting to these limitations to preserve quality of life and functional participation. Education regarding available support groups is the first step. Many of these patients need to reach out for help. Asking for help and delegating tasks can be difficult for those who have been fiercely independent or are used to running the household; therefore providing techniques that help patients adjust to these needs is a vital part of rehabilitation. Often medications prescribed by physicians that target anxiety and depression can be beneficial in maintaining a patient's ability to participate in rehabilitation. Alternative methods that may offer some relief with regard to psychosocial issues include meditation, guided imagery, and use of scented candles. Education regarding positive self-image is important for many people, especially those facing complications from chemotherapy.

SIGNATURE CASE

A 59-year-old woman initially was seen by a chiropractor with a complaint of neck pain that had lasted for a period of several weeks. The chiropractor felt a mass and ordered a CT scan, which showed a neck mass involving the C4 vertebral body, consistent with chordoma. The subsequent diagnosis was a massive cervical chordoma involving C2-7, and the patient was scheduled for two-stage spine surgery. The first stage involved an occiput-to-T3 fusion through a transpedicular approach, with a posterior spinal osteotomy at C3-6, vertebral artery mobilization bilaterally from C2-7, nerve root rhizotomy bilaterally at C4 and right C5, nerve neurolysis of C3-6, and laminectomy for an extradural tumor at C2-T1. Eight days later, the patient returned to the operating room for an anterior spine fusion of C2-7, anterior cervical cage placement at C2-7, anterior spinal osteotomy at C3-6, anterior spinal corpectomy for tumor at C3-6 and en bloc resection, vertebral artery skeletonization, and mobilization, and C2-3 and C6-7 discectomies. The hospital course was complicated by respiratory failure requiring a tracheostomy, methicillin-sensitive *Staphylococcus aureus*, ventilator-associated pneumonia, and *Escherichia coli* urinary tract infection with sepsis. The patient's tracheostomy was successfully capped, but approximately 3 weeks after the second surgery she developed respiratory distress secondary to bleeding from the tracheostomy site, with aspiration prompting a return to the intensive care unit, where she was placed on a ventilator.

A physical therapist was initially consulted on postoperative day 10, and on day 11 the patient was seen by an occupational therapist who prescribed bed rest, the wearing of a Miami J collar (Fig. 8-7) at all times for 6 months, and cervical spine precautions of no neck flexion, extension, or rotation, no lifting, pushing, or pulling more than 10 pounds, and no shoulder flexion greater than 90 degrees. The patient was evaluated by a physical therapist and an occupational therapist in the intensive care unit; she was

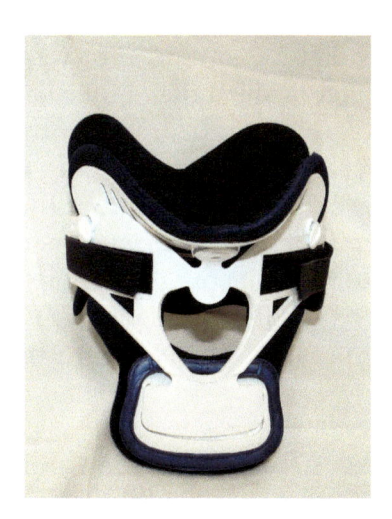

Fig. 8-7 Miami J collar.

communicating with eye blinks, distal hand gestures, and mouthing words because of her inability to speak as a result of the tracheostomy and diffuse bilateral upper extremity weakness, which limited her to writing and the use of a communication board.

Before admission, the patient was living with her husband and was completely independent in terms of functional mobility, ADLs, and independent ADLs. At the time of the initial evaluation, she was alert, oriented, dependent on two persons for bed mobility, including rolling and scooting, required maximum assistance for all ADLs, and reported no pain. The patient had full passive ROM in the bilateral upper extremities within the confines of cervical precautions. A manual muscle test produced the following results: bilateral shoulder flexion/extension 0 to 1/5, bilateral shoulder abduction 0 to 1/5, right shoulder adduction 2+/5, left shoulder adduction 2/5, right biceps 2+/5, left biceps 2/5, bilateral triceps 2+/5, bilateral supination/pronation 3/5, bilateral wrist extension 3+/5, bilateral digital flexion/extension 3/5, bilateral lower extremities proximal weakness noted in hip flexion 3+/5, hip abduction 3/5, hip extension and adduction 4/5, and knee, ankle, and extensor hallucis longus 5/5. No abnormal tone or clonus was noted, and sensation was intact to light touch in the bilateral upper and lower extremities.

Throughout this initial evaluation, vital signs (heart rate, arterial blood pressure, and oxygen saturation) were stable, and the patient had no pain. Physical therapy and occupational therapy assessments noted that postoperative upper extremity weakness was limiting the patient's ability to perform ADLs, whereas proximal weakness at the hips was anticipated to affect balance and mobility once she was out of bed. A plan of care was established to continue treatment for therapeutic activities, mobility progression when she was taken off of bed rest, and retraining for ADLs. Frequency was set at three to five therapeutic treatment sessions per week while she was on bed rest, progressing to once daily when her activity level was upgraded to activity out of bed. The recommendation was discharge to an acute rehabilitation center to improve functional independence before discharge home.

The patient was seen five to seven times a week for a total of 5 weeks by occupational and physical therapists during her hospital stay. Three days after the initial evaluation, the patient was cleared for activity out of bed, and mobility status included supine to sitting with moderate assistance and sitting to standing and two steps to a chair with moderate assistance from two persons. Throughout the hospital stay, rehabilitation treatments were limited by episodes of hypertension, tachycardia, and oxygen desaturation with activity, fatigue from sleeping poorly, left shoulder subluxation, pain, psychosocial issues, and various medical procedures. The patient's communication progressed to writing and eventually to speech once the tracheostomy was capped with a Passy-Muir valve.

Physical therapy interventions provided education about bilateral lower extremity therapeutic exercises in supine, sitting, and standing positions, including handouts for compliance with the program. Functional mobility training, progressing from bed level to edge-of-bed transfers was introduced in compliance with spinal precautions. The physical therapist educated the patient on environmental modifications to allow for successful mobility and safety, such as altering seat height and energy conservation and pacing techniques, including the use of a rate of perceived exertion (RPE) journal. Gait training focused on balance, cadence, stride length, step length, proper weight shifting for contralateral limb advancement, initial contact with heel strike, and use of assistive devices, including a front-wheeled walker and a single-point cane.

Occupational therapy treatment focused on upper extremity function, including passive and active assistive ROM, participation in ADLs, progressing from bed level to sitting to standing, with the use of adaptive devices, as needed, and functional mobility. The patient was educated on bilateral upper extremity therapeutic exercises to be performed outside of the treatment sessions, alone and with family assistance, cervical precautions as they applied to ADLs, functional mobility and safety, adaptive equipment for ADLs and provision of same, positioning and handling of the left upper extremity because of shoulder subluxation, as well as proper fitting of a GivMohr sling (GivMohr Corp., Albuquerque, NM), diaphragmatic breathing during activity, and energy conservation techniques because of overall deconditioning. The patient's home environment was reviewed and simulated, and suggestions were made to increase safety, including use of a 3-in-1 commode in the bathroom.

On occupational and physical therapy reassessment 1 month after the initial evaluation, the patient was performing grooming and hygiene with minimum assistance, upper extremities were supported with minimum assistance, upper body dressing including cervical collar with moderate assistance, lower body bathing, dressing, and toileting were performed independently, the patient was ambulating independently for 300 feet with a single-point cane and rest breaks, maintaining cervical precautions during all activities without cues, and performing all prescribed upper and lower extremities without difficulty. A manual muscle test revealed the following scores: right shoulder 2/5, left shoulder 1/5, bilateral biceps/triceps 3/5, bilateral grip 4/5, and bilateral lower extremities 4/5 to 5/5 throughout.

Because of these significant functional gains, discharge recommendations were changed to home with family, a 3-in-1 commode, and follow-up outpatient occupational and physical therapy to continue strength and endurance training, along with retraining in ADLs and independent ADLs, high-level balance activities, and advanced functional mobility training. Forty-eight days after the patient was admitted to the hospital, she was discharged home with family.

CONCLUSION

Collaboration between all team members is vital for a successful outcome. Use of physical and occupational therapy specialists postoperatively improves functional outcomes and significantly affects neurologic recovery. Through intensive training, therapeutic exercises, environmental modifications, activity analysis, and adaptations, physical therapists and occupational therapists offer patients the opportunity to improve function. Rehabilitation plays a valuable role in the recovery of patients after spine surgery by providing them with the skills they need to regain independence and participate fully in life.

TIPS FROM THE MASTERS

A physical or occupational therapist should:
- Be proactive, concise with evaluation, and creative with interventions.
- Be positive and optimistic with postsurgical management.
- Collaborate with all team members.
- Engage and empower the patient, family members, and caregivers.

References (With Key References in Boldface)

1. Abrahm JL, Banffy MB, Harris MB. Spinal cord compression in patients with advanced metastatic cancer. JAMA 299:937-946, 2008.
2. **Thomas CL, ed. Taber's Cyclopedic Medical Dictionary. Philadelphia: FA Davis, 1981.**
3. Ruff RL, Ruff SS, Wang X. Persistent benefits of rehabilitation on pain and life quality for nonambulatory patients with spinal epidural metastasis. J Rehabil Res Dev 44:271-278, 2007.
4. **Tang V, Garvey D, Dorsay JP, et al. Prognostic indicators in metastatic spinal cord compression: using functional independence measure and Tokuhashi scale to optimize rehabilitation planning. Spinal Cord 45:671-677, 2007.**
5. Today's Physical Therapist: A Comprehensive Review of a 21st Century Health Care Professional. Prepared by the American Physical Therapy Association I, January 2011. Available at *www.apta.org*.
6. Guide to Physical Therapist Practice, 2nd ed. Alexandria, VA: American Physical Therapy Association, 2001.
7. American Spinal Injury Association (ASIA). International Standards for Neurological Classification of Spinal Cord Injury. Atlanta, GA: American Spinal Injury Association, 2002.
8. Hirsh MA, Toole T, Maitland C, et al. The effects of balance training and high-density resistance training on persons with idiopathic Parkinson's disease. Arch Phys Med Rehabil 84:1009-1017, 2003.

9. Van Peppen RPS, Kwakkel G, Wood-Dauphinee S, et al. The impact of physical therapy on functional outcomes after stroke: what's the evidence? Clin Rehabil 18:833-862, 2004.
10. Sullivan KJ, Knowlton BJ, Dobkin BH. Step training with body weight support: effect of treadmill speed and practice paradigms on poststroke locomotor recovery. Arch Phys Med Rehabil 83:683-691, 2002.
11. Behrman AL, Bowden MG, Nair PM. Neuroplasticity after spinal cord injury and training: an emerging paradigm shift in rehabilitation and walking recovery. Phys Ther 86:1406-1425, 2006.
12. Sherrington CS. On the proprioceptive system, especially in its reflex aspect. Brain 29:467-485, 1907.
13. American Occupational Therapy Association. The Occupational Therapy Practice Framework: Domain and Process, 2nd ed (Framework-II). American Journal of Occupational Therapy, Vol. 62, No. 6, November/December 2008.
14. Crepeau EB, Cohn ES, Boyt Schell BA. Willard and Spackman's Occupational Therapy, 10th ed. Philadelphia: Lippincott Williams & Wilkins, 2003.
15. Watson DE, Wilson SA. Task Analysis: An Individual and Population Approach, 2nd ed. American Occupational Therapy Association, 2003.
16. Pedretti LW, Pendleton HM, Schultz-Krohn W. Pedretti's Occupational Therapy Practice Skills for Physical Dysfunction, 6th ed. St Louis: Mosby/Elsevier, 2006.
17. **Conway R, Graham J, Kidd J; Scottish Cord Compression Group. What happens to people after malignant cord compression? Survival, function, quality of life, emotional well-being and place of care 1 month after diagnosis. Clin Oncol 19:56-62, 2007.**
18. World Federation of Occupational Therapists, online forum. Available at *http://www.wfot.org*.
19. Bear MF, Connors BW. Neuroscience: Exploring the Brain, 2nd ed. New York: Lippincott Williams & Wilkins, 2001.
20. Morris M. Movement disorders in people with Parkinson's disease: a model for physical therapy. Phys Ther 80:578-597, 2000.
21. Schoeggl A, Reddy M, Matula C. Neurological outcome following laminectomy in spinal metastases. Nature 40:363-366, 2002.
22. O'Sullivan SB, Schmitz TJ. Physical Rehabilitation: Assessment and Treatment, 5th ed. Philadelphia: FA Davis, 2007.
23. **Guo Y, Young B, Palmer JL, et al. Prognostic factors for survival in metastatic spinal cord compression: a retrospective study in a rehabilitation setting. Am J Phys Med Rehabil 82:665-668, 2003.**

Chapter 9

Speech and Swallow Management

Sara G. Bennett, Jennifer Moore

The overall objective of swallow management is to optimize a person's ability to swallow safely, thereby improving quality of life. It includes the evaluation and treatment of swallowing disorders to ensure safe oral feeding or determine the need for alternative means of nutrition in patients with dysphagia. Dysphagia is defined as difficulty moving food or liquids from the oral cavity to the stomach. It is generally the result of an underlying disease that is commonly neurogenic or mechanical in origin.[1,2] Swallowing problems may involve the oral, pharyngeal, and/or esophageal phases of the swallow.[1] In patients with cervical spine and spinal cord tumors, the swallowing disorder is often pharyngeal or esophageal in nature, and a disturbance to these phases of the swallow can result in impaired transfer of the bolus from the oral cavity to the stomach, with the risk of misdirection of food, liquid, or secretions into the airway.

Patients with cervical spine and spinal cord tumors often have dysphagia both preoperatively and postoperatively. A spine tumor that impinges on the pharynx or esophagus may result in dysphagia, including difficulty managing secretions and oral intake and odynophagia. In patients undergoing spine tumor resection, dysphagia may occur during recovery. Postoperatively dysphagia may be caused by pharyngeal or laryngeal edema or injury from surgery and/or intubation, cranial nerve damage, or overall deconditioning of the swallow. The goal of dysphagia therapy is to optimize swallow function and improve the quality of life in these patients.

OROPHARYNGEAL SWALLOW

To simplify the act of deglutition, swallowing has often been described in the following four stages: oral preparatory, oral transit, pharyngeal, and esophageal.[1,3]

ORAL PREPARATORY PHASE

The oral preparatory phase is the initial phase of the swallow in which food is mixed with saliva, and the necessary mastication occurs for a consistency to be swallowed. There is no time frame for this phase of the swallow, and the swallow can be voluntarily stopped during this phase. During oral preparation, a labial seal prevents material from spilling out of the oral cavity. The strength and tension of the buccal muscles prevent food particles from falling into the buccal cavity. Rotary tongue and jaw movements occur, and material is pulled into a cohesive bolus and held between the surfaces of the tongue and the hard palate. During this time the larynx is at rest, the airway is open, and nasal breathing occurs.[1-3]

ORAL TRANSIT PHASE

The oral transit phase begins once the bolus has been moved posteriorly, by the tongue, from the anterior oral cavity to the faucial pillars. The tongue movement has been described as an anterior-to-posterior rolling action of the midline of the tongue; the elevation and posterior movement of the tongue move the bolus backward. The sides of the tongue are secured on the alveolar ridge, and the tongue forms a central chute to allow food to move posteriorly. The pressure of the tongue increases with the viscosity of the bolus; more viscous consistencies require increased strength to move the bolus. The duration of this phase ranges from less than 1 second to 1½ seconds. The duration increases as bolus viscosity increases.

When the bolus travels to the level between the anterior faucial arches and the ramus of the mandible, the oral transit of the swallow is completed and the pharyngeal phase of the swallow is initiated.[1]

PHARYNGEAL PHASE

During the pharyngeal phase of the swallow, the bolus passes through the pharynx to the opening of the esophagus. This phase of the swallow is involuntary. Coordination of swallowing and respiration must occur because respiration halts during this phase. This phase is initiated when the bolus reaches the point where the mandible crosses the tongue base. In elderly patients presbyphagia may occur in which normal delays resulting from aging may allow the bolus to fill the valleculae before triggering the pharyngeal swallow.[1] The following is a list of the main components of a normal pharyngeal phase of the swallow[1,3]:

1. Velar elevation to allow closure of the velopharyngeal port and prevent food or liquid from entering the nasal cavity.
2. Elevation and anterior movement of the hyoid bone and larynx. The larynx and hyoid bone elevate and move anteriorly by the contraction of the floor of the mouth muscles.
3. Laryngeal closure at the following three levels: (1) the true vocal cords, (2) the false cords, and (3) the anterior movement of the arytenoids to the epiglottis, closing the larynx in an anterior/posterior manner. When the larynx has elevated to approximately 50% of the highest elevation, vocal cord closure is completed.[1,4]

4. Base of tongue retraction and pharyngeal wall contraction. The base of the tongue makes complete contact with the pharyngeal wall during the swallow, which builds pressure and allows for bolus propulsion down the pharynx.
5. Cricopharyngeal relaxation to allow the bolus to pass from the pharynx to the esophagus.

Esophageal Phase

The esophageal phase of the swallow begins once the bolus has passed through the cricopharyngeus and into the esophagus. Consultation with a gastroenterologist is recommended to further assess this phase of the swallow, which is usually managed medically or surgically.

ASSESSMENT OF DYSPHAGIA

The speech-language pathologist has an important role in evaluating and managing dysphagia resulting from cervical spine tumors. When dysphagia is not diagnosed or treated, the patient may be at risk for aspiration, malnutrition, and/or dehydration. A swallow assessment will help determine whether the patient is able to safely maintain oral feeding and whether there is a need for an alternative means of nutrition.

A swallow assessment should be ordered when the patient is medically stable and able to maintain adequate alertness to participate in feeding trials. Once the referral is received, the speech-language pathologist will conduct a clinical evaluation of swallowing to determine the safety of the patient's oral intake. A treatment plan is developed according to the results of the assessment. This will include dietary recommendations or further instrumental testing as appropriate.

The speech-language pathologist will begin the assessment process with a clinical evaluation to determine whether the patient is exhibiting signs of an oropharyngeal dysphagia and whether an instrumental assessment is indicated. Speech-language pathologists typically use one of two types of instrumental evaluations, a modified barium swallow study (MBSS) or a fiberoptic endoscopic evaluation of swallowing (FEES).[5-7]

CLINICAL EVALUATION OF SWALLOWING

The clinical evaluation of swallowing is an assessment performed at bedside to determine the presence or absence of a swallowing disorder. The evaluation will determine the possible cause of the dysphagia, the risk of aspiration, and the need for an alternative means of nutrition or dietary modifications. This initial evaluation will allow the clinician to recommend additional assessments, as appropriate, to further evaluate the oropharyngeal swallow, such as the MBSS or the FEES.[1,5]

The speech-language pathologist will begin the assessment with a medical history and clinical observations. The clinician will also take note of the patient's vital signs, respiratory status, and ability to manage oropharyngeal secretions. Patients with oral and/or pharyngeal swallowing disorders may have decreased secretion management requiring frequent oral hygiene and suctioning.

The clinical examination will include an oral-motor examination and a laryngeal function examination. This includes assessment of strength, range of motion, and rate of labial, lingual, and velar structure. The clinician will assess the patient's vocal quality and ability to protect the airway by coughing and clearing the throat. Once the anatomic evaluation is complete, the clinician will begin the functional assessment. Depending on the patient's ability to swallow, the clinician will present substances with various consistencies, which can include the following:

1. Ice chips
2. Water
3. Nectar-thick liquid
4. Honey-thick liquid
5. Puree
6. Ground/soft solids
7. Regular solids

The speech-language pathologist will assess the patient's oral preparation of the bolus. During the swallow, the clinician will assess the timing of the pharyngeal swallow and laryngeal elevation while observing the patient for clinical signs of aspiration, such as coughing, throat clearing, increased work of breathing, and/or a wet vocal quality. The clinician must take into consideration the possibility of silent aspiration, in which outward signs of aspiration, such as coughing, are not demonstrated. Research has shown that silent aspiration may be associated with central or local weakness, in coordination of the pharyngeal musculature, reduced laryngopharyngeal sensation, and impaired ability to produce a reflexive cough.[8]

MODIFIED BARIUM SWALLOW STUDY

The MBSS is a videofluoroscopic procedure that is used to assess the oropharyngeal swallow (Figs. 9-1 and 9-2).[1,7] Given the limitations of a clinical swallow evaluation, the MBSS is an instrumental examination that identifies oropharyngeal dysphagia by allowing the viewing of a bolus in relation to structural movement throughout the oropharynx in real time.[9] The MBSS is completed in collaboration with a radiologist and a speech-language pathologist. Images are observed in lateral and anteroposterior views. The MBSS evaluates the oropharyngeal swallow before, during, and after the swallow to determine the nature of a swallow disorder and the presence or absence of penetration or aspiration.[7] During the study the clinician evaluates postural modifications, swallowing maneuvers, bolus modifications, and sensory enhancements.[1] The MBSS enables the clinician to identify normal and abnormal anatomy and physiology of the swallow to determine appropriate therapeutic techniques for oral, pharyngeal, and laryngeal disorders. The speech-language pathologist will present a representative variety of barium consistencies to reach conclusions about the state of a patient's swallowing and safety for oral intake.

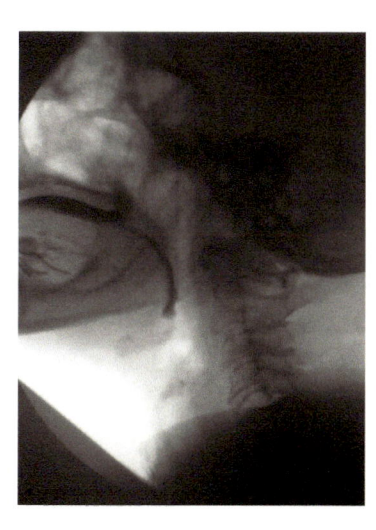

Fig. 9-1 Radiographic view of modified barium swallow study.

Fig. 9-2 Radiology suite for modified barium swallow study.

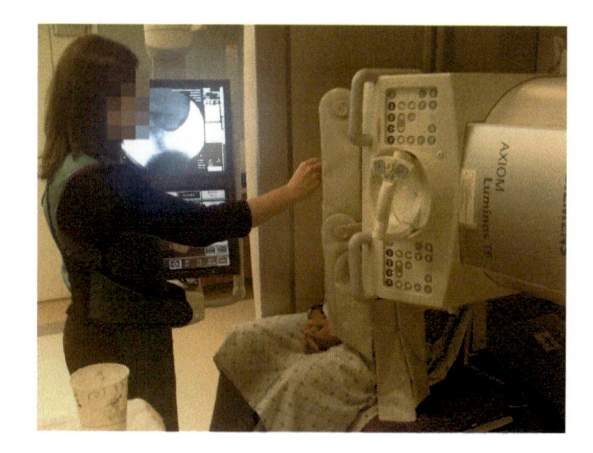

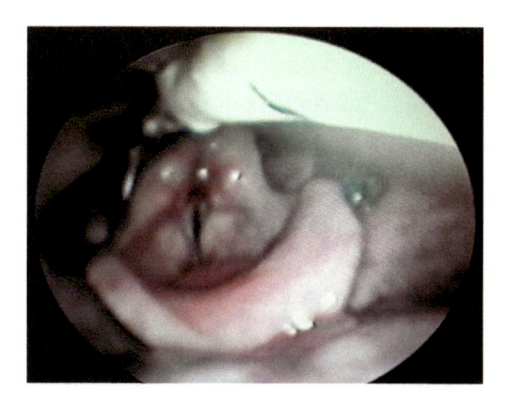

Fig. 9-3 View of the larynx during fiberoptic endoscopic evaluation of swallowing.

FIBEROPTIC ENDOSCOPIC EVALUATION OF SWALLOWING

The FEES is an instrumental assessment that involves the use of an endoscope, light source, and camera to view the pharyngeal swallow (Fig. 9-3). The procedure involves inserting the endoscope through the nares, into the nasopharynx, and remaining above the epiglottis. This study allows the clinician to view the pharynx before and after the swallow. During the pharyngeal phase of the swallow, a whiteout occurs because of epiglottic retroflexion and a pharyngeal squeeze, eliminating the view during the swallow. An anatomic physiologic assessment is completed that looks at velopharyngeal closure, the hypopharynx and the larynx at rest, secretion management and swallow frequency, base of tongue and pharyngeal muscles, laryngeal function (respiratory, phonation, and airway protection), and sensory testing.[6,10] Solids and liquids are mixed with blue or green dye, which allows an enhanced view to determine whether pharyngeal residue, laryngeal penetration, and/or aspiration are present before or after the swallow. Trials with a variety of food or liquid consistencies may be attempted depending on the patient's needs and the pharyngeal disorders observed. Compensatory strategies, such as postural modification, swallowing maneuvers, bolus modifications, and sensory enhancements, may be used as needed. A multitude of studies have shown a high level of agreement between the MBSS and the FEES.[6]

PHARYNGEAL PHASE DISORDERS

The following pharyngeal disorders may be observed preoperatively:

1. A tumor on the anterior cervical spine can produce symptoms similar to those of an osteophyte impinging on the pharynx or upper esophagus, resulting in reduced bolus propulsion, pharyngeal contraction, and cricopharyngeal relaxation.[11,12] In a case of an anterior C1-2 osteochondroma, the patient had dysphagia preoperatively.[13]
2. Reduced velopharyngeal closure can result in nasal backflow, during the swallow, into the nasal cavity. This can occur if a spine tumor is located at the level of the velopharyngeal port.
3. A tumor on the anterior cervical spine can result in decreased deflection of the epiglottis because of the obstruction. This may result in decreased closure of the laryngeal vestibule causing laryngeal penetration or aspiration during the swallow.

The following pharyngeal phase disorders may be observed after resection of cervical spine tumors (Table 9-1).[1,10] Included are the strategies and recommendations for each specific pharyngeal disorder. Some of the barriers in this patient population are limitations to performing postural strategies, such as the chin tuck, head turn, and head tilt, because these patients must follow cervical spine precautions and wear a cervical collar.

Table 9-1 **Status After Resection of Cervical Spine Tumors**

Pharyngeal Disorder	Potential Strategies and Recommendations
Delayed swallow initiation. Premature spillage of bolus to the pharynx may result in aspiration before pharyngeal swallow is initiated.[1,10]	Thickened liquids, supraglottic swallow
Reduced velopharyngeal closure can result in nasal regurgitation into the nasal cavity during the swallow. This may occur as a result of hardware placement following surgery. Also, if reduced pharyngeal contraction occurs, food or liquid may move upward toward the velopharyngeal port.[1]	Palatal lift, thickened liquids
Reduced posterior movement of the tongue base (often caused by cranial nerve damage), can result in the deconditioned patient with an overall weak swallow, causing residue in the valleculae and/or along the pharyngeal wall.[1] Residue in the valleculae after the swallow may place the patient at risk for aspiration.	Effortful swallows, thin liquids, tongue base retraction exercises, alternate solids and liquids, multiple swallows, smaller bolus volumes
Reduced pharyngeal wall contraction as a result of pharyngeal edema and/or weakness from surgery. This can result in residue in the pharynx. This places the patient at risk for aspiration after the swallow.[1] This can be unilateral or bilateral.	Thin liquids, effortful swallows, multiple swallows, alternating solids and liquids, smaller bolus volumes, supraglottic swallow followed by a repeat swallow
Reduced closure of the laryngeal vestibule from cranial nerve damage. Reduced laryngeal closure can result in laryngeal penetration and/or aspiration before or during the swallow. In most patients with abnormal closure, the closure is delayed. Closure of the laryngeal vestibule is crucial for adequate airway protection.[10]	Supraglottic and super-supraglottic swallows, thickened liquids
Reduced true vocal cord closure resulting from cranial nerve damage postoperatively or injury from intubation. This may result in aspiration during the swallow. Vocal cord paresis can be unilateral or bilateral. An ear, nose, and throat specialist should be consulted for further assessment and treatment of vocal cord dysfunction.	Supraglottic swallow, super-supraglottic swallow, pitch exercises, pushing/pulling exercises

DYSPHAGIA TREATMENT AND STRATEGIES

The following swallow strategies, maneuvers, and exercises are used to improve specific areas of the pharyngeal swallow (Table 9-2)[1]:

Table 9-2 Dysphagia Treatment and Strategies

Maneuvers and Strategies	Pharyngeal Disorder	Rationale
Effortful swallow: Patient is instructed to swallow hard with increased effort, squeezing all the throat muscles while swallowing.	Reduced base of tongue retraction	An effortful swallow increases retraction of the tongue to help bolus propulsion and bolus clearance.
Mendelsohn maneuver: Patient is instructed to hold the larynx at its highest point midway through the swallow for several seconds. Patient is directed to squeeze all throat and neck muscles and then to complete the swallow.	Reduced laryngeal elevation Discoordinated swallow	Laryngeal elevation opens the cricopharyngeus. Prolonging laryngeal elevation will allow the cricopharyngeus to remain open for a prolonged time. Improve timing of the oropharyngeal swallow
Supraglottic swallow: Patient is instructed to hold breath, swallow, and then cough. In the super-supraglottic swallow, patient is instructed to hold breath, bear down, swallow, and then cough, but with increased effort compared with the supraglottic swallow.	Reduced true vocal cord closure and laryngeal closure	A breath hold closes the true vocal cords. An effortful breath hold tilts the arytenoids forward, which closes the airway entrance before and during the swallow.
Double swallows: Patient is instructed to swallow two (or multiple) times.	Reduced pharyngeal contraction Reduced cricopharyngeal relaxation	To clear residue in pharyngeal spaces
Alternating solids/liquids: Patient alternates a solid and a liquid bolus.	Weak pharyngeal contraction	To clear pharyngeal residue by the liquid bolus helping move the solids through the pharynx and into the esophagus.
Masako maneuver: Patient holds the tip of the tongue between the front teeth and swallows.	Reduced posterior movement of the tongue base	Intended to increase base of tongue strength

Data from Logemann JA. Evaluation and Treatment of Swallowing Disorders, 2nd ed. Austin, TX: Pro-Ed Publishers, 1998.

POTENTIAL COMPLICATIONS

Potential complications include the following (Box 9-1):

1. Hardware displacements, such as late screw migration, can result in dysphagia. Cases of pharyngeal diverticulum or fistula have also been a rare complication after hardware displacement in anterior cervical discectomy and fusion.[14-16]
2. Vocal cord paresis from surgery or intubation can result in aspiration during the moment of the swallow, given that this first level of airway protection is not complete.[17]
3. Overall generalized weakness or deconditioning from surgery may result in decreased secretion management and inability to tolerate oral intake.
4. Edema of the posterior pharyngeal wall may result in dysphagia, including reduced pharyngeal wall movement.[1]
5. Poor respiratory support may result from surgery. Decreased breath support and/or pain while coughing may result in a weak throat clear, cough, or swallow.
6. Radiation alone or concurrent chemotherapy and radiation can result in dysphagia, most likely because of fibrosis. A recent study was completed in which patients had some dysphagia at baseline, which was likely related to the presence of the tumor. At 3 months after treatment, frequency of reduced tongue base retraction, slow or delayed laryngeal closure, and reduced laryngeal elevation were increased from baseline values. Some disorders continued for 12 months after treatment.[18]
7. Postoperatively a patient may require a tracheostomy because of decreased respiratory support or an inability to tolerate extubation. A tracheostomy can result in decreased subglottic pressure, reduced laryngeal sensation, and reduced laryngeal elevation.
8. Postoperatively patients may require long-term alternative feeding measures, such as a percutaneous endoscopic gastrostomy tube, for long-term nutritional support.

Box 9-1 Definitions

Aspiration: Entry of food or liquid into the airway below the true vocal folds
Laryngeal penetration: Entry of food or liquid into the laryngeal vestibule at some level down to but not below the true vocal cords
Odynophagia: Pain during swallowing
Presbyphagia: Characteristic changes in the swallowing mechanism of otherwise healthy older adults
Residue: Food or liquid that is left behind in the oral cavity or pharynx after the swallow
Silent aspiration: Entry of food or liquid into the airway below the true vocal folds without demonstrating outward signs of aspiration such as coughing or throat clearing

SIGNATURE CASES

A 21-year-old woman was admitted to the hospital with a 3-month history of neck pain, arm tingling, and neck flexion. A CT scan showed a C2-5 intradermal tumor with rostral, caudal syrinx formation. The patient underwent a C1 laminectomy and occipital craniectomy, laminoplasty at C2-4, and midline myelotomy. She wore a Miami J cervical collar after surgery (Ossur Americas Holdings, Inc., 27051 Towne Center Drive, Foothill Ranch, CA 92610).

A clinical swallow evaluation was completed, which revealed a functional oropharyngeal swallow. A diet of pureed foods and thin liquids was recommended for this patient because of her fluctuating level of alertness. The patient was upgraded to regular solids and thin liquids 3 days later, as her alertness and endurance improved, and dysphagia services were no longer indicated.

A 60-year-old woman with a C3-6 chordoma was admitted to the hospital. The tumor and the adjacent vertebrae of C3-6 were resected. To support the spinal cord, a metal tube was inserted with four titanium rods attaching to C2 and C7. Postoperatively the patient had respiratory failure requiring a tracheotomy; she also developed a urinary tract infection with sepsis. She also had episodes of decreased mental status with increased work of breathing and respiratory support and transient hypotension. A percutaneous endoscopic gastrostomy tube was placed for long-term nutritional support. She was advised to wear an Aspen cervical collar (Aspen Medical Products, Inc., Irvine, CA) at all times for approximately 6 months postoperatively.

The FEES was completed to further assess the patient's pharyngeal swallow function. The patient had a No. 4 Shiley cuffed tracheostomy tube in place during this assessment. She had a weak voice, characterized by a hoarse, breathy quality. The results of this assessment showed a functional oral swallow and severe pharyngeal dysphagia characterized by the following:
1. A pharyngeal delay resulting in premature spillage of thin/nectar/honey-thick liquids to the level of the lateral channels/piriform sinus. Thin and nectar-thick liquids spilled into the laryngeal vestibule before the swallow.
2. Suspected reduced true vocal cord/laryngeal closure resulting in laryngeal penetration and aspiration with thin/nectar/honey-thick liquids during the swallow. After the swallow, residue was observed coating the laryngeal vestibule.
3. Reduced bolus propulsion resulting in residue of puree after the swallow, which was aspirated, and a weak cough resulted. An effortful swallow, multiple dry swallows, and alternating solids and liquids were not successful in eliminating this residue.

Recommendations were to continue alternative tube feeding with a repeat FEES after laryngeal and base-of-tongue exercises were completed with the speech-language pathologist. The otolaryngology department was consulted, which resulted in a diagnosis of unilateral vocal cord paralysis.

A repeat FEES was completed approximately 2 weeks later. At that time the patient had a tracheostomy button in place. The patient's voice continued to be weak and low in volume. The results of the assessment revealed a functional oral swallow and moderate-to-severe pharyngeal dysphagia characterized by the following:

1. Pharyngeal delay resulting in premature spillage of nectar-thick liquids to the level of the laryngeal vestibule with laryngeal penetration.
2. Reduced laryngeal closure given the recent diagnosis of unilateral vocal cord paralysis, which resulted in suspected aspiration during the swallow with nectar-thick liquids.
3. Reduced bolus propulsion resulting in mild-to-moderate residue in the pharynx; however, this was cleared with a double, effortful swallow. Alternating solids and honey-thick liquids helped to clear the pharyngeal residue as well. It was recommended that the patient continue main nutritional support through a tube feeding and initiate small amounts of pureed solids and honey-thick liquids for pleasure feeding with the speech-language pathologist and use of compensatory strategies.

On discharge from the hospital, the patient received home health speech therapy for dysphagia. The patient continued to safely tolerate pureed solids and honey-thick liquids, and by approximately 6 months after discharge she was on a regular diet with the strategy of alternating solids and liquids. The patient continued to have difficulty with thin liquids and required very careful intake.

CONCLUSION

Swallowing dysfunction is common in the patient population with cervical spine and spinal cord tumors. The aim of the speech-language pathologist is to evaluate and manage the patient's swallow function to ensure safe oral intake, to strengthen swallow function, and ultimately to improve the patient's quality of life.

TIPS FROM THE MASTERS

Continued assessment and treatment are recommended given the evolving swallow function of the postsurgical patient

References (With Key References in Boldface)

1. **Logemann JA. Evaluation and Treatment of Swallowing Disorders, 2nd ed. Austin, TX: Pro-Ed Publishers, 1998.**
2. **Groher ME. Dysphagia: Diagnosis and Management, 2nd ed. Oxford, UK: Butterworth-Heinemann, 1992.**
3. Leonard R, Kendall K. Dysphagia Assessment and Treatment Planning: A Team Approach, 2nd ed. San Diego, CA: Plural Publishing, 2008.

4. Gilbert RJ, Daftary S, Woo P, et al. Echo-planar magnetic resonance imaging of deglutitive vocal fold closure: normal and pathologic patterns of displacement. Laryngoscope 106(5 Pt 1):568-572, 1996.
5. Langmore SE, Schatz K, Olson N. Endoscopic and videofluoroscopic evaluations of swallowing and aspiration. Ann Otol Rhinol Laryngol 100:678-681, 1991.
6. Langmore SE. Evaluation of oropharyngeal dysphagia: which diagnostic tool is superior? Curr Opin Otolaryngol Head Neck Surg 11:485-489, 2003.
7. Logemann JA. Manual for the Videofluorographic Study of Swallowing, 2nd ed. Austin, TX: Pro-Ed Publishers, 1993.
8. Ramsey D, Smithard D, Kalra L. Silent aspiration: what do we know? Dysphagia 20:218-225, 2005.
9. Martin-Harris B, Brodsky MB, Michel Y, et al. MBS measurement tool for swallow impairment–MBSImp: establishing a standard. Dysphagia 23:392-405, 2008.
10. Langmore SE. Endoscopic Evaluation and Treatment of Swallowing Disorders. New York: Thieme, 2001.
11. Deutsch EC, Schild JA, Mafee MF. Dysphagia and Forestier's disease. Arch Otolaryngol 111:400-402, 1985.
12. Mal RK, Biswas D. Dysphagia secondary to osteoid osteoma of the transverse process of the second cervical vertebra. Dysphagia 22:73-75, 2007.
13. Wang V, Chou D. Anterior C1-2 osteochondroma presenting with dysphagia and sleep apnea. J Clin Neurosci 16:581-582, 2009.
14. Lee WJ, Sheehan JM, Stack BC Jr. Endoscopic extruded screw removal after anterior cervical disc fusion: technical case report. Neurosurgery 58:E589; discussion E589, 2006.
15. Allis TJ, Grant NN, Davidson BJ. Hypopharyngeal diverticulum formation following anterior discectomy and fusion: case series. Ear Nose Throat 89:E4-E9, 2010.
16. Kuo YC, Levine MS. Erosion of anterior cervical plate into pharynx with pharyngotracheal fistula. Dysphagia 25:334-337, 2010.
17. Blitzer A, Brin MF, Sasaki C, et al. Neurological Disorders of the Larynx. New York: Thieme, 1992.
18. Logemann JA, Pauloski BR, Rademaker AW, et al. Swallowing disorders in the first year after radiation and chemoradiation. Head Neck 30:148-158, 2008.

SECTION II

Oncology

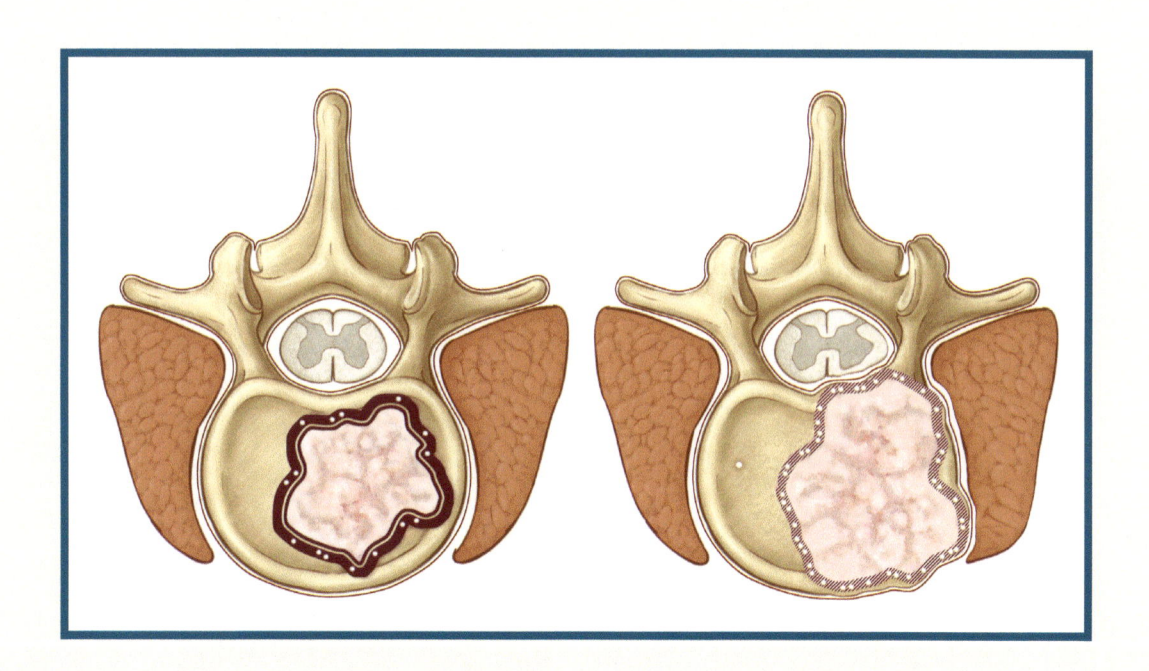

Chapter 10

Chordoma

Jamal McClendon, Jr., Christopher P. Ames,
Frank L. Acosta, Jr.

Chordomas are rare, relatively slow-growing, locally aggressive and invasive, low-grade malignant neoplasms that are thought to be derived from embryonic remnants of the notochord.[1-10] Chordomas of the spinal neuroaxis arise from ectopic notochordal cells and tissue, and have an ectodermal origin.[4,10-12] The notochord is a structure that appears during the fourth week of embryonic life and ultimately regresses by the seventh week. It is associated with the formation and development of the axial skeleton.[1,13] The spinal column is formed from condensation of mesoderm around the notochord.[1] The cephalic portion of the notochord approaches the inner surface of the future sphenoid bone in the region of the dorsum sellae and extends caudally in the midline on the pharyngeal surface of the developing occipital bone.[1] Although the centrum of the nucleus pulposus is thought to be the only derivative of this structure, tissue remnants of the notochord can persist in the adult from the clivus to the coccyx.[1] After reaching maturity in the embryo, the notochord disappears, but microscopic foci remain in the vertebral bodies at the cranial and caudal ends of the embryo.[4]

Chordomas occur almost entirely in the axial skeleton and histologically resemble embryonic notochordal remnants on light and electron microscopy.[1,11,14,15] They have a dual epithelial-mesenchymal differentiation. They are soft, jelly like, lobulated tumors that may have areas of hemorrhage, cystic changes, or calcification.[16] These tumors typically have a proclivity for the spheno-occipital region of the skull base and the sacrococcygeal regions.[4,16] Intracranial chordomas typically arise in the midline from the clivus and posterior part of the sella and invade the underlying bone.[16,17] These neoplasms may occur anywhere along the vertebral spinal column but commonly appear in the clivus or the sacrum and less often in the vertebrae.[16,18-21]

Chordomas are rare, relatively uncommon primary bone tumors with an incidence rate of less than 0.1 per 100,000 per year, with approximately 250 affected persons diagnosed in the United States annually.[1,4,6,22] Chordomas are low-grade malignant tumors that account for approximately 1% to 4% of all primary malignant bone tumors.[4,6,23-28] Chordomas account for more than 4% of all bone tumors. Excluding plasmacytomas, chordomas are the most frequent primary and malignant tumors of the mobile spine, and they occur mainly in elderly men.[5,9,25] Chordomas are not sarcomas but are traditionally classified and approached as sarcomas because they are considered primary bone tumors.[4,29] Although they can be observed in children, chordomas are typically seen in late middle-aged adults, and the elderly.[18,19,25,30] They are uncommon in patients less than 30 years of age, but all age groups may be affected.[1,6,28,31,32] The median age at presentation is approximately 60 years.[4,24] The male/female ratio is 2:1.[1,6,28,31]

Chordomas of the mobile spine originate within ectopic chordal rests in the vertebral body, usually the posterior aspect of the affected vertebral body.[6,16,25,32] At the time of radiographic detection, chordomas demonstrate infiltrative growth that often occupies most of the vertebral body.[25] Chordomas are destructive in their evolution, slowly infiltrating cancellous bone, but intervertebral discs are rarely involved.[6,25,32] The course of the disease is slow, extending over a period of many years. Death can result from complications related to local extension of the disease.[25] Local recurrence is frequent when chordomas are not treated adequately.[9]

In adults approximately 50% of chordomas originate in the sacrococcygeal region, 35% in the clivus, 10% in the cervical vertebrae, and 5% in the thoracolumbar vertebrae.* Chordomas often recur locally and metastasize late, progressing to the lungs, liver, brain, bone, skin, and soft tissues.[7,19,25] Both initial symptoms and recurrences after treatment arise later.[5] In the lumbar spine the disease is four- to fivefold more common in men.[6,39,40] Also, in men in the fifth decade of life, the lesions appear to have a predilection for the L4 and L5 vertebrae, whereas L3 is favored in the seventh decade of life.[6,40] The sacrum is one of the most common sites in the axial skeleton, and these tumors often grow to large sizes before they are detected.[11] Chordomas of the sacrum occur approximately twice as frequently in men compared with women, and they are uncommon in persons less than 40 years of age.[10,41,42]

Treatment of chordomas involves en bloc surgical resection, surgical excision with radiation, or palliative radiation. Wide en bloc resection or radical extralesional surgery affords an opportunity for total cure.[6,10,31,39,43-49] Local recurrence is the most important predictor of death in patients with chordomas and is related to the extent of the initial resection.[10,44,50-53] The tumor should be excised with a wide margin, and the specimen should include the route of the previous biopsy tract. However, long-term survival has been documented in cases where the needle biopsy tract was not included because the site was unknown.[6,49,54] Chordomas have a marked tendency to recur after intralesional excision or biopsy contamination, seeding of tumors along the wound, or intradurally.[5,50,55,56] Kaiser et al[52] reported that local recurrence rates correlated significantly with violation of the tumor margins at the initial surgery.[10]

---

*References 1, 2, 4, 10, 24, 33-38.

These investigators found that the local recurrence rate for patients who underwent complete en bloc resection without contamination of the surgical wound was 28%.[10,52] Among patients in whom the tumor capsule was entered at the time of surgery, the recurrence rate was 64%.[10,52] York et al[44] found that the time from surgery to local recurrence in patients undergoing radical resection was 2.27 years, and the time to local recurrence in patients undergoing subtotal resection was 8 months.[10] Bergh et al[50] showed that local recurrence was significantly associated with an increased risk of metastasis and tumor-related death.[10] Intralesional or subtotal resection will lead to local recurrence, which is usually more aggressive in its behavior and only amenable to palliative treatment, often causing the death of the patient.[6,31,54]

INDICATIONS AND CONTRAINDICATIONS

Chordomas are invasive. Without timely treatment, patients can develop metastasis and die of disease progression.[57-60] At the time of diagnosis, patients should be offered a treatment plan consisting of surgical resection, with or without radiation, and possibly chemotherapy or palliative radiation therapy. Operative approach–related morbidity should be at a minimum to improve postsurgical functional outcomes. Total excision offers the best chance of cure and is the optimal treatment to achieve prolonged disease-free survival. However, the effectiveness of treatment is greatly affected by the size and location of the chordoma.[25,58] Although the ideal treatment goal in the management of chordomas is wide en bloc excision of the tumor, the proximity to neural, vascular, and visceral structures creates significant challenges.[58] If the tumor is quite large at the time of diagnosis, because of an insidious clinical course, en bloc resection may not be feasible. The functional costs for the patient, with respect to anorectal and urogenital dysfunction, are significantly increased when the tumor involves the high sacral levels.[10]

Contraindications include large tumor size, which prevents oncologically appropriate surgical resection. Palliative radiation should be offered to these patients. Biopsy and radiosurgery may be considered in patients who have too many comorbid conditions to undergo a major operation, or when the extent of the tumor makes total resection unlikely. The combination of palliative and/or debulking surgery with high-energy radiation is being used in recurrent tumors or tumors that are not suitable for en bloc resection.[5,61-64] Neurologic deterioration is a key indication for surgery and/or palliative radiation.

BIOLOGY

Although chordomas are slow-growing tumors, surgical cure is rare.[1] Chordomas are locally invasive, destroy bone, and infiltrate soft tissues.[3,16,34,65] In most instances chordomas of the mobile spine occur directly from the vertebral body, often expanding to the whole vertebra.[5] Tumor extension is the major criterion that negatively impacts the possibility of performing an en bloc resection and therefore can significantly affect prognosis.[5] The tendency for chordomas to recur locally is known, but their propensity to metastasize is unclear.[1,66,67] Chordomas have been considered to have low metastatic potential, but distant metastasis to lung, bone, soft tissue, lymph nodes, liver, skin, brain, and other intraabdominal viscera has been reported in up to 43% of patients.[1,4,18,68,69] Occasionally widely disseminated metastases that include the heart, pleura, and brain have been seen.[1] Metastasis to the continuous spine is rare.[5,70-73] Clinically this diverse behavior is demonstrated by obvious indolent growth of the tumors in some patients, in contrast to rapid and massive recurrences with disseminated metastases in others.[1] Metastatic sites usually occur late in the course of the disease.[4] The incidence of metastasis ranges from 5% to as high as 43%, although the presence of metastasis does not significantly affect survival.[1,18,34,36,38] Rates of metastasis can be as high as 65% at autopsy.[25,69] Metastasis is infrequent at presentation, but significant extracompartmental growth is often seen at the time of diagnosis.[10] Metastasis is usually a late event, after long periods of slow local progression of the disease.[9,10,52,69]

Chordomas are divided into conventional, chondroid, and dedifferentiated types, but conventional types are the most common.[4] Conventional chordomas are characterized by the absence of cartilaginous or additional mesenchymal components.[4] Chondroid chordomas contain both chordomatous and chondromatous features, and they have a predilection for the spheno-occipital region of the skull base.[4] This variant accounts for 5% to 15% of all chordomas and up to 33% of cranial chordomas.[4] Dedifferentiation or sarcomatous transformation, which can develop at the onset of disease or much later, occurs in 2% to 8% of chordomas.[4] Although the biological activity of chordomas may be highly variable, the most conventional chordomas are slow growing.[10,74] Chordomas show varying degrees of histologic atypia, but the relationship between histologic features and biological behavior is unclear.[10,75] Dedifferentiated chordoma is a very rare variant of chordoma that is clinicopathologically analogous to dedifferentiated chondrosarcoma.[10] The sarcomatous component of dedifferentiated chordomas may demonstrate more aggressive biological behavior and has high metastatic potential.[10,76,77] Bergh et al[50] found that the presence of microscopic tumor necrosis and/or evidence of high proliferative activity (>5% of cells staining positive for Ki-67) were adverse prognostic factors, the former correlated with local recurrence and the latter with metastasis.[10] Other morphologic features, such as cellularity, pleomorphism, number of spindle cells, predominance of physaliphorous compared with epithelioid tumor cells, and rate of mitosis did not correlate with the clinical course.[10,50]

Resection of sacral chordomas is associated with significant morbidity, but the rate of local recurrence has been correlated with survival.[11] Chemotherapy and conventional radiation therapy have not been proved to be effective treatment methods for sacral chordomas.[11] Local recurrence of disease is not unusual, even after total en bloc resection of sacral chordomas.[10,78] Yonemoto et al[47] reported that local recurrences may be the result of residual chordoma infiltrating the gluteal muscles.[10] Preoperative magnetic resonance imaging (MRI) for assessment of the dorsal musculature is important for complete tumor removal and, if muscle is involved, a radical wide posterior margin of gluteal muscle should be obtained.[10,74]

Genetic studies have yielded various cytogenetic and molecular findings that show 1p36 loss as a consistent change in sporadic and inherited chordomas.[4,79] Microsatellite instability at one or more loci and loss of heterozygosity have been seen in some patients.[4,80] Numerical and structural alterations in chromosomes 3 and 21 have also been observed.[4] Some patients have also shown hypodiploid or near-diploid chromosome numbers.[4,81] Bridge et al[81] and Sandberg and Bridge[82] found that half of all chordomas show chromosomal aberrations of a diverse nature, suggesting that these alterations occur as late events in tumor progression.[4] Eisenberg et al[83] found that chordomas have demonstrated loss of heterozygosity at intron 17 of the retinoblastoma gene, a tumor suppressor gene with protein that binds to nuclear DNA to control cell cycle regulation.[4] Clonality studies in eight cases of sacral chordoma indicated a polyclonal origin for the tumor.[4,84] Malignant transformation typically occurs in the third or fourth decade of life for spheno-occipital lesions and in the fifth or sixth decade for sacrococcygeal lesions.[4,84]

CLINICAL PRESENTATION

Symptoms of spinal chordomas vary according to the location and size or extent of the tumor.[1] Pain is usually the cardinal symptom, which may be incapacitating, and neurologic deficits vary based on tumor location.[4,5] The slow and gradual onset of pain is the most consistent complaint in the mobile spine.[5,25] Pain typically is noted in the involved region of the spine.[1,10] Persistent low back pain or posterior pelvic pain is commonly the presenting complaint for lumbar or sacrococcygeal tumors.*

Chordomas may be discovered incidentally while patients are being evaluated for unrelated medical issues.[11] Chordomas are a frequent cause of cord compression, which causes myelopathy because of the silent and slow rate of tumor growth that frequently expands toward the spinal canal and encroaches on the spinal cord.[5,25] Radiculopathy, paresthesia, or weakness occurs when the tumor burden extends to nerve roots or the neural foramina causing irritation.[1,10]

Patients with cervical chordomas have been known to complain of dysphagia or throat discomfort when there is retropharyngeal involvement. Neurogenic claudication, paraparesis, paraplegia, incomplete cord, and cauda equina compression can be features of stenosis caused by a lumbar chordoma.[9,25] Bladder or bowel function may be compromised, depending on the location of the tumor, and a mass may be palpable presacrally on rectal or gynecologic examination.[10,16] Additional symptoms include pain in the buttocks or perineum, or an abnormal gait. Rectal dysfunction manifesting as a change in bowel habits, tenesmus, or bleeding per rectum has been noted as well.[1] Urinary incontinence has been reported by some patients.[1] Saddle anesthesia can be a presenting complaint as well.[1,25]

---

*References 1, 6, 11, 32, 54, 85.

PREOPERATIVE EVALUATION

The importance of preoperative evaluation cannot be overstated. Diagnostic workup begins with plain radiographs of the involved area. The usual radiographic pattern is lytic with frequent calcifications and seldom appearing as an ivory vertebra.[6,25,86,87] Radiographs can show calcification, osteosclerosis, or bone erosion caused by the lesion, with or without a soft tissue component.[16] Chordomas appear late on standard radiographs as radiolucencies.[5] They may have minimal lytic and sclerotic changes in the vertebral body, and possibly scanty ossifications.[5,6,25] Computed tomography (CT) is a radiologic modality that is used to diagnose chordomas and evaluate the extent of disease. The pattern is radiolucent with permeation of cancellous bone, but it may feature bone destruction or a soft tissue mass.[5,16] Calcifications are present in 30% to 70% of cases.[10,88] Myelography can be employed as well and may feature epidural block or epidural compression.[16] CT and MRI scans have allowed for the development of oncologic and surgical staging systems.[8,25,89-91] MRI studies are useful in detecting lesions that do not appear on plain radiographs.[5] The magnetic resonance signal is isointense or hypointense on T1-weighted images and hyperintense on T2-weighted images.[10,25,88] Unlike most bone tumors, chordomas may show reduced uptake or normal distribution of radioisotopes on bone scans.[10,92] Although chordomas are relatively avascular lesions, a tumor stain can often be identified by angiography with subtraction techniques.[1] Angiograms can be useful in patients with cervical chordomas to identify dominance of the vertebral arteries. Balloon test occlusion is carried out before surgery if a vertebral artery needs to be ligated. The preoperative sedimentation rate may be elevated.

CLINICAL DECISION-MAKING

Treatments for spinal chordomas include surgical excision alone, combined surgical resection with radiation, or isolated low-dose or high-voltage radiation therapy.* In light of the unpredictable nature of spinal column chordomas, surgical resection should be attempted. En bloc resection of chordomas is the principal treatment modality used to achieve long-term survival and disease-free intervals in patients.† Studies have demonstrated that negative surgical margins are the most important predictors of local recurrence and survival associated with chordomas and chondrosarcomas.[10,44,58,97-101] The goal of surgery is en bloc tumor removal, spinal decompression, if needed, and reconstruction and stabilization of the spine.[6,102-104] Before deciding on radical excision, the full extent of tumor involvement with the spine and surrounding structures should imperatively be determined. Planning includes proper assessment of the surgical approach—anterior, posterior, or combined. Furthermore, depending on the number of levels involved and the possibility of instability, provisions should be made for stabilization of the spine.[1] Early and complete surgical excision of the tumor is the only curative procedure.[3,19,25] Treatment outcome is significantly influenced by the size and location of the chordoma.[7,19,25] These tumors are often so large at diagnosis that their size prevents oncologically adequate treatments.[5,105] Efforts to perform

---

*References 2, 5, 19, 25, 50, 95, 96.
†References 3, 16, 18, 19, 21, 25, 63, 93, 94.

margin-free en bloc tumor resection of the cervical, thoracic, and lumbar spine should be considered.[5] Multilevel chordomas pose challenges because of the need to remove multiple segments of the spine in one piece without violating the tumor. En bloc resection of chordomas with wide margins, or even marginal margins, has a significantly better rate of control than intralesional resection.[19,25,50,96,97] En bloc spondylectomy techniques have been well described for the lumbar, thoracic, and cervical spine.[25,95,106-109]

Advances in imaging techniques have improved the prognosis for chordomas because they allow detection of smaller tumors, which are more amenable to en bloc resection.[5,110-113] A biopsy procedure is usually indicated for diagnostic purposes.[10] The minimally invasive nature of fine-needle aspiration biopsy makes it the most oncologically sound technique because it allows for an accurate diagnosis that uses the cytomorphologic features of chordomas.[10,114] Many surgeons believe that the same person should perform both the biopsy and the definitive tumor resection, or should at least direct the choice of biopsy procedure.[10] Poorly planned incisional biopsies or incomplete debulking operations performed before a patient is referred to a major tumor center have been shown to increase the risk of local recurrence and metastasis.[10,50]

Radiation therapy has been advocated for the treatment of chordomas, either in conjunction with surgery or as the sole treatment.[1,115-117] Most patients undergoing surgery are offered radiation therapy unless the tumor resection is deemed complete. Despite the radioresistance of spinal column chordomas, the value of radiation therapy is significant.[117-120] Objective evidence of tumor regression is difficult to evaluate in the vast majority of patients.[1] Radiation affords palliation in most cases. When adequate excision is not possible, radiation therapy may provide at least a short-term benefit and can be used to treat recurrences.[16,19,25,43,93]

The role of radiation therapy in the management of these tumors is not well established, and the optimum dose, fractionation, and quality of radiation therapy are not well known.[16] Doses can range from 5000 cGy delivered over a 5-week period to 6600 cGy over a 6.5-week period, with a daily fraction of 180 to 200 cGy given 5 days per week and all fields treated daily.[16] Radiation therapy has proved valuable for local control, particularly with the advent of charged particle radiation therapy.[4]

SURGICAL TREATMENT

The goal of surgery for chordoma is en bloc resection at the initial surgery. Surgical techniques have allowed for wide or marginal en bloc tumor excision with judicious preservation of nerve roots and surrounding structures, thereby improving functional outcome without compromising oncologic results.[58] Complete tumor excision on the basis of oncologic criteria can be hampered by extension of the tumor and anatomic constraints in the mobile spine.[25] If, during surgical staging, only intralesional margins can be achieved, the risk-benefit ratio for performing en bloc resection must be carefully weighed by the surgeon.[5] En bloc resection of a recurrence often poses a surgical risk that exceeds the benefits, as planes of dissection are not well demarcated because of the formation of scar tissue.[5] An intralesional excision combined with high-dose radiation seems to be the best treatment for recurrent lesions.[5] En bloc excision, even if marginal, is the treatment of choice for chordomas of the spine.[25] Lesions with a rim of normal tissue surrounding the tumor are considered wide excisions, tumors with a pseudocapsule identified at the margin are considered marginal excisions, and tumors with violation of the capsule or neoplastic cells seen at the margin are considered contaminated/intralesional resections.[58]

Although different treatment approaches exist, including radiation and surgery, the only curative treatment is early and complete surgical excision.[1,6,18,19,121] The treatment of choice for spinal column chordomas is wide-margin surgical resection combined with radiation therapy, because intralesional or marginal resection can lead to local recurrence.[9,25,122] Control of the primary disease remains the major therapeutic challenge.[4] Careful planning is essential before any surgical intervention.[19] Traditionally surgery facilitates local control and therapeutic intervention.[4] Wide en bloc resection is the primary modality in the management of chordomas and long-term local control.[9] Wide or marginal en bloc excision of sacral chordomas is associated with significant improvement in disease-free survival with acceptable perioperative morbidity rates.[58] The challenge lies in obtaining en bloc resection to achieve negative margins, and this can be technically challenging depending on the location and expansion of the tumor.[4] Patients may be offered surgical fusion if instability is entertained preoperatively. Immediate spinal stability must be achieved with appropriate replacement or bone graft with rigid fixation.[19] Chemotherapy, although suboptimal, can be used for either recurrent or disseminated disease, although the response is regarded as minimal. Chordomas are relatively refractory to cytotoxic chemotherapy.[4] When the tumor permeates the dura, resection, not including the dura, is intralesional, with a high risk of local recurrence.[9] Therefore a proper wide resection consists of vertebrectomy with removal of the dura infiltrated by the chordoma.[9]

Careful and complete preoperative planning is based on oncologic and surgical staging.[25] When total surgical excision is not feasible, decompressive laminectomy combined with removal of all gross tumor from the spinal canal in the epidural space, along with involved bone, can provide patients with valuable short-term benefits that may be extended by repeated operations.[1] Late diagnosis often makes complete surgical resection challenging because of widespread extension into soft tissue and bone at the time of diagnosis.[1,25] Surgical resection with wide margins has been shown to be the most reliable means of curing sacral chordomas and is an important predictor of local recurrence and survival.[11,97] Surgical removal of sacral chordomas is associated with significant morbidity affecting bowel, bladder, and sexual function.[11,98,123,124]

TECHNIQUE

The surgical techniques for margin-free, en bloc tumor resection have been proved to be effective in terms of local control and long-term prognosis for chordomas occurring in the cervical, thoracic, and lumbar spine.[4,6,19,50,125-127] Patients who undergo en bloc resection achieve better long-term survival, improved quality of life, and generally have less pain. Spinal instrumentation for reconstruction has been performed immediately when surgery has caused instability or reconstruction was inevitable.[25] Critical to reconstruction after vertebrectomy is restoration of the anterior column and three-dimensional balance.[5]

For posterior approaches requiring reconstruction, patients are positioned on a Jackson table after endotracheal intubation where all contact points are padded. The incision encompasses the area of interest, and subperiosteal dissection is carried out to the appropriate levels. Posterior exposure is performed to access the rostral, caudal, posterior, and lateral segments of the tumor. Soft tissue dissection is commenced away from the margins of the tumor, leaving a cuff of normal tissues on the neoplasm, when possible. Pedicle screws and/or lateral mass screws are placed two segments above and below the level of the area in need of resection and/or decompression. Aggressive laminectomies are performed, if needed, for decompression. If en bloc resection can be safely performed posteriorly, removal of the articular processes, pedicles, intervertebral discs, and posterior longitudinal ligament allows for dural exposure and disconnection of the column. This can be accomplished by medial facetectomy and osteotome disconnection of the pedicles flush to the vertebral body under direct vision. The intervening disc spaces above and below the corpectomy can be excised partially at this point. Osteotomies are performed with an AM-8 matchstick drill bit and Kerrison rongeurs around the tumor to detach it from the spine. Nerve roots are sacrificed as needed, with double suture ligation if involved and needed for en bloc resection. If needed, the vertebral arteries are appropriately ligated above and below the appropriate levels.

Total en bloc spondylectomy may be combined with dural resection occasionally for wide margins. However, in practice, a marginal margin is usually obtained at the dura. The added benefit of an extralesional dural margin may be negated by possible contamination of the intradural space and issues relating to cerebrospinal fluid leakage. Chondrosarcomas have a greater propensity for dural invasion than chordomas.

The dura containing tumor should be resected, and lyophilized bovine pericardium double wrapping or another dural substitute should be placed to form a dural cylindrical robe.[9] Lyophilized pericardium is easily sutured to be watertight by using standard suture material. It is relatively inexpensive, forms a good barrier for tumoral invasion, is strong, and has low antigenicity and toxicity; in addition, adhesions are minimal in the adjacent anatomic structures.[9,128] Therefore, in the event of local recurrences, it cannot permeate the nearby anatomic structures and it also remains bordered by the pericardium, making it easier to excise. If only the inner dural layer is involved with the tumor, the outer layer is stripped away from the inner layer that is surrounding the tumor base.[9] The tumor is then resected together with the inner layer alone, outside the arachnoid membrane, and the outer layer is simply closed.[9] This allows the outer part of the dura mater not invaded by the tumor to be preserved so that dural reconstruction is not necessary.[9] This lowers the risk of postoperative cerebrospinal fluid fistulas in comparison to when the dura is completely resected together with the tumor.[9] Posterior stabilization with rod fixation to pedicular and/or lateral mass screws is then performed. With completion of the osteotomies, the tumor and its surrounding bone are circumferentially detached from their bony attachments with the spine. If feasible, tumor specimens are removed in an en bloc fashion, and the surgeon performs an examination to assess the integrity of the tumor capsule and margins. The surgical specimen is sent to the pathology laboratory for detailed histopathologic examination of the tumor margins. The wound is then closed in a layered fashion.

If en bloc removal is unsafe posteriorly, usually because of anterior vascular involvement, the patient is then placed in a supine or lateral decubitus position, and vertebrectomy is completed. The vertebral body or bodies involved are removed en bloc. An expandable cage is placed in the defect. Circumferential detachment of the tumor from the surrounding bone and soft tissues can allow for safe dissection of the tumor away from the ventral vascular and visceral structures to achieve en bloc tumor resection by means of a posterior-only approach.[58] An anterior approach is often used for large presacral tumors that extend above the L5-S1 disc space or for tumors with rectal invasion that require possible colonic resection and/or colostomy.[58] If a partial sacrectomy is performed, after the tumor is excised, lumbosacropelvic instrumented fusions are performed if more than 50% of the S1 body or sacroiliac joint is removed.[58] In these cases, segmental pedicle screws are placed in the lumbar spine, and the pelvis is reconstructed with double iliac screw/bolt fixation, a transiliac bar with an interbody cage and iliac bolts, or a modified Galveston technique. This features the posterior pelvic rim reconstituted with cages, allografts, or transiliac bar for translational and rotational stability.[58]

Anterior retroperitoneal approach or lateral retroperitoneal approach can be used for resection of chordomas confined to lumbar vertebral bodies.[19] The assistance of a vascular surgeon or general surgeon may be necessary for access or vascular reconstruction or bypass. Special attention is paid to lumbar vertebrectomies because of the relative proximity of the great vessel bifurcation. For a lateral retroperitoneal approach, a left paramedian or oblique incision is performed to approach the lumbar spine retroperitoneally. Division of the median sacral, as well as the iliolumbar and L4 segmental vessels on the left, allow for adequate exposure of the L4-S1 disc space.[6] The L5-S1 intervertebral disc can be removed with the iliac vessels retracted cehalad.[6] The L4-5 disc can be removed by retracting the great vessels laterally and to the right.[6] The usual approach for an L5 corpectomy is anterior retroperitoneal because of the anatomic position of the major vessels. The L5 vertebral body can be levered out of its anatomic position if the pedicles have been disconnected during the posterior approach.[6] An expandable cage can be placed after the corpectomy procedure.

En bloc resection of a chordoma in the lumbar spine is achieved anteriorly by freeing the vertebral body from the pedicles after posterior disarticulation, posterior pedicular osteotomies, and removal of known or suspected tumor involvement.[19] An interbody device is often placed in the area of the defect, and posterior segmental instrumentation is placed above and below the resection for stabilization by a screw and rod system.[5] Interbody devices may include a femoral shaft allograft or cage. If extraosseous soft tissues are involved, the surgical resection should incorporate these areas.[19] If the psoas muscles are involved, resection must be seriously considered.[19] Internal segmental instrumentation is augmented with posterolateral arthrodesis and fusion with the use of an autograft.[19] In the cervical spine, complex reconstructive systems can feature a vascularized fibula strut graft for cervical body reconstruction.[5,129]

For chordomas involving the cervical spine, and after a posterior approach, an anterior approach can be performed to remove the tumor en bloc. Anterior cervical discectomies are performed cephalad and caudad to the area to be resected, along with the posterior longitudinal ligament. A parasagittal osteotomy can be performed to circumferentially remove the tumor en bloc. This can be accomplished with a high-speed drill and an AM-8 matchstick burr with a Kerrison rongeur punch. An expandable cage and anterior plating system can be used to reconstruct the anatomy. This approach may require unilateral vertebral artery ligation. For lateralized tumors, an alternative to performing multilevel spondylectomies may be the use of parasagittal osteotomies for en bloc resection of chordomas.[95] Although these resections are not spondylectomies, they adhere to the oncologic principle of marginal en bloc resection.[95] Parasagittal osteotomy may be used to achieve en bloc resection of multiple vertebral bodies without intralesional resection and without excessive operative time and morbidity of multilevel spondylectomy.[95] Parasagittal osteotomy is less demanding technically than multilevel spondylectomies.

All specimens obtained from en bloc resections should be carefully evaluated and submitted immediately for critical review by the pathology team and the surgeon.[5] Margins are submitted for both gross examination and histologic studies. Care should be taken to ensure that the adjacent soft tissues around the wound do not get seeded on resection and to prevent damage to the intraabdominal organs or ureters during dissection while performing a vertebrectomy, if needed. The wound should be irrigated with copious amounts of antibiotic irrigation before closure to prevent wound infections, which are a frequent complication.

OUTCOMES WITH EVALUATION OF RESULTS

Early postoperative care is of the utmost importance. Severe respiratory failure can be an issue with removal of upper cervical chordomas, and disseminated intravascular coagulation can be an issue after long operations with significant blood loss.[5] Cardiac complications have also been seen after these major operations, including myocardial infarction and dysrhythmias.[5] Because of the prevalence of chordomas in older adults and elderly patients, loosening of the screws in osteoporotic bone must be considered as a possible risk after complex vertebral resections and reconstructions.[5] Wound infection is a common complication. For patients with sacral chordomas, preservation of ambulatory function and bladder and bowel function is important for patient satisfaction.

On gross specimens, the consistency of a chordoma can vary from firm and focally ossified or calcified to soft, myxoid, gelatinous, or even semifluid, and the tumor often appears lobulated.[1,19] These lesions are gray, partially translucent, cystic, or solid masses resembling a cartilage tumor or occasionally a mucin-producing adenocarcinoma.[1]

These lesions often are well circumscribed with formation of a pseudocapsule only in the soft tissues but absent in the region of bone extension by tumor.[1] Microscopically the lesions are characterized by a distinctly lobular architecture formed by the mucin-producing physaliphorous (e.g., dewdrop-like) cells with ample vacuolated cytoplasm, and "signet ring"–type cells.[1,19]

Histologically the lesions are composed of cords or masses of large cells with abundant eosinophilic cytoplasm and round nuclei.[16] They have nests of variable, moderately atypical, epithelioid, neoplastic cells in a myxoid stroma background matrix separated by fibrous bands.[4,11,130] Physaliphorous cells have cytoplasmic vacuolation and granules of glycogen and abundant intercellular mucoid material or mucous droplets.[16,19] A thick layer of peripheral fibrous investment can appear to be focally incomplete and is often invaded by infiltrating tumor cells.[1] The incomplete encapsulation and microscopic involvement by strands of chordoma cells at some distance from the major tumor mass may explain the high rates of local recurrence of this neoplasm.[1] The intracytoplasmic mucus droplets vary greatly in size and show a positive staining reaction for both glycogen and mucin.[1] The smaller, better-preserved, tumor nodules demonstrate oval or polygonal cells in close proximity to each other, with a distinct resemblance to carcinoma cells with mucin production.[1] The larger tumor lobules show ample extracellular mucin production, with only a few cells scattered about, especially in the peripheral areas.[1] Differences in nuclear size and chromatin are features of this tumor type.[1] Binucleate forms and multinucleated giant cells can be seen, but mitotic figures are rarely discerned.[1] Cellular anaplasia and an increased rate of mitosis are not necessarily indicative of a more virulent clinical course.[1] These large mucin-producing cells containing vacuoles are positive for cytokeratin, which excludes the diagnosis of chondrosarcoma.[25,131]

As with other slow-growing neoplasms, evaluation of the efficacy of various modes of therapy is difficult because of the length of follow-up necessary.[1] Thus the natural history of patients with chordomas is poorly understood.[1] Surgical outcomes are dependent on the location and size of the tumor at diagnosis.[4] The number of vertebral chordomas potentially amenable to radical surgical excision is smaller than for those occurring in the sacrococcygeal area.[1] En bloc surgical excision of chordomas with negative tumor margins is the ideal treatment.[10,31,58,60] Bulky tumors adjacent to critical structures frequently preclude margin-negative resections, and treatment consists only of decompression or tumor debulking.[4,105,121,132] Chordomas have a minimal response to chemotherapy and conventional radiation therapy.[10,31,58-60]

The largest challenge in the treatment of chordomas is local control, and the uncontrolled growth of this tumor is commonly the cause of death.[5] Inadequate tumor margins are the main factor negatively affecting prognosis and are also the cause of seeding of the tumor.[5,50,55] Negative surgical margins are the single most important predictor of tumor recurrence rates and long-term survival, with recurrence rates on the order of 70% in cases where negative margins are not achieved.[4,10,58,59] Boriani et al[5] found a group of 52 patients who had a 100% local recurrence rate within 17 to 20 months when treated with radiation alone, palliative therapy, or intralesional intracapsular excision.[4] However, only 20% had local recurrences at 56 to 94 months after en bloc resection with appropriate margins.[4,5] The combination of palliative and/or debulking surgery with high-energy radiation seems promising for recurrent tumors and tumors that are not suitable for en bloc resection.[4,61-64] Park et al[57] found, in a series of 21 patients, that local control of sacral chordomas treated with surgery and radiation was achieved in 86% for primary lesions and 14% for recurrent lesions.[4] Boriani et al[5] found that the rate of local recurrence after intralesional extracapsular excision, even if associated with conventional radiation therapy (independently from the usual range of dose and fractions), is consistently higher and earlier (8 of 12 cases at an average of 37 months). Wide or marginal en bloc excision of sacral chordomas results in a significant increase in disease-free survival.[58]

Chordomas are considered relatively resistant to radiation therapy, but large doses of radiation may achieve some degree of local control.[16,18] Radiation therapy has been used for incomplete resections and for palliation.[6,28,48,54,121] Radiation therapy is strongly recommended as an adjuvant.[16,25] Chordomas require doses in excess of 60 Gy, but radiation therapy appears to prolong survival in approximately 30% of patients treated with 56.5 Gy.[4,25,133] Conventional radiation therapy with high-energy photons, up to a dosage of 50 to 55 Gy, does not provide a high local control rate.[4,68,93,134] Tewfik et al[135] recommended a total dosage of 6000 to 6500 cGy after surgical resection of chordomas and 7000 to 7500 cGy if the tumor is unresectable.[16] Reddy et al[136] suggested the combined use of surgery and supervoltage radiation consisting of 6500 to 7000 cGy over 6 or 7 weeks using careful treatment planning to minimize normal tissue damage.[16] Between 60 and 65 Gy is considered the minimum useful dose, but higher doses have been favored in some series, particularly when particle radiation is used.[4,137,138] Conventional radiation therapy is reasonable when en bloc resection is not feasible or feasible with a concrete possibility of contamination or intralesional margins.[5] Several forms of radiation therapy have been described, including proton beam therapy, which may have specific advantages over other forms.[25,93,139] The objective is to concentrate high doses of radiation to the tumor itself without affecting neighboring tissues. Conventional radiation therapy alone can relieve symptoms for short periods, unless high doses (e.g., 70 Gy) are used.[25,119,140] Different radiation therapy techniques, especially proton beam radiation therapy, have improved the outcome for skull base chordomas.[6] When compared with conventional radiation therapy, proton beam radiation therapy improves the dose distribution, and it has increased the disease-free 5-year survival rate to 76%, and the local control rate to 82%.[6,134,141] Proton beam radiation therapy permits the delivery of higher doses to significantly more tumor.[6,142]

Dahlin and MacCarty[34] first reported on the beneficial role of radiation therapy in patients with chordomas located in the base of the skull in 1952.[16] Patients may experience nausea, diarrhea, and erythema of the skin as side effects of radiation. Suit et al[139] treated patients with chordomas of the clivus and cervical spine with high-energy photon beam and 16 MV proton beam radiation. The advent of advanced imaging, planning, and the delivery of photon radiation therapy has provided opportunities for safe delivery of high doses of radiation to patients.[143,144] Improvements have been made regarding the physical dose distribution of radiation treatment for chordomas by use of charged particles, especially protons.[4] This has improved tumor control and reduced radiation-induced second malignancies.[4] Berson et al[145] reported a 5-year local control rate of 54% for 10 patients with chordomas and chondrosarcomas of the cervical spine treated with charged particles.[4] Hug et al[146] treated 14 patients with spinal and sacral chordomas with protons and reported a 5-year local control rate of 53%.[4] Proton beam radiation therapy can be used for patients with contaminated intralesional tumor excisions or after detection of a tumor recurrence in patients undergoing wide or marginal en bloc tumor excisions.[58] Even with adjuvant therapy with proton beam radiation, Hsieh et al[58] showed that patients with contaminated intralesional tumor excisions had a significantly decreased disease-free survival compared with patients with wide or marginal en bloc excisions. Supplementary radiation treatment is a useful adjunct to surgical care but is not sufficient as stand-alone therapy.[10,44,45,68] York et al[44] reported the results of a 40-year series investigating the addition of radiation therapy to subtotal resection in which it significantly prolonged the disease-free survival for patients undergoing subtotal resection—2.12 years compared with 8 months.[10] Catton et al[68] found no differences between conventional and hyperfractionated radiation therapy regimens for chordomas, with respect to both the degree or duration of symptomatic responses and progression-free survival.[10] They also showed no survival advantage for patients receiving radiation in doses greater than 50 Gy compared with those receiving doses less than 50 Gy.[10,68] Results of brachytherapy techniques for recurrent sacral chordomas have been reported in small numbers of patients.[10,147]

Low-grade chordomas are not reported to be sensitive to chemotherapy, which has been of little value in the management of these tumors.* Patients with high-grade dedifferentiated chordomas (<5% of all chordomas) may have a response to chemotherapy.[4,76] Chondroid histology exhibits low-grade behavior and a favorable long-term outcome and prognosis.[4]

Dedifferentiated chordomas, which are observed in less than 5% of cases, have features of high-grade spindle cell sarcoma and an aggressive clinical course.[4] Anecdotal reports of responses to chemotherapy, such as vinca alkaloids and alkylating agents, have been limited to case reports.[4,51,148-150] Molecular targets, such as platelet-derived growth factor receptor-beta and epidermal growth factor receptor, have been targets for adjuvant therapy.[4] Intraoperative use of cryosurgery with liquid nitrogen has been advocated as well.[11,151,152] Marcove[153] described the use of cryosurgery and guidelines for usage featuring three freeze cycles interrupted by periods of thawing.[11]

Deaths from chordomas are often the result of the neurologic effects produced by the tumor (e.g., paraplegia-induced sepsis, urinary tract infection, pneumonia, and so forth).[1] Aggressive initial therapy for dedifferentiation or sarcomatous transformation of chordomas improves overall outcome.[4] Local relapse is associated with a poor prognosis, but both radiation therapy and surgery can be used as salvage therapy.[4] Subtotal resection can result in stable or improved status in as many as 50% of patients who have relapses after primary therapy.[4] Chordomas found in the vertebral bodies are of-

---

*References 4, 6, 10, 44, 48, 51, 54.

ten more malignant than those arising in the clivus or the sacrum.[18,19] Metastases have been reported in 80% of vertebral body chordomas, as compared with an overall rate of 43% for all chordomas.[18,19] Recurrent tumors can be treated with local excision, which can achieve good palliation, or with radiation therapy.[6,28,31,48]

The differential diagnosis of sacral tumors is very comprehensive and includes metastasis, giant cell tumors, chordomas, and chondrosarcomas.[10] Sacrifice of the sacral nerve roots produces varying degrees of bladder, bowel, and sexual dysfunction.[10,154-156] High sacral amputation may jeopardize lumbopelvic stability, and total sacrectomy requires stabilization of the dissociated lumbar spine and pelvis.[10,157,158] Sexual dysfunction, bowel dysfunction, or the need for self-catheterization are issues patients may face after resection of sacral chordomas, depending on nerve root involvement.[11] Bowel, bladder, and sexual function have been reported to rely on the presence of at least one if not both S3 nerve roots.[11,50,123,124,159] Larger sacral tumors can involve the pudendal nerve, and sacrifice of the pudendal nerves bilaterally abrogates any bowel, bladder, or sexual function, even when all of the sacral roots are spared.[11] If resection involves sacrifice of both S2 nerve roots, urinary and bowel incontinence may ensue.[4]

Schwab et al[11] observed a higher rate of local recurrence for patients with prior resections in a retrospective study analyzing patients who had undergone surgical resection for sacral chordomas. Local adjuvant therapy was used in all cases, with wide surgical resections with "contaminated" or positive margins.[11] The use of a rectus abdominis myocutaneous flap was statistically significant with regard to reducing wound complications for resection of sacral chordomas. Schwab et al[11] published 5-year and 10-year overall survival rates of 59% and 35%, respectively, for 42 patient undergoing surgical resection with or without cryosurgery, and with or without adjuvant radiation therapy, for sacral chordoma. The magnitude of sacral resections for chordomas and the often slow recovery period afterward predispose patients to development of hospital-acquired infections. The surgical management of sacral chordomas is associated with significant morbidity.[11] The 5-year survival rate for patients with vertebral chordomas is approximately 50%, and with early diagnosis and effective treatment the disease-free interval at 5 years should be 30% to 50%.[1,6,31] The mortality rate for lumbar chordomas is lower than mortality rates for thoracic or cervical lesions. The lower the spinal level, the better the prognosis.[6,54,160]

Aggressive and thorough resection is important. Chordomas are very difficult to resect completely, often because of their size and the challenge of operating around the spine without injuring the adjacent vital neural and vascular tissues.[7,19,25] Survival seems to be more frequently affected by the local progression of the tumor rather than by metastases.[19,25] These tumors have a 50% survival rate at 5 years, but the rate drops to 28% at 10 years.[19,21,25,63,93] Pena et al,[29] in a series of 28 patients with chordomas, found that metastatic disease may be considered to have adverse prognostic significance because the median survival time was reported to be less than 12 months after the development of distant metastasis.[4] Another study showed that the overall median survival time for patients with chordomas is approximately 6 years, with a survival rate of 70% at 5 years, which falls to 40% at 10 years.[4]

SIGNATURE CASES

Cervical chordoma (Fig. 10-1). A 55-year-old male patient, in good health, with no history of malignancy, presented with a palpable neck mass. CT-guided needle biopsy of the mass over a sheath demonstrated a chordoma. The patient underwent a staged parasagittal osteotomy and circumferential reconstruction. Postoperatively the patient demonstrated new left deltoid weakness (4/5) and was maintained on a jejunostomy tube for 4 months. The patient underwent proton beam therapy 6 months postoperatively.

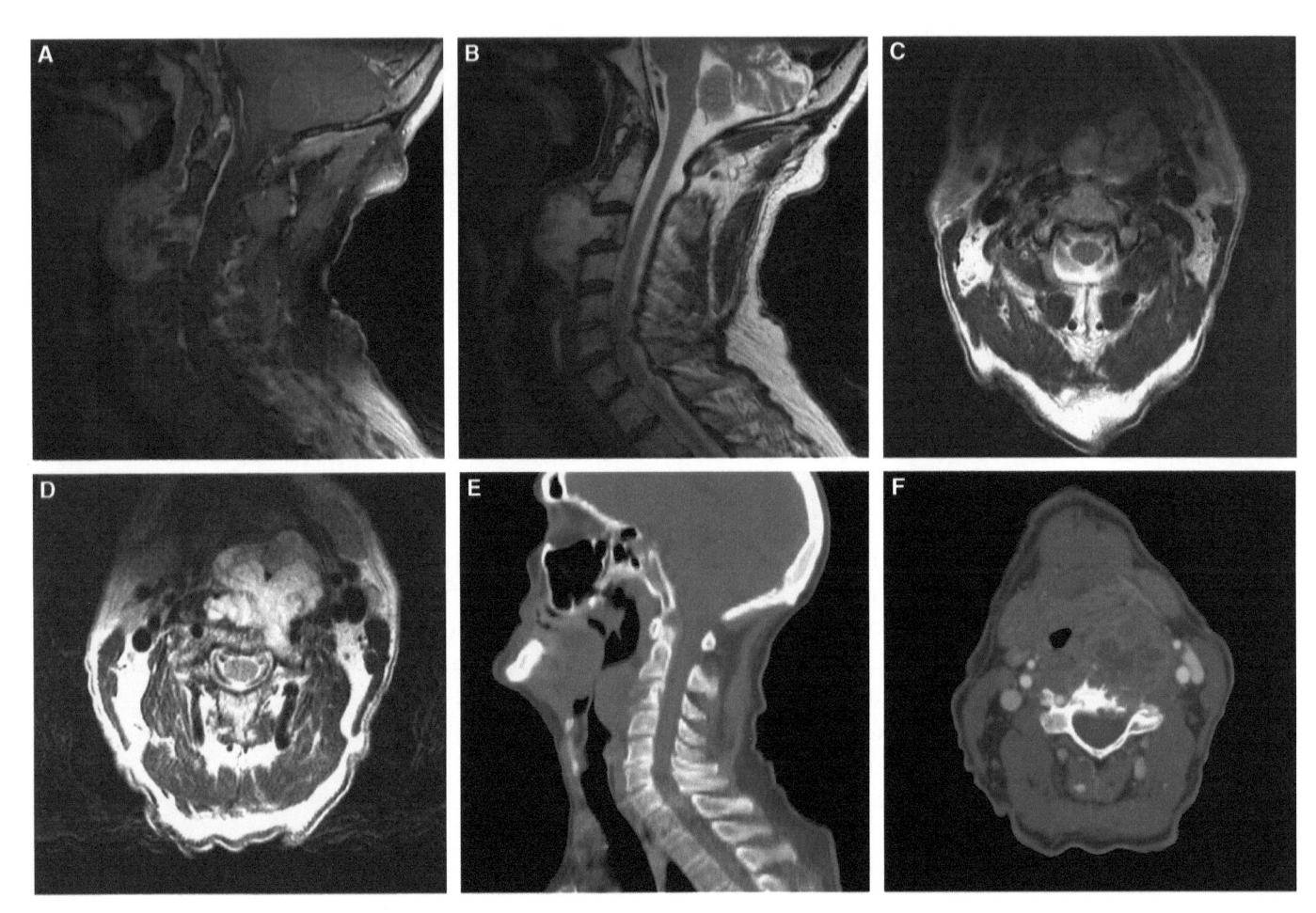

Fig. 10-1 **A,** Sagittal T1 postcontrast MRI scan of the cervical spine demonstrating a multilevel, nonhomogeneously enhancing chordoma. **B,** Sagittal T2-weighted MRI scan of the cervical spine demonstrating a multilevel chordoma involving cervical vertebral bodies. **C** and **D,** Axial MRI scans of a multilevel cervical chordoma with extensive soft tissue involvement. **E,** Sagittal CT scan of the cervical spine demonstrating a significant prevertebral mass causing local bone destruction of the vertebral spine and significant airway compromise. **F,** Axial CT scan with contrast enhancement demonstrating a significant cervical chordoma with local tissue invasion and bony destruction.

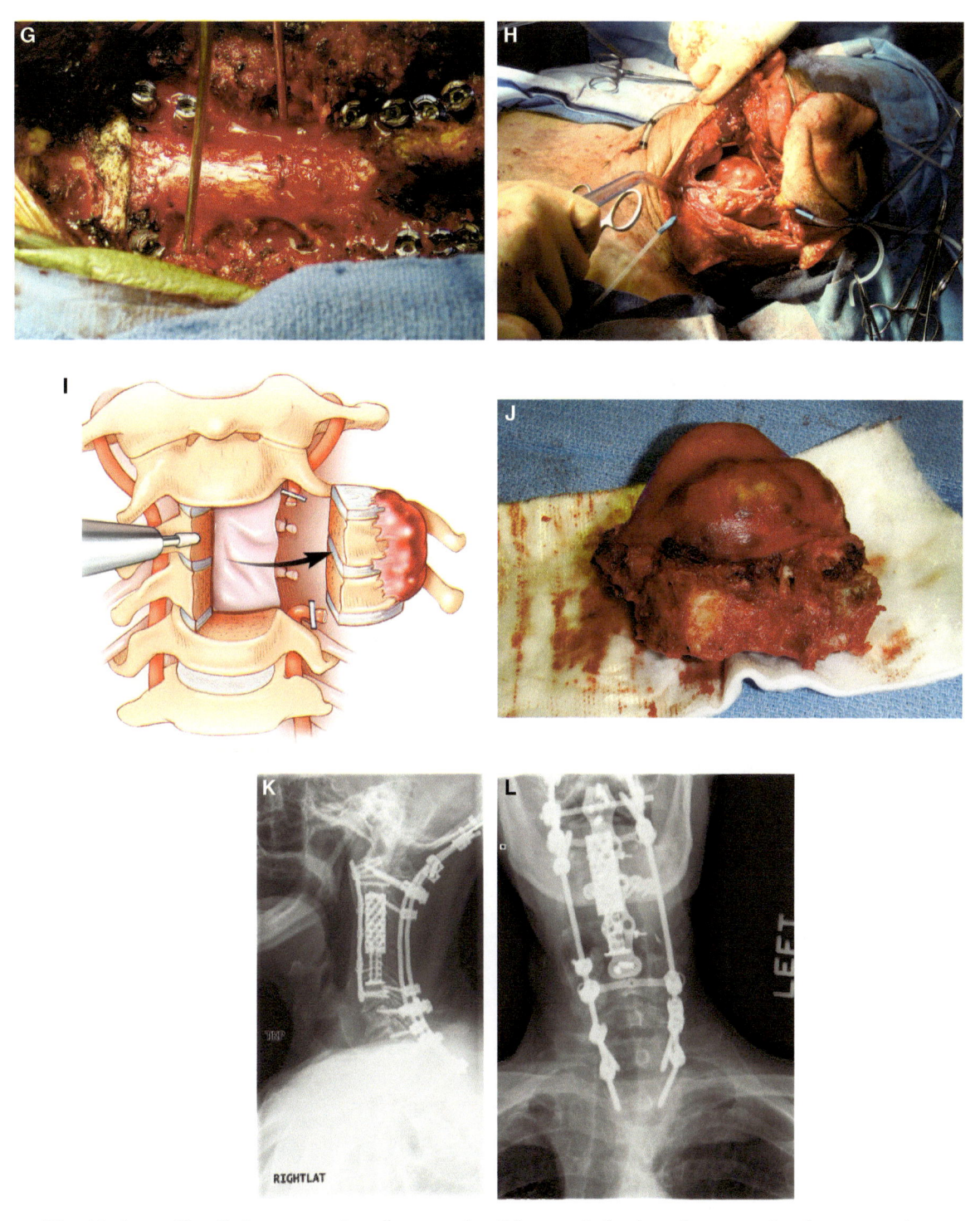

Fig. 10-1, cont'd **G,** Intraoperative photograph of the cervical spine after posterior decompression, segmental instrumentation, and nerve root ligation. **H,** Intraoperative photograph after anterior exposure of the tumor. **I,** Parasagittal osteotomy procedure performed to maintain oncologic margins while removing multiple cervical levels featuring the chordoma en bloc. Nerve root and vertebral artery ligation are featured. **J,** Photograph of en bloc cervical specimen after removal of the multilevel chordoma en bloc. **K,** Postoperative lateral and **L,** anteroposterior plain radiographs demonstrating spinal reconstruction after tumor removal.

Sacral chordoma (Fig. 10-2). A 52-year-old woman presented with sacral pain. Diagnostic workup, including CT-guided sheath biopsy, was consistent with a diagnosis of chordoma. She underwent en bloc sacrectomy and posterior reconstruction.

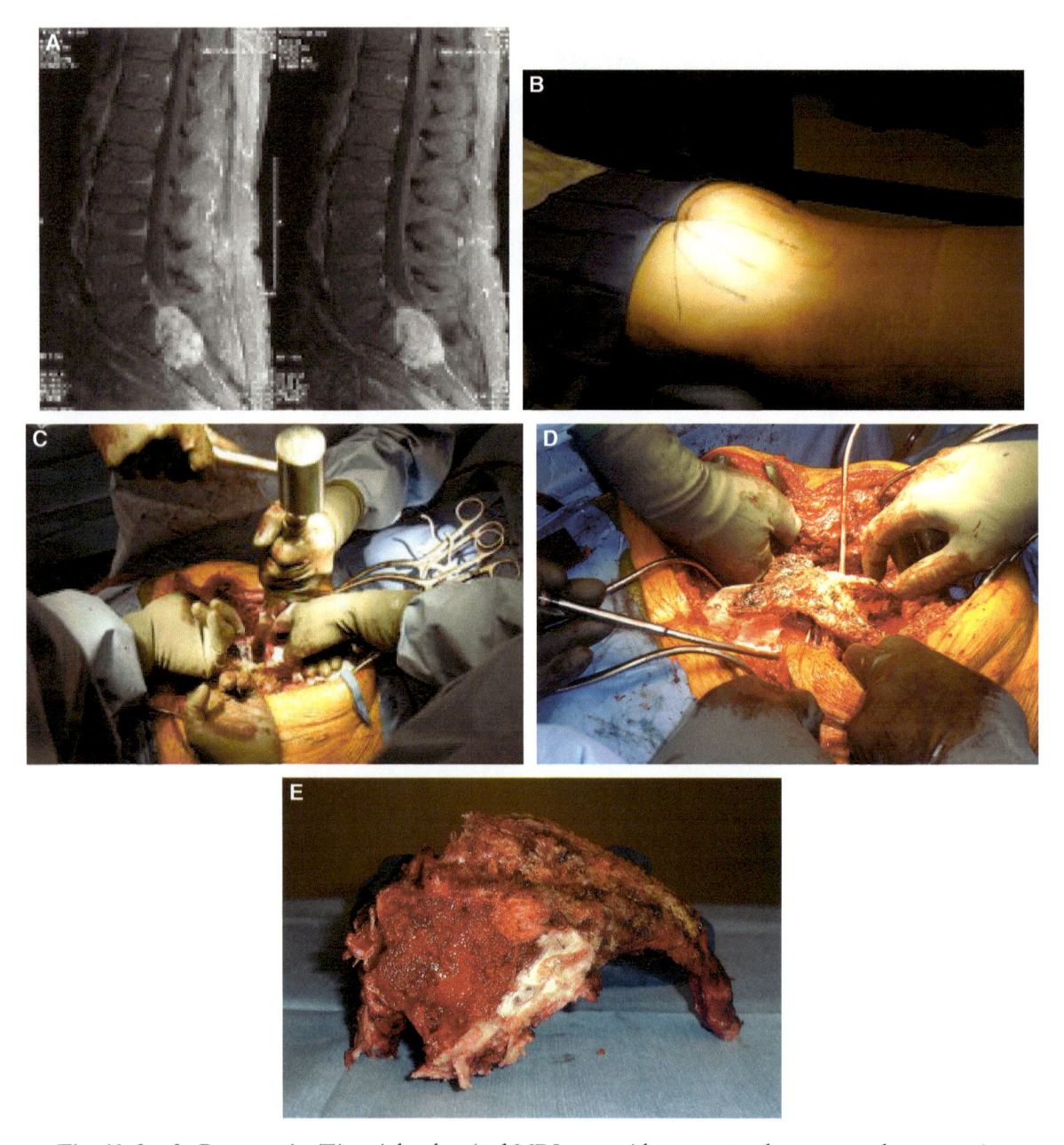

Fig. 10-2 **A,** Preoperative T1-weighted sagittal MRI scan with contrast enhancement demonstrating a sacral mass. **B,** Incision planning for en bloc sacrectomy. **C,** Intraoperative photograph during sacral osteotomy. Osteotomes are used rather than drills to maintain the integrity of the margins. **D,** Blunt dissection of a ventral tumor during sacrectomy. **E,** Photograph of a sacrectomy specimen.

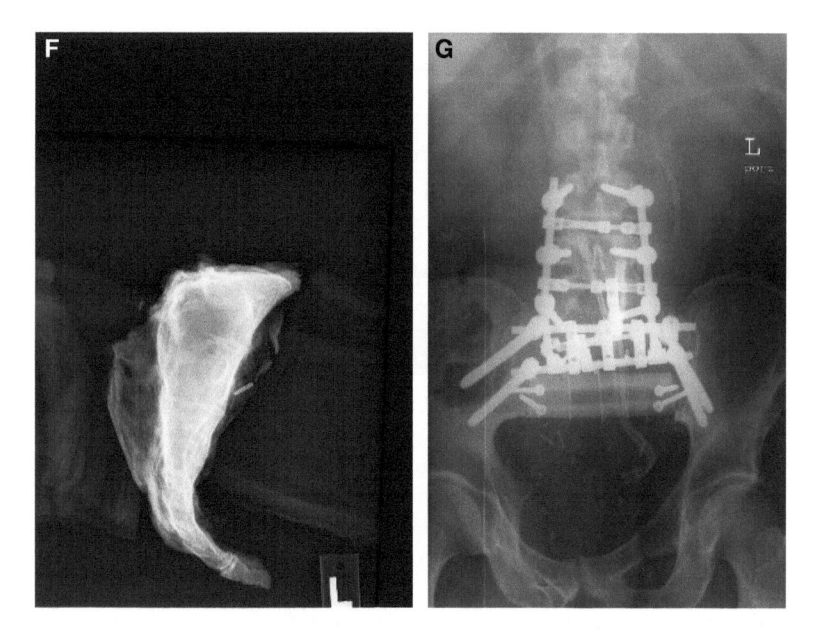

Fig. 10-2, cont'd **F,** Intraoperative radiograph demonstrating en bloc sacral resection. **G,** Postoperative radiograph demonstrating reconstruction after sacrectomy, including transiliac strut graft (Gokaslan technique).

CONCLUSION

Chordomas are rare primary bone tumors with a high risk of local recurrence and a modest propensity for distant metastasis.[4] All patients who have lesions with imaging characteristics resembling a chordoma of the vertebral column should be evaluated by a multidisciplinary group of physicians. Biopsy followed by resection of all gross tumor, when feasible, should be done followed by elective radiation therapy.[16] Margin-free en bloc resection is the only treatment that allows long-term disease-free survival.[5] The effectiveness of en bloc resection for recurrent tumors or tumors with intralesional margins is comparable to that of intralesional extracapsular excision combined with adjuvant treatment. Precise treatment planning and accurate radiation may prolong, and even permanently control, the local regrowth of chordomas.[16] Unfortunately local recurrence of chordoma is not uncommon after en bloc resection.[10,44,47,78] Refinements in treatment techniques, including hyperfractionation, proton beam irradiation, and particle-beam therapy, may further improve results.[4,16] Conventional radiation therapy has a proven role, but the high doses required for these tumors can lead to significant toxicity to surrounding normal tissues and limit its therapeutic value.[4] Charged-particle therapy can achieve adequate dose delivery and good disease control.[4] Chemotherapy has a limited role, but molecular targeted therapy has shown some promise and potential.[4] It is important to work closely with the surgical pathologist to correctly identify the location and quality of the surgical resection.[11]

TIPS FROM THE MASTERS

- Dedifferentiated chordomas often have very high local recurrence rates and behave differently from conventional chordomas despite en bloc resection.
- Aggressive adjuvant treatment is critical in this subtype, but local recurrence rates are still high.

References (With Key References in Boldface)

1. Sundaresan N, Galicich JH, Chu FCH, et al. Spinal chordomas. J Neurosurg 50:312-319, 1979.
2. Beaugie JM, Mann CV, Butler ECB. Sacrococcygeal chordoma. Br J Surg 56:586-588, 1969.
3. Mindell ER. Chordoma: current concepts review. J Bone Joint Surg Am 63:501-505, 1981.
4. Chugh R, Tawbi H, Lucas DR, et al. Chordoma: the nonsarcoma primary bone tumor. Oncologist 12:1344-1350, 2007.
5. **Boriani S, Bandiera S, Biagini R, et al. Chordoma of the mobile spine: fifty years of experience. Spine 31:493-503, 2006.**
6. Bosma JJ, Pigott TJ, Pennie BH, et al. En bloc removal of the lower lumbar vertebral body for chordoma. Report of two cases. J Neurosurg 94 (2 Suppl):S284-S291, 2001.
7. Mirra JM. Bone Tumors: Diagnosis and Treatment. Philadelphia: JB Lippincott, 1980, pp 243-253.
8. Weinstein JN. Spine neoplasms. In Weinstein SL, ed. The Pediatric Spine: Principles and Practice. New York: Raven Press, 1994, pp 887-916.
9. Biagini R, Casadei R, Boriani S, et al. En bloc vertebrectomy and dural resection for chordoma: a case report. Spine 83:E368-E372, 2003.
10. Fourney DR, Gokaslan ZL. Current management of sacral chordoma. Neurosurg Focus 15:E9, 2003.
11. Schwab JH, Healey JH, Rose P, et al. The surgical management of sacral chordomas. Spine 34:2700-2704, 2009.
12. Yamaguchi T, Yamoto M, Saotome K. First histologically confirmed case of a classic chordoma arising in a precursor benign notochordal lesion: differential diagnosis of benign and malignant notochordal lesions. Skeletal Radiol 31:413-418, 2002.
13. Willis RA. Pathology of Tumours, 4th ed. London: Butterworth, 1967, p 937.
14. Spjut HJ, Luse SA. Chordoma: an electron microscopic study. Cancer 17:643-656, 1964.
15. Vujovic S, Henderson S, Presneau N, et al. Brachyury, a crucial regulator of notochordal development, is a novel biomarker for chordomas. J Pathol 209:157-165, 2006.
16. Amendola BE, Amedola MA, Oliver E, et al. Chordoma: role of radiation therapy. Radiology 158:839-843, 1986.
17. Firooznia H, Pinto RL, Lin PJ, et al. Chordoma: radiologic evaluation of 20 cases. AJR Am J Roentgenol 127:797-805, 1976.
18. Higinbotham NL, Phillips RF, Farr HW, et al: Chordoma. Thirty-five-year study at Memorial Hospital. Cancer 20:1841-1850, 1967.
19. Hsu KY, Zucherman JF, Mortensen N, et al. Follow-up evaluation of resected lumbar vertebral chordoma over 11 years: a case report. Spine 25:2537-2540, 2000.
20. Krol G, Sundaresan N, Deck M. Computed tomography of axial chordomas. J Comput Assist Tomogr 7:286-289, 1983.
21. Sundaresan N, Rosenthal DI, Schiller AK, et al. Chordomas. In Sundaresan SN, Schmidek JJ, Schiller AL, eds. Tumors of the Spine: Diagnosis and Clinical Management. Philadelphia: WB Saunders, 1990.
22. Jemal A, Siegel R, Ward E, et al. Cancer statistics. CA Cancer J Clin 57:43-66, 2007.

23. McMaster ML, Goldstein AM, Bromley CM, et al. Chordoma. Incidence and survival in the United States, 1973-1995. Cancer Causes Control 12:1-11, 2001.
24. Mirra J, Nelson S, Della Rocca C, et al. Chordoma. In Fletcher CD, Unni K, Mertens F, eds. Pathology and Genetics of Tumours of Soft Tissue and Bone. Lyon, France: IARC Press, 2002, pp 316-317.
25. **Boriani S, Chavalley F, Weinstein JN, et al. Chordoma of the spine above the sacrum: treatment and outcome in 21 cases. Spine 21:1569-1577, 1996.**
26. Campanacci M. Bone and Soft Tissue Tumors. Berlin: Springer-Verlag/Bologna, Aulo Gaggi, 1990.
27. Healey JH, Lane JM. Chordoma: a critical review of diagnosis and treatment. Orthop Clin North Am 20:3-9, 1989.
28. Dahlin DC. Bone Tumors. General Aspects and Data on 8,542 Cases. Springfield, IL: Charles C Thomas, 1986.
29. Pena CE, Horvat BL, Fisher ER. The ultrastructure of chordoma. Am J Clin Pathol 53:544-551, 1970.
30. Sebag G, Dubois J, Beniamnovitz A, et al. Extraosseous spinal chordoma: radiographic appearance. Am J Neuroradiol 14:205-207, 1993.
31. Sundaresan N. Chordomas. Clin Orthop Relat Res 204:135-142, 1986.
32. Jaffe HL. Tumors and Tumorous Conditions of the Bone and Joints. Philadelphia: Lea & Febiger, 1974, pp 451-462.
33. Birrell JHW. Chordomata: a review of nineteen cases of chordomata including five vertebral cases. Aust NZ J Surg 22:258-267, 1953.
34. Dahlin DC, MacCarty CS. Chordoma. Cancer 5:1170-1178, 1952.
35. Forti E, Venturini G. [Contribution to the knowledge of notochord neoplasms] Riv Anat Patol Oncol 17:317-396, 1960 (in Italian).
36. Faust DB, Gilmore HR Jr, Mudgett CS. Chordomata: a review of the literature with report of a sacrococcygeal case. Ann Intern Med 21:678-698, 1944.
37. Gray SW, Singhabhandhu B, Smith RA, et al. Sacrococcygeal chordoma: report of a case and review of the literature. Surgery 78:573-582, 1975.
38. Mabrey RE. Chordoma: a study of 150 cases. Am J Cancer 25:501-517, 1935.
39. Hartofilakidis-Garofalidi SG, Papathanassiou BT, Kamabouroglou G. Chordoma of the lumbar spine. Int Surg 50:566-570, 1968.
40. Portmann J. [Chordoma of the spine] Z Orthop Ihre Grenzgeb 111:755-763, 1973 (in German).
41. Anson KM, Byrne PO, Robertson ID, et al. Radical excision of sacrococcygeal tumours. Br J Surg 81:460-461, 1994.
42. Smith J, Ludwig RL, Marcove RC. Sacrococcygeal chordoma. A clinicoradiological study of 60 patients. Skeletal Radiol 16:37-44, 1987.
43. Cheng EY, Ozerdemoglu AA, Transfeldt EE, et al. Lumbosacral chordoma, prognostic factors, and treatment. Spine 24:1639-1645, 1999.
44. York JE, Kaczaraj A, Abi-Said D, et al. Sacral chordoma: 40-year experience at a major cancer center. Neurosurgery 44:74-79; discussion 79-80, 1999.
45. Samson IR, Springfield DS, Suit HD, et al. Operative treatment of sacrococcygeal chordoma. A review of twenty-one cases. J Bone Joint Surg Am 75:1476-1484, 1993.
46. Sundaresan N, Huvos AG, Krol G, et al. Surgical treatment of spinal chordomas. Arch Surg 122:1479-1482, 1987.
47. Yonemoto T, Tatezaki S, Takenouchi T, et al. The surgical management of sacrococcygeal chordoma. Cancer 85:878-883, 1999.
48. Chevalier X, Voisin MC, Brugières P, et al. [Chordoma of the mobile spine. Report of 9 cases. Review of the literature] Rev Rhum Mal Osteoartic 57:767-778, 1990 (in French).
49. Stener B. Complete removal of vertebrae for extirpation of tumors. A 20-year experience. Clin Orthop 245:72-82, 1989.

50. Bergh P, Kindblom LG, Gunterberg B, et al. Prognostic factors in chordoma of the sacrum and mobile spine: a study of 39 patients. Cancer 88:2122-2134, 2000.
51. Azzarelli A, Quagliuolo V, Cerasoli S, et al. Chordoma: natural history and treatment results in 33 cases. J Surg Oncol 37:185-191, 1988.
52. Kaiser TE, Pritchard DJ, Unni KK. Clinicopathologic study of sacrococcygeal chordoma. Cancer 53:2574-2578, 1984.
53. Stener B, Gunterberg B. High amputation of the sacrum for extirpation of tumors. Principles and technique. Spine 3:351-366, 1978.
54. Benoit J, Videcoq P, Hardy P, et al. [Spinal chordoma. A case report on chordoma of the L3 vertebra] Rev Rhum Mal Osteoartic 57: 557-561, 1990 (in French).
55. Arnautovic KI, Al Mefty O. Surgical seeding of chordomas. J Neurosurg 95:798-803, 2001.
56. Kirshenbaum AH, Yang WC. Cervical chordoma with intradural invasion. A case report. Bull Hosp Jt Dis Orthop Inst 43:38-48, 1983.
57. Park L, Delaney TF, Liebsch NJ, et al. Sacral chordomas: impact of high-dose proton/photon-beam radiation therapy combined with or without surgery for primary versus recurrent tumor. Int J Radiat Oncol Biol Phys 65:1514-1521, 2006.
58. **Hsieh PC, Xu R, Sciubba DM, et al. Long-term clinical outcomes following en bloc resections for sacral chordomas and chondrosarcomas: a series of twenty consecutive patients. Spine 34:2233-2239, 2009.**
59. Sciubba DM, Chi JH, Rhines LD, et al. Chordoma of the spinal column. Neurosurg Clin N Am 19:5-15, 2008.
60. McLoughlin GS, Sciubba DM, Wolinsky JP. Chondroma/chondrosarcoma of the spine. Neurosurg Clin N Am 19:57-63, 2008.
61. Bilsky MH, Yamada Y, Yenice KM, et al. Intensity-modulated stereotactic radiotherapy of paraspinal tumors: a preliminary report. Neurosurgery 54:823-830; discussion 830-831, 2004.
62. Noël G, Habrand JL, Jauffret E, et al. Radiation therapy for chordoma and chondrosarcoma of the skull base and the cervical spine. Prognostic factors and patterns of failure. Strahlenther Onkol 179:241-248, 2003.
63. Bjornsson J, Wold LE, Ebersold MJ, et al. Chordoma of the mobile spine. A clinicopathologic analysis of 40 patients. Cancer 71:735-740, 1993.
64. Logroscino CA, Astolfi S, Sacchettoni G. Chordoma: long-term evaluation of 15 cases treated surgically. Chir Organi Mov 83:87-103, 1998.
65. Saxton JP. Chordoma. Int J Radiat Oncol Biol Phys 7:913-915, 1981.
66. Chalmers J, Coulson WF. A metastasizing chordoma. J Bone Joint Surg Br 42:556-559, 1960.
67. Congdon CC. Benign and malignant chordomas. A clinico-anatomical study of twenty-two cases. Am J Pathol 28:793-822, 1952.
68. Catton C, O'Sullivan B, Bell R, et al. Chordoma: long-term follow up after radical photon irradiation. Radiother Oncol 41:67-72, 1996.
69. Chambers PW, Schwinn CP. Chordoma. A clinicopathologic study of metastasis. Am J Clin Pathol 72:765-776, 1979.
70. Abdelwahab IF, O'Leary PF, Steiner GC, et al. Case report 357: chordoma of the fourth lumber vertebra metastasizing to the thoracic spine and ribs. Skeletal Radiol 15:242-246, 1986.
71. Delank KS, Kriegsmann J, Drees P, et al. Metastasizing chordoma of the lumbar spine. Eur Spine J 11:167-171, 2002.
72. Jenny J, Sulser H. [Metastasizing chordoma of the lumbar spine] Schweiz Med Wochenschr 103:697-701, 1973 (in German).
73. Jones RB. Chordoma of the third lumbar vertebra simulating carcinoma of the prostate with vertebral metastasis. Report of a case. Br J Surg 48:162-165, 1960.
74. Berven S, Zurakowski D, Mankin HJ, et al. Clinical outcome in chordoma: utility of flow cytometry in DNA determination. Spine 27:374-379, 2002.
75. Naka T, Fukuda T, Chuman H, et al. Proliferative activities in conventional chordoma: a clinicopathologic, DNA flow cytometric, and immunohistochemical analysis of 17 specimens with

special reference to anaplastic chordoma showing a diffuse proliferation and nuclear atypia. Hum Pathol 27:381-388, 1996.
76. Fleming GF, Heimann PS, Stephens JK, et al. Dedifferentiated chordoma. Response to aggressive chemotherapy in two cases. Cancer 72:714-718, 1993.
77. Meis JM, Raymond AK, Evans HL, et al. "Dedifferentiated" chordoma. A clinicopathologic and immunohistochemical study of three cases. Am J Surg Pathol 11:516-525, 1987.
78. Ishii K, Chiba K, Watanabe M, et al. Local recurrence after S2-3 sacrectomy in sacral chordoma. Report of four cases. J Neurosurg 97(1 Suppl):98-101, 2002.
79. Riva P, Crosti F, Orzan F, et al. Mapping of candidate region for chordoma development to 1p36.13 by LOH analysis. Int J Cancer 107:493-497, 2003.
80. Klingler L, Shooks J, Fiedler PN, et al. Microsatellite instability in sacral chordoma. J Surg Oncol 73:100-103, 2000.
81. Bridge JA, Pickering D, Neff JR. Cytogenetic and molecular cytogenetic analysis of sacral chordoma. Cancer Genet Cytogenet 75:23-25, 1994.
82. Sandberg AA, Bridge JA. Updates on the cytogenetics and molecular genetics of bone and soft tissue tumors: chondrosarcoma and other cartilaginous neoplasms. Cancer Genet Cytogenet 143:1-31, 2003.
83. Eisenberg MB, Woloschak M, Sen C, et al. Loss of heterozygosity in the retinoblastoma tumor suppressor gene in skull base chordomas and chondrosarcomas. Surg Neurol 47:156-160; discussion 160-161, 1997.
84. Klinger L, Trammell R, Allan DG, et al. Clonality studies in sacral chordoma. Cancer Genet Cytogenet 171:68-71, 2006.
85. Macnab I, McCulloch J. Backache, 2nd ed. Baltimore: Williams & Wilkins, 1990, pp 72-74.
86. Meyer JE, Lepke RA, Lindfors KK, et al. Chordomas: their CT appearance in the cervical, thoracic and lumbar spine. Radiology 153:693-696, 1984.
87. Schwarz SS, Fisher WS, Pulliam MW, et al. Thoracic chordoma in a patient with paraparesis and ivory vertebral body. Neurosurgery 16:100-102, 1985.
88. Lauger J, Palmer J, Amores S, et al. Primary tumors of the sacrum: diagnostic imaging. AJR Am J Roentgenol 174:417-424, 2000.
89. Campanacci M, Boriani S, Savini R. Staging, biopsy, surgical planning of primary spine tumors. Chir Organi Mov 75 (Suppl 1):99-103, 1983.
90. Enneking WF, Spanier SS, Goodman MA. A system for the surgical staging of musculoskeletal sarcoma. Clin Orthop Relat Res 153:106-120, 1980.
91. Weinstein JN, Hart R, Boriani S, et al. Spine tumors—surgical staging and clinical outcome: application to giant cell tumors of the spine. Presented at the Twenty-First Annual Meeting of the International Society for the Study of the Lumbar Spine, Seattle, WA, June 22-25, 1994.
92. Rossleigh MA, Smith J, Yeh SD. Scintigraphic features of primary sacral tumors. J Nucl Med 27:627-630, 1986.
93. Cummings BJ, Hodson DI, Bush RS. Chordoma: the results of megavoltage radiation therapy. Int J Radiat Oncol Biol Phys 9:633-642, 1983.
94. Pearlman AW, Friedman M. Radical radiation therapy: chordoma. AJR Am J Roentgenol 53:544-551, 1970.
95. **Chou D, Acosta F Jr, Cloyd JM. Parasagittal osteotomy for en bloc resection of multilevel cervical chordomas. J Neurosurg Spine 10:397-403, 2009.**
96. Currier BL, Papagelopoulos PJ, Krauss WE, et al. Total en bloc spondylectomy of C5 vertebra for chordoma. Spine 32:E294-E299, 2007.
97. Fuchs B, Dickey ID, Yaszemski MJ, et al. Operative management of sacral chordoma. J Bone Joint Surg Am 87:2211-2216, 2005.
98. Hulen CA, Temple HT, Fox WP, et al. Oncologic and functional outcome following sacrectomy for sacral chordoma. J Bone Joint Surg Am 88:1532-1539, 2006.
99. Fourney DR, Rhines LD, Hentschel SJ, et al. En bloc resection of primary sacral tumors: classification of surgical approaches and outcome. J Neurosurg Spine 3:111-122, 2005.
100. York JE, Berk RH, Fuller GN, et al. Chondrosarcoma of the spine: 1954 to 1997. J Neurosurg 90:73-78, 1999.

101. Bergh P, Gunterberg B, Meis-Kindblom JM, et al. Prognostic factors and outcome of pelvic, sacral, and spinal chondrosarcomas: a center-based study of 69 cases. Cancer 91:1201-1212, 2001.
102. Findlay GFG. Tumors of the lumbar spine. In Jayson MIV, ed. The Lumbar Spine and Back Pain, 4th ed. Edinburgh: Churchill Livingstone, 1992, pp 355-369.
103. Senning A, Weber G, Yaşargil MG. Zur operativen Behandlung von Tumoren der Wirbelsäule. Schweiz Med Wochenschr 48:1574-1576, 1962.
104. Verbiest H. Giant-cell tumors and aneurismal bone cysts of the spine. With special reference to the problems related to the removal of a vertebral body. J Bone Joint Surg Br 47:699-713, 1965.
105. Cotler HB, Cotler JM, Cohn HE, et al. Intrathoracic chordoma presenting as a posterior superior mediastinal tumor. Spine 8:781-786, 1983.
106. Fujita T, Kawahara N, Matsumoto T, et al. Chordoma of the cervical spine managed with en bloc excision. Spine 24:1848-1851, 1999.
107. Boriani S, Weinstein JN, Biagini R. Primary bone tumors of the spine. Terminology and surgical staging. Spine 22:1036-1044, 1997.
108. Cohen ZR, Fourney DR, Marco RA, et al. Total cervical spondylectomy for primary osteogenic sarcoma. Case report and description of operative technique. J Neurosurg 97:386-392, 2002.
109. **Tomita K, Kawahara N, Baba H, et al. Total en bloc spondylectomy. A new surgical technique for primary malignant vertebral tumors. Spine 22:324-333, 1997.**
110. Anegawa T, Rai M, Hara K, et al. An unusual cervical chordoma: CT and MRI. Neuroradiology 38:466-467, 1996.
111. Ducou le Pointe H, Brugieres P, Chevalier X, et al. Imaging of chordomas of the mobile spine. J Neuroradiol 18:267-276, 1991.
112. Murphy JM, Wallis F, Toland J, et al. CT and MRI appearances of a thoracic chordoma. Eur Radiol 8:1677-1679, 1998.
113. Smolders D, Wang X, Drevelengas A, et al. Value of MRI in the diagnosis of non-clival, non-sacral chordoma. Skeletal Radiol 32:343-350, 2003.
114. Crapanzano JP, Ali SZ, Ginsberg MS, et al. Chordoma: a cytologic study with histologic and radiologic correlation. Cancer 93:40-51, 2001.
115. Murad TM, Murthy MSN. Ultrastructure of a chordoma. Cancer 25:1204-1215, 1970.
116. Ribbert H. Ueber die Ecchondrosis physalifora sphenoccipitalis. Z Allg Path Path Anat 5:457-461, 1894.
117. Windeyer BW. Chordoma. President's address. Proc R Soc Med 52:1088-1100, 1959.
118. Kamrin RP, Potanos JN, Pool JL. An evaluation of the diagnosis and treatment of chordoma. J Neurol Neurosurg Psychiatry 27:157-165, 1964.
119 Pearlman AW, Friedman M. Radical radiation therapy of chordoma. Am J Roentgenol Radium Ther Nucl Med 108:333-341, 1970.
120. Sennet EJ. Chordoma: its roentgen diagnostic aspects and its response to roentgen therapy. Am J Roentgenol Radium Ther Nucl Med 69:613-622, 1953.
121. Rich TA, Schiller A, Suit HD, et al. Clinical and pathologic review of 48 cases of chordoma. Cancer 56:182-187, 1985.
122. Enneking WF. Musculoskeletal Tumor Surgery. New York: Churchill Livingstone, 1983.
123. Gunterberg B, Kewenter J, Petersen I, et al. Anorectal function after major resections of the sacrum with bilateral or unilateral sacrifice of sacral nerves. Br J Surg 63:546-554, 1976.
124. Gunterberg B, Petersen I. Sexual function after major resections of the sacrum with bilateral or unilateral sacrifice of sacral nerves. Fertil Steril 27:1146-1153, 1976.
125. Bas T, Bas P, Prieto M, et al. A lumbar chordoma treated with a wide resection. Eur Spine J 3:115-117, 1994.
126. Heary RF, Vaccaro AR, Benevenia J, et al. "En-bloc" vertebrectomy in the mobile lumbar spine. Surg Neurol 50:548-556, 1998.
127. Sundaresan N, Steinberger AA, Moore F, et al. Indications and results of combined anterior-posterior approaches for spine tumor surgery. J Neurosurg 85:438-446, 1996.
128. Anson JA, Marchand EP. Bovine pericardium for dural grafts: clinical results in 35 patients. Neurosurgery 39:764-768, 1996.

129. Wright NM, Kaufman BA, Haughey BH, et al. Complex cervical spine neoplastic disease: reconstruction after surgery by using a vascularized fibular strut graft. Case report. J Neurosurg Spine 90:133-137, 1999.
130. Baratti D, Gronchi A, Pennacchioli E, et al. Chordoma: natural history and results in 28 patients treated at a single institution. Ann Surg Oncol 10:291-296, 2003.
131. Walaas L, Kindblom LG. Fine-needle aspiration biopsy in the preoperative diagnosis of chordoma: a study of 17 cases with application of electron microscopic, histochemical, and immunocytochemical examination. Hum Pathol 22:22-28, 1991.
132. Keisch ME, Garcia DM, Shibuya RB. Retrospective long-term follow-up analysis in 21 patients with chordomas of various sites treated at a single institution. J Neurosurg 75:374-377, 1991.
133. Lybert MLM, Meerwalddt JH. Chordoma: report on treatment results in eighteen cases. Acta Radiol Oncol 25:41-43, 1986.
134. Austin-Seymour M, Munzenrider J, Goitein M, et al. Fractionated proton radiation therapy of chordoma and low-grade chondrosarcoma of the base of the skull. J Neurosurg 70:13-17, 1989.
135. Tewfik HH, McGinnis WL, Nordstrom DG, et al. Chordoma: evaluation of clinical behavior and treatment modalities. Int J Radiat Oncol Biol Phys 2:959-962, 1977.
136. Reddy EK, Mansfield CM, Hartman GV. Chordoma. Int J Radiat Oncol Biol Phys 7:1709-1711, 1981.
137. Igaki H, Tokuuye K, Okumura T, et al. Clinical results of proton beam therapy for skull base chordoma. Int J Radiat Oncol Biol Phys 60:1120-1126, 2004.
138. **Noel G, Feuvret L, Calugaru V, et al. Chordomas of the base of the skull and upper cervical spine. One hundred patients irradiated by a 3D conformal technique combining photon and proton beams. Acta Oncol 44:700-708, 2005.**
139. Suit HD, Goitein M, Munzenrider J, et al. Definitive radiation therapy for chordoma and chondrosarcoma of base of skull and cervical spine. J Neurosurg 56:377-385, 1982.
140. Walsh TM, Mayer PJ. Chordoma of the thoracic spine presenting as a second primary malignant lesion: a case report. Spine 17:1524-1528, 1992.
141. Suit HD, Goitein M, Munzenrider J, et al. Increased efficacy of radiation therapy by use of proton beam. Strahlenther Onkol 166:40-44, 1990.
142. Tatsuzaki H, Urie MM. Importance of precise positioning for proton beam therapy in the base of skull and cervical spine. Int J Radiat Oncol Biol Phys 21:757-765, 1991.
143. Crockard A. Chordomas and chondrosarcomas of the cranial base: results and follow-up of 60 patients. Neurosurgery 38:420, 1996.
144. Foweraker KL, Chantler HJ, Geater AR, et al. Conformal versus IMRT for chordoma of the skull base and cervical spine. Clin Oncol (R Coll Radiol) 19:S28-S29, 2007.
145. Berson AM, Castro JR, Petti P, et al. Charged particle irradiation of chordoma and chondrosarcoma of the base of skull and cervical spine: the Lawrence Berkeley Laboratory experience. Int J Radiat Oncol Biol Phys 15:559-565, 1988.
146. Hug EB, Loredo LN, Slater JD, et al. Proton radiation therapy for chordomas and chondrosarcomas of the skull base. J Neurosurg 91:432-439, 1999.
147. Kumar PP, Good RR, Skultety FM, et al. Local control of recurrent clival and sacral chordoma after interstitial irradiation with iodine-125: new techniques for treatment of recurrent or unresectable chordomas. Neurosurgery 22:479-483, 1988.
148. Scimeca PG, James-Herry AG, Black KS, et al. Chemotherapeutic treatment of malignant chordoma in children. J Pediatr Hematol Oncol 18:237-240, 1996.
149. Razis DV, Tsatsaronis A, Kyriazides I, et al. Chordoma of the cervical spine treated with vincristine sulfate. J Med 5:274-277, 1974.
150. McSweeney AJ, Sholl PR. Metastatic chordoma use of mechlorethiamine (nitrogen mustard) in chordoma therapy. Arch Surg 79:152-155, 1959.
151. de Vries J, Oldhoff J, Hadders HN. Cryosurgical treatment of sacrococcygeal chordoma. Report of four cases. Cancer 58:2348-2354, 1986.
152. Kollender Y, Meller I, Bickels J, et al. Role of adjuvant cryosurgery in intralesional treatment of sacral tumors. Cancer 97:2830-2838, 2003.

153. Marcove RC. A 17-year review of cryosurgery in the treatment of bone tumors. Clin Orthop Relat Res 163:231-234, 1982.
154. Biagini R, Ruggieri P, Mercuri M, et al. Neurologic deficit after resection of the sacrum. Chir Organi Mov 82:357-372, 1997.
155. Nakai S, Yoshizawa H, Kobayashi S, et al. Anorectal and bladder function after sacrifice of the sacral nerves. Spine 25:2234-2239, 2000.
156. Todd LT Jr, Yaszemski MJ, Currier BL, et al. Bowel and bladder function after major sacral resection. Clin Orthop Relat Res 397:36-39, 2002.
157. Gokaslan ZL, Romsdahl MM, Kroll SS, et al. Total sacrectomy and Galveston L-rod reconstruction for malignant neoplasms. Technical note. J Neurosurg 87:781-787, 1997.
158. Jackson RJ, Gokaslan ZL. Spinal-pelvic fixation in patients with lumbosacral neoplasms. J Neurosurg 92(1 Suppl):61-70, 2000.
159. Gunterberg B, Norlen L, Stener B, et al. Neurourologic evaluation after resection of the sacrum. Invest Urol 13:183-188, 1975.
160. Wellinger C. [Spinal chordoma. II. Review of the literature since 1960] Rev Rhum Mal Osteoartic 42:195-204, 1975 (in French).

Chapter 11

Chondrosarcoma of the Spine

Daniel M. Sciubba, Jean-Paul Wolinsky,
Ziya L. Gokaslan

Chondromas and chondrosarcomas are cartilage-forming tumors of mesenchymal origin. In the spine such lesions are very rare. Similar to most primary tumors of the spine, these lesions can be locally aggressive both at presentation and after resection from residual tumor cells. Unlike most other sarcomas, the grade of a chondrosarcoma has prognostic significance. Therefore a preoperative biopsy can help prognosticate the growth potential of the lesion. Nonetheless, definitive treatment is complete en bloc resection, because conventional chemotherapy and radiation therapy are relatively ineffective modalities for chondrosarcomas.

EPIDEMIOLOGY

Chondromas account for approximately 5% of all primary bone tumors,[1] but they are extremely rare in the spinal column. Chondrosarcomas are estimated to comprise 7% to 12% of all primary spine tumors and account for 25% of primary malignant neoplasms of the spine.[2,3] Although more common than chondromas, chondrosarcomas of the spine are also considered rare, with only 21 cases encountered over a 43-year period at a major cancer center.[4] Both types of tumors can occur anywhere along the mobile spine, although most commonly they occur in the thoracic spine (up to 60% for chondrosarcomas).[5] The remaining distribution of chondrosarcomas is divided between the lumbar spine (20% to 40%) and the cervical spine (20%).[6] Both benign and malignant tumors are more common in males, with a ratio of 2:1 to 4:1. Age at diagnosis is typically between 30 and 50 years and varies depending on the chondrosarcoma subtype.[3,5,7]

PATHOLOGY AND STAGING

Chondrosarcomas are malignant cartilage-forming tumors; they are more locally aggressive than chondromas, which are benign tumors of cartilage that appear in the spine. Chondrosarcomas have the ability to distantly metastasize. Chondromas can be labeled according to their site of origin; namely, from the medullary cavity (enchondroma) or the cortical surface (periosteal chondroma).[8] Enchondromas tend to produce an expansible growth pattern, whereas periosteal chondromas are exophytic. Any part of the vertebra can be affected, including the spinous process, lamina, pedicles, and body.

With regard to the pathologic characteristics of chondromas, these tumors resemble lobules of firm, mature cartilage with grittiness from internal mineralization that is well circumscribed from the adjacent bone.[5] Chondromas are typically small tumors, and a diameter greater than 7 cm may be suggestive of malignancy.[9] Histologically these tumors are composed of neoplastic chondrocytes dispersed within an abundant hyaline or myxoid background. The tumor cells are small and do not exhibit cellular pleomorphism or nuclear atypia.[10] Multinucleated cells are rare and mitoses are absent. Foci of calcifications may be present. It is of critical importance that the entire histologic specimen be closely examined, because sarcomatous cells may occupy a small nest of an otherwise benign tumor.[2,11]

Although cytogenetic aberrations may not be detectable for some chondromas, nonrandom genomic abnormalities have been linked to chromosomes 4, 5, 6, 7, 11, 12, and 15.[12,13] Monosomies of chromosomes 9, 19, and 22 have also been reported, as well as 12q13-15 rearrangements.[14,15] Most chondromas grown in cell culture do not exhibit chromosomal aberrations.[14] These properties are in contrast to chondrosarcomas, which consistently demonstrate complex mutations. It is interesting to note that c-Myc oncogene amplification and polysomy 8 have been associated with malignant transformation of a benign chondroma into a dedifferentiated chondrosarcoma.[9,16]

Pathologic assessment and staging are more complex with regard to chondrosarcomas. The World Health Organization (WHO) defines chondrosarcomas as mesenchymal, nonmeningothelial tumors and grades them from low (grade I) to high (grade IV).[10,17] The grade is based on histologic features, such as tumor cellularity, nuclear atypia, stromal content (chondroid or myxoid), and mitoses. The WHO grading definitions have been shown to be one of the most important prognostic features of chondrosarcomas.[6] The 10-year survival for grade I chondrosarcomas is 90%, declining to 65% to 80% for grade II tumors. The 10-year survival for high-grade chondrosarcomas is 30% to 40%.[6]

Histologically, grade I chondrosarcomas closely resemble chondromas, and it may prove difficult to differentiate the two entities pathologically. Both tumors resemble mature cartilage on microscopic examination. Distinguishing features of low-grade chondrosarcomas include invasion or entrapment of surrounding tissues, penetration of the bony cortex, and a prominent myxoid stroma, supporting the suggestion that the entire specimen be reviewed closely.[2,18] The neoplastic cells are small and exhibit minimal nuclear atypia, and mitosis is absent.[19] If the stroma is predominantly myxoid in nature, the tumor grade is increased to grade II. In addition, grade II lesions exhibit a relative increase in cellularity as compared with grade I tumors, and they demonstrate greater nuclear pleomorphism. Mitoses rarely occur in grade II lesions.[6]

Grade III and IV lesions possess increasingly cellular and pleomorphic features compared with lower grade tumors. The neoplastic cells are often multinucleated with prominent nucleoli and must exhibit at least two mitotic figures per 10 high-power fields.[6] As the cellularity increases, the proportion of stromal substance decreases, producing a softer and more friable tumor, which is in contrast to the hard cartilaginous matrix of low-grade lesions. The likelihood of distant metastasis is also directly linked to grade (grade I chondrosarcomas do not metastasize), whereas grade III and IV tumors metastasize 70% of the time.[6]

In addition to the WHO grading system, chondrosarcomas are subclassified into subtypes based on stereotypical histologic features, including conventional, mesenchymal, clear cell, and dedifferentiated categories.[2] The origin of the tumor (primary or secondary), imaging features, pathologic findings, and immunohistochemical profiles are unique to each subtype. Conventional chondrosarcomas compose 80% to 90% of the chondrosarcoma subtypes, and almost all of these tumors are low grade, with less than 10% grade III or IV lesions.[20] These lobulated tumors demonstrate lytic extension into the surrounding bone. They can arise from the medullary cavity or cortical surface of normal bone (primary chondrosarcoma) or from a preexisting benign cartilaginous or osseous tumors (secondary chondrosarcoma).[19] Also, low-grade typical chondrosarcomas may produce a stroma resembling mature cartilage similar to that of a chondroma.[18] These tumors are reactive to vimentin and S100, which are often reactive in other low-grade chondrosarcoma subtypes.[9]

Dedifferentiated chondrosarcomas are characterized as malignant degeneration of a conventional, low-grade chondrosarcoma.[21] Histologically this pattern is recognized as an abrupt shift in the microscopic appearance of the lesion, and specimens will demonstrate a clear demarcation between the low-grade and high-grade areas.[26] Dedifferentiated chondrosarcomas are extremely aggressive, with frequent metastases, and 5-year survival can be less than 10%.[22] These tumors may also harbor foci of neoplastic tissues resembling other sarcomas, including osteosarcoma, leiomyosarcoma, rhabdomyosarcoma, or malignant fibrous histiocytoma, which are identifiable by immunostaining that follows the profile of the embryologic origin of neoplasms.[6]

Similar to dedifferentiated chondrosarcomas, mesenchymal chondrosarcomas are composed of two separate cell populations. Low-grade chondrocytes are interspersed among small, undifferentiated neoplastic cells.[23] However, these biomorphic collections lack the clear margins of dedifferentiated chondrosarcomas.[24] In some instances the undifferentiated small cells may express desmin and myogenin, which suggests a skeletal muscle lineage.[23] Caution must be used when interpreting CT-guided biopsy samples of mesenchymal chondrosarcomas, because a small sample of low-grade tumor may lead to the incorrect diagnosis of conventional chondrosarcoma. Mesenchymal chondrosarcomas are also associated with a relatively poor prognosis—that is, the 5-year survival rate is estimated to be approximately 50%.[6]

The last type of chondrosarcoma is the clear cell chondrosarcoma, which is characterized by dense collections of neoplastic cells with abundant cytoplasm. This cytoplasm is rich in glycogen and therefore stains strongly for periodic acid–Schiff.[25] Each cell shares a discrete border with its neighbors. Lobules of cells are dispersed among bony trabeculae, and foci of conventional chondrosarcomas may be present. Necrosis can sometimes occur. These tumors are immunoreactive to S100.[25] In general, clear cell chondrosarcomas have a better prognosis than mesenchymal or dedifferentiated chondrosarcomas.[26]

In addition to the histologic assessment of chondrosarcomas being associated with prognosis, some cytogenetic abnormalities of chondrosarcomas may also be associated with outcome. A variety of nonrandom genetic aberrations occur, and allelic losses are seen in almost 70% of tumors.[6] The mutations responsible for the malignant degeneration of a chondroma may occur in a stepwise fashion, including amplification of the c-Myc oncogene and/or the addition of chromosome 8.[6,27] Other genomic mutations include the loss of chromosome 6 and the gain of 12q12, which correlate with high-grade chondrosarcomas[28]; 6q13-21 chromosome aberrations also occur in aggressive tumors.[29] Medullary (central) chondrosarcomas may be diploid, whereas surface (peripheral) tumors may be aneuploid. Dedifferentiated tumors can have a (9;22)(q22-31;q11-12) translocation[27] and may also overexpress p53.[20] The addition of chromosome 7 has been associated with high-grade lesions, as have 17p1 alterations.[28] Aberrant platelet-derived growth factor receptor-α (PDGFR-α) and PDGFR-β expression have been shown to occur in chondrosarcomas.[22] In addition, estrogen hormone signaling, matrix metalloproteinsase-1 expression, histone dysregulation, and methylthioadenosine phosphorylase (MTAP) deletions have also been discovered.[6] Some have hypothesized that the blood supply to the tumor may result from vascular endothelial growth factor A (VEGF-A) overexpression.[6] Targeted therapy directed at such proteins and their receptors may provide potential novel chemotherapeutic agents in the future.[30]

CLINICAL PRESENTATION

Patients with a spinal chondroma typically present with local tenderness at the site of the tumor. In addition, a palpable mass may be present as the tumor expands into the surrounding paraspinous tissues.[1] Because chondromas are slow-growing tumors, neurologic symptoms and signs may develop gradually, if at all. Rarely, a radiculopathy or myelopathy can result from direct neural compression.[5] Remodeling or erosion of bone can occur, causing widening of the neural foramen and impingement of the exiting nerve.[8] Occasionally a pathologic fracture will occur in the affected bone, leading to local and mechanical spine pain. In a review of 11 patients with chondromas, Gaetani et al[31] noted that the mean duration of symptoms before diagnosis was 13.8 ± 3.4 months.

Because chondromas usually occur as isolated lesions, the presence of multiple chondromas may suggest a multiple chondromatosis syndrome, identified as Ollier disease and Maffucci syndrome.[32] These rare conditions are characterized by multiple chondromas in childhood. The exact cause is unknown, but it has been suggested that multiple somatic mutations play a role in the development of the lesions.[33] Multiple chondromas occur throughout the skeleton, creating skeletal deformities, limb-length discrepancies, and pathologic fractures. Maffucci syndrome can be differentiated from Ollier disease by the presence of cutaneous hemangiomata.[34]

Compared with patients with isolated tumors, patients with the chondromas of Ollier disease or Maffucci syndrome are at greater risk for sarcomatous degeneration, which can occur in up to 25% of patients with these conditions.[2] The overall incidence of malignant degeneration for isolated chondromas is low, and it is impossible to predict which patients are at risk. Therefore all patients require careful assessment of syndromic anomalies and should undergo complete resection, if possible. Cytologic analysis may also be prognostic, inasmuch as (9;12)(q22;q24) translocation has been associated with malignant degeneration of a chondroma.[35]

Although more locally aggressive, chondrosarcomas usually exhibit an indolent growth pattern, and symptoms may present gradually. The most common symptom is focal pain.[4] Because these tumors are larger and invade or encroach on surrounding tissues, neurologic deficits are common and can manifest as radiculopathy, myelopathy, or cauda equina syndrome.[36] Up to 50% of all patients may have a neurologic deficit at the time of presentation.[6] In addition, a palpable mass may be present in the neck or back as the tumor expands outward from the posterior elements.

IMAGING

Radiologic assessment of chondromas and chondrosarcomas includes the use of plain radiographs, CT scans, MRI, and bone scans. Although plain radiographs of spine tumors can be helpful, the imaging findings for chordomas may be subtle, and CT scans are usually necessary to view these lesions. A plain radiograph may demonstrate a well-circumscribed lytic lesion without reactive sclerosis.[1] Once such a lesion is noted on plain radiographs, CT scans should be used to define the location of the tumor and characterize its growth. CT scans of chondromas will often correspondingly reveal a radiolucent erosive lesion. Cartilage will appear as regions of low attenuation on CT scans, with stippled areas where calcification may be present.[37] CT images of chondrosarcomas often reveal lytic destruction of lesions of varying density. Local deformity may occur, and the neural foramen may be wide if the tumor is intraforaminal.[8] Radiologic differentiation between a chondroma and a low-grade chondrosarcoma can be challenging. MRI studies with gadolinium contrast material can be useful to help distinguish between benign and malignant lesions, because an enhancing cartilaginous tumor is more likely to be consistent with a chondrosarcoma.[5,31]

Imaging features can sometimes be suggestive of particular chondrosarcoma subtypes.[37] A peripheral chondrosarcoma may produce thickening of the vertebral cortex with exophytic extension into the soft tissue.[38] The water content in the cartilage matrix of such lesions will appear as a focus of low attenuation on a CT image.[37] Clear cell chondrosarcomas specifically may appear as rounded, lytic lesions with calcifications and surrounding sclerosis.[25] Dedifferentiated and mesenchymal chondrosarcomas may demonstrate more substantial destruction of local bone.[27] "Ring and arc" calcifications may indicate the chondroid matrix of a conventional chondrosarcoma.[37]

MRI scans are useful to assess the extent of soft tissue invasion and neural compromise. T1-weighted images often demonstrate a hypointense lesion, whereas T2-weighted images will be hyperintense; both of these are consistent with the high water content of neoplastic cartilage[37] (Fig. 11-1). Mineralization, if present, will appear as a low signal. Intravenous gadolinium can reveal a peripheral ring of enhancement or heterogeneous enhancement of the entire tumor. If used, a bone scan may demonstrate increased uptake of radiotracer in the vicinity of the tumor.[37]

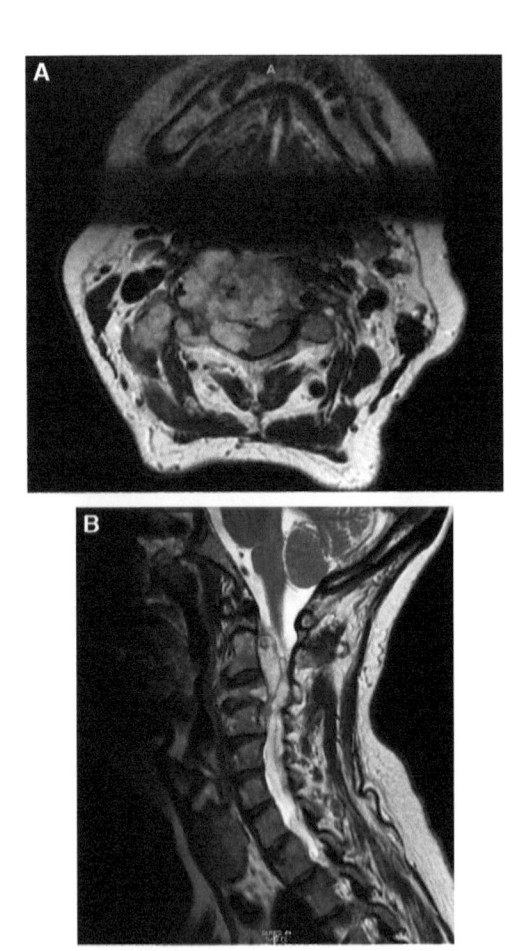

Fig. 11-1 **A,** Axial T1-weighted MRI image and **B,** sagittal T2-weighted image of a cervical chondrosarcoma showing extension into soft tissues and the spinal canal.

TREATMENT

The treatment goal for chondromas and chondrosarcomas is complete surgical resection[1,17,22] (Figs. 11-2 and 11-3). In this way, surgery is used to establish a histologic diagnosis, prevent sarcomatous degeneration, and preserve neurologic function.[5] Furthermore, these tumors are resistant to conventional chemotherapy and radiation, and their role in treatment is limited. It is highly recommended that the results of CT-guided biopsies be evaluated with caution, because sampling errors may lead to a false-positive diagnosis of a benign tumor.[2,11] Because of the heterogeneity of chondrosarcoma cytoarchitecture, the false-negative rate for malignancy can approach 24%.[11] The entire specimen should be histologically examined for areas of malignant degeneration. After complete resection of a chondroma, the recurrence rate has been reported to be less than 10%.[5]

It is well established that a complete en bloc resection is the ideal surgical technique for resecting chondrosarcomas, because en bloc vertebrectomy and spondylectomy have been associated with prolonged recurrence-free survival, and local curettage of a chondrosarcoma virtually guarantees recurrence.[4,22,39-42] However, such procedures

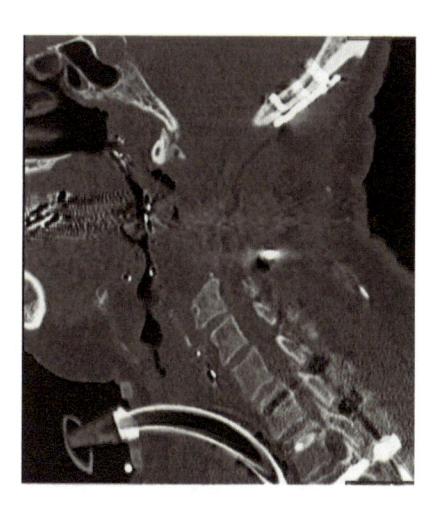

Fig. 11-2 Sagittal CT reconstruction after en bloc resection of the cervical chondrosarcoma shown in Fig. 11-1. The patient underwent a preoperative tracheostomy and required an occipitocervical fusion.

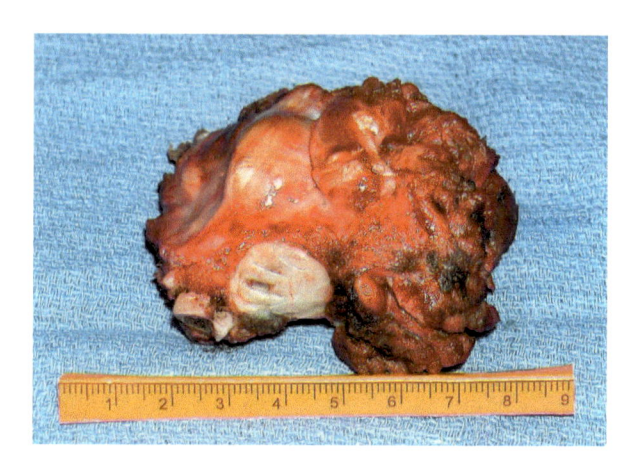

Fig. 11-3 Specimen removed en bloc from the patient shown in Figs. 11-1 and 11-2.

may be technically challenging to perform. Complete en bloc resections require careful planning, an experienced multidisciplinary team, and meticulous surgical technique (Figs. 11-4 through 11-6).[43,44] It has been shown that even minor contamination of the margin of an en bloc specimen with tumor has a worse prognosis.[4] Complete en bloc resections have yielded recurrence rates of 20% or lower, and in some instances survival of 5 years or more.[22]

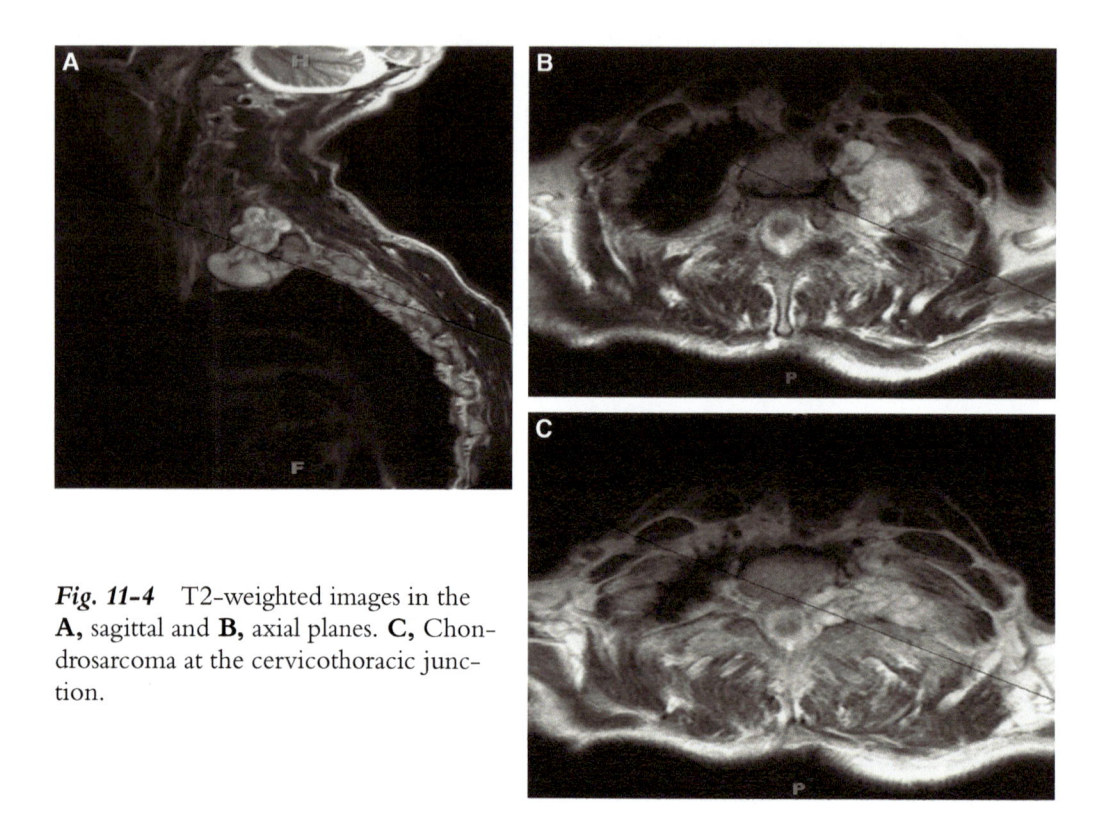

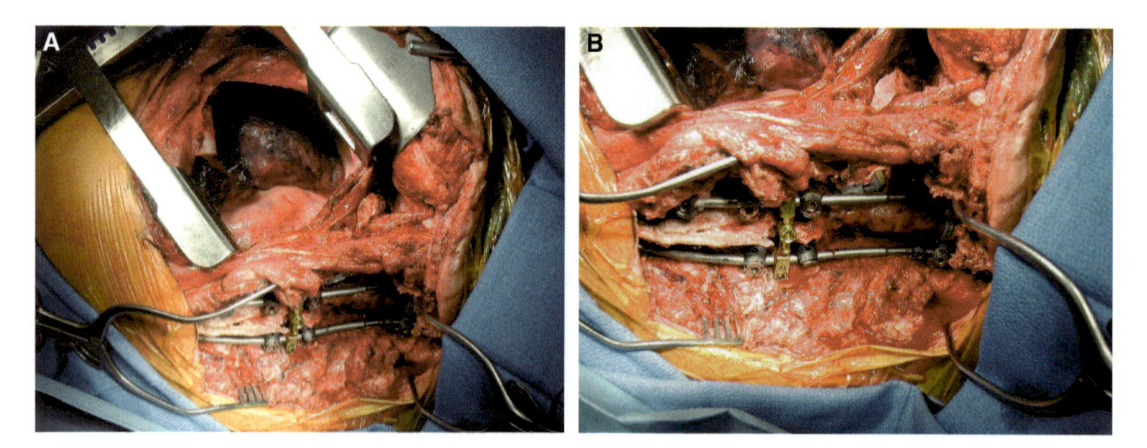

Fig. 11-4 T2-weighted images in the **A,** sagittal and **B,** axial planes. **C,** Chondrosarcoma at the cervicothoracic junction.

Fig. 11-5 **A** and **B,** Intraoperative photographs showing simultaneous thoracotomy and posterior midline incision to allow delivery of the tumor and placement of an anterior titanium cage and posterior instrumentation.

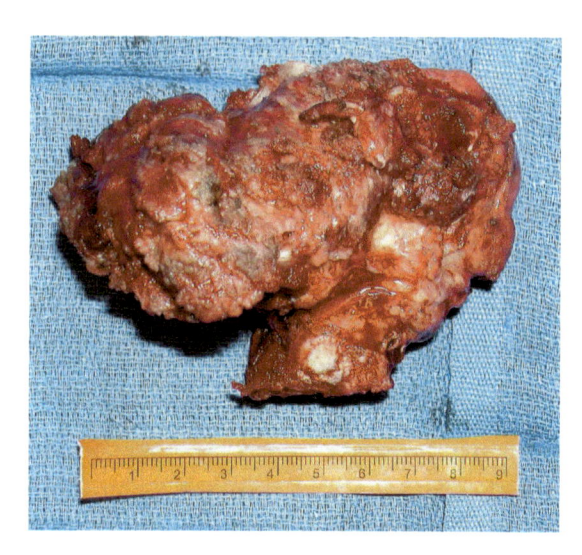

Fig. 11-6 En bloc specimen delivered from the patient shown in Figs. 11-4 and 11-5.

Local tumor recurrence is associated with a dismal prognosis, with more than 50% of patients dying of their disease within less than 2 years.[2,45] The role of aggressive surgical resection for local recurrence has yet to be defined, although Weber et al[46] reported a 50% long-term survival rate in 12 patients treated surgically for recurrent pelvic chondrosarcomas. It remains to be seen whether these findings can be generalized to recurrent chondrosarcomas of the mobile spine. Although metastases do occur with chondrosarcomas, local recurrence is a stronger negative prognostic factor for survival.[45]

High-dose radiation therapy or proton beam therapy may slow tumor progression. Therefore this modality should be considered for tumor recurrences and palliation.[47,48] Specifically, hypofractionated stereotactic radiation therapy has provided some evidence of a therapeutic response, but the long-term results of this treatment are unknown.[48,49] Novel radiosensitizers may hold some promise for improving the efficacy of these therapies.[47]

The prognosis for low-grade chondrosarcomas is good with wide en bloc excision. Intralesional excision is to be avoided, except in cases of spinal cord compression with metastatic disease.

Solitary high-grade chondrosarcomas are also best treated with wide excision, but many of these patients may have undetected metastatic disease at presentation. Thorough preoperative evaluation for distant metastasis is recommended, and patients should be informed of differences in biological behavior as they make decisions with their surgeons regarding functional sacrifice for wider margins.

CONCLUSION

Chondromas and chondrosarcomas are rare primary tumors of the vertebral column that indolently cause focal pain and, occasionally, progressive neurologic deficits. To achieve long-term local control, these lesions must be completely resected. Histologic diagnosis (chondroma versus chondrosarcoma), subtype of chondrosarcoma, and tumor grade are the most important prognostic factors. Because these tumors are resistant to adjuvant chemotherapy and radiation therapy, a complete en bloc resection offers the best chance of a prolonged and recurrence-free survival.

TIPS FROM THE MASTERS

- CT-guided biopsy to establish the diagnosis for a primary bone tumor is critical. Pathology dictates the treatment plan, and if an en bloc resection is to be undertaken, given the potential morbidity of the procedure, the pathology needs to be known with a high degree of certainty.
- Surgical planning for an en bloc resection requires involvement of many different surgical disciplines. The surgical strategy for the en bloc resections of the mobile spine is to visualize the spine as a ring with the neural elements incarcerated within the ring. The first stage of the operation is designed to open the ring so that the specimen and spine can be safely delivered away from the neural elements. In addition, spinal reconstruction is performed during the first stage. The second stage consists of delivery of the specimen and completion of the reconstruction.
- Careful assessment of the pathology and the surgical margins will determine whether adjuvant chemotherapy or radiation therapy will be needed.

References (With Key References in Boldface)

1. Palaoglu S, Akkas O, Sav A. Chondroma of the cervical spine. Clin Neurol Neurosurg 90:253-255, 1988.
2. Coons S. Pathology of tumors of the spinal cord, spine, and paraspinous soft tissue. In Dickman CA, Fehlings MG, Gokaslan Z, eds. Spinal Cord and Spinal Column Tumors: Principles and Practice. New York: Thieme, 2006, pp 41-110.
3. **Boriani S, De Iure F, Bandiera S, et al. Chondrosarcoma of the mobile spine: report on 22 cases. Spine (Phila Pa 1976) 25:804-812, 2000.**
4. **York JE, Berk RH, Fuller GN, et al. Chondrosarcoma of the spine: 1954 to 1997. J Neurosurg 90(1 Suppl):73-78, 1999.**
5. Morard M, De Tribolet N, Janze RC. Chondromas of the spine: report of two cases and review of the literature. Br J Neurosurg 7:551-556, 1993.
6. Chow WA. Update on chondrosarcomas. Curr Opin Oncol 19:371-376, 2007.
7. Antić B, Roganović Z, Tadić R, et al. Chondroma of the cervical spinal canal. Case report. J Neurosurg Sci 36:239-241, 1992.
8. Baber WW, Numaguchi Y, Kenning JA, et al. Periosteal chondroma of the cervical spine: one more cause of neural foramen enlargement. Surg Neurol 29:149-152, 1988.
9. Staals EL, Bacchini P, Mercuri M, et al. Dedifferentiated chondrosarcomas arising in preexisting osteochondromas. J Bone Joint Surg Am 89:987-993, 2007.

10. Paulus W, Scheithauer B. Mesenchymal, non-meningothelial tumours. In Kleihues P, Cavanee WK, eds. Pathology and Genetics: Tumours of the Nervous System. New York: World Health Organization, 2000, pp 185-189.
11. **Lis E, Bilsky MH, Pisinski L, et al. Percutaneous CT-guided biopsy of osseous lesion of the spine in patients with known or suspected malignancy. AJNR Am J Neuroradiol 25:1583-1588, 2004.**
12. Buddingh EP, Naumann S, Nelson M, et al. Cytogenetic findings in benign cartilaginous neoplasms. Cancer Genet Cytogenet 141:164-168, 2003.
13. Dal Cin P, Qi H, Sciot R, et al. Involvement of chromosomes 6 and 11 in a soft tissue chondroma. Cancer Genet Cytogenet 93:177-178, 1997.
14. Gunawan B, Weber M, Bergmann F, et al. Solitary enchondroma with clonal chromosomal abnormalities. Cancer Genet Cytogenet 104:161-164, 1998.
15. Mandahl N, Willén H, Rydholm A, et al. Rearrangement of band q13 on both chromosomes 12 in a periosteal chondroma. Genes Chromosomes Cancer 6:121-123, 1993.
16. Gunawan B, Weber M, Bergmann F, et al. Clonal chromosome abnormalities in enchondromas and chondrosarcomas. Cancer Genet Cytogenet 120:127-130, 2000.
17. McLoughlin GS, Sciubba DM, Wolinsky JP. Chondroma/chondrosarcoma of the spine. Neurosurg Clin N Am 19:57-63, 2008.
18. Rozeman LB, Cleton-Jansen AM, Hogendoorn PC. Pathology of primary malignant bone and cartilage tumours. Int Orthop 30:437-444, 2006.
19. Sandberg AA. Cytogenetics and molecular genetics of bone and soft-tissue tumors. Am J Med Genet 115:189-193, 2002.
20. Sandberg AA. Genetics of chondrosarcoma and related tumors. Curr Opin Oncol 16:342-354, 2004.
21. Dahlin DC, Beabout JW. Dedifferentiation of low-grade chondrosarcomas. Cancer 28:461-466, 1971.
22. Jacobs WB, Fehlings M. Primary vertebral column tumors. In Dickman CA, Fehlings MG, Gokaslan Z, eds. Spinal Cord and Spinal Column Tumors: Principles and Practice. New York: Thieme, 2006, pp 369-386.
23. Matsuda Y, Sakayama K, Sugawara Y, et al. Mesenchymal chondrosarcoma treated with total en bloc spondylectomy for 2 consecutive lumbar vertebrae resulted in continuous disease free survival for more than 5 years: case report. Spine 31:E231-E236, 2006.
24. Lloret I, Server A, Bjerkehagen B. Primary spinal chondrosarcoma: radiologic findings with pathologic correlation. Acta Radiol 47:77-78, 2006.
25. Collins MS, Koyama T, Swee RG, et al. Clear cell chondrosarcoma: radiographic, computed tomographic, and magnetic resonance findings in 34 patients with pathologic correlation. Skeletal Radiol 32:687-694, 2003.
26. Donati D, Yin JQ, Colangeli M, et al. Clear cell chondrosarcoma of bone: long time follow-up of 18 cases. Arch Orthop Trauma Surg 128:137-142, 2008.
27. Tarkkanen M, Wiklund T, Virolainen M, et al. Dedifferentiated chondrosarcoma with t(9;22)(q34;q11-12). Genes Chromosomes Cancer 9:136-140, 1994.
28. Bridge JA, Bhatia PS, Anderson JR, et al. Biologic and clinical significance of cytogenetic and molecular cytogenetic abnormalities in benign and malignant cartilaginous lesions. Cancer Genet Cytogenet 69:79-90, 1993.
29. Sawyer JR, Swanson CM, Lukacs JL, et al. Evidence of an association between 6q13-21 chromosome aberrations and locally aggressive behavior in patients with cartilage tumors. Cancer 82:474-483, 1998.
30. Tallini G, Dorfman H, Brys P, et al. Correlation between clinicopathological features and karyotype in 100 cartilaginous and chordoid tumours. A report from the Chromosomes and Morphology (CHAMP) Collaborative Study Group. J Pathol 196:194-203, 2002.
31. Gaetani P, Tancioni F, Merlo P, et al. Spinal chondroma of the lumbar tract: case report. Surg Neurol 46:534-539, 1996.
32. Silve C, Jüppner H. Ollier disease. Orphanet J Rare Dis 1:37, 2006.

33. Ahmed SK, Lee WC, Irving RM, et al. Is Ollier's disease an understaging of Maffucci's syndrome? J Laryngol Otol 113:861-864, 1999.
34. McDermott AL, Dutt SN, Chavda SV, et al. Maffucci's syndrome: clinical and radiological features of a rare condition. J Laryngol Otol 115: 845-847, 2001.
35. Lee FY, Zawadsky M, Parisien M, et al. Novel translocation (9;12)(q22;q24) in secondary chondrosarcoma arising from hereditary multiple exostosis. Cancer Genet Cytogenet 132:68-70, 2002.
36. Yünten N, Calli C, Zileli M, et al. Chondrosarcoma causing cervical neural foramen widening. Eur Radiol 7:1028-1030, 1997.
37. Ross J, Brant-Zawadski M, Moore K. Chondrosarcoma. In Ross J, Brant-Zawadski M, Moore K, eds. Diagnostic Imaging: Spine. Salt Lake City: Amirsys, 2005, pp 1-39.
38. Shives TC, McLeod RA, Unni KK, et al. Chondrosarcoma of the spine. J Bone Joint Surg Am 71:1158-1165, 1989.
39. Marmor E, Rhines LD, Weinberg JS, et al. Total en bloc lumbar spondylectomy. Case report. J Neurosurg 95(2 Suppl):264-269, 2001.
40. Mandelli C, Bernucci C, Mortini P, et al. Chondrosarcoma of the thoracic spine: total en bloc sagittal resection. A case report. J Neurosurg Sci 45:114-119, 2001.
41. Hasegawa K, Homma T, Hirano T, et al. Margin-free spondylectomy for extended malignant spine tumors: surgical technique and outcome of 13 cases. Spine (Phila Pa 1976) 32:142-148, 2007.
42. **Tomita K, Kawahara N, Baba H, et al. Total en bloc spondylectomy. A new surgical technique for primary malignant vertebral tumors. Spine (Phila Pa 1976) 22:324-333, 1997.**
43. Zileli M, Hoscoskun C, Brastianos P, et al. Surgical treatment of primary sacral tumors: complications associated with sacrectomy. Neurosurg Focus 15:E9, 2003.
44. Rawlins JM, Batchelor AG, Liddington MI, et al. Tumor excision and reconstruction of the upper cervical spine: a multidisciplinary approach. Plast Reconstr Surg 114:1534-1538, 2004.
45. Ozaki T, Hillmann A, Blasius TS, et al. Skeletal metastases of intermediate grade chondrosarcoma without pulmonary involvement. A case report. Int Orthop 22:131-133, 1998.
46. **Weber KL, Pring ME, Sim FH. Treatment and outcome of recurrent pelvic chondrosarcoma. Clin Orthop Relat Res 397:19-28, 2002.**
47. Foweraker KL, Burton KE, Maynard SE, et al. High-dose radiotherapy in the management of chordoma and chondrosarcoma of the skull base and cervical spine: Part 1—Clinical outcomes. Clin Oncol (R Coll Radiol) 19:509-516, 2007.
48. Foweraker KL, Burton KE, Maynard SE, et al. High-dose photon radiotherapy in the management of chordoma and chondrosarcoma of the skull base and cervical spine. Clin Oncol (R Coll Radiol) 19(3 Suppl):S28, 2007.
49. Gwak HS, Yoo HJ, Youn SM, et al. Hypofractionated stereotactic radiation therapy for skull base and upper cervical chordoma and chondrosarcoma: preliminary results. Stereotact Funct Neurosurg 83:233-243, 2005.

Chapter 12

Giant Cell Tumors

Rosanna Wustrack, Shane Burch

Giant cell tumors (GCTs) are benign but locally aggressive tumors of bone that have a high rate of local recurrence. Although categorized as benign lesions, GCTs are known to metastasize to the lungs in 1% to 3% of cases with a mortality rate of 15% to 20% for patients with benign lung metastases.[1] Although GCTs often occur at the ends of long bones and rarely occur in the spine, they pose a significant treatment challenge for spine surgeons and must be approached differently from GCTs of long bones.

CLINICAL PRESENTATION

Only 2% to 3% of GCTs are found in the spine and sacrum. GCTs account for less than 5% of all primary bone tumors of the spine. Within the spine the upper sacrum is the most common location. In the spinal column 70% of GCTs occur in the vertebral body with variable involvement of the pedicle. Only 15% are isolated within the posterior elements.[2] Multifocal presentation is rare.

GCTs typically occur in the second to fourth decade of life and are rare in persons less than 10 or more than 60 years of age. There is a slight preponderance of females with a female-to-male ratio of 1.5:1. Pain or localized backache is the most common symptom. A high proportion of patients have radicular pain down the legs or around the thorax. Among published case series, 20% to 50% of patients have neurologic symptoms, including weakness and numbness in the lower extremities and urinary incontinence.[2,3] There may be a delay of several months before patients are seen in the clinic.

IMAGING
RADIOGRAPHS

Unlike GCTs in long bones, where purely lytic, eccentric lesions are characteristic of GCTs, radiographs of the spine show areas of bone rarefaction without any distinguishable features (Fig. 12-1).[4] There can be a variable amount of cortical expansion and local remodeling. However, a rim of cortex usually remains, which easily distinguishes these lesions from more aggressive malignant tumors. There is usually no periosteal reaction and minimal surrounding sclerosis. GCTs of the sacrum are more distinguished than GCTs of the spine. These lesions may be eccentric, although they often cross the midline and the sacroiliac joint. The sacral foraminal lines are usually obliterated by the tumor.

COMPUTED TOMOGRAPHY SCANS

Computed tomography (CT) scans are useful to characterize the extent of these lesions and the involvement of the pedicles or posterior elements. Axial images are often necessary for preoperative planning (Fig. 12-2).

MAGNETIC RESONANCE IMAGING

Magnetic resonance imaging (MRI) can be a helpful adjunctive study in evaluating patients for nerve root involvement and soft tissue expansion, especially in the sacrum where an anterior soft tissue mass is not uncommon. GCTs appear as an expansile

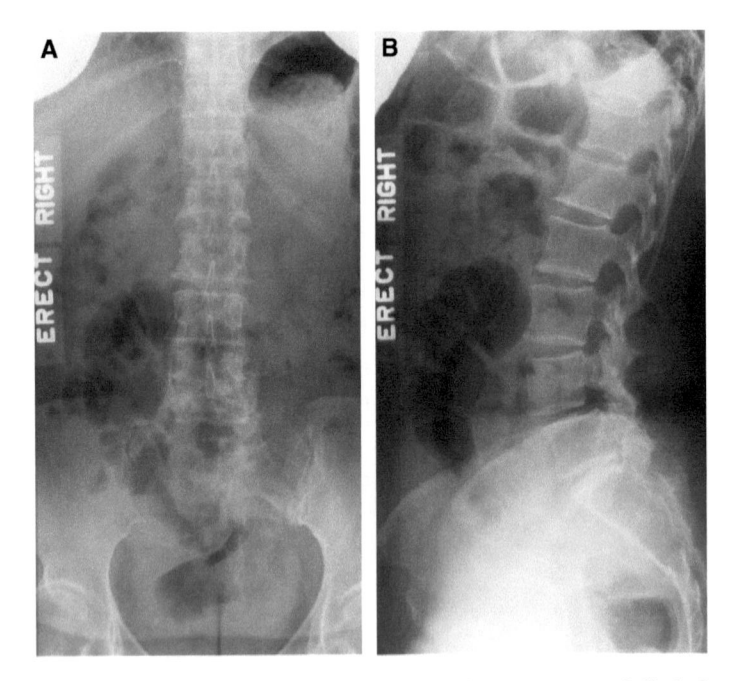

Fig. 12-1 **A,** Anteroposterior view of the lumbar spine showing area of ill-defined lucency in the right sacrum in a 56-year-old woman. **B,** Lateral view of the lumbar spine again showing a lytic lesion in the sacrum (S1-3).

mass with a heterogeneous signal on all sequences. T1-weighted images show a low-to-intermediate signal intensity; T2-weighted images show an intensity that is low or similar to that of the spinal cord[5] (Fig. 12-3).

RADIOGRAPHIC DIFFERENTIAL DIAGNOSIS

Other lytic lesions of the spine, such as aneurysmal bone cysts and osteoblastomas, can appear similar to GCTs of the spine. However, if the lesion occurs exclusively within the posterior elements, a diagnosis of aneurysmal bone cysts is more likely.

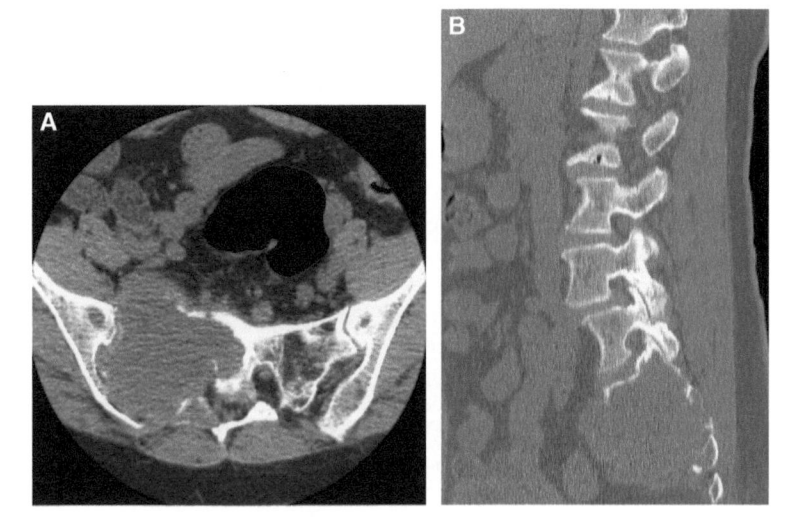

Fig. 12-2 **A,** Axial CT scan of the sacrum of patient shown in Fig. 12-1. Note destruction of the right sacroiliac joint along with anterior cortical disruption. **B,** Sagittal CT scan of the same patient.

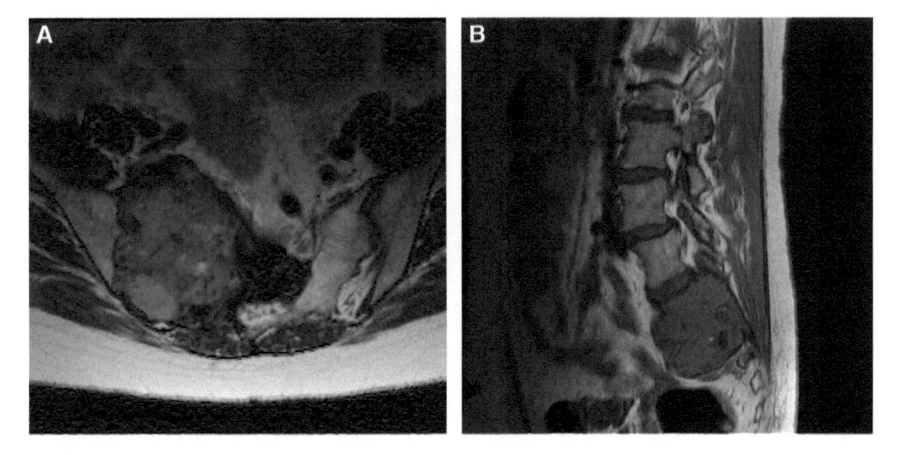

Fig. 12-3 **A,** Axial MRI. T2-weighted fast-recovery fast spin-echo sequence shows heterogeneity of the mass, disruption through the anterior cortex, and the extent of the anterior soft tissue mass. **B,** Sagittal MRI. T1-weighted sequence showing low-to-moderate intensity lesion of the sacrum.

GROSS PATHOLOGY

Grossly, GCTs are soft, friable masses with a reddish-brown color because of the high vascularity within the tumor. The amount of yellow and gray areas may vary depending on the amount of necrosis, hemorrhage, and fatty degeneration.

HISTOLOGIC FINDINGS

Numerous multinucleated giant cells uniformly dispersed among a field of mononuclear stromal cells characterize GCTs. There are typically 40 to 60 nuclei per giant cell. These giant cells have characteristics that are similar to those of osteoclasts and contain enzymes for bone resorption. Two types of mononuclear stromal cells are present: spindle-shaped cells (type I cells) and benign, rounded cells (type II cells). Type I cells resemble interstitial fibroblasts and share features of mesenchymal stem cells. Type I cells have the capacity to proliferate and are believed to be the tumor component. Type II cells resemble the monocyte/macrophage lineage and are the precursors of giant cells, which are the reactive component.[6] Although abundant mitotic figures may be seen in the nuclei of the stromal cells, pleomorphism and cellular atypia are not present, which distinguishes GCTs from sarcomas (Fig. 12-4). In some histologic sections, aneurysmal bone cyst formation may be seen as a secondary feature.[7]

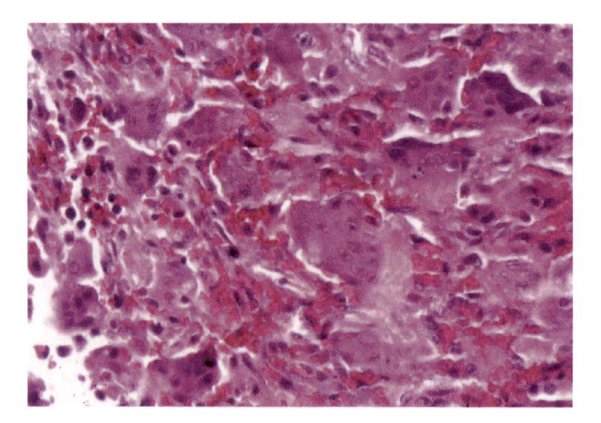

Fig. 12-4 Histology of GCT. Note multinucleated giant cells and benign-appearing mononuclear stroma. (Courtesy Dr. James O. Johnston.)

Table 12-1 Enneking Musculoskeletal Surgical Tumor Staging System for Benign Bone Tumors

Stage	Description	Site	Metastasis
1	Latent	T0	M0
2	Active	T0	M0
3	Aggressive	T1 or T2	M0 or M1

GENETICS

There does not appear to be an inherited pattern or any specific genetic translocation.

CLASSIFICATION

The Enneking surgical classification of benign bone tumors is used to describe these lesions. This system describes the local aggressiveness of the tumor and the risk of local recurrence. Most GCTs of the spine are Enneking stage 2 (active lesions with a thinned cortex) or stage 3 (active and aggressive lesions of large volume, with or without metastases, and a high frequency of local recurrence) (Table 12-1).

STAGING

Once a lesion is identified in the spine or sacrum, a full staging workup should be initiated. In addition to plain radiographs, CT or MRI scans of the affected area are required to characterize the local involvement of the tumor. A total-body bone scan rules out additional asymptomatic bony lesions. A chest radiograph or CT scan rules out lung metastases and is the accepted strategy. Basic laboratory tests, including calcium, phosphorous, and parathyroid hormone levels, should be used to rule out brown tumors. A biopsy is mandatory to confirm the diagnosis. In the spine, CT-guided core biopsy is the safest and most accurate approach to obtaining an adequate sample.

TREATMENT

The goal of treatment of GCTs in the spine is to eradicate these lesions while preserving the stability of the spinal column and minimizing complications. The literature is limited to small case series and reviews, making conclusive treatment recommendations difficult (Table 12-2).

Table 12-2 Outcomes From Select Series of Giant Cell Tumor Treatment

Reference	N	Site	Follow-up	Treatment	LR	Mets	SM	Functional Outcome	DOD
Sanjay[8] (1993)	24	Spine	149	En bloc, intralesional excision	10	0	1/7	3/4 improved strength	2
Chakravarti et al[9] (1999)	20	Sacrum (5) Spine (7) Long bones (5) Skull (2) Pubis (1)	112	Megavoltage radiation therapy	3 (progression)	3	0	5/5 improved neurologic symptoms	0
Lin et al[10] (2002)	18	Sacrum	106	Embolization	3 (with disease progression)	1	2	3 with new lower extremity weakness, 3 with improved bladder/bowel funtion	4
Fidler[11] (2001)	9	Spine	100	En bloc, intralesional excision	1	1	0	3 with new weakness	1
Marcove et al[12] (1994)	7	Sacrum	121	Intralesional excision plus cryotherapy	2	2	0	No new neurologic symptoms	0
Ozaki[13] (2002)	6	Spine (3) Sacrum (3)	69	Marginal excision, en bloc, embolization (1)	1 (disease progression)	1	0	1 with new bowel/bladder dysfunction, 1 continued bladder/bowel dysfunction	1
Di Lorenzo et al[4] (1980)	6	Spine (5) Sacrum (1)	140	Subtotal resection (5), en bloc (1)	2	0	0	4 with improved paraparesis	0

DOD, Died of disease; *LR,* local recurrence; *SM,* secondary metastases.

INTRALESIONAL PROCEDURES

Intralesional procedures include curettage of the tumor and packing of the remaining cavity with bone graft or cement. Intralesional treatment alone has a high rate of local recurrence, up to 50% in some series.[2,12,14] Radiation therapy or cryotherapy can be used with intralesional procedures to reduce recurrence rates.

RADIATION THERAPY

Radiation therapy alone is no longer used to treat GCTs because of high recurrence rates and reported cases of malignant transformation. However, radiation therapy is often necessary to reduce local recurrences in lesions that are treated with intralesional procedures, incompletely resected lesions, or GCTs that have already recurred. Leggon et al[14] conducted a literature review of 166 sacral GCTs. Radiation-induced sarcoma occurred in 11% (10 of 95) of patients at 5-year follow-up, and nine of those patients died of the disease. Chakravarti et al[9] used megavoltage radiation therapy to treat 20 patients with GCTs that could not be completely resected. After a mean follow-up of 9 years, only 3 of 20 patients had progression of the disease, and only 1 of 20 had new metastases. None of the patients in that series developed secondary malignancies, possibly because of the newer technique of megavolt radiation instead of standard techniques. Current recommendations favor an initial en bloc resection that is as aggressive as possible, followed by radiation therapy only when complete resection is not feasible or in cases of recurrent lesions. Intraoperative radiation therapy is a new technology that has been used frequently to treat marginally excised sarcomas. This may be an alternative treatment to reduce the recurrence rate for GCTs without increasing the morbidity associated with high-dose radiation.

EMBOLIZATION

GCTs of the spine are highly vascularized tumors and can cause extensive intraoperative blood loss. Preoperative embolization has been used to minimize intraoperative hemorrhage and shorten the operating time. Some surgeons have reported using embolization as a primary treatment to halt tumor progression when the tumor cannot be addressed surgically. Lin et al[10] treated 18 patients with selective arterial embolization for GCTs of the sacrum. Fourteen of 18 patients responded favorably with stabilization and reossification of the tumor. Three patients had recurrent disease in the sacrum. Kaplan-Meier analysis showed a 31% risk of disease recurrence at 10 years and a 43% risk of recurrence at 15 years. Three patients had neurologic complications, but none had bowel or bladder dysfunction.[10]

CRYOTHERAPY

Cryosurgery involves removal of most of the tumor by curettage or intralesional excision followed by freezing of the tumor bed with liquid nitrogen or another freezing agent. Limited excision with adjuvant therapies is an important method to spare the upper sacral nerve roots and preserve bowel, bladder, and sexual functions. Marcove et al[12] treated seven patients with sacral GCTs by means of either curettage and cryosurgery or limited excision and cryosurgery. At a mean of 10.1 years, two patients had local recurrences, two patients had pulmonary metastases, and none of the patients had neurologic deterioration or transient nerve dysfunction. Four patients had wound complications, and three of them required wound revision.[12] Cryotherapy has a necrotizing effect on surrounding tissue, so a wide exposure must be used to prevent wound complications. Althausen et al[15] published a case report in which argon-based cryotherapy was used to treat a large sacral defect. These investigators achieved a good result with no wound complications.

New biologic therapies are also being evaluated against giant cell tumors with success. Denosumab is a monoclonal antibody that inhibits the RANK ligand. Treatment of patients with giant cell tumors with denosumab 120 mg every 4 weeks showed reduction in 90% of RANK-positive tumor cells in 100% of patients with giant cell tumors at week 25 of treatment. Furthermore, 65% of these patients had either an increase in woven bone or dense fibrous tissue. The safety profile of these medications continues to be evaluated with arthralgias and infection being the most common and most serious complications associated with the oncologic use of denosumab, respectively.[16,17]

EN BLOC RESECTION

En bloc resection with wide margins yields the lowest recurrence rates but may be technically difficult because of the location and size of the tumor in the spine. Leggon et al[14] found no statistical difference in recurrences among patients treated with radiation therapy alone (49%), those treated with excision with intralesional margins (47%), and those treated with surgery with intralesional margins plus radiation therapy (46%). However, the recurrence rate was 0% (0 of 23) when wide margins were achieved.[14]

SURGICAL TECHNIQUES

Cervical Spine

A variety of approaches are used to resect the tumor and stabilize the cervical spine. Gille et al[18] published a case report of three-level total cervical vertebrectomy performed in two stages with fibular strut grafts posteriorly and autogenous iliac crest graft anteriorly, plus plate and screw osteosyntheses for recurrent GCTs. Although this procedure was technically difficult, preoperative neurologic symptoms improved and stability was achieved.[18]

Thoracolumbar Spine

Lièvre et al[19] first described complete spondylectomy in 1968. Currently reconstruction of the large defect can be achieved with the use of strut grafts, metal cages, and posterior instrumentation. Newer surgical techniques allow for greater postresection stability, but neurologic damage is still a concern when attempting to attain wide margins. Abe et al[20] described the use of a detailed approach to complete spondylectomy in the thoracolumbar spine in six patients. All patients underwent anterior and posterior stabilization either in two stages or in a one-stage combined anterior and posterior approach. At an average follow-up of 3.2 years, one patient was alive with disease, five patients had no evidence of disease, and the hardware was intact in all cases with no failures.[20]

Sacrum

Total sacrectomy is often necessary to achieve wide margins but is associated with bowel and bladder dysfunction, pelvic instability, and a high rate of intraoperative blood loss. Smaller lesions that have not crossed the midline can be treated with hemisacrectomy, which can preserve sphincter function. Most investigators agree that high sacrectomies do not require internal fixation if at least 50% of the sacroiliac joint remains intact. Similarly, many surgeons will not perform lumbopelvic reconstruction in cases of unilateral sacroiliac joint removal.[21] Complete sacrectomies or larger resections crossing the midline or violating both sacroiliac joints require spinopelvic stabilization or lumbosacral reconstruction to allow earlier mobilization and stability.[22] Lumbar, and sacral when available, pedicle screws and Galveston rods or iliac bolts that purchase to the ilium have been shown through biomechanical testing to provide a stable construct that transmits compression forces from the spine to the pelvis.[2]

OUTCOMES
FUNCTIONAL OUTCOMES
En bloc resection of sacral tumors necessitates sacrifice of the sacral nerve root. Fourney et al[21] reviewed 29 cases of sacral tumors in which en bloc resection with wide margins was attempted. All patients who underwent low or middle sacrectomy or unilateral resection of the sacroiliac joint were able to walk without external support. Nine of 12 patients who underwent total or high sacrectomy were able to walk without the use of external support 6 to 12 months after surgery. Three required external support long term. It was concluded that sectioning of S1 roots may result in clinically relevant motor disability requiring assistive devices.[21] Abe et al[20] performed total spondylectomy for primary tumors of the thoracolumbar spine. In this series of patients, two had GCTs. Pain was diminished in all six patients; however, only two patients showed improvement by one Frankel grade, and one patient worsened. Four patients underwent unilateral or bilateral nerve root ligation at the level of resection.[20]

BOWEL AND BLADDER FUNCTION
Bowel and bladder outcomes depend on the level of the sacrectomy and the number of nerve roots sectioned. In a series of 29 patients with primary localized sacral tumors, Fourney et al[21] found that amputations distal to S3 preserved sphincter function in most patients. Those who underwent a high sacrectomy, with sectioning of one or both S1 or S2 nerve roots, had severe bowel and bladder dysfunction.[21] Todd et al[23] published similar results in 53 patients who underwent sacral resection for primary tumors. Bowel and bladder function was preserved in 89% and 87% of patients, respectively, in whom a hemisacrectomy was performed preserving the contralateral nerve roots. However, when only bilateral S1 nerve roots were spared, no patient retained normal bowel and bladder function. When bilateral S1 and S2 roots were spared, 40% retained bowel function and 25% retained bladder function. Preservation of bilateral S1-S3 nerve roots gave near-normal results; 100% had normal bowel function and 69% had normal bladder function. The investigators concluded that either unilateral resection or preservation of at least one S3 nerve root in bilateral resection is essential to providing normal bowel and bladder function in most patients.[23]

SEXUAL FUNCTION

Similar to the preceding findings, higher sacrectomy resulted in decreased sexual function and perineal sensation. If both S1 roots are sacrificed, complete sexual dysfunction along with bowel and bladder dysfunction can be expected.

SIGNATURE CASE

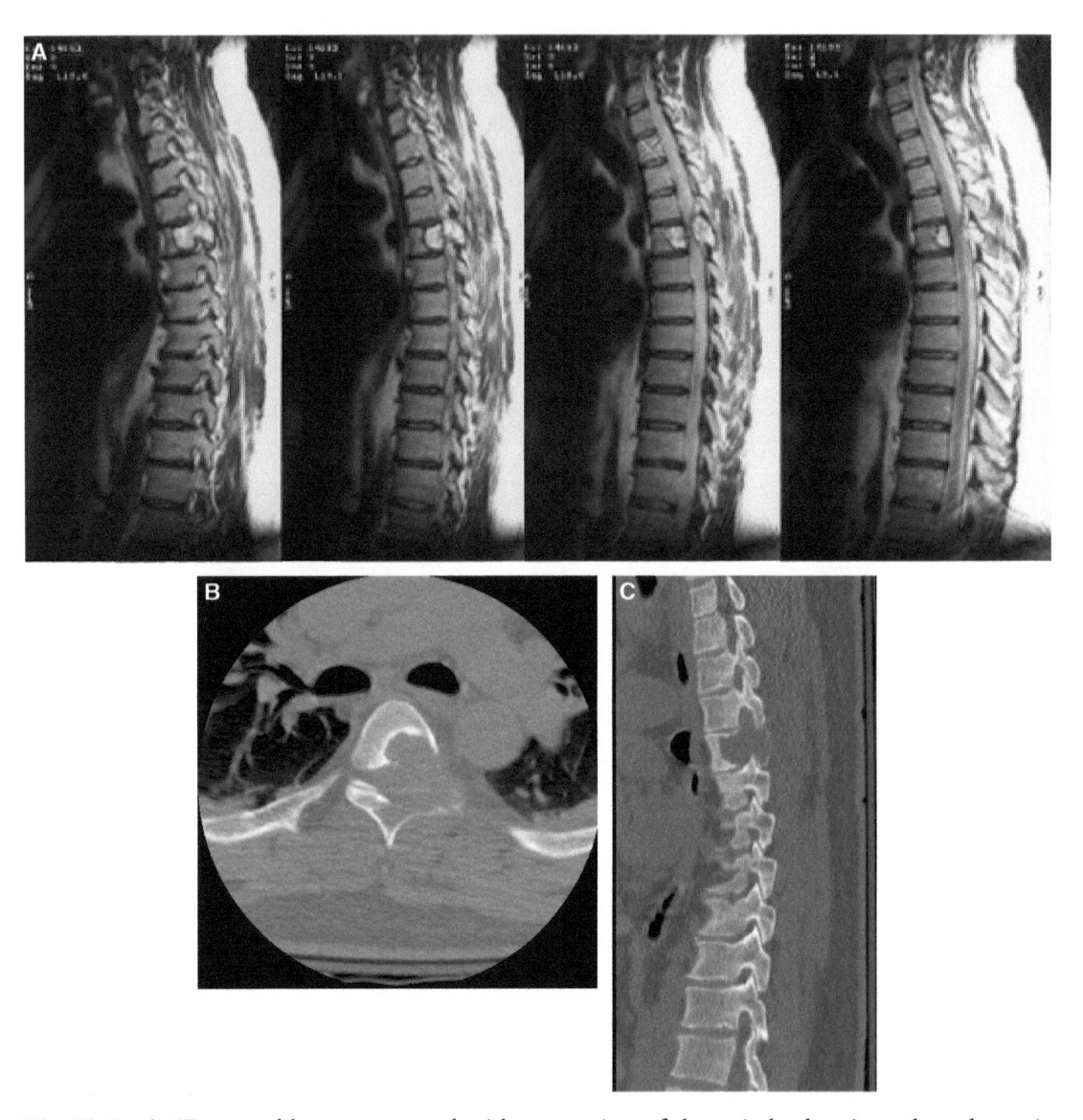

Fig. 12-5 A 47-year-old man presented with worsening of thoracic back pain and weakness in lower extremities. **A,** MRI of the thoracic spine demonstrating a lesion at T4 involving the posterior elements and posterior aspect of the vertebral body. **B,** Axial CT of the thoracic spine demonstrates an expansile lytic vertebral lesion with erosion of the posterior wall of the vertebral body. **C,** Sagittal CT of the thoracic spine of the same lesion showing loss of posterior elements at T4. Biopsy of the lesion confirmed a diagnosis of giant cell tumor.

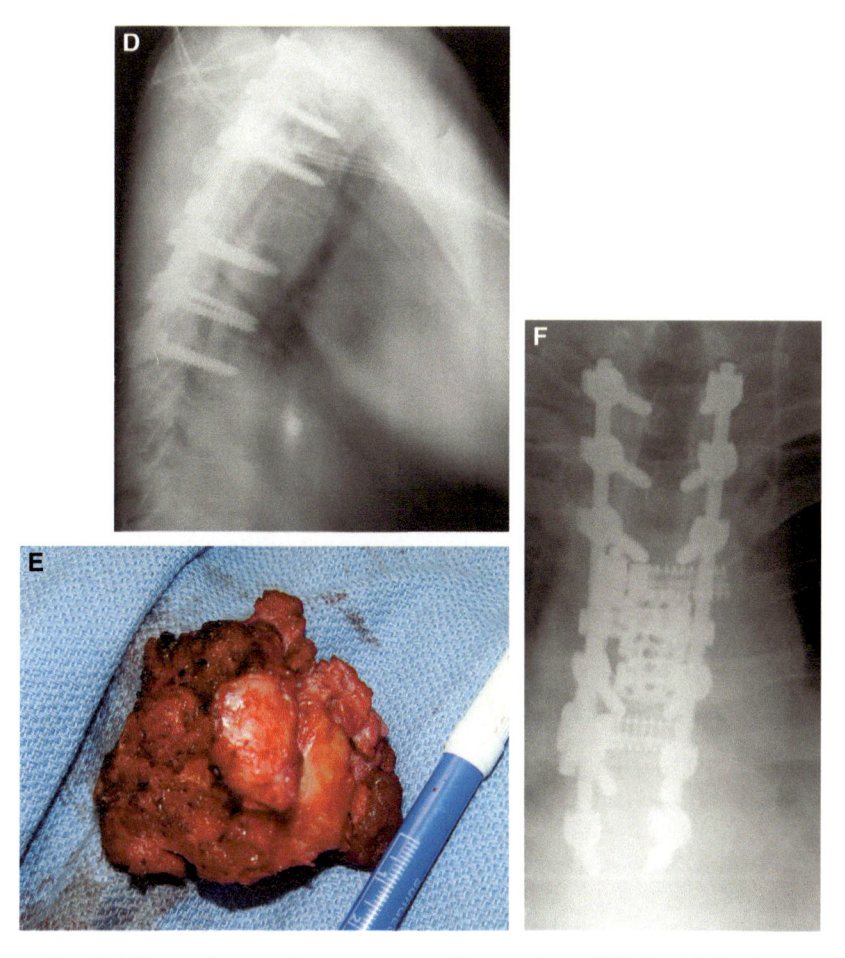

Fig. 12-5, cont'd **D,** The patient underwent a staged posterior of T1-7 with laminectomy at T3 and T4, followed by posterior instrumentation of T1-7. **E,** Gross specimen resected at T4. **F,** Anterior and posterior reconstruction of the thoracic spine following reconstruction.

CONCLUSION

Treatment of GCTs in the spine and sacrum remains challenging. Although en bloc resection with wide margins is the goal, to prevent local recurrences, it can cause significant morbidity with lasting neurologic deficits along with bowel, bladder, and sexual dysfunction in many cases. Therefore marginal resection with adjuvant radiation, cryotherapy, or embolization may provide the best combined oncologic and functional outcomes. Newer stabilization techniques in the spine and sacrum provide surgeons with better options and may allow for more aggressive tumor resection.

TIPS FROM THE MASTERS

- Only wide en bloc excision seems to offer a substantial clinical benefit in disease-free survival. Recurrences after intralesional resection can be quite severe and difficult to treat.
- Long-term cure rates need to be carefully weighed against expected functional deficits after en bloc resection, especially for sacral lesions in younger patients.

References (With Key References in Boldface)

1. McDonald DJ, Weber KL. Giant cell tumor of bone. In Schwartz H, ed. Orthopaedic Knowledge Update Musculoskeletal Tumors 2 (Orthopedic Knowledge Update Series). Rosemont, IL: American Academy of Orthopedic Surgeons, 2007, pp 133-140.
2. Luther N, Bilsky MH, Härtl R. Giant cell tumor of the spine. Neurosurg Clin N Am 19:49-55, 2008.
3. Shikata J, Yamamuro T, Shimzu K, et al. Surgical treatment of giant-cell tumors of the spine. Clin Orthop Relat Res 278:29-36, 1992.
4. Di Lorenzo N, Spallone A, Nolletti A, et al. Giant cell tumors of the spine: a clinical study of six cases, with emphasis on the radiological features, treatment and follow-up. Neurosurgery 6:29-34, 1980.
5. **Kwon JW, Chung HW, Sang KY. MRI findings of giant cell tumor of the spine. AJR Am J Roentgenol 189:246-250, 2007.**
6. Turcotte RE. Giant cell tumor of bone. Orthop Clin North Am 37:35-51, 2006.
7. Verbiest H. Giant-cell tumours and aneurysmal bone cysts of the spine. With special reference to the problems related to the removal of a vertebral body. J Bone Joint Surg Br 47:699-713, 1965.
8. **Sanjay BK, Sim FH, Unni KK, et al. Giant-cell tumours of the spine. J Bone Joint Surg Br 75:148-154, 1993.**
9. Chakravarti A, Spiro IJ, Suit HD. Megavoltage radiation therapy for axial and inoperable giant-cell tumor of bone. J Bone Joint Surg Am 81:1566-1573, 1999.
10. Lin PP, Guzel VB, Yasko AW, et al. Long-term follow-up of patients with giant cell tumor of the sacrum treated with selective arterial embolization. Cancer 95:1317-1325, 2002.
11. Fidler MW. Surgical treatment of giant cell tumours of the thoracic and lumbar spine: report of nine patients. Eur Spine J 10:69-77, 2001.
12. Marcove RC, Sheth DS, Brien EW, et al. Conservative surgery for giant cell tumors of the sacrum. The role of cryosurgery as a supplement to curettage and partial excision. Cancer 74:1253-1260, 1994.
13. Ozaki T, Liljenqvist U, Halm H, et al. Giant cell tumor of the spine. Clin Orthop Relat Res 401:194-201, 2002.
14. **Leggon RE, Zlotecki R, Reith J, et al. Giant cell tumor of the pelvis and sacrum: 17 cases and analysis of the literature. Clin Orthop Relat Res 423:196-207, 2004.**
15. Althausen PL, Schneider PD, Boid RJ, et al. Multimodality management of a giant cell tumor arising in the proximal sacrum: case report. Spine (Phila Pa 1976) 27:E361-E365, 2002.
16. Branstetter DB, Nelson SD, Manivel JC, et al. Denosumab induces tumor reduction and bone formation in patients with giant-cell tumor of bone. Clin Cancer Res 18:4415-4425, 2012.
17. Thomas D, Henshaw R, Skubitz K, et al. Denosumab in patients with giant-cell tumour of bone: an open-label, phase 2 study. Lancet Oncol 11:275-280, 2010.
18. Gille O, Soderlund C, Berge J, et al. Triple total cervical vertebrectomy for a giant cell tumor: case report. Spine (Phila Pa 1976) 30:E272-E275, 2005.
19. Lièvre JA, Darcy M, Pradat P, et al. Giant cell tumor of the lumbar spine; total spondylectomy in two states. Rev Rhum Mal Osteoartic 35:125-130, 1968.
20. Abe E, Sto K, Tazawa H, et al. Total spondylectomy for primary tumor of the thoracolumbar spine. Spinal Cord 38:146-152, 2000.
21. **Fourney DR, Rhines LD, Hentschel SJ, et al. En bloc resection of primary sacral tumors: classification of surgical approaches and outcome. J Neurosurg Spine 3:111-122, 2005.**
22. McCord DH, Cunningham BW, McAfee PC. Biomechanical analysis of lumbosacral fixation. Spine 17(Suppl 8):S235-S243, 1992.
23. Todd LT, Yaszemski MJ, Sim FH, et al. Bowel and bladder function after major sacral resection. Clin Orthop Relat Res 397:36-39, 2002.

Chapter 13

Aneurysmal Bone Cysts

Joseph H. Schwab, Luigi Simonetti, Alessandro Gasbarrini, Stefano Bandiera, Luca Amendola, Stefano Boriani

Aneurysmal bone cysts represent less than 2% of all primary bone tumors. However, between 10% and 30% occur in the spine.[1-5] As implied by the name, these tumors can be quite vascular, making surgical resection challenging.[6] Typically patients with these tumors have pain, and treatment options include surgery, radiation, and embolization.[1,3,7,8-11]

Before 1942, when Lichtenstein and Jaffe[12] described aneurysmal bone cysts, they were grouped under various names with giant cell tumors, hemangiomas, and bone cysts. After their description, aneurysmal bone cysts were frequently referred to as Jaffe-Lichtenstein disease.[13] Subsequently aneurysmal bone cysts were reported to occur along with other tumors, including giant cell tumors, osteoblastomas, chondroblastomas, and some bone sarcomas.[14] More recently genetic studies have shown that aneurysmal bone cysts are indeed neoplasms that are driven, in some cases, by the oncogene ubiquitin-specific protease 6 (USP6).[15] A recurrent translocation t(16;17)(q22;p13) has also been identified.[16] It is perhaps more interesting that these genetic changes seem to be absent in "secondary" aneurysmal bone cysts, suggesting that they are, in fact, different entities.[15] On gross inspection, blood-filled cavities are noted within expanded bone. Histologically the cysts are lined with fibrous tissue, as well as macrophages and giant cells.[17] An important histologic diagnosis that can be ruled out is telangiectatic osteogenic sarcoma, because these tumors have a high rate of metastatic disease and should be treated with chemotherapy.[18]

INDICATIONS AND CONTRAINDICATIONS

The key to the management of aneurysmal bone cysts is the diagnosis. Aneurysmal bone cysts can be quite enigmatic, and they are often colocalized with other tumors. In addition, they can appear to be radiographically similar to telangiectactic osteogenic sarcomas, requiring an adequate histologic diagnosis before surgical intervention.[14] Treatment of osteogenic sarcomas typically begins with chemotherapy followed by wide resection, although neither is necessary for aneurysmal bone cysts, where intralesional resection is sufficient. If doubt remains, a tissue biopsy should be performed. Once the diagnosis has been established, appropriate treatment can proceed. Indications for surgery include an unstable or potentially unstable spine and spinal cord compression. Pain and radicular symptoms are indications for treatment but not necessarily surgery.

PREOPERATIVE EVALUATION

The vast majority of patients with aneurysmal bone cysts in the spine are less than 18 years of age, and the most common presenting complaint is pain, which is present in more than 95% of patients.[1,6] Neurologic symptoms are present in 10% to 40% of patients.[1,6] One third of these patients have a palpable mass.[1] Coronal and sagittal deformities are also relatively common.

Plain radiographs should be the first tests ordered for these patients. Pathologic fractures can be detected in 10% to 20% of these patients,[1,6] and kyphosis and/or scoliosis are present in nearly 50%.[1] The lesions almost always involve the posterior elements and often involve both the posterior elements and the vertebral body.[1,6] Aneurysmal bone cysts involve adjacent bones (ribs or vertebrae) in 10% to 50% of patients.[6,7] The bone is often expanded and/or ballooned out with a thin rim of bone reaming. Complete collapse of the vertebrae, also known as *vertebra plana*, has also been reported.[19,20]

The lesions almost always display increased uptake on bone scans. They have also been described as having a central region with decreased uptake.[21] MRI typically demonstrates lobulated, cystic structures separated by septa with fluid/fluid lines within the cysts. The lesions typically show peripheral enhancement with gadolinium. CT scans show the bone to be expanded with a thin border. Little or no matrix is noted within the cystic areas, and fluid/fluid lines can also be detected on CT scans.

Most aneurysmal bone cysts are active Enneking stage 2 or locally aggressive Enneking stage 3 tumors.[22] The Weinstein-Boriani-Biagini staging system has been applied to aneurysmal bone cysts, and the results demonstrate that all aneurysmal bone cysts in the spine have posterior element involvement (zone 10-3), and more than half have vertebral body involvement.[1,23]

Once appropriate imaging studies have been obtained and a differential diagnosis has been formulated, a biopsy should be considered before treatment is begun. Either an open biopsy or a CT-guided biopsy can be performed. CT biopsies are associated with less morbidity, but the accuracy of the diagnosis may be diminished because less tissue is obtained. An open biopsy has the advantage of allowing the surgeon to obtain a larger amount of tissue to establish a diagnosis, but there is a greater risk of hemorrhage.

CLINICAL DECISION-MAKING
TREATMENT DECISIONS

Once the diagnosis is established, treatment options for aneurysmal bone cysts include the following: surgery, radiation, and arterial embolization. The goals of treatment are to relieve pain and prevent neurologic dysfunction, eradicate the tumor, and prevent local recurrences.

Surgery

Surgery has classically been the primary treatment modality. Intralesional resection has been the mainstay of treatment. En bloc resection of spine tumors has become increasingly more common,[24] but most investigators do not advocate en bloc excision for aneurysmal bone cysts unless the tumor is localized to the posterior elements, where an en bloc resection can be performed with morbidity that is comparable to intralesional resection.[1,6,25] When feasible, en bloc resection is essentially curative with very low local recurrence rates for aneurysmal bone cysts in the extremities and spine.[1,17] However, en bloc resection carries with it a known level of morbidity that may be unacceptably high for the management of a benign tumor.[26] Local recurrence rates after intralesional resection range from 10% to 60%.[1,3,6,25,27] In addition, aneurysmal bone cysts can be quite vascular, and intralesional excision can result in significant hemorrhaging. Most investigators advocate preoperative embolization to help with this problem.[1,6,25]

Another factor to consider before treatment of aneurysmal bone cysts of the spine is biomechanical instability. When patients have neurologic compromise resulting from vertebral collapse, it may not be possible to embolize the lesion preoperatively. However, it may be possible to stabilize the spine without violating the tumor in the acute stage as the first intervention. Then the patient can undergo embolization and subsequent resection.

Radiation

Radiation therapy has been used alone and more commonly as an adjuvant to surgery for aneurysmal bone cysts. This method of treatment has been advocated when surgical resection is not possible or complete removal of the tumor is unlikely. Doses given range from 2000 to 5000 cGy.[3,7] The use of radiation in children with benign bone tumors is discouraged because of the risk of radiation-induced sarcoma during the patient's lifetime.[3,28-30] In addition, the presumed benefit of radiation is that it will reduce local recurrence in these patients; however, this has not been supported in the literature.[3,7] The risk of local recurrence after radiation therapy with or without surgery ranges from 14% to 50%.[7,31]

Embolization

Selective arterial embolization was introduced as a preoperative measure in the treatment of aneurysmal bone cysts to facilitate safer surgical excision.[32] Subsequently it was shown to be an effective treatment for pelvic aneurysmal bone cysts without the need for surgery.[33,34] This method of selective arterial embolization without surgery was then applied to aneurysmal bone cysts in the spine.[1,35-37] The risk of local recurrence after embolization of aneurysmal bone cysts ranges from 0% to 14%.[38-42] Furthermore, we have conducted a prospective study of seven patients who were treated with selective arterial embolization for aneurysmal bone cysts in the spine with no local recurrences.[43]

CHOICE OF TECHNIQUE

In general we advocate selective embolization as the first line of treatment for aneurysmal bone cysts in the spine if no spinal instability or spinal cord compression exists (Fig. 13-1). The rationale for this method of treatment is based on the properties of

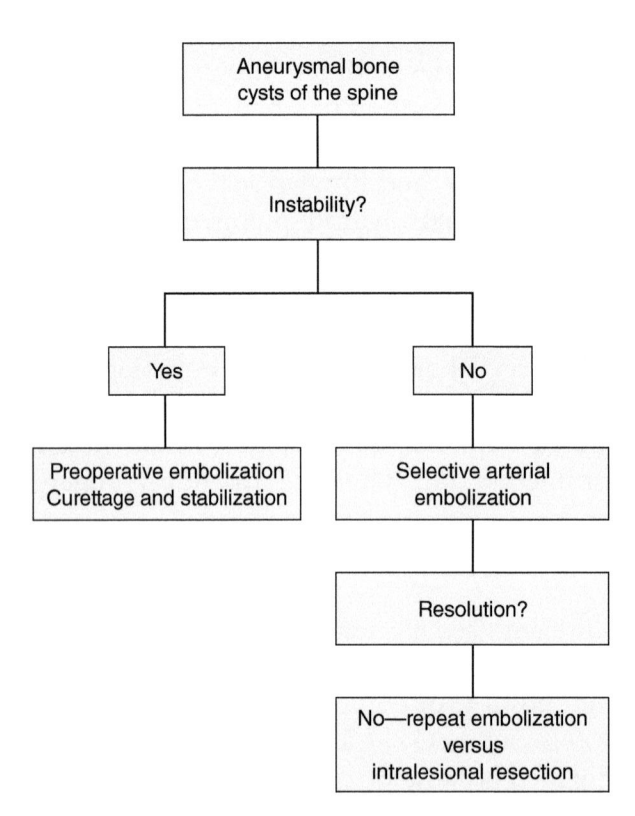

Fig. 13-1 Algorithm demonstrating the basic thought process behind the treatment of aneurysmal bone cysts of the spine. Surgery is mandated when the spine has been rendered unstable by the tumor. Selective arterial embolization should be used preoperatively or as a definitive treatment modality.

aneurysmal bone cysts and the population in which they arise. These tumors generally occur in children, and although they do have the genetic makeup of a neoplasm,[15,16,44] they should not be considered malignant. These tumors do not normally metastasize, and the risks presented by the tumor must be weighed against the risks of the therapeutic intervention. Both en bloc excision and intralesional excision of aneurysmal bone cysts of the spine pose a risk of perioperative death.[1,6]

Although selective arterial embolization is not without risk,[45] it is less invasive than surgery. In the setting of aneurysmal bone cysts of the spine without myelopathy or instability, it is reasonable to proceed with selective arterial embolization followed by careful clinical and radiographic follow-up. We do not usually recommend radiation as treatment for these tumors because the local recurrence rate does not seem to be improved with radiation, and there is a risk of radiation-induced sarcoma.[28-30] Embolization can be repeated, if necessary. In recalcitrant cases, intralesional excision with careful removal of the tumor capsule is an effective means of treating these tumors.

TECHNIQUE

Selective arterial embolization is attempted as a curative measure in aneurysmal bone cysts of the spine. When surgery is required (after failure of selective arterial embolization or in cases of spinal instability), we prefer to have the tumor embolized before surgery to help control bleeding. As in all cases of spinal embolization, it is important to pay particular attention to the preembolization angiogram. When an artery under consideration for embolization is found to be critical to the blood supply of the spinal cord, embolization of that segment is avoided. After embolization, patients should also be followed with periodic imaging in the clinic. We prefer plain radiographs, as well as CT or MRI scans. Clinical resolution of symptoms is the first measure of treatment success. However, one must look for signs of tumor resolution as well. Radiographic signs of tumor resolution include decreased tumor volume on axial imaging. Disappearance of the fluid/fluid lines is indicative of cyst resolution, and mineralization of the previously lytic areas is also a mark of tumor resolution. Embolization can be repeated and, in fact, is commonly needed before resolution occurs. However, if embolization is unsuccessful or contraindicated, surgery may be required.

When aneurysmal bone cysts of the spine are treated surgically, massive blood loss must be anticipated and requires adequate central venous access for intraoperative resuscitation. In all cases of aneurysmal bone cysts of the spine, the posterior elements are involved. If spinal stabilization is needed, it is better to place the instruments before entering the tumor. This will allow the surgeon to quickly place rods and close the patient if uncontrolled bleeding occurs. Once the screws are in place and the rods have been contoured to the desired position, the tumor can be removed with the use of curettes and Kerrison rongeurs, as indicated. Care must be taken to identify and protect important neurovascular structures when removing the tumor. Efforts should be made to remove the capsule of the tumor. It is important to note that the bleeding will often diminish significantly once the lining of the tumor has been removed. It is also important to remember that aneurysmal bone cysts have been shown to resolve even after a biopsy, and complete excision should be performed when it can be done safely.

OUTCOMES

The most common presenting complaint among patients with aneurysmal bone cysts of the spine is pain. Some patients have radicular symptoms or myelopathy, but pain is present in nearly all patients. Although aneurysmal bone cysts are tumors, they are not malignant and do not metastasize. Thus eradication of pain and treatment of instability should be the goals of treatment. However, local recurrence is often the metric used to assess the success or failure of treatment. There are no published prospective studies assessing local treatment failures, and the data available from retrospective reports demonstrate that local control is quite variable (Table 13-1). We have conducted a prospective study in which selective arterial embolization was the primary treatment modality in patients with aneurysmal bone cysts of the spine.[43] At the conclusion of our study, all patients demonstrated radiographic signs of tumor regression. All patients had complete relief of axial back pain, and both of the patients with radicular pain had complete resolution of their symptoms. No complications occurred during this study. Although serious complications are possible with embolization, our experience shows that embolization is both effective and safe. One of the risks associated with embolization is death, as has been reported; however, death is also one of the complications of surgery and/or radiation. Furthermore, the reported rates of local recurrence after embolization are lower compared with surgery or radiation alone. Only a randomized, clinical trial could fully elucidate whether embolization is indeed safer and more effective than surgery or radiation. Still, we find the available evidence and our own anecdotal experience to be compelling.

Table 13-1   Rates of Local Treatment Failure

Treatment	Local Recurrence
Intralesional resection	10% to 60%[1,3,6,25,27]
Radiation alone	14% and 50%[7,31]
Selective arterial embolization	0% to 14%[38-42]

SIGNATURE CASES

A 13-year-old girl was first seen with pain and muscle spasms. An axial CT scan demonstrated a lytic lesion within the cervical spine. She was treated with four selective embolizations within a period of 12 months. Postoperatively she is symptom free (Fig. 13-2).

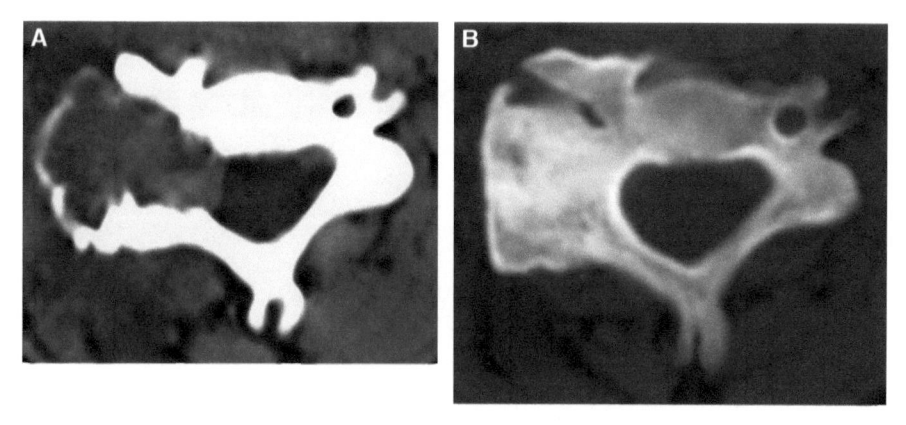

Fig. 13-2 **A** and **B,** Axial CT scans demonstrating a lytic lesion within the cervical spine in a 13-year-old girl who was first seen with pain and muscle spasms. She was treated with four selective embolizations within a period of 12 months. The last CT scan was obtained at the final follow-up control 30 months after the diagnosis. She is symptom free.

An 18-year-old man had pain and weakness in the left quadriceps. He was treated with three selective arterial embolizations and seven direct injections of acrylic glue. Postoperatively the patient had no pain, and he has full strength in the quadriceps (Fig. 13-3).

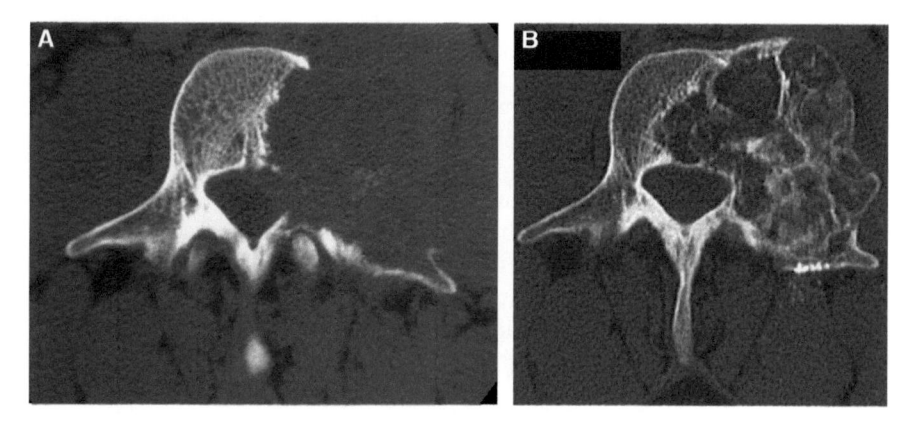

Fig. 13-3 **A** and **B,** Axial CT scans from an 18-year-old man with pain and weakness in the left quadriceps. Surgery would have posed a high risk of morbidity, and the L4 nerve root would have been in jeopardy. An anteroposterior approach would have been required with a large reconstruction and the possibility for life-threatening blood loss. This patient was treated with three selective arterial embolizations and seven direct injections of acrylic glue between June 2007 and April 2008. The most recent radiograph (June 2009) shows interval bony healing. The patient is pain free and has full strength in the quadriceps.

A 32-year-old man had a recurrence of aneurysmal bone cysts. Axial CT and MRI scans showed that the facet joint has been destroyed by the tumor, and the neck was unstable. The patient was treated with preoperative selective arterial embolization followed by anterior and posterior intralesional resection and reconstruction. Postoperatively he had no complications and is pain free 8 years later.

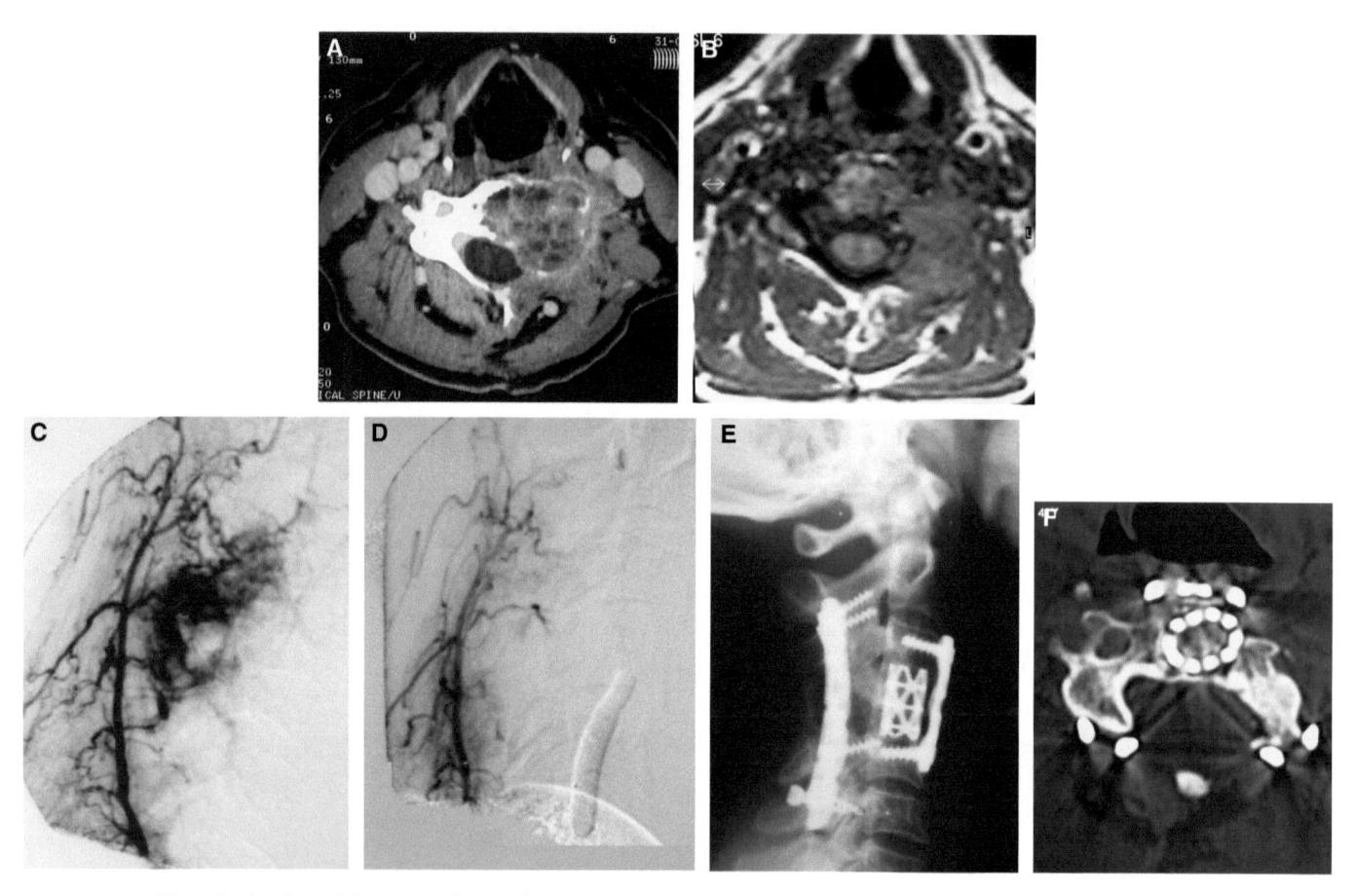

Fig. 13-4 **A** and **B,** Axial CT and MRI scans from a 32-year-old man with a recurrent aneurysmal bone cyst. The facet joint had been destroyed by the tumor, leaving the patient with an unstable neck. He was treated with preoperative selective arterial embolization **C** and **D,** followed by **E** and **F,** anterior and posterior intralesional resection and reconstruction. The patient had no complications from surgery and is pain free 8 years later.

BAILOUT TECHNIQUES

- If embolization is not possible, direct injection of the tumor can be performed. We have used this for patients in whom we were unable to safely embolize the tumor because of potential compromise of the blood supply to the spinal cord. Polyvinyl alcohol can be directly injected, as would be the case in embolization procedures.
- When pathologic fractures occur and the spinal cord is threatened or compressed, there may not be sufficient time for embolization. Entering the tumor without preoperative embolization is potentially dangerous. In these cases one might opt for closed reduction and instrumented stabilization in the acute setting. Once the spine is stable and the spinal cord is protected, the tumor can be managed in a more elective fashion, which may allow for embolization. Percutaneous stabilization of the fracture may also be considered without any attempt at fusion. If the tumor is treated with embolization, and the affected vertebrae are reconstituted, then the instrumentation can be removed. This is a particularly relevant strategy in the pediatric patient population.

TIPS FROM THE MASTERS

- Aneurysmal bone cysts in the spine can be effectively treated with selective arterial embolization.
- Surgery should be reserved for those cases that are not amenable to selective arterial embolization, such as patients with spinal instability.
- When surgery is necessary, an intralesional resection after preoperative embolization provides adequate local control. We do not routinely perform en bloc resections or radiation in our management of aneurysmal bone cysts of the spine.

References (With Key References in Boldface)

1. **Boriani S, De Iure F, Campanacci L, et al. Aneurysmal bone cyst of the mobile spine: report on 41 cases. Spine 26:27-35, 2001.**
2. Tillman BP, Dahlin DC, Lipscomb PR, et al. Aneurysmal bone cyst: an analysis of ninety-five cases. Mayo Clinic Proc 43:478-495, 1968.
3. **Vergel De Dios AM, Bond JR, Shives TC, et al. Aneurysmal bone cyst. A clinicopathologic study of 238 cases. Cancer 69:2921-2931, 1992.**
4. Ameli NO, Abbassioun K, Saleh H, et al. Aneurysmal bone cysts of the spine. Report of 17 cases. J Neurosurg 63:685-690, 1985.
5. Dahlin DC, McLeod RA. Aneurysmal bone cyst and other nonneoplastic conditions. Skeletal Radiol 8:243-250, 1982.

6. Papagelopoulos PJ, Currier BL, Shaughnessy WJ, et al. Aneurysmal bone cyst of the spine. Management and outcome. Spine 23:621-628, 1998.
7. Capanna R, Albisinni U, Picci P, et al. Aneurysmal bone cyst of the spine. J Bone Joint Surg Am 67:527-531, 1985.
8. Scott I, Connell DG, Duncan CP. Regression of aneurysmal bone cyst following open biopsy. Can Assoc Radiol J 37:198-200, 1986.
9. Saglik Y, Kapicioglu MI, Guzel B. Spontaneous regression of aneurysmal bone cyst. A case report. Arch Orthop Trauma Surg 112:203-204, 1993.
10. Delloye C, De Nayer P, Malghem J, et al. Induced healing of aneurysmal bone cysts by demineralized bone particles. A report of two cases. Arch Orthop Trauma Surg 115:141-145, 1996.
11. Malghem J, Maldague B, Esselinckx W, et al. Spontaneous healing of aneurysmal bone cysts. A report of three cases. J Bone Joint Surg Br 71:645-650, 1989.
12. Jaffe HL, Lichtenstein L. Solitary unicameral bone cyst, with emphasis on the roentgen picture, the pathologic appearance and the pathogenesis. Arch Surg 44:1004-1025, 1942.
13. Mankin HJ. Pathophysiology of Orthopaedic Diseases. Rosemont, IL: The American Academy of Orthopedic Surgery, 2009.
14. **Campanacci M. Bone and Soft Tissue Tumors, 2nd ed. New York: Springer Verlag, 1999.**
15. Oliveira AM, Perez-Atayde AR, Inwards CY, et al. USP6 and CDH11 oncogenes identify the neoplastic cell in primary aneurysmal bone cysts and are absent in so-called secondary aneurysmal bone cysts. Am J Pathol 165:1773-1780, 2004.
16. Oliveira AM, Perez-Atayde AR, Dal Cin P, et al. Aneurysmal bone cyst variant translocations upregulate USP6 transcription by promoter swapping with the ZNF9, COL1A1, TRAP150, and OMD genes. Oncogene 24:3419-3426, 2005.
17. Mankin HJ, Hornicek FJ, Ortiz-Cruz E, et al. Aneurysmal bone cyst: a review of 150 patients. J Clin Oncol 23:6756-6762, 2005.
18. Bacci G, Ferrari S, Ruggieri P, et al. Telangiectatic osteosarcoma of the extremity: neoadjuvant chemotherapy in 24 cases. Acta Orthop Scand 72:167-172, 2001.
19. Codd PJ, Riesenburger RI, Klimo P Jr, et al. Vertebra plana due to an aneurysmal bone cyst of the lumbar spine. Case report and review of the literature. J Neurosurg 105(6 Suppl):490-495, 2006.
20. Papagelopoulos PJ, Currier BL, Galanis EC, et al. Vertebra plana of the lumbar spine caused by an aneurysmal bone cyst: a case report. Am J Orthop (Belle Mead NJ) 28:119-124, 1999.
21. Wang K, Allen L, Fung E, et al. Bone scintigraphy in common tumors with osteolytic components. Clin Nucl Med 30:655-671, 2005.
22. Enneking WF. A system of staging musculoskeletal neoplasms. Clin Orthop Relat Res 204:9-24, 1986.
23. Hart RA, Boriani S, Biagini R, et al. A system for surgical staging and management of spine tumors. A clinical outcome study of giant cell tumors of the spine. Spine 22:1773-1782; discussion 1783, 1997.
24. Stener B, Johnsen OE. Complete removal of three vertebrae for giant-cell tumour. J Bone Joint Surg Br 53:278-287, 1971.
25. de Kleuver M, van der Heul RO, Veraart BE. Aneurysmal bone cyst of the spine: 31 cases and the importance of the surgical approach. J Pediatr Orthop B 7:286-292, 1998.
26. Boriani S, Bandiera S, Donthineni R, et al. Morbidity of en bloc resections in the spine. Eur Spine J 19:231-241, 2010.
27. Koskinen EV, Visuri TI, Holmstrom T, et al. Aneurysmal bone cyst: evaluation of resection and of curettage in 20 cases. Clin Orthop Relat Res 118:136-146, 1976.
28. Sim FH, Cupps RE, Dahlin DC, et al. Postradiation sarcoma of bone. J Bone Joint Surg Am 54:1479-1489, 1972.
29. Huvos AG, Woodard HQ, Cahan WG, et al. Postradiation osteogenic sarcoma of bone and soft tissues. A clinicopathologic study of 66 patients. Cancer 55:1244-1255, 1985.
30. Palmerini E, Ferrari S, Bertoni F, et al. Prognosis of radiation-induced bone sarcoma is similar to primary osteosarcoma. Clin Orthop Relat Res 462:255; author reply 256, 2007.

31. Nobler MP, Higinbotham NL, Phillips RF. The cure of aneurysmal bone cyst. Irradiation superior to surgery in an analysis of 33 cases. Radiology 90:1185-1192, 1968.
32. Dick HM, Bigliani LU, Michelsen WJ, et al. Adjuvant arterial embolization in the treatment of benign primary bone tumors in children. Clin Orthop Relat Res 139:133-141, 1979.
33. Murphy WA, Strecker EB, Schoenecker PL. Transcatheter embolisation therapy of an ischial aneurysmal bone cyst. J Bone Joint Surg Br 64:166-168, 1982.
34. Wallace S, Granmayeh M, deSantos LA, et al. Arterial occlusion of pelvic bone tumors. Cancer 43:322-328, 1979.
35. DeRosa GP, Graziano GP, Scott J. Arterial embolization of aneurysmal bone cyst of the lumbar spine. A report of two cases. J Bone Joint Surg Am 72:777-780, 1990.
36. Boriani S, De Cristofaro R, Ruggieri P, et al. Selective arterial embolization in the treatment of lesions of the musculoskeletal apparatus. Chir Organi Mov 76:99-112, 1991.
37. De Cristofaro R, Biagini R, Boriani S, et al. Selective arterial embolization in the treatment of aneurysmal bone cyst and angioma of bone. Skeletal Radiol 21:523-527, 1992.
38. Suby-Long T, Bos GD, Rösch J. Biopsy proven eradication of an aneurysmal bone cyst treated by superselective embolization: a case report. Cardiovasc Intervent Radiol 11:292-295, 1988.
39. Cigala F, Sadile F. Arterial embolization of aneurysmal bone cysts in children. Bull Hosp Jt Dis 54:261-264, 1996.
40. Radanovic B, Simunic S, Stojanovic J, et al. Therapeutic embolization of aneurysmal bone cyst. Cardiovasc Intervent Radiol 12:313-316, 1989.
41. Misasi N, Cigala F, Iaccarino V, et al. Selective arterial embolisation in aneurysmal bone cysts. Int Orthop 6:123-128, 1982.
42. Green JA, Bellemore MC, Marsden FW. Embolization in the treatment of aneurysmal bone cysts. J Pediatr Orthop 17:440-443, 1997.
43. Amendola L, Simonetti L, Simoes CE, Bandiera S, De Iure F, Boriani S. Aneruysmal bone cyst of the mobile spine: the therapeutic role of embolization. Eur Spine J. 2012 Nov 8. [Epub ahead of print]
44. Oliveira AM, Hsi BL, Weremowicz S, et al. USP6 (Tre2) fusion oncogenes in aneurysmal bone cyst. Cancer Res 64:1920-1923, 2004.
45. Peraud A, Drake JM, Armstrong D, et al. Fatal ethibloc embolization of vertebrobasilar system following percutaneous injection into aneurysmal bone cyst of the second cervical vertebra. AJNR Am J Neuroradiol 25:1116-1120, 2004.

Chapter 14

Hemangiomas

Jamal McClendon, Jr., Stephen L. Ondra,
Frank L. Acosta, Jr.

Vertebral hemangiomas are relatively common entities affecting the vertebral spinal column. They have been recognized as pathologic lesions since 1863.[1] This benign dysplasia or vascular tumor accounts for approximately 2% to 3% of all spine tumors and occurs with an estimated incidence of 10% to 12% of the population. This rate was determined on the basis of findings by workers in Schmorl's laboratory, who provided three large autopsy studies and reviews of plain radiographs of the spine.[2-8] These lesions are usually asymptomatic and have characteristic radiographic striations and trabeculations, which were described in 1927.[9] They often appear as incidental findings on plain radiographs and/or MRI.[7] Rarely they may become enlarged and cause local or regional pain, pathologic fractures, expansion of the vertebral body or posterior arch, and/or compression of the spinal cord.[8,10,11] These lesions have been managed surgically and nonsurgically with adjunctive analgesic medication and/or radiation therapy.

INDICATIONS AND CONTRAINDICATIONS

The vast majority of tumors are asymptomatic and do not require surgery. Indications for intervention include pain that is unrelieved by conservative measures, symptomatic burst or compression fractures, and/or high-grade spinal cord compression with or without neurologic deficits. There are no absolute contraindications to invasive procedures for treatment of vertebral hemangiomas. Acosta et al[12] provided data from 16 patients with a diagnosis of symptomatic vertebral hemangiomas causing pain or neurologic deficits, who underwent therapeutic intervention based on recommendations from a multidisciplinary team of radiologists and neurosurgeons.

PREOPERATIVE EVALUATION

It is difficult to make a diagnosis of hemangioma causing pain or neurologic compromise because it is often asymptomatic. However, patients who do have symptoms may have a variety of complaints, including pain, paresthesia, weakness, myelopathy, and incontinence. The clinical onset of spinal compression is often progressive, over a period of several months, but the onset can also be sudden.[6] Fox and Onofrio[7] described 10 of 11 patients who had neck or back pain that preceded the onset of neurologic symptoms. Thoracic myelopathy is the most common presenting syndrome.

Numerous radiographic studies demonstrate common entities that are seen in vertebral hemangiomas. Plain radiographs of the spine may demonstrate coarse vertical vertebral striations or a "honeycomb" appearance.[7] This positive finding on plain radiographs is seen in only 41% of patients.[13] This imaging finding will often suggest the diagnosis.[7] In cases where hemangiomatous vertebral body involvement is not extensive, plain radiographs are unrevealing. It has been stated that up to one third of the body must be involved for the classic findings to be present.[7,14,15] The disc spaces are generally intact.[16] The presence of pain or neurologic symptoms usually dictates additional imaging modalities.

CT with or without myelography has been performed for further evaluation and is the diagnostic procedure of choice.[17-19] The characteristic "polka-dot" appearance within the vertebral body represents transverse or axial cuts through thickened vertical trabeculae.[20] Myelography can confirm the existence of an extradural block at the level of cord compression but contributes little to the differential diagnosis.[10,13] Myelograms can show the extent of vertebral body involvement and, if present, myelograms can also show the location of this spinal cord compression.

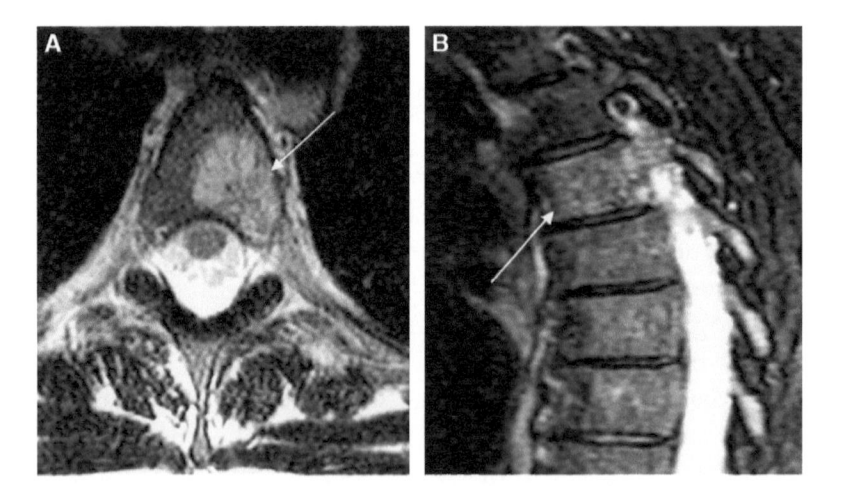

Fig. 14-1 **A,** Axial fast-spin echo (FSE) T2-weighted MRI performed without fat saturation demonstrates a vertebral hemangioma, with pedicular extension, with increased signal representing the adipocyte, edema, and vascular content. **B,** Sagittal FSE T2-sequence with fat saturation highlights mild increase signal corresponding to the vascular and water content *(arrows).*[12]

Bone scans may be helpful in differentiating multiple hemangiomas from metastatic disease of the spinal column.[6,10] MRI scans have been used selectively to discern cord compression or other bone or soft tissue lesions. MRI scans can also provide additional information regarding the aggressiveness of the hemangioma (Fig. 14-1).[21] Stable intraosseous lesions have a mottled appearance and increased "fat" (signal intensity on both T1- and T2-weighted MRI scans).[17,20,22] Symptomatic osseous or extraosseous lesions more commonly have isointense signals on T1-weighted images, with increased signal intensity on T2-weighted images.[22]

Angiography of the spine has been used in selected cases (e.g., symptomatic lesions) when other imaging modalities have suggested large feeding or draining vessels, or when embolization is considered a presurgical adjunct (Fig. 14-2).[7,10,23] Arteriography is particularly useful in determining the vascularity of the osseous and extraosseous components of the lesion, to identify feeding and draining vessels, and to identify the blood supply to the spinal cord.[23] It may aid in the diagnosis in some cases. Asymptomatic lesions often show a normal or slightly increased vascularity, whereas hemangiomas causing pain or spinal compression are associated with moderate-to-intense hypervascularization.[7]

Vertebral hemangiomas have a dysembryogenic origin, which causes secondary resorption of underlying bone and produces a honeycomb mass within the bone.[6,10,24-26] Although most trabeculae are atrophic because of the abnormal blood vessels, some trabeculae become thickened and sclerotic. Microscopically there are two main types of vertebral hemangiomas that are characterized by cavernous or capillary vessels. The cavernous type consists of multiple, large, wall-to-wall, thin-walled vascular spaces lined by flat endothelial cells.[7] The capillary type is composed of numerous capillary channels lined with plump uniform endothelial cells and separated by reactive fibrous tissue.[7]

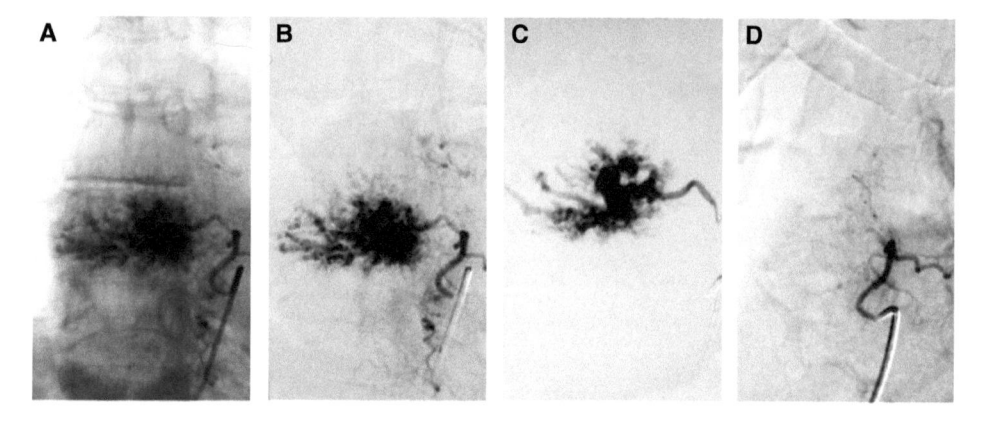

Fig. 14-2   **A** and **B,** Selected anteroposterior spot views from a spine angiogram through the left T8 intercostal artery show a prominent vascular stain with large venous pools predominantly within the left T8 vertebra. **C,** The vertebral body is not well visualized after microcatheterization and embolization performed with 250 to 350 μm polyvinyl acetate particles. **D,** Postembolization angiogram shows no residual vascular supply.[12]

CLINICAL DECISION-MAKING

Asymptomatic lesions or lesions that are incidentally found as a result of imaging for another reason may remain asymptomatic for years or even decades.[8,27,28] Fox and Onofrio[7] reported 35 asymptomatic cases among their 59 patients who had a diagnosis of vertebral hemangiomas. Only 2 of 35 patients with incidental hemangiomas later had symptoms.[7] Both patients developed localized back pain, which progressed to thoracic myelopathy in one patient.[7] Additional studies are often obtained at the appropriate spine level if asymptomatic lesions eventually cause pain or neurologic symptoms (Fig. 14-3).

Asymptomatic vertebral hemangiomas are generally intraosseous only without osseous expansion.[29] They are often discovered in the thoracic or lumbar spine and are localized to the vertebral body without involvement of the posterior element. Asymptomatic lesions are slightly more common in females and are usually discovered in middle-aged patients.

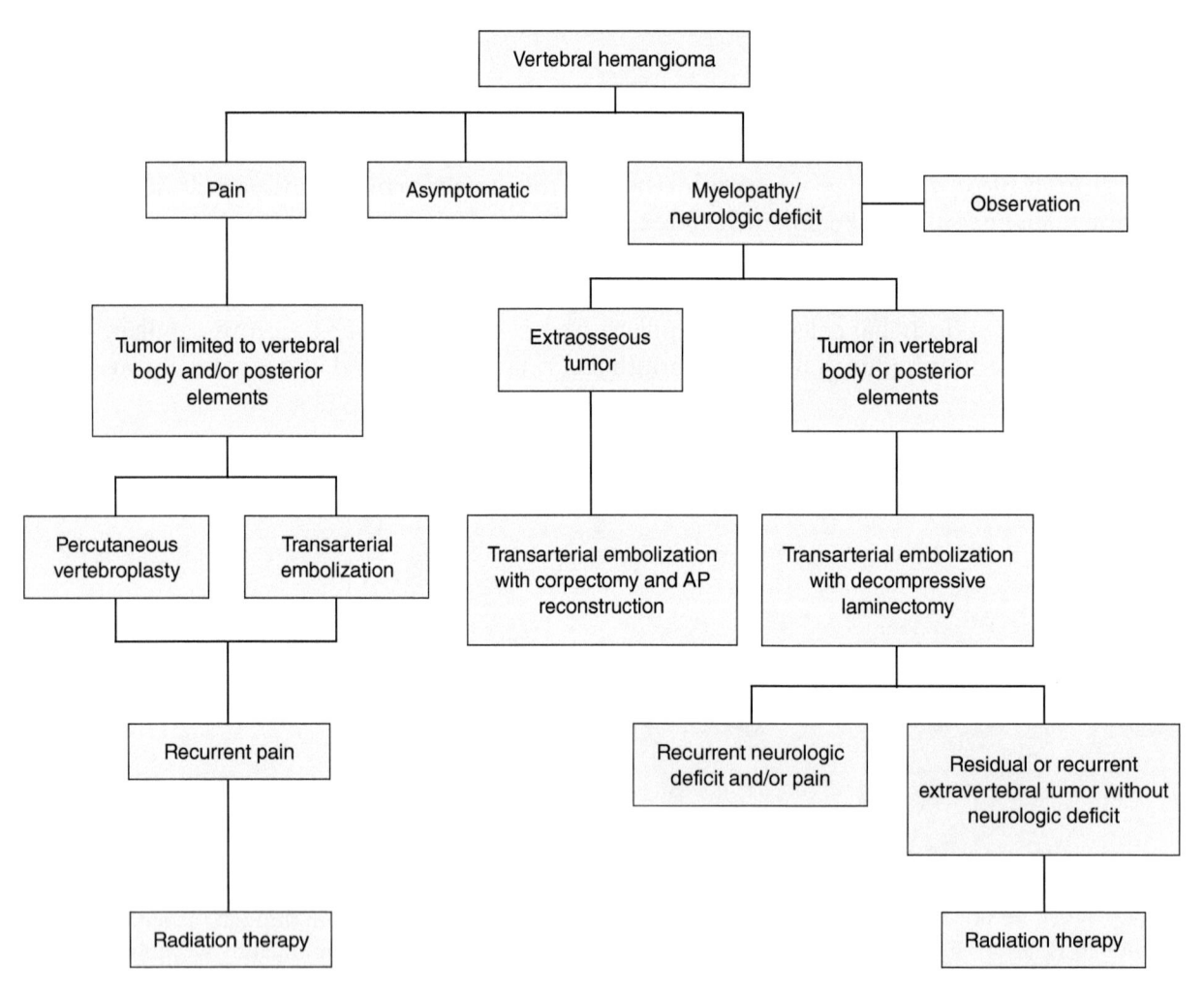

Fig. 14-3 Treatment algorithm for symptomatic vertebral hemangiomas. Surgical decompression, resection, vertebroplasty, transarterial embolization, and radiation therapy *(XRT)* are included.

Patients with pain as a presenting complaint may have other causes for their pain, including spondylosis, spondylolisthesis, degenerative joint disease, vertebral disc herniation, or other musculoskeletal disorders.[15,30,31] Reizine et al[29] suggested that if a painful vertebral hemangioma is localized to the cervical or lumbar spine but has no posterior element involvement or cortical disruption, it should be stable. However, if the painful lesion involves a thoracic vertebra, especially in a young female patient, and includes posterior element disease, cortical blistering, or soft tissue extension, the lesion must be considered evolving, and it may have the potential to cause future spinal cord compression.[29] Spinal cord compression may be the result of direct neural compression by epidural tumor tissue as an extension from the vertebral body or posterior elements, expanded vascular bone, epidural hematomas, compression fractures of the hemangiomatous vertebra, or anomalous vessels draining or feeding the lesion.[5,6,27,30-36]

Surgical management may be offered if a significant or progressive neurologic deficit is present.[7,11,16] The surgical approach, whether anterior or posterior, is determined by the location of the hemangioma and the rate of neurologic decline.[7,10,11,37,38] Emergency surgery consisting of a decompression with laminectomy, and possible segmental instrumentation, should be performed in all instances of a rapid and progressive neurologic deficit.[7,10,16,39] Some investigators have reported surgical resection leading to cure with rates as high as 70% to 80% with the use of laminectomy alone to treat lesions involving only the posterior element without soft tissue extension.[6-8,10,16,40,41]

When there is vertebral body involvement, with or without extraosseous extension of the tumor into the spinal canal causing cord or thecal sac compression and neurologic deficits, surgical resection through a corpectomy or vertebrectomy has been advocated.[7,32,33,42-44] Although patients undergoing corpectomy for vertebral body hemangiomas traditionally underwent reconstruction with interbody grafts placed anteriorly (e.g., strut grafts) without posterior stabilization,[7,45] advancements in pedicle screw-rod segmental instrumentation supplemented with posterolateral arthrodesis and fusion can provide increased spinal stability after anterior column reconstruction to facilitate the fusion process.[46-48]

With surgical resection of these lesions, there is the potential for significant intraoperative blood loss and postoperative epidural hematomas.[7,10,33,42,45,49] Preoperative transarterial embolization reduces these complications.[6,32,39,45,49] This technique has also been used as the sole therapy for vertebral hemangiomas.[50-53] There are a few studies with long-term follow-up that evaluated outcomes in vertebral hemangiomas treated with transarterial embolization alone. Smith et al[53] reported on two patients who were treated with transarterial embolization alone for vertebral hemangiomas causing neurologic symptoms but failed to improve clinically; thus transarterial embolization is recommended as an adjunct to surgical treatment for symptomatic vertebral hemangiomas. However, in 1972, Hekster et al[54] showed that transarterial embolization could relieve spinal cord compression from vertebral hemangiomas. Additional studies have demonstrated that embolization alone can decrease the size of the hemangioma, provide significant pain relief, and relieve subarachnoid blockage.[51,53,55,56] Acosta et al[12] showed that three of four patients who underwent transarterial embolization for vertebral hemangiomas had resolution of pain without further treatment, thus showing the effectiveness of one type of therapy in treating pain referable to an interosseous vertebral hemangioma in selected patients. Those with extensive lesions causing neurologic compromise, more than pain, require embolization only in preparation for operative intervention. If the feeding vessel does not also supply the anterior spinal artery, it can potentially be embolized as a presurgical adjunct, thereby reducing intraoperative hemorrhages.[10,32,56] The feeding vessel is usually a branch of a lumbar or intercostal artery that arises proximal to the radicular branches.[57]

Percutaneous vertebroplasty is a relatively new technique that has been shown to provide pain relief in patients with symptomatic vertebral hemangiomas.[58-65] It consists of injecting an acrylic cement, typically polymethyl methacrylate (PMMA), into the vertebral body affected by the hemangioma. The mechanism by which vertebroplasty results in pain relief is unknown, but it may be related to stabilization of microfractures and prevention of further compression or deformity. In addition, theoretically PMMA induces a chemical response in the vertebral body that ablates pain-sensitive nerve endings.[59,66-68] Unfortunately, vertebroplasty does not obliterate the hemangioma, and progressive expansion of the lesion in the spinal canal can cause symptomatic cord compression.[69] During vertebroplasty, care is taken to avoid retropulsion of PMMA into the spinal canal, because there have been reports of spinal cord compression resulting from leakage.[61,67] Acosta et al[12] reported that three of four patients showed subjective improvement in pain after PMMA vertebroplasty; thus it was recommended as a potentially effective treatment for pain. Vertebroplasty is not indicated for patients with neurologic deficits resulting from vertebral hemangiomas causing cord compression. The long-term efficacy of this procedure is unknown and requires further research.

Vertebral hemangiomas are radiosensitive lesions that have been shown to respond to low doses of radiation, typically 30 to 40 Gy.[7,70] Although highly effective and most often used to treat lesions causing pain, radiation therapy has also been reported to effectively reverse neurologic deficits from vertebral hemangiomas.[7,70-72] However, the use of radiation therapy as the sole treatment for vertebral hemangiomas causing neurologic symptoms remains controversial, and most investigators recommend surgical decompression.[7,11,41,56] Others believe that radiation therapy is as effective as embolization of feeding vessels without the hazards of an invasive technique.[73] The appearance of the affected bone may not change after radiation, despite symptomatic relief, or the bone may show increased density indicating sclerosis.[10,16,70]

Because of the unacceptably high operative morbidity and mortality associated with complete tumor resection in the past, subtotal tumor removal for spinal cord decompression followed by postoperative irradiation was advocated by some as treatment for these types of lesions.* However, modern techniques in preoperative transarterial embolization, advances in anesthesia and perioperative care, and improvements in the design and safety of spinal instrumentation have made aggressive surgical resection and reconstruction more feasible as treatment for spine tumors. Radiation therapy is

---

*References 7, 10, 16, 32, 36, 39, 45, 49, 71, 74, 75.

not always offered because of the potential risk of radiation necrosis and the slow, benign nature of vertebral hemangiomas. However, fractionated doses of less than 4000 Grays are considered to carry minimal risk.* Skin ulceration has been the only reported complication in a minority of patients.[78]

In 1994, Heiss et al[79] reported relief of spinal cord compression from vertebral hemangiomas after percutaneous ethanol injections in two patients. Because of these reported cases, there were additional successful cases of ethanol vertebroplasty effectively treating both pain and neurological deficit from vertebral hemangioma.[69,80-82] However, serious complications have been noted with ethanol vertebroplasty, including posttreatment Brown-Sequard syndrome and pathologic fracture.[80,81,83]

TECHNIQUE

Surgical decompression should be used for intraosseous lesions causing progressive neurologic decline.[10,11,23] It features placing the patient supine on a Wilson frame in the operating theater after general endotracheal intubation. Subperiosteal dissection is performed after identification of the appropriate level by means of fluoroscopy and after an incision has been made. Laminectomy is performed at the appropriate level using a high-speed drill or Leksell rongeurs (Fig. 14-4). Adequate decompression is facilitated by means of Kerrison rongeurs. After hemostasis is achieved, the fascia is closed with 0-Vicryl sutures, the dermis is reapproximated with 2-0 Vicryl sutures, and staples are used to close the skin.

Patients undergoing limited decompressive laminectomies do not need fusion procedures. But patients undergoing aggressive transpedicular or lateral extracavitary ap-

---

*References 11, 24, 28, 36, 56, 70, 72, 76, 77.

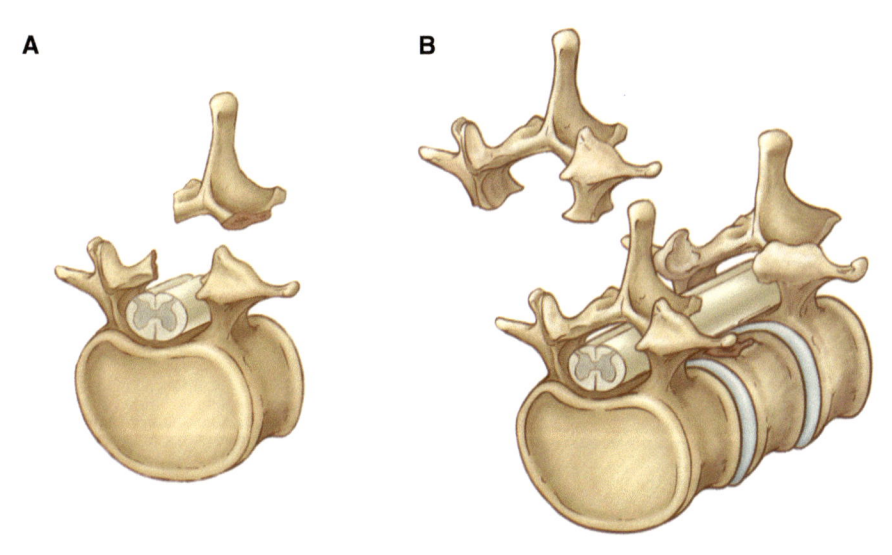

Fig. 14-4 **A** and **B**, Laminectomy for decompression.[7]

proaches, retroperitoneal approaches, or extensive laminectomies require posterior instrumentation for stabilization.[7] Patients undergoing vertebral body resection or corpectomy through posterior approaches or lateral retroperitoneal approaches require anterior struts, such as an autologous and allograft iliac crest or a cage packed with bone for stabilization (Fig. 14-5). If a lateral retroperitoneal approach is used for vertebrectomy or corpectomy, an open surgical procedure or minimally invasive surgery may be used under the same anesthesia or at a later date for posterior spinal column stabilization for the segments rostral and caudal to the corpectomy site.

Posterior approaches for corpectomy through transpedicular or lateral extracavitary methods require that patients be placed in the prone position on a Jackson table after general endotracheal intubation. Subperiosteal dissection is performed after the correct levels needed are confirmed and an incision is made. Segmental instrumentation by means of pedicle screws is performed after all rostral, caudal, and lateral exposure is completed. Transpedicular and lateral extracavitary approaches for corpectomy are facilitated by means of a high-speed drill after sacrifice of the nerve root at the corpectomy level. The rostral and caudal intervertebral discs are identified, and vertebrectomy is performed with a high-speed drill. The graft or cage is placed in the interspace. After hemostasis is achieved, the rods are placed bilaterally. Posterolateral arthrodesis is performed to facilitate fusion, and the incision is closed after the fascia and dermis are reapproximated.

For lateral retroperitoneal approaches, patients are placed on a bean bag after endotracheal intubation, with the hips and knees flexed, and a pillow is placed between the thighs. Mobilization of the psoas muscle for visualization of the appropriate level confirmed by fluoroscopy allows for initiation of corpectomy. The intervertebral disc is removed after vertebrectomy is performed above and below the vertebral body of interest. A graft or cage is inserted where vertebral body screw-rod instrumentation is placed in the levels above and below the corpectomy site for added stability. Attention is then turned toward posterior stabilization (minimally invasive or open surgical), after hemostasis is achieved plus closure of the thoracolumbar incision.

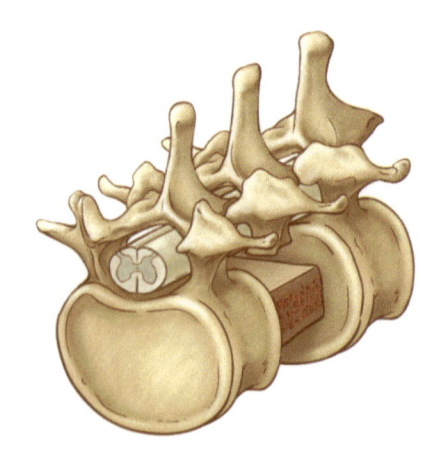

Fig. 14-5 Corpectomy and strut grafting.[7]

COMPLICATIONS

- The greatest surgical risk is the potential for intraoperative blood loss and postoperative epidural hematomas.
- Preoperative embolization and radiosurgery have been used as adjuncts to minimize these complications.
- Intraoperative hemostasis techniques (e.g., monopolar and bipolar electrocautery, bone wax, Surgifoam [Johnson & Johnson, New Brunswick, NJ], and Gelfoam [Baxter Healthcare, Deerfield, IL]) are used to minimize blood loss and achieve meticulous hemostasis.
- Blood products should be available intraoperatively, and a cell saver may be used in these cases.

OUTCOMES WITH EVALUATION OF RESULTS

In a review with a 52-month follow-up period,[41] laminectomy followed by radiation therapy, when used to treat vertebral hemangiomas involving the entire vertebra, was reported to yield a rate of 93% for recovery of neurologic function without a recurrence.

Acosta et al[12] reported a total of nine patients who underwent surgery for symptomatic vertebral hemangiomas (eight with neurologic deficits and one with pain). Six patients with neurologic deficits underwent decompressive laminectomy, and the other two underwent vertebrectomy. Seven of nine patients had complete resolution of both neurologic symptoms and pain after the initial surgical treatment.[12] None of the patients undergoing corpectomy had recurrent or new symptoms.[12] Rarely hemangiomas may behave more aggressively with involvement of the anterior and posterior columns and significant soft tissue extension into the spinal canal. Partial resection and stabilization are not often effective in this subgroup, and complete removal of the involved vertebral segment is recommended.[84]

SIGNATURE CASES

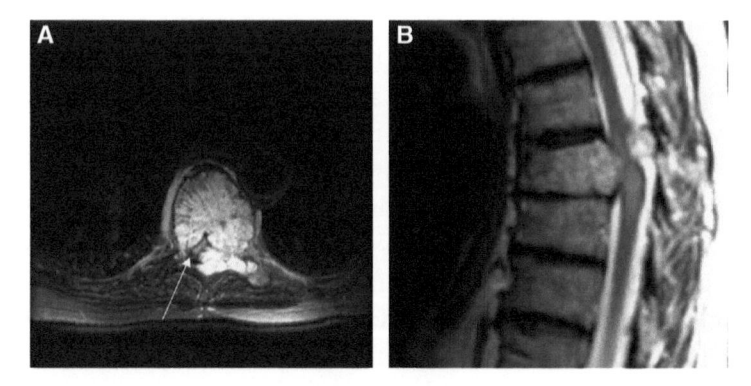

Fig. 14-6 **A,** Axial and **B,** sagittal T2-weighted MRI scans showing a T8 hemangioma with pedicular extension bilaterally and invasion of the left lamina and transverse process, and the left T8 rib. Posterior vertebral body expansion and epidural extension results in severe cord compression with cord signal change.[12]

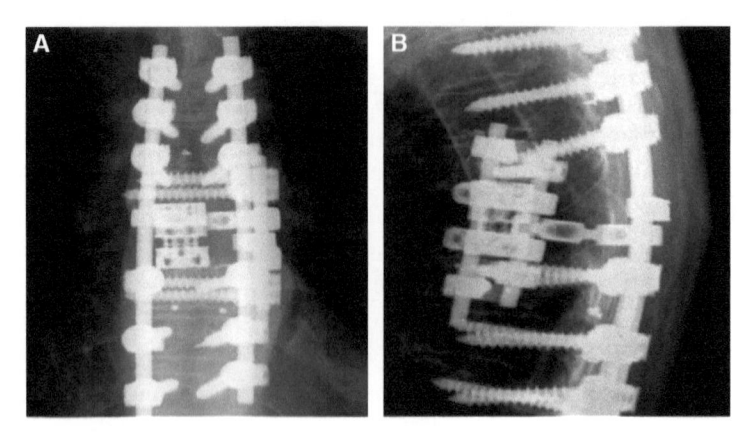

Fig. 14-7 **A,** Anteroposterior and **B,** lateral plain radiographs after T8 corpectomy with placement of an expandable interbody cage, T7 to T9 lateral fusion plate, and T5 to T11 pedicle screws and bilateral rods.[12]

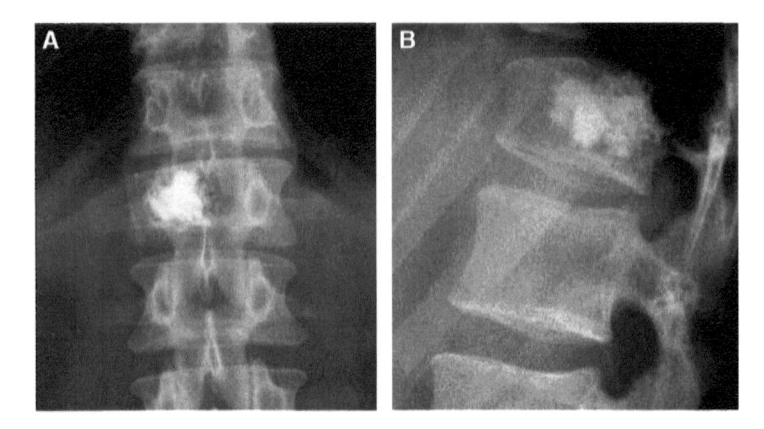

Fig. 14-8 **A,** Anteroposterior and **B,** lateral plain radiographs showing high-density methylmethacrylate within the right L1 vertebral body after vertebroplasty. Note there is an associated mild compression fracture of the right L1 vertebral body.

CONCLUSION

Vertebral hemangioma is a clear pathologic entity that may occur with pain or neurologic injury, or rarely from an incidental lesion progressing to spinal cord compression.[7] Patients with incidentally discovered lesions do not need serial evaluation unless pain or a neurologic deficit develops at the appropriate spine level.[7] Patients with pain should be followed with an annual examination, including CT and MRI scans to look for potential progression.[7] Painful lesions may be managed conservatively with radiation therapy or embolization.[7] Transarterial embolization can be used without decompression to effectively alleviate pain symptoms only.[12] Vertebroplasty is useful in improving back pain in the immediate acute period but is less effective in providing complete and long-term pain relief.[12] Radiation surgery can be used as a second line of treatment for painful intraosseous lesions.[12] Surgical intervention in patients with vertebral hemangiomas associated with spinal cord compression can be performed safely, with successful neurologic recovery. Transarterial embolization followed by laminectomy is a safe and effective procedure for the treatment of spinal cord compression caused by intraosseous vertebral bodies and posterior element hemangiomas.[12] Transarterial embolization should be performed in all patients with large feeding vessels to reduce intraoperative blood loss.[7] Vertebral corpectomy or spondylectomy, preceded by embolization, is used to treat spinal cord compression from vertebral body and neural arch expansion with epidural or extraosseous tumor extension, pathologic fracture, and kyphotic deformity.[12] Gross total resection obviates the need for postoperative irradiation, but radiation therapy reduces the risk of tumor recurrence in patients undergoing subtotal tumor removal.[7,12] Simultaneous anterior column reconstruction with an expandable cage and anterolateral plate fixation, supplemented with a posterior pedicle screw-rod construct segmental instrumentation, makes extraosseous tumor involvement surgically feasible.[12] Reoperation with circumferential vertebrectomy should be used to treat recurrent myelopathy, progressive deformities, or refractory painful lesions.[12]

TIPS FROM THE MASTERS

- The surgical approach depends on many factors but, most important, the decision will be made on the basis of what is in the best interests of the patient and which surgical techniques the neurosurgeon is most familiar with.
- If applied appropriately according to the patient's symptoms, radiation surgery, vertebroplasty, and embolization are safe procedures. For patients in whom the aforementioned treatments are unsuccessful, for patients with neurologic deficits, and/or for patients who have spinal instability, surgery remains the best therapeutic intervention.
- For aggressive lesions involving the anterior and posterior columns of the spine, complete removal by means of intralesional spondylectomy will best prevent a recurrence.

References (With Key References in Boldface)

1. Virchow R. Die Krankhasten Geschwulste, vol III. Berlin: Hirschwald, 1967, pp 306-496.
2. Junghanns H. Uber die Haufigkeit gutartiger Geschwulste in den Wirkbelkorpern (Angiome. Lipome. Osteome). Arch Klin Chir 169:204-212, 1932.
3. Junghanns H. Hamangiom des 3: Brust wirbelkorpers mit Ruckenmarkkompression: Laminektomie. Heilung. Arch Klin Chir 169:321-330, 1932.
4. Topfer DI. Uber eininfiltrierend wachsendes Hamangiom der Haut and Multiple Kapillarektasien der Haut und inneren: Organe-II Zur Kenntnis der Wirbelangiome. Frank Z Pathol 36:337-345, 1928.
5. Blankstein A, Spiegelmann R, Shacked I, et al. Hemangioma of the thoracic spine involving multiple adjacent levels: case report. Paraplegia 26:186-191, 1988.
6. Dagi TF, Schmidek HH. Vascular tumors of the spine. In Sundaresan N, Schmidek HH, Schiller AL, et al, eds. Tumors of the Spine: Diagnosis and Clinical Management. Philadelphia: WB Saunders, 1990, pp 181-191.
7. Fox MW, Onofrio BM. The natural history and management of symptomatic and asymptomatic vertebral hemangiomas. J Neurosurg 78:36-45, 1993.

8. **Krueger EG, Sobel GL, Weinstein C. Vertebral hemangioma with compression of spinal cord. J Neurosurg 18:331-338, 1961.**
9. **Perman E. On haemangiomata in the spinal column. Acta Chir Scand 61:91-105, 1927.**
10. McAllister VL, Kendall BE, Bull JW. Symptomatic vertebral haemangiomas. Brain 98:71-80, 1975.
11. Nguyen JP, Djindjian M, Gaston A, et al. Vertebral hemangiomas presenting with neurologic symptoms. Surg Neurol 27:391-397, 1987.
12. **Acosta FL, Dowd CF, Chin C, et al. Current treatment strategies and outcomes in the management of symptomatic vertebral hemangiomas. Neurosurgery 58:287-295, 2005.**
13. Padovani R, Poppi M, Pozzati E, et al. Spinal epidural hemangiomas. Spine 6:336-340, 1981.
14. Schlezinger NS, Ungar H. Hemangioma of the vertebra with compression myelopathy. AJR 42:192-216, 1939.
15. Healy M, Herz DA, Pearl L. Spinal hemangiomas. Neurosurgery 13:689-691, 1983.
16. Mohan V, Gupta SK, Tuli SM, et al. Symptomatic vertebral haemangiomas. Clin Radiol 31:575-579, 1980.
17. Larendo JD, Reizine D, Bard M, et al. Vertebral hemangiomas: radiologic evaluation. Radiology 161:183-189, 1986.
18. Nguyen JP, Djindjian M, Gaston A, et al. Vertebral hemangiomas presenting with neurologic symptoms. Surg Neurol 27:391-397, 1987.
19. Schnyder P, Fankhauser H, Mansouri B. Computed tomography in spinal hemangioma with cord compression. Report of two cases. Skeletal Radiol 15:372-375, 1986.
20. **Ross JS, Masaryk TJ, Modic MT, et al. Vertebral hemangiomas: MR imaging. Radiology 165:165-169, 1987.**
21. Laredo JD, Assouline E, Gelbert F, et al. Vertebral hemangiomas: fat content as a sign of aggressiveness. Radiology 177:467-472, 1990.
22. Laredo JD, Assouline E, Gaston A, et al. [Radiological features differentiating compressive and asymptomatic vertebral hemangiomas] Neurochirgurgie 35:284-288, 1989.
23. Baker ND, Klein MJ, Greenspan A, et al. Symptomatic vertebral hemangiomas: a report of four cases. Skeletal Radiol 15:458-463, 1986.
24. Raco A, Ciappetta P, Artico M, et al. Vertebral hemangiomas with cord compression: the role of embolization in five cases. Surg Neurol 34:164-168, 1990.
25. Gray F, Gherardi R, Benhaiem-Sigaux N. [Vertebral hemangiomas: definition and pathologic features] Neurochirurgie 35:267-269, 1989.
26. Unni KK, Ivins JC, Beabout JW, et al. Hemangioma, hemangiopericytoma, and hemangioendothelioma (angiosarcoma) of bone. Cancer 27:1403-1414, 1971.
27. Bergstrand A, Hook O, Lidvall H. Vertebral hemangiomas compressing the spinal cord. Acta Neurol Scand 39:59-66, 1963.
28. Wara WM, Phillips TL, Sheline GE, et al. Radiation tolerance of the spinal cord. Cancer 35:1558-1562, 1975.
29. Reizine D, Laredo JD, Riche MC, et al. Vertebral hemangiomas. In Jeanmart L, ed. Radiology of the Spine. Tumors. Berlin: Springer-Verlag, 1986, pp 73-80.
30. Kosary IZ, Braham J, Shacked I, et al. Spinal epidural hematoma due to hemangioma of vertebra. Surg Neurol 7:61-62, 1977.
31. Lang EF Jr, Peserico L. Neurologic and surgical aspects of vertebral hemangiomas. Surg Clin North Am 40:817-823, 1960.
32. Esparza J, Castro S, Portillo JM, et al. Vertebral hemangiomas: spinal angiography and preoperative embolization. Surg Neurol 10:171-173, 1978.
33. Feuerman T, Dwan PS, Young RF. Vertebrectomy for treatment of vertebral hemangioma without preoperative embolization. Case report. J Neurosurg 65:404-406, 1986.
34. Leehey P, Naseem M, Every P, et al. Vertebral hemangioma with compression myelopathy: metrizamide CT demonstration. J Comput Assist Tomogr 9:985-986, 1985.
35. ter Spill HW, Tijssen CC. Spinal epidural hematoma due to a vertebro-epidural hemangioma. Clin Neurol Neurosurg 91:91-93, 1989.
36. Bell RL. Hemangioma of a dorsal vertebra with collapse and compression myelopathy. J Neurosurg 12:570-576, 1955.

37. Sar C, Eralp L. Double thoracic vertebral hemangioma causing complete paraplegia. Am J Orthop 33:81-84, 2004.
38. Shah KC, Chacko AG. Extensive vertebral hemangioma with cord compression in two patients: review of the literature. Br J Neurosurg 18:250-252, 2004.
39. Bandiera S, Gasbarrini A, De Iure F, et al. Symptomatic vertebral hemangioma: the treatment of 23 cases and a review of the literature. Chir Organi Mov 87:1-15, 2002.
40. Djindjian M, Nguyen JP, Gaston A, et al. Multiple vertebral hemangiomas with neurological signs. Case report. J Neurosurg 76:1025-1028, 1992.
41. Nguyen JP, Djindjian M, Pavlovitch JM, et al. [Vertebral hemangioma with neurologic signs. Therapeutic results. Survey of the French Society of Neurosurgery] Neurochirurgie 35:299-303; 305-308, 1989.
42. Murugan L, Samson RS, Chandy MJ. Management of symptomatic vertebral hemangiomas: review of 13 patients. Neurol India 50:300-305, 2002.
43. Nassar SI, Hanbali FS, Haddad MC, et al. Thoracic vertebral hemangioma with extradural extension and spinal cord compression. Case report. Clin Imaging 22:65-68, 1998.
44. Ogura T, Mori M, Hayashida T, et al. Spinal reconstruction for symptomatic thoracic haemangioma using a titanium cage. Postgrad Med J 78:559-561, 2002.
45. Graham JJ, Yang WC. Vertebral hemangioma with compression fracture and paraparesis treated with preoperative embolization and vertebral resection. Spine 9:97-101, 1984.
46. Oda I, Cunningham BW, Abumi K, et al. The stability of reconstruction methods after thoracolumbar total spondylectomy. An in vitro investigation. Spine 24:1634-1638, 1999.
47. Singh K, Vaccaro AR, Kim J, et al. Biomechanical comparison of cervical spine reconstructive techniques after a multilevel corpectomy of the cervical spine. Spine 28:2352-2358, 2003.
48. Vahldiek MJ, Panjabi MM. Stability potential of spinal instrumentations in tumor vertebral body replacement surgery. Spine 23:543-550, 1998.
49. Hemmy DC, McGee DM, Armbrust FH, et al. Resection of vertebral hemangioma after preoperative embolization. Case report. J Neurosurg 47:282-285, 1977.
50. Hekster RE, Endtz L. Spinal-cord compression caused by vertebral haemangioma relieved by percutaneous catheter embolisation: 15 years later. Neuroradiology 29:101, 1987.
51. Jayakumar PN, Vasudev MK, Srikanth SG. Symptomatic vertebral haemangioma: endovascular treatment of 12 patients. Spinal Cord 35:624-628, 1997.
52. MacErlean DP, Shanik DG, Martin EA. Transcatheter embolisation of bone tumour arteriovenous malformations. Br J Radiol 51:414-419, 1978.
53. Smith TP, Koci T, Mehringer CM, et al. Transarterial embolization of vertebral hemangioma. J Vasc Interv Radiol 4:681-685, 1993.
54. Hekster RE, Luyendijk W, Tan TI. Spinal-cord compression caused by vertebral haemangioma relieved by percutaneous catheter embolisation. Neuroradiology 3:160-164, 1972.
55. Gaston A, Nguyen JP, Djindjian M, et al. Vertebral haemangioma: CT and arteriographic features in three cases. J Neuroradiol 12:21-33, 1985.
56. Gross CE, Hodge CH Jr, Binet EF, et al. Relief of spinal block during embolization of a vertebral body hemangioma. Case report. J Neurosurg 45:327-330, 1976.
57. Hemmy DC. Vertebral hemangiomas. In Wilkins RH, Rengachary SS, eds. Neurosurgery. New York: McGraw-Hill, 1985, pp 1076-1079.
58. Barr JD, Barr MS, Lemley TJ, et al. Percutaneous vertebroplasty for pain relief and spinal stabilization. Spine 25:923-928, 2000.
59. Cohen JE, Lylyk P, Ceratto R, et al. Percutaneous vertebroplasty: technique and results in 192 procedures. Neurol Res 26:41-49, 2004.
60. Cotton A, Deramond H, Cortet B, et al. Preoperative percutaneous injection of methyl methacrylate and N-butyl cyanoacrylate in vertebral hemangiomas. AJNR Am J Neuroradiol 17:137-142, 1996.
61. Deramond H, Despriester C, Galibert P, et al. Percutaneous vertebroplasty with polymethylmethacrylate. Technique, indications, and results. Radiol Clin North Am 36:533-546, 1998.
62. Gabal AM. Percutaneous technique for sclerotherapy of vertebral hemangioma compressing spinal cord. Cardiovasc Intervent Radiol 25:494-500, 2002.

63. Galibert P, Deramond H, Rosat P, et al. Preliminary note on the treatment of vertebral angioma by percutaneous acrylic vertebroplasty. Neurochirurgie 33:166-168, 1987.
64. Larsen D. Percutaneous vertebroplasty. Nurs Stand 18:33-37, 2004.
65. Peh WC, Gilula LA. Percutaneous vertebroplasty: indications, contraindications, and technique. Br J Radiol 76:69-75, 2003.
66. Amar AP, Larsen DW, Esnaashari N, et al. Percutaneous transpedicular polymethylmethacrylate vertebroplasty for the treatment of spinal compression fractures. Neurosurgery 49:1105-1114, 2001.
67. Cotton A, Boutry N, Cortet B, et al. Percutaneous vertebroplasty: state of the art. Radiographics 18:311-320, 1998.
68. San Millan Ruiz D, Burkhardt K, Jean B, et al. Pathology findings with acrylic implants. Bone 25:85S-90S, 1999.
69. Bas T, Aparisi F, Bas JL. Efficacy and safety of ethanol injections in 18 cases of vertebral hemangioma: a mean follow-up of 2 years. Spine 26:1577-1582, 2001.
70. Faria SL, Schlupp WR, Chimnazzo H Jr. Radiotherapy in the treatment of vertebral hemangiomas. Int J Radiat Oncol Biol Phys 11:387-390, 1985.
71. Glanzmann C, Rust M, Horst W. Irradiation therapy of vertebral angionomas: results in 62 patients during the years 1939 to 1975 (author's translation). Strahlentherapie 153:522-525, 1977.
72. Yang ZY, Zhang LJ, Chen ZX, et al. Hemangioma of the vertebral column. A report on twenty-three patients with special reference to functional recovery after radiation therapy. Acta Radiol Oncol 24:129-132, 1985.
73. Eisenstein S, Spiro F, Browde S, et al. The treatment of a symptomatic vertebral hemangioma by radiotherapy. A case report. Spine 11:640-642, 1986.
74. Miszczyk L, Ficek K, Trela K, et al. The efficacy of radiotherapy for vertebral hemangiomas. Neoplasma 48:82-84, 2001.
75. Sakata K, Hareyama M, Oouchi A, et al. Radiotherapy of vertebral hemangiomas. Acta Oncol 36:719-724, 1997.
76. Benati A, Da Pian R, Mazza C, et al. Preoperative embolisation of a vertebral haemangioma compressing the spinal cord. Neuroradiology 7:181-183, 1974.
77. Pavlovitch JM, Nguyen JP, Djindjian M, et al. [Radiotherapy of compressive vertebral hemangiomas] Neurochirurgie 35:296-298, 1989.
78. Zito G, Kadis GN. Multiple vertebral hemangiomas resembling metastases with spinal cord compression. Arch Neurol 37:247-248, 1980.
79. Heiss JD, Doppman JL, Oldfield EH. Brief report: relief of spinal cord compression from vertebral hemangioma by intralesional injection of absolute ethanol. N Engl J Med 331:508-511, 1994.
80. Doppman JL, Oldfield EH, Heiss JD. Symptomatic vertebral hemangiomas: treatment by means of direct intralesional injection of ethanol. Radiology 214:341-348, 2000.
81. Goyal M, Mishra NK, Sharma A, et al. Alcohol ablation of symptomatic vertebral hemangiomas. AJNR Am J Neuroradiol 20:1091-1096, 1999.
82. Munk PL, Marotta TR. Intralesional injection of absolute alcohol into vertebral hemangiomas: a new treatment option? AJNR Am J Neuroradiol 20:959-960, 1999.
83. Niemeyer T, McClellan J, Webb J, et al. Brown-Sequard syndrome after management of vertebral hemangioma with intralesional alcohol. A case report. Spine 24:1845-1847, 1999.
84. Acosta FL Jr, Sanai N, Cloyd J, Deviren V, Chou D, Ames CP. Treatment of Enneking stage 3 aggressive vertebral hemangiomas with intralesional spondylectomy: report of 10 cases and review of the literature. J Spinal Disord Tech 24: 268-275, 2011.

Chapter 15

Osteoid Osteomas and Osteoblastomas

Shane Burch

Osteoid osteomas and osteoblastomas are benign osseous lesions that generally appear in young patients. Osteoid osteomas were first described by Bergstrand in 1930 and further characterized by Jaffe in 1935.[1] These lesions were described as having a nidus of vascularized osseous tissue with surrounding sclerosis. It was not until 1956 that Jaffe[2] described osteoblastomas as a separate entity. However, they may represent a continuum of the same process, because they share a common histologic appearance and are often differentiated solely on the basis of size and radiographic appearance. Osteoid osteomas are common, accounting for approximately 10% of all benign bone tumors. Osteoblastomas are less common and represent less than 1% of all bone tumors.[3]

In 1977 Jackson et al[4] reviewed the English literature and found reports of 860 cases of osteoid osteoma and 184 cases of osteoblastoma. In this series approximately 10% of the reported cases of osteoid osteoma and 35% of osteoblastomas were localized to the spine. In a large series osteoblastomas occurred throughout the skeleton, although the spine was the most common location followed by the femur. Osteoid osteomas have been described in the cervical, thoracic, and lumbar spine, with a predominance in the lumbar region (59%), with the cervical region accounting for approximately 25% of cases, whereas the lesions occur in the thoracic region in 12% and the sacrum in 2%.[5,6] In contrast, osteoblastomas have been described with equal distribution throughout the spine.[7] Kirwan et al[8] described a series of 18 osteoid osteomas in the thoracolumbar spine in which 83% were noted in the pedicle, whereas in a report by Kroon and Schurmans[7] 94% of osteoblastomas occurred in the spinous processes and "arches." Both lesions are localized primarily to the posterior elements, including the pedicle, facets, and lamina, although there are reports of lesions occurring in the vertebral body.[5,9]

HISTOLOGY

The histologic findings of osteoid osteomas and osteoblastomas appear similar and may represent a continuum of the same process.[10] The gross appearance of osteoid osteomas includes a red or pink nidus surrounded by sclerotic bone. In 1977 Jackson et al[4] described nine cases of osteoid osteomas and three cases of osteoblastomas; these investigators noted that "each lesion had trabeculae of osteoid containing a variable amount of mineralization supported by a very vascular connective tissue stroma." Osteoclasts are present within the lesion but are relatively few. The osteoblasts within the lesion are larger than those identified outside the lesion, although they contain irregular indented nuclei and other ultrastructural irregularities.[6] The host bone around these lesions contains woven and lamellar bone.

The gross appearance of osteoblastomas includes red or tan tissue at the nidus. Microscopic pathologic findings demonstrate a sharp, tumor-host interface. The lesion can contain immature woven bone. Extraosseous tumors showed soft tissue with a reactive layer of surrounding bone.[11] Characteristic histologic findings include a nidus of osteoblasts surrounded by trabecular and woven bone in a fibrovascular stroma. A subtype carries epithelioid osteoblasts, which have an elongated morphologic appearance, and these lesions tend to be more aggressive than those without this histologic subtype. In contrast to osteoid osteomas, osteoblastomas showed greater cellularity, minimal mitosis within the osteoblasts, and the ability to form soft tissue masses outside the cortex. Thus a main difference between osteoid osteomas and osteoblastomas is less sclerosis and a greater propensity to form an expansile mass in the latter.[12] In addition, a small portion of osteoblastomas contain tissue consistent with aneurysmal bone cysts. Paus and Kim[9] reported similar findings. Furthermore, the histologic appearance of osteoid osteoblastomas can be difficult to distinguish from osteosarcomas. One key feature is a lack of destructive permeation into adjacent tissues, which differentiates it from osteosarcomas.[11] Bertoni et al[13] described a lesion they called *osteoblastoma-like osteosarcoma*, which was differentiated from osteoblastomas by the invasion of the surrounding host tissue despite 9 of 11 cases being considered benign based on initial biopsy specimens. In one series two osteoblastomas with initially benign histologic findings became malignant after several recurrences.[11] Multifocal lesions were identified in 14% of patients and had higher recurrence rate.

Despite similar histologic properties, osteoblastomas are differentiated from osteoid osteomas by radiographic appearance and size. By convention, lesions larger than 1.5 to 2 cm are considered to be osteoblastomas.[10] Similar to other osseous tumors of the spine, the Enneking and Weinstein-Boriani-Biagini[14] classification can be applied to these lesions for classification and staging purposes. They are considered benign active lesions, but osteoblastomas may display benign aggressive behavior. Lesions are considered stage 2 if they remain within the osseous compartment and stage 3 if they have an extraosseous component.[15] Boriani et al[10] described a series of 30 osteoblastomas that were localized to the spine; 14 were stage 2 and 16 were stage 3, with an average diameter of 3.5 cm and a range of 2 to 6.5 cm.

NATURAL HISTORY AND CLINICAL PRESENTATION

Both osteoid osteomas and osteoblastomas are benign lesions that occur in young patients, with a male:female predominance of 2:1. Typically they are described in patients less than 30 years of age. The course can be insidious, and the diagnosis can be delayed for many years.[16] In one study the youngest patient with a spinal osteoid osteoma was 3 years old.[1] The natural history described by reports in the early literature and the clinical course of osteoid osteomas differs from that of osteoblastomas. Osteoid osteomas produce night pain that is relieved by nonsteroidal antiinflammatory agents. In part this may be due to the increased production of prostaglandins in these tumors.[17] There is also a high association between scoliosis and both osteoid osteomas and osteoblastomas. Scoliosis was present in 63% of the patients in one metaanalysis of osteoid osteomas.[18] Curves occur less frequently in patients with osteoblastomas but can be found, especially if the lesion is situated asymmetrically in the posterior elements.[10,18] Likewise, cervical lesions are known to produce torticollis.

The symptoms are insidious, with pain being described as starting as a dull ache. The time to diagnosis in one study was approximately 15 months, indicating the slow but steady onset of symptoms. In 1956, in the series described by Sabanas et al,[1] night pain was described in only 8 of 30 patients with osteoid osteomas. However, Pettine and Klassen[12] described pain related to evening and activity, which was present in 95% of their patients, but only 29% of their patients reported being awakened by the pain. Night pain is not associated with osteoblastomas. Aspirin has been shown to effectively treat pain stemming from osteoid osteomas, whereas it is not as effective for osteoblastomas.[19] All patients in the series described by Sabanas et al[1] reported pain on palpation, and scoliosis was identified in 18 of 30 cases reviewed. Swelling also occurred, although this was a late finding. Lesions were typically localized at the apex of the deformity and on the concavity of the curve with all curves being less than 30 degrees. If the lesion occurs in the lumbar spine, the apex is proximal and pelvic obliquity is noted.[20] The cause of the scoliosis is thought to be muscle spasms secondary to the effects of the lesion. Kawahara et al[21] identified two patients with scoliosis resulting from osteoid osteomas, with MRI scans showing increased gadolinium uptake and edema within the muscles. Subsequent biopsy findings of muscles at the time of tumor resection identified replacement of the muscle fibers with fatty tissue and inflammatory cells.[21] Once the lesion is removed, the inflammatory component causing changes in the paraspinal musculature usually resolves. However, if significant myolysis occurs, scoliosis may persist.

Although osteoid osteomas have been shown to spontaneously regress, osteoblastomas typically continue to progress and expand from stage 2 to stage 3 and in doing so may cause paresis or paralysis. In the series of osteoblastomas reported by Boriani et al,[10] 13 of 30 patients had a neurologic deficit. However, early reports of the natural history of osteoid osteomas also described patients with radiculopathy, hyperreflexia, and associated weakness caused by the lesion.[1] Results of laboratory tests, including complete blood count, erythrocyte sedimentation rate, C-reactive protein, and alkaline phosphatase levels, have been shown to be normal in several reports.

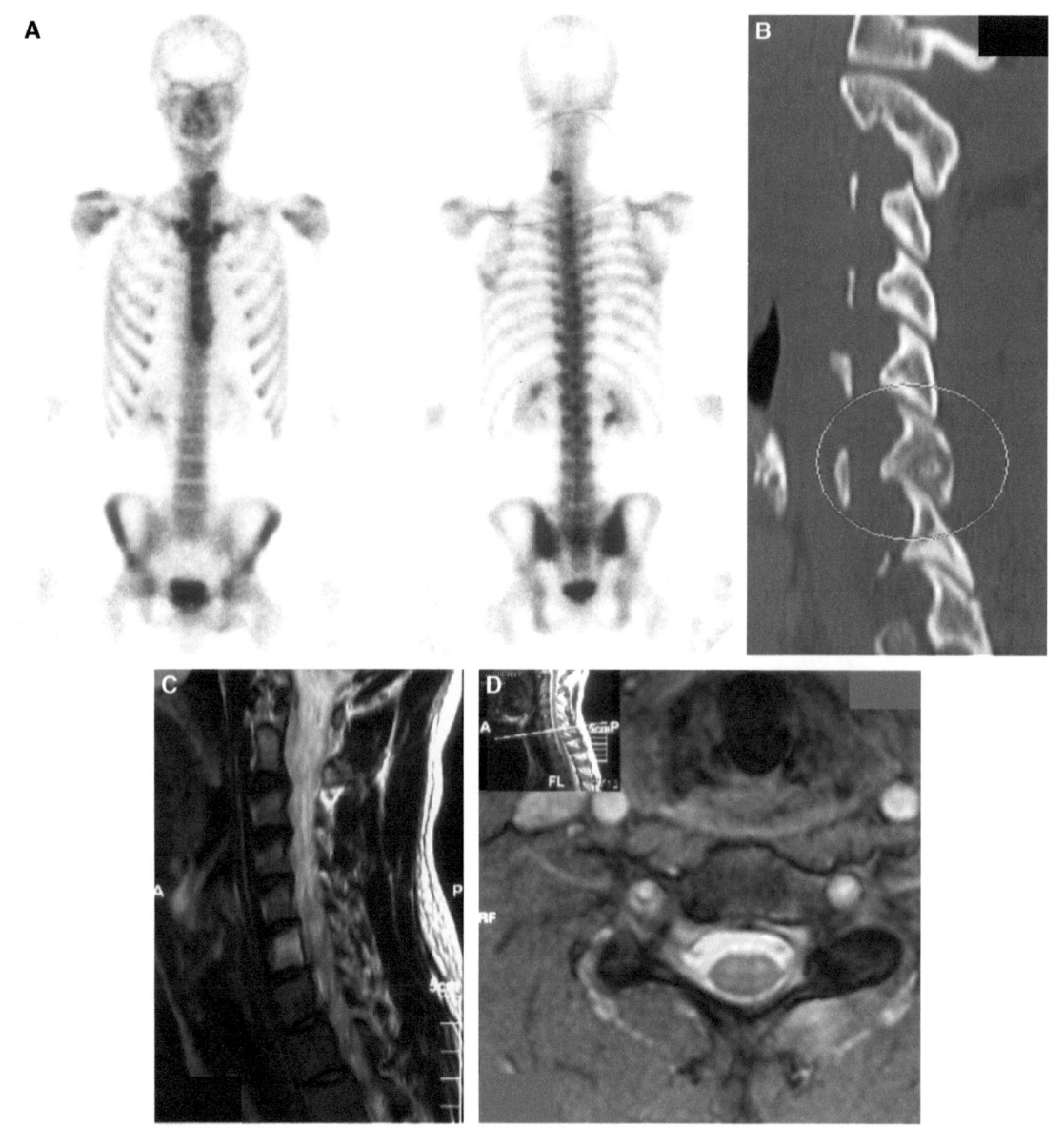

Fig. 15-1 Osteoid osteoma of the cervical spine. **A,** Technetium-99m scan indicating increased uptake on the left C6 vertebra. **B,** Sagittal fine-cut CT image showing the nidus of the lesion in the lateral mass of C6. **C,** T2-weighted sagittal MRI scan of the cervical spine depicting a diffuse increase in signal intensity in the C6 vertebra. **D,** T2-weighted MRI scan of C6 vertebra in the axial plane showing paraspinal edema and diffusely enlarged lateral mass on the left.

IMAGING

Historically, osteoid osteomas and osteoblastomas were diagnosed on roentgenograms. Radiographically, immature osteoid osteomas appear radiolucent compared with more mature lesions, which are radiopaque. Therefore osteoid osteomas may have a radiolucent or sclerotic nidus surrounded by a sclerotic rim. The lesions are small (<1.5 to 2 cm), and the lack of sclerosis early on makes the diagnosis impossible by plain radiography alone.[22] The appearance of an osteoblastoma is that of a well-circumscribed, expansile lytic lesion that is larger than 1.5 to 2 cm, with or without matrix mineralization, surrounded by a region of sclerosis.[7,23] Azouz et al[24] described technetium bone scanning as an effective tool for localizing these lesions (Fig. 15-1). In a series by Pettine and Klassen,[12] the use of technetium-99m scans was estimated to reduce the time to diagnosis by approximately two thirds.

Both computed tomography (CT) and magnetic resonance imaging (MRI) scans have been used to identify osteoid osteomas, with CT scans being more specific (see Fig. 15-1).[22] Thin-slice CT scans were shown to be diagnostic in 71% of patients compared with 19% for MRI scans.[25] Comparing these two modalities, in 1993, Assoun et al[26] determined that MRI scans were less specific than CT scans. In their report of 19 patients, 12 had decreased signal intensity on all pulse sequences with some increased signal intensity after gadolinium. This has also been reported elsewhere.[5] In the remaining patients, low T1 signal intensity was noted along with high T2 signal intensity. The nidus, which contains sclerotic bone, is typically low on T1 imaging. In this present study, 11 of 12 patients with a bone marrow response shown on MRI scans had not taken salicylates, whereas six of seven patients who had no bone marrow response had taken salicylates. Similarly, there was a statistical difference between those with soft tissue masses who had not taken salicylates and those without soft tissue masses who had taken salicylates.

TREATMENT

Treatment of osteoid osteomas and osteoblastomas includes pain management secondary to the inflammatory component of the tumor, the structural aberrations induced by the tumor, muscle spasms, and resultant scoliosis. Initial management of osteoid osteomas includes the use of salicylates. Up to 75% of patients with osteoid osteomas achieve some pain relief with aspirin. Treatment is less effective in patients with osteoblastomas.

Osteoid osteomas in the lumbar and thoracic spine are also amenable to radiofrequency ablation, which was described by Osti and Sebben[27] in 1998. A radiofrequency probe is directed under CT guidance into the lesion. If the lesion is localized in the cervical spine, because of the proximity of the vertebral artery and spinal cord, or no cortex shields the spinal cord in other locations, radiofrequency is not recommended.[28] Nevertheless, Laus et al[29] reported using radiofrequency ablation in the cervical spine with no neurologic deficit. However, in a series of 10 patients reported by Martel et al,[28] treatment was performed within 2 mm of the adjacent nerve root. Treatment consisted of introducing the radiofrequency probe through an 11-gauge biopsy needle, heated to 90° C for 4 minutes.[28] These lesions, along with lesions that do not respond to radiofrequency ablation, are treated with excision. A challenge of treatment includes identifying the lesion at the time of surgery. To that end, computer-assisted surgery has been described to reduce the difficulty in finding the nidus.[30] If this is unsuccessful, or if the lesion recurs, treatment involves complete excision of the nidus. The recurrence rate with the use of this technique is 4% for osteoid osteomas. In contrast, osteoblastomas have a higher recurrence rate, which ranges from 9% to 19%. Stage 2 lesions have a lower recurrence rate than stage 3 lesions, equating to a more aggressive approach to their resection. Because of the recurrence rate and the propensity for osteoblastomas to invade the central canal, a marginal resection is indicated for all osteoblastomas, if feasible.

Depending on the location of the lesion, a posteroanterior or combined surgical approach may be required. Depending on the size and location of the lesion, a radiopaque marker may be placed before surgery to mark the tumor. The selection of the approach is on a case-by-case basis that uses the principles of musculoskeletal oncology. Lamina, facets, pars interarticularis, pedicles, and vertebral bodies may all be involved, which may require a fusion in addition to excision of the tumor. In cases where the osteoblastoma appears radiographically or histologically similar to an osteosarcoma, a wide resection may be required, especially if the lesion has invasive margins.

OUTCOMES

Several investigators have reported immediate relief in patients after radiofrequency ablation of osteoid osteomas, with visual analog scores dropping dramatically.[27,31-33] In a series by Martel et al,[28] 2 of 10 patients had a recurrence after radiofrequency ablation.

In a series reported by Zileli et al[34] of 16 patients who underwent surgical resection of their lesions, 15 had complete relief in accordance with other reports in the literature.[35] In patients with scoliosis resulting from osteoid osteomas, Ransford et al[36] described the magnitude of the curve as being associated with the interval between the onset of symptoms and the time of surgical treatment. Several investigators described the resolution of scoliosis once the lesion had been removed. Persistent scoliosis has been noted in patients who have been treated after a long course of the disease at a younger age.

The recurrence rate for osteoblastomas is quite different from that for osteoid osteomas. In the series by Lucas et al,[11] a recurrence rate of 19% was noted. Other investigators have noted fewer recurrences after intralesional curettage. In a series from the Mayo Clinic, tumor size and location were not associated with recurrences, but the lesions with epithelioid osteoblasts (24%) were recognized as having a greater risk of recurrence.[11] However, this was not substantiated by other studies.[37]

CONCLUSION

Osteoid osteomas and osteoblastomas are benign neoplasms of bone and are common to the spine. They share some histologic features but differ radiographically and clinically. Most important, osteoid osteomas are small lesions that have an inflammatory component that can induce scoliosis. Treatment is simple and straightforward, and includes the use of salicylates, radiofrequency ablation, and complete resection, if possible. One challenge that remains is localizing the lesion during surgery. In contrast, osteoblastomas are larger lesions that can cause pain, but because of their size and expansile nature, they can produce neural deficits. These lesions are more aggressive and may be invasive, multifocal, and have a higher rate of recurrence. Rare occurrences of malignant transformation have been reported. The treatment is aimed at excising the tumor en bloc to reduce the recurrence rate, if feasible. The success rate is high, greater than 90%, with respect to treating the patient's symptoms. Different approaches are required based on the location and elements involved.

TIPS FROM THE MASTERS

- Intraoperative CT navigation can be quite helpful in localizing small completely intraosseous lesions to ensure complete resection.
- For osteoid osteomas, radiofrequency ablation is the treatment of choice for lesions that are anatomically accessible for this technique.
- Intralesional gross total marginal resection is recommended for osteoblastomas to decrease the risk of recurrence, even if reconstruction would be required.

References (With Key References in Boldface)

1. Sabanas AO, Bickel WH, Moe JH. Natural history of osteoid osteoma of the spine: review of the literature and report of three cases. Am J Surg 91:880-889, 1954.
2. **Jaffe HL. Benign osteoblastoma. Bull Hosp Joint Dis 17:141-151, 1956.**
3. Frassica FJ, Waltrip RL, Sponseller PD, et al. Clinicopathologic features and treatment of osteoid osteoma and osteoblastoma in children and adolescents. Orthop Clin North Am 27:559-574, 1996.
4. **Jackson RP, Reckling FW, Mants FA. Osteoid osteoma and osteoblastoma. Similar histologic lesions with different natural histories. Clin Orthop Relat Res 128:303-313, 1977.**
5. Houang B, Grenier N, Gréselle JF, et al. Osteoid osteoma of the cervical spine. Misleading MR features about a case involving the uncinate process. Neuroradiology 31:549-551, 1990.
6. Greenspan A. Benign bone-forming lesions: osteoma, osteoid osteoma, and osteoblastoma. Clinical, imaging, pathologic, and differential considerations. Skeletal Radiol 22:485-500, 1993.
7. Kroon HM, Schurmans J. Osteoblastoma: clinical and radiologic findings in 98 new cases. Radiology 175:783-790, 1990.
8. Kirwan EO, Hutton PA, Pozo JL, et al. Osteoid osteoma and benign osteoblastoma of the spine. Clinical presentation and treatment. J Bone Joint Surg Br 66:21-26, 1984.
9. Paus BC, Kim TK. Osteoid osteoma of the spine. Acta Orthop Scand 33:24-29, 1963.
10. **Boriani S, Capanna R, Donati D, et al. Osteoblastoma of the spine. Clin Orthop Relat Res 278:37-45, 1992.**
11. Lucas DR, Unni KK, McLeod RA, et al. Osteoblastoma: clinicopathologic study of 306 cases. Hum Pathol 25:117-134, 1994.
12. **Pettine KA, Klassen RA. Osteoid-osteoma and osteoblastoma of the spine. J Bone Joint Surg Am 68:354-361, 1986.**
13. Bertoni F, Bacchini P, Donati D, et al. Osteoblastoma-like osteosarcoma. The Rizzoli Institute experience. Mod Pathol 6:707-716, 1993.
14. Boriani S, Weinstein JN, Biagini R. Primary bone tumors of the spine. Terminology and surgical staging. Spine (Phila Pa 1976) 22:1036-1044, 1997.
15. Enneking WF. Musculoskeletal tumor staging: 1988 update. Cancer Treat Res 44:39-49, 1989.
16. Sapkas G, Efstathopoulos NE, Papadakis M. Undiagnosed osteoid osteoma of the spine presenting as painful scoliosis from adolescence to adulthood: a case report. Scoliosis 4:9, 2009.
17. Mungo DV, Zhang X, O'Keefe RJ, et al. COX-1 and COX-2 expression in osteoid osteomas. J Orthop Res 20:159-162, 2002.

18. Saifuddin A, White J, Sherazi Z, et al. Osteoid osteoma and osteoblastoma of the spine. Factors associated with the presence of scoliosis. Spine (Phila Pa 1976) 23:47-53, 1998.
19. Saccomanni B. Osteoid osteoma and osteoblastoma of the spine: a review of the literature. Curr Rev Musculoskelet Med 2:65-67, 2009.
20. Crist BD, Lenke LG, Lewis S. Osteoid osteoma of the lumbar spine. A case report highlighting a novel reconstruction technique. J Bone Joint Surg Am 87:414-418, 2005.
21. Kawahara C, Tanaka Y, Kato H, et al. Myolysis of the erector spinae muscles as the cause of scoliosis in osteoid osteoma of the spine. Spine (Phila Pa 1976) 27:E313-E315, 2002.
22. Yamamoto K, Asazuma T, Tsuchihara T, et al. Diagnostic efficacy of thin slice CT in osteoid osteoma of the thoracic spine: report of two cases. J Spinal Disord Tech 18:182-184, 2005.
23. Kransdorf MJ, Stull MA, Gilkey FW, et al. Osteoid osteoma. Radiographics 11:671-696, 1991.
24. Azouz EM, Kozlowski K, Marton D, et al. Osteoid osteoma and osteoblastoma of the spine in children. Report of 22 cases with brief literature review. Pediatr Radiol 16:25-31, 1986.
25. Hosalkar HS, Garg S, Moroz L, et al. The diagnostic accuracy of MRI versus CT imaging for osteoid osteoma in children. Clin Orthop Relat Res 433:171-177, 2005.
26. Assoun J, Richardi G, Railhac JJ, et al. Osteoid osteoma: MR imaging versus CT. Radiology 191:217-223, 1994.
27. Osti OL, Sebben R. High-frequency radio-wave ablation of osteoid osteoma in the lumbar spine. Eur Spine J 7:422-425, 1998.
28. Martel J, Bueno A, Nieto-Morales ML, et al. Osteoid osteoma of the spine: CT-guided monopolar radiofrequency ablation. Eur J Radiol 71:564-569, 2009.
29. Laus M, Albisinni U, Alfonso C, et al. Osteoid osteoma of the cervical spine: surgical treatment or percutaneous radiofrequency coagulation? Eur Spine J 16:2078-2082, 2007.
30. Van Royen BJ, Baayen JC, Pijpers R, et al. Osteoid osteoma of the spine: a novel technique using combined computer-assisted and gamma probe-guided high-speed intralesional drill excision. Spine (Phila Pa 1976) 30:369-373, 2005.
31. Hadjipavlou AG, Tzermiadianos MN, Kakavelakis KN, et al. Percutaneous core excision and radiofrequency thermo-coagulation for the ablation of osteoid osteoma of the spine. Eur Spine J 18:345-351, 2009.
32. Hadjipavlou AG, Lander PH, Marchesi D, et al. Minimally invasive surgery for ablation of osteoid osteoma of the spine. Spine (Phila Pa 1976) 28:E472-E477, 2003.
33. Cové JA, Taminiau AH, Obermann WR, et al. Osteoid osteoma of the spine treated with percutaneous computed tomography-guided thermocoagulation. Spine (Phila Pa 1976) 25:1283-1286, 2000.
34. Zileli M, Cagli S, Basdemir G, et al. Osteoid osteomas and osteoblastomas of the spine. Neurosurg Focus 15:E5, 2003.
35. Lin HH, Yu CT, Chang IL, et al. Painful scoliosis secondary to osteoid osteoma of the lumbar spine in adolescents. Int Surg 93:32-36, 2008.
36. Ransford AO, Pozo JL, Hutton PA, et al. The behaviour pattern of the scoliosis associated with osteoid osteoma or osteoblastoma of the spine. J Bone Joint Surg Br 66:16-20, 1984.
37. Della Rocca C, Huvos AG. Osteoblastoma: varied histological presentations with a benign clinical course. An analysis of 55 cases. Am J Surg Pathol 20:841-850, 1996.

Chapter 16

Osteosarcoma

Lee Jae Morse, Vedat Deviren

Osteosarcoma is the most common primary malignancy of bone. It has a bimodal distribution, with most of these tumors being diagnosed in adolescence during the growth spurt, and a second peak in the fourth decade of life. Most osteosarcomas arise in the appendicular skeleton, whereas osteosarcomas in the spine are rare. Ozaki et al[1] looked at osteosarcomas in the axial skeleton and found that 7% to 9% of all osteosarcomas arose in the pelvis, and only 0.85% to 3% were detected in the spine. Relatively large case series of osteosarcoma in the appendicular skeleton have been reported, but most series of primary osteosarcoma of the spine are composed of only 10 to 30 patients. One of the largest series was reported by Ilaslan et al,[2] who retrospectively reviewed 4887 cases of osteosarcoma registered at the Mayo Clinic between 1915 and 2001. Among these cases, 198 patients had primary vertebral osteosarcomas (4%). Age at onset of osteosarcomas of the spine was significantly more advanced than that of osteosarcomas in the appendicular skeleton. The median age of patients with osteosarcomas of the spine was 34.5 years of age, and there was no statistically significant difference between male and female patients. These investigators found that most of the tumors were located in the thoracic and lumbar spine, 66 and 64 patients, respectively, whereas only 27 patients had involvement of the cervical spine, and 41 patients had sacral tumors. Forty-four of 56 patients (79%) with adequate imaging had tumors that arose in the posterior elements. Histologically the most common subtypes were osteoblastic (68%), chondroblastic (17%), telangiectatic (6%), fibroblastic (6%), small cell (1%), and epithelioid (1%). Another large series, the Leeds Regional Bone Tumour Registry, consisted of a cohort of 2750 patients with bone tumors of the spine, who were registered from 1958 to 2000.[3] Of the 2750 patients, 126 (4.6%) had primary vertebral tumors. The most common diagnoses were multiple myeloma and plasmacytoma. Osteosarcomas ranked third (12 patients) behind chordomas (28 patients). Among those 12 patients, six (50%) had preexisting Paget's disease. The National Cancer Data Base reported 11,961 cases of osteosarcoma from 1985 to 2003 and found that only 2.5% involved the vertebral column.[4]

The exact cause of osteosarcomas of the spine is unknown, but some risk factors have been identified. Examples are patients with metabolic bone disorders, such as Paget's disease of the bone, fibrous dysplasia, hereditary multiple exostoses, and enchondromatosis. Patients with hereditary retinoblastoma are at significant risk for developing a second tumor, 50% of which are osteosarcomas. Radiation exposure for treatment of cancer increases the risk of axial osteosarcoma, which typically has a 5- to 20-year latency period.

In general, the age of onset and the location of tumors in the spine have been shown to be predictors of potential malignancy. Approximately two thirds of spine tumors diagnosed in patients less than 18 years of age are benign. This trend is reversed in adults. The location of the tumor within the spine is also prognostic where more than two thirds of tumors within the vertebral body are malignant, as opposed to tumors in the posterior elements, which tend to be benign with only one third being malignant.

The prognosis for osteosarcomas of the limbs has dramatically improved from a universally fatal disease to a relatively curable one. Bielack et al[5] found the overall 5-year relapse-free survival rate for osteosarcomas of the limbs to be 65%. The prognosis for osteosarcomas of the spine has also significantly improved but lags far behind that of osteosarcomas of the limbs. The Cooperative Osteosarcoma Study Group reported results from a cohort of 22 patients with osteosarcomas of the spine.[1] Six patients had metastases at the time of diagnosis. Twelve of the 22 patients underwent surgical resections (2 wide excisional, 3 marginal, and 7 intralesional). The overall median survival was 23 months, with only three patients living longer than 6 years.

CLINICAL PRESENTATION

Most patients with primary vertebral osteosarcomas initially have pain. Patients often complain of chronic progressive back or neck pain that has no exacerbating or relieving factors, persists despite rest, and will often wake them up at night. In the *Leeds Regional Bone Tumor Registry*, more than 95% of patients with malignant tumors had pain, whereas 76% of patients with benign tumors had pain.[3] Similarly, many of these patients have some neurologic deficit caused by tumor invasion into the dural space or retropulsion of fragments resulting from a pathologic fracture leading to compression of the spinal canal or the spinal roots. In the Leeds tumor registry, 51 of 98 patients (52%) with malignant spine tumors had evidence of cord compression or radicular symptoms versus 5 of 29 patients (17%) with benign lesions.[3] Patients with significant loss of vertebral body height or pathologic fractures may develop severe kyphosis. Focal swelling or a palpable mass is reported in less than 10% of patients.

DIAGNOSTIC IMAGING

Imaging is integral to all facets of diagnosis, staging, surgical planning, and posttreatment monitoring of patients with osteosarcomas of the spine. The first step in radiographic evaluation is plain radiography. Osteosarcomas usually present as a mix of osteolytic and sclerotic lesions. Because the vertebral body is often involved, the first indication of a tumor is a compression fracture that, on further evaluation, has a pathologic cause. After the initial plain radiographs of the spine are obtained, there are many imaging modalities available for further diagnostic studies. The major advantage of CT scans is that they allow evaluation of bony involvement. CT scans have also proved useful for improving the accuracy of biopsies and intraoperative pedicle screw placement. MRI with contrast allows further assessment of tumor invasion into soft tissues. The amount of mineralization in the tumor will dictate the appearance on MRI scans. Mineralized tumors will be dark on both T1- and T2-weighted images, whereas nonmineralized lesions will be dark on T1-weighted images but bright on T2-weighted images. MRI scans also allow the tumor to be viewed in multiple planes, which is critical to surgical planning.

Nuclide bone scans are frequently used to stage both primary and metastatic bone tumors of the spine and to monitor treatment. Caution must be used when monitoring treatment responses to avoid misinterpretations resulting from the *flare phenomenon*. Discovered in the 1980s, the flare phenomenon is a paradoxical increase in tumor uptake of radiotracer when the tumor is actually very chemoresponsive.[6-8] This uptake is thought to be the result of robust bone healing.

Positron emission tomography (PET) has been shown to be extremely accurate in staging disease and monitoring therapy Franzius et al[9] compared 18F-labeled 2-deoxy-2-fluoro-D-glucose (FDG-PET) scans with bone scans in patients with Ewing's sarcoma and found that FDG-PET scans were more accurate (97% versus 82%), sensitive (100% versus 68%), and specific (96% versus 87%) than bone scans in detecting metastases. In a recent review, Sundaresan et al[10] stated that the use of PET scans to stage bone and soft part sarcomas and to monitor treatment is now the standard of care.

BIOPSY

It is extremely important to have complete imaging of the tumor before proceeding with biopsy because of the potential artifact created by tract lines, local inflammation, or hematoma formation. The three major types of biopsies are needle or trocar aspiration, open incisional, and excisional biopsy. A biopsy-confirmed diagnosis is especially important in osteosarcoma where surgery is often delayed in order to start early neoadjuvant chemotherapy. An excisional biopsy can be diagnostic as well as therapeutic for tumors confined to the posterior elements. Ozsarlak et al[11] showed that the diagnostic accuracy of CT-guided percutaneous needle biopsy can be as high as 80% to 90% in experienced hands. But one of the most common complications continues to be a nondiagnostic biopsy. Many experienced investigators report that 25% of their biopsies are nondiagnostic.

> **Box 16-1** **Principles for Performing Safe Incisional or Needle Biopsy**
>
> 1. The incision or needle tract must be positioned so that it will be excised when the definitive surgery is performed.
> 2. Approach the biopsy target through the most direct route possible, and avoid entering other compartments. The epidural space should not be compromised because this may cause extracompartmental spread of cancerous cells.
> 3. Meticulous hemostasis is paramount in preventing unwanted hematomas, which could disseminate tumor cells along fascial planes or by hematogenous spread.
> 4. Use small bone windows that are carefully planned out to prevent destabilization of the spine, which may contribute to pathologic fractures. Bone wax and Gelfoam should be used liberally to prevent localized spread of tumor.
> 5. Because of the high risk associated with a biopsy, if resources are available it is advantageous to have an intraoperative histopathologic evaluation to ensure that an adequate specimen is obtained. Always treat the specimen with absolute care so that it does not get crushed or distorted in any way.

Biopsies carry significant risk for dissemination of a currently localized tumor. Therefore thoughtful planning and meticulous execution are imperative (Box 16-1). Mankin et al[12] stressed that biopsies be performed at high-volume centers to reduce the unwanted spread of tumor cells and resultant poor outcomes.

PATHOLOGY

There are several classifications of osteosarcomas, but common to all subtypes is that they contain neoplastic osteoblasts that produce bone. The four major subdivisions are osteoblastic osteosarcoma, chondroblastic osteosarcoma, fibroblastic osteosarcoma, and secondary osteosarcoma (Fig. 16-1). Osteosarcomas are usually very well vascularized and will often have areas of hemorrhage and necrosis. Combined with staining of blood and osteoid production, many tumors have a red, gritty quality. Mineralized tumors have areas of rock-hard density, whereas fibrogenic or chondrogenic tumors have areas of grayish-white or blue tissues that are often slimy in texture. Microscopically all osteosarcomas have disorganized bony spicules in a well-vascularized stroma surrounded by spindle or polygonal mitotic cells. Usually the osteoid production is obvious, and no special stains are needed. Polarized light microscopy can be used to identify woven bone within the tumor if it is not present with normal staining. If no bone is detected and the spindle cell tumor is arranged in whorls, resembling a pinwheel pattern, malignant fibrous histiocytoma should be considered as the diagnosis.

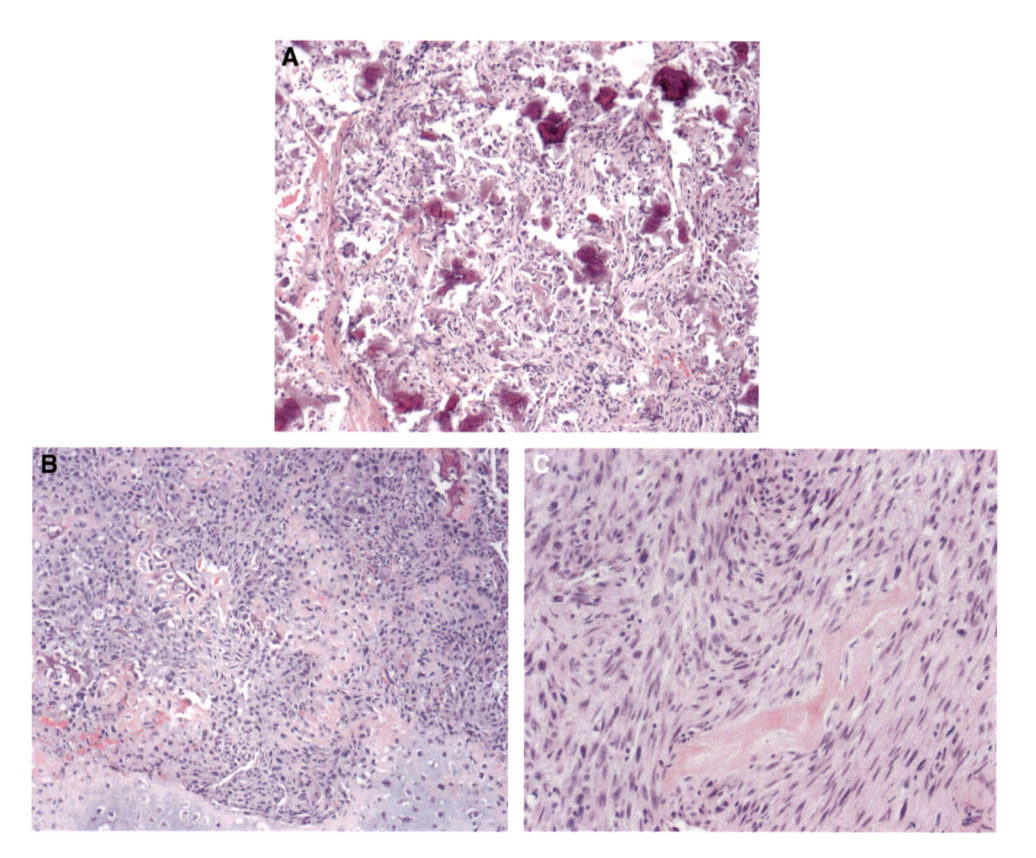

Fig. 16-1 **A,** Osteoblastic osteosarcoma. **B,** Chondroblastic osteosarcoma. **C,** Fibroblastic osteosarcoma. (Courtesy Andrew E. Horvai, MD, PhD, Department of Pathology, University of California San Francisco.)

MEDICAL MANAGEMENT

A complete medical evaluation must be performed before chemotherapy and surgery are initiated. This should include a full cardiac workup consisting of an electrocardiogram and echocardiogram, as well as an audiogram, because of the potential cardiac and auditory toxicities associated with certain chemotherapeutic agents. Currently there are no specific laboratory markers for osteosarcoma, although higher levels of alkaline phosphatase and lactate dehydrogenase have been correlated with a poorer outcome.[13,14]

Unless there is spinal instability with neurologic deficits or impending collapse, neoadjuvant chemotherapy should be initiated immediately after the diagnosis is established. It is almost certain that micrometastases exist, which makes clean surgical margins extremely difficult to achieve. Preoperative chemotherapy may reduce the tumor burden requiring less aggressive resections. In addition, the preoperative tumor response gives prognostic indications and allows for appropriate postoperative chemotherapeutic planning.

Currently doxorubicin, cisplatin, high-dose methotrexate with leucovorin rescue, and ifosfamide are considered the most active agents against osteosarcoma.[15] The best chemotherapeutic regimen has yet to be determined. Different histologic subtypes have been shown to have varying responses to chemotherapy. With the use of methotrexate, cisplatin, and adriamycin, Bacci et al[16] showed telangiectatic tumors to have the best response rate (86.7% showed a good response) followed by osteoblastic (63.9%), fibroblastic (61.7%), chrondroblastic (50.6%), and small cell tumors (25%). These investigators defined a good response as at least 90% tumor necrosis after chemotherapy. Multivariate analysis in this study correlated a poor chemotherapeutic response with a worse prognosis.

Optimal dosages and timing of chemotherapy are also being aggressively researched. A recent study of 497 patients with nonmetastatic high-grade appendicular osteosarcoma showed that there is an improved histologic response with dose-intense chemotherapy (six 2-week cycles of cisplatin and doxorubicin) compared with a standard regimen (six 3-week cycles).[17] Surgery was performed at 6 weeks in both arms of the study. Fifty percent of patients treated with dose-intense chemotherapy showed a good tumor response (>90% tumor necrosis) versus 36% treated with the standard regimen. Unfortunately 5-year survival with dose-intense chemotherapy was not improved when compared with the standard regimen, 58% (95% confidence interval 51% to 65%) versus 55% (95% confidence interval 48% to 62%), respectively.

Unlike Ewing's sarcoma, which is radiosensitive, osteosarcoma has proved to be highly resistant to radiation therapy. Currently radiation therapy is used to treat osteosarcoma of the spine when the tumor is unresectable, and it is also used as palliative treatment. Ozaki et al[1] and DeLaney et al[18] have shown a possible benefit in achieving local control with adjuvant radiation therapy. Improvements in image-guided photon and proton beam radiation therapy have decreased radiation exposure to healthy tissues, allowing for more precise localization in radiation treatment of tumor cells, particularly near radiosensitive normal structures.

Basic scientists and clinicians are researching several molecular biomarkers for their prognostic and therapeutic potential. Some examples are P-glycoprotein (P-gp), CXCR4, and the apoptotic inhibitor, survivin. P-gp is encoded by the multiple-drug–resistant-1 *(MDR1)* gene. One of the functions of this protein is the active efflux of drugs. Baldini et al[19] suggested that increased levels of P-gp in osteosarcoma cells were responsible for resistance to doxorubicin and resulted in a significant reduction in recurrence-free survival. Ferrari et al[20] showed that pulmonary metastatic cells had higher levels of P-gp than cells from primary osteosarcoma, suggesting that P-gp levels correlated with malignant potential. CXCR4 is a chemokine receptor that is implicated in the metastatic pathway of several cancers including osteosarcoma. Laverdiere et al[21] showed a correlation of CXCR4 mRNA levels with the presence of metastasis at diagnosis and reduced survival. Animal models have shown that CXCR4 and its ligand, stromal cell–derived factor 1 (SDF-1), to be potential therapeutic targets. Perissinotto et al[22] used the T134 peptide to inhibit CXCR4 in mice with pulmonary metastases. All six mice with pulmonary metastases that were treated with T134 had complete elimination of their pulmonary tumors. Another molecular marker of interest is survivin, which is an antiapoptotic protein known to bind and inhibit procaspases. With the use of reverse transcription–polymerase chain reaction (RT-PCR), Osaka et al[23] found survivin mRNA in all 16 osteosarcoma samples, whereas none of the normal samples contained survivin. This study and others have also suggested a relationship between high survivin levels and reduced overall survival.

STAGING AND GRADING

Once the diagnosis and the extent of the tumor have been determined, the tumor is staged and graded. Boriani et al[24] have successfully applied the oncologic staging system devised by Enneking[25,26] to primary vertebral tumors. This new system categorizes spine tumors into stages I, II, and III. Stages I and II are low-grade and high-grade tumors, respectively (Fig. 16-2). Low-grade tumors are relatively slow growing and form a layer of "reactive tissue" called a *pseudocapsule,* which contains microscopic islands of tumor. Examples of low-grade tumors are chordomas and chondrosarcomas. Osteosarcoma is a high-grade tumor, stage II. High-grade neoplasms tend to not have a pseudocapsule because they proliferate so rapidly that a reactive layer does not have time to form. This explosion of growth may disseminate tumor cells locally, resulting in the formation of satellite lesions. If these satellite lesions occur even farther away, they are called *skip metastases* and are considered stage III tumors. A letter designation is added to define the spread of the tumor. The letter *A* means there is no tumor extension beyond the vertebral cortex. The letter *B* signifies that the tumor has spread beyond the vertebra into the paravertebral compartments. Thus osteosarcoma that has spread into the epidural space without metastasis would be classified as a stage IIB tumor. Stage IIIA and IIIB tumors are high-grade tumors that have distant metastases.

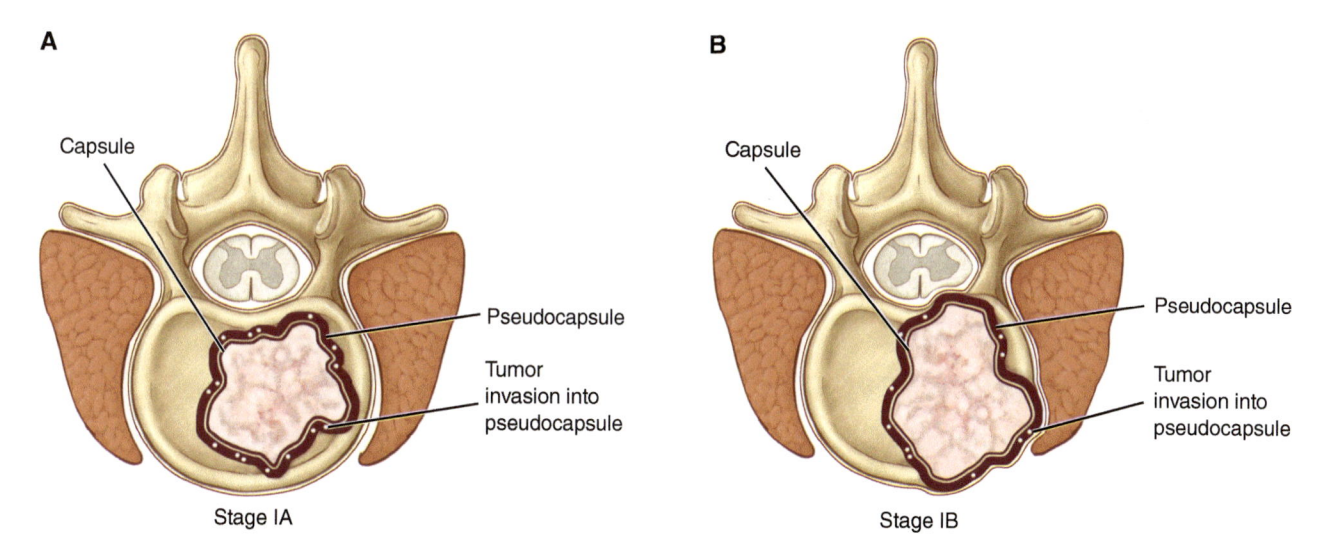

Fig. 16-2 Tumor grades and stages. **A,** Low-grade tumor (i.e., chordoma or chondrosarcoma), stage IA, confined to the vertebra. **B,** Low-grade tumor (i.e., chordoma or chondrosarcoma), stage IB, showing expansion beyond the vertebral cortex into the paravertebral soft tissues. (Modified from Boriani S, Weinstein JN, Biagini R. Primary bone tumors of the spine. Terminology and surgical staging. Spine [Phila Pa 1976] 22:1036-1044, 1997.)

Continued

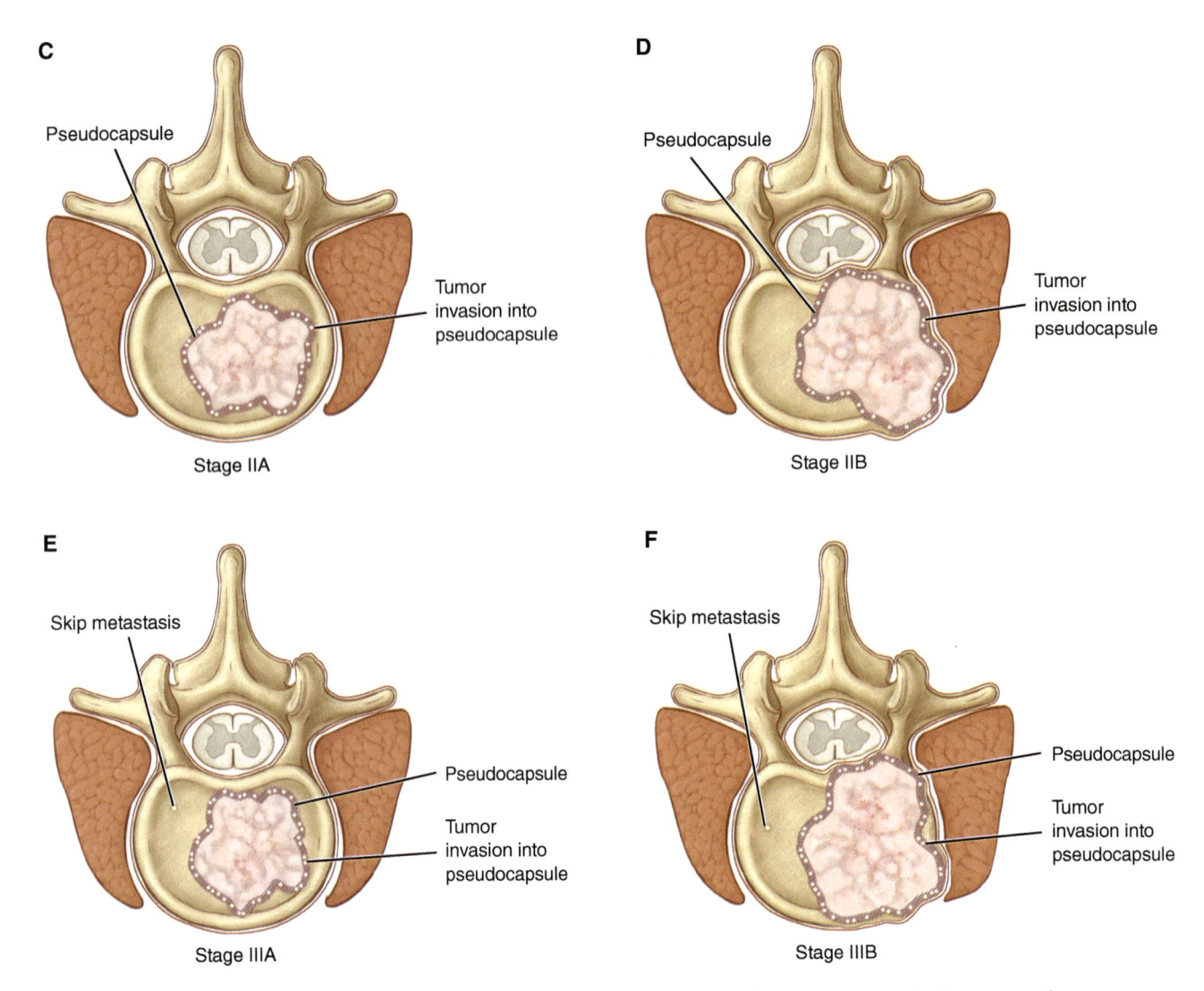

C Pseudocapsule — Tumor invasion into pseudocapsule — Stage IIA

D Pseudocapsule — Tumor invasion into pseudocapsule — Stage IIB

E Skip metastasis — Pseudocapsule — Tumor invasion into pseudocapsule — Stage IIIA

F Skip metastasis — Pseudocapsule — Tumor invasion into pseudocapsule — Stage IIIB

Fig. 16-2, cont'd **C,** High-grade tumor (i.e., osteosarcoma or other sarcoma, Ewing's sarcoma, lymphoma), stage IIA, confined to the vertebra. **D,** High-grade tumor (i.e., osteosarcoma or other sarcoma, Ewing's sarcoma, lymphoma), stage IIB, showing expansion beyond the vertebral cortex into the paravertebral soft tissues. **E,** High-grade tumor, stage IIIA, with distant metastasis confined to the vertebra. **F,** High-grade tumor, stage IIIB, with distant metastasis showing expansion beyond the vertebral cortex into the paravertebral soft tissues.

SURGICAL PLANNING

Once the spine tumor has been anatomically defined, graded, and staged, a careful well-thought-out surgical plan must be devised. Every attempt should be made to attain wide margins. In a retrospective series, Talac et al[27] evaluated the risk of local recurrence after wide, marginal, and intralesional resections and the impact on survival. Thirty patients with sarcoma of the mobile spine underwent wide (7 patients), marginal (3 patients), or intralesional (20 patients) resections. The patients with positive margins had a fivefold increase in local recurrences, and 92% of those patients died of sequelae related to their recurrences. The median survival for patients treated with en bloc resection was 62 months versus 37 months for patients who underwent piecemeal resection.

As recently as 20 years ago, many spine tumors were thought to be unresectable because of the close proximity to crucial neurovascular structures and the difficult approaches required to achieve wide margins. Spine tumors still present a formidable surgical challenge, but improved techniques and better instrumentation are allowing spine surgeons to successfully treat larger and more difficult tumors. It is essential that a multidisciplinary team approach be used for every patient. Radiologists, oncologists, radiation oncologists, and spine surgeons are necessary components of the team. Occasionally, cardiothoracic or general surgeons are necessary to assist with attaining adequate exposures and in cases of anterior vascular involvement.

Boriani et al[24] developed a surgical staging system that has been validated in previous studies and is now widely used.[28-31] To anatomically define the tumor, these investigators divided the transverse cross-section of a vertebra into 12 consecutive radiating zones with 1 being at the spinous process and 2 through 12 following in a clockwise direction (Fig. 16-3). Starting from the extraosseous soft tissues, there are five zones (A through E), with zone A being outside the vertebrae in the soft tissues and zone E involving the dura. Longitudinal extension refers to the spine levels involved as determined by imaging.

It is important to use appropriate terms when describing the surgical resection of spine tumors. It can be confusing to state that a resection was radical when the capsule was compromised. Many investigators have now developed terms that can be universally

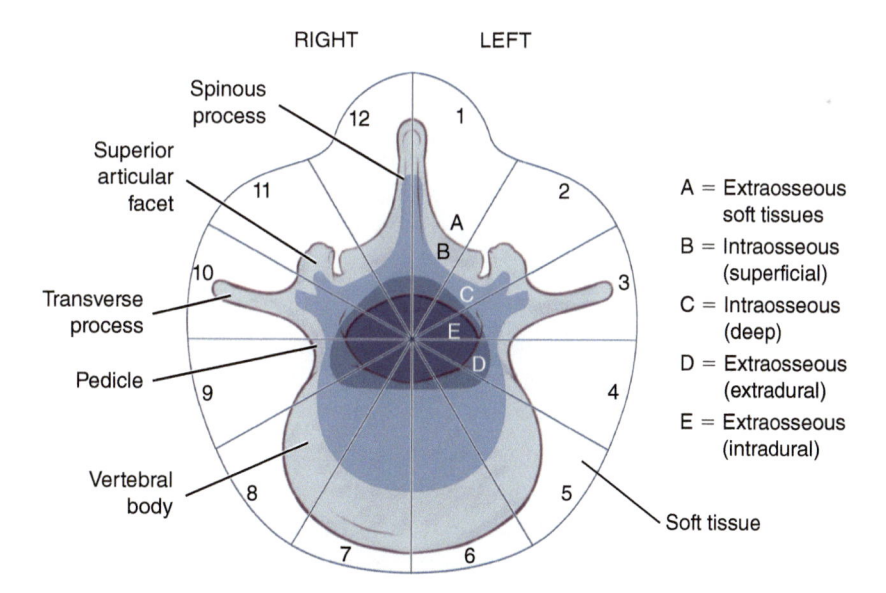

Fig. 16-3 The Weinstein-Boriani-Biagini surgical staging system divides the transverse section of a vertebra into 12 radiating zones arranged in a clockwise manner. Concentric layers *A* through *E* are arranged from extraosseous to intradural, respectively. (Modified from Boriani S, Weinstein JN, Biagini R. Primary bone tumors of the spine: terminology and surgical staging. Spine [Phila Pa 1976] 22:1036-1044, 1997.)

understood. En bloc resection describes removal of the entire tumor in one piece. Vertebrectomy or spondylectomy is an en bloc resection of the entire vertebral body with portions of the affected posterior elements. With the use of the Weinstein-Boriani-Biagini staging system, a tumor can be resected if at least one pedicle is free of disease. Thus a resectable tumor would fall into zones 4 to 8 or 5 to 9.

An alternative surgical staging system was devised by Tomita et al[32,33] for the classification of metastatic vertebral tumors, but it can also be applied to primary tumors of the spine. There are seven types, with types I, II, and III being intracompartmental and types IV, V, VI, and VII being extracompartmental. Type I tumors are confined within the vertebral body, type II tumors invade one or both pedicles, type III tumors have laminar extension, type IV tumors involve the epidural space, type V tumors infiltrate the extraosseous soft tissues, type VI tumors are multilevel, and type VII tumors have multiple skip lesions on more than one level. The histologic classification of a resection is defined as intralesional if the tumor has been violated, marginal if the tumor is whole but the margins are within the reactive layer or pseudocapsule, and wide for surgical dissections in which healthy tissue completely encompasses the tumor and its reactive layer.

SURGICAL APPROACHES

One of the pioneers of surgical spinal oncology is Bertil Stener.[34,35] In 1971 he described the use of a total spondylectomy for a chondrosarcoma arising from the thoracic spine.[36] En bloc spondylectomy is now considered the benchmark procedure in the surgical treatment of primary vertebral osteosarcomas. Tumors in the spine can be approached posteriorly or anteriorly, and they can be treated in one or two stages. Although midline posterior tumors can be resected by means of a traditional posterior approach, many surgeons use a posterolateral approach to gain access to involved lateral structures, such as the transverse processes, facets, and ribs. Roy-Camille et al,[37] Stener,[36] and Tomita et al[32] performed thoracic en bloc spondylectomies in one stage using a posterolateral approach. The vertebra is rotated around its longitudinal axis so that it can be removed. This one-stage approach can be used in the thoracic spine because spinal nerve roots may be sacrificed with no consequent motor deficit and the sensory loss is clinically acceptable. A posterior one-stage approach may not be technically feasible in the lumbar spine, given that the L2 to L5 nerve roots are crucial for ambulation. The risks of complications and consequent morbidity increase substantially with multilevel disease. A two-stage posterior approach followed by an anterior approach allows for easier control of hemostasis of the epidural venous plexus and posterior stabilization. Depending on the level of the tumor, an anterior approach can be employed with the use of a transpleural thoracotomy, a retroperitoneal approach, or a thoracoabdominal approach. An anterior approach has the advantage of allowing a direct view of the anterior vertebra and surrounding soft tissues, which aids in defining tumor margins. This approach also allows easier ligation of segmental vessels above and below the affected vertebra or any vessels incorporated within the tumor. Fig. 16-4 shows how the Weinstein-Boriani-Biagini surgical staging system is used to plan surgical approaches.

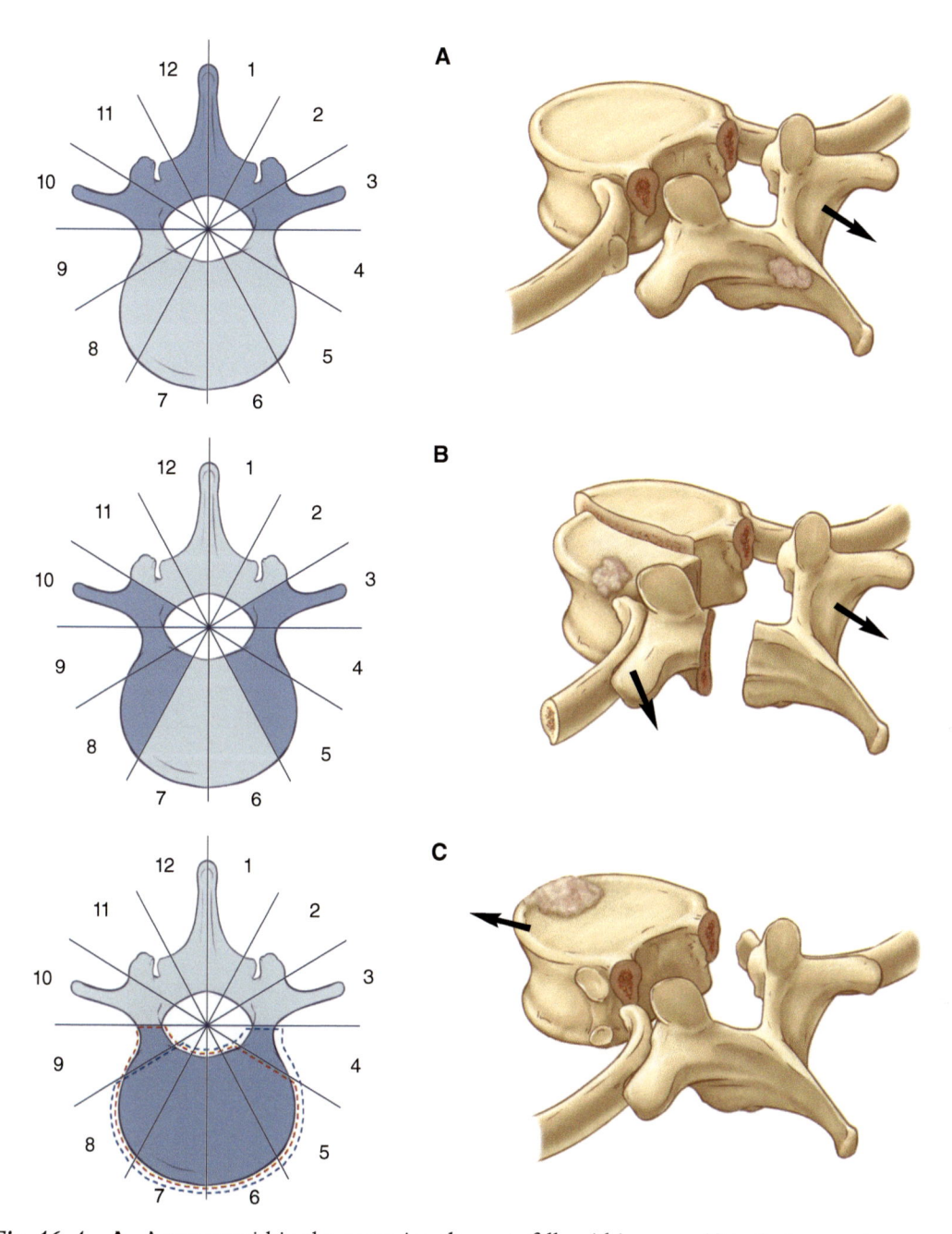

Fig. 16-4 **A,** A tumor within the posterior elements falls within zones 10 to 3. A posterior approach is used to perform an en bloc excision. **B,** Tumors located within zones 3 to 5 or 8 to 10 require a combined posterior and anterior approach to safely obtain clean margins. **C,** Tumors within the vertebral body and confined to one pedicle require vertebrectomy to obtain appropriate margins. This can be achieved in one stage for tumors located in the thoracic vertebrae or a combined approach for cervical and lumbar involvement. (Modified from Boriani S, Weinstein JN, Biagini R. Primary bone tumors of the spine. Terminology and surgical staging. Spine [Phila Pa 1976] 22:1036-1044, 1997.)

After spondylectomy, the vertebral body can be reconstructed with the use of an expandable titanium or carbon fiber cage filled with autologous or bone allograft (Fig. 16-5). It is essential that the cartilage be removed from the vertebral endplates to allow cortical contact. It is recommended that at least two levels above and below the resection be fused posteriorly with the addition of cancellous bone graft to achieve spondylodesis.[38,39]

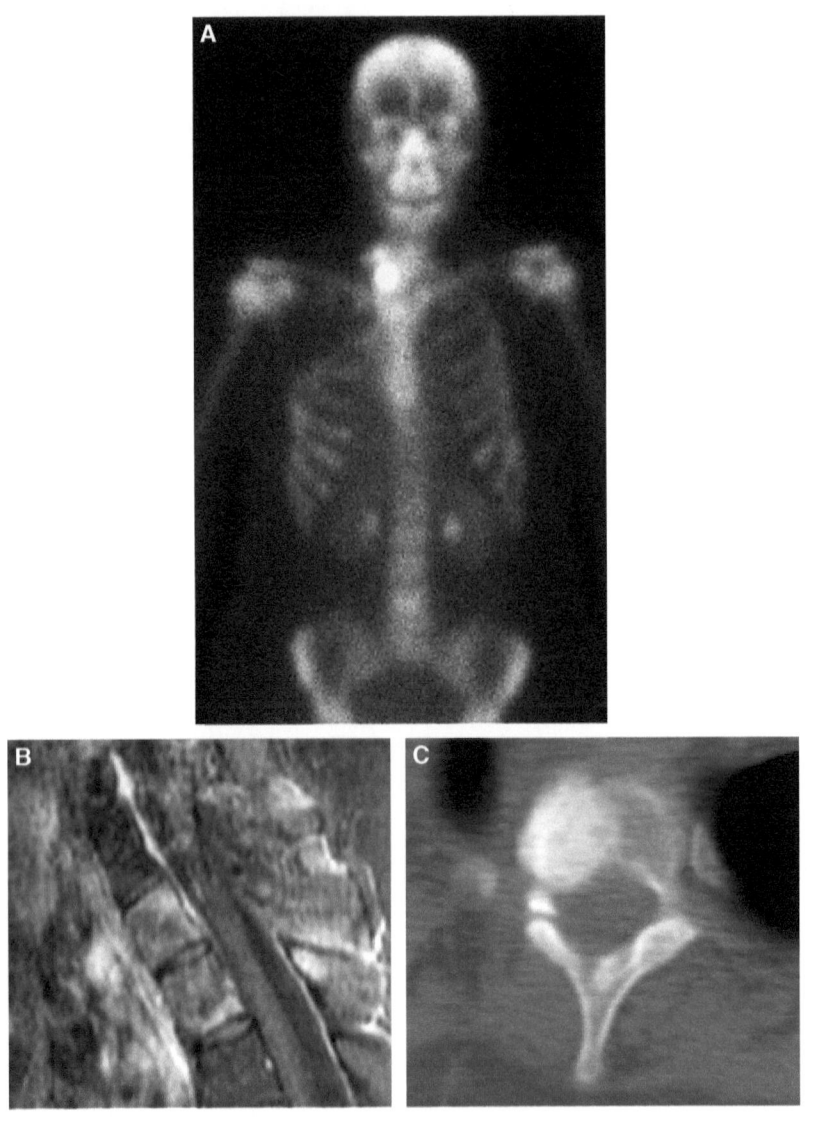

Fig. 16-5 Osteosarcoma at the cervicothoracic junction in a 22-year-old woman. **A,** Bone scan demonstrating increased uptake at T1-2. **B,** Enhancement of T1 and T2 vertebral bodies on T1-weighted MRI scan with gadolinium. **C,** Axial CT scan showing tumor within the T1 vertebral body. (Courtesy Dean Chou, MD, Department of Neurological Surgery, and Andrew E. Horvai, MD, PhD, Department of Pathology, University of California San Francisco.)

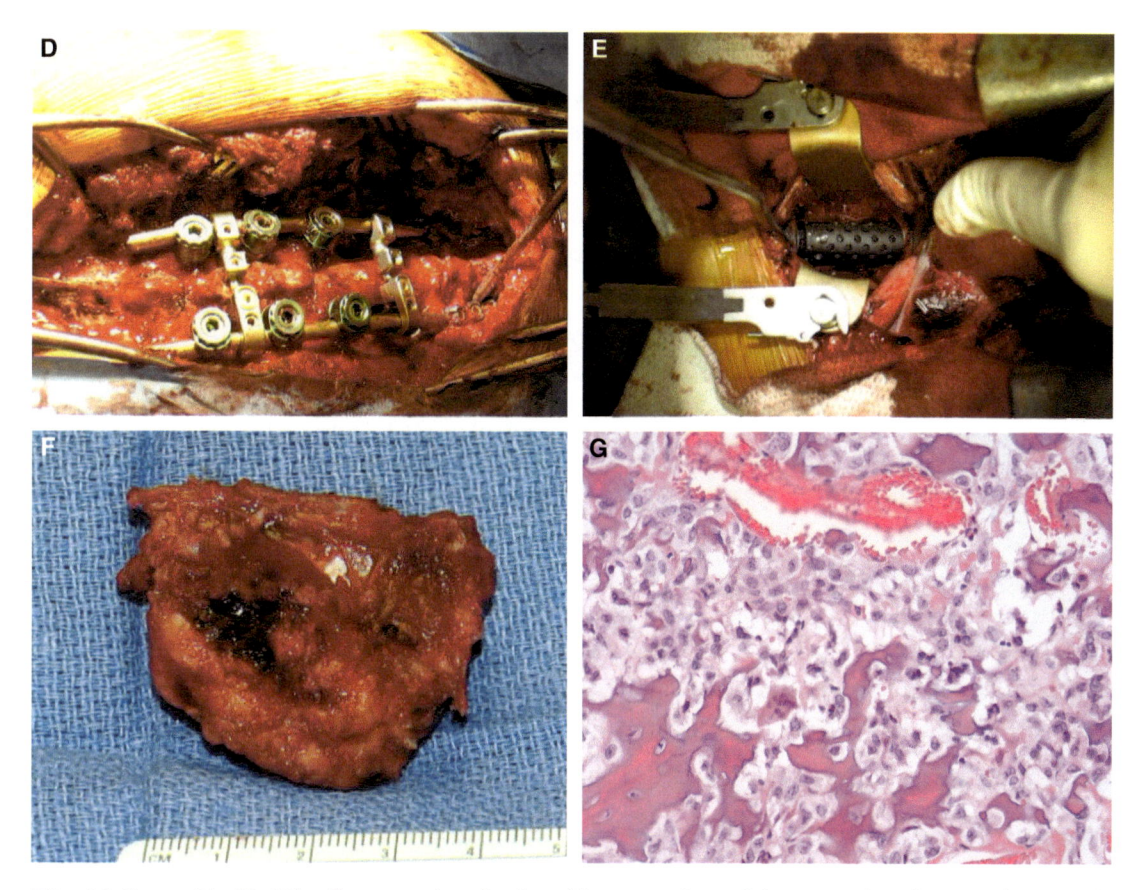

Fig. 16-5, cont'd **D,** The first stage involved en bloc resection of the posterior elements by pedicle amputation followed by posterior spine fusion from C5 to T5 with allograft. **E,** A transcervical approach was used for the second stage. The T1 and T2 vertebral bodies were removed en bloc followed by reconstruction with an expandable titanium cage with allograft. **F,** Gross specimen of T1 and T2 vertebral bodies resected en bloc. **G,** Pathology specimen showing osteosarcoma (original magnification ×200).

CONCLUSION

Osteosarcoma of the spine is a rare entity and is therefore difficult to study. Significant improvements in surgical technique and chemotherapeutic regimens have transformed what was once a universally terminal disease into a potentially curable one. Discoveries in basic science have given us additional understanding into the pathology of osteosarcoma and identified potential therapeutic molecular targets. There is still significant room for improvement. It is essential that a full clinical, imaging, and laboratory evaluation be completed before biopsy, initiation of chemotherapy, and surgery. A biopsy must be carefully planned in conjunction with surgical planning to prevent inadvertent spread of microscopic disease. The standard of care for definitive treatment of osteosarcoma of the spine is neoadjuvant polychemotherapy followed by total en bloc spondylectomy, with postoperative radiation therapy possibly having some benefit in controlling local disease. Because of the rarity of osteosarcoma of the spine, the complexity of the treatment, and the need for a multidisciplinary team approach to provide optimal care for patients with osteosarcoma of the spine, we recommend that these patients be managed at specialized musculoskeletal treatment centers.

TIPS FROM THE MASTERS

- Preoperative chemotherapy is extremely beneficial, especially when combined with subsequent en bloc resection. Preoperative adjuvant treatment will often render a lesion much more amenable to wide resection. Multiple rounds of chemotherapy may be used before surgery in challenging cases.
- For aggressive lesions in young patients who are already severely neurologically compromised, en bloc resection including the spinal canal and spinal cord may be considered.

References (With Key References in Boldface)

1. **Ozaki T, Flege S, Liljenqvist U, et al. Osteosarcoma of the spine: experience of the Cooperative Osteosarcoma Study Group. Cancer 94:1069-1077, 2002.**
2. **Ilaslan H, Sundaram M, Unni KK, et al. Primary vertebral osteosarcoma: imaging findings. Radiology 230:697-702, 2004.**
3. **Kelley SP, Ashford RU, Rao AS, et al. Primary bone tumours of the spine: a 42-year survey from the Leeds Regional Bone Tumour Registry. Eur Spine J 16:405-409, 2007.**
4. Damron TA, Ward WG, Stewart A. Osteosarcoma, chondrosarcoma, and Ewing's sarcoma: National Cancer Data Base Report. Clin Orthop Relat Res 459:40-47, 2007.
5. Bielack SS, Kempf-Bielack B, Delling G, et al. Prognostic factors in high-grade osteosarcoma of the extremities or trunk: an analysis of 1,702 patients treated on neoadjuvant cooperative osteosarcoma study group protocols. J Clin Oncol 20:776-790, 2002.
6. Johns WD, Garnick MB, Kaplan WD. Leuprolide therapy for prostate cancer. An association with scintigraphic "flare" on bone scan. Clin Nucl Med 15:485-487, 1990.
7. Rossleigh MA, Lovegrove FT, Reynolds PM, et al. The assessment of response to therapy of bone metastases in breast cancer. Aust N Z J Med 14:19-22, 1984.
8. Schneider JA, Divgi CR, Scott AM, et al. Flare on bone scintigraphy following Taxol chemotherapy for metastatic breast cancer. J Nucl Med 35:1748-1752, 1994.
9. Franzius C, Sciuk J, Daldrup-Link HE, et al. FDG-PET for detection of osseous metastases from malignant primary bone tumours: comparison with bone scintigraphy. Eur J Nucl Med 27:1305-1311, 2000.
10. **Sundaresan N, Rosen G, Boriani S. Primary malignant tumors of the spine. Orthop Clin North Am 40:21-36, 2009.**
11. Ozsarlak O, De Schepper AM, Wang X, et al. CT-guided percutaneous needle biopsy in spine lesions. JBR-BTR 86:294-296, 2003.
12. Mankin HJ, Mankin CJ, Simon MA. The hazards of the biopsy, revisited. Members of the Musculoskeletal Tumor Society. J Bone Joint Surg Am 78:656-663, 1996.

13. Bacci G, Longhi A, Ferrari S, et al. Prognostic significance of serum alkaline phosphatase in osteosarcoma of the extremity treated with neoadjuvant chemotherapy: recent experience at Rizzoli Institute. Oncol Rep 9:171-175, 2002.
14. Gonzalez-Billalabeitia E, Hitt R, Fernandez J, et al. Pre-treatment serum lactate dehydrogenase level is an important prognostic factor in high-grade extremity osteosarcoma. Clin Transl Oncol 11:479-483, 2009.
15. Bielack S, Carrle D, Casali PG. Osteosarcoma: ESMO clinical recommendations for diagnosis, treatment and follow-up. Ann Oncol 20 (Suppl 4):137-139, 2009.
16. Bacci G, Longhi A, Versari M, et al. Prognostic factors for osteosarcoma of the extremity treated with neoadjuvant chemotherapy: 15-year experience in 789 patients treated at a single institution. Cancer 106:1154-1161, 2006.
17. Lewis IJ, Nooij MA, Whelan J, et al. Improvement in histologic response but not survival in osteosarcoma patients treated with intensified chemotherapy: a randomized phase III trial of the European Osteosarcoma Intergroup. J Natl Cancer Inst 99:112-128, 2007.
18. DeLaney TF, Park L, Goldberg SI, et al. Radiotherapy for local control of osteosarcoma. Int J Radiat Oncol Biol Phys 61:492-498, 2005.
19. Baldini N, Scotlandi K, Serra M, et al. P-glycoprotein expression in osteosarcoma: a basis for risk-adapted adjuvant chemotherapy. J Orthop Res 17:629-632, 1999.
20. Ferrari S, Bertoni F, Zanella L, et al. Evaluation of P-glycoprotein, HER-2/ErbB-2, p53, and Bcl-2 in primary tumor and metachronous lung metastases in patients with high-grade osteosarcoma. Cancer 100:1936-1942, 2004.
21. Laverdiere C, Hoang BH, Yang R, et al. Messenger RNA expression levels of CXCR4 correlate with metastatic behavior and outcome in patients with osteosarcoma. Clin Cancer Res 11:2561-2567, 2005.
22. Perissinotto E, Cavalloni G, Leone F, et al. Involvement of chemokine receptor 4/stromal cell-derived factor 1 system during osteosarcoma tumor progression. Clin Cancer Res 11 (2 Pt 1):490-497, 2005.
23. Osaka E, Suzuki T, Osaka S, et al. Survivin expression levels as independent predictors of survival for osteosarcoma patients. J Orthop Res 25:116-121, 2007.
24. **Boriani S, Weinstein JN, Biagini R. Primary bone tumors of the spine. Terminology and surgical staging. Spine (Phila Pa 1976) 22:1036-1044, 1997.**
25. **Enneking WF. A system of staging musculoskeletal neoplasms. Clin Orthop Relat Res 204:9-24, 1986.**
26. Enneking WF, Spanier SS, Goodman MA. A system for the surgical staging of musculoskeletal sarcoma. Clin Orthop Relat Res 153:106-120, 1980.
27. Talac R, Yaszemski MJ, Currier BL, et al. Relationship between surgical margins and local recurrence in sarcomas of the spine. Clin Orthop Relat Res 397:127-132, 2002.
28. Bohinski RJ, Rhines LD. Principles and techniques of en bloc vertebrectomy for bone tumors of the thoracolumbar spine: an overview. Neurosurg Focus 15:E7, 2003.
29. Boriani S, De Iure F, Bandiera S, et al. Chondrosarcoma of the mobile spine: report on 22 cases. Spine (Phila Pa 1976) 257:804-812, 2000.
30. **Hart RA, Boriani S, Biagini R, et al. A system for surgical staging and management of spine tumors. A clinical outcome study of giant cell tumors of the spine. Spine (Phila Pa 1976) 22:1773-1782; discussion 1783, 1997.**
31. Sundaresan N, Boriani S, Rothman A, et al. Tumors of the osseous spine. J Neurooncol 69:273-290, 2004.
32. **Tomita K, Kawahara N, Baba H, et al. Total en bloc spondylectomy. A new surgical technique for primary malignant vertebral tumors. Spine (Phila Pa 1976) 22:324-333, 1997.**
33. **Tomita K, Kawahara N, Murakami H, et al. Total en bloc spondylectomy for spinal tumors: improvement of the technique and its associated basic background. J Orthop Sci 11:3-12, 2006.**

34. Stener B. Complete removal of vertebrae for extirpation of tumors. A 20-year experience. Clin Orthop Relat Res 245:72-82, 1989.
35. Stener B. Musculoskeletal tumor surgery in Goteborg. Clin Orthop Relat Res 191:8-20, 1984.
36. Stener B. Total spondylectomy in chondrosarcoma arising from the seventh thoracic vertebra. J Bone Joint Surg Br 53:288-295, 1971.
37. Roy-Camille R, Saillant G, Mazel CH, et al. Total vertebrectomy as treatment of malignant tumors of the spine. Chir Organi Mov 75 (1 Suppl):94-96, 1990.
38. Disch AC, Luzzati A, Melcher I, et al. Three-dimensional stiffness in a thoracolumbar en-bloc spondylectomy model: a biomechanical in vitro study. Clin Biomech (Bristol, Avon) 22:957-964, 2007.
39. Disch AC, Melcher I, Luzatti A, et al. [Surgical technique of en bloc spondylectomy for solitary metastases of the thoracolumbar spine] Unfallchirurg 110:163-170, 2007.

Chapter 17

Soft Tissue Sarcomas and Malignant Peripheral Nerve Sheath Tumors

Azadeh Farin, Jacqueline Benjamin, Christopher P. Ames

SOFT TISSUE SARCOMAS

Soft tissue sarcomas are extremely rare tumors. In adults with solid malignancies, less than 1% are identified as soft tissue sarcomas. These tumors originate from mesenchymal cells of viscera, integument, and various connective tissue structures and then spread hematogenously, especially to the lungs. More than 50 separate subtypes of soft tissue sarcomas have been identified from such origins as fat, muscle (striated and smooth), vasculature, lymphatic vessels, synovial tissue, peripheral nerves, cartilage and bone-forming tissue, and fibrous tissue. On average, approximately 9530 new cases of soft tissue sarcoma are diagnosed each year in the United States; one third of the tumors are located in the abdomen, retroperitoneum, or trunk, and two thirds are found in an extremity. Risk factors for soft tissue sarcoma include inherited retinoblastoma, Gardner's syndrome, Li-Fraumeni syndrome, neurofibromatosis type 1 (NF1), exposure to vinyl chloride, and prior lymphadenectomy. Previous irradiation may be responsible for 5% of sarcomas.

Staging is used to determine tumor extension and is the most significant factor determining prognosis and treatment options. Biopsies as well as local and surveillance imaging are helpful. The tumor-node-metastasis (TNM) system of the American Joint

Table 17-1 **Staging for Soft Tissue Sarcomas**

Primary Tumor (T)

TX	Primary tumor cannot be assessed
T0	No evidence of primary tumor
T1	Tumor 5 cm or less in greatest dimension
T1a	Superficial tumor*
T1b	Deep tumor*
T2	Tumor more than 5 cm in greatest dimension
T2a	Superficial tumor*
T2b	Deep tumor*

Regional Lymph Nodes (N)

NX	Regional lymph nodes cannot be assessed
N0	No regional lymph node metastasis
N1	Regional lymph node metastasis

Distant Metastasis (M)

MX	Presence of metastasis cannot be assessed
M0	No distant metastasis
M1	Distant metastasis

Histopathologic Grade (G)†

GX	Grade of differentiation cannot be assessed
G1	Well differentiated
G2	Moderately differentiated
G3	Poorly differentiated
G4	Undifferentiated

Staging Group

IA	G1,2, T1a, N0, M0
	G1,2, T1b, N0, M0
IB	G1,2, T2a, N0, M0
IIA	G1,2, T2b, N0, M0
IIB	G3,4, T1a, N0, M0
	G3,4, T1b, N0, M0
IIC	G3,4, T2a, N0, M0
III	G3,4, T2b, N0, M0
IV	Any G, any T, N1, M0
	Any G, any T, any N, M1

Adapted from Sobin LH, Fleming ID, eds. Tumors of the bone and soft tissues. In TNM Classification of Malignant Tumors, 5th ed. New York: Wiley, 1997, p 101.

*Superficial tumors are located exclusively above the superficial fascia without invasion of the fascia; deep tumors are located either exclusively beneath the superficial fascia or superficial to the fascia with invasion of or through the fascia. Retroperitoneal, mediastinal, and pelvic sarcomas are classified as deep tumors.

†After the histologic type has been determined, the tumor should be graded according to the accepted criteria, which include cellularity, cellular pleomorphism, mitotic activity, and necrosis. The amount of intercellular substance, such as collagen or mucoid material, should be considered as a favorite factor in assessing the grade.

Table 17-2 Enneking System of Oncologic Staging of Primary Spine Tumors

Tumor	Type	Stage
Benign	SI (latent or inactive stage)	Tumor not growing; few symptoms; true capsule (e.g., incidental vertebral hemangioma)
	SII (active stage)	Slow growth; confined to bone; pseudocapsule (e.g., osteoblastomas)
	SIII (aggressive stage)	Not confined to bone; may invade epidural space or surrounding soft tissue structures (e.g., locally aggressive giant cell tumor)
Malignant	Low grade (I)	
	IA	Confined to vertebra
	IB	Extension into paravertebral compartment
	High grade (II)	
	IIA	Intracompartmental; no capsule
	IIB	Invasion of surrounding structures; extensive bone destruction; pathologic fracture
	High grade with distant metastasis (III)	

From Vincent F, Fehlings MG. Spinal column tumors. In Bernstein M, Berger MS. Neuro-oncology: The Essentials. 2nd ed. New York: Thieme, 2008, pp 391-402.

Committee on Cancer is commonly used to stage sarcomas, as shown in Table 17-1.[1] An alternative is the Enneking system for oncologic staging of primary spine tumors, as depicted in Table 17-2.[2] The Weinstein-Boriani-Biagini (WBB) system is used to strategize resection of primary spine tumors.[3-5] The WBB staging system divides the involved vertebrae into 12 radiating zones in the axial plane, numbered 1 to 12 in clockwise order, and five layers, A through E, from prevertebral to dural involvement, as indicated in Fig. 17-1.[6] Identifying the specific vertebra or vertebrae involved indicates the longitudinal extent of the tumor. This system enables preoperative planning for en bloc resection of spine tumors, whereby the involved vertebrae are rested along the proposed planes.

Survival rates depend on the type of sarcoma, stage, location, and patient age. The overall survival rate is approximately 30% to 50% at 5 years after surgery in combination with other treatment modalities. According to the National Cancer Institute, the survival rate is 83% for localized sarcomas, 54% for regional sarcomas, and 16% for sarcomas with distant spread. According to data from Memorial Sloan-Kettering Cancer Center, the 5-year survival rates are better for sarcomas of the limbs: stage I (90%); stage II (81%); stage III (56%); and stage IV (only a small percentage of patients survive

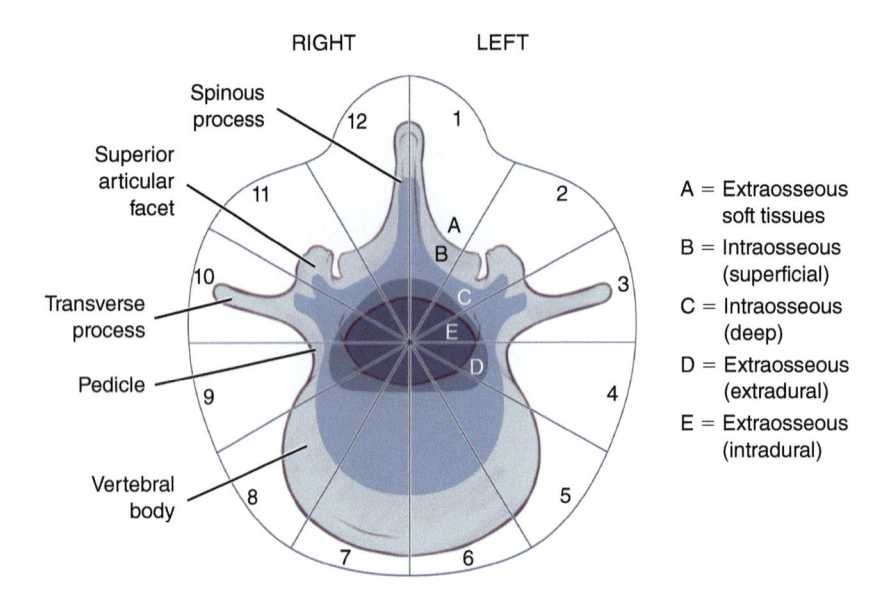

Fig. 17-1 The Weinstein-Boriani-Biagini surgical staging system divides the transverse section of a vertebra into 12 radiating zones arranged in a clockwise manner. Concentric layers *A* through *E* are arranged from extraosseous to intradural, respectively. (Modified from Boriani S, Weinstein JN, Biagini R. Primary bone tumors of the spine: terminology and surgical staging. Spine 22:1036-1044, 1997.)

5 years).* The 10-year relative survival rate is only slightly worse for these stages, meaning that most patients who survive for 5 years are cured. Local recurrence does not necessarily mean that the sarcoma will spread to other parts of the body. Fewer data are available specifically for primary soft tissue sarcomas of the spine, which are extremely rare. The major subtypes are described herein.

Malignant Fibrous Histiocytomas

These malignant mesenchymal neoplasms, also known as malignant fibrous xanthomas, fibrosarcomas, and xanthosarcomas, are derived from fibroblastic or myofibroblastic cells.[7,8] The lesions commonly arise in soft tissue and directly extend to bone. Although malignant fibrous histiocytomas (MFHs) account for only 2% of primary bone malignancies, they are the most common primary soft tissue sarcomas of bone. Tubular bones of the lower extremities are most commonly involved, with spine involvement being extremely rare. MFHs are one of the most common sarcomas to develop after radiation therapy. Epidemiologic studies show that the highest incidence of MFHs is in patients older than 50 years, with less than 10% in patients younger than 20. Twice as many men are affected as women.[9,10]

---

*Additional information can be found in the AJCC Cancer Staging Manual, 7th ed. New York: Springer, 2010.

On gross examination, erosion, destruction, invasion, and expansion of bone and surrounding soft tissue may be observed. MFHs are lobulated tumors with a circumscribed appearance. However, invasion of surrounding soft tissue extends beyond the obvious circumscribed borders. Most of these tumors are grayish-tan and have a fleshy appearance. Yellow indicates the presence of histiocytes, and hemorrhagic foci may also be observed.

Subtypes include storiform-pleomorphic, giant cell, myxoid, and inflammatory. The storiform-pleomorphic variant is the most common; it is composed of primarily pleomorphic histiocytoid cells and, to lesser extent, fibroblastic spindle cells. Osteoclast-like giant cells may be seen without bony involvement. Although they are usually rich in collagenous stroma, focal myxoid stroma may also predominate. Neutrophils and lymphocytes define the inflammatory subtype. Atypia and mitoses may be observed, and a higher rate of mitosis is associated with more extensive necrosis. Tumor grades are based on atypia, mitotic activity, and necrosis but may bear little relevance to prognosis.

Immunohistochemical analysis is used to exclude other types of tumors.[8] MFHs are positive for vimentin, but this is not a pathognomonic characteristic. They do not stain for S100 (chondrosarcoma, liposarcoma, melanoma), desmin (rhabdomyosarcoma), smooth muscle actin (leiomyosarcoma), or cytokeratins (metastatic carcinoma). Furthermore, demonstrating that these tumors do not originate from histiocytes, MFHs are negative for specific markers of histiocytes, including CD68 and Ham-56. Overexpression of p53 protein has been implicated in 40% of tumors, and MDM2 protein has been identified in 45% of tumors.[11,12] A recent study found both proteins in 8 of 10 patients with detectable p53 protein but without p53 gene mutation. The presence of both proteins was associated with poor survival. Expression of p53 alone was not a negative prognostic factor.

FIBROSARCOMA

Because fibroblastic tumors with prominent nuclear pleomorphism are classified as MFHs, fibrosarcomas are limited to low-grade and well-differentiated variants. Both MFHs and fibrosarcomas are collagen-forming tumors composed of myofibroblastic cells, and they are diagnoses of exclusion. A recent Mayo Clinic review identified only 92 cases of primary fibrosarcoma of bone during an 85-year period.[13] Adults are primarily affected, with the peak incidence from the fourth to sixth decade of life. Men and women are affected with equal frequency. Long bones are most frequently involved, with spine involvement being extremely rare.[10]

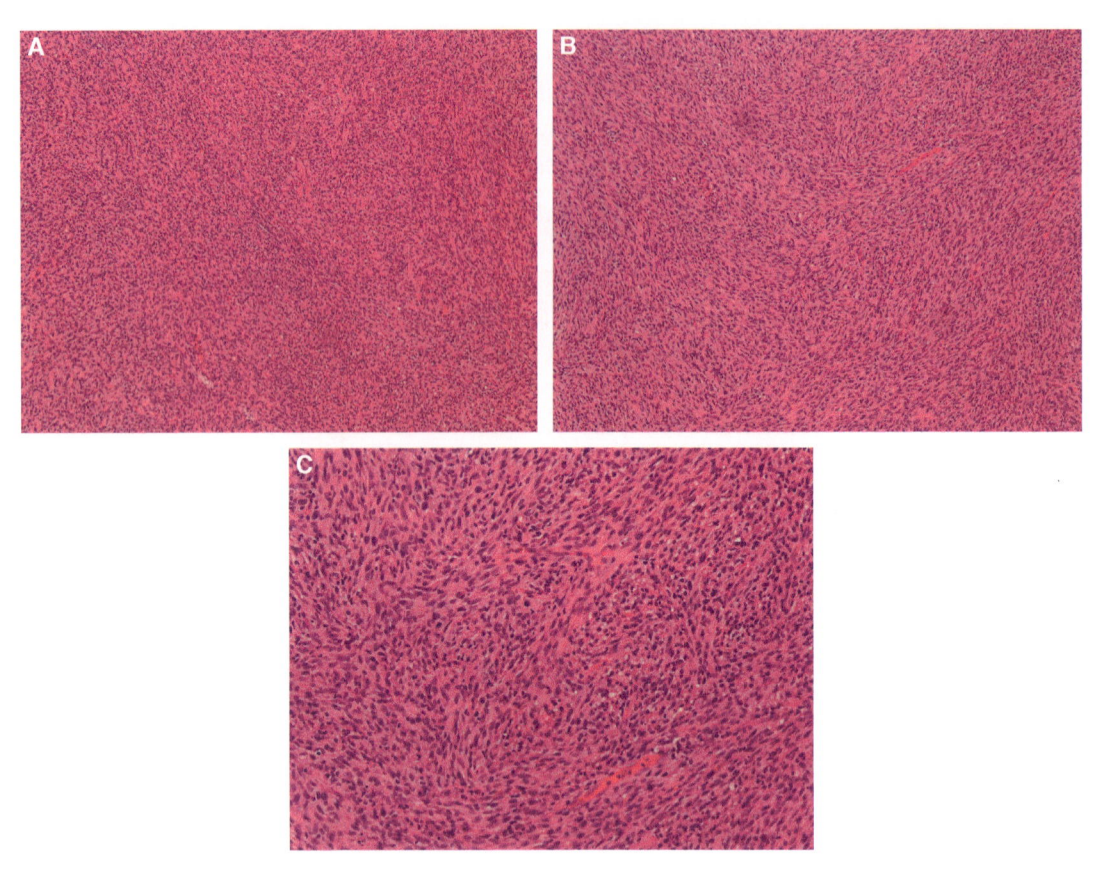

Fig. 17-2 **A** and **B**, Low-power magnification (×100) showing tumor cells arranged in intersecting fascicles. **C**, High-power magnification (×200) showing a densely cellular, mitotically active neoplasm with a fascicular growth pattern.

Fibrosarcomas are composed of spindle cells with eosinophilic cytoplasm, indistinct cytoplasmic borders, and fusiform nuclei (Fig. 17-2). Interweaving fascicles classically create a herringbone pattern. Cellularity and stromal collagen vary within and between tumors. Most are well differentiated with few mitotic figures and little atypia. High-grade fibrosarcomas have a higher rate of mitosis, show greater atypia, and exhibit necrosis. In general, fibrosarcomas lack the marked pleomorphism and size variation that is classic for MFHs.

These firm, lobulated tumors have a fleshy appearance and fibrous texture. Although seemingly well circumscribed, the tumors can extend into surrounding soft tissue beyond obvious tumor borders. The typical whitish-tan cross-section can become gray when myxoid stroma is prominent. Hemorrhage and necrosis may be present. Immunohistochemical analysis is used to exclude other diagnoses. Fibrosarcomas are positive for vimentin, which is nonspecific and weakly positive for muscle actin. They are negative for S100 and cytokeratins.

LEIOMYOSARCOMA

Leiomyosarcomas generally originate in retroperitoneal soft tissue and extend into surrounding bone.[9,10] Tubular bones are most commonly affected, and spine involvement is extremely rare.[13] Leiomyosarcomas presenting as primary bone tumors have been reported in approximately 50 patients. Retroperitoneal leiomyosarcomas have a 2:1 female predominance, primarily affecting older adults.[14]

On gross inspection, leiomyosarcomas are firm and appear well circumscribed, although the latter may be misleading. Cross-sections are usually white, with areas of necrosis and discoloration. Most primary bone tumors are high-grade myxoid/round cell or pleomorphic variants. Leiomyosarcomas are characterized by greater cellularity, atypia, pleomorphism, and necrosis compared with leiomyomas. Five mitoses per 10 high-power fields are sufficient to classify a tumor as malignant. Diagnosis is by immunohistochemical analysis, the results of which are positive for the muscle markers smooth muscle actin (SMA) and muscle-specific actin (MSA) in almost all cases and desmin in 50% of cases.[15-17] Aggressive tumor behavior has been associated with glucose transporter type 1 (GLUT1) and Bcl-2 positivity, p53 protein overexpression, and CD44 negativity.[12,18,19] Some specimens have also been found to be reactive to markers of drug resistance, including P-glycoprotein and multidrug-resistant protein.[20]

LIPOSARCOMA

Liposarcomas are the most common soft tissue sarcomas, but in extremely rare instances they present as primary bone tumors.[21] Spinal presentation is even rarer.[22] Median age at diagnosis is approximately 50 years for soft tissue liposarcomas and younger for primary bone tumors. Spine involvement is generally by extension from retroperitoneal tumors, which carry a worse prognosis than liposarcomas at other sites.[23,24]

On gross examination, the tumors appear multilobular. Histologic analysis defines the following three subgroups of liposarcomas: well differentiated/dedifferentiated, round cell/myxoid (Fig. 17-3), and pleomorphic.[25] Depending on the histologic subtype, tumors may be soft and gelatinous, firm or fleshy, and the color may be off-white, yellow, gray, or translucent. Microscopic diagnosis by means of hematoxylin-eosin staining is usually sufficient for diagnosis, and immunohistochemical analysis is not required. Most specimens are vimentin positive, and some are S100 positive. In one study of 42 soft tissue liposarcomas, 21% demonstrated overexpression of p53 protein, which was also found more often in pleomorphic rather than well-differentiated subtypes and was associated with a worse prognosis.[12] Soft tissue sarcomas with abnormalities of MDM2 are considered aggressive.[12] Aggressive tumor growth is also associated with a high MIB-1 labeling index.[26] Low p27 protein expression was significantly associated with poor outcomes in a study of 47 myxoid liposarcomas.[27]

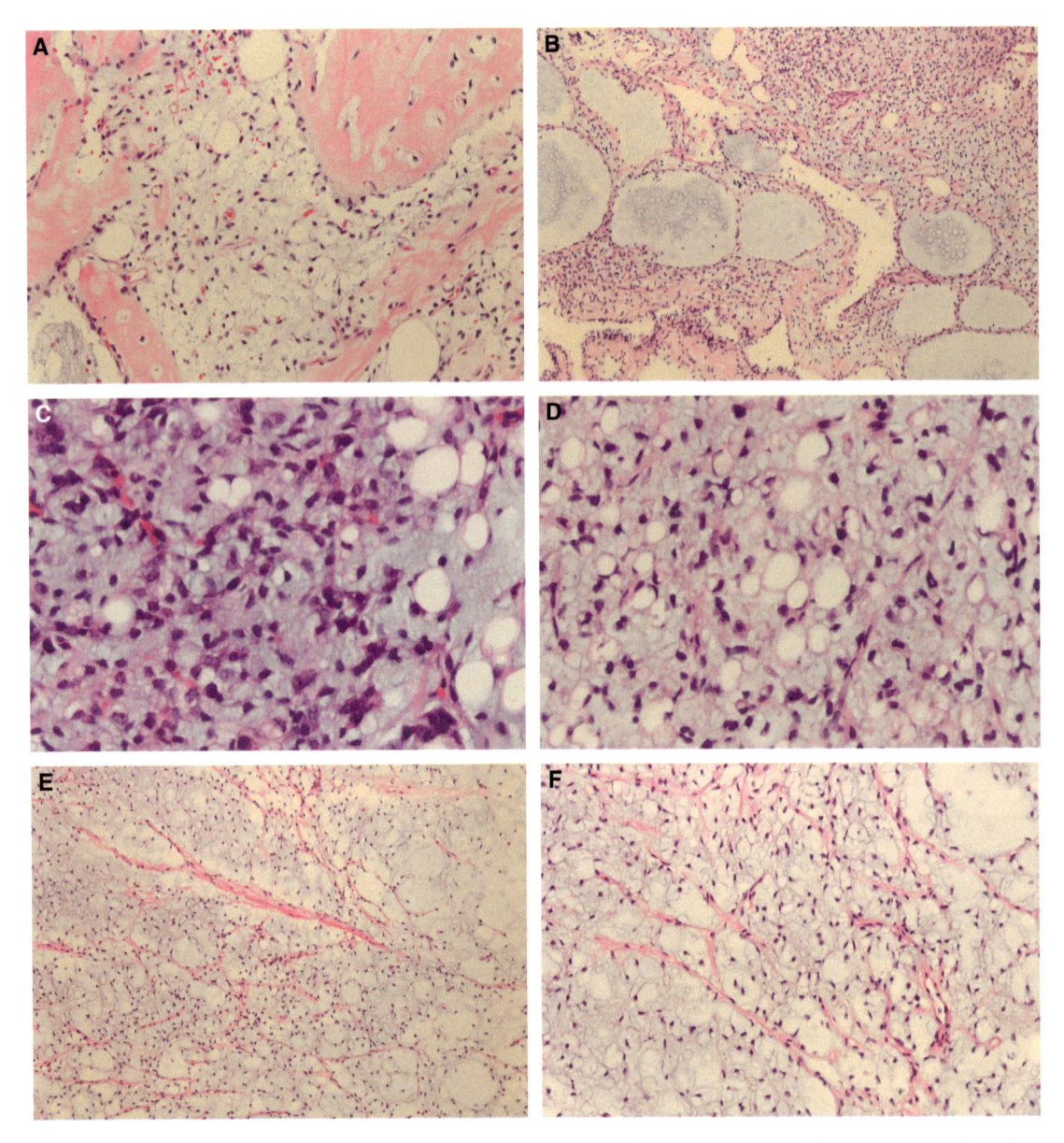

Fig. 17-3 **A,** Medium-power view of lipoblasts invading bone. **B,** Myxoid liposarcomas showing lipoblasts in myxoid background and large mucin pools. **C,** High-power view of neoplastic lipoblasts with pleomorphic nuclei in myxoid background. **D** and **E,** Classic appearance of myxoid liposarcoma showing thin stromal blood vessels. **F,** Another typical view showing plexiform capillaries.

ANGIOSARCOMA

These rare malignant neoplasms have a rapid proliferative capacity, which accounts for the aggressive nature of these tumors. Some reports describe tumor invasion of cord and nerve roots, as well as extension to and destruction of surrounding bone and soft tissues, along with high rates of local recurrence and distant metastases. Typical sites of origin include skin, soft tissue, liver, and cardiac tissue. Only a handful of case reports exist, most of which describe extensive tumor vascularity, which makes surgical resection extremely challenging, as manifested by vascular differentiation or intratumoral hemorrhage. Some have compared primary cardiac angiosarcomas metastatic to the spine with high-flow arteriovenous malformations.[28] A few case reports describe the epithelioid variant of angiosarcoma of bone, a high-grade lesion associated with a bleeding diathesis, although angiosarcomas, in general, have been linked with coagulopathy from tumor-related disseminated intravascular coagulopathy and fibrinolysis. One case report of primary sacral epithelioid angiosarcoma was found to be associated with a large epidural hematoma and a severe bleeding diathesis requiring massive transfusions.[29] Preoperative embolization followed by en bloc resection, where possible, with epsilon-aminocaproic acid drip and then adjuvant chemotherapy/radiation has been employed to prevent local recurrence and distant metastasis, although the prognosis is poor. As an exception, the first case report of primary thoracic angiosarcoma successfully treated with en bloc spondylectomy and postoperative chemotherapy documented no signs of local recurrence or metastasis 5 years postoperatively.[30] The risk of postirradiation sarcoma at long-term follow-up is thought to be 0.03% to 0.8%. A few cases of radiation-induced angiosarcoma of the spine several years after radiation to surrounding regions have been reported.[31]

OSTEOGENIC SARCOMA (OSTEOSARCOMA)

Osteosarcomas are the second most common primary bone malignancy after multiple myelomas, constituting approximately 20% of all cases. Osteosarcomas may arise de novo or, more commonly, evolve as the late stage of another process, including progression from one of the following: preexisting primary bone disease (Paget's disease, osteogenesis imperfect, fibrous dysplasia, or osteoblastoma); malignant evolution of a prior benign lesion (germ cell tumor or osteoblastoma); or an irritative process (radiation therapy after several years' latency, chronic osteomyelitis, or infarction).[32-35]

Approximately half of all cases occur in the distal femur or proximal tibia.[36,37] Less than 4% are in the spine, with the anterior lumbosacral region as the most common location.[35,38-42] Osteosarcoma secondary to radiation is more common in the spine than in the limbs.[43] As is indicative of their aggressive nature and frequent bony metastases, osteosarcomas of the spine usually occur secondary to metastases from another skeletal source of osteosarcoma. Primary osteosarcomas of the spine account for only 2% to 3% of the total cases of osteosarcoma and 5% of primary malignant spine tumors.[38,40,42] In these cases it usually originates in the vertebral body and extends centrally into the canal or laterally into the paraspinous soft tissues. Approximately 80% of patients present with a neurologic deficit.[38] Spine involvement is a negative prognostic factor.[36,37,44-47] Osteosarcomas typically appear in the second decade of life in the appendicular skeleton and during the second to fourth decades of life for spine lesions.[35]

A pathognomonic feature of osteosarcomas is the production of bone in a woven pattern by anaplastic osteoblasts. Large angular atypical nuclei produce irregular foci of osteoids, which require calcification before becoming bone. Microfoci of chondrosarcoma are common in osteosarcoma and should not justify classification as the chondroblastic subtype. Intramedullary osteosarcomas are telangiectatic and well differentiated. Surface osteosarcomas are parosteal and periosteal. A third type is small cell

Table 17-3 Osteosarcoma: Epidemiologic, Pathologic, and Microscopic Details

Subtype	Frequency (%)	Frequency in Spine (%)	Age at Diagnosis	M:F Ratio
Conventional	>90	<4; older patients	Second decade; 50+ yr	1.3:1
Telangiectatic	4	<4	Second decade; 50+	9:1
Well-differentiated	1	Rare	Third decade	1:1
Parosteal	3	Rare	Third to fourth decade	F/M
Periosteal	1	Not reported	Second decade	1:17
Small cell	1–4	Not reported	First to second decade	1:13

Modified from Coons SW. Pathology of tumors of the spinal cord, spine, and paraspinous soft tissue. In Dickman CA, Fehlings MG, Gokaslan ZL, eds. Spinal Cord and Spinal Column Tumors: Principles and Practice. New York: Thieme, 2006, pp 41–110.

osteosarcoma, which shares translocation t(11;22) (q24:q21) with the group of Ewing's primitive neuroectodermal tumors.[48]

Microscopic features of major variants are summarized in Table 17-3.[49] Conventional osteosarcomas, constituting more than 90% of osteosarcomas and considered to be high grade, are composed of highly atypical spindle or angular cells in a fibrous stroma. Malignant osteoids are usually prominent. The lack of osteoblastic rimming is critical

Grade	Gross Features	Microscopic Features
Low-high	Soft or bony due to osteolytic and osteoblastic areas; hemorrhage or necrosis may be present; white/yellow/translucent/tan	Various
High	Vascular, hemorrhagic, similar to aneurysmal bone cyst. Cystic, spongy. Well demarcated. Cortical invasion with erosion into soft tissue.	Vascular; cystic. Tumor cells in contact with blood-filled spaces. High-grade tumors with atypia and pleomorphism. Numerous atypical mitoses. Multinucleate sarcomatous giant cells and benign osteoclast-like giant cells. Rare and focal osteoid.
Low; dedifferentiation with recurrence	Contained within medullary cavity; fleshy and gritty with poor demarcation versus adjacent medullary bone	Features of low-grade tumor (uncommon mitoses) but may dedifferentiate to high-grade tumor in recurrences; mature bone trabeculae coursing through tumor
Low	Firm polypoid exophytic lesion extending into soft tissue with well-defined margins; attached to cortex and medullary bone	Well-differentiated bony trabeculae; lack of atypia and mitoses may result in misdiagnosis as benign reactive process; disordered cartilage with atypical chondrocytes
Low-intermediate	Fusiform and well-demarcated subperiosteal tumors attached to cortex but elevating perisoteum. Reactive bone extending through tumor.	Immature bone and osteoid in poorly differentiated spindle cell stroma. Predominance of malignant cartilage is common.
High	Same as high-grade conventional sarcoma	Hypercellular sheets of undifferentiated appearing cells; branching blood vessels; osteoid production sparse; cartilaginous differentiation; mitoses may not be frequent and may not correlate with aggressive behavior

in recognizing osteoid and bone formation as malignant in differentiated areas. Mitotic figures, as well as areas of necrosis and hemorrhage, are typical. Conventional osteosarcomas have several histologic subtypes, all of which are more common than any variant. Subtypes of conventional osteosarcomas include chondroblastic, osteoblastic, fibroblastic giant cell–rich, fibrosarcomatous, and malignant fibrous histiocytoma-like.

No specific immunohistochemical markers identify osteosarcomas. Microfoci of chondroid differentiation are S100 positive (Fig. 17-4). Abnormalities in protein expression

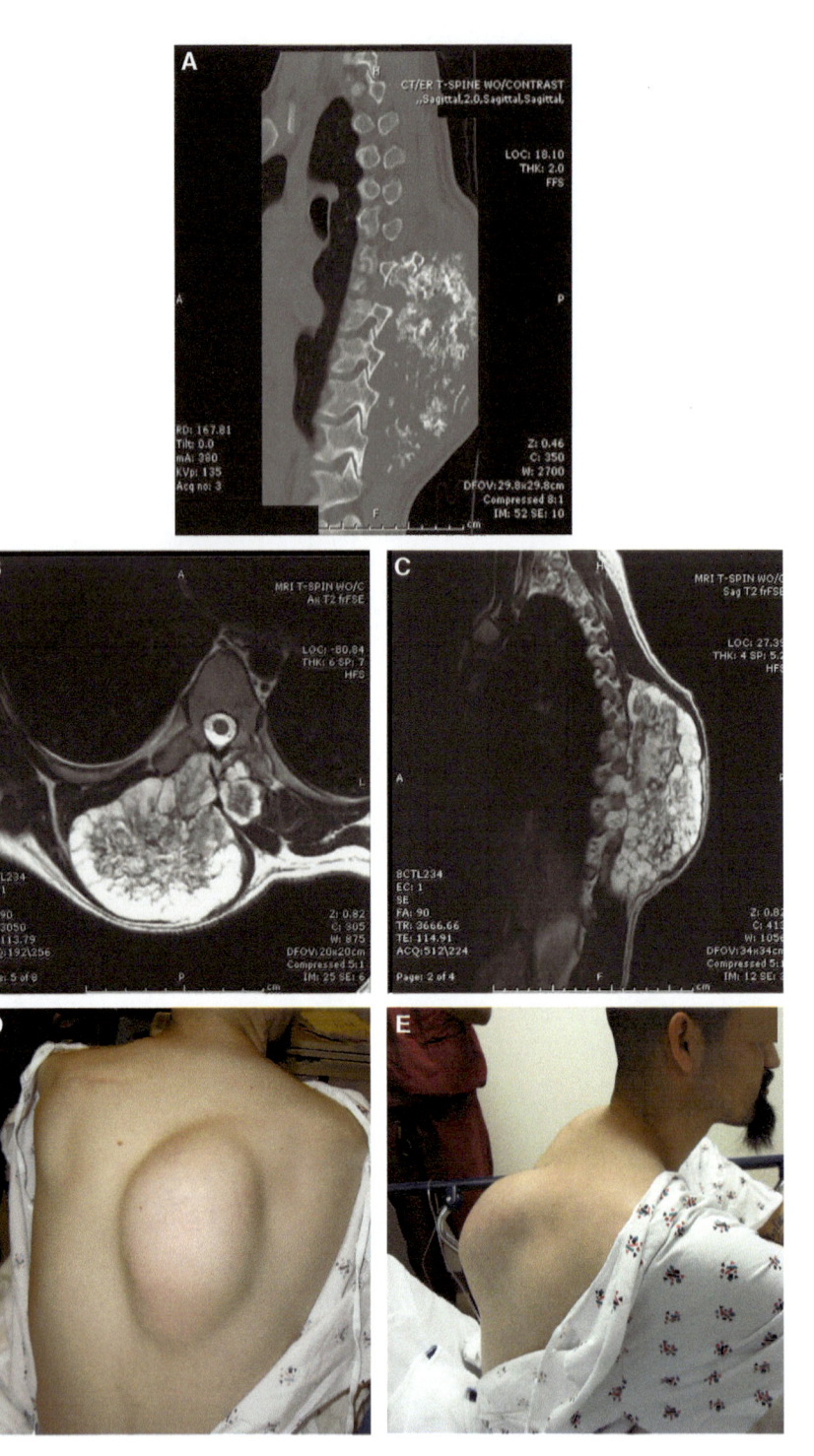

Fig. 17-4 A 32-year-old man with familial osteochondroma presented with a slow-growing painful thoracic mass. As a child he had undergone resection of a scapular mass and bilateral femoral masses consistent with osteochondroma. Given the risk of malignant transformation to chondrosarcoma, which occurs in up to 25% of patients with osteochondroma, especially those with hereditary osteochondroma, the mass was removed en bloc. **A,** Parasagittal CT scan demonstrating calcified mass abutting posterior elements from T5-11. **B,** Axial T2-weighted MRI scan demonstrating a right parasagittal mass abutting posterior elements and ribs. **C,** Parasagittal T2-weighted MRI scan demonstrating a mass. **D** and **E,** Preoperative clinical photographs.

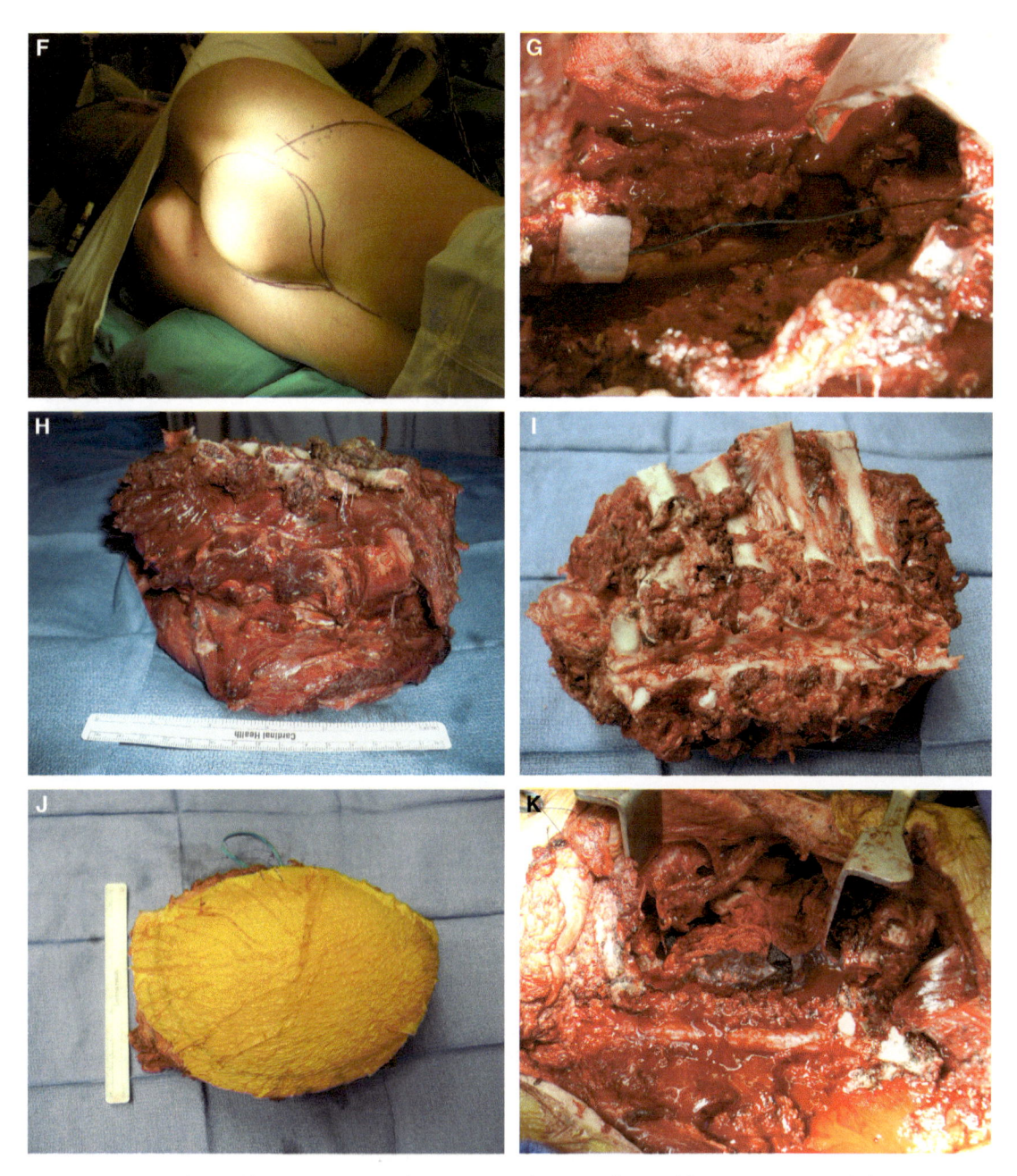

Fig. 17-4, cont'd **F,** Skin incision and operative planning for en bloc resection and thoracotomy. **G,** Intraoperative photograph showing the mass being peeled off of the thoracic spinal cord (marked by cottonoid) after thoracotomy and osteotomies, which have been carried out from inside the pleural cavity through bilateral pedicles T7-10. **H,** En bloc specimen, right-sided view, demonstrating cut through the ribs. **I,** En bloc specimen, ventral view, demonstrating ribs 7 to 10, pedicles, and bony posterior spinal canal. **J,** En bloc specimen, dorsal view, including skin. **K,** Intraoperative photograph of postresection cavity, demonstrating thoracic cord and deflated right lung underneath the rib spreader.

of p53, MDM2, or both are associated with metastatic disease.[50,51] Human epidermal growth factor receptor 2 (HER2) is identified in more than 40% of patients with osteosarcoma. The 5-year disease-free survival rate is 47% for HER2-positive tumors and 79% for HER2-negative tumors. HER2 is also associated with a significant decrease in the response to chemotherapy, the most important prognostic factor for osteosarcomas.[52] Tenascin-C is an extracellular matrix protein associated with cellular motility and is expressed in almost all osteosarcomas. Increased expression is associated with metastasis and decreased length of survival.[53] Increased expression of P-glycoprotein is also associated with earlier recurrence and death.[54]

Radiographs and CT scans demonstrate dense mineralization of involved vertebrae ("ivory vertebrae").[55] More osteoblastic than osteolytic processes are apparent, with the osteoblastic process responsible for mineralization. However, purely lytic osteosarcomas have been documented. Mineralized lesions have low intensity on T1- and T2-weighted sequences, whereas nonmineralized areas are hyperintense on T2-weighted sequences. The lesions are enhanced with contrast medium. Technetium-99m bone scans show skip or satellite lesions. Bone scans may also be used in follow-up surveillance for residual, persistent, and recurrent tumors. Vertebral body collapse and adjacent soft tissue invasion may be present but not disc space invasion. Osteosarcomas should be distinguished from osteoblastomas or aneurysmal bone cysts.

Osteosarcomas of the axial skeleton are more refractory to treatment than limb tumors.[56] A noncontaminating core-sheathed biopsy, usually CT guided, is the first step in diagnosis.[57] This should be performed at an institution with experience in primary spine tumors. Long-term survival is influenced by how well standardized diagnostic and treatment plans are followed, and very few institutions have experience treating primary bone tumors.[5] Pulmonary and other metastases should be ruled out on CT scans of the chest and on bone scans; they are detected at diagnosis in 10% to 20% of patients but do not necessarily obviate long-term survival. Aggressive resection of pulmonary metastases is indicated, even through multiple thoracotomies. In the population with pulmonary metastases, 40% have been reported to be disease free with long-term survival.[58]

Treatment includes en bloc surgical resection to maximize tumor-free survival, and possibly chemotherapy and radiation.[59-62] En bloc resection is critical, because these lesions are aggressive and often radioresistant and sometimes chemoresistant.[63,64] However, in some cases local radiation therapy and chemotherapy alone may be appropriate for those with multiple noncontiguous metastases or when surgical risks do not outweigh the benefits.[65] The prognosis can be poor. One series found a 23-month median survival, despite maximal management. In the Mayo Clinic series of 27 cases of primary osteogenic sarcoma of the vertebrae, between 1909 and 1975, a total of 21 patients received radiation therapy and five received chemotherapy.[59] All but one patient died of disease. The study found only a 10-month median survival, with less than 25% of patients surviving for more than 1 year.[35] Even fewer survive for more than 5 years.[35,38,66] In a series of 10 patients with osteosarcoma reported by Barwick et al,[42] nine underwent resection and postoperative radiation therapy, with doses ranging from 25 to 36 Gy. Of these 10 patients, nine died of disease within 2 years.

By modern-day standards the dose of radiation used to treat osteogenic sarcomas in prior series may have been inadequate. More contemporary data demonstrate that highly conformed high-dose radiation volumes can be associated with long-term local control and survival in a subset of patients with spinal osteosarcoma. A recent series reported local control in 11 of 15 patients and a 5-year survival rate of 44% associated with combined photon-proton radiation therapy with a three-dimensional approach to treatment planning. The mean dose was 69.8 cobalt gray equivalents.[67]

Some advocate delaying surgery in favor of starting chemotherapy preoperatively. Their rationale is the combination of neoadjuvant chemotherapy and radiation may improve survival and facilitate a more thorough resection, because a true en bloc resection at the time a patient is first seen, when the tumor is at its most voluminous, can be particularly challenging in the spine.[68-70] Chemotherapy can reduce the systemic tumor burden, because systemic micrometastases are typically present by the time a patient is first seen, and primary tumor regression resulting from chemotherapy can facilitate en bloc resection.

The ideal chemotherapy regimen has not yet been outlined.[71] Formulas that were previously tried include combined methotrexate, bleomycin, cyclophosphamide, actinomycin-D, and adriamycin; adriamycin alone; and high-dose methotrexate alone.[70] The MAID combination (adriamycin, ifosfamide, dacarbazine, and mesna) resulted in a 26% response rate when used as adjuvant therapy only.[72] The addition of cisplatinum and adriamycin to high-dose methotrexate, bleomycin, and cyclophosphamide preoperatively did not increase survival.[73] Occasional case reports demonstrate remission with intraarterial adriamycin, followed by systemic combined cyclophosphamide, vincristine, methotrexate, phenylalanine mustard, and adriamycin, with the combination of adriamycin, carboplatin, and etoposide, and with the combination of adriamycin and epirubicin.[66,69,74]

Preoperatively irradiated patients had 42% of all complications and 70% of all major complications.[75] One series found 18% to have wound infections, 18% to have vascular injuries, and 36% to have transient neurologic deficits. Other complications from radiation include sarcomatous degeneration, neurologic deterioration, and failed growth.[76] Progressive neurologic dysfunction, not only in this subset of patients, may result from instability and deformity stemming from inadequate reconstruction or delayed construct failure caused by disease progression or hardware failure. Harrington,[77] in a series of 77 patients treated with posterior stabilization and methylmethacrylate, found failed fixation in five patients who required restabilization.[78] Six patients developed instability because of metastatic disease at adjacent levels. In the series reported by McAfee et al,[79] 5 of 24 complications occurred after anterior stabilization by means of methylmethacrylate. Construct failure was identified in 15 of 19 patients who underwent posterior stabilization, including progressive kyphosis. Half of those with deep infections had significant neurologic deterioration. Kostuik et al[80] reported three construct failures in their series of 100 patients. Failure to recognize the extent of bony involvement by the tumor at an adjacent level was relevant in one case. The other two failures involved the use of Harrington instrumentation without sublaminar wires in the thoracic spine, which resulted in hook pullout. Autologous bone grafts and synthetic cages are recommended over methylmethacrylate.[78,81,82] Eventually the advent of pedicle screws provided the opportunity to resect more tumor and create a more stable construct involving fewer segments, compared with hooks and sublaminar wires; however, complications still arise.[75,83] These include pseudarthrosis, tumor progression resulting in late instability, and construct failure resulting in thecal compression in a delayed manner. Treatment failure is associated with any construct that does not address pathologic conditions in the anterior column.

MALIGNANT PERIPHERAL NERVE SHEATH TUMORS

Malignant peripheral nerve sheath tumors (MPNSTs) include any malignant tumor arising from or differentiating toward cells of the peripheral nerve sheath. With an incidence of 1 per 10,000 (0.0001%) in the general population, MPNSTs account for 3% to 10% of all soft tissue sarcomas.[84-87] They include malignant schwannomas, malignant neurofibromas, nerve sheath fibrosarcomas, and neurofibrosarcomas.[86,88] They may arise de novo or, in half of the cases, from sarcomatous degeneration of a preexisting plexiform neurofibroma. Malignant progression is thought to result from additional mutations involving tumor suppressor genes, such as p53. Approximately half to two thirds of sporadic and NF1-associated tumors are found in men.[84,86,89,90] Only 10% occur in children. The average age is 29 years for NF1-associated tumors and 40+ years for sporadic tumors. The sciatic nerve and the brachial plexus are the most common sites, followed by proximal spinal nerves. Lumbar and sacral tumors are 2.5 times more common than thoracic tumors, and tumors arising in the torso are three times more common than those in the head and neck.[86,90] Half of all paraspinous tumors encroach on the spine, and 10% have foraminal or intradural involvement.[90] Paraspinous tumors have a worse prognosis because complete resection is rare.

Diagnosis is based on patients meeting at least one of the following criteria: origin from a nerve, contiguity with a benign neurofibroma, or presentation in a patient who has NF1. Approximately half to two thirds of MPNSTs arise from neurofibromas in patients with NF1, or von Recklinghausen's disease.[86,87,90] In this subgroup of patients, large plexiform neurofibromas are at risk for malignant progression at a rate of 3% to 15% over the patient's lifetime because of secondary mutations of tumor suppressor genes.[86,91-94] Malignant derangement of dermal or subcutaneous neurofibromas or schwannomas does not occur. In addition to those with the plexiform neurofibroma subtype, patients with intraneural neurofibromas are also at risk for malignant progression to MPNST.[95] Accelerated growth and neurologic deficits are suggestive of malignant conversion of a preexisting neural lesion.

Prior irradiation, with an average latency period of 15 years, is another risk factor for MPNSTs, accounting for as many as 10% of all MPNSTs and as many as 20% of paraspinous MPNSTs.[84,96,97] Radiation-induced tumors are not associated with neurofibromatosis or preexisting neurofibromas. The remaining MPNSTs are sporadic and stem from peripheral nerves, although MPNSTs arise rarely from benign schwannomas or ganglioneuromas.[84,86,90,98,99]

Imaging and histochemical analysis are not specific for MPNSTs, as opposed to soft tissue sarcomas and other peripheral nerve tumors. Therefore suspicion of malignant transformation to MPNSTs is increased in patients with a history of rapid clinical presentation, increasing pain, increasing growth clinically or radiographically, or a neurologic deficit in association with a preexisting plexiform neurofibroma, especially in patients with NF1. A suspicious history may also point to secondary involvement of a nerve from an underlying primary neoplasm, such as Pancoast tumor. Distinguishing MPNSTs from other soft tissue sarcomas and atypical peripheral nerve tumors can be a diagnostic challenge that requires detailed review of evidence from many sources. Confirmation of the pathologic diagnosis is critical so that appropriate management decisions can be made. If a peripheral nerve tumor is suspected of being malignant, a thorough regional and general physical examination accompanied by chest radiographs should be undertaken to rule out overt metastasis.

MRI or CT scans cannot definitively determine whether a tumor is benign or malignant, because no homogeneous enhancement on CT or MRI scans suggestive of intratumoral necrosis or hemorrhage can indicate MPNSTs, as well as benign lesions. A small study suggests that a positive gallium scan may be specific for MPNSTs.[100-104] Some reports indicate that physiologic imaging with 18F-fluorodeoxyglucose positron emission tomography (18F-FDG PET), a technique for dynamic imaging of glucose metabolism, may differentiate benign neurofibromas from MPNSTs and, in general, identify soft tissue sarcomas, metastases, and potentially malignant transformation of a benign plexiform neurofibroma to an MPNST.[105,106]

If malignant transformation is suspected, on the basis of history, physical examination, or imaging, the patient should be referred to a tertiary center for biopsy of the lesion before definitive surgery. Diagnostic needle biopsies performed blindly may leave the patient with disabling neuropathic pain and may not be representative of pathologically heterogeneous tumors. Open four-quadrant biopsy is preferred because of the pathologic heterogeneity of MPNSTs, the requirement of adequate tissue for diagnosis, and the potential for induction of severe neuropathic pain. Surgery should be undertaken without neuromuscular paralysis to allow intraoperative electrophysiologic evaluation, including nerve action potentials. Draping should allow accessibility and evaluation of the distal muscles supplied by the nerve in question. Exposure should extend proximally and distally over the entire length of the peripheral nerve tumor. Frozen-section analysis by an experienced pathologist should be performed very early to facilitate the subsequent surgical plan. Proximal and distal segments of the nerve in question are dissected and wrapped in vessel loops. Electrical stimulation of the tumor should show no neurophysiologic function, and a small biopsy specimen from the electrically silent region should be sent for pathologic verification. Pathologic findings, along with gross and microscopic observations, will determine the feasibility of total removal versus limited resection. If the frozen-section specimen is consistent with benign neurofibroma or schwannoma, the tumor is excised microsurgically. If the frozen-section findings are consistent with MPNST, the incision should be closed without further manipulation of the tumor to await final pathologic verification. After pathologic confirmation of MPNST, a metastatic survey that includes CT or MRI scans of the chest is performed. The presence of metastases is an indication for palliative radiation locally, and possibly to the metastases, combined with chemotherapy and occasionally surgery for debulking, although long-term control is limited. Most patients do not present with metastases, and radical surgery is performed by a neurosurgeon and an orthopedic oncologist, with wide oncologic resection of the tumor, nerves, and adjacent muscle and fascial planes with clean tumor margins. Simple excision alone leads to recurrence and an increased possibility of systemic metastases, a dangerous phenomenon, because sarcomatous cells spread extensively within fascial plans.[107] Previous studies have shown that negative margins were obtained at the cost of limb amputations and disarticulation; contemporary surgery involves wide oncologic limb-sparing procedures in conjunction with neoadjuvant and adjuvant radiation or chemotherapy, which are as effective without necessitating limb sacrifice.[108,109] Chemotherapy alone has not proved to be very effective.[99] Two studies, each consisting of more than 100 patients with MPNSTs, some of whom had received adjuvant chemotherapy, demonstrated no benefit with regard to overall survival and control of local or distant metastases.[86,89,110,111] One long-term responder and 10-year disease-free survivor, who had unsuccessful surgery and did not respond to radiation therapy, responded well to an adriamycin-based combination chemotherapy, but this is an exception.[84] The ideal management of MPNSTs that is meant to minimize the risk of ultimately fatal systemic metastases remains unclear, because these lesions are not very sensitive to radiation and chemotherapy. Centers with pathologists experienced in peripheral nerve abnormalities and multidisciplinary teams involving neurosurgeons, orthopedic surgeons, reconstructive surgeons, radiation and medical oncologists, and occupational therapists should manage these patients.

Macroscopically, MPNSTs appear firm to rubbery and fleshy and are light colored, reddish-blue or yellow, corresponding to areas of hemorrhage and necrosis; they are observed in 60% of specimens and portend a poor prognosis.[87,89] Benign nerve sheath tumors may share similar characteristics. The lesions are well circumscribed, with a fibrous pseudocapsule and a fascicular pattern. Fusiform enlargement of the involved parent nerve can be present in 32% of cases according to one series.[89] A lobulated mass can be observed when nerve involvement cannot be identified. Most are 2 to 40 cm; tumors larger than 5 cm have a worse prognosis. Similar to other sarcomas, MPNSTs are graded microscopically on the basis of cellularity, nuclear pleomorphism, anaplasia, mitotic rate, microvascular proliferation, and degree of necrosis and invasion.[112] The lesions are hypercellular with spindle-shaped cells with high mitotic activity, atypia, necrosis, and infiltration. In fact, 4 and 6 mitoses per 10 high-power fields have been reported.[86,89,90] Based on these characteristics, most MPNSTs are World Health Organization (WHO) grade III or IV.[86,89,90,95] The tumor cells may be arranged in fascicles, resulting in a herringbone pattern, similar to that of fibrosarcomas or a storiform pattern, as in malignant fibrous histiocytomas. When the involved parent nerve is identified, tumor invasion courses parallel to the axons.

There are no pathognomonic immunohistochemical or imaging markers for MPNSTs, making it challenging to differentiate these lesions from benign peripheral nerve tumors or other soft tissue sarcomas. Fifty percent to 80% of MPNSTs demonstrate S100 immunoreactivity.[90,99,113,114] Schwannomas and neurofibromas stain even more commonly for S100; however, the stain distinguishes MPNSTs from other soft tissue sarcomas. Two other Schwann cell markers, leu-7 and myelin basic protein, enhance the diagnosis of MPNSTs, although they are not diagnostic because of false-positive and false-negative rates resulting from tumor dedifferentiation.[114] Transformed Schwann cells may lose S100 staining and neurofibromin expression, while exhibiting loss of the p53 tumor suppressor gene and overexpression of epidermal growth factor receptor.[115] Approximately 16% to 27% of MPNSTs contain areas of divergent malignant differentiation, a feature most commonly associated with NF1 tumors.[84,86,89,90] The most common patterns are rhabdomyosarcoma, chondrosarcoma, osteosarcoma, epithelioid, and angiosarcoma. MPNSTs with rhabdomyosarcomatous elements are also known as *triton tumors*. Dedifferentiation can lead to expression of muscle in malignant triton tumors. CD99 stains positively in 86% of MPNSTs, and p53 overexpression occurs in 50% to 87% of patients, whereas p53 immunoreactivity is rare in benign neurofibromas.[99,113,116-118] An MIB-1 labeling index greater than 25% is associated with shorter life expectancy.[117]

Cytogenetic studies demonstrate hypodiploid and triploid chromosome numbers, as well as chromosome loss, rearrangement, and translocation. NF1 patients with MPNSTs often carry structural abnormalities of chromosome 17 and chromosome 22.[119-121] There are no known differences in karyotypes of tumors arising sporadically compared to those associated with NF1. In patients with NF1, both NF1 alleles are missing or inactivated, resulting in the development of neurofibromas.[122] Sporadic tumors that have alterations at the NF1 locus require additional changes to transform the tumors into MPNSTs. Malignant progression to MPNSTs is associated with alterations in the p53 gene and in p53 protein expression.[123-125] Half of MPNSTs also have a homozygous deletion of the CDKN2A gene, which encodes the p16 cell cycle inhibitory molecule.[126,127] Those genetic derangements not observed in benign neurofibromas are associated with malignant transformation of neurofibromas.

CONCLUSION

Soft tissue sarcomas and malignant peripheral nerve sheath tumors are extremely rare tumors originating from mesenchymal cells of viscera, integument, and various connective tissue structures, with hematogenous spread. More than 50 separate subtypes of soft tissue sarcomas have been identified from such origins as fat, muscle, vasculature, lymphatic vessels, synovial tissue, peripheral nerves, cartilage and bone-forming tissue, and fibrous tissue. Just under 10,000 cases are identified in the US annually; two-thirds are found in an extremity. Risk factors for soft tissue sarcoma include inherited retinoblastoma, Gardner's syndrome, Li-Fraumeni syndrome, neurofibromatosis type 1 (NF1), exposure to vinyl chloride, and prior lymphadenectomy. Previous irradiation may be responsible for 5% of sarcomas. Staging is used to determine tumor extension and is the most significant factor determining prognosis and treatment options. The tumor node metastasis (TNM) system of the American Joint Committee on Cancer is commonly used to stage sarcomas. The Weinstein-Boriani-Biagini (WBB) system is used to strategize resection of primary spine tumors.[3-5] The overall survival rate is approximately 30% to 50% at 5 years after surgery in combination with other treatment modalities.

Malignant peripheral nerve sheath tumors include any malignant tumor arising from or differentiating toward cells of the peripheral nerve sheath. These rare tumors may arise de novo or, in half of the cases, from sarcomatous degeneration of a preexisting plexiform neurofibroma. Malignant progression is thought to result from additional mutations involving tumor suppressor genes, such as p53. The sciatic nerve and the brachial plexus are the most common sites, followed by proximal spinal nerves. Lumbar and sacral tumors are 2.5 times more common than thoracic tumors, and tumors arising in the torso are three times more common than those in the head and neck.[86,90] Diagnosis is based on patients meeting at least one of the following criteria: origin from a nerve, contiguity with a benign neurofibroma, or presentation in a patient who has NF1. Approximately half to two thirds of MPNSTs arise from neurofibromas in patients with NF1. Accelerated growth and neurologic deficits are suggestive of malignant conversion of a preexisting neural lesion. Prior irradiation, with an average latency period of 15 years, is another risk factor for MPNSTs. Imaging and histochemical analysis are not specific for MPNSTs. Therefore suspicion of malignant transformation to MPNSTs is increased in patients with a history of rapid clinical presentation, increasing pain, increasing growth clinically or radiographically, or a neurologic deficit in association with a preexisting plexiform neurofibroma, especially in patients with NF1. Care should be undertaken at a tertiary facility with relevant experience. Most MPNSTs are World Health Organization (WHO) grade III or IV.[86,89,90,95] There are no pathognomonic immunohistochemical or imaging markers for MPNSTs, making it challenging to differentiate these lesions from benign peripheral nerve tumors or other soft tissue sarcomas.

TIPS FROM THE MASTERS

- Staging is the most significant factor determining prognosis and treatment options.
- The WBB system enables preoperative planning for en bloc resection of spine tumors.
- Most patients who survive for 5 years are considered cured.
- Malignant fibrous histiocytomas are the most common primary soft tissue sarcomas of bone.

- Osteosarcomas are the second most common primary bone malignancy after multiple myelomas. No specific immunohistochemical markers identify osteosarcomas.
- The sciatic nerve and the brachial plexus are the most common sites for MPNSTs.
- Imaging and histochemical analysis are not specific for MPNSTs.
- Suspicion of malignant transformation to MPNSTs is increased with a history of rapid clinical presentation, increasing pain, increasing growth, or a neurologic deficit in association with a preexisting plexiform neurofibroma.
- If a peripheral nerve tumor is suspected of being malignant, a thorough regional and general physical examination accompanied by chest radiographs should be undertaken to rule out overt metastasis.
- A tertiary center should perform biopsy of the lesion before definitive surgery. Pathologic findings, along with gross and microscopic observations, will determine the feasibility of total removal versus limited resection.
- Simple excision alone leads to recurrence and an increased possibility of systemic metastases. Tumors larger than 5 cm have a worse prognosis.
- There are no pathognomonic immunohistochemical or imaging markers for MPNSTs.

References (With Key References in Boldface)

1. Sobin LH, Fleming ID, eds. Tumors of the bone and soft tissues. In TNM Classification of Malignant Tumors, 5th ed. New York: Wiley, 1997, p 101.
2. Vincent F, Fehlings MG. Spinal column tumors. In Bernstein M, Berger MS. Neuro-oncology: The Essentials, 2nd ed. New York: Thieme, 2008, pp 391-402.
3. **Weinstein JN, McLain RF. Primary tumors of the spine. Spine 12:843-851, 1987.**
4. **Boriani S, De Iure F, Bandeiera S, et al. Chondrosarcoma of the mobile spine. Report on 22 cases. Spine 25:804-812, 2000.**
5. **Boriani S, Weinstein JN. Differential diagnosis and surgical treatment of primary benign and malignant neoplasms. In Frymoyer JW, ed. The Adult Spine: Principles and Practice, 2nd ed. Philadelphia: Lippincott-Raven, 1997, pp 951-987.**
6. Boriani S, Weinstein JN, Biagini R. Primary bone tumors of the spine: terminology and surgical staging. Spine 22: 1036-1044, 1997.
7. Fu YS, Gabbini G, Kaye GI, et al. Malignant soft tissue tumors of probable histiocytic origin (malignant fibrous histiocytomas): general considerations and electron microscopic and tissue culture studies. Cancer 35:176-198, 1975.
8. Roholl PJM, Kleyne J, Elbers H, et al. Characterization of tumor cells in malignant fibrous histiocytomas and other soft tissue tumours in comparison with malignant histiocytes. I. Immunohistochemical study on paraffin sections. J Pathol 147:87-95, 1985.
9. Weiss SW, Goldblum JR. Enzinger and Weiss's Soft Tissue Tumors, 4th ed. St Louis: Mosby–Year Book 2001.
10. Dorfman H, Czerniak B. Bone Tumors. St Louis: Mosby–Year Book, 1998.
11. Molina P, Pellin A, Navarro S, et al. Analysis of p53 and MDM2 proteins in malignant fibrous histiocytoma in absence of gene alteration: prognostic significance. Virchows Arch 435:596-605, 1999.

12. Rieske P, Bartkowiak JK, Szadowska AM, et al. A comparative study of P53/MDM2 genes alterations and P53/MDM2 proteins immunoreactivity in soft-tissue sarcomas. J Exp Clin Cancer Res 18:403-416, 1999.
13. Ochiai H, Yamakawa Y, Fukushima T, et al. Primary leiomyosarcoma of the cervical spine causing spontaneous compression fracture: report of an autopsy case. Neuropathology 20:60-64, 2000.
14. Shmookler BM, Lauer DH. Retroperitoneal leiomyosarcoma. A clinicopathologic analysis of 36 cases. Am J Surg Pathol 7:269-280, 1983.
15. De Saint Aubain Somoerhausen N, Fletcher CD. Leiomyosarcoma of soft tissue in children: clinicopathologic analysis of 20 cases. Am J Surg Pathol 23:755-763, 1999.
16. Wirbel RJ, Verelst S, Hanselmann R, et al. Primary leiomyosarcoma of bone: clinicopathologic, immunohistochemical, and molecular biologic aspects. Ann Surg Oncol 5:635-641, 1998.
17. Lopez-Barea F, Rodriguez-Peralto JL, Sanchez-Herrera S, et al. Primary epithelioid leiomyosarcoma of bone. Case report and literature review. Virchows Arch 434:367-371, 1999.
18. Rao UN, Finkelstein SD, Jones MW. Comparative immunohistochemical and molecular analysis of uterine and extrauterine leiomyosarcomas. Mod Pathol 12:1001-1009, 1999.
19. Konomoto T, Fukuda T, Hayashi K, et al. Leiomyosarcoma in soft tissue: examination of p53 status and cell proliferating factors in different locations. Hum Pathol 29:74-81, 1998.
20. Plaat BE, Hollema H, Molenaar WM, et al. Soft tissue leiomyosarcomas and malignant gastrointestinal stromal tumors: differences in clinical outcome and expression of multidrug resistance proteins. J Clin Oncol 18:3211-3220, 2000.
21. Addison AK, Payne SR. Primary liposarcoma of bone. Case report. J Bone Joint Surg Am 64:301-304, 1982.
22. Turanli S, Ozer H, Ozyurekoglu T, et al. Liposarcoma in the epidural space. Spine 25:1733-1735, 2000.
23. Nijhuis PH, Sars PR, Plaat BE, et al. Clinico-pathological data and prognostic factors in completely resected AJCC stage I-III liposarcomas. Ann Surg Oncol 7:535-543, 2000.
24. Linehan DC, Lewis JJ, Leung D, et al. Influence of biologic factors and anatomic site in completely resected liposarcoma. J Clin Oncol 18:1637-1643, 2000.
25. Dei Tos AP. Liposarcoma: new entities and evolving concepts. Ann Diagn Pathol 4:252-266, 2000.
26. Schneider-Stock R, Ziegeler A, Haeckel C, et al. Prognostic relevance of p53 alterations and Mib-1 proliferation index in subgroups of primary liposarcomas. Clin Cancer Res 5:2830-2835, 1999.
27. Oliveira AM, Nascimento AG, Okuno SH, et al. p27 (kip1) protein expression correlates with survival in myxoid and round-cell liposarcoma. J Clin Oncol 18:2888-2893, 2000.
28. Shapiro S, Scott J, Kaufman K. Metastatic cardiac angiosarcoma of the cervical spine. Case report. Spine (Phila Pa 1976) 24:1156-1158, 1999.
29. Sanchez-Mejia RO, Ojemann SG, Simko J, et al. Sacral epithelioid angiosarcoma associated with a bleeding diathesis and spinal epidural hematoma: case report. J Neurosurg Spine 4:246-250, 2006.
30. Kawashima H, Ishikawa S, Fukase M, et al. Successful surgical treatment of angiosarcoma of the spine: a case report. Spine (Phila Pa 1976) 29:E280-E283, 2004.
31. Zidan J, Stayerman C, Turani H. [Perisacral angiosarcoma after radiotherapy for sigmoid carcinoma] Harefuah 134:353-355, 423, 1998.
32. Unni KK, Dahlin DC. Premalignant tumors and conditions of bone. Am J Surg Pathol 3:47-60, 1979.
33. Friedlaener GE, Southwick WO. Tumors of the spine. In Rothman RH, Simeone FA, eds. The Spine. Philadelphia: WB Saunders, 1982, pp 1022-1040.
34. Fielding JW, Fietti VG Jr, Hughes JE, et al. Primary osteogenic sarcoma of the cervical spine: a case report. J Bone Joint Surg Am 58:892-894, 1976.
35. Shives TC, Dahlin DC, Sim FH, et al. Osteosarcoma of the spine. J Bone Joint Surg Am 68:660-668, 1986.
36. Dorfman HD, Czerniak B. Epidemiology of bone tumors: SEER population-based data. 1973-1987. Cancer 75:223-227, 1995.
37. Dorfman HD, Czerniak B. Bone cancers. Cancer 75(1 Suppl):203-210, 1995.

38. Tasdermiroglu E, Bagatur E, Ayan I, et al. Primary spinal column sarcomas. Acta Neurochir (Wien) 138:1261-1266, 1996.
39. Uribe-Botero G, Russell WD, Sutow WW, et al. Primary osteosarcoma of bone. A clinical pathological investigation of 243 cases, and the necroscopy studies in 54. Am J Clin Pathol 67:427-435, 1977.
40. Flemming DJ, Murphey MD, Carmichael BB, et al. Primary tumors of the spine. Semin Musculoskelet Radiol 4:299-320, 2000.
41. Patel DV, Hammer RA, Levin B, et al. Primary osteogenic sarcoma of the spine. Skeletal Radiol 12:276-279, 1984.
42. Barwick KW, Huvos AG, Smith J. Primary osteogenic sarcoma of the vertebral column: a clinicopathologic correlation of ten patients. Cancer 46:595-604, 1980.
43. Weinfeld MS, Dudley HR Jr. Osteogenic sarcoma. A follow-up study of the ninety-four cases observed at the Massachusetts General Hospital from 1920 to 1960. J Bone Joint Surg Am 44:269-276, 1962.
44. Unni KK. Dahlin's Bone Tumors. General Aspects and Data on 11,087 Cases, 5th ed. Philadelphia: Lippincott-Raven, 1996.
45. Huvos AG, Sundaresan N, Bretsky SS, et al. Osteogenic sarcoma of the skull. A clinicopathologic study of 19 patients. Cancer 56:1214-1221, 1985.
46. Huvos AG. Osteogenic sarcoma of bones and soft tissues in older persons. A clinicopathologic analysis of 117 patients older than 60 years. Cancer 57:1442-1449, 1986.
47. Tigani D, Pignatti G, Picci P, et al. Vertebral osteosarcoma. Ital J Orthop Traumatol 14:5-13, 1988.
48. Burger PC, Scheithauer BW. Tumors of the Central Nervous System. Washington, DC: Armed Forces Institute of Pathology, 1994.
49. Coons SW. Pathology of tumors of the spinal cord, spine, and paraspinous soft tissue. In Dickman CA, Fehlings MG, Gokaslan ZL, eds. Spinal Cord and Spinal Column Tumors: Principles and Practice. New York: Thieme, 2006, pp 41–110.
50. Ladanyi M, Cha C, Lewis R, et al. MDM2 gene amplification in metatastic osteosarcoma. Cancer Res 53:16-18, 1993.
51. Toguchida J, Yamaguchi T, Dayton SH, et al. Prevalence and spectrum of germline mutations of the p53 gene among patients with sarcoma. N Engl J Med 326:1301-1308, 1992.
52. Morris CD, Gorlick R, Hugos AG, et al. Human epidermal growth factor receptor 2 as a prognostic indicator in osteogenic sarcoma. Clin Orthop 382:59-65, 2001.
53. Tanaka M, Yamazaki T, Araki N, et al. Clinical significance of tenascin-C expression in osteosarcoma: tenascin-C promotes distant metastases of osteosarcoma. Int J Mol Med 5:505-510, 2000.
54. Baldini N, Scotlandi K, Barbanti-Brodano G, et al. Expression of P-glycoprotien in high-grade osteosarcomas in relation to clinical outcome. N Engl J Med 333:1380-1385, 1995.
55. Fenton D, Czervionke L. Image-Guided Spine Intervention. Philadelphia: WB Saunders, 2003.
56. Bielack SS, Wulff B, Delling G, et al. Osteosarcoma of the trunk treated by multimodal therapy: experience of the Cooperative Osteosarcoma Study Group (COSS). Med Pediatr Oncol 24:6-12, 1995.
57. Erlemann R, Reiser MF, Peters PE, et al. Musculoskeletal neoplasms: static and dynamic Gd-DTPA-enhanced MR imaging. Radiology 171:767-773, 1989.
58. Goorin AM, Delorey MJ, Lack EE, et al. Prognostic significance of complete surgical resection of pulmonary metastases from osteogenic sarcoma: analysis of 32 patients. J Clin Oncol 2:425-431, 1984.
59. Ozaki T, Flege S, Lilienqvist U, et al. Osteosarcoma of the spine: experience of the Cooperative Osteosarcoma Study Group. Cancer 94:1069-1077, 2002.
60. Takaishi H, Yabe H, Fujimuyra Y, et al. The results of surgery on primary malignant tumors of the spine. Arch Orthop Trauma Surg 115:49-52, 1996.
61. Talac R, Yaszemski MJ, Currier BL, et al. Relationship between surgical margins and local recurrence in sarcomas of the spine. Clin Orthop Relat Res 397:127-132, 2002.
62. Sundaresan N, Rosen G, Huvox AG, et al. Combined treatment of osteosarcoma of the spine. Neurosurgery 23:714-719, 1988.
63. Ferguson WS, Goorian AM. Current treatment of osteosarcoma. Cancer Invest 19:292-315, 2001.

64. Spiegel DA, Richardson WJ, Scully SP, et al. Long-term survival following total sacrectomy with reconstruction for the treatment of osteosarcoma of the spine. Neurosurgery 23:714-719, 1988.
65. Sim F, Frassica F, Wold L, et al. Chondrosarcoma of the spine: Mayo Clinic experience. In Sundaresan N, Schmidek H, Schiller A, et al, eds. Tumors of the Spine. Philadelphia: WB Saunders, 1990, pp 155-162.
66. Ogihara Y, Sekiguchi K, Tsureta T. Osteogenic sarcoma of the fourth thoracic vertebra. Long term survival by chemotherapy only. Cancer 46:595-604, 1984.
67. Hug EB, Fitzek MM, Liebsch NJ, et al. Locally challenging osteo- and chondrogenic tumors of the axial skeleton: results of combined proton and photon radiation therapy using three-dimensional treatment planning. Int J Radiat Oncol Biol Phys 15:559-565, 1988.
68. Rosen G, Marcove RC, Huvos AG, et al. Primary osteogenic sarcoma: eight-year experience with adjuvant chemotherapy. J Cancer Res Clin Oncol 106:55-67, 1983.
69. Bauernhofer T, Stoger H, Kasparek AK, et al. Combined treatment of metastatic osteosarcoma of the spine. Oncology 57:265-268, 1999.
70. Sundaresan N, Rosen G, Fortner JG, et al. Preoperative chemotherapy and surgical resection in the management of posterior paraspinal tumors. Report of three cases. J Neurosurg 58:446-450, 1983.
71. Malawer MM, Lin MP, Donaldson SS. Sarcomas of the soft tissue and bone. In DeVita VTJ, Hellman S, Rosenberg SA, eds. Cancer Principles and Practice of Oncology, 6th ed. Philadelphia: Lippincott Williams & Wilkins, 2001, pp 1891-1935.
72. Antman K, Corwley J, Balcerzak SP, et al. A Southwest Oncology Group and Cancer and Leukemia Group B phase II study of doxorubicin, dacarbazine, ifosfamide, and mesna in adults with advanced osteosarcoma, Ewing's sarcoma, and rhabdomyosarcoma. Cancer 82:1288-1295, 1998.
73. Myers PA, Gorlick R, Heller G, et al. Intensification of preoperative chemotherapy for osteogenic sarcoma: results of the Memorial Sloan-Kettering (T12) protocol. J Clin Oncol 16:2452-2458, 1998.
74. Kebudi R, Ayan I, Darendeliler E, et al. Primary osteosarcoma of the cervical spine: a pediatric case report and review of the literature. Med Pediatr Oncol 23:162-165, 1994.
75. McLain R, Kabins M, Weinstein J. VSP stabilization of lumbar neoplasms: technical considerations and complications. J Spinal Disord 56:294-306, 1991.
76. Weatherby RP, Dahlin DC, Ivins JC. Postradiation sarcoma of bone: review of 78 Mayo Clinic cases. Mayo Clin Proc 56:294-306, 1981.
77. Harrington KD. Metastatic disease of the spine. In Harrington KD, ed. Orthopaedic Management of Metastatic Bone Disease. St Louis: Mosby-Year Book, 1988, pp 309-383.
78. Scoville WB, Palmer AH, Samra K, et al. The use of acrylic plastic for vertebral replacement and fixation in metastatic disease of the spine. Technical note. J Neurosurg 27:274-281, 1967.
79. McAfee P, Bohlman H, Ducker T, et al. Failure of stabilization of the spine with methylmethacrylate. A retrospective analysis of twenty-four cases. J Bone Joint Surg Am 68:1145-1157, 1986.
80. Kostuik JP, Errico TJ, Gleason TF, et al. Spinal stabilization for vertical tumors. Spine 13:250-256, 1988.
81. Kaneda K, Takeda N. Reconstruction with a ceramic vertebral prosthesis and Kaneda device following subtotal or total vertebrectomy in metastatic thoracic and lumbar spine. In Bridwell KH, DeWald RL, eds. The Textbook of Spinal Surgery, 2nd ed. Philadelphia: Lippincott Williams & Wilkins, 1997, pp 2071-2087.
82. Steffee AD, Sitkowski DJ, Topham LS. Total vertebral body and pedicle arthroplasty. Clin Orthop 203:203-208, 1986.
83. Oda I, Cunningham BW, Abumi K, et al. The stability of reconstruction methods after thoracolumbar total spondylectomy. An in vitro investigation. Spine 24:1634-1638, 1999.
84. Wanebo JE, Malik JM, VandenBerg SR, et al. Malignant peripheral nerve sheath tumors. A clinicopathologic study of 28 cases. Cancer 71:1247-1253, 1993.
85. Lewis JJ, Brennan MF. Soft tissue sarcomas. Curr Probl Surg 33:817-872, 1996.
86. Ducatman BS, Scheithauer BW. Malignant peripheral nerve sheath tumors: a clinicopathologic study of 120 cases. Cancer 57:2006-2021, 1986.

87. Hruban RH, Shiu MH, Senie RT, et al. Malignant peripheral nerve sheath tumors of the buttock and lower extremity. A study of 43 cases. Cancer 66:1253-1265, 1990.
88. Thiele CJ, McKeon C, Triche TJ, et al. Differential protooncogene expression characterizes histopathologically indistinguishable tumors of the peripheral nervous system. J Clin Invest 80:804-811, 1987.
89. Wong WW, Hirose T, Scheithauer BW, et al. Malignant peripheral nerve sheath tumor: analysis of treatment outcome. Int J Radiat Oncol Biol Phys 42:351-360, 1998.
90. Kourea HP, Bilsky MH, Leung DH, et al. Subdiaphragmatic and intrathoracic paraspinal malignant peripheral nerve sheath tumors: a clinicopathologic study of 25 patients and 26 tumors. Cancer 82:2191-2203, 1998.
91. **Enneking WF, Spanier SS, Goodman MA. Current concepts review: the staging of musculoskeletal sarcoma. J Bone Joint Surg Am 62:1027-1030, 1980.**
92. Von Deimling A, Foster R, Krone W. Neurofibromatosis type 1. In Kleihues P, Cavenee WK, eds. Pathology and Genetics of Tumours of the Nervous System (World Health Organization Classification of Tumours). Lyon: IARC Press, 2000, pp 216-218.
93. McMenamin ME, Fletcher CDM. Expanding the spectrum of malignant change in schwannomas. Epithelioid malignant change, epithelioid malignant peripheral nerve sheath tumor, and epithelioid angiosarcoma: a study of 17 cases. Am J Surg Pathol 25:13-25, 2001.
94. Sorensen SA, Mulvihill JJ, Nielsen A. Long-term follow-up on von Recklinghausen neurofibromatosis: survival and malignant neoplasms. N Engl J Med 314:1010-1015, 1986.
95. Woodruff JM. Pathology of tumors of the peripheral nerve sheath in type I neurofibromatosis. Am J Med Genet 89:23-30, 1999.
96. Ducatman BS, Scheithauer BW. Postirradiation neurofibrosarcoma. Cancer 51:1028-1033, 1983.
97. Foley KM, Woodruff JM, Ellis FT, et al. Radiation-inducing malignant and atypical peripheral nerve sheath tumors. Ann Neurol 7:311-318, 1980.
98. Russell DS, Rubinstein LJ. Pathology of Tumors of the Nervous System. Baltimore: Williams & Wilkins, 1989.
99. Stark AM, Buhl R, Hugo HH, et al. Malignant peripheral nerve sheath tumours—report of 8 cases and review of the literature. Acta Neurochir (Wien) 143:357-364, 2001.
100. Cerofolini E, Landi A, DeSantis G, et al. MR of benign peripheral nerve sheath tumors. J Comput Assist Tomogr 15:593-597, 1991.
101. Levine E, Huntrakoon M, Wetzel LH. Malignant-nerve sheath neoplasms in neurofibromatosis: distinctions from benign tumors by using imaging techniques. Am J Roentgenol 149:1059-1064, 1987.
102. Stull M, Moser R, Kransdorf M, et al. Magnetic resonance appearance of peripheral nerve sheath tumors. Skeletal Radiol 20:9-14, 1991.
103. Suh J, Abenoza P, Galloway H, et al. Peripheral (extracranial) nerve tumors: correlation of MR imaging and histological findings. Radiology 183:341-346, 1992.
104. Fuchs B, Spinner RJ, Rock MGH. Malignant peripheral nerve sheath tumors: an update. J Surg Orthop Adv 14:168-174, 2005.
105. Dyck P, Wilson C. Anterior sacral meningocele. J Neurosurg 53:548-552, 1980.
106. Ferner RE, Lucas JD, O'Doherty MJ, et al. Evaluation of (18) fluorodeoxyglucose positron emission tomography ([18]FDG PET) in the detection of malignant peripheral nerve sheath tumours arising from within plexiform neurofibromas in neurofibromatosis 1. J Neurol Neurosurg Psychiatry 68:353-357, 2000.
107. Simon MA, Enneking WF. The management of soft-tissue sarcomas of the extremities. J Bone Joint Surg Am 58:317-327, 1976.
108. Sadoski C, Suit HD, Rosenberg A, et al. Preoperative radiation, surgical margins, and local control of extremity sarcomas of soft tissues. J Surg Oncol 52:223-230, 1993.
109. Bell RS, O'Sullivan B, Liu FF, et al. The surgical margin in soft-tissue sarcoma. J Bone Joint Surg Am 71:370-375, 1989.
110. Stefanko SZ, Vuzevski VD, Maas AI, et al. Intracerebral malignant schwannoma. Acta Neuropathol (Berl) 71:321-325, 1986.

111. Singh RV, Suys S, Campbell DA, et al. Malignant schwannoma of the cerebellum: case report. Surg Neurol 39:128-132, 1993.
112. Russell WO, Cohen J, Enzinger F, et al. A clinical and pathological staging system for soft tissue sarcomas. Cancer 40:1562-1570, 1977.
113. O'Sullivan MJ, Kyriakos M, Zhu X, et al. Malignant peripheral nerve sheath tumors with t(X:18). A pathologic and molecular genetic study. Mod Pathol 13:1253-1265, 2000.
114. Wick MR, Swanson PE, Scheithauer BW, et al. Malignant peripheral nerve sheath tumor: an immunohistochemical study of 62 cases. Am J Clin Pathol 87:425-433, 1987.
115. Perry A, Roth KA, Banerjee R, et al. NF1 deletions in S-100 protein-positive and negative cells of sporadic and neurofibromatosis-1 (NF1)-associated plexiform neurofibromas and malignant peripheral nerve sheath tumors. Am J Pathol 159:57-61, 2001.
116. Halling KC, Scheithauer BW, Halling AC, et al. p53 expression in neurofibroma and malignant peripheral nerve sheath tumor. An immunohistochemical study of sporadic and NF1-associated tumors. Am J Clin Pathol 106:282-288, 1996.
117. Watanabe T, Oda Y, Tamiya S, et al. Malignant peripheral nerve sheath tumour arising within neurofibroma. An immunohistochemical analysis in the comparison between benign and malignant components. J Clin Pathol 54:631-636, 2001.
118. McCarron KF, Goldblum JR. Plexiform neurofibroma with and without associated malignant peripheral nerve sheath tumor: a clinicopathologic and immunohistochemical analysis of 54 cases. Mod Pathol 11:612-617, 1998.
119. Mertens F, Rydholm A, Bauer HF, et al. Cytogenetic findings in malignant peripheral nerve sheath tumors. Int J Cancer 61:793-798, 1995.
120. Jhanwar SC, Chen Q, Li FP, et al. Cytogenetic analysis of soft tissue sarcomas. Recurrent chromosome abnormalities in malignant peripheral nerve sheath tumors (MPNST). Cancer Genet Cytogenet 78:138-144, 1994.
121. Rao UN, Surti U, Hoffner L, et al. Cytogenetic and histologic correlation of peripheral nerve sheath tumors of soft tissue. Cancer Genet Cytogenet 88:17-25, 1996.
122. Legius E, Marchuk DA, Collins FS, et al. Somatic deletion of the neurofibromatosis type 1 gene in a neurofibrosarcoma supports a tumour suppressor gene hypothesis. Nat Genet 3:122-126, 1993.
123. Legius E, Dierick H, Wu R, et al. TP53 mutations are frequent in malignant NF1 tumors. Genes Chromosomes Cancer 10:250-255, 1994.
124. Lothe RA, Slettan A, Saeter G, et al. Alterations at chromosome 17 loci in peripheral nerve sheath tumors. J Neuropathol Exp Neurol 54:65-73, 1995.
125. Menon AG, Anderson KM, Riccardi VM, et al. Chromosome 17p deletions and p53 gene mutations associated with the formations of malignant neurofibrosarcomas in von Recklinghausen neurofibromatosis. Proc Natl Acad Sci USA 87:5435-5439, 1990.
126. Kourea HP, Orlow I, Scheithauer BW, et al. Deletions of the INK4A gene occur in malignant peripheral nerve sheath tumors but not in neurofibromas. Am J Pathol 155:1855-1860, 1999.
127. Neilson GP, Stemmer-Rachamimov AO, Ino Y, et al. Malignant transformation of neurofibromas in neurofibromatosis 1 is associated with CDKN2A/p16 inactivation. Am J Pathol 155:1879-1884, 1999.

Chapter 18

Systemic Treatment of Advanced Lung Cancer

Thierry M. Jahan

Lung cancer is a major health concern as a leading cause of morbidity and mortality. It is the second leading cause of new cancer in both men and women, behind prostate cancer and breast cancer, respectively, but it has consistently been the single most common cause of cancer death by far for both sexes. There were 219,440 new cases and 159,390 deaths in the United States in 2009.[1] More than half of all patients with lung cancer are seen at an advanced stage,[2-4] so the 5-year overall survival rate for patients diagnosed with lung cancer, all stages combined, is only 16%.[1] Thirty to 40% of all patients with lung cancer will develop bone metastases at some point during the course of their illness, with up to 66% of these patients exhibiting bone metastases at the initial diagnosis.[3,5] The probability of developing an invasive lung cancer with spinal metastases has been estimated to be as high as 1 in 16 among patients 60 to 79 years of age,[6] and the median survival for these patients has been estimated at approximately 7 months.[7] Consequently it is critical that the multidisciplinary team of physicians caring for these patients have an understanding of the nonsurgical therapeutic options available to patients with metastatic lung cancer, as well as an understanding of the prognosis that these patients face with or without intervention.

Lung cancer is generally divided into two major categories: non–small cell lung cancer (NSCLC) and small cell lung cancer (SCLC). NSCLC accounts for the vast majority of cases of lung cancer, at more than 80%. It also accounts for most of the cases associated with bone and spinal metastases. SCLC, on the other hand, represents less than 20% of all cases, with a declining incidence over the past few years.[8] Seventy-five percent of patients with NSCLC[4] and 53% to 70% of patients with SCLC[2,9] are first seen with advanced disease. The mainstay of therapeutic options for both groups involves systemic therapy.

THERAPEUTIC MANAGEMENT OF ADVANCED SMALL CELL LUNG CANCER

Sixty percent of patients with SCLC have advanced or extensive-stage disease, with distant metastases to organs such as the brain, lungs, liver, adrenal glands, and bones, among others.[8] Among patients with advanced disease, it is estimated that 10% to 20% will have spinal metastases, with either epidural metastases (more than 80% of all patients with spinal metastases) or intramedullary lesions (approximately 17% of all patients with SCLC with spinal metastases).[10,11]

SCLC appears to be sensitive to systemic chemotherapy, with strong initial complete responses. Unfortunately the duration of the response is limited, and most patients have relapses despite initial excellent responses. The standard regimen of cis-platinum or carboplatinum plus etoposide,[12,13] which is used in the United States and most of Western Europe, has remained the same for the past three decades, with no clear improvement despite multiple phase III clinical trials to try to advance response rates and improve survival.[14] The combination of cis-platinum and irinotecan was shown to be superior to platinum and etoposide in Japan.[15] These promising results were never duplicated in Western populations.[16,17] The combination of a platinum and etoposide, although initially effective, has significant side effects that include nausea, vomiting, leukopenia, anemia, and thrombocytopenia. It should be noted that the addition of prophylactic cranial irradiation to prevent future brain metastases is recommended for all patients with SCLC who respond to their chemotherapy regimens, because this has been shown to improve survival.[18]

The prognosis for patients with extensive-stage SCLC is, in part, determined by their performance status (see Tables 18-2 and 18-3), which is not surprising, given that SCLC is a rapidly progressing disease, and most patients come to therapy fairly debilitated. Age is a less important determinant of outcome than performance status for patients with SCLC who are being treated with chemotherapy. It is clear that fit elderly patients who otherwise have no prohibitive comorbid conditions can be treated as aggressively as their younger counterparts.[19]

Ultimately patients with advanced SCLC are likely to benefit from systemic therapy, but they are not likely to be cured or to survive beyond 2 years from the time of diagnosis.

THERAPEUTIC MANAGEMENT OF ADVANCED NON–SMALL CELL LUNG CANCER

ROLE OF CYTOTOXIC CHEMOTHERAPY

Until the mid-1990s, the management of advanced NSCLC focused primarily on the use of supportive care to ease the suffering endured by these patients. Systemic cytotoxic chemotherapy was thought to be an investigational option, reserved for patients who participated in clinical trials. Many such trials were undertaken, and a number of these compared chemotherapy regimens with the best supportive care. Two landmark reports examined the role of chemotherapy in patients with NSCLC. In the first report

Souquet et al[20] carried out a meta-analysis with individual patient data from seven trials and more than 700 patients. The trials were included because they compared multiagent chemotherapy with supportive care. The analysis clearly showed a benefit in survival and in quality of life at 6 months in favor of chemotherapy. The second report, authored by the Non-Small Cell Lung Cancer Collaborative Group, consisted of a meta-analysis of more than 50 trials that compared chemotherapy and supportive care with supportive care alone. This analysis determined that platinum-based chemotherapy yielded a 27% reduction in the risk of death from lung cancer, which translated into a 10% survival difference at 1 year in favor of chemotherapy.[21] Taken together, both of these reports dispelled the prevailing notion that systemic therapy was not effective for lung cancer and opened the door to additional investigations on the optimal combination of chemotherapy for patients with advanced NSCLC. Although the benefit of chemotherapy determined in these analyses was small, it was on the same order of magnitude as the benefits seen in patients with other common cancers in whom chemotherapy was readily accepted and endorsed, namely, breast cancer.

In the months and years that followed these reports, several of the second-generation chemotherapy compounds listed in Table 18-1 became available for testing in patient populations with lung cancer. These newer agents were thought to be less toxic and more active than their predecessors. Many trials were carried out that yielded clear advances in the treatment of patients with advanced disease. Through these efforts we identified certain key factors to help define which patients with lung cancer might be best suited for aggressive intervention. In particular we realized that a patient's performance status, as defined in Tables 18-2 and 18-3,[22,23] is more important than age when it comes tolerating cytotoxic chemotherapy.[24,25] In the case of patients with bone and spinal metastases, it is clear that patients whose performance status allow for surgical interventions to manage their spine lesions should also allow them to be considered candidates for systemic therapy at some point in their management.

Additional trials performed during this time period helped define the role that platinum compounds (cis-platinum and carboplatinum) play in the first-line management of advanced NSCLC. Several trials have shown that the platinum compounds are ideal partners to the drugs listed in Table 18-1.

The Eastern Cooperative Oncology Group (ECOG) carried out a seminal clinical trial in the late 1990s that compared four platinum-based regimens. The trial revealed that none of these regimens was superior, in terms of efficacy or toxicity, to the others, and one could expect a median survival of 8 months, along with a response rate of approximately 30% with these agents.[26]

Additional studies performed by other investigative groups during that same period allowed us to reach some conclusions defining to whom and how cytotoxic chemotherapy should be delivered to patients with advanced lung cancer. It became clear that performance status is more important than age in determining whether a patient receives chemotherapy. In other words, a fit elderly patient with minor comorbidity is a better candidate for chemotherapy than a chronically ill younger patient with multiple

Table 18-1 Second-Generation Cytotoxic Compounds Used to Treat Patients With Lung Cancer

Agent	Active Alone	Commonly Combined With	FDA Approved for Lung Cancer
Vinorelbine	Yes	Cis-platinum Carboplatinum Gemcitabine Docetaxel Cetuximab	Yes
Gemcitabine	Yes	Cis-platinum Carboplatinum Vinorelbine Bevacizumab	Yes
Paclitaxel	Yes	Cis-platinum Carboplatinum Bevacizumab	Yes
Docetaxel	Yes	Cis-platinum Carboplatinum Vinorelbine	Yes
Irinotecan	Yes	Cis-platinum Carboplatinum	No
Pemetrexed	Yes	Cis-platinum Carboplatinum Bevacizumab	Yes

comorbid conditions. More debilitated patients can be treated with chemotherapy, but they should be offered single-agent therapy in combination with one of the partner agents (see Table 18-1) commonly combined with platinum, while avoiding platinum. Conversely, patients who are physically fit are likely to respond better and survive longer with a platinum-based pair than with a single drug.[27,28] Finally, a meta-analysis of studies exploring the addition of a third cytotoxic drug to a platinum-based combination showed convincingly that the third cytotoxic drug, while raising the response rate, increased the toxicity without improving survival.[27] So the bottom line is that fit patients with advanced NSCLC who have spinal metastases should be considered for chemotherapy with a platinum-containing doublet after they have recovered from spine surgery. Patients who are not as fit can be offered non-platinum–containing single agents. Severely debilitated patients who are not surgical candidates should be treated with comfort care measures.

Table 18-2 Karnofsky Performance Status Scale Definitions Rating (%) Criteria

Criteria	Rating	Description
Able to carry on normal activity and to work; no special care needed	100	Normal, no complaints; no evidence of disease
	90	Able to carry on normal activity; minor signs or symptoms of disease
	80	Normal activity with effort; some signs or symptoms of disease
Unable to work; able to live at home and care for most personal needs; varying amount of assistance needed	70	Able to care for self; unable to carry on normal activity or do active work
	60	Requires occasional assistance but is able to care for most personal needs
	50	Requires considerable assistance and frequent medical care
Unable to care for self; requires equivalent of institutional or hospital care; disease may be progressing rapidly	40	Disabled; requires special care and assistance
	30	Severely disabled; hospital admission is indicated although death not imminent
	20	
	10	Very sick; hospital admission necessary; active supportive treatment necessary
	0	Moribund; fatal processes progressing rapidly Dead

Table 18-3 ECOG/WHO Zubrod Scale

Zubrod Scale	Equivalent Karnofsky Scale
0 = Asymptomatic	100
1 = Symptomatic but completely ambulant	90-70
2 = Symptomatic, <50% in bed during the day	60-50
3 = Symptomatic, >50% in bed, but not bed bound	40-30
4 = Bed bound	20-10
5 = Death	0

A few groups also investigated the optimal duration of treatment as it became clear that an indefinite duration of treatment could be associated with significant toxicity. Several studies compared the use of longer regimens versus shorter ones and showed that the shorter regimens were just as effective and were associated with a better quality of life than the longer ones.[29-33] Consequently it has become accepted practice to limit the duration of chemotherapy to four to six cycles.

ROLE OF SECOND-LINE CYTOTOXIC CHEMOTHERAPY

With all of these improvements in first-line treatment options, patients have clearly been living longer, yet their disease still progresses because the initial treatment has limited efficacy. Furthermore, many of these patients who have recently progressed still possess the kind of strong performance status that could allow further treatment. So we have seen a great many clinical investigating second-line treatments for patients with progressing lung cancer. Docetaxel was the first agent approved by the United States Food and Drug Administration (FDA) for use in lung cancer as a second-line drug. It was studied in two large phase III randomized clinical trials; one of the trials compared docetaxel with the best supportive care to show that patients who received the drug had a longer time to progression and survival as well as higher 1-year survival rates.[34] Docetaxel is not without significant side effects that can have a negative impact on quality of life, such as asthenia and neuropathy, both of which can be severely debilitating; thus additional efforts have led to a comparison of docetaxel and pemetrexed. Although both drugs prolong survival in a similar manner, pemetrexed is clearly better tolerated,[35] which led to its approval as a second-line option for patients with progressing NSCLC. It should be noted that although the actual radiographic response rate for these patients is low, the degree of clinical benefit is the result of clear disease stabilization, which allows patients to have an improved quality of life as well as a longer survival. Patients whose spinal metastases may be evident once they have completed their first-line chemotherapy are still candidates for these second-line chemotherapy interventions, as long as their performance status allows it.

BEYOND CHEMOTHERAPY ALONE

Targeting the Vascular Endothelial Growth Factor Pathway

Cytotoxic chemotherapy quickly reaches a therapeutic plateau when patients are treated with the conventional doublet strategy. Furthermore, the addition of another cytotoxic drug does not produce enough of a clinical benefit to make the increased toxicity of the new combination worth the risk. To improve the results of the current combinations, we needed to develop combinations without additive toxic effects. As our understanding of cancer biology has grown dramatically in recent years, it has become clear that the growth of a lung cancer tumor may depend, in part, on acquiring the ability to secure an adequate blood supply to support that growth.[36] The concept that cancer cells will drive neoangiogenesis, or the formation of new blood vessels, is now recognized as one of several characteristics that define cancer cells.[37] Vascular endothelial growth factor (VEGF) has been identified as an essential molecule to stimulate angiogenesis.[38] In addition, the overexpression of VEGF, as well as the excessive growth of new vessels in a tumor, has been negatively linked to prognosis in many types of cancer, including lung cancer.[39] Consequently targeting VEGF or its receptors has been an area of intense investigation. Bevacizumab became the first monoclonal antibody directed against VEGF and its isoforms to be approved by the FDA for the treatment of first-line NSCLC. Sandler et al[40] reported improvements in response rates, median survival, and overall survival among 878 patients randomized in a phase III clinical trial of platinum chemotherapy plus or minus bevacizumab. The improvement in survival comes at a cost, however. Bevacizumab is associated with a number of toxic effects, such as hypertension (an effect seen as a class effect with other VEGF/VEGF receptor inhibitors), wound-healing delays, and fatal tumor-related bleeding. However, these effects can be mitigated with judicious patient selection. Therefore it is crucial to treat only those patients with nonsquamous histologic findings who do not have centrally located tumors that could be involving large mediastinal blood vessels and who have not had hemoptysis as a presenting symptom. When dealing with patients with spinal metastases who may require extensive surgical repair, it is imperative to observe at least a 4-week delay between the administration of the last dose of bevacizumab and the need for surgical intervention. The recent use of a drug such as bevacizumab could lead to disastrous postoperative wound dehiscence, hardware failure, and added postoperative morbidity. Additional compounds that are being developed to target the VEGF pathway are listed in Table 18-4.[41] Some of these agents are administered intravenously, whereas others are administered orally. The oral agents belong to a class of small molecules, the tyrosine kinase inhibitors. Generally they tend to target several important pathways at once. All agents listed in Table 18-4 are still in clinical trials for use in patients with NSCLC. Three of these agents have been approved by the FDA for other cancer-related indications: sorafenib, sunitinib, and pazopanib for the treatment of renal cell carcinoma and sorafenib for the treatment of hepatocellular carcinoma.

Table 18-4 Promising Oral Anti-VEGF Inhibitors in Development for Treatment of Advanced Non–Small Cell Lung Cancer

Agent	Targets	Phase of Development	Comments
Sorafenib	VEGFR, RAF, PDGFR, C-KIT	III	FDA approved for treatment of RCC and HCC
Motesanib	VEGFR, PDGFR, C-KIT	II/III	Developed in combination with chemotherapy
Sunitinib	VEGFR, PDGFR, C-KIT	II	FDA approved for treatment of GIST
Axitinib	VEGFR, PDGFR, C-KIT	II	
Pazopanib	VEGFR, PDGFR, C-KIT	II	Developed in combination with chemotherapy
ABT-869	VEGFR, PDGFR	II	
BIBF1120	VEGFR, PDGFR, FGFR	I	Developed in combination with chemotherapy
BMS-690514	VEGFR, EGFR	I	In combination with chemotherapy

Adapted from Pallis AG, Serfass L, Dziadziusko R, et al. Targeted therapies in the treatment of advanced/metastatic NSCLC. Euro J Cancer 45:2473-2487, 2009.
C-KIT, C-KIT receptor; *EGFR,* epidermal growth factor receptor; *FGFR,* fibroblast growth factor receptor; *GIST,* gastrointestinal stromal tumor; *HCC,* hepatocellular carcinoma; *PDGFR,* platelet-derived growth factor receptor; *RAF,* rapidly accelerated fibrosarcoma; *RCC,* renal cell carcinoma; *VEGFR,* Vascular endothelial growth factor receptor.

Although these oral agents are generally well tolerated, they can cause hypertension and proteinuria similar to that seen with bevacizumab. In addition, these drugs may also affect wound healing in a manner similar to bevacizumab. Their half-lives tend to be much shorter than that of bevacizumab, so they may be easier to integrate in the care of patients who might require spine surgery.

Targeting the Epidermal Growth Factor Pathway

The epidermal growth factor pathway is involved in cell growth, neoangiogenesis, and cell survival. Endothelial growth factor activates the pathway through binding to the epidermal growth factor receptor (EGFR). Once the ligand binds the receptor, the receptor dimerizes, which in turn activates a tyrosine kinase enzyme, which phosphorylates a secondary protein that, in turn, activates an additional protein in this particular pathway, leading to the end result of cell amplification. Lung cancer cells can harness the power of this pathway in several ways. They can amplify the gene coding for the receptors, which will result in overexpression of the receptor. They can also mutate the gene that codes for the receptor in such a way as to yield an activating mutation. This activating mutation generally results in a growth and expansion advantage for the cancer cells. The mutations that lead to this activating and advantageous result usually occur in a portion of the gene that codes for amino acids in an adenosine triphosphate binding region of the tyrosine kinase associated with the EGFR.[42,43] In effect, the mutated cancer cells become very dependent on the activated EGFR pathway, and disruption of the activity of the tyrosine kinase yields impressive cancer control effects in patients with advanced NSCLC harboring these mutations. Phase II and phase III clinical trials of these tyrosine kinase inhibitors have established the effectiveness of gefitinib and erlotinib.[44,45] Both of these drugs are oral agents, with modest toxicity profiles; the major side effects include an acneiform rash and easily controlled diarrhea. It is noteworthy that the intensity of the rash does correlate with the response to the agent.[46] Erlotinib is currently approved as a second-line or third-line option for patients with advanced NSCLC in North America and Europe, whereas gefitinib is approved in Asia. Furthermore, investigations into the mechanisms of activity have allowed us to define the population likely to harbor a favorable mutation that could lead to a positive result. These drugs are most likely to work effectively in nonsmoking female Asian patients with adenocarcinoma of the lungs, because a high percentage of this particular group of patients is likely to harbor an activating mutation. A recent study, the Iressa Pan-Asia Study coordinated by Mok et al[47] in Hong Kong, included primarily patients who were light smokers or who had never smoked, in an effort to increase the proportion of patients harboring activating mutations. Patients were then randomized to either upfront standard, platinum doublet chemotherapy or gefitinib. The trial showed convincingly that patients who harbored mutations benefited from gefitinib therapy, whereas patients without mutations benefited from standard chemotherapy. The results of the Iressa Pan-Asia Study established a standard of care for a very narrow patient population that harbors a specific molecular defect, rendering it vulnerable to a precisely targeted therapeutic approach. However, such precision is not yet possible for the vast majority of patients with lung cancer.

A great deal of effort has been focused on trying to identify new therapeutic targets that would apply to a broader segment of the population. Until such new targets and their corresponding inhibitors are identified and validated, standard chemotherapeutic combinations will continue to apply.

Preventing/Neutralizing Bone Metastases?

As patients with lung cancer continue to survive longer through the use of more effective therapies, their risk of developing complications from bone metastases increases. Metastatic disease of bone is generally considered less sensitive to chemotherapy than metastases at other common sites.[48] Skeletal-related events, such as pathologic fractures or spinal cord compression, are associated with tremendous impact on quality of life and general impairment of function. The bone microenvironment releases growth factors during osteolysis,[49] which accentuate further osteoclast activity.[50] In addition, the microenvironment can also release tumor growth factors that will, in turn, cause further osteoclast activation and so on, aggressively driving the process forward.[51] Bisphosphonates are pyrophosphate analogues that bind to the bony matrix and inhibit the activity of osteoclasts, with zoledronic acid having the broadest activity profile as it can inhibit the activity of both osteolytic and osteoblastic metastases. Its effectiveness at decreasing the annual incidence of skeletal complications of bone metastases has been demonstrated in a phase III randomized placebo-controlled trial in patients with nonbreast and nonprostate cancers.[52] In addition, zoledronic acid has been demonstrated to be superior to prior generation bisphosphonates such as pamidronate.[53] Clinical trials to determine whether zoledronic acid can prevent the onset of bone metastases are presently underway.

Further insight into the molecular pathophysiology of bone remodeling reveals that it is under the control of the receptor activator of nuclear factor kB (RANK), the RANK ligand, and the osteoprotegerin pathway. In the setting of bone metastases, that pathway is disrupted and tumor cells can induce severe osteolysis through the unregulated expression of RANK or through the production of parathyroid hormone–related peptide (PTH-rp).[54] The RANK ligand binds to RANK on the surface of pro-osteoclasts to induce their differentiation to osteoclasts, which in turn actively causes bone resorption that leads to bone weakening and bone damage. Denosumab, a monoclonal antibody directed against RANK, is effective at suppressing bone resorption. Denosumab is being actively studied to define its role in the treatment of bone metastases caused by lung cancer.[54] Finally, the anti-EGFR tyrosine kinase that can be so effective in certain patients with NSCLC, Gefitinib, appears to reverse the damage caused by NSCLC spinal metastases.[55] In addition, gefitinib also appears to decrease the secretion of PTH-rp, which results also in decreased bone resorption.[56] Gefitinib has been reported also to inhibit the induction of osteoclast differentiation by decreasing the level of the RANK ligand expression.[57]

CONCLUSION

Although advanced lung cancer remains a daunting disease, with limited overall survival, novel therapeutic approaches are benefiting patients not only in terms of lengthening patient survival but also improving quality of life. Modern treatments more than double the traditional median survival expected from either best supportive care or traditional treatment strategies. Because spine and spinal cord lesions can dramatically compromise the quality of life and length of life that these patients might otherwise have, it is imperative that these patients be managed in a concerted multidisciplinary fashion if they are to reap all of the benefits of advances in neurospine surgery techniques and modern medical oncology interventions.

References (With Key References in Boldface)

1. Jemal A, Siegel R, Ward E, et al. Cancer statistics, 2009. CA Cancer J Clin 59:225-249, 2009.
2. Yang P, Allen MS, Aubry MC, et al. Clinical features of 5,628 primary lung cancer patients: experience at Mayo Clinic from 1997 to 2003. Chest 128:452-462, 2005.
3. Al Husaini H, Wheatley-Price P, Clemons M, et al. Prevention and management of bone metastases in lung cancer: a review. J Thorac Oncol 4:251-259, 2009.
4. Dubey S, Powell CA. Update in lung cancer 2008. Am J Respir Crit Care Med 179:860-868, 2009.
5. **Tsuya A, Kurata T, Tamura K, et al. Skeletal metastases in non-small cell lung cancer: a retrospective study. Lung Cancer 57:229-232, 2007.**
6. Aebi M. Spinal metastases in the elderly. Eur Spine J 12 (Suppl 2):S202-S213, 2003.
7. **Coleman, R. Skeletal complications of malignancy. Cancer 80:1588-1594, 1997.**
8. **Govindan R, Page N, Morgensztern D, et al. Changing epidemiology of small-cell lung cancer in the United States over the last 30 years: analysis of the surveillance, epidemiologic, and end results database. J Clin Oncol 24:4539-4544, 2006.**
9. Dowell J. Small cell lung cancer: are we making progress? Am J Med Sci 339:68-76, 2010.
10. Sculier JP, Feld R, Evans WK, et al. Neurologic disorders in patients with small cell lung cancer. Cancer 60:2275-2283, 1987.
11. **van Oosterhout AG, van de Pol M, ten Velde GP, et al. Neurologic disorders in 203 consecutive patients with small cell lung cancer. Results of a longitudinal study. Cancer 77:1434-1441, 1996.**
12. Ihde D. Small cell lung cancer. State-of-the-art therapy 1994. Chest 107 (Suppl):S243-S248, 1995.
13. Ihde D, Pass H. Small cell lung cancer. In DeVita V, Hellman S, Rosenberg S, eds. Cancer: Principles and Practice of Oncology, 5th ed. Philadelphia: Lippincott-Raven, 1997, pp 911-949.
14. Oze I, Hotta K, Katsuyuki K, et al. Twenty-seven years of phase III trials for patients with extensive disease small-cell lung cancer: disappointing results. PLoS One 4:e7835, 2009.
15. Noda K, Nishiwaki Y, Kawahara M, et al; Japan Clinical Oncology Group. Irinotecan plus cisplatin compared with etoposide plus cisplatin for extensive small-cell lung cancer. N Engl J Med 346:85-91, 2002.
16. Hanna N, Bunn PA Jr, Langer C, et al. Randomized phase III trial comparing irinotecan/cisplatin with etoposide/cisplatin in patients with previously untreated extensive-stage disease small-cell lung cancer. J Clin Oncol 24:2038-2043, 2006.
17. Lara PN Jr, Natale R, Crowley J, et al. Phase III trial of irinotecan/cisplatin compared with etoposide/cisplatin in extensive-stage small-cell lung cancer: clinical and pharmacogenomic results from SWOG S0124. J Clin Oncol 27:2530-2535, 2009.
18. **Slotman B, Faivre-Finn C, Kramer G, et al; EORTC Radiation Oncology Group and Lung Cancer Group. Prophylactic cranial irradiation in extensive small-cell lung cancer. N Engl J Med 357:664-672, 2007.**

19. Sekine I, Yamamoto N, Kunitoh H, et al. Treatment of small cell lung cancer in the elderly based on a critical literature review of clinical trials. Cancer Treat Rev 30:359-368, 2004.
20. Souquet PJ, Chauvin F, Boissel JP, et al. Polychemotherapy in advanced non small cell lung cancer: a meta-analysis. Lancet 342:19-21, 1993.
21. **Chemotherapy in non-small cell lung cancer: a meta-analysis using updated data on individual patients from 52 randomised clinical trials. Non-small Cell Lung Cancer Collaborative Group. BMJ 311:899-909, 1995.**
22. Oken MM, Creech RH, Tormey DC, et al. Toxicity and response criteria of the Eastern Cooperative Oncology Group. Am J Clin Oncol 5:649-655, 1982.
23. Schag CC, Heinrich RL, Ganz PA. Karnofsky performance status revisited: reliability, validity, and guidelines. J Clin Oncol 2:187-193, 1984.
24. Pfister DG, Johnson DH, Azzoli CG, et al. American Society of Clinical Oncology treatment of unresectable non-small-cell lung cancer guideline: update 2003. J Clin Oncol 22:330-353, 2004.
25. Socinski M, Crowell R, Hensing TE, et al. Treatment of non-small cell lung cancer, stage IV: ACCP evidence-based clinical practice guidelines (2nd edition). Chest 132:S277-S289, 2007.
26. **Schiller JH, Harrington D, Belani CP, et al; Eastern Cooperative Oncology Group. Comparison of four chemotherapy regimens for advanced non-small-cell lung cancer. N Engl J Med 346:92-98, 2002.**
27. Delbaldo C, Michiels S, Syz N, et al. Benefits of adding a drug to a single-agent or a 2-agent chemotherapy regimen in advanced non-small-cell lung cancer: a meta-analysis. JAMA 292:470-484, 2004.
28. **Lilenbaum RC, Herndon JE II, List MA, et al. Single-agent versus combination chemotherapy in advanced non-small-cell lung cancer: the cancer and leukemia group B (study 9730). J Clin Oncol 23:190-196, 2005.**
29. Smith I, O'Brien M, Talbot DC, et al. Duration of chemotherapy in advanced non-small cell lung cancer: A randomized trial of 3 versus 6 courses of mitomycin, vinblastine, cisplatin. J Clin Oncol 19:1336-1343, 2001.
30. Socinski MA, Schell MJ, Peterman A, et al. Phase III trial comparing a defined duration of therapy versus continuous therapy followed by second-line therapy in advanced-stage IIIB/IV non-small-cell lung cancer. J Clin Oncol 20:1335-1343, 2002.
31. von Plessen C, Bergman B, Andresen O, et al. Palliative chemotherapy beyond three courses conveys no survival or consistent quality-of-life benefits in advanced non-small-cell lung cancer. Br J Cancer 95:966-973, 2006.
32. Barata FJ, Parente B, Teixeira E, et al. Optimal duration of chemotherapy in non-small lung cancer: multicenter, randomized, prospective clinical trial comparing 4 vs. 6 cycles of carboplatinum and gemcitabine. J Thorac Oncol 2:S666, 2007.
33. Park JO, Kim SW, Ahn JS, et al. Phase III trial of two versus four additional cycles in patients who are nonprogressive after two cycles of platinum-based chemotherapy in non small-cell lung cancer. J Clin Oncol 25:5233-5239, 2007.
34. Shepherd FA, Dancey J, Ramlau R, et al. Prospective randomized trial of docetaxel versus best supportive care in patients with non-small-cell lung cancer previously treated with platinum-based chemotherapy. J Clin Oncol 18:2095-2103, 2000.
35. Hanna N, Shepherd FA, Fossella FV, et al. Randomized phase III trial of pemetrexed versus docetaxel in patients with non-small-cell lung cancer previously treated with chemotherapy. J Clin Oncol 22:1589-1597, 2004.
36. **Folkman J. Tumor angiogenesis. Adv Cancer Res 43:175-203, 1985.**
37. Hanahan D, Weinberg R. The hallmarks of cancer. Cell 100:57-70, 2000.
38. Ferrara N, Gerber HP, LeCouter J. The biology of VEGF and its receptors. Nat Med 9:669-676, 2003.
39. Jain RK, Duda DG, Clark JW, et al. Lessons from phase III clinical trials on anti-VEGF therapy for cancer. Nat Clin Pract Oncol 3:24-40, 2006.
40. **Sandler A, Gray R, Perry MC, et al. Paclitaxel-carboplatin alone or with bevacizumab for non-small-cell lung cancer. N Engl J Med 355:2542-2550, 2006.**

41. Pallis AG, Serfass L, Dziadziusko R, et al. Targeted therapies in the treatment of advanced/metastatic NSCLC. Euro J Cancer 45:2473-2487, 2009.
42. Lynch TJ, Bell DW, Sordella R, et al. Activating mutations in the epidermal growth factor receptor underlying responsiveness of non-small-cell lung cancer to gefitinib. N Engl J Med 350:2129-2139, 2004.
43. Paez JG, Jänne PA, Lee JC, et al. EGFR mutations in lung cancer: correlation with clinical response to gefitinib therapy. Science 304:1497-1500, 2004.
44. Kris MG, Natale RB, Herbst RS, et al. Efficacy of gefitinib, an inhibitor of the epidermal growth factor receptor tyrosine kinase, in symptomatic patients with non-small cell lung cancer: a randomized trial. JAMA 290:2149-2158, 2003.
45. Shepherd FA, Rodrigues Pereira J, Ciuleanu T, et al; National Cancer Institute of Canada Clinical Trials Group. Erlotinib in previously treated non-small-cell lung cancer. N Engl J Med 353:123-132, 2005.
46. Perez-Soler R, Chachoua A, Huberman M, et al. Final results from a phase II study of erlotinib (Tarceva) monotherapy in patients with advanced non-small cell lung cancer following failure of platinum-based chemotherapy. Lung Cancer 41 (Suppl 2):S246, 2003.
47. Mok TS, Wu YL, Thongprasert S, et al. Gefitinib or carboplatin-paclitaxel in pulmonary adenocarcinoma. N Engl J Med 361:947-957, 2009.
48. Langer C, Hirsh V. Skeletal morbidity in lung cancer patients with bone metastases: demonstrating the need for early diagnosis and treatment with bisphosphonates. Lung Cancer 67:4-11, 2010.
49. Mundy G. Mechanisms of bone metastasis. Cancer 80:1546-1556, 1997.
50. Saad F, Schulman CC. Role of bisphosphonates in prostate cancer. Eur Urol 45:26-34, 2004.
51. Kaukonen S, Mundy G. Mechanisms of osteolytic bone metastases in breast carcinoma. Cancer 97:834-839, 2003.
52. Rosen LS, Gordon D, Tchekmedyian NS, et al. Long-term efficacy and safety of zoledronic acid in the treatment of skeletal metastases in patients with nonsmall cell lung carcinoma and other solid tumors: a randomized, Phase III, double-blind, placebo-controlled trial. Cancer 100:2613-2621, 2004.
53. Lipton A, Small E, Saad F, et al. The new bisphosphonate, Zometa (zoledronic acid), decreases skeletal complications in both osteolytic and osteoblastic lesions: a comparison to pamidronate. Cancer Invest 20(Suppl 2):S45-S54, 2002.
54. Neville-Webbe HL, Coleman RE. Bisphosphonates and RANK ligand inhibitors for the treatment and prevention of metastatic bone disease. Eur J Cancer 46:1211-1222, 2010.
55. Zukawa M, Nakano N, Hirano N, et al. The effectiveness of gefitinib on spinal metastases of lung cancer—report of two cases. Asian Spine J 2:109-113, 2008.
56. Normanno N, Gullick WJ. Epidermal growth factor receptor tyrosine kinase inhibitors and bone metastases: different mechanisms of action for a novel therapeutic application? Endocr Relat Cancer 13:3-6, 2006.
57. Normanno N, De Luca A, Aldinucci D, et al. Gefitinib inhibits the ability of human bone marrow stromal cells to induce osteoclast differentiation: implications for the pathogenesis and treatment of bone metastasis. Endocr Relat Cancer 12:471-482, 2005.

Chapter 19

Renal Cell Carcinoma

Matthew Mei, Andrea L. Harzstark

Renal cell carcinoma (RCC) arises from the epithelial cells of the kidney and represents the large majority of kidney neoplasms in adults. There were 54,390 estimated new cases of kidney and renal pelvic cancers in the United States in 2008,[1] the large majority of which were RCCs, and the incidence continues to increase over time. RCC has always represented a clinical challenge, with respect to both diagnosis and management, given the variety of potential clinical presentations and a relative resistance to chemotherapy. Moreover, late recurrences of RCC many years after surgical resection are frequently observed.

Recent years have seen better classification of the cytogenetics of RCC, as well as the development of multiple new biological agents with proved efficacy against RCC. Previously patients with metastatic disease had few options for systemic therapy, aside from immunotherapy with either interleukin-2 (IL-2) or interferon alfa (IFN-α). A small but significant minority of patients who were able to tolerate the severe toxicities of IL-2 treatment experienced significant responses, and in a small proportion of patients, remissions lasting decades were observed. Moreover, the past 5 years have seen a dramatic change in the therapies available for RCC, with the application of targeted therapies to metastatic disease.

EPIDEMIOLOGY

RCC is primarily a disease of older persons, with an average age of onset in the seventh decade of life. Men are more likely to develop RCC than women, and RCC is more common in African-Americans than in persons of other ethnicities. The incidence of RCC has increased over time from 8.6 to 11.2 cases per 100,000 individuals between 1988 and 2002.[2] Although improved abdominal imaging is likely partially responsible for some of this trend, late-stage disease is also becoming more common, suggesting that the true overall incidence is increasing.[3] The specific cause is unknown, although the increased prevalence of obesity has been cited as a potential etiologic factor.[4]

Many risk factors for the development of RCC have been identified. Modifiable risk factors include smoking,[5] obesity, hypertension, and acquired cystic disease of the kidney (usually in patients on chronic dialysis).[6] Various studies have examined the link between occupational toxins, including asbestos, trichloroethylene solvent, gasoline, and cadmium, with somewhat mixed results. Moderate alcohol consumption may decrease the risk of RCC.[7]

DIAGNOSIS

Traditionally, RCC is associated with the triad of hematuria, flank pain, and a palpable abdominal mass, although this classic presentation is becoming less common over time. Other clinical manifestations, such as scrotal varicoceles from gonadal vein obstruction and lower extremity edema from inferior vena cava invasion, are associated with locally advanced disease. Distant metastatic disease is present at the time of diagnosis in approximately 20% of patients.[8] RCC has been associated with a wide variety of paraneoplastic syndromes, including anemia and erythrocytosis, weight loss, fever, hepatic dysfunction (Stauffer's syndrome), hypercalcemia, and polymyalgia rheumatica. With the development of advanced imaging techniques, RCC is being detected incidentally with increasing frequency; in one study the percentage of RCCs detected incidentally rose from 13% in 1982 to 1983 to 60% in 1996 to 1997.[9]

HISTOPATHOLOGY

At present, RCC is divided into six histopathologic subtypes: clear cell, papillary, chromophobe, collecting duct (also known as Bellini duct), oncocytoma, and unclassified.[10] Although there are rare reports of metastatic oncocytoma,[11] in general, its behavior is benign. Clear cell carcinoma accounts for more than 70% to 80% of cases of RCC, whereas the frequency of the other histologic subtypes is as follows: papillary 9% to 19%, chromophobe 2% to 6%, oncocytoma 7%, and collecting duct less than 1%.[12-14]

Pathologists have formulated numerous grading systems for RCC; of those, the Fuhrman system (Table 19-1), which is based on nuclear morphology and has four tiers, is the most widely used.[15] However, RCC grading is problematic because of a lack of interobserver reliability,[16] as well as histologic heterogeneity, with areas of different grades in the same tumor.[15] Nonetheless, tumor grade has been found to be an independent prognostic factor in RCC.

GENETIC SYNDROMES

Although the overwhelming majority of RCCs is thought to be sporadic, multiple familial genetic syndromes that convey a predisposition toward developing RCC have been identified. Indications that patients may have an inherited syndrome that predisposes them to RCC include early age of onset, bilaterality of RCC, and multiple tumors. The most well-known genetic disease associated with RCC is von Hippel-

Table 19-1 Fuhrman Grading System

Grade	Histologic Features
1	Small nuclei (<10 μm); nucleoli are invisible
2	Larger nuclei (approximately 15 μm) with irregularities in outline; nucleoli are invisible at low power
3	Even large nuclei (>20 μm) with irregularities in outline; nucleoli are visible at low power
4	Bizarrely shaped nuclei with clumped irregular chromatin; nucleoli are large

Table 19-2 Inherited Renal Cell Carcinoma (RCC) Syndromes

Syndrome	RCC Subtype	Genetic Defect	Other Clinical Features
VHL	Clear cell	VHL	Hemangioblastoma, pheochromocytoma
HPRCC	Papillary, type 1	MET	None
HLRCC	Papillary, type 2	FH	Cutaneous and uterine leiomyomas
BHD	Chromophobe	FLCN	Hair follicle hamartomas, spontaneous pneumothorax[21]

BHD, Birt-Hogg-Dubé; *FH*, fumarate hydratase; *FLCN*, folliculin; *HLRCC*, hereditary leiomyomatosis and RCC; *HPRCC*, hereditary papillary RCC; *VHL*, von Hippel-Lindau.

Lindau disease (VHLD), which is an autosomal dominant disease caused by mutation of the tumor suppressor gene VHL on chromosome 3p. Affected patients are prone to develop hemangioblastoma, clear cell RCC, pheochromocytoma, and other neoplasms. The prevalence is approximately 1 in 36,000 live births, and the incidence of RCC in these patients is approximately 25% to 60%, with an average age of onset of 39 years.[17] Chromosome 3 translocations have been identified as the cause in non-VHLD familial clear RCC as well.

Other inherited RCC syndromes include hereditary papillary RCC (HPRCC), hereditary leiomyomatosis RCC (HLRCC), and Birt-Hogg-Dubé (BHD) syndrome. HPRCC is caused by a germline mutation in MET, a protooncogene located on chromosome 7q, and is characterized by multiple bilateral type 1 papillary RCCs.[18] HLRCC is the result of a germline mutation in a gene located on chromosome 1q, which codes for fumarate hydratase, an enzyme involved in the Krebs cycle. Affected patients also develop cutaneous and uterine leiomyomas.[19] Finally, BHD syndrome arises from a mutation in a gene on chromosome 17p encoding the protein folliculin, the function of which is unknown.[20] Table 19-2 lists four of the most well-known inherited syndromes associated with RCC, all of which are characterized by an autosomal dominant mode of transmission.

Table 19-3 American Joint Committee on Cancer Staging TNM Stages for Renal Cell Carcinoma

Primary Tumor (T)

TX	Primary tumor cannot be assessed
T0	No evidence of primary tumor
T1	Tumor 7 cm or less in diameter and limited to the kidney
T1a	Tumor 4 cm or less in greatest dimension and limited to kidney
T1b	Tumor more than 4 cm but not more than 7 cm and limited to kidney
T2	Tumor more than 7 cm in greatest dimension limited to the kidney
T3	Tumor extends into major veins or invades the adrenal gland or perinephric tissues but not beyond Gerota's fascia
T3a	Tumor directly invades the adrenal gland or perinephric tissues but not beyond Gerota's fascia
T3b	Tumor grossly extends into the renal vein or its segmental (muscle-containing) branches, or vena cava below the diaphragm
T3c	Tumor grossly extends into the vena cava above the diaphragm or invades the wall of the vena cava
T4	Tumor invades beyond Gerota's fascia

Regional Lymph Nodes (N)*

NX	Regional lymph nodes cannot be assessed
N0	No regional lymph node metastases
N1	Metastasis in a single regional lymph node
N2	Metastases in more than one regional lymph node

Distant Metastasis (M)

MX	Distant metastasis cannot be assessed
M0	No distant metastasis
M1	Distant metastasis

Used with permission from the American Joint Committee on Cancer (AJCC), Chicago, Illinois. The original source for this material is the AJCC Cancer Staging Manual, 7th ed. Springer Science and Business Media, LLC, 2010.
*Laterality does not affect the node classification.

STAGING

The most commonly used staging method for RCC is the American Joint Committee on Cancer (AJCC) staging system, which is based on the tumor node metastasis (TNM) classification (Tables 19-3 and 19-4).[22]

Abdominal CT is the imaging modality of choice to evaluate the extent of local disease. Although administration of intravenous contrast material is ideal, renal insufficiency is very common in patients with RCC; a noncontrast CT scan or MRI performed without gadolinium is a reasonable alternative. CT scans of the chest are typically used to evaluate patients for pulmonary metastases because the sensitivity of chest radiographs is low. Although bony metastases are common, a bone scan is rarely positive when there is only limited-stage disease (T1-3aN0M0) and lack of bone pain.[23] A reasonable approach is to obtain a bone scan in the setting of either bone pain or an elevated alkaline phosphatase level.

Table 19-4 Stage Grouping for Renal Cell Carcinoma Based on the American Joint Committee on Cancer TNM Stages

Stage	T	N	M
Stage I	T1	N0	M0
Stage II	T2	N0	M0
Stage III	T1	N1	M0
	T2	N1	M0
	T3	N0	M0
	T3	N1	M0
	T3a	N0	M0
	T3a	N1	M0
	T3b	N0	M0
	T3b	N1	M0
	T3c	N0	M0
	T3c	N1	M0
Stage IV	T4	N0	M0
	T4	N1	M0
	Any T	N2	M0
	Any T	Any N	M1

Used with permission from the American Joint Committee on Cancer (AJCC), Chicago, Illinois. The original source for this material is the AJCC Cancer Staging Manual, 7th ed. Springer Science and Business Media, LLC, 2010.

TREATMENT

Surgery is the treatment of choice for limited-stage disease in stages I, II, and III and offers the best chance for a cure. Although late recurrences can appear many years after resection of initially limited disease, no therapy has yet been shown to have clinical efficacy in the adjuvant setting.[24] In the presence of metastatic disease, cytotoxic nephrectomy has been shown to improve overall survival in patients subsequently treated with IFN-α.[25,26] Randomized studies to evaluate the benefit of targeted therapy in the adjuvant setting are ongoing. There are no randomized prospective trials examining the role of nephrectomy before the administration of high-dose IL-2, and there are no data specifically examining the clinical effect of nephrectomy in the era of molecularly targeted therapy.

CHEMOTHERAPY

Cytotoxic chemotherapy has been shown to have poor response rates in metastatic RCC[27] and is rarely used. Many agents have been studied, but none has demonstrated a response rate that merits its use as a first-line therapy.[28]

IMMUNOTHERAPY

Immunotherapy with IL-2 and IFN-α has been shown to induce significant responses in a specific minority of patients. In particular, high-dose IL-2 therapy has been associated with sustained complete tumor regression in a small number of patients,[29]

although it also causes severe toxicity, including severe hemodynamic perturbations,[30] and requires a high level of monitoring during administration. IFN-α has been studied both as monotherapy and in combination with other agents; although it has an acceptable toxicity profile, the response rate is modest at best,[31] and it is no longer considered first-line therapy.

MOLECULAR AGENTS

Advances in understanding the molecular basis of RCC have led to the application of molecularly targeted agents to RCC therapy, and a number of these biological agents have demonstrated efficacy in metastatic RCC.

Overproduction of vascular endothelial growth factor (VEGF) has been implicated in the pathogenesis of many clear cell RCCs. Two tyrosine kinase inhibitors that target VEGF receptors have demonstrated efficacy in metastatic RCC. Sunitinib (Sutent; Pfizer, New York, NY) was demonstrated to prolong overall survival compared with IFN-α in a randomized phase III study.[32] Sorafenib (Nexavar; Bayer, Pittsburgh, PA) has been shown to prolong progression-free survival in metastatic RCC compared with placebo in a phase III study, although overall survival was unchanged.[33] Both agents can cause significant hypertension,[34,35] and sunitinib has also been linked to diminished left ventricular function,[36] with one series reporting the development of symptomatic grade III or IV heart failure in 15% of patients taking sunitinib.[37] The mechanism of the hypertension is not entirely clear, but decreased levels of nitric oxide as well as reduced numbers of small vessels have been postulated.[38] Compensatory increases in VEGF levels may also play a role. Hand-foot syndrome, diarrhea, fatigue, and bone marrow suppression are also well-described side effects.[39] Abnormal thyroid function tests consistent with hypothyroidism were reported in 85% of patients receiving sunitinib in one series[40]; hypothyroidism appears to be significantly less common with sorafenib administration.[41] Bevacizumab (Avastin; Genentech/Roche, San Francisco, CA), a monoclonal antibody against the VEGF protein, has shown to improve progression-free survival in conjunction with IFN-α, compared to IFN-α alone, in metastatic RCC in two separate phase III studies.[42,43] Although it has not been approved by the FDA thus far for treatment of RCC, approval is expected to be granted soon for use in combination with IFN-α.

Mammalian target of rapamycin (mTOR) is a serine/threonine protein kinase with an important role in cell proliferation,[44] as well as in response to hypoxia-induced stress.[45] Two small-molecule inhibitors of mTOR have demonstrated clinical activity against RCC. In a recent phase III trial, temsirolimus was shown to prolong both overall survival and progression-free survival, compared with IFN-α, in patients with previously untreated, poor-prognosis metastatic RCC. Notable toxicities included peripheral edema, rash, hyperglycemia, and hyperlipidemia.[46] Another phase III trial showed that everolimus prolonged progression-free survival compared with placebo in patients who had metastatic RCC that had been previously treated with sunitinib, sorafenib, or both. Significant toxicities included stomatitis, infections, and noninfectious pneumonitis.[47] The latter typically appears as either dyspnea on exertion or a dry cough, with radiographic findings of ground-glass opacities or pulmonary consolidation. Pulmonary function tests may also demonstrate restrictive physiology or a decreased diffusing capacity for carbon monoxide, and the drug should be withheld if evidence of pneumonitis is present, although it can often be restarted at a lower dose.[48]

Adjuvant Therapy

Data are currently lacking regarding molecular targeted therapy in the adjuvant setting, and at least three phase III trials are being conducted to examine the role of adjuvant sorafenib or sunitinib after resection of high-risk RCC: ASSURE (sorafenib or sunitinib versus placebo), S-TRAC (sunitinib versus placebo), and SORCE (sorafenib versus placebo). Preoperative VEGF TRIs and bevacizumab apparently do not increase surgical morbidity,[49] and prospective studies are under way to evaluate multiple VEGF TRIs in the neoadjuvant setting.[50,51]

THERAPIES FOR BONE METASTASES

Up to 30% of patients with advanced RCC will develop bone metastases, which are usually osteolytic in nature. The most common sites for bony disease are the pelvis, ribs, and spine. These are a significant source of pain and can also result in pathologic fractures and spinal compression.[52] Potential therapies for bony lesions that have been shown to be beneficial in RCC include bisphosphonate therapy with zoledronic acid, rank liquid inhibitor therapy with denosumab, radiation therapy, and surgery. A phase III study of zoledronic acid in metastatic solid tumors, excluding breast and prostate cancer, demonstrated a decreased number of patients with skeletal-related events, defined as pathologic fracture, spinal cord compression, radiation to bone, and surgery to bone. Although not stratified to examine patients with RCC separately, zoledronic acid significantly reduced the number of patients suffering at least one skeletal-related event in the RCC subset.[53]

PROGNOSIS

Prognosis in RCC is influenced by many factors; the TNM stage is the most important. The 5-year survival rate for patients with stage I disease is more than 90%, and stage II disease is associated with a survival rate of approximately 75% to 95% at 5 years.[54] Stage III disease confers a 5-year survival of approximately 60% to 70%, and the prognosis of patients with stage IV disease is poor, with 5-year survival ranging from 15% to 30%. Distant metastatic disease is associated with an extremely poor prognosis with a 5-year survival of less than 10%.

Histopathologic grade is also an important determinant of prognosis in RCC, with nuclear morphology being the key component. The histologic subtype itself has not been definitively established as an independent prognostic variable in RCC when controlled for other clinical variables.[14]

Numerous prognostic factors have been found to significantly affect survival in stage IV RCC. These include low Karnofsky performance status, a high serum lactate dehydrogenase level, anemia, hypercalcemia, and lack of prior nephrectomy. Patients at high risk (defined as having three or more risk factors), moderate risk (defined as having two or more risk factors), and low risk (defined as no risk factors) have median survival rates of 4 months, 10 months, and 20 months, respectively,[55] although these data were obtained before the advent of targeted therapy. A newer model exists that includes data from the targeted therapies, but it has not been externally validated. Other clinical factors with prognostic relevance include thrombocytosis[56] and the presence of clinical symptoms, such as hematuria, flank pain, and weight loss.[57]

CONCLUSION

Much progress has been made in the field of RCC in recent years. Refinements in molecular biology have allowed more precise classification of RCC subtypes, and the advent of molecularly targeted therapies has resulted in a significant improvement in clinical outcomes. Although the new developments in RCC are very exciting, we should not lose sight of the fact that advanced-stage disease still portends a poor prognosis, while the overall incidence of RCC continues to increase. Challenges abound in all aspects of RCC research, and further advances are urgently needed to combat this disease.

TIPS FROM THE MASTERS

- RCC is one of the more common types of tumors to require surgery for spinal metastatic disease. This is due, in part, to its relative resistance to radiation therapy and variable response to chemotherapy.
- High-dose single-fraction stereotactic radiosurgery has recently shown promising results with doses ranging from 16 to 24 Gy in single fractions.
- A combination of surgical stabilization with spinal cord decompression and spinal radiosurgery should be considered, especially in patients with spinal cord compression.
- More aggressive surgical strategies, including radical gross total intralesional resection or even en bloc spondylectomy, may be used for truly isolated spinal metastatic disease for better long-term control.

References (With Key References in Boldface)

1. Jemal A, Siegel R, Ward E, et al. Cancer statistics, 2008. CA Cancer J Clin 58:71-96, 2008.
2. Nguyen MM, Gill IS, Ellison LM. The evolving presentation of renal carcinoma in the United States: trends from the Surveillance, Epidemiology, and End Results program. J Urol 176 (6 Pt 1): 2397-2400, 2006.
3. Hock LM, Lynch J, Balaji KC. Increasing incidence of all stages of kidney cancer in the last 2 decades in the United States: an analysis of surveillance, epidemiology and end results program data. J Urol 167:57-60, 2002.
4. Decastro GJ, McKiernan JM. Epidemiology, clinical staging, and presentation of renal cell carcinoma. Urol Clin North Am 35:581-592, 2008.
5. Hunt JD, van der Hel OL, McMillan GP, et al. Epidemiology, clinical staging, and presentation of renal cell carcinoma. Int J Cancer 114:101-108, 2005.
6. Truong LD, Krishnan B, Cao JT. Renal neoplasm in acquired cystic kidney disease. Am J Kidney Dis 26:1-12, 1995.
7. Greving JP, Lee JE, Wolk A, et al. Alcoholic beverages and risk of renal cell cancer. Br J Cancer 97:429-433, 2007.
8. Horner MJ, Ries LAG, Krapcho M, et al. SEER Cancer Statistics Review, 1975-2006. *Available at: http://seer.cancer.gov/csr/1975_2006.*
9. Luciani LG, Cestari R, Tallarigo C. Incidental renal cell carcinoma-age and stage characterization and clinical implications: study of 1092 patients (1982-1997). Urology 56:58-62, 2000.
10. Kovacs G, Akhtar M, Beckwith BJ, et al. The Heidelberg classification of renal cell tumours. J Pathol 183:131-133, 1997.
11. Perez-Ordonez B, Hamed G, Campbell S, et al. Renal oncocytoma: a clinicopathologic study of 70 cases. Am J Surg Pathol 21:871-883, 1997.
12. Amin MB, Amin MB, Tamboli P, et al. Prognostic impact of histologic subtyping of adult renal epithelial neoplasms: an experience of 405 cases. Am J Surg Pathol 26:281-291, 2002.
13. Cheville JC, Lohse CM, Zincke H, et al. Comparisons of outcome and prognostic features among histologic subtypes of renal cell carcinoma. Am J Surg Pathol 27:612-624, 2003.
14. Patard J, Leray E, Rioux-Leclercq N, et al. Prognostic value of histologic subtypes in renal cell carcinoma: a multicenter experience. J Clin Oncol 23:2763-2771, 2005.
15. Novara G, Martignoni G, Artibani W, et al. Grading systems in renal cell carcinoma. J Urol 177:430-436, 2007.
16. Lanigan D, Conroy R, Barry-Walsh C. A comparative analysis of grading systems in renal adenocarcinoma. Histopathology 24:473-476, 1994.
17. Lonser RR, Glenn GM, Walther M, et al. von Hippel-Landau disease. Lancet 361:2059-2067, 2003.
18. Schmidt L, Duh FM, Chen F, et al. Germline and somatic mutations in the tyrosine kinase domain of the MET proto-oncogene in papillary renal carcinomas. Nat Genet 16:68-73, 1997.
19. Cohen D, Zhou M. Molecular genetics of familial renal cell carcinoma syndromes. Clin Lab Med 25:259-277, 2005.
20. Linehan WM, Pinto PA, Bratslavsky G, et al. Hereditary kidney cancer: unique opportunity for disease-based therapy. Cancer 115 (10 Suppl):S2252-S2261, 2009.
21. Nickerson ML, Warren MB, Toro JR, et al. Mutations in a novel gene lead to kidney tumors, lung wall defects, and benign tumors of the hair follicle in patients with the Birt-Hogg-Dubé syndrome. Cancer Cell 2:157-164, 2002.
22. Edge SB, Byrd DR, Compton CC, et al, eds. AJCC Cancer Staging Manual, 7th ed. New York: Springer, 2010.
23. Koga S, Tsuda S, Nishikido M, et al. The diagnostic value of bone scan in patients with renal cell carcinoma. J Urol 166:2126-2128, 2001.
24. Haas NB, Uzzo R. Adjuvant therapy for renal cell carcinoma. Curr Oncol Rep 10:245-252, 2008.
25. Flanigan RC, Salmon SE, Blumenstein BA, et al. Nephrectomy followed by interferon alfa-2b compared with interferon alfa-2b alone for metastatic renal-cell cancer. N Engl J Med 345:1655-1659, 2001.

26. Mickisch GH, Garin A, van Poppel H, et al; European Organisation for Research and Treatment of Cancer (EORTC) Genitourinary Group. Radical nephrectomy plus interferon-alfa-based immunotherapy compared with interferon alfa alone in metastatic renal-cell carcinoma: a randomised trial. Lancet 358:966-970, 2001.
27. Yagoda A, Petrylak D, Thompson S. Cytotoxic chemotherapy for advanced renal cell carcinoma. Urol Clin North Am 20:303-321, 1993.
28. Motzer RJ, Russo P. Systemic therapy for renal cell carcinoma. J Urol 163:408-417, 2000.
29. Klapper JA, Downey SG, Smith FO, et al. High-dose interleukin-2 for the treatment of metastatic renal cell carcinoma: a retrospective analysis of response and survival in patients treated in the surgery branch at the National Cancer Institute between 1986 and 2006. Cancer 113:293-301, 2008.
30. Schwartz RN, Stover L, Dutcher J. Managing toxicities of high-dose interleukin-2. Oncology (Williston Park) 16 (11 Suppl 13):11-20, 2002.
31. McDermott DF. Immunotherapy of metastatic renal cell carcinoma. Cancer 115 (10 Suppl): 2298-2305, 2009.
32. Motzer RJ, Hutson TE, Tomczak P, et al. Overall survival and updated results for sunitinib compared with interferon alfa in patients with metastatic renal cell carcinoma. J Clin Oncol 27:3584-3590, 2009.
33. Escudier B, Eisen T, Stadler WM, et al; TARGET Study Group. Sorafenib in advanced clear-cell renal-cell carcinoma. N Engl J Med 356:125-134, 2007.
34. Zhu X, Stergiopoulos K, Wu S. Risk of hypertension and renal dysfunction with an angiogenesis inhibitor sunitinib: systematic review and meta-analysis. Acta Oncol 48:9-17, 2009.
35. Wu S, Chen JJ, Kudelka A, et al. Incidence and risk of hypertension with sorafenib in patients with cancer: a systematic review and meta-analysis. Lancet Oncol 9:117-123, 2008.
36. Motzer RJ, Hutson TE, Tomczak P, et al. Sunitinib versus interferon alfa in metastatic renal-cell carcinoma. N Engl J Med 356:115-124, 2007.
37. Telli ML, Witteles RM, Fisher GA, et al. Cardiotoxicity associated with the cancer therapeutic agent sunitinib malate. Ann Oncol 19:1613-1618, 2008.
38. van Heeckeren WJ, Ortiz J, Cooney MM, et al. Hypertension, proteinuria, and antagonism of vascular endothelial growth factor signaling: clinical toxicity, therapeutic target, or novel biomarker? J Clin Oncol 25:2993-2995, 2007.
39. Motzer RJ, Rini BI, Bukowski RM, et al. Sunitinib in patients with metastatic renal cell carcinoma. JAMA 295:2516-2524, 2006.
40. Rini BI, Tamaskar I, Shaheen P, et al. Hypothyroidism in patients with metastatic renal cell carcinoma treated with sunitinib. J Natl Cancer Inst 99:81-83, 2007.
41. Tamaskar I, Bukowski R, Elson P. Thyroid function test abnormalities in patients with metastatic renal cell carcinoma treated with sorafenib. Ann Oncol 19:265-268, 2008.
42. Rini BI, Halabi S, Rosenberg JE, et al. Bevacizumab plus interferon alfa compared with interferon alfa monotherapy in patients with metastatic renal cell carcinoma: CALGB 90206. J Clin Oncol 26:5422-5428, 2008.
43. Escudier B, Pluzanska A, Koralewski P, et al; AVOREN Trial investigators. Bevacizumab plus interferon alfa-2a for treatment of metastatic renal cell carcinoma: a randomised, double-blind phase III trial. Lancet 370:2103-2111, 2007.
44. Hay N, Sonenberg N. Upstream and downstream of mTOR. Genes Dev 18:1926-1945, 2004.
45. Hudson CC, Liu M, Chiang GG, et al. Regulation of hypoxia-inducible factor 1alpha expression and function by the mammalian target of rapamycin. Mol Cell Biol 22:7004-7014, 2002.
46. Hudes G, Carducci M, Tomczak P, et al; Global ARCC Trial. Temsirolimus, interferon alfa, or both for advanced renal-cell carcinoma. N Engl J Med 356:2271-2281, 2007.
47. Motzer RJ, Escudier B, Oudard S, et al; RECORD-1 Study Group. Temsirolimus, interferon alfa, or both for advanced renal-cell carcinoma. Lancet 372:449-456, 2008.
48. Sankhala K, Mita A, Kelly K, et al. The emerging safety profile of mTOR inhibitors, a novel class of anticancer agents. Target Oncol 4:135-142, 2009.
49. Margulis V, Matin SF, Tannir N, et al. Surgical morbidity associated with administration of targeted molecular therapies before cytoreductive nephrectomy or resection of locally recurrent renal cell carcinoma. J Urol 180:94-98, 2008.

50. Rini BI, Garcia J, Elson P, et al. Neoadjuvant sunitinib in patients with unresectable primary renal cell carcinoma (RCC). 2009 American Society of Clinical Oncology Genitourinary Cancers Symposium, Abstract 288.
51. Rathmell K, Amin C, Wallen E, et al. Neoadjuvant therapy with sorafenib for locally advanced renal cell carcinoma (RCC). 2008 American Society of Clinical Oncology Genitourinary Cancers Symposium, Abstract 370.
52. Zekri J, Ahmed N, Coleman RE, et al. The skeletal metastatic complications of renal cell carcinoma. Int J Oncol 19:379-382, 2001.
53. Rosen LS, Gordon D, Tchekmedyian S, et al. Zoledronic acid versus placebo in the treatment of skeletal metastases in patients with lung cancer and other solid tumors: a phase III, double-blind, randomized trial—the Zoledronic Acid Lung Cancer and Other Solid Tumors Study Group. J Clin Oncol 21:3150-3157, 2003.
54. Pantuck AJ, Zisman A, Belldegrun AS. The changing natural history of renal cell carcinoma. J Urol 166:1611-1623, 2001.
55. Motzer RJ, Mazumdar M, Bacik J, et al. Survival and prognostic stratification of 670 patients with advanced renal cell carcinoma. J Clin Oncol 17:2530-2540, 1999.
56. Suppiah R, Shaheen PE, Elson P, et al. Thrombocytosis as a prognostic factor for survival in patients with metastatic renal cell carcinoma. Cancer 107:1793-1800, 2006.
57. Patard JJ, Dorey FJ, Cindolo L, et al. Symptoms as well as tumor size provide prognostic information on patients with localized renal tumors. J Urol 172 (6 Pt 1):2167-2171, 2004.

Chapter 20

Breast Cancer

Sally Greenberg, Hope S. Rugo

EPIDEMIOLOGY

Breast cancer is the most common noncutaneous cancer in women.[1] More than one million cases are diagnosed worldwide, and 500,000 women die of the disease each year.[2] Approximately 1% of breast cancers occur in men.

In the United States breast cancer is second only to lung cancer as a cause of cancer-related deaths in women. It is estimated that in 2013, more than 230,000 new cases will be diagnosed, representing 29% of all cancers, and approximately 40,000 women will die of this disease, representing 14% of all cancer deaths. The lifetime risk of developing breast cancer for an American woman is 12% (1 in 8).[1] There are now more than 2.9 million breast cancer survivors in North America.[2,3]

The incidence of breast cancer has been relatively stable since 2005, with variations worldwide, following a marked decline from 2003 to 2005 in postmenopausal women, coinciding with the decrease in the use of hormone replacement therapy after the release of results from the Women's Health Initiative study.[4] There has been a sustained decline in mortality rates over the past five decades, with more stable rates over the past 10 years. Longer follow-up has emphasized the corresponding long natural history of this disease, with recurrences out to 15 years or more in patients with the most common hormone receptor–positive subtype.

PATHOGENESIS

The multistep model describes the pathogenesis of breast cancer. This hypothesis portrays the development of breast cancer through a process of sequential genetic mutations resulting in dedifferentiation and enhanced proliferation of cells. Initial genetic alterations result in hyperplasia, with or without atypia. With additional genetic changes, there is progression to in situ carcinoma. Subsequently invasive localized carcinoma occurs, and eventually metastatic disease may develop.[5]

RISK FACTORS

Only one fourth of women diagnosed with breast cancer have any identifiable risk factors other than age.[6] Risks are summarized in Table 20-1. A small number of breast cancers are attributed to inherited genetic mutations (see p. 327).

Table 20-1 Risk Factors for Breast Cancer

Risk Factors	**Lower Risk**	**Higher Risk**
Sex	Male	Female
Age	Younger	Older
Socioeconomic status	Lower	Higher
Race	Nonwhite	White
Endogenous hormonal factors	Late menarche Early menopause Early first pregnancy Breast-feeding No hormone replacement therapy	Early menarche (<12 years) Late menopause Nulliparity
Exogenous hormonal factors	No hormone replacement therapy	Hormone replacement therapy with estrogen and progesterone
Family history of breast cancer	Absent	Present
History of radiation to chest	Absent	Present
Weight (postmenopausal)	Minimal weight gain with menopause	Obesity
Personal history of breast cancer (in situ or invasive)	Absent	Present
Personal history of benign proliferative breast disease	Absent	Present
Alcohol use	Moderate	Minimal

DEMOGRAPHICS

Ninety-nine percent of breast cancers occur in women. Apart from sex, age is the biggest risk factor. The median age at diagnosis is 61 years. Overall, the incidence rises from the mid-30s and plateaus at 80 years of age. The age at diagnosis varies according to hormone receptor status. Hormone receptor–negative tumors have a peak incidence at 50 years, whereas the frequency of new cases of hormone receptor–positive tumors is highest at age 70.[6]

White women have a higher risk of developing breast cancer but a lower risk of death compared with black women.[7] Breast cancer is also less common in other minority groups in the United States. Premenopausal black women are more likely to be diagnosed with a biologically more aggressive phenotype of breast cancer, which is associated with a worse prognosis. The reason for this is unclear, but it is probably related to a combination of factors.[8] Breast cancer is more common in women from a higher socioeconomic class, in an urban environment, and among those who have never been married, along with the risk factors listed in Table 20-1.

HORMONAL FACTORS

Cumulative lifetime exposure to endogenous estrogens is an important risk factor.[6] For every 2-year delay in menarche, there is approximately a 10% reduction in the likelihood of cancer. A delay in menopause of 5 years increases the risk by approximately 10%. Having a first pregnancy before 20 years of age is associated with a reduced risk, and nulliparous women are at increased risk.

In postmenopausal women, large observational and randomized trials have shown that exogenous hormones, and in particular combined estrogen and progesterone, increase the incidence of invasive breast cancer.[9,10] Hormone replacement therapy doubles the risk of recurrence in breast cancer survivors.[11]

GENETIC FACTORS

A family history of breast cancer, reported in 15% to 20% of women, increases the risk of breast cancer. Women who have a first-degree relative with breast cancer (on either the maternal or paternal side) have a two to three times higher lifetime risk of developing breast cancer.[12]

Five percent of breast cancers are associated with inherited genetic mutations.[13] Breast cancer susceptibility genes 1 and 2 (*BRCA1* and *BRCA2*) are tumor suppressor genes that were first identified in the Ashkenazi Jewish population, which has autosomal dominant inheritance with variable penetrance. Genetic mutations in the *BRCA* genes account for approximately 75% of hereditary breast cancers. Such mutations result in at least a 30% risk of breast cancer by age 50 and a 56% risk by age 70.[14] The risk has been suggested to be as high as 85% by 70 years.[14] These mutations are also associated with an increase in other types of cancer, most notably ovarian cancer.

BRCA-associated cancers can occur in women or men who inherit this mutation, and these cancers are associated with specific phenotypes depending on the mutation. Patients who should be considered for genetic counseling and possible testing include the following: those who are premenopausal at diagnosis, those who have bilateral breast cancer, men, those who have a family history of premenopausal breast cancer and/or ovarian cancer, and those of Ashkenazi Jewish ethnicity. Testing is particularly important for prevention and screening.

Other rare genetic mutations resulting in a predisposition to an increased risk of breast cancer along with other malignancies include Li-Fraumeni (loss of the *p53* tumor suppressor gene, recently associated with increased risk of HER2-positive breast cancer in young women[15] and Peutz-Jeghers syndromes, among others.[16]

PERSONAL HISTORY OF BREAST CANCER

A personal history of invasive or in situ breast cancer incurs substantial risk of subsequent breast cancer development. Over 20 years of follow-up, approximately 10% of patients treated for a primary early-stage breast cancer will be diagnosed with a new, contralateral breast cancer.[17]

Ductal carcinoma in situ (DCIS) refers to a neoplastic proliferation of ductal epithelial cells that do not invade through the basement membrane. Left untreated, there is a 35% chance of progression to invasive breast cancer.[18] With optimal local therapy approximately 10% of patients have a recurrence, 50% of these with invasive cancer.[19] Lobular carcinoma in situ (LCIS) is also associated with an increased incidence of breast cancer.[20] Rather than being a precursor for subsequent cancer, it may be a proliferative disorder that identifies women who are at risk of developing subsequent breast cancer.

BENIGN BREAST DISEASE

Women with benign proliferative breast disease have a slightly increased risk (1.5- to twofold) for subsequent development of cancer.[21,22] Those with typical ductal and lobular hyperplasia (hyperplasia with cellular atypia) incur approximately a twofold to fourfold increase in risk when compared with the general population.[22,23]

LIFESTYLE AND RADIATION

Recently there has been an interest in lifestyle or modifiable risk factors for breast cancer. Moderate alcohol consumption, obesity (particularly in postmenopausal women), and lack of exercise increase the risk of breast cancer.[24] Moderate exercise (up to 7 hours per week) reduces the likelihood by up to 20%.[6] Chest wall exposure to ionizing radiation, especially before 20 years of age, increases risk after a latency of at least 15 years.[12]

DIAGNOSIS

Breast cancer may appear as a palpable breast mass or axillary mass, or radiographically as either a spiculated density or abnormal calcification. Three fourths of women with symptomatic breast cancer will have a discrete, palpable mass.[6]

Diagnostic mammography may show a spiculated mass or microcalcification. Mammography is an important procedure, because it can also show a nonpalpable synchronous second primary tumor.[6] False-negative rates range from 2% to 35%, depending on the type of breast cancer, the age of the patient, and other factors. In women with dense breasts, the sensitivity may be as low as 30% to 48%.[25]

Ultrasound imaging of the breast increases the diagnostic accuracy of mammography. Combined with clinical examination and mammography for suspicious lesions, the sensitivity of detection improves up to 93.2%. Ultrasonography can differentiate between solid and cystic masses, estimate the size of the tumor, and facilitate image-guided biopsy. It can also be used to detect pathologic axillary lymphadenopathy.[25]

Magnetic resonance imaging of the breast is a very sensitive imaging modality for breast cancer (91% to 100%). MRI can detect occult synchronous tumors that are not detected by clinical examination or mammography in 16% to 37% of patients.[26] The lack of specificity, however, results in a high number of false-positive findings. In addition, there are significant differences in the quality of MRI scans of the breast, as well as in the accuracy of interpretation. For these reasons, this imaging modality is not currently recommended as a part of routine evaluation for all patients. However, it is recommended, along with mammography and clinical examination, for women who are at particularly high risk for developing breast cancer, such as those with known *BRCA* mutations or a strong family history of breast cancer. Further studies are underway to clarify the role of MRI in screening, diagnosis, and management of the broader population.

STAGING

Breast cancer is staged on the basis of clinical and/or pathologic features. Similar to other cancers, the manner of staging is referred to as *c* for clinical staging, or *p* for pathologic staging. The American Joint Committee on Cancer publishes a periodically updated tumor, node, metastasis (TNM) staging system that is used internationally to stage most solid tumors, including breast cancer. Tables 20-2 and 20-3 display a summary of TNM staging for breast cancer.[27]

Although a universally accepted staging system allows a common language for clinical trials and treatment guidelines, it does not include other important prognostic information, such as hormone and HER2 receptors, tumor grade, and so forth (discussed later).

Detection of malignancy in an axillary node measuring less than 0.2 mm is called an *isolated tumor cell* or ITC. For treatment purposes this would be considered node negative until further data are available. A *micrometastasis* is defined as a tumor deposit ranging from 0.2 to 2 mm. The significance of these deposits is not known.[2]

Table 20-2 **TNM Staging for Breast Cancer**

Tumor (T)

T0	No evidence of primary tumor
Tis	Carcinoma in situ
T1	Tumor <20 mm
T2	Tumor 20-50 mm
T3	Tumor >50 mm
T4	Direct extension of tumor into chest wall or skin

Node (N)

N0	No regional lymph node involvement
N1	Metastases in moveable ipsilateral level I or II axillary lymph node or node(s)
N2	Metastases in ipsilateral level I or II axillary lymph node(s) fixed to one another or to other structures *or* ipsilateral internal mammary lymph node(s) in absence of axillary lymph node metastasis
N3	Metastases in ipsilateral infraclavicular lymph node(s) or ipsilateral internal mammary lymph node(s) with level II *or* III axillary lymph node metastases *or* metastases in ipsilateral supraclavicular lymph node(s) involvement

Metastases (M)

M0	No distant metastases
cM0(i+)	Deposits of microscopically detected tumor cells in circulating blood, bone marrow, or other nonregional lymph node(s) less than 0.2 mm in patients without clinical or radiographic evidence of distant metastases
M1	Distant metastases detected by classical clinical or radiographic methods

Adapted from the American Joint Committee on Cancer Staging Manual, 7th ed. Available at *http://www.cancerstaging.org*.

Table 20-3 **Staging for Breast Cancer**

Stage 0	Carcinoma in situ
Stage I	T1N0
Stage II	T0-1N1 T2N0-1 T3N0
Stage III	T0-2N2-3 T3-4N1-3
Stage IV	M1

Adapted from the American Joint Committee on Cancer Staging Manual, 7th ed. Available at *http://www.cancerstaging.org*.

CHARACTERIZATION OF BREAST CANCER

Breast cancer refers to a very heterogeneous disease. Differences between tumors are important for prognostication and to predict responses to the various systemic treatments available.

HISTOLOGY

Most malignant breast tumors arise from mammary ductal epithelial cells. Infiltrating ductal carcinoma accounts for approximately 75% of all diagnoses.[29] There are various subclassifications of infiltrating ductal carcinoma, although most are classified as *not otherwise specified*.

Lobular carcinoma accounts for 5% to 15% of invasive breast cancers.[29] Compared with ductal cancer, detection can be difficult, with higher rates of false-negative mammograms and fine needle aspiration. When detected, lobular tumors are often larger, more likely to be low grade, and have hormone receptor positivity.[30]

Other less common epithelial cell breast tumors, all with particular pathologic and prognostic features, include tubular, cribriform, mucinous, papillary, apocrine, neuroendocrine, medullary, secretory, adenoid cystic, acinic cell, small cell neuroendocrine, micropapillary, metaplastic, and lipid rich.[29]

Inflammatory breast cancer composes 1.3% of breast cancers. Classically, there is evidence of dermal lymphatic invasion by tumor cells. A higher histologic grade is often seen, and estrogen receptors are usually negative. Inflammatory breast cancer is associated with a significantly worse prognosis than noninflammatory, locally advanced breast cancer.[31]

ESTROGEN AND PROGESTERONE RECEPTORS

Hormone receptor status, including the estrogen and progesterone receptors, is determined by immunohistochemical (IHC) staining. The degree of positivity is generally reported by the intensity and proportion of staining. Approximately 80% of breast cancers diagnosed in postmenopausal women are hormone receptor positive.[32] Hormone receptor–positive tumors are less common in younger women.

Relapse rates vary considerably depending on hormone receptor status. It is substantially higher during the first 5 years after diagnosis for hormone receptor–negative tumors.[33] Only 50% of recurrences in hormone receptor–positive tumors will occur within this time frame, with the other 50% occurring 5 to 15 years after diagnosis.[34]

Hormone receptor status is also associated with responses to therapy. Tumors that are hormone receptor–negative do not respond to hormonal therapy.[33] The benefits of chemotherapy are greater in hormone receptor–negative tumors.[35]

HUMAN EPIDERMAL GROWTH FACTOR RECEPTOR TYPE 2

Human epidermal growth factor receptor type 2 (HER2) is a tyrosine kinase involved in cell growth and proliferation. It is overexpressed in 20% to 25% of breast cancers as a result of amplification of the *erbB2* gene.[36] These tumors are referred to as HER2-positive regardless of hormone receptor status; 50% also express hormone receptors.

Overexpression of HER2 is detected by IHC staining, which determines the degree of plasma membrane staining for HER2. A score of 0 to 3 is given depending on the relative intensity of staining. A score of 0 to 1 is negative for HER2 overexpression, a score of 2 is indeterminate, and a score of 3 is positive. Fluorescent in situ hybridization (FISH) measures amplification of the *erbB2* gene[37] and is used as a primary measure of HER2 status as well as a reflex test to assess tumors with 2+ staining by IHC.[34]

Tumors with overexpression of HER2 are associated with an aggressive phenotype. They have increased invasive and metastatic capabilities, and also more stimulation of angiogenesis. These tumors are usually higher grade and have lymph node involvement.[38] Until the introduction of trastuzumab, a monocolonal antibody directed against the extracellular domain of HER2, HER2-positive breast cancers were associated with a significantly worse prognosis than HER2-negative cancers.[6]

False-negative and false-positive results may be seen for hormone receptors or for HER2. In addition, receptor status may change over time and with progression of the disease. Generally, receptor status should be rechecked in the metastatic tumor, because the results may have a significant impact on the choice of therapy.

TRIPLE-NEGATIVE TUMORS

Triple-negative breast cancer refers to tumors that are defined on the basis of negative estrogen and progesterone receptors and lack of HER2 amplification. These tumors are often higher grade and occur in younger women. When metastases occur, they are more likely to be in visceral organs or in the central nervous system. Triple-negative tumors have higher response rates to chemotherapy; however, they are associated with inferior survival and a short time from diagnosis of early-stage disease to the development of metastases.[39-41]

TUMOR PROLIFERATION

Tumor grade refers to the particular histologic characteristics of a tumor and is an estimate of the proliferation of the cells. Two systems are most commonly used to

Table 20-4 Grading of Breast Tumors

Composite Grade
1	Well differentiated	Low grade
2	Moderately well differentiated	Intermediate grade
3	Poorly differentiated	High grade

assess grade; the Nottingham system may be more objective than the Scarff-Bloom-Richardson grading system. Grade is determined by assigning an individual score to each of the following three histologic features of tumors: tubule formation, mitotic count, and nuclear pleomorphism. These scores are combined to derive a composite assessment of grade (Table 20-4). Grade is variably correlated with tumor proliferation, which is used to assess prognosis and determine treatment in the early-stage setting.[42]

Ki-67 is a nuclear protein expressed in proliferating tissues. Expression of Ki-67 can be determined through antibodies, including MIB-1, and is perhaps a more reproducible marker of proliferation than grade. The prognostic utility of Ki-67 in predicting recurrence is not clear, although breast tumors with higher Ki-67 levels have improved responses to chemotherapy.[43] Newer tests focusing on gene expression may provide a more accurate assessment of proliferation.

Gene Expression

Analysis of gene expression patterns has led to the classification of breast cancers into a number of subsets that have been correlated with biological behavior, outcomes, and responses to specific therapies. Gene expression profiling may be superior to traditional clinical and pathologic markers at predicting breast cancer outcomes.[44] Originally four distinct subtypes of breast cancer were described: luminal, basal-like, HER2 overexpressors, and normal breast type.[45] Subsequently there have been additional subclassifications.

Commercially available molecular assays of gene signatures include Oncotype DX and MammaPrint. In particular circumstances these tests provide additional information concerning predicted benefits of treatment.[46]

PROGNOSIS
Early-Stage Breast Cancer

Prognostic factors are summarized in Table 20-5.

Outcomes for women with breast cancer have improved considerably over the past 30 years[47] (Fig. 20-1).

Table 20-5 Key Factors Affecting Breast Cancer Prognosis

Prognostic Factor	Lower Risk	Higher Risk
Size	Smaller	Larger
Axillary node involvement	Negative	Positive
Grade	Low grade	High grade
Hormone receptor status	Positive	Negative
HER2 status	Negative	Positive*
Stage	Earlier	Later

*The use of adjuvant trastuzumab has altered the relative prognostic significance of HER2 positivity, since treatment markedly improves outcome.

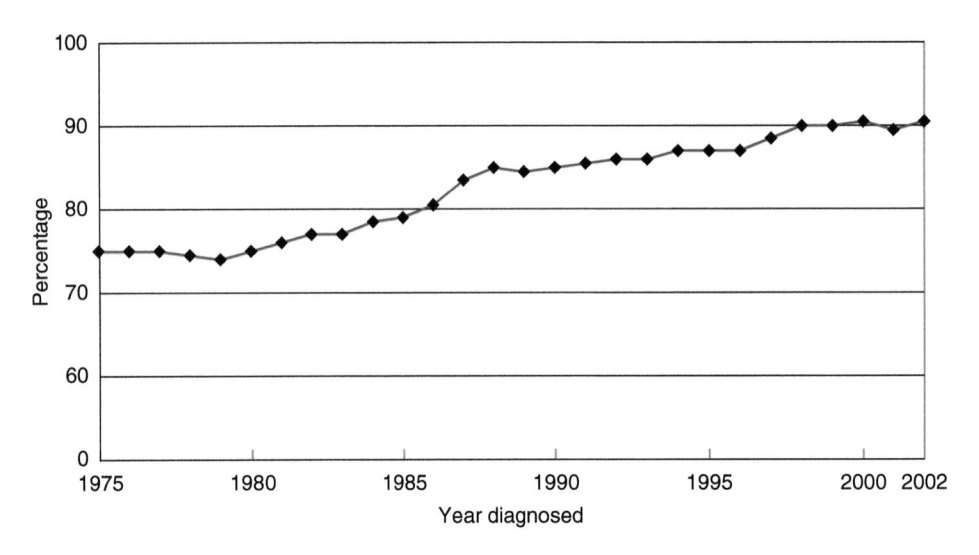

Fig. 20-1 Breast cancer 5-year survival by year of diagnosis. (Adapted from the National Cancer Institute: Surveillance, Epidemiology and End Results [SEER]. Available at *http://www.seer.cancer.gov.*)

ADVANCED BREAST CANCER

For patients with recurrent breast cancer, a number of factors affect survival. In addition to estrogen receptor, progesterone receptor, and HER2 status, other prognostic factors include response to therapy and site of recurrence[48,49] (Table 20-6).

The median survival for women diagnosed with advanced breast cancer improved significantly between 1991 and 2001.[49,50] This is demonstrated by a study analyzing the British Columbia Cancer Agency's Breast Cancer Outcomes Database involving more than 2000 patients with breast cancer[50]; the results are summarized in Table 20-7. This improvement is probably the result of the development and use of more effective systemic treatment, as well as a better understanding of tumor biology. Trials

Table 20-6 Additional Prognostic Factors in Advanced Breast Cancer

Prognostic Factor	Better Prognosis	Worse Prognosis
Disease-free interval	Longer	Shorter
Site of recurrence	Local/contralateral breast	Distant
Site of metastases	Nonvisceral dominant/bone only	Visceral dominant

Table 20-7 Changes in Median Survival for Patients With Metastatic Breast Cancer From 1991 to 2009

Year Diagnosed	Median Survival (mo)	1-Year Survival (mo)	2-Year Survival (mo)
1991–1992	14.5	55	33
1999–2001	20.4	71	45
1999–2009	22	NA	NA

NA, Not available.

conducted in patients receiving first-line chemotherapy for metastatic breast cancer between 1999 and 2009 have demonstrated an average median overall survival of 22 months, with significant variation, depending on biologic subtype and response to therapy. For example, patients with advanced triple-negative disease generally survive less than 2 years, whereas patients with hormone-sensitive hormone receptor disease might live 5 years or more.[51]

As noted above, survival after a diagnosis of metastatic breast cancer varies by biological tumor subtype. For example, patients with low-grade, hormone receptor–positive breast cancer with metastasis to bone and/or soft tissue sites alone have a more favorable prognosis,[52] as do some patients with HER2–positive metastatic disease. In these cases, long-term disease stability may be seen with targeted biological therapy.[51,53]

MANAGEMENT OF EARLY BREAST CANCER

Early breast cancer is a disease found only in the breast or locoregional lymph nodes, which can be fully surgically resected.

LOCOREGIONAL TREATMENT

Locoregional treatments that reduce local recurrence significantly improve the overall survival of patients with breast cancer.[54]

> **Box 20-1 Contraindications to Breast-Conserving Surgery**
>
> - Multifocal breast cancer
> - Inflammatory breast cancer
> - Prior radiation therapy to the area
> - Persistent positive surgical margins
> - Unfavorable breast-to-tumor ratio
> - Large tumors (relative contraindication)
> - History of scleroderma or systemic lupus erythematosus (relative contraindication to radiation therapy)
> - Pregnancy (if radiation therapy has to be performed before delivery)
>
> Data from Morrow M, Strom EA, Bassett LW, et al; American College of Radiology; American College of Surgeons; Society of Surgical Oncology; College of American Pathology. Standard for breast conservation therapy in the management of invasive breast carcinoma. CA Cancer J Clin 52:277-300, 2002.

Surgery

Breast conservation surgery is the preferred method of surgery in most patients.[6] It involves removing the tumor without removing excess amounts of normal breast tissue. When a local excision is combined with radiation therapy, the long-term survival is equivalent to that of mastectomy.

More than 60% of patients are eligible for breast-conserving surgery as opposed to mastectomy. Reexcision to obtain clear margins is required in up to 25% of patients.[6] Some patients chose to have a mastectomy. Contraindications to breast-conserving surgery are shown in Box 20-1.[55] Neoadjuvant systemic treatment can be considered with the aim of reducing the size of a tumor to allow breast-conserving surgery in the case of a larger tumor.

Sentinel node biopsy is now the standard of care for axillary node staging in patients who are clinically node negative.[28] It is based on the theory that when tumor cells migrate, they colonize one or a few nodes before involving others. Dye or radioactive colloid is injected around the tumor to determine which node or nodes drain the area of the tumor. It is possible to identify the sentinel node in up to 90% of patients.[55] There is a false-negative result in less than 5% to 10%. Full axillary dissection is recommended in all women who have either macroscopic metastasis or micrometastasis in their sentinel lymph nodes and in those who have clinical evidence of axillary disease.[55]

Radiation Therapy

There is clear evidence of increased ipsilateral breast cancer recurrence when breast-conserving surgery is conducted without radiation therapy. This is illustrated in the results of a 2005 meta-analysis involving 7300 patients enrolled in trials assessing the benefit of radiation therapy compared with breast-conserving therapy (Table 20-8).[54]

A typical course of radiation therapy is 45 to 50 Gy in 25 to 30 fractions. It usually begins 4 to 6 weeks after surgery, or after adjuvant chemotherapy, if it is given.[56]

Table 20-8 Benefit of Radiation Therapy in Addition to Breast-Conserving Surgery

	Breast-Conserving Surgery Alone	Breast-Conserving Surgery Combined With Radiation Therapy
5-year local recurrence	26%	7%
Risk of death at 15 years (node-negative women)	35.9%	30.4%
Risk of death at 15 years (node-positive women)	55%	48%

Data from Clarke M, Collins R, Darby S, et al; Early Breast Cancer Trialists' Collaborative Group (EBCTCG). Effects of radiotherapy and of differences in the extent of surgery for early breast cancer on local recurrence and 15-year survival: an overview of the randomised trials. Lancet 366:2087-2106, 2005.

There are methods of local breast radiation therapy that may be as effective as total breast irradiation. However, these are not used routinely in many institutions.[56] One method is brachytherapy, in which implants are placed at the tumor bed, allowing local radiation therapy over a 1-week period. Intraoperative radiation therapy and brachytherapy through a balloon catheter are other methods of accelerated partial breast irradiation.[6] A recent review found that a shorter duration of localized radiation therapy is not inferior to the standard treatment for tumors smaller than 5 cm with no lymph node involvement.[57]

Indications for postmastectectomy radiation therapy are evolving. There is evidence for a reduction in local recurrence by up to 75% when the primary tumor is larger than 5 cm, or if more than four axillary nodes are involved. It is uncertain whether there is a mortality benefit, and there are conflicting trial results.[6]

SYSTEMIC THERAPY

Early hematogenous spread of malignant cells results in a proportion of women developing metastatic disease despite adequate local therapy. In some women with early-stage breast cancer, micrometastases can be detected as circulating tumor cells in peripheral blood or disseminated tumor cells in other tissues.[58,59] When detected, these micrometastases do not always result in the development of clinically apparent metastatic disease; presumably some are destroyed by natural host defense mechanisms. Current methods used for detection of micrometastases do not allow these cells to be detected in all women who will develop distant recurrence.[59] Therefore other prognostic indicators, including those outlined in Table 20-5, are used to determine risk of recurrence in individual patients. The aim of systemic adjuvant therapy is to eradicate these circulating or disseminated cells before they proliferate into overt metastatic disease, for which there is currently no cure.

> **Box 20-2** Factors Affecting Systemic Treatment Choices in Early-Stage Breast Cancer
>
> **Cancer Factors**
> Size of tumor
> Lymph node status
> Grade/histopathology
> Hormone receptor status
> HER-2 expression
> Gene expression profile
>
> **Patient Factors**
> Preference
> Age
> Menopausal status
> Comorbidities
> Performance status

Table 20-9 Hormone Therapies Commonly Used in Breast Cancer

Mechanism	Example	Menopausal State
Estrogen receptor blockage	Tamoxifen	Premenopausal and postmenopausal
Reduction in ovarian production of estrogen	Medical: LHRH agonists Surgical: Oophorectomy	Premenopausal
Reduction in nonovarian production of estrogen	Aromatase inhibitors: anastrozole, letrozole, and exemestane	Postmenopausal

Adapted from Rugo HS. The breast cancer continuum in hormone-receptor-positive breast cancer in postmenopausal women: evolving management options focusing on aromatase inhibitors. Ann Oncol 19:16-27, 2008.
LHRH, Luteinizing hormone–releasing hormone.

The addition of adjuvant systemic therapies, including chemotherapy, hormonal therapy, and biological therapy, to localized treatment has improved disease-free and overall survival rates for early breast cancer.[60]

Systemic treatment for early-stage breast cancer has changed significantly in recent years. As more is understood about the biology of the cancer, treatment has become more individualized. The choice of treatment is a balance of risk versus benefit. The chances of an individual tumor's recurrence are weighed against the predicted toxicity, and the expected benefit, of particular treatments to each individual patient. Thus there are both patient factors and tumor factors to consider (Box 20-2).

Hormonal Therapy

Antiestrogen or hormonal treatment can target estrogen receptor–positive tumors. These drugs are not effective in hormone receptor–negative cancer.[33] Menopausal state is a key determinant in the choice of hormonal therapy. The hormonal treatments commonly used are shown in the Table 20-9.[61]

Tamoxifen is a nonsteroidal antiestrogen that antagonizes estrogen at its receptor site.[62] For more than 20 years, tamoxifen was the standard hormonal treatment for all women with hormone receptor–positive breast cancer. It is associated with a 41% to 47% relative reduction in risk of recurrence and a 26% to 34% relative reduction in the risk of death for women with estrogen receptor–positive or unknown tumors.[60] Five years of tamoxifen therapy is the standard treatment and is superior, in terms of tumor recurrence and overall survival, compared with 1 to 2 years of tamoxifen.

Hormonal treatment in premenopausal women can also be achieved through ovarian suppression. This can be achieved either surgically with an oophorectomy or chemically through treatment with a luteinizing hormone–releasing hormone analog. This is usually in addition to either tamoxifen or an aromatase inhibitor.

Aromatase inhibitors (anastrozole, letrozole, and exemestane) are effective agents in postmenopausal women. They suppress the peripheral conversion of androgens to estrogens.[34] They are not effective in premenopausal women because a lower circulating estrogen level indirectly stimulates the ovaries to produce estrogen and maintain regular levels.[16] A recently published meta-analysis found that 5 years of adjuvant aromatase inhibitor therapy in postmenopausal women is superior to 5 years of tamoxifen, in terms of tumor recurrence, when given either as up-front therapy or after 2 to 3 years of tamoxifen.[63]

Five years of hormonal treatment is standard, yet 50% of hormone receptor–positive tumors relapse after this period.[60] Trials with extended tamoxifen have been inconclusive.[34] The addition of an aromatase inhibitor, after the completion of 5 years of tamoxifen, has shown promising results, including improved disease-free survival.[64] There may also be a survival benefit in high-risk patients, such as those with positive axillary lymph nodes. There are ongoing trials to further assess the benefits of extended aromatase inhibitor therapy.

The side effects of hormonal treatment include hot flashes and decreased sexual function. Women who develop hot flashes may have a better outcome.[34] Aromatase inhibitors can reduce bone density and increase the risk of fractures. Osteopenia and osteoporosis can be treated successfully with bisphosphonate therapy. Arthralgia is also more common with aromatase inhibitors. Tamoxifen is associated with an age-related modest increase in the risk of endometrial cancer and venous thrombotic events.[34]

Chemotherapy

Adjuvant chemotherapy improves overall and disease-free survival in breast cancer.[60] A meta-analysis of almost 200 randomized trials found that 6 months of polychemotherapy reduced annual breast cancer death rates by 38% for women less 50 years of age at diagnosis and 20% for women 50 to 69 years of age. The benefits were greater in younger women irrespective of lymph node or hormone receptor status.[32] Table 20-10 summarizes the benefits of chemotherapy for women younger than 50 seen in this meta-analysis.[32]

Table 20-10 Effects of Chemotherapy in Women Younger Than 50 Years With Resected Early-Stage Breast Cancer

	Chemotherapy	No Chemotherapy
10-year recurrence	33%	45%
Breast cancer mortality	24%	32%
Death from any cause	25%	33%

Data from Early Breast Cancer Trialists' Collaborative Group (EBCTCG). Effects of chemotherapy and hormonal therapy for early breast cancer on recurrence and 15-year survival: an overview of the randomised trials. Lancet 365:1687-1717, 2005.

The meta-analysis was updated in 2008: 46 trials for estrogen receptor–negative women were conducted, and again significant reductions were found in recurrences, breast cancer deaths, and deaths from any cause in women up to 69 years of age. The benefits seen were once again greater in younger women, and trial data were insufficient for women older than 70.[33]

The use of chemotherapy in women with low-grade, node-negative, hormone-responsive tumors is less defined. These tumors respond well to hormonal therapy. These are examples of cases where newer, biologic tests of the tumor, such as Oncotype DX, may be used to predict the potential benefit from chemotherapy plus hormone therapy versus hormone therapy alone.

The chemotherapeutic agents that have been shown to be most beneficial in the adjuvant setting are the anthracycline-based (doxorubicin) and taxane-based (paclitaxel, docetaxel) regimens.[32] A combination of anthracycline-based chemotherapy, followed by a taxane-based treatment, improves survival over anthracycline treatment alone in node-positive tumors.[65] The duration and timing of each cycle of treatment varies with different protocols, and the best protocol is not currently known. Gene expression profile studies are underway, with the aim of detecting particular genes, to predict improved responses to different types of chemotherapy.

Chemotherapy is usually given over a 3- to 6-month period. Side effects include bone marrow suppression, nausea, vomiting, alopecia, fatigue, ovarian suppression, cardiac toxicity, hypersensitivity reactions, and neuropathy.

Biologic Therapy

Trastuzumab is a humanized monoclonal antibody that targets the extracellular domain of the HER2 protein.[36] It is given intravenously, either weekly or every 3 weeks. In women with HER2-positive tumors, trastuzumab improves disease-free and overall survival independent of age, axillary node, or hormone receptor status.[38] The most serious side effect of trastuzumab, seen in 0.5% to 4% of patients, is cardiotoxicity, which is often reversible by discontinuing the drug. Cardiac assessment is routine before and during treatment with trastuzumab. A summary of treatment decisions in early breast cancer is given in Fig. 20-2.

Chapter 20 ■ *Breast Cancer* **341**

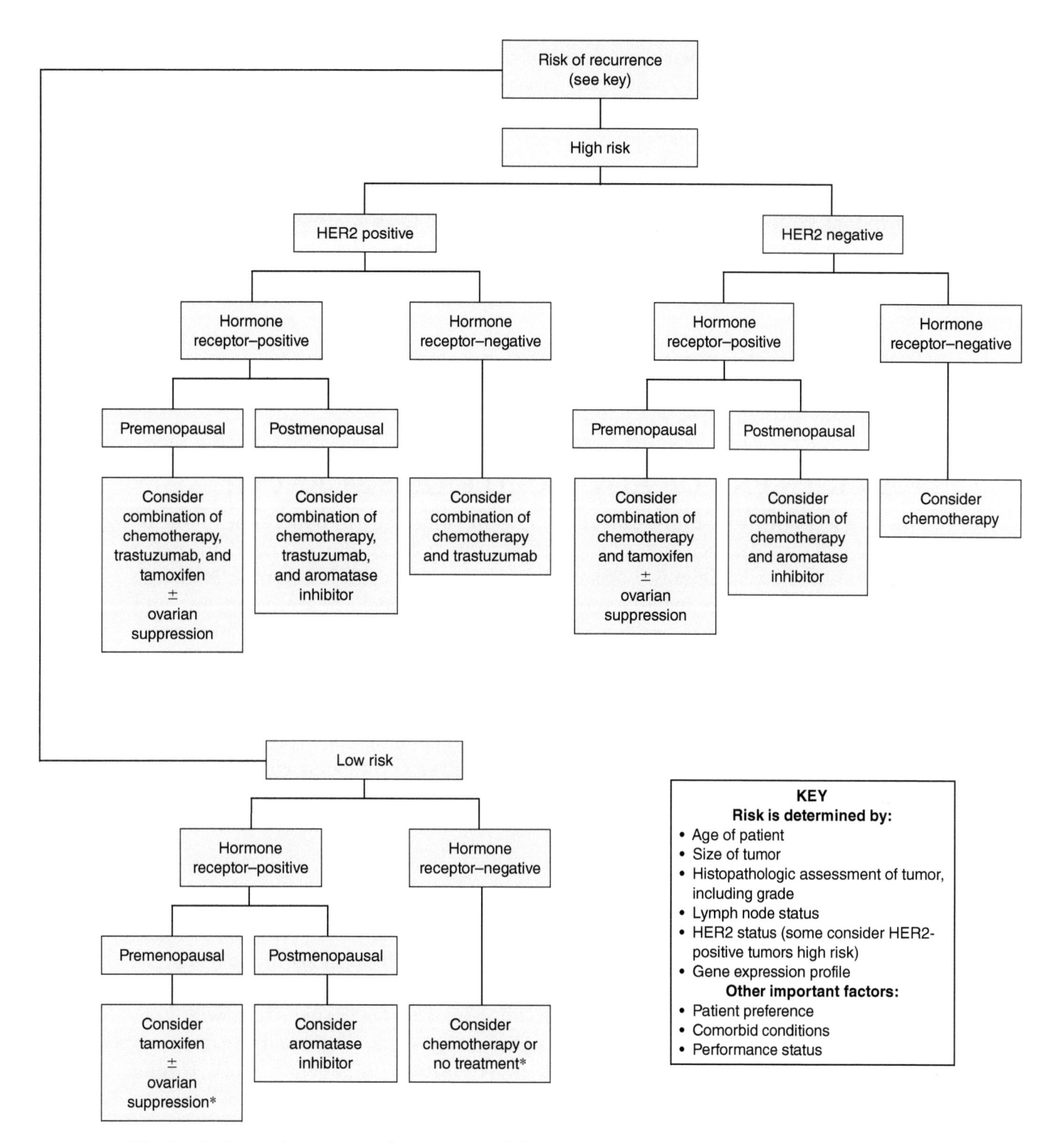

Fig. 20-2 Systemic treatment decisions in early breast cancer. (*, Indicates that few patients fit into these categories because young age and hormone receptor status are important prognostic factors.)

Neoadjuvant Therapy

Systemic treatment is given before surgery in certain situations. Usually this is either because the cancer is inoperable at diagnosis or has a poor prognosis with locoregional treatment alone.[31] Neoadjuvant therapy may also be used to reduce the size of a tumor to allow breast-conserving surgery rather than mastectomy. The advantages of neoadjuvant therapy include earlier systemic treatment of subclinical micrometastasis and an in vivo assessment of the response to a particular systemic treatment.[31]

Hormonal, standard chemotherapeutic, and biologic treatments are all given in the neoadjuvant setting. There is a significant clinical response that includes a complete pathologic response of the tumor in 19% to 36% of patients and a partial response in 43% to 66%.[66]

Trials comparing adjuvant and neoadjuvant therapy for breast cancer in a primary operable cancer have yielded similar outcomes.[31] The risk of disease progression during neoadjuvant therapy is low at 1% to 3%.[66]

MANAGEMENT OF ADVANCED BREAST CANCER

Distant metastases from breast cancer occur most commonly in bone, either alone or in combination with liver, lung, pleura, or soft tissue.[67] Breast cancer can relapse many years after the initial diagnosis, especially hormone receptor–positive cancer. Although it is not possible to cure metastatic breast cancer, hormonal, chemotherapeutic, and biological therapies can all prolong survival and improve symptoms. There are many active agents, including those that are used in early breast cancer. The first agent to improve response to hormone therapy was recently approved for the second-line treatment of metastatic hormone receptor–positive breast cancer. Everolimus inhibits mTOR, the mammalian target of rapamycin, and in combination with the aromastase inhibitor exemestane, improves PFS and response rates compared with exemestane alone.[68] Multiple new medications are in clinical trials, with the goal of improving response to hormone therapy, most with unique toxicities distinct from those seen with hormone therapy.

The choice of initial systemic therapy depends on the extent of the disease, hormone receptor and HER2 status of the tumor, and comorbid conditions, performance status, and personal preferences of the patients. A review of the trials in hormone receptor–positive tumors found that using hormonal treatment initially, as compared with upfront chemotherapy, did not alter survival, and there were fewer side effects with hormonal treatment. However, there was a higher response rate in patients treated with chemotherapy.[69] Hormone therapy is often used initially in patients with hormone receptor–positive cancer when there is a low volume of metastatic disease.

In HER2–positive metastatic breast cancer, the use of HER2 targeted therapy improves survival compared with the use of chemotherapy alone and is the standard of care for treatment of this subset of breast cancer. In comparison with chemotherapy alone, the combination of trastuzumab and chemotherapy has been shown to significantly improve median survival, time to disease progression, and responses to treatment.[70]

Recently, the addition of a second antibody, pertuzumab, to trastuzumab and chemotherapy as first-line therapy for advanced, HER2-positive breast cancer was shown to improve both progression-free survival (PFS) and overall survival (OS) compared with the standard of trastuzumab and chemotherapy.[71] Based on these data, pertuzumab was approved as treatment of advanced HER2-positive breast cancer. Several studies are evaluating the use of pertuzumab in combination with trastuzumab and chemotherapy for early-stage breast cancer.

Lapatanib is an oral tyrosine kinase inhibitor directed against HER2 and epidermal growth factor. The combination of lapatinib with capecitabine, an oral fluorouracil prodrug chemotherapy, was superior to capecitabine alone as treatment for patients with trastuzumab-refractory HER2-positive metastatic breast cancer, with an improvement in PFS, but not OS.[72] The combination of lapatinib and trastuzumab has also been shown to improve survival compared with treatment with lapatinib alone.[73]

A novel immunotoxin called *trastuzumab derivative of maytansine-1* (TDM-1) or *emtansine* was recently approved for the treatment of trastuzumab-resistant disease, based on superior PFS and OS compared with treatment with lapatinib and capecitabine.[74] TDM-1 is composed of trastuzumab linked to a potent toxin, allowing trastuzumab to deliver the toxin directly to the HER2-positive cancer cell. TDM-1 is given intravenously every 3 weeks, has an excellent safety profile, and is now considered the standard of care for second-line treatment for HER2-positive advanced disease.

Angiogenesis plays a critical role in cancer progression.[75] Vascular endothelial growth factor is an important regulator of angiogenesis.[76] Antibodies to vascular endothelial growth factor, such as bevacizumab, are active agents in metastatic breast cancer. When used in combination with chemotherapy, bevacizumab (Avastin) has been shown to improve response rates and progression-free survival, but without improvement in overall survival.[77] Bevacizumab is no longer approved for the treatment of breast cancer.

CENTRAL NERVOUS SYSTEM METASTASES

Metastasis from breast cancer can occur in the brain and leptomeninges. It is the second most common cancer to have central nervous system (CNS) metastases, and the most common solid malignancy is leptomeningeal involvement. Parenchymal metastases are clinically apparent in 10% to 16% of patients with metastatic breast cancer and are found at autopsy in up to 30%.[78] An increasing incidence has been reported in more recent studies. This is likely the result of the improvement in survival, which is a result of more effective systemic treatments.[79] Leptomeningeal deposits are less common and are found in 5% to 16% of patients at postmortem examination.[78]

The well-established risk factors for CNS metastases include young age, hormone receptor negativity, and an increase in the number of metastatic sites of disease.[79]

HER2–positive tumors have been recognized as having an increased risk in more recent studies, particularly in patients receiving trastuzumab therapy. The increased survival resulting from trastuzumab and the inability of this antibody to adequately penetrate the blood-brain barrier are likely reasons for this observation.[80,81]

CNS metastases most commonly present with headaches (24% to 48% of patients). They may also present with states of altered consciousness, motor and sensory deficits, seizures, ataxia, nausea, and vomiting.[78]

Magnetic resonance imaging is more sensitive than computed tomography in detecting parenchymal and leptomeningeal metastasis. Cerebrospinal fluid cytology has equivalent sensitivity and greater specificity compared with MRI for the diagnosis of leptomeningeal metastasis.[78]

Solitary brain metastases alone are uncommon. They more often occur late, when there is widespread metastatic disease to other organs, such as the lungs, liver, or bone.[82] One large study found that young women with no other sites of metastatic disease who had good performance status had the most favorable prognosis, with a median survival of 7.1 months. Patients with a worse performance status had a median survival of 2.3 months.[84]

Approximately 50% of women with brain metastasis will die as a result of their CNS disease. This is why local control of CNS disease is so important.[82,83]

The treatment of parenchymal metastases includes corticosteroids, which reduce edema within hours. Whole-brain radiation therapy improves symptoms, especially headaches and seizures.[78] There is improved survival with radiation therapy, up to approximately 5 to 6 months, when compared with corticosteroids alone.[85] The most common schedule is 30 Gy delivered in 10 fractions.[78] Surgical resection has been shown to result in an improved outcome compared with whole-brain radiation therapy. This may only be for women with solitary parenchymal metastasis, good performance status, and well-controlled systemic disease.

The role of surgery when there are multiple parenchymal cerebral metastases is less clear. There is possibly a role with a single symptomatic dominant lesion. Stereotactic radiosurgery is also considered, especially in patients with one to three small metastases.[78]

Many chemotherapeutic agents that are active in breast cancer do not cross the blood-brain barrier and therefore may not be useful in CNS metastases. Patients with cerebral disease are often excluded from clinical trials for this reason. Response rates to combination chemotherapy of up to 50% have been reported in small trials.[80] One theory is that the tumor may disrupt the usually impermeable barrier.[78]

Leptomeningeal metastases are treated differently. The median survival after diagnosis is only 12 weeks. Radiation therapy is used to control local symptoms. Intrathecal chemotherapy, through an Ommaya reservoir or a lumbar puncture, is considered for patients with good performance status and low-volume or well-controlled systemic metastases. This can result in improved median survival in various case reports and small trials of up to 7 months.

BONE METASTASES

Half of the patients with breast cancer will develop bone metastases.[86] These metastases are commonly painful. The management of cancer pain starts with an assessment of the symptoms, intensity, likely etiologic factors, and impact on the patients' lives.

A combination of short-acting and long-acting opioids is often necessary to control cancer-related pain. Frequent follow-up, assessment, and a timely response are required if pain control is inadequate. Options include changing the dose, switching or adding medication, radiation therapy, and procedures such as nerve blocks and intrathecal opiates or local anesthesia.[86]

Either bisphosphonates[87] or an inhibitor of RANK ligand[88] is used to reduce pain from and delay progression of bone metastases. These agents are usually used in combination with chemotherapy or hormonal therapy. Zoledronic acid is given by monthly intravenous infusion, and denosumab is given by monthly subcutaneous injection.

A single fraction of radiation therapy is often very effective for bone pain. A meta-analysis has shown there is no advantage, in terms of pain control, between single or multiple fractions of radiation therapy.[89] Contraindications include prior radiation therapy, pathologic fractures, spinal cord involvement, or cauda equina syndrome.

Indications for surgery for bone metastases include pathologic fractures, impending pathologic fractures, spinal neurologic deficits, and pain. A population-based study of 641 patients showed that surgical intervention improved pain in 77% and improved performance status in 65% of patients.[90]

The spine is the most common site of bone metastases, and metastases occur in up to 40% of patients.[90] Spinal cord compression is common with metastatic vertebral disease. It is found in 5% to 20% of cancer patients at autopsy.[86] In 90% of patients, cord compression is associated with pain and 50% have other neurologic symptoms.[91]

The treatment options are surgery or radiation therapy. A 2005 meta-analysis found that patients undergoing surgical treatment are 1.3 times more likely to ambulate after treatment (85% versus 64%).[92] Surgical management has become the preferred option in most cases. Radiation therapy is usually preferred when the patient has an estimated life expectancy of less than or up to 4 months or is unable to tolerate an operation.

SPECIAL TOPICS

BREAST CANCER IN MEN

Only 1% of breast cancer occurs in men. In the United States the incidence is relatively stable at approximately 1500 men per year. The median age at diagnosis is 68, which is slightly older than in women. Approximately 80% of cancers are estrogen receptor positive.[92,93] The prognostic factors and prognoses are similar to those in women. Men have a lower overall survival rate than women, but when matched for age, stage of tumor, and death from intercurrent illness, these differences are probably insignificant.[94]

With regard to treatment, there is very little evidence from trials. Recommended surgery is usually a modified radical mastectomy, and adjuvant radiation therapy is often reserved for men with locally advanced disease. Adjuvant systemic therapies are similar to those used in women.[94]

First-line therapy for metastatic disease is usually hormonal manipulation. A 69% response rate has been shown in hormone receptor–positive tumors but no response in receptor-negative tumors. Medical treatments include tamoxifen, aromatase inhibitors, androgens, antiandrogens, steroids and progestins. Surgical options include orchiectomy, adrenalectomy, and hypophysectomy. Chemotherapy is usually reserved for second-line treatment, with an overall response rate of 40%.[95,96]

PREVENTION OF BREAST CANCER

Screening mammography in postmenopausal women, with or without clinical breast examination, can reduce breast cancer mortality by up to 20%. For women older than 40 years, the sensitivity of mammography ranges from 71% to 96%. Mammography is much less sensitive for younger women. Suspicious findings on mammography have a specificity of 94% to 97%.[97] MRI of the breast is recommended annually for women with a lifetime risk of breast cancer of 20% or greater. This includes women with a strong family history including the *BRCA* mutations.[26] Trials have not shown that breast self-examination is beneficial.[6]

Some women are at very high risk of developing cancer, including those with *BRCA* mutations. In such cases prophylactic chemoprevention or surgical intervention is often considered. Tamoxifen given in the adjuvant setting results in a 47% reduction in contralateral breast cancer.[32] Trials using prophylactic tamoxifen in premenopausal and postmenopausal women with a high risk of developing breast cancer have shown up to a 50% reduction in cancer, but the reduction is seen only in estrogen receptor–positive disease. Interestingly, the benefit of tamoxifen lasts longer than the duration of the therapy. Similarly, there is a 50% reduction in cancer risk after oophorectomy in women who are *BRCA* carriers. Prophylactic bilateral mastectomy is also considered for women who are considered particularly high risk.[16]

ON THE HORIZON

There is substantial interest in improving the individualization of breast cancer treatments. The aim is to further develop ways to enhance predictions regarding the prognosis and efficacy of various treatments for individual tumors, thus minimizing toxicity from ineffectual therapies. Gene expression profiling has provided the most recent step in individualizing breast cancer treatments.

References (With Key References in Boldface)

1. American Cancer Society. Cancer Facts & Figures 2013. Available at *www.cancer.org/research/cancerfactsfigures/acspc-036845*.
2. **Siegel R, Naishadham D, Jemal A. Cancer statistics, 2013. CA Cancer J Clin 63:11-30, 2013.**
3. De Angelis R, Tavilla A, Verdecchia A, et al. Breast cancer survivors in the United States: geographic variability and time trends, 2005-2015. Cancer 115:1954-1966, 2009.
4. Ravdin PM, Cronin KA, Howlader N, et al. The decrease in breast-cancer incidence in 2003 in the United States. N Engl J Med 356:1670-1674, 2007.
5. **Stephens PJ, Tarpey PS, Davies H, et al. The landscape of cancer genes and mutational processes in breast cancer. Nature 486:400-404, 2012.**
6. Benson JR, Jatoi I, Keisch M, et al. Early breast cancer. Lancet 373:1463-1479, 2009.
7. Stead LA, Lash TL, Sobieraj JE, et al. Triple-negative breast cancers are increased in black women regardless of age or body mass index. Breast Cancer Res 11:R18, 2009.
8. Trivers KF, Lund MJ, Porter PL, et al. The epidemiology of triple-negative breast cancer, including race. Cancer Causes Control 20:1071-1082, 2009.
9. Chlebowski RT, Hendrix SL, Langer RD, et al; WHI Investigators. Influence of estrogen plus progestin on breast cancer and mammography in healthy postmenopausal women: the Women's Health Initiative Randomized Trial. JAMA 289:3243-3253, 2003.
10. Chlebowski RT, Kuller LH, Prentice RL, et al; WHI Investigators. Breast cancer after use of estrogen plus progestin in postmenopausal women. N Engl J Med 360:573-587, 2009.
11. Holmberg L, Iversen OE, Rudenstam CM, et al; HABITS Study Group. Increased risk of recurrence after hormone replacement therapy in breast cancer survivors. J Natl Cancer Inst 100:475-482, 2008.
12. Kelsey JL, Gammon MD. The epidemiology of breast cancer. CA Cancer J Clin 41:146-165, 1991.
13. Lynch HT, Snyder CL, Lynch JF, et al. Hereditary breast-ovarian cancer at the bedside: role of the medical oncologist. J Clin Oncol 21:740-753, 2003.
14. Masciari S, Dillon DA, Rath M, et al. Breast cancer phenotype in women with TP53 germline mutations: a Li-Fraumeni syndrome consortium effort. Breast Cancer Res Treat 133:1125-1130, 2012.
15. Struewing JP, Hartge P, Wacholder S, et al. The risk of cancer associated with specific mutations of BRCA1 and BRCA2 among Ashkenazi Jews. N Engl J Med 336:1401-1408, 1997.
16. Morrow M, Gradishar W. Breast cancer. BMJ 324:410-414, 2002.
17. Rosen PP, Groshen S, Kinne DW, et al. Contralateral breast carcinoma: an assessment of risk and prognosis in stage I (T1N0M0) and stage II (T1N1M0) patients with 20-year follow-up. Surgery 106:904-910, 1989.
18. Collins LC, Tamimi RM, Baer HJ, et al. Outcome of patients with ductal carcinoma in situ untreated after diagnostic biopsy: results from the Nurses' Health Study. Cancer 103:1778-1784, 2005.
19. Julien JP, Bijker N, Fentiman IS, et al. Radiotherapy in breast-conserving treatment for ductal carcinoma in situ: first results of the EORTC randomised phase III trial 10853. EORTC Breast Cancer Cooperative Group and EORTC Radiotherapy Group. Lancet 355:528-533, 2000.
20. Carson W, Sanchez-Forgach E, Stomper P, et al. Lobular carcinoma in situ: observation without surgery as an appropriate therapy. Ann Surg Oncol 1:141-146, 1994.

21. Hartmann LC, Sellers TA, Frost MH, et al. Benign breast disease and the risk of breast cancer. N Engl J Med 353:229-237, 2005.
22. Santen RJ, Mansel R. Benign breast disorders. N Engl J Med 353:275-285, 2005.
23. Degnim AC, Visscher DW, Berman HK, et al. Stratification of breast cancer risk in women with atypia: a Mayo cohort study. J Clin Oncol 25:2671-2677, 2007.
24. Renehan AG, Tyson M, Egger M, et al. Body-mass index and incidence of cancer: a systematic review and meta-analysis of prospective observational studies. Lancet 371:569-578, 2008.
25. Berg WA, Gutierrez L, NessAiver MS, et al. Diagnostic accuracy of mammography, clinical examination, US, and MR imaging in preoperative assessment of breast cancer. Radiology 233:830-849, 2004.
26. Orel S. Who should have breast magnetic resonance imaging evaluation? J Clin Oncol 26:703-711, 2008.
27. American Joint Committee on Cancer Staging Manual, 7th ed. Available at *http://www.cancerstaging.org*.
28. Singletary SE, Allred C, Ashley P, et al. Revision of the American Joint Committee on Cancer staging system for breast cancer. J Clin Oncol 20:3628-3636, 2002.
29. Yerushalmi R, Hayes MM, Gelmon KA. Breast carcinoma—rare types: review of the literature. Ann Oncol 20:1763-1770, 2009.
30. Molland JG, Donnellan M, Janu NC, et al. Infiltrating lobular carcinoma—a comparison of diagnosis, management and outcome with infiltrating duct carcinoma. Breast 13:389-396, 2004.
31. Chia S, Swain SM, Byrd DR, et al. Locally advanced and inflammatory breast cancer. J Clin Oncol 26:786-790, 2008.
32. Early Breast Cancer Trialists' Collaborative Group (EBCTCG). Effects of chemotherapy and hormonal therapy for early breast cancer on recurrence and 15-year survival: an overview of the randomised trials. Lancet 365:1687-1717, 2005.
33. Clarke M, Coates AS, Darby SC, et al; Early Breast Cancer Trialists' Collaborative Group (EBCTCG). Adjuvant chemotherapy in oestrogen-receptor-poor breast cancer: patient-level meta-analysis of randomised trials. Lancet 371:29-40, 2008.
34. Lin NU, Winer EP. Advances in adjuvant endocrine therapy for postmenopausal women. J Clin Oncol 26:798-805, 2008.
35. **Berry DA, Cirrincione C, Henderson IC, et al. Estrogen-receptor status and outcomes of modern chemotherapy for patients with node-positive breast cancer. JAMA 295:1658-1667, 2006.**
36. Hudis C. Trastuzumab—mechanism of action and use in clinical practice. N Engl J Med 357:39-51, 2007.
37. Bartlett JM, Going JJ, Mallon EA, et al. Evaluating HER2 amplification and overexpression in breast cancer. J Pathol 195:422-428, 2001.
38. Mackey J, McLeod D, Ragaz J, et al. Adjuvant targeted therapy in early breast cancer. Cancer 115:1154-1168, 2009.
39. Carey LA, Perou CM, Livasy CA, et al. Race, breast cancer subtypes, and survival in the Carolina Breast Cancer Study. JAMA 295:2492-2502, 2006.
40. Rakha EA, El-Sayed ME, Green AR, et al. Prognostic markers in triple-negative breast cancer. Cancer 109:25-32, 2007.
41. Dent R, Trudeau M, Pritchard KI, et al. Triple-negative breast cancer: clinical features and patterns of recurrence. Clin Cancer Res 13(15 Pt 1):4429-4434, 2007.
42. Elston CW, Ellis IO. Pathological prognostic factors in breast cancer. I. The value of histological grade in breast cancer: experience from a large study with long-term follow-up. Histopathology 19:403-410, 1991.
43. Urruticoechea A, Smith IE, Dowset M. Proliferation marker Ki-67 in early breast cancer. J Clin Oncol 23:7212-7220, 2005.
44. van't Veer LJ, Paik S, Hayes DF. Gene expression profiling of breast cancer: a new tumor marker. J Clin Oncol 23:1631-1635, 2005.
45. Perou CM, Sørlie T, Eisen MB, et al. Molecular portraits of human breast tumours. Nature 406:747-752, 2000.

46. Sotiriou C, Pusztai L. Gene-expression signatures in breast cancer. N Engl J Med 360:790-800, 2009.
47. National Cancer Institute: Surveillance, Epidemiology and End Results [SEER]. Available at http://www.seer.cancer.gov.
48. Rugo HS. The importance of distant metastases in hormone-sensitive breast cancer. Breast (17 Suppl 1):S3-S8, 2008.
49. Giordano SH, Buzdar AU, Smith TL, et al. Is breast cancer survival improving? Cancer 100:44-52, 2004.
50. **Chia SK, Speers CH, D'yachkova Y, et al. The impact of new chemotherapeutic and hormone agents on survival in a population-based cohort of women with metastatic breast cancer. Cancer 110:973-979, 2007.**
51. **Kiely BE, Soon YY, Tattersall MH, et al. How long have I got? Estimating typical, best-case, and worst-case scenarios for patients starting first-line chemotherapy for metastatic breast cancer: a systematic review of recent randomized trials. J Clin Oncol 29:456-463, 2011.**
52. James JJ, Evans AJ, Pinder SE, et al. Bone metastases from breast carcinoma: histopathological-radiological correlations and prognostic features. Br J Cancer 89:660-665, 2003.
53. Sherry MM, Greco FA, Johnson DH, et al. Metastatic breast cancer confined to the skeletal system. An indolent disease. Am J Med 81:381-386, 1986.
54. Clarke M, Collins R, Darby S, et al; Early Breast Cancer Trialists' Collaborative Group (EBCTCG). Effects of radiotherapy and of differences in the extent of surgery for early breast cancer on local recurrence and 15-year survival: an overview of the randomised trials. Lancet 366:2087-2106, 2005.
55. Morrow M, Strom EA, Bassett LW, et al; American College of Radiology; American College of Surgeons; Society of Surgical Oncology; College of American Pathology. Standard for breast conservation therapy in the management of invasive breast carcinoma. CA Cancer J Clin 52:277-300, 2002.
56. Buchholz TA. Radiation therapy for early-stage breast cancer after breast-conserving surgery. N Engl J Med 360:63-70, 2009.
57. James ML, Lehman M, Hider PN, et al. Fraction size in radiation treatment for breast conservation in early breast cancer. Cochrane Database Syst Rev Jul 16, 2008 CD003860.
58. Sandri MT, Zorzino L, Cassatella MC, et al. Changes in circulating tumor cell detection in patients with localized breast cancer before and after surgery. Ann Surg Oncol 17:1539-1545, 2010.
59. Braun S, Vogl FD, Naume B, et al. A pooled analysis of bone marrow micrometastasis in breast cancer. N Engl J Med 353:793-802, 2005.
60. Early Breast Cancer Trialists' Collaborative Group (EBCTCG). Effects of chemotherapy and hormonal therapy for early breast cancer on recurrence and 15-year survival: an overview of the randomised trials. Lancet 365:1687-1717, 2005.
61. Rugo HS. The breast cancer continuum in hormone-receptor-positive breast cancer in postmenopausal women: evolving management options focusing on aromatase inhibitors. Ann Oncol 19:16-27, 2008.
62. Smith IE, Dowsett M. Aromatase inhibitors in breast cancer. N Engl J Med 348:2431-2442, 2003.
63. **Dowsett M, Cuzick J, Ingle J, et al. Meta-analysis of breast cancer outcomes in adjuvant trials of aromatase inhibitors versus tamoxifen. J Clin Oncol 28:509-518, 2010.**
64. **Goss PE, Ingle JN, Martino S, et al. Randomized trial of letrozole following tamoxifen as extended adjuvant therapy in receptor-positive breast cancer: updated findings from NCIC CTG MA.17. J Natl Cancer Inst 97:1262-1271, 2005.**
65. Mamounas EP, Bryant J, Lembersky B, et al. Paclitaxel after doxorubicin plus cyclophosphamide as adjuvant chemotherapy for node-positive breast cancer: results from NSABP B-28. J Clin Oncol 23:3686-3696, 2005.
66. Wolff AC, Davidson NE. Primary systemic therapy in operable breast cancer. J Clin Oncol 18:1558-1569, 2000.
67. Fossati R, Confalonieri C, Torri V, et al. Cytotoxic and hormonal treatment for metastatic breast cancer: a systematic review of published randomized trials involving 31,510 women. J Clin Oncol 16:3439-3460, 1998.

68. Baselga J, Campone M, Piccart M, et al. Everolimus in postmenopausal hormone-receptor-positive advanced breast cancer. N Engl J Med 366:520-529, 2012.
69. Wilcken N, Hornbuckle J, Ghersi D. Chemotherapy alone versus endocrine therapy alone for metastatic breast cancer. Cochrane Database Syst Rev 2003 CD002747.
70. Slamon DJ, Leyland-Jones B, Shak S, et al. Use of chemotherapy plus a monoclonal antibody against HER2 for metastatic breast cancer that overexpresses HER2. N Engl J Med 344:783-792, 2001.
71. Swain SM, Kim SB, Cortés J, et al. Pertuzumab, trastuzumab, and docetaxel for HER2-positive metastatic breast cancer (CLEOPATRA study): overall survival results from a randomised, double-blind, placebo-controlled, phase 3 study. Lancet Oncol 14:461-471, 2013.
72. Geyer CE, Forster J, Lindquist D, et al. Lapatinib plus capecitabine for HER2-positive advanced breast cancer. N Engl J Med 355:2733-2743, 2006.
73. Blackwell KL, Burstein HJ, Storniolo AM, et al. Overall survival benefit with lapatinib in combination with trastuzumab for patients with human epidermal growth factor receptor 2-positive metastatic breast cancer: final results from the EGF104900 Study. J Clin Oncol 30:2585-2592, 2012.
74. **Verma S, Miles D, Gianni L, et al. Trastuzumab emtansine for HER2-positive advanced breast cancer. N Engl J Med 367:1783-1791, 2012.**
75. Folkman J. Tumor angiogenesis: therapeutic implications. N Engl J Med 285:1182-1186, 1971.
76. Bando H. Vascular endothelial growth factor and bevacizumab in breast cancer. Breast Cancer 14:163-173, 2007.
77. Miller K, Wang M, Gralow J, et al. Paclitaxel plus bevacizumab versus paclitaxel alone for metastatic breast cancer. N Engl J Med 357:2666-2676, 2007.
78. Lin NU, Bellon JR, Winer EP. CNS metastases in breast cancer. J Clin Oncol 22:3608-3617, 2004.
79. Saip P, Cicin I, Eralp Y, et al. Factors affecting the prognosis of breast cancer patients with brain metastases. Breast 17:451-458, 2008.
80. **Walbert T, Gilbert MR. The role of chemotherapy in the treatment of patients with brain metastases from solid tumors. Int J Clin Oncol 14:299-306, 2009.**
81. Chien AJ, Rugo HS. Emerging treatment options for the management of brain metastases in patients with HER2-positive metastatic breast cancer. Breast Cancer Res Treat 137:1-2, 2013.
82. Park BB, Uhm JE, Cho EY, et al. Prognostic factor analysis in patients with brain metastases from breast cancer: how can we improve the treatment outcomes? Cancer Chemother Pharmacol 63:627-633, 2009.
83. Melisko ME, Moore DH, Sneed PK, De Franco J, Rugo HS. Brain metastases in breast cancer: clinical and pathologic characteristics associated with improvements in survival. J Neurooncol 88:359-365, 2008.
84. Gaspar L, Scott C, Rotman M, et al. Recursive partitioning analysis (RPA) of prognostic factors in three Radiation Therapy Oncology Group (RTOG) brain metastases trials. Int J Radiat Oncol Biol Phys 37:745-751, 1997.
85. Rosner D, Nemoto T, Lane WW. Chemotherapy induces regression of brain metastases in breast carcinoma. Cancer 58:832-839, 1986.
86. **Dy SM, Asch SM, Naeim A, et al. Evidence-based standards for cancer pain management. J Clin Oncol 28:3879-3885, 2008.**
87. Kohno N, Aogi K, Minami H, et al. Zoledronic acid significantly reduces skeletal complications compared with placebo in Japanese women with bone metastases from breast cancer: a randomized, placebo-controlled trial. J Clin Oncol 23:3314-3321, 2005.
88. Lipton A, Fizazi K, Stopeck AT, et al. Superiority of denosumab to zoledronic acid for prevention of skeletal-related events: a combined analysis of 3 pivotal, randomised, phase 3 trials. Eur J Cancer 48:3082-3092, 2012.
89. Wu JS, Wong R, Johnston M, et al; Cancer Care Ontario Practice Guidelines Initiative Supportive Care Group. Meta-analysis of dose-fractionation radiotherapy trials for the palliation of painful bone metastases. Int J Radiat Oncol 55:594-605, 2003.
90. Walcott BP, Cvetanovich GL, Barnard ZR, et al. Surgical treatment and outcomes of metastatic breast cancer to the spine. J Clin Neurosci 18:1336-1339, 2011.

91. Loblaw DA, Perry J, Chambers A, et al. Systematic review of the diagnosis and management of malignant extradural spinal cord compression: the Cancer Care Ontario Practice Guidelines Initiative's Neuro-Oncology Disease Site Group. J Clin Oncol 23:2028-2037, 2005.
92. **Klimo P Jr, Thompson CJ, Kestle JR, et al. A meta-analysis of surgery versus conventional radiotherapy for the treatment of metastatic spinal epidural disease. Neuro Oncol 7:64-76, 2005.**
93. **Veeravagu A, Lieberson RE, Mener A, et al. CyberKnife stereotactic radiosurgery for the treatment of intramedullary spinal cord metastases. J Clin Neurosci 19:1273-1277, 2012.**
94. Giordano SH, Buzdar AU, Hortobagyi GN. Breast cancer in men. Ann Intern Med 137:678-687, 2002.
95. Thomas DB, Jimenez LM, McTiernan A, et al. Breast cancer in men: risk factors with hormonal implications. Am J Epidemiol 135:734-748, 1992
96. Jaiyesimi IA, Buzdar AU, Sahin AA, et al. Carcinoma of the male breast. Ann Intern Med 117:771-777, 1992.
97. Humphrey LL, Helfand M, Chan BK, et al. Breast cancer screening: a summary of the evidence for the US Preventive Services Task Force. Ann Intern Med 137(5 Part 1):347-360, 2002.

Chapter 21

Prostate Cancer

Sumanta Kumar Pal, Susan Onami,
David Josephson, Przemyslaw Twardowski

Prostate cancer represents the most common malignancy in men, with an estimated 192,280 cases diagnosed in 2009.[1] As illustrated in Fig. 21-1, the incidence of prostate cancer rose sharply between 1990 and 1995, which is likely attributable to more widespread adoption of prostate-specific antigen (PSA) screening. PSA screening has also resulted in a drastic stage migration in prostate cancer, with far fewer patients presenting with de novo metastatic disease.[2] With a preponderance of early-stage disease, deaths from prostate cancer have declined—recent data suggest that prostate cancer–related deaths decreased by 36% between 1990 and 2005, with a total of 27,360 deaths estimated in 2009.[1] Also contributing to this decline is a continual advancement in therapeutic approaches for prostate cancer. In the setting of metastatic disease, a greater understanding of tumor biology and immunology has led to the development of numerous targeted therapies. In this chapter, paradigms for the management of advanced prostate cancer, including the use of androgen deprivation therapy (ADT) and chemotherapy, are described and used as a framework for discussion of novel agents in clinical development. Updated strategies for preserving bone integrity and homeostasis are also discussed. These are of particular relevance to neurosurgeons who frequently treat skeletal events related to prostate cancer and associated therapy.

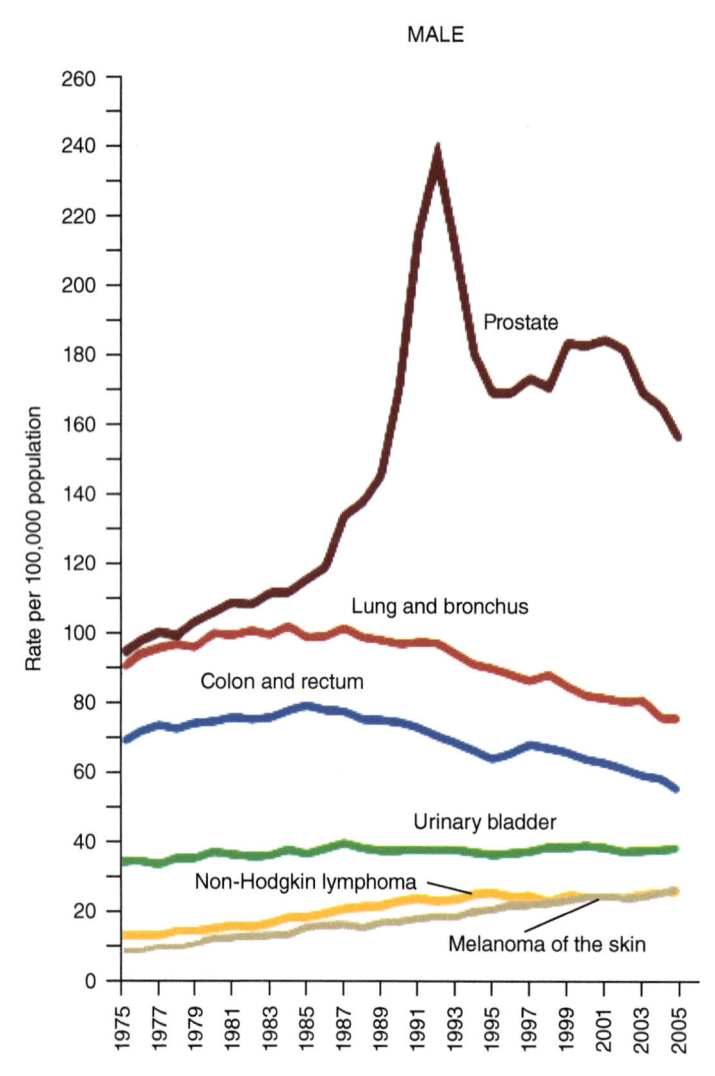

Fig. 21-1 Age-adjusted incidence of prostate cancer derived from the Surveillance, Epidemiology, and End Results (SEER) program. Note the sharp increase in the incidence of prostate cancer between 1989 and 1995, coinciding with adoption of PSA screening. (From Jemal A, Siegel R, Ward E, et al. Cancer Statistics, 2009. CA Cancer J Clin 59:225-249, 2009. © 2009 American Cancer Society.)

EXISTING PARADIGMS: ANDROGEN DEPRIVATION THERAPY AND CHEMOTHERAPY

Since publication of the seminal work by Huggins et al,[3,4] in 1941, the pivotal role of testosterone in prostate cancer growth and the antitumor effect of castration have been recognized. Bilateral simple orchiectomy remains a valid option for patients with newly diagnosed metastatic disease, depleting circulating testosterone within 24 hours. Pharmacologic suppression of testosterone is another alternative. The luteinizing hormone–releasing hormone (LHRH) agonists (including leuprolide, goserelin, and triptorelin) alter pituitary signaling, thereby decreasing gonadal steroid synthesis.[5,6] A distinct class of agents, the antiandrogens, bind directly to the androgen receptor and inhibit downstream mitogenic pathways. The antiandrogens include bicalutamide, flutamide, and nilutamide, and these are primarily used in combination with LHRH agonists.[7] If this combination, which is called *combined androgen blockade* (CAB) is employed, a strategy of antiandrogen withdrawal can be attempted after clinical progression is observed because, over time, antiandrogens can begin exerting an agonistic effect on the androgen receptor.[8] The greatest benefit of CAB for bony metastases is seen in patients with prostate cancer who have not previously undergone hormonal therapy.[9] Although ADT spares the patient many adverse effects associated with cytotoxic therapy, the toxicity panel still warrants extensive discussion. Hot flashes, fatigue, and decreased libido are among the well-documented adverse effects associated with ADT. In addition, it is increasingly recognized that ADT can affect endocrine axes (thereby leading to greater risk of diabetes) and heighten the risk of osteoporotic fracture.[10] Strategies to mitigate the latter are discussed elsewhere in this chapter.

After failure of ADT, therapy with ketoconazole may be attempted. In high doses this antifungal agent leads to decreases in adrenal steroid synthesis and testosterone secretion from Leydig cells. However, the utility of the agent is compromised by its relatively short duration of activity and extensive side effect profile (including lethargy, weakness, and hepatic dysfunction).[11]

An established standard after failure of ADT is docetaxel-based chemotherapy, which has been validated in two large prospective trials. Docetaxel is an antimitotic agent with documented activity across a wide spectrum of malignancies.[12-14] In the Southwest Oncology Group (SWOG) 9916 clinical trial, a total of 770 patients with advanced prostate cancer that had progressed while the patients were on ADT were randomized to the combination of docetaxel and estramustine or mitoxantrone and prednisone. Treatment with docetaxel-based therapy was associated with an improved rate of PSA response (50% decline in 50% versus 27% of patients, $P = 0.01$), time to progression (6.3 months versus 3.2 months [$P < 0.001$]), and improved overall survival (17.5 months versus 15.6 months [$P = 0.02$]).[15] The combination of docetaxel and estramustine also led to a greater incidence of neutropenic fever ($P = 0.01$), nausea, and vomiting ($P < 0.01$) and cardiovascular events ($P < 0.001$).

A second larger trial, the TAX 327 study, omitted the use of estramustine (a cytotoxic conjugate of estradiol and nitrogen mustard) as used in the SWOG 9916 study. In this study, a total of 1006 men whose disease had progressed on ADT were randomized to either docetaxel and prednisone or mitoxantrone and prednisone.[16] Once again, superior survival was observed with docetaxel chemotherapy (19.2 months versus 16.3 months). Similar trends in survival were observed irrespective of the presence or absence of pain at baseline, age greater than or less than 65 years, and for PSA values greater than or less than the median value (115 ng/ml). Thus the combination of docetaxel and prednisone now represents an accepted standard for patients who have progression of their disease on ADT.

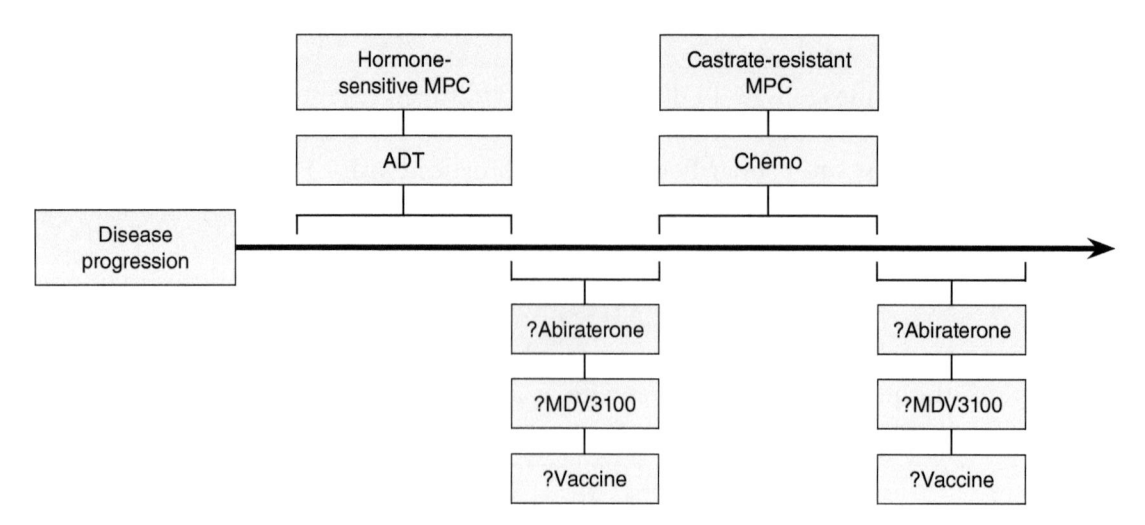

Fig. 21-2 Changing paradigms in prostate cancer. The traditional approach to metastatic prostate cancer (MPC) involves use of ADT in the hormone-sensitive state, followed by addition of chemotherapy in the castrate-resistant state. Novel agents, including abiraterone, MDV3100, and vaccine therapies, may find a role between or subsequent to these states.

EXPLOITING HORMONAL AXES: BEYOND ANDROGEN DEPRIVATION THERAPY

Beyond docetaxel chemotherapy, existing guidelines suggest only the use of supportive care strategies.[17] However, numerous agents currently under evaluation hold substantial promise (Fig. 21-2). For some of these agents, that promise is predicated on the fact that the androgen receptor still plays a critical role in prostatic carcinogenesis beyond failure of ADT. In this "castrate-resistant" state, there appears to be upregulation of the androgen receptor, facilitating androgen-driven pathways at low serum concentrations of testosterone or through other costimulatory molecules.[18,19] The prognostic value of the androgen receptor is being increasingly recognized—that is, increased levels of nuclear androgen receptor may correlate with survival in the setting of advanced disease.[20]

ABIRATERONE AFTER CHEMOTHERAPY

Harnessing these scientific findings, the agent abiraterone inhibits cytochrome P 17 (CYP17) in an irreversible fashion, leading to depletion of both testosterone and estradiol through the feedback loop described in Fig. 21-3.[21] In rodent models abiraterone decreased plasma testosterone levels to less than 0.1 nmol/L and led to a decline in ventral prostatic and testicular weight.[22] It should be noted that abiraterone

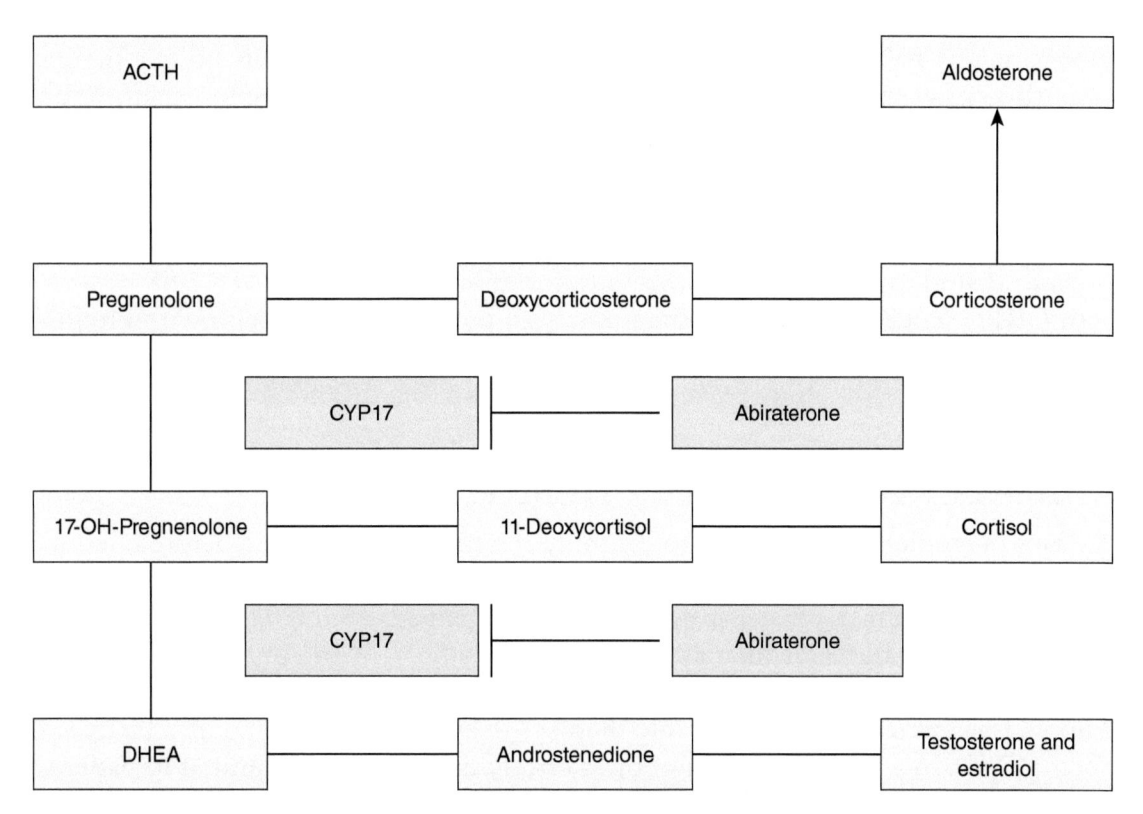

Fig. 21-3 Mechanism of abiraterone. (Reprinted from Pal SK, Twardowski P, Josephson DY. Beyond castration and chemotherapy: novel approaches to targeting androgen-driven pathways. Maturitas 64:61-66, 2009.)

monotherapy does lead to increases in deoxycorticosterone. Clinical consequences of deoxycorticosterone production include hypokalemia, hypertension, and fluid retention. To mitigate these effects, abiraterone can be coadministered with glucocorticoids. Several of the clinical trials examined herein explore abiraterone with or without concomitant steroid therapy.

Two phase II experiences have characterized the activity of abiraterone in the postchemotherapy setting. In the first study, 47 patients with castrate-resistant prostate cancer (CRPC) were treated with abiraterone, 1000 mg per day by mouth, with or without glucocorticoids, after the failure of docetaxel chemotherapy.[23] Only six patients (14%) in this study had received prior ketoconazole therapy. A decline in PSA of greater than 50% was noted in 24 patients (51%), and patients were treated for a median of 167 days. In the second phase II experience, 58 patients were treated after failure of up to two cytotoxic regimens.[24] An identical dose of abiraterone was used, but was combined with a standardized dose of prednisone (5 mg by mouth twice daily). Similar to the previous phase II experience, nearly half of patients (45%) experienced a decline in PSA of more than 50%. Abiraterone led to an improvement in global functioning (assessed by Eastern Cooperative Oncology Group [ECOG] performance status) in approximately half of the patients in an exploratory analysis. In this study a higher proportion of patients (41%) had prior ketoconazole therapy, allowing for stratification by prior receipt of this agent. Those patients previously treated with ketoconazole had a much shorter time to PSA progression (99 days versus 198 days).

Given the impressive activity of abiraterone after failure of docetaxel chemotherapy, a phase III study was launched in this setting.[25] This study randomized 1158 patients with CRPC in a 2:1 fashion to abiraterone with prednisone or placebo with prednisone and was powered to detect a 25% improvement in survival with abiraterone. With the accrual goal of the study recently met, results are eagerly anticipated.

ABIRATERONE BEFORE CHEMOTHERAPY

A series of studies has attempted to examine the role of abiraterone before chemotherapy, potentially inserting the agent between ADT and docetaxel in the current treatment algorithm. A phase I analysis included 33 patients with CRPC and identified a PSA response of greater than 50% in 18 patients (55%).[26] In contrast to the postchemotherapy setting, an appreciable rate of response was observed in those patients who had received prior ketoconazole therapy (decline in PSA >50% in 7 of 15 patients [47%]). In a phase II extension of the study, enrollment was limited to patients who had not received prior ketoconazole.[27] In 27 evaluable patients, a decline in PSA of greater than 50% was noted in 15 patients (71%).

A parallel phase I/II study was conducted by a different group that enrolled 21 chemotherapy-naïve patients with CRPC in the phase I component. Decreases in PSA levels of more than 50% were observed in 12 patients (57%).[28] Correlative studies performed in this analysis suggested that the ERG gene rearrangement could predict the response to abiraterone. Fusion of the TMPRSS2 and ERG genes is estimated to occur in up to 60% of patients with prostate cancer, and the resultant gene product plays a putative role in androgen-driven mitogenesis.[29] TMPRSS2-ERG fusion is now being studied more extensively as a biomarker of abiraterone response. The phase II expansion of this phase I experience included a total of 42 patients.[30] A decline in PSA of more than 50% was observed in 28 patients (67%). It is worth noting that treatment with dexamethasone (instituted at the time of progression on abiraterone monotherapy) appeared to reverse resistance to abiraterone therapy in one third of the patients.

The cumulative experience from early-phase trials suggests that abiraterone may actually have slightly higher activity in chemotherapy-naïve patients with CRPC. Thus a phase III trial has been devised to evaluate abiraterone in this setting. The schema of the study is similar to that evaluating abiraterone chemotherapy–refractory patients, with the exception that patients will be randomized in a 1:1 fashion to either abiraterone and prednisone or placebo and prednisone.[31] Powered to detect a 20% increase in overall survival, this study could potentially change the current algorithm of advanced prostate cancer management, inserting abiraterone between ADT and docetaxel.

MDV3100

Similar to abiraterone, the androgen receptor antagonist MDV3100 exploits the persistent functionality of testosterone-driven pathways in CRPC. MDV3100 binds to the androgen receptor with substantially higher affinity compared with bicalutamide and has also been shown to inhibit nuclear translocation of the receptor.[32] The agent leads to increased apoptosis and growth inhibition in preclinical models of CRPC.[32,33] In terms of clinical assessment, a phase I/II experience that included 140 patients was recently reported.[34] Within this group approximately half had received prior chemotherapy (75 patients [54%]). As two seizures were observed at doses of 360 mg and 600 mg daily, a dosage of 240 mg daily was selected for further assessment. The toxicity profile of MDV3100 was otherwise minimal. The most common moderate-to-severe toxicity was fatigue, which occurred in 9% of patients. As in the abiraterone experience, the frequency of PSA decline of more than 50% was slightly greater among chemotherapy-naïve patients as compared with chemotherapy-refractory patients (62% versus 51%). Similarly, soft tissue responses were higher in the chemotherapy-naïve population (36% versus 12%). Nonetheless, the impressive overall activity of the agent and the reasonable side effect profile have led to the implementation of a phase III trial assessing the agent. In the AFFIRM trial, 1170 patients with chemotherapy-refractory CRPC will be randomized in a 2:1 fashion to MDV3100 or placebo.[35] It remains to be seen how MDV3100 will compete in treatment algorithms with abiraterone; presumably a combination of the agents could be attempted given their distinct mechanisms of activity.

EVOLUTION OF VACCINE THERAPY

Vaccine therapy has long since been postulated as a potential anticancer strategy. However, only recently has the therapeutic potential of this strategy been realized (Table 21-1). In the setting of prostate cancer, one vaccine therapy has been immersed in controversy since its initial stages of development; that drug is sipuleucel-T. Sipuleucel-T represents an autologous cell product, derived from host APCs cultured with the fusion protein PA2024.[36] PA2024 is composed of prostatic acid phosphatase linked to granulocyte-macrophage colony-stimulating factor (GM-CSF).[37] In the phase III

Table 21-1 Available Vaccine Therapies for Prostate Cancer and Associated Levels of Evidence

Vaccine	Type	Evidence
Sipuleucel-T	Autologous cellular immunotherapy, activated in vitro by recombinant fusion protein	Phase III
G-VAX	Whole-cell vaccine composed of irradiated PC3 and LNCaP secreting G-CSF	Phase III
PROSTVAC-VF	Two viral vectors encoding PSA and three immune costimulatory molecules (B7.1, ICAM-1, and LFA3)	Phase II

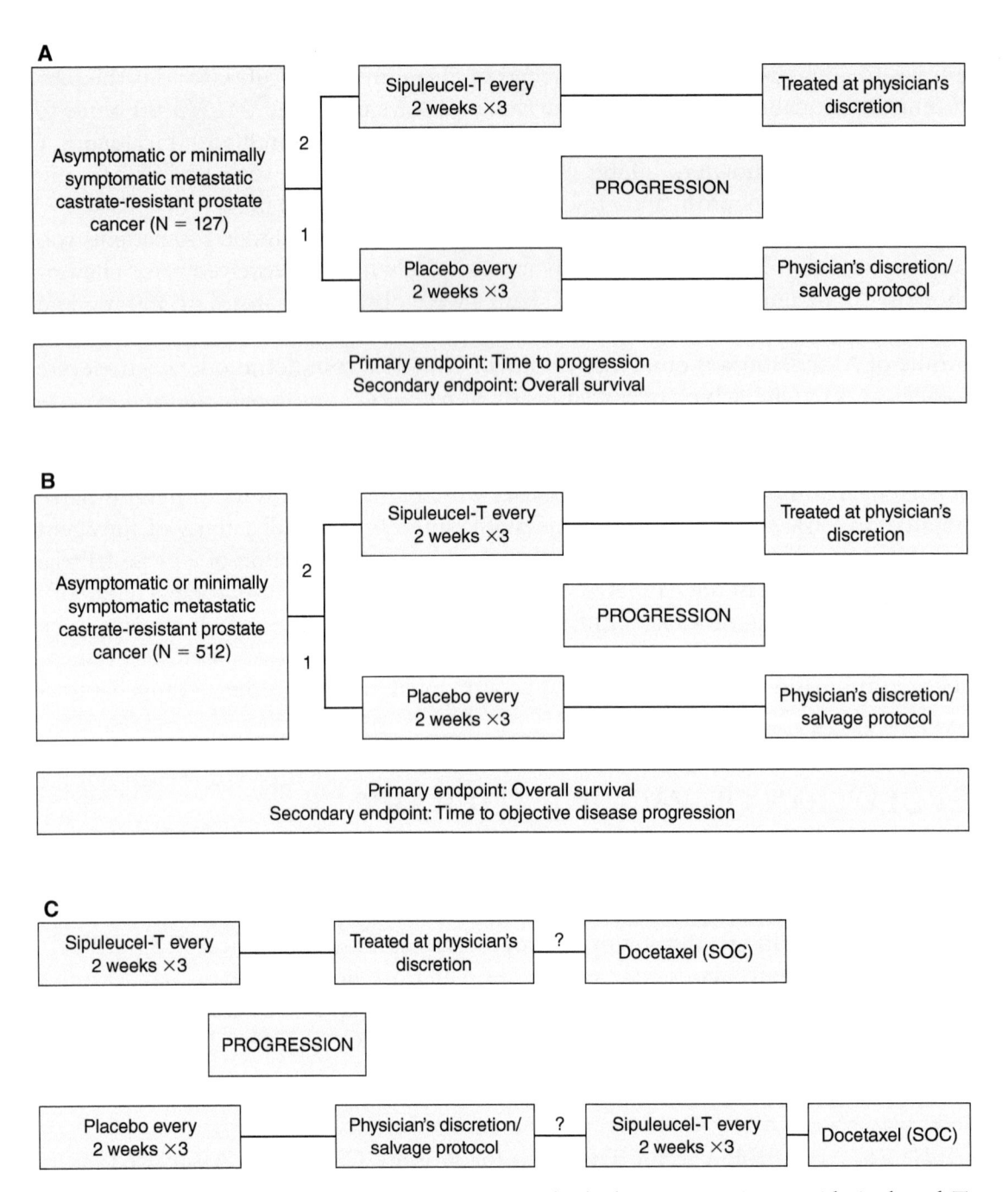

Fig. 21-4 Schema for the **A,** D9901 and **B,** IMPACT, both phase III experiences with sipuleucel-T. **C,** A problem frequently cited with the "salvage protocol" offered in both experiences is the potential delay in docetaxel chemotherapy incurred as a result.

D9901 trial, 127 patients with asymptomatic metastatic prostate cancer were randomized in a 2:1 fashion to receive three infusions of sipuleucel-T or placebo (Fig. 21-4, *A*). At the time of progression, patients could receive salvage therapy with a cryopreserved product. The study failed to improve time-to-progression but did lead to a significant improvement in overall survival (25.9 versus 21.4 months, $P = 0.01$). Although approval from the United States Food and Drug Administration was sought on the basis of this trial, the dataset was heavily criticized for several reasons, including failure to meet its primary endpoint (improvement in time-to-progression), small sample size, and methodologic variations in administration of salvage therapy at crossover.

A more robust experience ensued in trial D9901. The phase III IMPACT study randomized 512 patients with CRPC in a 2:1 fashion to receive sipuleucel-T or placebo every 2 weeks for a total of three cycles (Fig. 21-4, *B*).[38] At the time of progression, patients were eligible to receive sipuleucel-T derived from cryopreserved cells. The trial achieved its primary endpoint of improved overall survival (25.8 versus 21.7 months, $P = 0.032$). However, this improvement in overall survival was not paralleled by a change in disease-free survival ($P = 0.63$). The toxicity profile of sipuleucel-T in this experience was modest, with the most common side effects being chills (54%) and pyrexia (29%). Despite these compelling results, several questions remain. As observed in D9901, with no difference in disease-free survival, could the improved survival observed with sipuleucel-T simply be the result of delayed administration of cytotoxic chemotherapy (Fig. 21-4, *C*)? Alternatively it has been posited that a latent immune effect could account for this phenomenon, as delineated in Fig. 21-5. As these debates proceed, the place of sipuleucel-T in current algorithms remains controversial.

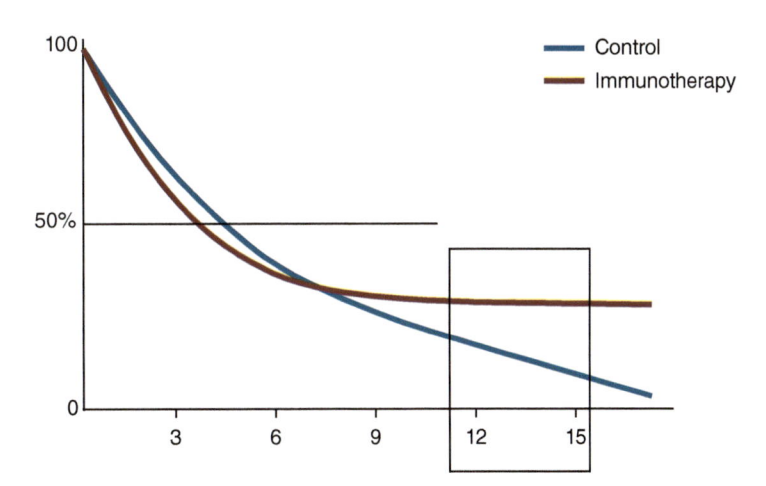

Fig. 21-5 A proposed latent of vaccine therapy. This hypothetical model demonstrates how vaccine therapy could potentially prolong survival without having an impact on intermediate endpoints, such as time-to-progression (TTP). (Courtesy M. Eisenberger. Discussion presented at the 2009 Annual Meeting of the American Society of Clinical Oncology).

Several other forays into vaccine therapy have been met with lesser success. G-VAX represents a whole-cell vaccine that consists of two fused prostate cancer cell lines, PC3 and LN-CaP, modified to secrete GM-CSF and irradiated to prevent further cell division.[39] In a phase I/II assessment, the agent appeared to be immunogenic, and dosing was correlated with survival.[40] Unfortunately, phase III results from the VITAL-2 study were more sobering.[41] In this study, patients with symptomatic CRPC and one prior nontaxane regimen were randomized to either G-VAX with docetaxel or docetaxel and prednisone. The study ultimately demonstrated a survival advantage favoring docetaxel and prednisone (14.8 versus 12.4 months, $P = 0.02$). Although the study design has been criticized for omission of steroid therapy on the treatment arm, these results are nonetheless discouraging.

Other vaccine therapies are currently in earlier phases of testing. Data from a randomized phase II trial of PROSTVAC-VF were recently presented.[42] PROSTVAC-VF represents a fusion of two recombinant viral vectors, each encoding PSA and three costimulatory molecules (B7.1, ICAM-1, and LFA3). A total of 122 patients with chemotherapy-naïve metastatic prostate cancer were randomized in a 2:1 fashion to receive either vaccine therapy or empty vector. Reflecting the experience with sipuleucel-T, the vaccine prolonged survival (24.5 versus 15 months, $P = 0.016$) but did not lead to any difference in progression-free survival. The common themes emerging from vaccine-based trials (i.e., improved survival but no change in progression-free survival) underscore the need to better understand the mechanisms of these agents. With multiple vaccines in development, results of additional studies are eagerly anticipated.

PRESERVING BONE INTEGRITY

As noted previously, ADT is associated with a number of potential risks, including osteoporosis.[43] As a result, guidelines from the National Comprehensive Cancer Network (NCCN) suggest that all patients receiving ADT be screened by means of the fracture risk assessment tool (FRAX), a clinically validated algorithm that can stratify the risk of skeletal events.[17,44] Although all patients more than 50 years of age who are on ADT are advised to take supplemental calcium (1200 mg/day) and vitamin D_3 (800 to 1000 IU daily), more aggressive approaches are recommended for those men with a higher 10-year risk of hip fracture (>3%) or major osteoporosis-related fracture (>20%). These approaches frequently include bisphosphonate therapy. Bisphosphonates primarily inhibit osteoclast function, thereby decreasing bone turnover and preserving bone homeostasis (Fig. 21-6).[45] Prospective studies assessing patients with nonmetastatic prostate cancer on ADT suggest that the bisphosphonate zoledronic acid can lead to substantial improvements in bone mineral density (BMD).[46]

Smaller series have identified a potential benefit of zoledronic acid therapy in hormone-sensitive metastatic disease. A Veterans Administration study randomized 93 patients to either placebo or 4 mg of zoledronic acid intravenously every 3 months for 1 year.[47] Patients were stratified by the prior duration of ADT (less than or greater than 1 year). In this prospective effort, patients had an improvement in BMD with zoledronic acid therapy at the 12-month assessment, whether they had been previ-

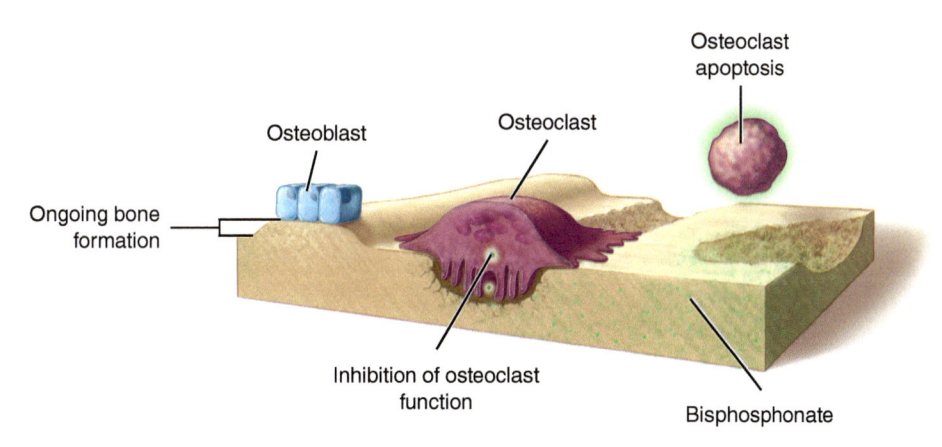

Fig. 21-6 Mechanism of bisphosphonates. (From Solomon CG. Bisphosphonates and osteoporosis. N Engl J Med 346:642, 2002. © 2002 Massachusetts Medical Society. Reprinted with permission.)

ously treated with less than 1 year of ADT (+5.95% versus −3.23% change in BMD; $P = 0.004$) or more than 1 year of ADT (+6.08 versus +1.57% change in BMD; $P = 0.005$). More follow-up is necessary to determine whether the agent can lead to a decline in skeletal-related events in this setting. The optimal frequency of therapy also needs to be defined. A prospective trial of 58 men with hormone-sensitive prostate cancer treated every 3 months with intravenous zoledronic acid identified an increase in BMD at 12 months as compared with baseline values.[48] However, 1 year after the completion of zoledronic acid therapy, there was a significant decline in BMD, suggesting that annual therapy with zoledronic acid may not be sufficient.

Patients with CRPC and bony metastases may benefit substantially from bisphosphonate therapy as well. Zoledronic acid has been examined in this setting in a pivotal phase III trial.[49] In this study 643 patients with CRPC and bone metastases were randomized to receive one of two dosage levels of zoledronic acid or placebo intravenously every 3 weeks for 15 months. Compliance with this regimen was somewhat poor, with only approximately one third of patients on each arm completing the prescribed regimen. Nonetheless, compared with those patients who received placebo, patients receiving zoledronic acid at a standard dose (4 mg) had fewer skeletal-related events (44.2% versus 33.2%; $P = 0.021$). Furthermore, time to a skeletal event was prolonged in those patients receiving zoledronic acid. Correlative studies assessing markers of bone turnover demonstrated a decrease in marker levels with either dose of zoledronic acid. However, treatment on the experimental arms did not lead to improvements in clinical endpoints, such as disease progression, performance status, or quality of life. Also, the elevated dose of zoledronic acid in this study (8 mg) was associated with deterioration of renal function.

Outside of bisphosphonate therapy, a novel approach to improving bone homeostasis is inhibition of the RANK ligand (RANK-L). RANK-L is a critical mediator in osteoclast differentiation and activation.[50] Therefore agents such as denosumab (a monoclonal antibody antagonizing RANK-L) can lead to decreased bone resorption. Denosumab has been evaluated in a large, randomized phase III experience. In this study 734 patients with nonmetastatic prostate cancer on ADT were randomized to receive either denosumab, 60 mg subcutaneously every 6 months, or placebo. At the 24-month follow-up, BMD had improved by 5.6% in the denosumab group but decreased by 1.0% in the placebo group. At the 36-month follow-up, those patients on denosumab had a decreased incidence of new vertebral fractures (1.5% versus 3.9%; $P = 0.006$). With respect to management of metastatic prostate cancer, results from a trial comparing zoledronic acid and denosumab in patients with CRPC are eagerly anticipated.[51] Ongoing scientific and clinical developments in the area of bone metabolism have already made a substantial impact on the care and management of patients with prostate cancer. Recent findings in the setting of breast cancer suggest that agents altering bone homeostasis can also have an impact on disease progression—similar outcomes are hoped for in prostate cancer.[52]

NONMEDICAL CONSIDERATIONS

Despite our greater understanding of tumor biology and immunology, and the development of numerous targeted medical therapies, it is estimated that up to one third of patients who ultimately die of prostate cancer have metastatic disease to the bone, with the spine being the most commonly affected site.[53] Spine lesions can cause neurologic deficits, pain, and mechanical instability, which subsequently require nonmedical interventions, such as radiation and/or surgery. Functional outlook is related to the degree of neurologic involvement at diagnosis, and treatment should be undertaken without delay. Radiation therapy alone is considered the mainstay of treatment for patients who are either ambulatory or moderately paretic at presentation.[54] When using conventional radiation therapy, it is recommended that the radiation plan include one or two vertebral bodies below and above the level of compression to decease the chance of local recurrences. The use of stereotactic radiosurgery has recently been reported to potentially offer advantages over conventional external beam radiation for prostate cancer metastases by giving larger radiobiological doses within a single day rather than over a period of several weeks, with less radiation exposure to surrounding structures.[55]

In carefully selected patients, aggressive surgical decompression and spinal reconstruction have been shown to improve neurologic outcomes and reduce the use of analgesics, even in the setting of previous radiation therapy to the site of neural compression.[56] Immediate surgical decompression approached through an anterior, posterior, or combined approach should be used for those with an expected life span of at least 3 months who fail or progress despite radiation treatment, and those with spinal instability. In patients with spinal cord compression (ambulatory, paraparetic, or paraplegic), surgical decompression followed by radiation therapy appears to be superior to radiation alone in restoring and preserving ambulation.[57] Other factors affecting outcomes and ultimately survival are histologic grade, metastatic burden, and degree of spinal canal compression and therefore should be considered carefully before opting for surgical management.

CONCLUSION

The landscape of prostate cancer therapy is rapidly changing. Beyond the standard approach to metastatic prostate cancer (i.e., ADT followed by the addition of chemotherapy, radiation, and/or surgical decompression), agents such as abiraterone and MDV3100 may substantially improve clinical outcomes. Vaccine therapies, although still controversial, have reported mixed results, and it remains to be seen where they will be incorporated into the current treatment algorithm. Beyond the novel treatments described in this chapter, a plethora of targeted agents and immunotherapies are in clinical development, as outlined in Table 21-2. An ongoing phase III trial comparing docetaxel and prednisone with and without bevacizumab merits particular mention, with the results of this study anticipated in the near future.[58] With the expected improvements in survival among patients with metastatic prostate cancer as a consequence of these novel therapies, issues pertaining to bone health gain prominence. Forthcoming studies will compare established standards for patients with CRPC and bony metastases (i.e., zoledronic acid) to novel therapies, such as denosumab, and inevitably these agents will become a critical component of the current treatment paradigm.[59]

Table 21-2 Novel Therapies for Prostate Cancer in Clinical Development

Target	Agent(s)
Immunotherapy	Sipuleucel-T, Prostvac, huJ591:177Lu (anti-PSMA), MK-4721 (anti-PSCA)
Endothelin receptor	Atrasentan, ZD4054
Androgen receptor	MDV3100
Estrogen receptor	Toremifene, tamoxifen, fulvestrant
VEGF, VEGFR, integrins, angiogenesis	Bevacizumab, sunitinib, sorafenib, IMC-1121B, thalidomide, DMXAA, cilengitide
mTOR	Temsirolimus, everolimus
HSP90	17 AAG
Microtubule	Epothilones, halichondrin B analog, SB0715992, abraxane
IGF-IR	IMC-A12
PKCβ, PI3k/AKT, GSK3	Enzastaurin
Apoptotic pathway	Gossypol, Bcl-2 antisense oligonucleotide, anticlusterin
IL-6	CNTO 328

TIPS FROM THE MASTERS

- Multiple levels of vertebral involvement are relatively common in prostate cancer metastatic to the spine on presentation.
- Radiation therapy, and particularly stereotactic radiosurgery, is initially the treatment of choice, except in cases of a rapidly progressive neurologic deficit or significant spinal instability.
- The other adjuvant treatments discussed in this chapter have a significant role in long-term control of bone disease.
- Given the often advanced age of patients with this type of tumor, patients' medical status should be considered when deciding on a specific surgical intervention, especially because the data from the Patchell study in Lancet seems to indicate less favorable outcomes with advanced age.[60]

References (With Key References in Boldface)

1. **Jemal A, Siegel R, Ward E, et al. Cancer Statistics, 2009. CA Cancer J Clin 59:225-249, 2009.**
2. Ryan CJ, Elkin EP, Small EJ, et al. Reduced incidence of bony metastasis at initial prostate cancer diagnosis: data from CaPSURE. Urol Oncol 24:396-402, 2006.
3. Huggins C, Hodges CV. Studies on prostatic cancer. I. The effect of castration, of estrogen and of androgen injection on serum phosphatases in metastatic carcinoma of the prostate. Cancer Res 1:293-297, 1941.
4. Huggins C, Stevens RE Jr, Hodges CV. Studies on prostatic cancer. II. The effects of castration on advanced carcinoma of the prostate gland. Arch Surg 43:209-223, 1941.
5. Aragon-Ching JB, Williams KM, Gulley JL. Impact of androgen-deprivation therapy on the immune system: implications for combination therapy of prostate cancer. Front Biosci 12:4957-4971, 2007.
6. Eisenberger M, O'Dwyer P, Friedman M. Gonadotropin hormone-releasing hormone analogues: a new therapeutic approach for prostatic carcinoma. J Clin Oncol 4:414-424, 1986.
7. Scher H, Liebertz C, Kelly W, et al. Bicalutamide for advanced prostate cancer: the natural versus treated history of disease. J Clin Oncol 15:2928-2938, 1997.
8. Scher H, Kelly W. Flutamide withdrawal syndrome: its impact on clinical trials in hormone-refractory prostate cancer. J Clin Oncol 11:1566-1572, 1993.
9. **Huddart RA, Rajan B, Law M, et al. Spinal cord compression in prostate cancer: treatment outcome and prognostic factors. Radiother Oncol 44:229-236, 1997.**
10. Alibhai SMH, Duong-Hua M, Sutradhar R, et al. Impact of androgen deprivation therapy on cardiovascular disease and diabetes. J Clin Oncol 27:3452-3458, 2009.
11. Small EJ, Halabi S, Dawson NA, et al. Antiandrogen withdrawal alone or in combination with ketoconazole in androgen-independent prostate cancer patients: a phase III trial (CALGB 9583). J Clin Oncol 22:1025-1033, 2004.
12. O'Shaughnessy J, Miles D, Vukelja S, et al. Superior survival with capecitabine plus docetaxel combination therapy in anthracycline-pretreated patients with advanced breast cancer: phase III trial results. J Clin Oncol 20:2812-2823, 2002.
13. Van Cutsem E, Moiseyenko VM, Tjulandin S, et al. Phase III study of docetaxel and cisplatin plus fluorouracil compared with cisplatin and fluorouracil as first-line therapy for advanced gastric cancer: a report of the V325 Study Group. J Clin Oncol 24:4991-4997, 2006.

14. Dreyfuss A, Clark J, Norris C, et al: Docetaxel: an active drug for squamous cell carcinoma of the head and neck. J Clin Oncol 14:1672-1678, 1996.
15. Petrylak DP, Tangen CM, Hussain MHA, et al. Docetaxel and estramustine compared with mitoxantrone and prednisone for advanced refractory prostate cancer. N Engl J Med 351:1513-1520, 2004.
16. Berthold DR, Pond GR, Soban F, et al. Docetaxel plus prednisone or mitoxantrone plus prednisone for advanced prostate cancer: updated survival in the TAX 327 study. J Clin Oncol 26:242-245, 2008.
17. Ramsey S, Aitchison M, Graham J, et al. The longitudinal relationship between the systemic inflammatory response, circulating T-lymphocytes, interleukin-6 and -10 in patients undergoing immunotherapy for metastatic renal cancer. BJU Int 102:125-129, 2008.
18. LaTulippe E, Satagopan J, Smith A, et al. Comprehensive gene expression analysis of prostate cancer reveals distinct transcriptional programs associated with metastatic disease. Cancer Res 62:4499-4506, 2002.
19. Sirotnak FM, She Y, Khokhar NZ, et al. Microarray analysis of prostate cancer progression to reduced androgen dependence: studies in unique models contrasts early and late molecular events. Mol Carcinog 41:150-163, 2004.
20. Donovan MJ, Osman I, Khan FM, et al. Androgen receptor expression is associated with prostate cancer-specific survival in castrate patients with metastatic disease. BJU Int 105:462-467, 2010.
21. Pal SK, Twardowski P, Josephson DY. Beyond castration and chemotherapy: novel approaches to targeting androgen-driven pathways. Maturitas 64:61-66, 2009.
22. Barrie SE, Potter GA, Goddard PM, et al. Pharmacology of novel steroidal inhibitors of cytochrome P450(17) alpha (17 alpha-hydroxylase/C17-20 lyase). J Steroid Biochem Mol Biol 50:267-273, 1994.
23. Reid AH, Attard G, Danila D, et al. A multicenter phase II study of abiraterone acetate (AA) in docetaxel pretreated castration-resistant prostate cancer (CRPC) patients (pts). J Clin Oncol 27(15s):[abstr] 5047, 2009.
24. Danila DC, Bono JD, Ryan CJ, et al. Phase II multicenter study of abiraterone acetate (AA) plus prednisone therapy in docetaxel-treated castration-resistant prostate cancer (CRPC) patients (pts): impact of prior ketoconazole (keto). J Clin Oncol 27(15s):[abstr] 5048, 2009.
25. Webster WS, Thompson RH, Harris KJ, et al. Targeting molecular and cellular inhibitory mechanisms for improvement of antitumor memory responses reactivated by tumor cell vaccine. J Immunol 179:2860-2869, 2007.
26. Ryan C, Smith MR, Rosenberg JE, et al. Impact of prior ketoconazole therapy on response proportion to abiraterone acetate, a 17-alpha hydroxylase C17,20-lyase inhibitor in castration resistant prostate cancer (CRPC). J Clin Oncol 26 (May 20 suppl):[abstr] 5018, 2008.
27. Ryan C, Efstathiou E, Smith M, et al: Phase II multicenter study of chemotherapy (chemo)-naive castration-resistant prostate cancer (CRPC) not exposed to ketoconazole (keto), treated with abiraterone acetate (AA) plus prednisone. J Clin Oncol 27(15s):[abstr] 5046, 2009.
28. Attard G, Reid AHM, Yap TA, et al. Phase I clinical trial of a selective inhibitor of CYP17, abiraterone acetate, confirms that castration-resistant prostate cancer commonly remains hormone driven. J Clin Oncol 26:4563-4571, 2008.
29. Tomlins SA, Rhodes DR, Perner S, et al. Recurrent fusion of TMPRSS2 and ETS transcription factor genes in prostate cancer. Science 310:644-648, 2005.
30. Attard G, Reid AHM, A'Hern R, et al. Selective inhibition of CYP17 with abiraterone acetate is highly active in the treatment of castration-resistant prostate cancer. J Clin Oncol 27:3742-3748, 2009.
31. Escudier B, Choueiri TK, Oudard S, et al. Prognostic factors of metastatic renal cell carcinoma after failure of immunotherapy: new paradigm from a large phase III trial with shark cartilage extract AE 941. J Urol 178:1901-1905, 2007.
32. Tran C, Ouk S, Clegg NJ, et al. Development of a second-generation antiandrogen for treatment of advanced prostate cancer. Science 324:787-790, 2009.

33. Liu W, Xie CC, Zhu Y, et al. Homozygous deletions and recurrent amplifications implicate new genes involved in prostate cancer. Neoplasia 10:897-907, 2008.
34. Scher HI, Beer TM, Higano CS, et al. Antitumor activity of MDV3100 in a phase I/II study of castration-resistant prostate cancer (CRPC). J Clin Oncol 27(15 suppl):[abstr] 5011, 2009.
35. Ito N, Eto M, Nakamura E, et al. STAT3 polymorphism predicts interferon-alfa response in patients with metastatic renal cell carcinoma. J Clin Oncol 25:2785-2791, 2007.
36. Burch PA, Breen JK, Buckner JC, et al. Priming tissue-specific cellular immunity in a phase I trial of autologous dendritic cells for prostate cancer. Clin Cancer Res 6:2175-2182, 2000.
37. Small EJ, Fratesi P, Reese DM, et al. Immunotherapy of hormone-refractory prostate cancer with antigen-loaded dendritic cells. J Clin Oncol 18:3894-3903, 2000.
38. Schellhammer P, Higano C, Berger E, et al. A randomized, double-blind, placebo-controlled, multi-center, phase III trial of sipuleucel-T in men with metastatic, androgen independent prostatic adenocarcinoma (AIPC). Presented at the Annual Meeting of the American Urological Association, San Francisco, CA, May 29-June 3, 2009.
39. Harzstark AL, Ryan CJ. Therapies in development for castrate-resistant prostate cancer. Expert Rev Anticancer Ther 8:259-268, 2008.
40. Higano CS, Corman JM, Smith DC, et al. Phase 1/2 dose-escalation study of a GM-CSF-secreting, allogeneic, cellular immunotherapy for metastatic hormone-refractory prostate cancer. Cancer 113:975-984, 2008.
41. Small E, Demkow T, Gerritsen WR, et al. A phase III trial of GVAX immunotherapy for prostate cancer in combination with docetaxel versus docetaxel plus prednisone in symptomatic, castration-resistant prostate cancer (CRPC). In ASCO Genitourinary Cancer Symposium, Orlando, FL, 2009.
42. Kantoff PW, Schuetz T, Blumenstein BA, et al. Overall survival (OS) analysis of a phase II randomized controlled trial (RCT) of a poxviral-based PSA targeted immunotherapy in metastatic castration-resistant prostate cancer (mCRPC). J Clin Oncol 27: (suppl):[abstr] 5013, 2009.
43. Stoch SA, Parker RA, Chen L, et al. Bone loss in men with prostate cancer treated with gonadotropin-releasing hormone agonists. J Clin Endocrinol Metab 86:2787-2791, 2001.
44. Kondo T, Nakazawa H, Ito F, et al. Favorable prognosis of renal cell carcinoma with increased expression of chemokines associated with a Th1-type immune response. Cancer Science 97:780-786, 2006.
45. Solomon CG. Bisphosphonates and osteoporosis. N Engl J Med 346:642, 2002.
46. Smith MR, Eastham J, Gleason DM, et al. Randomized controlled trial of zoledronic acid to prevent bone loss in men receiving androgen deprivation therapy for nonmetastatic prostate cancer. J Urol 169:2008-2012, 2003.
47. Bhoopalam N, Campbell SC, Moritz T, et al. Intravenous zoledronic acid to prevent osteoporosis in a veteran population with multiple risk factors for bone loss on androgen deprivation therapy. J Urol 182:2257-2264, 2009.
48. Wadhwa VK, Weston R, Parr NJ. Frequency of zoledronic acid to prevent further bone loss in osteoporotic patients undergoing androgen deprivation therapy for prostate cancer. BJU Int 105:1082-1088, 2009.
49. Saad F, Gleason D, Murray R, et al. Long-term efficacy of zoledronic acid for the prevention of skeletal complications in patients with metastatic hormone-refractory prostate cancer. J Natl Cancer Inst 96:879-882, 2004.
50. Saylor PJ, Smith MR. Bone health and prostate cancer. Prostate Cancer Prostatic Dis 13:20-27, 2010.
51. Fukuhara H, Matsumoto A, Kitamura T, et al. Neutralization of interleukin-2 retards the growth of mouse renal cancer. BJU Int 97:1314-1321, 2006.
52. Gnant M, Mlineritsch B, Schippinger W, et al. Endocrine therapy plus zoledronic acid in premenopausal breast cancer. N Engl J Med 360:679-691, 2009.
53. Bubendorf L, Schöpfer A, Wagner U, et al. Metastatic patterns of prostate cancer: an autopsy study of 1,589 patients. Hum Pathol 31:578-583, 2000.
54. Flynn DF, Shipley WU. Management of spinal cord compression secondary to metastatic prostatic carcinoma. Urol Clin North Am 18:145-152, 1991.

55. Gerszten PC, Welch WC. Cyberknife radiosurgery for metastatic spine tumors. Neurosurg Clin N Am 15:491-501, 2004.
56. Williams BJ, Fox BD, Sciubba DM, et al. Surgical management of prostate cancer metastatic to the spine. J Neurosurg Spine 10:414-422, 2009.
57. Tazi H, Manunta A, Rodriguez A, et al. Spinal cord compression in metastatic prostate cancer. Eur Urol 44:527-532, 2003.
58. NCT00110214. Docetaxel and prednisone with or without bevacizumab in treating patients with prostate cancer that did not respond to hormone therapy. Available at *www.clinicaltrials.gov* (last accessed December 3, 2009).
59. NCT00321620. Double-blind study of denosumab compared with zoledronic acid in the treatment of bone metastases in men with hormone-refractory prostate cancer. Available at *www.clinicaltrials.gov* (last accessed November 23, 2009).
60. Chi JH, Gokaslan Z, McCormick P. Selecting treatment for patients with malignant epidural spinal cord compression—does age matter?: results from a randomized clinical trial. Spine (Phila Pa 1976) 34:431-435, 2009.

Chapter 22

Plasmacytoma and Multiple Myeloma

Quang D. Ma, George Somlo, Mike Y. Chen

Plasmacytoma is a malignancy of plasma cell origin that may occur either at a solitary site or as part of the systemic disease multiple myeloma. Because plasmacytic lesions arise from bone marrow, both solitary plasmacytomas and plasmacytomas representing manifestations of systemic multiple myeloma have a predilection for spine involvement.[1] In fact, multiple myeloma is the most common primary malignancy of the spine.

The vast majority of spine lesions present as bony lesions arising from the marrow of the vertebral body. These lesions are distributed proportional to the amount of marrow in each segment of the spine. Consequently, the thoracic spine is the most commonly affected segment. Most surgical patients have extradural lesions in the thoracic spine. Intradural extramedullary and intramedullary lesions are rare.

The bone lesions associated with multiple myeloma and plasmacytoma are usually lytic. These lytic lesions are uniquely associated with considerable osteoclastic activity without severely depressed osteoblastic pathophysiology.[2] The pattern of involvement can be nodular, diffuse, or mixed.

As with most spine tumors, pain is the most common clinical manifestation. Most patients with multiple myeloma involving the spine can be managed nonoperatively with osteoclast inhibitors, such as pamidronate or zoledronic acid, and radiation. These treatment options are sufficient for most patients with solitary plasmacytomas. Current treatment strategies for patients with multiple myeloma include administration of novel drugs, such as bortezomib, thalidomide, or lenalidomide and steroids, followed by autologous stem cell transplants for younger and relatively healthy patients, or systemic therapy, including an older chemotherapeutic drug, melphalan, in combination with novel agents for patients who are not transplant candidates. Because most patients will benefit from systemic, steroid-containing therapy within weeks, radiation therapy may not be necessary for all cases of plasmacytoma in patients with myeloma.[3] Some patients with intractable pain resulting from compression fractures that do not compromise the spinal canal may eventually benefit from percutaneous kyphoplasty and vertebroplasty. Two percent to 10% of patients with multiple myeloma will require surgical intervention because of spinal cord compression resulting from vertebral compression fractures or growth of the tumor into the spinal canal.[4-6]

INDICATIONS AND CONTRAINDICATIONS

The role of the spine surgeon can be debatable in the early and acute settings, given the radiosensitivity of plasmacytoma and multiple myeloma and the success of systemic therapies. The median life expectancy for patients with newly diagnosed multiple myeloma is approaching 5 years, and 65% of patients with solitary bone plasmacytomas can be expected to be alive 10 years after the diagnosis.[3] Hence either in an acute situation or, paradoxically, because of improved systemic therapeutic results over the longer lifetime of patients surviving with myeloma, there may be an increasing role for surgical intervention.

In patients who are expected to survive at least 3 months, clear indications for surgery are as follows:
1. The requirement for acute decompression or stabilization because of progressive collapse or progressive neurologic deficit
2. Failure of radiation or systemic therapy to control tumor progression
3. Failure of radiation or systemic therapy to control pain from a pathologic fracture
4. To establish diagnosis

Contraindications to surgery or vertebroplasty include the following:
1. Patients who are expected to survive less than 3 months
2. Patients with cortical breach of the posterior vertebral body who are undergoing percutaneous vertebroplasty (a relative contraindication)
3. Patients with greater than 70% compression of the vertebral body who are undergoing percutaneous cement injection

PREOPERATIVE EVALUATION

The most characteristic findings on laboratory tests are a very highly elevated sedimentation rate and the presence of paraproteins in the serum and urine (Bence-Jones protein).[7] In addition, hypercalcemia, anemia, and elevated parathyroid hormone may be evident. In the later stages renal dysfunction may be seen, with rising levels of blood urea nitrogen and creatinine. More recently, levels of biomarkers of bone resorption and bone formation as an index of disease have been useful in predicting bony events and determining prognosis.[2,8]

A significant number of patients with multiple myeloma will show evidence of bony disease on radiographs.[9] Bone surveys of the skull, axial spine, and extremities are often the initial radiographic tests if multiple myeloma is suspected. Punched-out lytic lesions on plain radiographs are considered a hallmark of this disease. However, it is important to realize that at least 30% of cortical bone must be destroyed for plain radiographs to reflect disease.[5] Because of this lack of sensitivity, CT without contrast imaging, MRI, or PET/CT scans should be considered when there is a high suspicion of multiple myeloma and a negative bone survey.

CT scans are also particularly useful in assessing bone quality in adjacent levels for purposes of presurgical planning. Nonspecific findings on CT scans of patients with multiple myeloma include trabecular destruction of bony elements. The increasing availability of MRI has aided in the detection of multiple myelomas involving the spine and appears to be better at assessing marrow involvement and spinal cord compression compared with CT scans.[10] On MRI, T1- and T2-weighted sequences show low intensity and high signal intensity, respectively. Fludeoxyglucose PET/CT scans may show increased activity at lesion sites but may also represent areas of inflammation, thus increasing the rate of false-positive findings.

CLINICAL DECISION-MAKING

Patient history, physical examination, prior therapies, and preoperative performance status all guide clinical decisions. The type of surgery will largely depend on the extent and location of the lesion, the degree of spinal deformity, and patient suitability for extensive versus minimally invasive techniques. Surgical opinions will differ, but we use the following guidelines, because no others have been firmly established:

1. *Percutaneous vertebroplasty or kyphoplasty.*
   Patients with vertebral compression fractures with refractory pain and spinal deformity, without cord compromise, can benefit from percutaneous vertebroplasty or kyphoplasty if nonsurgical options are ineffective.
2. *Open vertebroplasty or kyphoplasty with unilateral pediculectomy.*
   In patients who have relative contraindications but who might otherwise benefit from a traditional percutaneous vertebroplasty or kyphoplasty, an open form of these procedures can be performed.
3. *Posterior decompression with or without instrumentation.*
   Posterior decompression with or without instrumentation should be performed in the less frequent event that clinically relevant spinal cord compression results from a posterior epidural component.
4. *Anterior and posterior decompression and reconstruction.*
   Most patients who undergo surgery for spinal cord compression should undergo this approach, because the epidural compression is usually ventral to the cord.

TECHNIQUE

It is beyond the scope of this chapter to discuss details of commonly used techniques, such as those for percutaneous cementing, posterior decompression with or without instrumentation, and anterior and posterior decompression and reconstruction. However, we will briefly describe our technique for thoracic open vertebroplasty.

The patient is placed in the prone position on a radiolucent table and a general anesthetic is administered. With the aid of fluoroscopy, an incision slightly off midline from the pedicle of interest to the one below is made. We prefer the right side to avoid aortic injury. A hemilaminectomy and facetectomy are then performed, exposing the exiting nerve root and pedicle of interest. The pedicle is then drilled away, and the nerve root is ligated, thus achieving exposure of the lateral aspect of the posterior vertebral body.

The injection cannula for the cement is then placed into the vertebral body under fluoroscopic guidance. Before injection, the flat surface of the curved end of a Penfield 3 elevator is placed between the thecal sac and the vertebral body, which will be cemented. This last maneuver decreases the risk of retropulsion and cement extravasation into the spinal canal while the methyl methacrylate is being injected. Because the pediculectomy was unilateral in the thoracic region, instrumentation was not required.

OUTCOMES

Multiple clinical trials have established the long-term benefits of kyphoplasty and vertebroplasty in osteolytic lesions, including those of multiple myeloma. Köse et al[11] showed that patients with multiple myeloma who have symptomatic compression fractures, who had undergone single-level and multiple-level vertebroplasty or kyphoplasty, had significantly less pain and need for analgesics at 6-week, 6-month, and 1-year follow-up visits. Furthermore, this study showed a superior effect for kyphoplasty at 6 months and 1 year compared with vertebroplasty, but not at the 6-week assessment. The average height restored in patients undergoing kyphoplasty in this group was approximately 54%. Similarly, Khanna et al[12] followed 211 patients (155 with osteoporosis and 55 with multiple myeloma) who underwent kyphoplasty for vertebral compression fractures. With a mean follow-up of 55 weeks, they achieved significant pain relief and decreased disability.

The well-known study of Patchell et al[13] demonstrated, in general, the value of anterior and posterior surgery for spine tumors causing cord compression. Nene et al[14] reported outcomes from a series of 13 patients with solitary plasmacytomas. Minimum follow-up was 5 years. Five patients with preoperative neurologic deficits improved after surgery, and all patients had marked relief of axial pain. Five patients developed multiple myeloma, three had no evidence of recurrence, three died, and two were lost to follow-up. McLain and Weinstein,[15] in an analysis of 12 patients along with 72 patients reported in the literature, found that the 5-year disease-free survival rate was 60%, and 44% of patients developed disseminated disease, emphasizing the need for close monitoring. Despite the reputed radiosensitivity of plasmacytomas, Mayr et al[16] showed that debulking is important for larger lesions, since radiation alone resulted in control of 100% of smaller lesions but in only 38% of lesions larger than 5 cm in the greatest dimension.

Although the overall prognosis for plasmacytoma is good, in general, the prognosis for patients who have multiple myeloma involving the spine is much worse, with a median survival of approximately 2 years. The percentage of patients who regain the ability to ambulate has been reported to range from 38% to 71% after surgical decompression, with results inversely proportional to the delay in diagnosis.[7,17]

SIGNATURE CASE

A 56-year-old man with recurrent plasmacytoma despite chemoradiation presented with excruciating low back pain and radiculopathy (Figs. 22-1, *A* and *B*). The patient was taken to the operating room for an L4 vertebrectomy using only a posterior approach (Fig. 22-1, *C*).

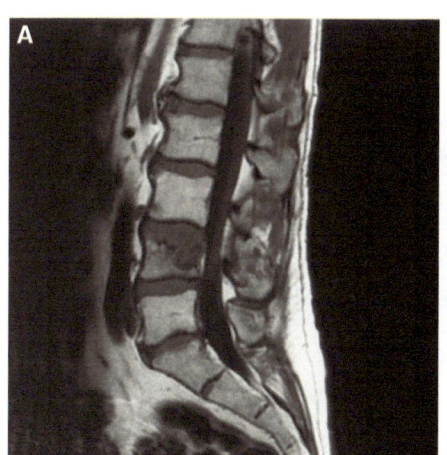

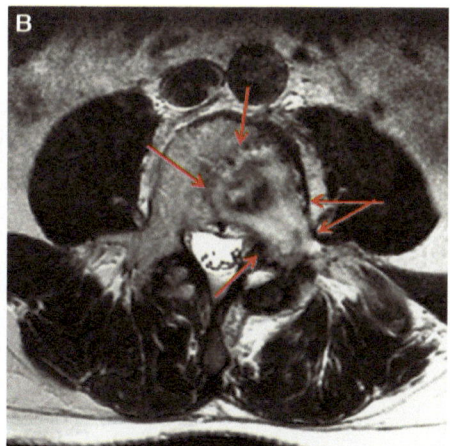

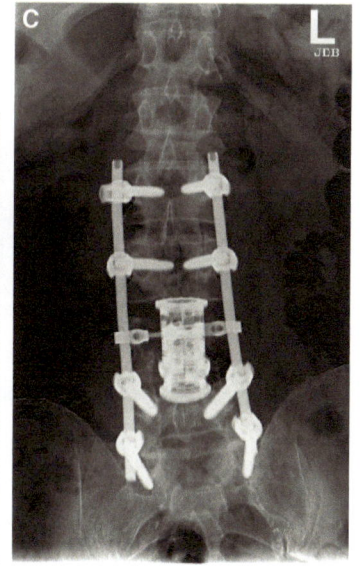

Fig. 22-1 **A,** Preoperative MRI. T1 sagittal MRI in which a hypointense L4 vertebral lesion is evident. **B,** Preoperative MRI. T2-weighted axial MRI of the same patient displaying hyperintense (outlined by red arrows), involving the vertebral body and pedicle. **C,** Postoperative radiograph. Using a lateral extracavitary approach through a midline posterior incision, L4 vertebrectomy and reconstruction were performed with sparing of all nerve roots.

CONCLUSION

Surgery should be performed for spinal cord decompression as rapidly as possible in nonmoribund patients. Kyphoplasty and vertebroplasty have been used successfully to treat pain that has not responded to radiation and conservative management.

BAILOUT TECHNIQUES

- Patients with multiple myeloma often have porotic bone that can be caused by the disease itself or by long-term steroid use. Poor purchase for pedicle screws and fracturing of the endplates from cage insertion are more likely to occur. Methylmethacrylate augmentation of the pedicle base and subchondral region can be used to address and/or repair problems arising from poor bone quality.
- Significant bleeding can occur during aggressive resection of these lesions. Because both plasmacytoma and multiple myeloma are radiosensitive, partial decompression is a viable option if patient instability occurs.

TIPS FROM THE MASTERS

- Preoperative tumor embolization may be helpful.
- For patients with myeloma, long constructs are often required because the bone is porotic.
- If the vertebral body is being replaced with a cage, a large-diameter cage should be used to prevent subsidence in patients with myeloma.
- The surgeon should be prepared to use cement in patients with myeloma.
- Because patients with myeloma are often immunosuppressed, a minimizing incision should be considered using a posterior-only approach or minimally invasive lateral approach with percutaneous posterior instrumentation.

References (With Key References in Boldface)

1. Dagan R, Morris CG, Kirwan J, et al. Solitary plasmacytoma. Am J Clin Oncol 32:612-617, 2009.
2. Yeh HS, Berenson JR. Treatment for myeloma bone disease. Clin Cancer Res 12:6279s-6284s, 2006.
3. Turesson I, Velez R, Kristinsson SY, et al. Patterns of improved survival in patients with multiple myeloma in the twenty-first century: a population-based study. J Clin Oncol 28:830-834, 2010.
4. Chataigner H, Onimus M, Polette A. [Surgical treatment of myeloma localized in the spine] Rev Chir Orthop Reparatrice Appar Mot 84:311-318, 1998.
5. Roodman GD. Skeletal imaging and management of bone disease. Hematology Am Soc Hematol Educ Program 2008:313-319.
6. Roodman GD. Pathogenesis of myeloma bone disease. Leukemia 23:435-441, 2009.

7. Rehak S, Maisnar V, Malek V, et al. Diagnosis and surgical therapy of plasma cell neoplasia of the spine. Neoplasma 56:84-87, 2009.
8. Abildgaard N, Brixen K, Kristensen JE, et al. Comparison of five biochemical markers of bone resorption in multiple myeloma: elevated pre-treatment levels of S-ICTP and U-Ntx are predictive for early progression of the bone disease during standard chemotherapy. Br J Haematol 120:235-242, 2003.
9. Kyle RA, Rajkumar SV. Multiple myeloma. Blood 111:2962-2972, 2008.
10. Lecouvet F, Richard BB, Vande J, et al. Long-term effects of localized spinal radiation therapy on vertebral fractures and focal lesions appearance in patients with multiple myeloma. Br J Haematol 96:743-745, 1997.
11. Köse KC, Cebesoy O, Akan B, et al. Functional results of vertebral augmentation techniques in pathological vertebral fractures of myelomatous patients. J Natl Med Assoc 98:1654-1658, 2006.
12. Khanna AJ, Reinhardt MK, Togawa D, et al. Functional outcomes of kyphoplasty for the treatment of osteoporotic and osteolytic vertebral compression fractures. Osteoporos Int 17:817-826, 2006.
13. Patchell RA, Tibbs PA, Regine WF, et al. Direct decompressive surgical resection in the treatment of spinal cord compression caused by metastatic cancer: a randomised trial. Lancet 366:643-648, 2005.
14. Nene A, Mumbai M, Bhojraj S, et al. Solitary Plasmacytomas of the Spine: Management & Outcomes. Abstract from the Scoliosis Research Society, 2006.
15. McLain RF, Weinstein JN. Solitary plasmacytomas of the spine: a review of 84 cases. J Spinal Disord 2:69-74, 1989.
16. Mayr NA, Wen BC, Hussey DH, et al. The role of radiation therapy in the treatment of solitary plasmacytomas. Radiother Oncol 17:293-303, 1990.
17. Onimus M, Schraub S, Bertin D, et al. Surgical treatment of vertebral metastasis. Spine (Phila Pa 1976) 11:883-891, 1986.

Chapter 23

Intradural Extramedullary Tumors

Agne Naujokas, Tarik Tihan

*I*ntradural extramedullary tumors constitute the largest group of primary neoplasms of the spinal cord. Peripheral nerve sheath tumors and meningiomas are the most common neoplasms and make up more than 80% of all tumors in this category. Other neoplasms that can occur as primary intradural extramedullary masses include an array of mesenchymal nonmeningothelial neoplasms, as well as rare examples of hemangioblastomas and ependymal tumors. These entities are unusual enough in appearance to be confused with metastases from neoplasms elsewhere.

Most intradural extramedullary tumors have the typical radiologic appearance, and it is critical to recognize these radiologic features for an accurate diagnosis. MRI and CT imaging are the methods of choice to narrow the preoperative differential diagnosis and guide surgical resection. Nevertheless, overlapping clinical and radiologic characteristics pose a challenge in the diagnosis of primary extramedullary neoplasms of the spinal cord, and pathologic correlation or verification becomes necessary. There is still much to be learned to better correlate the findings of new radiologic and pathologic assessment methods that are being used with increasing frequency in everyday practice.

Careful pathologic evaluation in close correlation with clinical and radiologic data provides the best information for neurosurgeons to appropriately manage patients during and after surgery. The effective use of intraoperative consultation is of significant benefit for this purpose and ensures sufficient material for pathologic diagnosis. It should always be remembered that in the current practice of pathology, intraoperative consultations provide a *preliminary diagnosis* but, more importantly, they are a tool for appropriate execution of the surgical plan. Active and open communication between neuropathologists and neurosurgeons is not only desirable but critical for the best possible patient care. This is certainly the case for the appropriate management of the tumors discussed in this chapter.

This chapter includes the major categories of primary neoplasms that occur in the intradural extramedullary space. Obviously one of the most common and critical groups of tumors that can involve this anatomic location are metastatic carcinomas. Metastases from common tumors, such as lung, breast, and prostate, often occur with much greater frequency and can pose significant challenges and certainly warrant a chapter of their own. In this section we focus on a select number of primary entities that can be encountered in spine surgery.

PERIPHERAL NERVE SHEATH TUMORS
SCHWANNOMAS
Definition/Clinical Presentation
Schwannomas are benign encapsulated neoplasms that are thought to originate from Schwann cells of the peripheral nervous system.[1] In the spinal cord these tumors preferentially affect sensory nerve roots and are most commonly located posterolaterally or anterolaterally. Less frequently, they can be seen in a purely ventral location.[2] Schwannomas of the spine show no predilection for either sex and affect mostly adults in the fourth to sixth decades of life. Multiple schwannomas are often associated with neurofibromatosis 2 (NF2) or schwannomatosis. Schwannomatosis, a disorder genetically distinct from NF2, also includes peripheral and intracranial schwannomas.[3,4] Schwannomas of the spinal cord can often present with radicular pain but also present with other sensory symptoms. Motor symptoms and incidental examples are rare. Some schwannomas can present acutely and may even be documented to increase in size within a relatively short period. Invariably this is related to intratumoral hemorrhage or cystic degeneration, but occasionally it is the result of the emergence of a malignant peripheral nerve sheath tumor.

Typical Macroscopic and Microscopic Findings
Most schwannomas are solid or heterogeneously solid tumors, and predominantly cystic schwannomas are uncommon.[5] Schwannomas are typically well-circumscribed firm to rubbery masses attached to peripheral nerves or nerve roots (Fig. 23-1). It is often possible to see the attachment to a nerve root, and some tumors can be easily detached from the nerve root or fascicle. Schwannomas are often grayish-tan, and they may have specks of yellow that correspond to foci of xanthomatous change. Hemorrhagic and cystic changes can also be observed in a minority of cases.

Schwannomas contain two distinct architectural patterns known as *Antoni A* and *Antoni B* areas (Fig. 23-2, *A*). Antoni A areas are characteristically cellular, composed of spindle cells with nuclear palisading, and whorled or nested arrangements called *Verocay bodies* (Fig. 23-2, *B*). Cells in Antoni B areas are loosely arranged and may show occasional bizarre hyperchromatic nuclei (Fig. 23-2, *C*). Typical schwannomas also include clustered hyalinized vessels (Fig. 23-2, *D*), a variable number of foamy

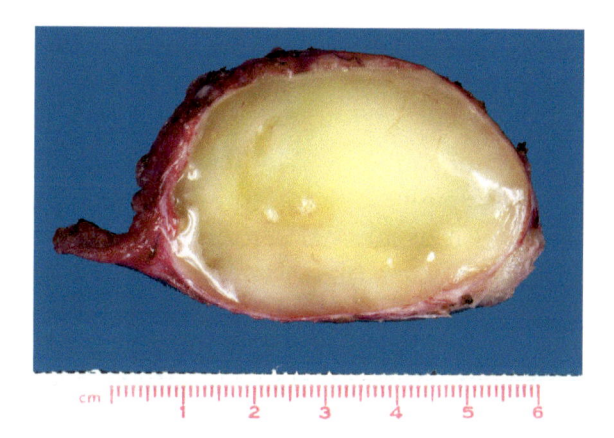

Chapter 23 ▪ *Intradural Extramedullary Tumors* **381**

Fig. 23-1 Schwannoma of the spinal cord. Macroscopic appearance.

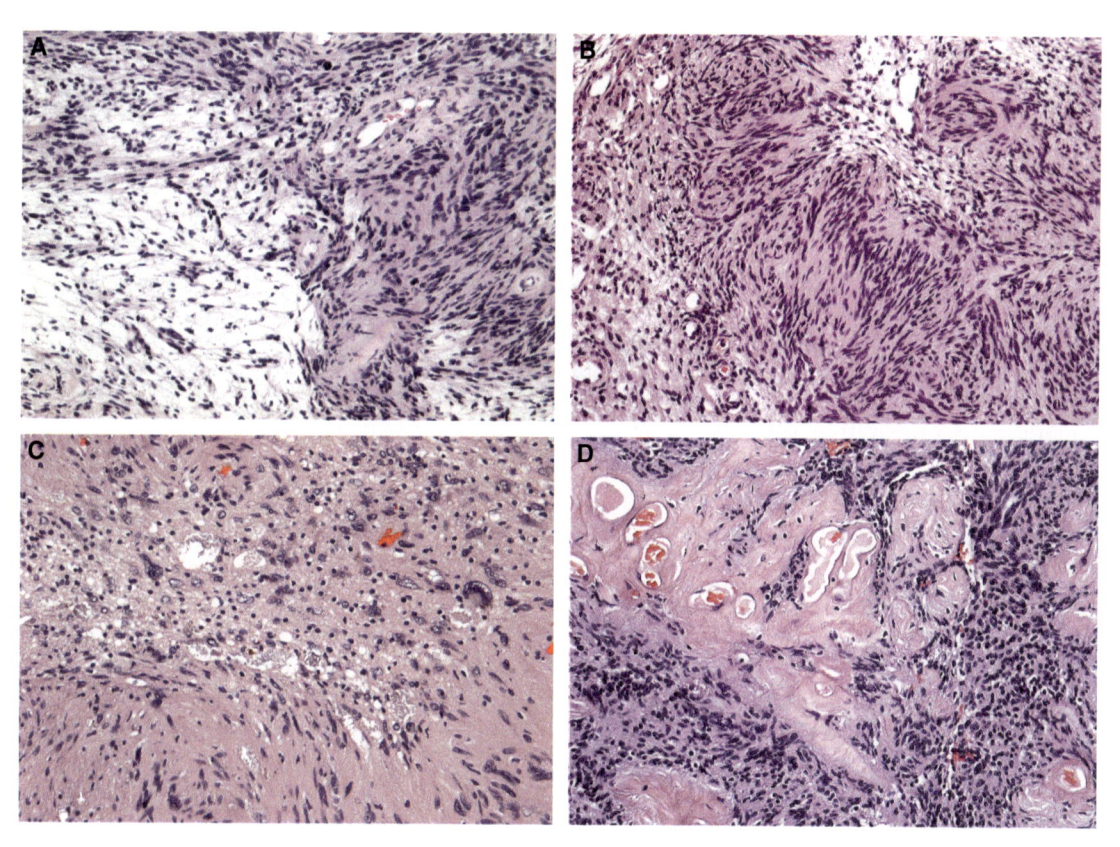

Fig. 23-2 Schwannoma of the spinal cord. Typical histologic characteristics include the following: **A,** biphasic architecture composed of Antoni A and Antoni B areas, **B,** Verocay bodies, **C,** bizarre cells, and **D,** hyalinized vessels.

macrophages, inflammatory cells, and hemosiderin pigment. Poorly formed whorls may be seen in NF2-associated schwannomas. Reticulin is abundant and distinctly pericellular in schwannomas.

A cellular schwannoma is an uncommon variant that often arises along the spinal cord. Cellular schwannomas lack the biphasic architecture and are composed predominantly of cellular Antoni A areas with occasional Verocay bodies, and they show variable mitotic activity.[6] These tumors have a higher rate of local recurrence compared with typical schwannomas.

Melanotic schwannoma is another variant that may affect the spinal cord and harbor melanin pigment, which can raise the differential diagnosis of melanoma or melanocytoma. Some melanotic schwannomas are seen in the Carney complex.[7]

Immunohistochemically, schwannomas are uniformly positive for the S100 protein antibody, and many are also positive for Leu-7 antibody. Positive staining for S100 protein, while universal, is not sufficient for the diagnosis because many other tumors can be S100 protein positive. Staining for laminin and collagen IV antibodies is typically uniform and membranous because schwannomas often harbor abundant basement membrane. Schwannomas are also reactive with calretinin,[8] demonstrate glucose-1 transporter (GLUT1) immunoreactivity, and have few CD34-positive cells within the Antoni B areas.[9] Cellular schwannomas have the same immunohistochemical characteristics as classic schwannomas. Ultrastructurally schwannomas contain spindle-shaped bipolar cells with abundant tangled processes and single or duplicated layers of pericellular basement membrane. Basement membrane formation is prominent and separates the cells that lack specialized intercellular junctions. Striated collections of long spacing collagen, also known as the *Luce body*, are typical in schwannomas.[10]

Pathologic Differential Diagnosis

The differential diagnosis of spinal cord schwannoma typically includes neurofibroma, meningioma, malignant peripheral nerve sheath tumors and other less common spindle cell tumors, such as solitary fibrous tumors. Neurofibromas can closely resemble schwannomas and both tumors may have areas that are indistinguishable from one another. Although neurofilament protein staining has been shown in a subset of both tumors, this staining is far more diffuse and stronger for neurofibromas. Both schwannomas and meningiomas are rich in collagen, and show xanthomatous cells, cellular elongation, and even palisading. Psammoma bodies and tight whorls are distinctive features of meningiomas and only a rare schwannoma may harbor an occasional psammoma body, except for the rare "psammomatous" variant in which these formations are abundant. Immunohistochemical staining for S100 protein and epithelial membrane antigen (EMA) can distinguish between these two tumors in most cases. Melanotic schwannoma can resemble melanocytoma or melanoma. Distinguishing between this tumor and malignant melanoma is of paramount importance, and melanocytic markers are unlikely to be helpful. Combined use of laminin and collagen type IV is valuable in distinguishing melanotic schwannomas from malignant melanoma.[11]

Diffuse strong laminin or collagen type IV staining, a uniform feature of schwannomas, is not a finding of meningiomas. Approximately 20% of meningiomas show immunoreactivity for this protein, albeit far less intensely than in schwannomas. Finally, meningiomas are reactive for EMA, whereas schwannomas are typically negative and, when positive, lack membranous staining.[12]

Genetics
Sporadic schwannomas demonstrate a high incidence of NF2 gene deletion.[13,14] Approximately 60% of schwannomas demonstrate inactivating mutations of the NF2 gene by both chromogenic in situ hybridization (CISH) and NF2 protein immunohistochemical analysis.[15] Loss of merlin (schwannomin) expression encoded by the NF2 gene has been universally found in all studied schwannomas.[16]

Radiologic/Pathologic Correlation
On MRI, schwannomas appear as well-circumscribed heterogeneously enhancing masses and can be difficult to distinguish from neurofibromas. Schwannomas are isointense to skeletal muscle on T1-weighted images and show slightly increased heterogeneous signal intensity on T2-weighted images. These tumors do not show a dural tail sign and may demonstrate bony scalloping with foraminal extension.[17] Schwannomas typically show avid contrast enhancement (Fig. 23-3). A classic appearance is the dumbbell-shaped lesion that expands the intervertebral foramen and extends both intradurally and extradurally. Schwannomas can grow into the paraspinal space, in which case gross total resection may be difficult. A sudden increase in the radiologic dimensions of a schwannoma is often accompanied by the emergence of central T1 hypointense areas, suggesting hemorrhagic or cystic degeneration.

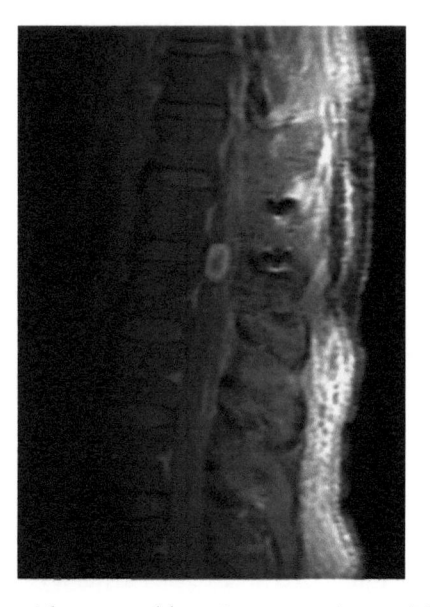

Fig. 23-3 Spinal schwannoma with a central hypointense region on T1-weighted contrast-enhanced MRI.

Prognosis

Treatment of schwannomas is dependent on the clinical and radiologic features of the tumors. Although some patients are followed without intervention, most tumors can be completely excised, and rare cases are treated with radiosurgery. Gross total resection of intradural extramedullary schwannomas is often curative and can be achieved in more than 90% of patients.[18] Subtotally excised conventional schwannomas recur in only about 5% of cases,[19] whereas more than 20% of gross totally excised cellular schwannomas recur.[20]

Practical Points

- Sudden signal changes on MRI, especially a central T1-hypointense region, are often associated with intratumoral hemorrhage or cystic degeneration. Only under exceptional circumstances does this change imply a malignancy.
- Frozen section analysis of spinal cord schwannomas is often straightforward, but occasional cases can be challenging. In such instances it is important to inform the pathologist of how much information is critical for the surgical plan.
- Malignant degeneration of schwannomas is exceptional and typically occurs in the setting of NF2.
- Melanotic schwannomas can mimic melanocytomas or melanomas. Occasionally melanomas can be misidentified as melanotic schwannomas. The critical issue is the presence of anaplastic histologic findings and mitotic figures, which should not be seen with melanotic schwannomas.
- It is important to refer patients with multiple spinal schwannomas to a genetics laboratory to determine the presence of NF2.
- Occasionally fragments of peripheral nerve or ganglion can be present in an excised schwannoma specimen. This feature has not been shown to correlate with any functional deficits either preoperatively or postoperatively.[21]
- In cases where the clinical presentation and radiologic findings are atypical, pathologic features can also be unusual.

NEUROFIBROMAS

Definition/Clinical Presentation

Neurofibromas are infiltrative and typically benign tumors arising within or in association with cranial or peripheral nerves. They can be solitary and intraneural or diffuse masses involving the subcutis or deep tissues. Neurofibromas are considered World Health Organization (WHO) grade I neoplasms. Multiple neurofibromas and especially the plexiform variants are typically seen in the setting of NF1. Most spinal neurofibromas are encountered in the context of NF1, but sporadic examples can be seen.

Most superficial neurofibromas present as slow-growing, painless masses that are freely movable under the skin. Spinal cord neurofibromas can present with sensory loss, weakness, and pain.[22] Some spinal neurofibromas can be entirely asymptomatic. Spinal neurofibromas in NF1 are more likely to result in sacrifice of the nerve root. A spinal neurofibroma can be the first manifestation of NF1. Although cutaneous neurofibromas are readily discovered, spinal neurofibromas are only recognized through radiologic studies.

Typical Macroscopic and Microscopic Findings

Most neurofibromas are solid with a gelatinous texture. Neurofibromas typically expand and distort the peripheral nerves and blend into the normal nerve tissue, where a clear separation may not be possible (Fig. 23-4, *A*). The relationship of the tumor to the spinal nerve roots is often clearly demonstrable intraoperatively. The histologic features are often characteristic enough for neurofibromas. One challenging issue is the diagnosis of neurofibroma during frozen section analysis. On frozen sections, neurofibromas can appear markedly pleomorphic and may not exhibit the typical monomorphous wavy nuclei. The smear preparation that is most often critical in the frozen section diagnosis of tumors is not as helpful because neurofibromas are quite difficult to smear. Some neurofibromas may mimic schwannomas or fibrous meningiomas.[22] Most neurofibromas contain scattered mast cells that can aid in the diagnosis, even though the true significance of this finding is unknown. Neurofibromas have a delicate vascular network and can be distinguished from the schwannomas that have markedly hyalinized vessels. The myxoid matrix in neurofibromas often stains positive with Alcian blue stain. The classic immunohistochemical staining profile for neurofibromas includes strong diffuse positivity with antibodies against vimentin and S100 protein, and focal positivity with CD34, CD56, and calretinin.[8,9,23] Neurofibromas incorporate numerous neurofilament-positive processes, and this stain can help to distinguish them from schwannomas and meningiomas. In addition, negative staining of neurofibromas for glial fibrillary acidic protein (GFAP) and EMA are helpful in distinguishing them from neuroepithelial and meningothelial tumors, respectively.

The histologic variants of neurofibromas include the following: localized intraneural neurofibroma, which is typically limited to a single nerve or nerve root; diffuse neurofibroma, a larger and poorly delineated tumor that often involves the soft tissues as well as the peripheral nerves[24]; and plexiform neurofibroma, a multilobular tumor har-

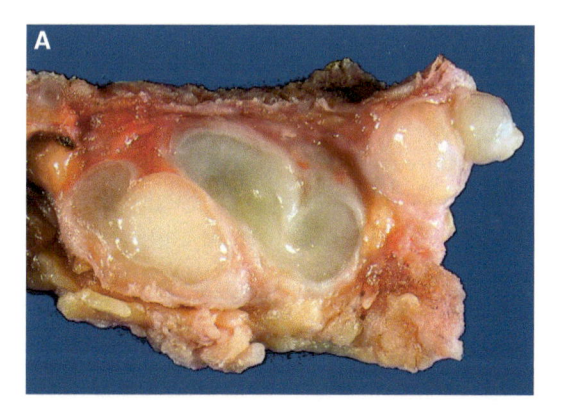

Fig. 23-4 Neurofibroma of the spinal cord. **A,** Macroscopic appearance of a plexiform neurofibroma.

Continued

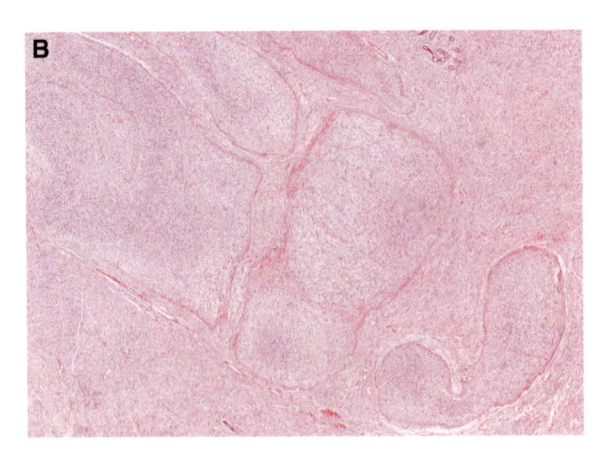

Fig. 23-4, cont'd **B,** Typical low-power image of a plexiform neurofibroma showing multiple nodular growths.

boring a complex set of abnormal fascicles and haphazard growth of tumor cells (Fig. 23-4, *B*) within a nerve root or spinal nerve.[25] Plexiform neurofibroma can extend beyond a nerve root or spinal nerve and can involve multiple levels of the spinal cord.[26]

Pathologic Differential Diagnosis

The differential diagnosis of neurofibroma often includes schwannoma, meningioma, and other rare mesenchymal lesions. Occasionally a metastatic low-grade sarcoma may be mistaken for a neurofibroma. Neurofibromas often blend with or infiltrate the peripheral nerves, whereas schwannomas are often solid with a well-defined fibrous rim/capsule. This is rarely a major challenge but may occasionally require the use of immunohistochemical stains such as neurofilament or calretinin. Rarely, a solitary fibrous tumor or a myxofibrosarcoma can be considered in the differential diagnosis of intradural extramedullary neurofibromas, but these can be easily distinguished by means of routine and specialized stains. The typical panel for the differential diagnosis of neurofibroma includes S100 protein, EMA, GFAP, CD34, calretinin, and neurofilament protein.

Genetics

Allelic loss of the NF1 gene region in chromosome 17 occurs in both NF1-related and sporadic neurofibromas. The NF1 gene and its product neurofibromin act as tumor suppressors in a negative regulator of the Ras proto-oncogene. A number of mechanisms had been postulated to account for biallelic inactivation of the NF1 gene. Loss of heterozygosity in the NF1 gene has been found in all types of neurofibromas regardless of their NF1 status. In addition, sporadic neurofibromas appear to have cytogenetic abnormalities similar to those arising in the setting of NF1. Although it is important to determine the presence of somatic mutations and NF1 in patients with multiple or plexiform neurofibromas, additional genetic analyses are not of practical benefit in the management of patients with sporadic neurofibromas.

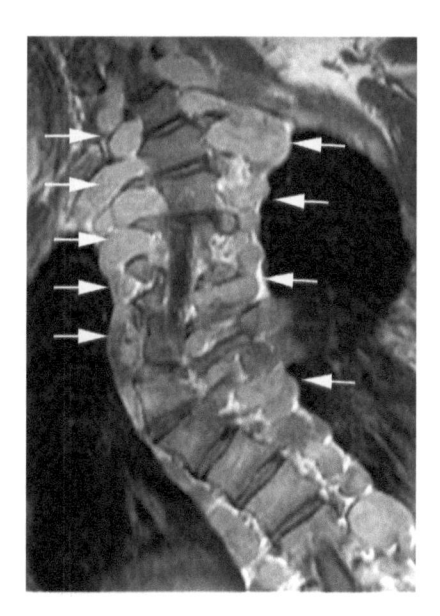

Fig. 23-5 Multiple spinal neurofibromas in a patient with NF1 on T1-weighted contrast-enhanced MRI *(arrows)*.

Radiologic/Pathologic Correlation

Neurofibromas are moderately to strongly enhancing masses with a wormlike appearance and may significantly expand the nerve roots, causing bony erosion. The overwhelming majority can be identified as intradural extramedullary, but some neurofibromas can also extend extradurally. Approximately one sixth of neurofibromas appear as dumbbell tumors, and only an exceptional example appears as a purely intramedullary mass. Plexiform neurofibromas are highly tortuous enhancing masses along the larger peripheral nerves and nerve roots (Fig. 23-5). The overwhelming majority of neurofibromas are isointense on T1-weighted and hyperintense on T2-weighted images and enhance strongly. Occasionally they can appear as simple enlargements of nerve roots.

Prognosis

Although a single neurofibroma is a benign neoplasm and is unlikely to undergo malignant degeneration, occasional cases of transformation into a malignant peripheral nerve sheath tumor have been reported. Almost all such cases of malignant degeneration have been reported in NF1. Large or plexiform neurofibromas are likely to cause nerve dysfunction that may persist or even worsen after resection. Multiplicity in the setting of NF1 poses a significant management problem that requires more than surgical intervention.

Practical Points

- Occasionally the frozen sample may not include all of the typical features that allow an accurate distinction between a neurofibroma and a schwannoma on frozen section.
- It is important to provide sufficient diagnostic tissue to the pathologist, if it is clinically important to distinguish between a neurofibroma and a schwannoma intraoperatively. Most often, the need for a more specific diagnosis should be clearly expressed if the preliminary diagnosis of *peripheral nerve sheath tumor* or *spindle cell neoplasm* is simply not sufficient.
- Care should be taken to avoid sending cauterized or crushed tissue for frozen section analysis. It is important to recognize that repeat surgical procedures will complicate interpretation during frozen section analysis.

MALIGNANT PERIPHERAL NERVE SHEATH TUMORS

Malignant peripheral nerve sheath tumors (MPNSTs) are extremely rare, aggressive sarcomas that account for approximately 5% to 10% of all soft tissue sarcomas. They occur either sporadically, in association with NF1, or subsequent to radiation therapy. Histologically, MPNSTs resemble fibrosarcomas in their basic organization (Fig. 23-6, *A*). Typically, low-grade and high-grade variants have been recognized on the basis of histologic features, such as mitotic rate, anaplastic nuclear morphology, and necrosis. A small number of MPNSTs are low grade and show moderate hypercellularity or nuclear pleomorphism but exhibit varied growth patterns, such as neurofibroma-like, low-grade myxofibrosarcoma–like, epithelioid, and hemangiopericytoma-like. Low-grade MPNSTs are more prominently positive for S100 protein and vimentin compared with high-grade MPNSTs. Immunohistochemical analysis, particularly S100 staining, plays an important role in the diagnosis but does not stain these tumors as avidly as their benign counterparts. Electron microscopy is often helpful if optimal tissue is available. At the molecular level, loss of the NF1 gene and high levels of Ras activity are the hallmarks of MPNSTs. Some studies suggest that distinct molecular classes of MPNSTs exist and that these tumors can be stratified on the basis of their gene expression profiles.[27] Patients with plexiform neurofibromas and with NF1 have a much higher risk of developing MPNSTs.[28] MRI is the most helpful imaging technique to clearly identify the extent of the tumor and its neurogenic origin and can also suggest malignant changes in these tumors (Fig. 23-6, *B*). Evidence of aggressive growth on certain MRI modalities may be valuable in indicating emergence of an MPNST and are helpful in the long-term follow-up of patients with plexiform neurofibromas.[29]

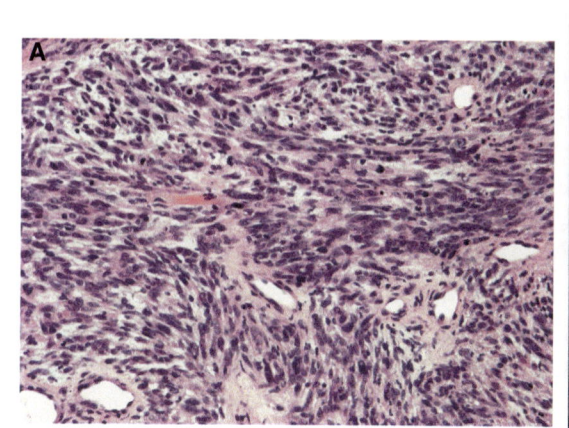

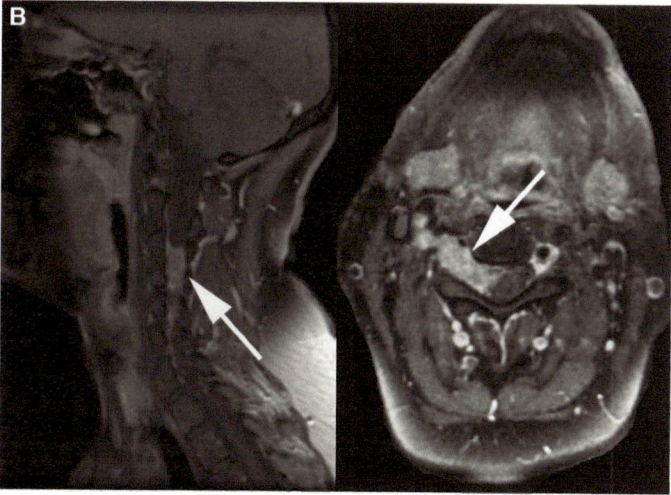

Fig. 23-6 Malignant peripheral nerve sheath tumor. **A,** Microscopic features of a malignant peripheral nerve sheath tumor showing a hypercellular, mitotically active area. **B,** Sagittal and axial images of a malignant peripheral nerve sheath tumor involving intradural and extradural spaces *(arrows)*.

Practical Points

- MPNSTs are most likely to be diagnosed in patients with well-established NF1 or in adults who have undergone radiation treatment.
- Typically there is a decade or longer lag time between radiation to the area and the emergence of MPNSTs.
- Most MPNSTs are high-grade tumors and need to be distinguished from other high-grade sarcomas.
- Immunohistochemical stains that are typically positive in neurofibromas or schwannomas in a diffuse fashion (such as S100 protein) can be focally or only weakly positive in high-grade MPNSTs.

MENINGIOMAS

Definition/Clinical Presentation

Meningiomas are the most common extra-axial tumors in adults and constitute approximately 15% of all adult primary CNS neoplasms. They also represent 20% to 25% of all primary spine neoplasms and are the second most common tumors in this location after peripheral nerve sheath tumors. Meningiomas are typically located around the thoracic spinal cord but can affect any level of the spine. Meningiomas are intradural, but concurrent intradural and extradural examples have been reported.[30] Although meningiomas can occur at any age, the incidence is highest among middle-aged women.[31,32] They are considerably rare in the pediatric population, comprising only 4.3% of all intraspinal tumors in children.[33] Spinal cord meningiomas can be one of the first manifestations of NF2. Increased risk of developing meningioma has also been linked to prior exposure to ionizing radiation.

Typical Macroscopic and Microscopic Findings

Most meningiomas are rubbery, firm, discrete, smooth, and round masses adherent to dura (Fig. 23-7, *A*). They can often erode the adjacent bone, a sign that is often taken to mean of long-standing presence. More than 15 distinct histologic types of meningiomas have been described in the literature, and they show a wide range of histologic patterns, ranging from epithelial to mesenchymal.[34] The three subtypes of meningiomas most commonly seen in the intradural extramedullary space are meningothelial meningiomas, fibrous (fibroblastic) meningiomas, and transitional (mixed) meningiomas.

Meningothelial meningiomas are composed of tightly packed whorls that are the microscopic hallmark of meningiomas (Fig. 23-7, *B*). Fibrous meningiomas have a distinct cellular spindling, with tumor cells arranged in a fascicular or storiform configuration in a variably rich collagenous background, and transitional meningiomas harbor both elements in varying proportions. The tumor cells typically have grooves or pseudoinclusions, and most tumors also harbor psammoma bodies that are laminated, calcified, basophilic extracellular structures.

Meningiomas are graded on the basis of their histologic features that reflect the risk of recurrence and aggressive growth.[35] Meningiomas with greater likelihood of aggressive behavior are classified as atypical (WHO grade II) or anaplastic (WHO grade III) tumors.[34] Four variants are automatically categorized into higher grades. Chordoid and clear cell meningiomas are considered atypical (WHO grade II), whereas the papillary and rhabdoid variants are considered anaplastic (WHO grade III). Ultrastructurally meningiomas have abundant intermediate filaments, elaborate interdigitating cell processes, and desmosome-like intercellular junctions.

Immunohistochemical markers for arachnoid cells, such as EMA and vimentin, are positive in most meningiomas.[36] Approximately two thirds of meningiomas also express progesterone receptors, and rare examples have estrogen receptor expression.

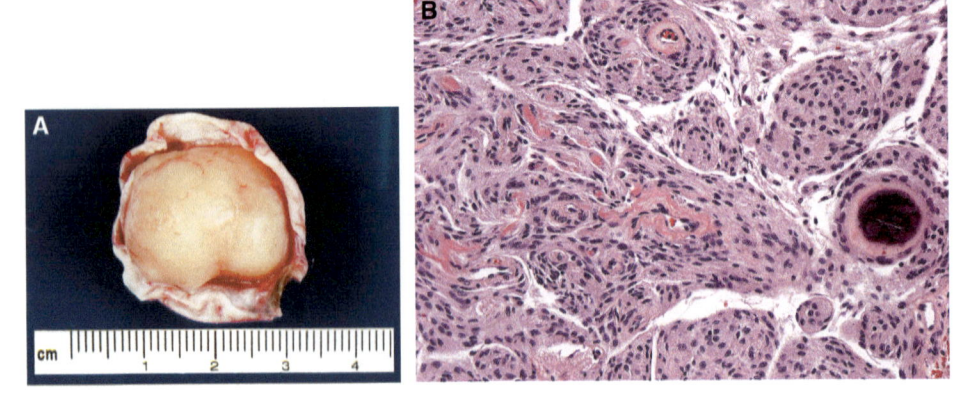

Fig. 23-7 Meningioma of the spinal cord. **A,** Macroscopic appearance of a meningioma with attached dura mater. **B,** Typical histologic characteristics of meningioma with meningothelial whorls and psammomatous calcification.

However, routine immunohistochemical stains may not be sensitive enough to recognize estrogen positivity.[37,38] Occasionally, meningiomas can stain for S100 protein, CD34 and CK18, and actin.

Pathologic Differential Diagnosis

Intraspinal meningiomas may look like schwannomas, hemangiopericytomas, solitary fibrous tumors, or other types of fibrous tumors. Although typical morphologic features are often sufficient in the vast majority of tumors, immunohistochemical analysis may become necessary in some cases. A panel of antibodies consisting of EMA, vimentin, progesterone, S100 protein, CD34, Bcl-2, and neurofilament protein is usually helpful in these unusual cases. Metastatic carcinoma may be a consideration in unusual or atypical meningiomas, and high-grade sarcomas or sarcomatoid carcinomas should be excluded for anaplastic meningiomas.

Genetics

Meningiomas are one the first types of solid tumors that were recognized as having cytogenetic alterations. Approximately 40% to 70% of meningiomas have loss of heterozygosity of markers from the chromosomal region 22q12.2 that encompasses the NF2 gene.[39] In general, chromosomal abnormalities are more extensive in atypical and anaplastic (malignant) meningiomas. Some anaplastic meningiomas are hyperploid with numerous chromosomal aberrations.

Radiologic/Pathologic Correlation

Characteristically meningiomas demonstrate radiologic evidence of changes in bones, such as hyperostosis and the typical dural tail sign, which is present in more than half of the tumors.[40] The tumors are often dark on noncontrast CT images and enhance intensely and homogeneously after contrast administration. On MRI, the tumors are isointense to brain parenchyma on T1-weighted images and display a darker rim. The tumors are isointense to slightly hyperintense to brain on T2-weighted images. Some markedly calcified or markedly fibrotic examples can be considerably hypointense. Meningiomas often enhance homogeneously on contrast (Fig. 23-8). Atypical menin-

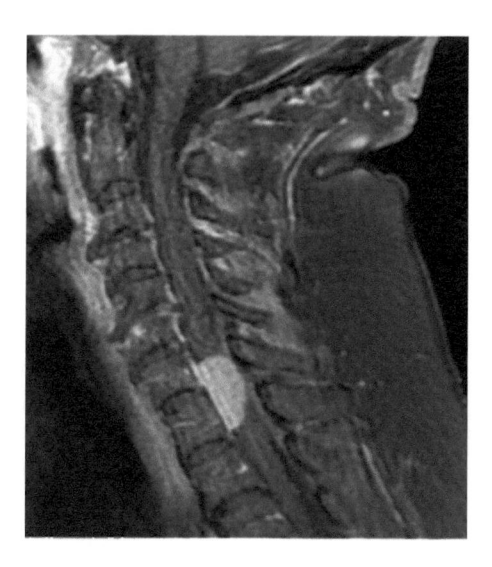

Fig. 23-8 Spinal meningioma with a dural tail on T1-weighted contrast-enhanced MRI.

giomas and some typical meningiomas elicit significant peritumoral edema. Anaplastic meningiomas often have irregular borders with the cord parenchyma.[41]

Prognosis

Because most meningiomas can be excised completely, surgery is the primary therapeutic modality. In addition, stereotactic radiosurgery may be used for primary treatment of spinal meningiomas.[42] Earlier reports suggest that despite the gross total resection, a significant percentage of meningiomas recur within 20 years.[43] Atypical meningiomas have even greater recurrence rates of 41% at 5 years and 48% at 10 years, even though gross total resection was achieved at the time of the initial surgery.[44] In general, the major factors predicting poor outcome are WHO grade, residual tumor, higher proliferative indices, loss of progesterone receptors, aneuploidy, and patient age.

Practical Points

- On frozen section analysis, atypical meningiomas are more likely to be undergraded, because the features that fulfill the criteria may not be readily observed in the frozen samples.
- Some meningiomas have minor (focal) clear cell or chordoid components. This is often not sufficient to consider these tumors higher grade.
- Immunohistochemical stains for EMA need to be titered specifically for meningiomas. If this is not done, the laboratory may report the stain as negative in many meningiomas. This may lead to an erroneous diagnosis.
- Spinal cord meningiomas in children often have a higher rate of aggressive variants.

MESENCHYMAL NONMENINGOTHELIAL NEOPLASMS

SOLITARY FIBROUS TUMORS

Definition/Clinical Presentation

Solitary fibrous tumors (SFTs) are well-circumscribed spindle cell tumors that are presumed to belong to the fibroblastic tumor category and were originally described in the pleura.[45] The literature on soft tissue considers SFTs to be neoplasms with clinical and pathologic features that overlap with the so-called hemangiopericytomas (HPCs) of soft tissue.[46,47] Both SFTs and HPCs show a marked resemblance to fibrous meningiomas in terms of their clinical and radiologic features. Although there have been some suggestions on how to distinguish SFTs from meningiomas radiologically, the definitive distinction is based on pathologic evaluation. SFTs in the spinal cord are rarely asymptomatic and are often associated with sensory or motor problems.[48]

Typical Macroscopic and Microscopic Findings

SFTs are described as tumors with a "patternless" pattern. They closely resemble fibrous meningiomas both macroscopically and microscopically. SFTs are composed of uniform spindle-shaped to oval cells invested in a variably collagenous background and are often arrayed in interlacing fascicles (Fig. 23-9). Most SFTs exhibit a biphasic pattern with areas rich in collagen that can attain a keloid-like appearance. Focal palisading or myxoid areas can be present, but these patterns are distinctly minor components.

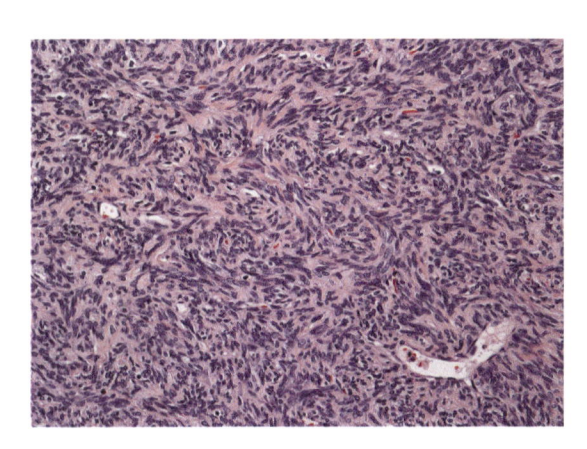

Fig. 23-9 Solitary fibrous tumors of the spinal cord. Typical histologic appearance with medium-power magnification.

The amount of vascularity varies from tumor to tumor and within a given tumor. The elaborate vascular network is composed of highly branching "staghorn"-type vessels. There is no established histologic grading scheme for SFTs, and most examples in the spine are low-grade tumors.

SFTs show positive staining with CD34, CD99, Bcl-2, and vimentin, and pertinent negative stains include S100 protein, EMA, collagen type IV, progesterone receptor, and desmin. Some SFTs can be focally and weakly positive for smooth muscle actin. Electron microscopy is of little value but can exclude other entities in the differential diagnosis.

Pathologic Differential Diagnosis

The principal differential diagnosis of SFTs includes meningioma, schwannoma, and HPC. Histologic features may give clues, but special stains and immunohistochemical analyses often become necessary to distinguish these tumors. Immunohistochemical studies for CD34 and EMA, as well as special stains for reticulin, are helpful to distinguish SFTs from meningioma. Other useful stains in differential diagnosis include S100 protein, calretinin, Bcl-2, and collagen type IV. SFTs with anaplastic histologic features are exceedingly rare in the spinal cord but should be distinguished from malignant meningiomas or other sarcomas. In such cases electron microscopy, in addition to immunohistochemical studies, can be helpful in determining the type of sarcoma.

Although the distinction between SFTs and HPCs may be trivial in soft tissue, there is evidence that they may behave differently in the central nervous system (CNS). Typically SFTs are diffusely and strongly positive for CD34, they often express CD99, and they display a poor reticulin network on collagen type IV staining. On the contrary, HPCs are negative or only focally positive for CD34, and they display a rich, elaborate, and delicate network of reticulin, wrapping individual or small groups of tumor cells.[49]

Genetics

No specific genetic alterations have been described for SFTs in the spinal cord or elsewhere in the CNS. Occasional reports of translocations have largely been restricted to case reports and have not been reproducible in larger studies.

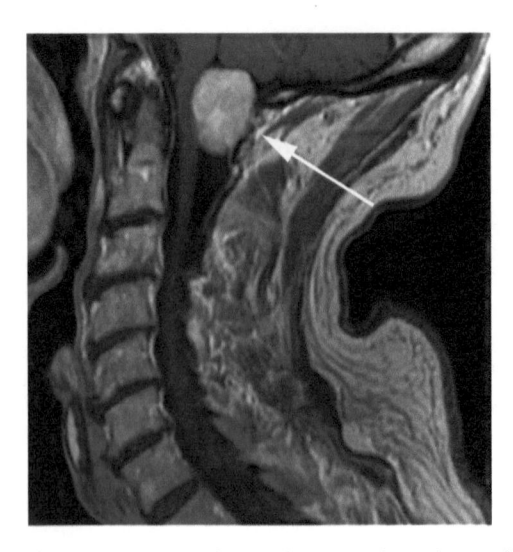

Fig. 23-10 Sagittal T1-weighted contrast-enhanced MRI of a solitary fibrous tumor involving the upper cervical spinal cord *(arrow)*.

Radiologic/Pathologic Correlation

SFTs are solid and diffusely enhancing tumors with a broad dural attachment and do not show the dural tail sign that is characteristic of meningiomas (Fig. 23-10). SFTs are isointense to hypointense on T2-weighted images and heterogeneous on T1-weighted images. Most SFTs enhance avidly after gadolinium injection and simulate meningiomas.

Prognosis

The overall prognosis of SFTs in the spinal cord is favorable after gross total resection, with only exceptional examples demonstrating local recurrence or aggressive behavior. The data on adjuvant therapy for subtotal resections are limited.

Practical Points

- Distinguishing solitary fibrous tumors from meningiomas is usually not possible with imaging, and there is little practical value for making this distinction preoperatively.
- The distinction between SFTs and HPCs is contentious. Soft tissue pathologists and neuropathologists have different perspectives on these two entities. Nevertheless, a tumor that looks like an HPC should be regarded as a sarcoma in the CNS.

Hemangiopericytoma

Definition/Clinical Presentation

In the 2007 edition of *Pathology of Tumours of the Central Nervous System*,[34] HPC is defined as a "highly cellular and vascularized mesenchymal tumor, exhibiting a characteristic monotonous low-power appearance and a well-developed, variably thick-walled, branching 'staghorn' vasculature; almost always attached to the dura and having a high tendency to recur and to metastasize outside the central nervous system." This definition is somewhat different from the one adopted by the WHO Soft Tissue and Tumor working group.[50] The symptoms and presentation of HPCs, as well as SFTs, are virtually indistinguishable from those of classic meningiomas. Tumors often present with sensory deficits and symptoms related to tumor location.

Typical Macroscopic and Microscopic Findings

Surgically, an HPC often appears as a well-circumscribed mass with a broad-based attachment to the dura. Some examples also have a highly vascular dural attachment that may be associated with bleeding. Erosion of the adjacent bones can be observed intraoperatively.

HPC in the CNS appears as a more epithelioid neoplasm with a classical "jumbled-up" architecture and vaguely nested appearance (Fig. 23-11, *A*). HPCs are often less obviously collagenous, but like SFTs, they show a biphasic pattern composed of paucicellular and hypercellular areas. The arborizing, "staghorn-like" vessels are typical of HPCs but occur in many other mesenchymal neoplasms (Fig. 23-11, *B*). Tumor cells have scant cytoplasm and monotonous nuclei. The tumor cells are often invested in a rich and delicate reticulin network, either individually or in small clusters. HPCs typically show strong diffuse staining with vimentin and Bcl-2 antibodies. Staining for

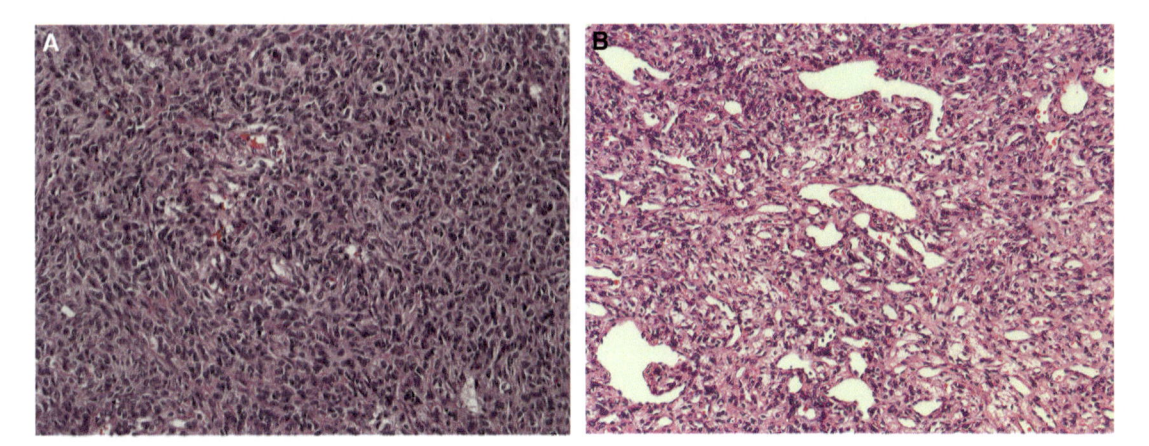

Fig. 23-11 HPC of the spinal cord. Typical histologic characteristics include **A,** jumbled architecture and **B,** staghorn vessels.

Continued

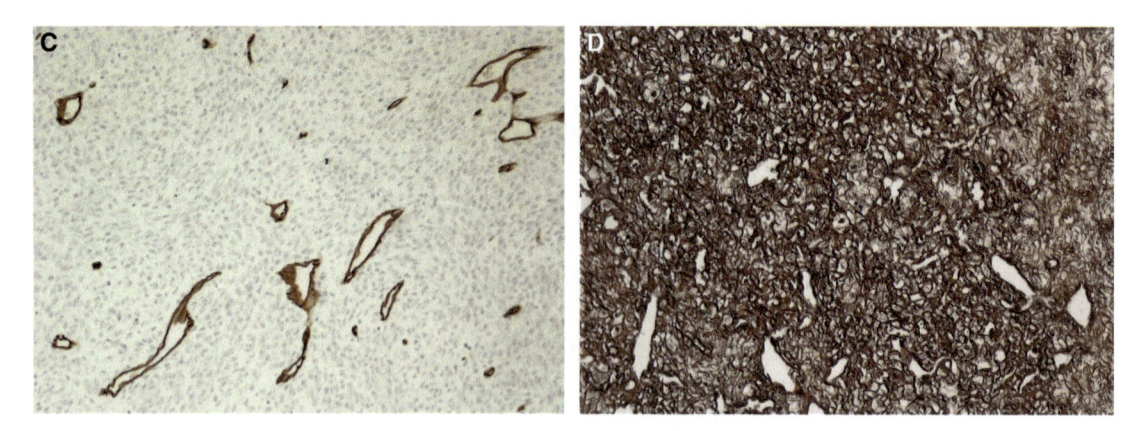

Fig. 23-11, cont'd **C,** CD34 immunohistochemistry, and **D,** reticulin stain.

EMA and S100 protein is negative, and the staining for CD34 is variable (Fig. 23-11, *C*). Typically CD34 highlights the vascular network with only rare positive tumor cells, but an occasional HPC can be strongly positive, making it quite difficult to distinguish from an SFT. Reticulin stain is often helpful in highlighting the delicate network in an HPC (Fig. 23-11, *D*). Anaplastic HPCs are rare and harbor increased mitosis, marked nuclear pleomorphism, and/or necrosis.

An uncommon variant, the lipomatous HPC, has been reported in the paranasal sinuses and exceptionally involves the base of the skull but not the spinal cord. These neoplasms are suggested to have less aggressive behavior than typical HPCs.

Pathologic Differential Diagnosis
The differential diagnosis of HPCs is identical to that of SFTs. There is good evidence that HPCs in the CNS may have a different biological behavior than either SFTs or meningiomas.[49] In addition, HPCs with anaplastic features may be quite difficult to distinguish from other high-grade undifferentiated sarcomas.[51]

Genetics
There is little known about the genetic alterations in HPCs. The typical genetic alterations of meningiomas, such as the mutations of the NF2 gene, were not found in HPCs. Rare case reports of translations in various chromosomes have been reported in HPCs, but none have been shown to occur with significant frequency.

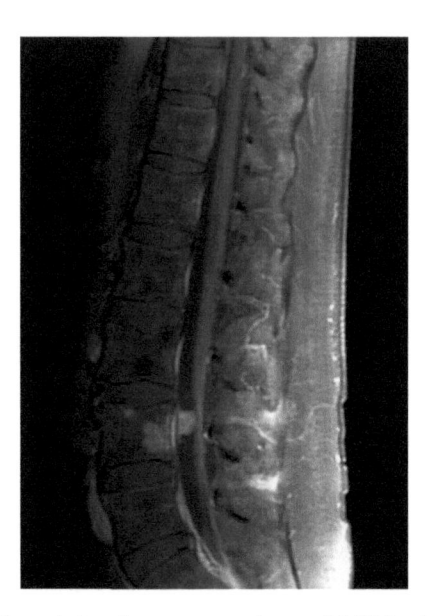

Fig. 23-12 Spinal HPC on T1-weighted contrast-enhanced MRI with associated signal changes in the adjacent vertebral body, suggesting bony involvement.

Radiologic/Pathologic Correlation
Rare examples of HPC exhibit the dural tail sign and are indistinguishable from meningiomas. On MRI scans, HPCs appear heterogeneous and predominantly isointense on both T1-weighted and T2-weighted images. These are often associated with vascular flow voids and variably enhance with gadolinium administration (Fig. 23-12).

Prognosis
HPCs are aggressive neoplasms and can often recur locally and metastasize.[52] Both recurrence and metastasis rates are much higher than for SFTs.[49] The most common metastatic sites are the lungs, liver, and bones. Metastases can occur many years after the initial resection. HPCs can also recur as poorly differentiated sarcomas. In rare instances, recurrent HPCs may be more akin to SFTs, which further supports the argument that these neoplasms are closely related.[49]

Practical Points
- HPCs should be considered an aggressive neoplasm, even if it does not have any anaplastic histology. Patients require follow-up over decades.
- HPC had been mistaken for "angioblastic meningioma" for many years before the recognition of its existence in the CNS. Therefore a tumor that was previously diagnosed as angioblastic meningioma with subsequent lung, liver, or bone metastases is most likely an HPC.
- There is significant overlap between HPCs and SFTs, and intermediate cases exist. The discrepancy between soft tissue classification and CNS classification is likely to remain until a uniform definition is adopted by the WHO.

PARAGANGLIOMAS

Definition/Clinical Presentation
Paragangliomas of the CNS are indolent, encapsulated neuroendocrine neoplasms that are assumed to originate from the paraganglionic chief cells. These tumors most commonly occur in the filum terminale[53] and affect adults in the fifth or sixth decade of life. The typical presenting symptoms are low back pain or sensorimotor deficits and, in rare cases, sphincter or erectile dysfunction, also known as *cauda equina syndrome*.[54]

Typical Macroscopic and Microscopic Findings
A paraganglioma is a soft, well-circumscribed, encapsulated tumor that occasionally shows calcification and is attached to the filum terminale. The tumor is composed of uniform spindle cells with a crisp nuclear membrane and well-defined cellular borders forming acinar structures and lobules. The smaller nests, often referred to as *Zellballen*, can be highlighted by reticulin stain. Rare isolated atypical cells with large hyperchromatic nuclei may be present. The neuroendocrine chief cells stain positive for chromogranin and synaptophysin, and the normal sustentacular cells are immunoreactive for S100 protein, and all of these can be positive in paragangliomas. Other positive antibodies include neuron-specific enolase, Leu-enkephalin, somatostatin, and GFAP.[53] Occasionally, paraganglioma may be weakly positive for cytokeratin, and should not be confused with epithelial tumors. Ultrastructurally, the chief cells have dense core neurosecretory granules and well-developed Golgi apparatus with both smooth and rough endoplasmic reticulum.[55] The sustentacular cells demonstrate elongated processes and occasional intermediate filaments. Unlike the chief cells, they lack dense core granules.

Pathologic Differential Diagnosis
The main pathologic differential diagnosis of paraganglioma is with ependymomas, as well as meningioma, but these are often easily distinguished on routine histologic and immunohistochemical studies. Primary paragangliomas in this area should be distinguished from an exceptional metastatic pheochromocytoma or paraganglioma.

Genetics
Paragangliomas of the spine are considered nonfamilial and have not been largely associated with familial syndromes. Unlike the paragangliomas elsewhere, spinal paragangliomas have not been associated with the Carney triad. Recent studies suggest germline succinate dehydrogenase mutations in sporadic cervical paragangliomas, and this has been observed in some spinal paragangliomas as well.[56,57]

Radiologic/Pathologic Correlation
Paragangliomas are well-defined masses that are hypointense to isointense on T1-weighted images and hyperintense on T2-weighted images. There is often intense but sometimes heterogeneous contrast enhancement.[58] Some examples show calcification, and they can appear as dumbbell lesions on imaging.

Prognosis

Spinal paragangliomas are categorized as WHO grade I; they are often slow growing and are managed by total excision. Rarely, spinal paragangliomas show cerebrospinal fluid seeding, and some can recur after subtotal or even gross total resection.[59] An exceptional paraganglioma can metastasize or be metastatic to the spinal cord.

Practical Points

- Frozen sections of paragangliomas can be confusing and alarming, but the discrete and noninfiltrative pattern should suggest the diagnosis.
- Diffuse GFAP staining in a tumor should raise the possibility of another diagnosis.
- Most laboratories do not routinely perform neurotransmitter immunohistochemical analysis, such as Leu-enkephalin, and it is not critical for the diagnosis.

EPENDYMAL TUMORS

Definition/Clinical Presentation

Although most ependymomas are intramedullary and therefore not covered in this chapter, rare examples of typical ependymomas and more frequently myxopapillary ependymomas can be extramedullary. The typical myxopapillary ependymoma is a well-circumscribed saclike tumor that is attached to the conus medullaris or cauda equina. This tumor typically occurs in adults and is extremely rare in children. Myxopapillary ependymoma is a WHO grade I neoplasm.

Typical Macroscopic and Microscopic Findings

The myxopapillary ependymoma is a discrete mass that often adheres to the nerve roots of the cauda equina or conus medullaris. The cut sections of the saclike mass can have a gelatinous gray appearance. Some patients can have multiple tumors.

Microscopic features of myxopapillary ependymoma are characteristic and consist of bland epithelial cells arranged around myxoid stroma, which in turn are layered around vascular structures, yielding a variably papillary architecture (Fig. 23-13). The epithelial

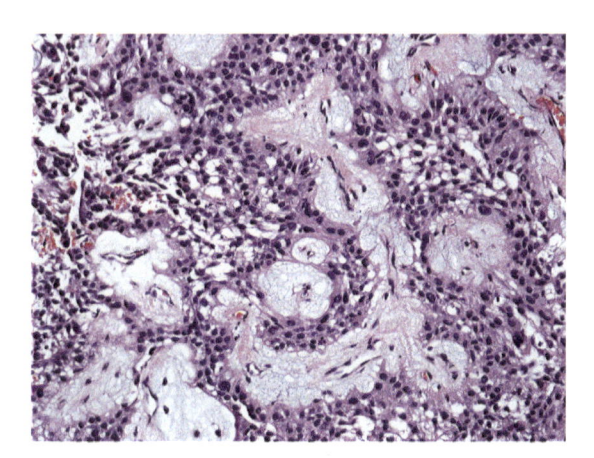

Fig. 23-13 Myxopapillary ependymoma. Typical low-power magnification of a tumor in the cauda equina.

cells appear vaguely as fibrillary and glial. The tumors are histologically identical to tumors described as *sacral ependymomas* that occur in the sacrum or parasacral soft tissues with no attachment to the spine or CNS.[60]

The immunohistochemical profile of myxopapillary ependymoma consists of positive GFAP, S100 protein, and vimentin staining. Staining for EMA that is typical of classic ependymomas is extremely rare, and most myxopapillary ependymomas are EMA negative.

Pathologic Differential Diagnosis

Myxopapillary ependymomas are quite distinctive in their overall histologic appearance and, despite some variations, have a short list of differential diagnosis. Schwannomas and paragangliomas in the spinal cord may simulate a myxopapillary ependymomas, and occasionally the myxoid background can be mistaken for a chordoma. In all of these instances, the histologic detail is helped by the positive GFAP staining on immunohistochemical studies.

Radiologic/Pathologic Correlation

Myxopapillary ependymomas are more commonly solitary but can be multiple. The typical location is the intradural extramedullary space, even though some may encroach on the epidural space. The typical MRI is isointense on T1-weighted images and hyperintense on T2-weighted images with uniform contrast enhancement[61] (Fig. 23-14).

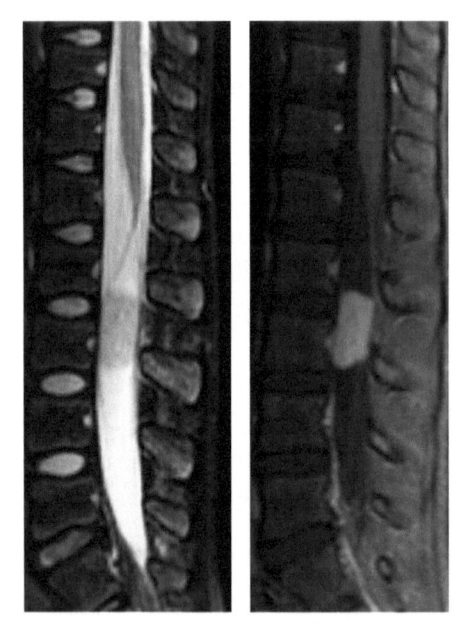

Fig. 23-14 Sagittal T2-weighted and contrast-enhanced T1-weighted images of a myxopapillary ependymoma involving the cauda equina.

Prognosis

Although most myxopapillary ependymomas are cured by gross total resection, rare examples may be aggressive with bone invasion. Multiplicity may also complicate patient management. Nevertheless, the overall outcome for this WHO grade I neoplasm is excellent.

Practical Points

- Myxopapillary ependymomas can be multiple and can erode bone, and the presence of multiple tumors with bone erosion does not exclude the diagnosis.
- A distinct giant cell pattern can occur in the cauda equina and may be difficult to diagnose.

HEMANGIOBLASTOMAS

Definition and Clinical Presentation

Hemangioblastomas are highly vascular, well-defined tumors with unclear tumorigenesis. They are rare and usually occur in adults at a mean age of approximately the third decade of life. Hemangioblastomas are slow-growing, benign neoplasms, classified as WHO grade I neoplasms, that predominantly arise in the cerebellum and can occur in the spinal cord either as an extramedullary or, less commonly, an intramedullary mass.[62,63]

Approximately 25% of hemangioblastomas are associated with von Hippel–Lindau (VHL) disease, an autosomal dominant inherited disorder that is characterized by a high incidence of renal cell carcinoma, visceral cysts, papillary cystadenoma of the epididymis or mesosalpinx, aggressive papillary middle ear tumor (endolymphatic sac tumor), and pheochromocytoma or extra-adrenal paraganglioma.[64] Hemangioblastomas associated with VHL disease can arise in the cerebellum, brainstem, or spinal cord and are often multifocal. Exceptional cases of diffuse spread throughout the spinal cord have been defined as *hemangioblastomatosis*[65] (Fig. 23-15).

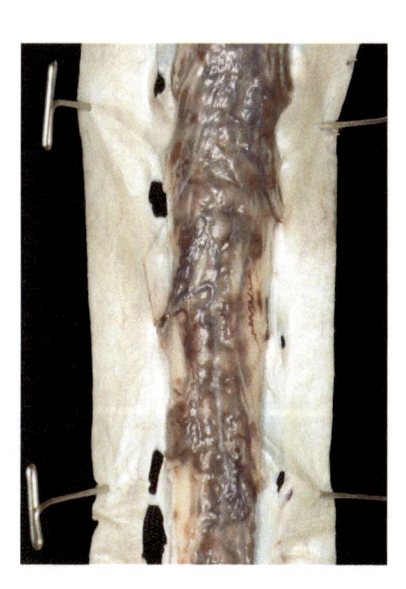

Fig. 23-15 Macroscopic appearance of multiple extradural intramedullary hemangioblastomas coating the surface of the spinal cord (hemangioblastomatosis).

Typical Macroscopic and Microscopic Findings

Hemangioblastomas are well-demarcated, reddish nodules with yellow specks or areas reflecting the presence of abundant vasculature and high lipid content within stromal cells, respectively. Hemangioblastomas are composed of lipid-filled so-called stromal cells and have an extensive network of large, often thin-walled, vessels. The classic cytologic triad that makes up the tumor consists of endothelial cells, stromal cells, and vacuolated cells (Fig. 23-16). Architecturally, hemangioblastomas can have either a loose appearance or more compact pattern with variable cellularity and HPC-like vasculature. Some cells can appear quite pleomorphic. Foci of extramedullary hematopoiesis can also be found in rare cases. This is possibly caused by erythropoietin synthesis found in the cystic component of approximately 10% of hemangioblastoma cases.[66] Mast cells, common in hemangioblastomas, are immunoreactive for erythropoietin and have been suggested to play a role in this process as well as angiogenesis.[67] On electron microscopy the stromal cells of hemangioblastomas contain abundant cytoplasmic lipid droplets. Hemagioblastoma stromal cells express neuron-specific enolase, neural cell adhesion molecule, vimentin, and ezrin. CD34 shows marked positivity because of the extensive tumor vascularity. In addition, they show cytoplasmic staining for inhibin alpha, a stain that can distinguish this tumor from metastatic renal cell carcinoma.[68] Although staining for neuron-specific enolase is not specific, it raises the possibility of a neuroepithelial origin for some tumor cells, a minority of which also stain for other neuronal markers.[69] Hemangioblastomas do not stain for factor VIII–related antigen (von Willenbrand factor), cytokeratin, EMA, or panepithelial antigen. Although glial fibrillary acidic protein is typically negative, some studies suggest positivity of this marker in hemangioblastoma.[70]

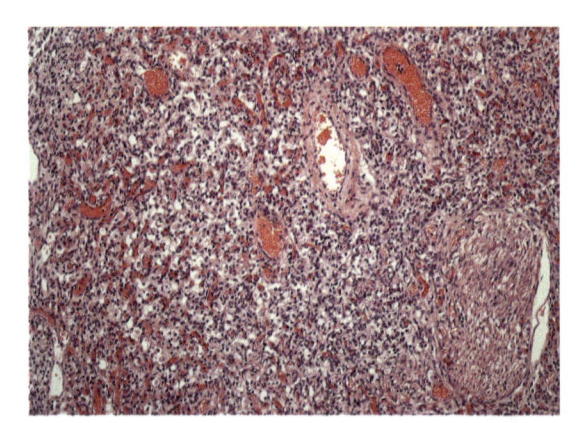

Fig. 23-16 Typical microscopic appearance of a hemangioblastoma.

Pathologic Differential Diagnosis

Because of its clear cell morphology and intracytoplasmic lipid-containing vacuoles, hemangioblastomas can be confused with metastatic renal cell carcinoma, a component of VHL disease. Hemangioblastomas can look similar to pilocytic astrocytomas or simple cysts, if the gliotic cyst wall is sampled. To further confound the issue, numerous case reports document metastatic renal cell carcinoma to hemangioblastoma in the setting of VHL disease. Hemangioblastomas have also been confused with so-called angioblastic meningiomas and hemangiopericytomas. Angiosarcoma can be mistaken for hemagioblastoma, especially in certain locations in the spine or in the setting of a highly aggressive tumor, such as hemangioblastomatosis.

Genetics

Vascular endothelial growth factor (VEGF) and VEGF receptors are upregulated in the stromal cells, seemingly because of the mutation in the VHL tumor suppressor gene, which is located on chromosome 3p25-26.[71,72] Mutations or deletions in the VHL gene have been found in the minority of sporadic hemangioblastomas.[73] On the other hand, in hemangioblastomas associated with VHL disease, VHL mutations are found in a larger percentage of tumors.[74]

Radiologic/Pathologic Correlation

Small hemangioblastomas tend to be isointense on T1-weighted images and hyperintense on T2-weighted images and show homogeneous enhancement, whereas larger tumors tend to be hypointense or isointense on T1-weighted images, heterogeneous on T2-weighted images, and show variable contrast enhancement. Recent changes in the radiologic appearance of hemangioblastomas are often due to cystic degeneration or an intratumoral hemorrhage. Multiple hemangioblastomas are more typical of VHL disease (Fig. 23-17). Exceptionally rare cases of metastatic renal cell carcinomas within spinal or posterior fossa hemangioblastomas have been reported.[75]

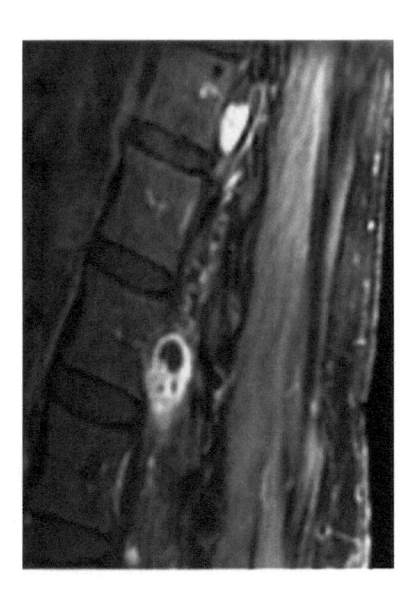

Fig. 23-17 Sagittal T1-weighted contrast-enhanced image of multiple spinal hemangioblastomas in the setting of von Hippel–Lindau disease.

Prognosis

Surgical excision is the treatment of choice inasmuch as complete resection is possible in most cases. Microsurgical technique has improved clinical outcomes. It is recommended that all patients with hemangioblastomas be investigated for evidence of VHL disease, especially those of younger age and with multiple lesions. Because of the slow-growing nature of this tumor, patients with hemangioblastomas have excellent outcomes, and permanent neurologic deficits are rare. The recurrence rates for hemangioblastoma are low, and gross total resection is considered curative. However, these tumors may recur if the excision is incomplete. Only in extremely rare instances, have hemangioblastomas been known to disseminate along the spinal cord. In contrast to sporadic cases, hemangioblastomas associated with VHL disease are the leading cause of morbidity and mortality. Exceptional cases demonstrate widespread involvement of the spinal cord, also known as *hemangioblastomatosis*.[65]

Practical Points

- When performing a biopsy, more solid areas should be targeted because biopsy of the gliotic cyst wall can be histologically confused with pilocytic astrocytoma or a simple cyst.
- The tendency for hemangioblastomas to bleed make them a poor candidate for incisional biopsy for frozen section sampling, because obtaining a small biopsy may require the use of cauterization, which can significantly complicate interpretation. In cases where this is absolutely necessary, incisional biopsy should be attempted with caution.
- Hemangioblastomas are more frequently intramedullary and less commonly purely extramedullary.

TIPS FROM THE MASTERS

- Although intraspinal nerve sheath tumors can present with radicular pain, the presence of severe recalcitrant pain from extraspinal or paraspinal lesions should raise the index of suspicion for a malignant subtype.
- Melanocytic schwannoma is an aggressive malignant tumor that should be treated like a cancerous lesion, with radiographic evaluation for metastatic disease, radical surgery, and early postoperative radiation or stereotactic radiosurgery.

References (With Key References in Boldface)

1. Mrugala MM, Batchelor TT, Plotkin SR. Peripheral and cranial nerve sheath tumors. Curr Opin Neurol 18:604-610, 2005.
2. Mahore A, Muzumdar D, Chagla A, et al. Pure ventral midline long segment schwannoma of the cervicodorsal spine: a case report. Turk Neurosurg 19:302-305, 2009.
3. **MacCollin M, Chiocca EA, Evans DG, et al. Diagnostic criteria for schwannomatosis. Neurology 64:1838-1845, 2005.**
4. MacCollin M, Woodfin W, Kronn D, et al. Schwannomatosis: a clinical and pathologic study. Neurology 46:1072-1079, 1996.
5. Kasliwal MK, Kale SS, Sharma BS, et al. Totally cystic intradural extramedullary schwannoma. Turk Neurosurg 18:404-406, 2008.
6. **Woodruff JM, Godwin TA, Erlandson RA, et al. Cellular schwannoma: a variety of schwannoma sometimes mistaken for a malignant tumor. Am J Surg Pathol 5:733-744, 1981.**
7. **Carney JA. Carney complex: the complex of myxomas, spotty pigmentation, endocrine overactivity, and schwannomas. Semin Dermatol 14:90-98, 1995.**
8. Fine SW, McClain SA, Li M. Immunohistochemical staining for calretinin is useful for differentiating schwannomas from neurofibromas. Am J Clin Pathol 122:552-559, 2004.
9. Hirose T, Tani T, Shimada T, et al. Immunohistochemical demonstration of EMA/Glut1-positive perineurial cells and CD34-positive fibroblastic cells in peripheral nerve sheath tumors. Mod Pathol 16:293-298, 2003.
10. Dickersin GR. The electron microscopic spectrum of nerve sheath tumors. Ultrastruct Pathol 11:103-146, 1987.
11. **Zhang HY, Yang GH, Chen HJ, et al. Clinicopathological, immunohistochemical, and ultrastructural study of 13 cases of melanotic schwannoma. Chin Med J (Engl) 118:1451-1461, 2005.**
12. Winek RR, Scheithauer BW, Wick MR. Meningioma, meningeal hemangiopericytoma (angioblastic meningioma), peripheral hemangiopericytoma, and acoustic schwannoma. A comparative immunohistochemical study. Am J Surg Pathol 13:251-261, 1989.
13. Bijlsma EK, Brouwer-Mladin R, Bosch DA, et al. Molecular characterization of chromosome 22 deletions in schwannomas. Genes Chromosomes Cancer 5:201-205, 1992.
14. Bijlsma EK, Merel P, Bosch DA, et al. Analysis of mutations in the SCH gene in schwannomas. Genes Chromosomes Cancer 11:7-14, 1994.
15. Begnami MD, Palau M, Rushing EJ, et al. Evaluation of NF2 gene deletion in sporadic schwannomas, meningiomas, and ependymomas by chromogenic in situ hybridization. Hum Pathol 38:1345-1350, 2007.
16. Huynh DP, Mautner V, Baser ME, et al. Immunohistochemical detection of schwannomin and neurofibromin in vestibular schwannomas, ependymomas and meningiomas. J Neuropathol Exp Neurol 56:382-390, 1997.
17. Bloomer CW, Ackerman A, Bhatia RG. Imaging for spine tumors and new applications. Top Magn Reson Imaging 17:69-87, 2006.
18. Gelabert-Gonzalez M. [Primary spinal cord tumours. An analysis of a series of 168 patients]. Rev Neurol 44:269-274, 2007.
19. Jeon JH, Hwang HS, Jeong JH, et al. Spinal schwannoma; analysis of 40 cases. J Korean Neurosurg Soc 43:135-138, 2008.
20. Casadei GP, Scheithauer BW, Hirose T, et al. Cellular schwannoma. A clinicopathologic, DNA flow cytometric, and proliferation marker study of 70 patients. Cancer 75:1109-1119, 1995.

21. Kim P, Ebersold MJ, Onofrio BM, et al. Surgery of spinal nerve schwannoma. Risk of neurological deficit after resection of involved root. J Neurosurg 71:810-814, 1989.
22. Levy WJ, Latchaw J, Hahn JF, et al. Spinal neurofibromas: a report of 66 cases and a comparison with meningiomas. Neurosurgery 18:331-334, 1986.
23. Kawahara E, Oda Y, Ooi A, et al. Expression of glial fibrillary acidic protein (GFAP) in peripheral nerve sheath tumors. A comparative study of immunoreactivity of GFAP, vimentin, S-100 protein, and neurofilament in 38 schwannomas and 18 neurofibromas. Am J Surg Pathol 12:115-120, 1988.
24. Pankratova ES, Chumachenko PA, Libiiainen TP, et al. [Diffuse neurofibroma invading the spinal cord channel and soft tissues of the chest] Arkh Patol 65:54-56, 2003.
25. van Sandick JW, van Coevorden F. Plexiform neurofibroma with intraspinal extension. J Am Coll Surg 195:572, 2002.
26. **Pollack IF, Colak A, Fitz C, et al. Surgical management of spinal cord compression from plexiform neurofibromas in patients with neurofibromatosis 1. Neurosurgery 43:248-255; discussion 255-256, 1998.**
27. Watson MA, Perry A, Tihan T, et al. Gene expression profiling reveals unique molecular subtypes of Neurofibromatosis Type I-associated and sporadic malignant peripheral nerve sheath tumors. Brain Pathol 14:297-303, 2004.
28. Tucker T, Wolkenstein P, Revuz J, et al. Association between benign and malignant peripheral nerve sheath tumors in NF1. Neurology 65:205-211, 2005.
29. **Friedrich RE, Kluwe L, Funsterer C, et al. Malignant peripheral nerve sheath tumors (MPNST) in neurofibromatosis type 1 (NF1): diagnostic findings on magnetic resonance images and mutation analysis of the NF1 gene. Anticancer Res 25:1699-1702, 2005.**
30. Weil SM, Gewirtz RJ, Tew JM Jr. Concurrent intradural and extradural meningiomas of the cervical spine. Neurosurgery 27:629-631, 1990.
31. Levy WJ Jr, Bay J, Dohn D. Spinal cord meningioma. J Neurosurg 57:804-812, 1982.
32. Solero CL, Fornari M, Giombini S, et al. Spinal meningiomas: review of 174 operated cases. Neurosurgery 25:153-160, 1989.
33. Fortuna A, Nolletti A, Nardi P, et al. Spinal neurinomas and meningiomas in children. Acta Neurochir (Wien) 55:329-341, 1981.
34. **Louis DN, Ohgaki H, Wiestler OD, et al. Pathology of Tumours of the Central Nervous System. Lyon: IARC Press, 2007.**
35. **Perry A, Stafford SL, Scheithauer BW, et al. Meningioma grading: an analysis of histologic parameters. Am J Surg Pathol 21:1455-1465, 1997.**
36. Meis JM, Ordonez NG, Bruner JM. Meningiomas. An immunohistochemical study of 50 cases. Arch Pathol Lab Med 110:934-937, 1986.
37. Moresco RM, Scheithauer BW, Lucignani G, et al. Oestrogen receptors in meningiomas: a correlative PET and immunohistochemical study. Nucl Med Commun 18:606-615, 1997.
38. Nagashima G, Aoyagi M, Wakimoto H, et al. Immunohistochemical detection of progesterone receptors and the correlation with Ki-67 labeling indices in paraffin-embedded sections of meningiomas. Neurosurgery 37:478-482; discussion 483, 1995.
39. Simon M, Bostrom JP, Hartmann C. Molecular genetics of meningiomas: from basic research to potential clinical applications. Neurosurgery 60:787-798; discussion 787-798, 2007.
40. Alorainy IA. Dural tail sign in spinal meningiomas. Eur J Radiol 60:387-391, 2006.
41. Liu WC, Choi G, Lee SH, et al. Radiological findings of spinal schwannomas and meningiomas: focus on discrimination of two disease entities. Eur Radiol 19:2707-2715, 2009.
42. Gerszten PC, Burton SA, Ozhasoglu C, et al. Radiosurgery for benign intradural spinal tumors. Neurosurgery 62:887-895; discussion 895-896, 2008.
43. Jaaskelainen J. Seemingly complete removal of histologically benign intracranial meningioma: late recurrence rate and factors predicting recurrence in 657 patients. A multivariate analysis. Surg Neurol 26:461-469, 1986.
44. Aghi MK, Carter BS, Cosgrove GR, et al. Long-term recurrence rates of atypical meningiomas after gross total resection with or without postoperative adjuvant radiation. Neurosurgery 64:56-60; discussion 60, 2009.

45. Klemperer P, Rabin CB. Primary neoplasms of the pleura. Arch Pathol 11:385-412, 1931.
46. Fletcher CD. The evolving classification of soft tissue tumours: an update based on the new WHO classification. Histopathology 48:3-12, 1986.
47. **Gengler C, Guillou L. Solitary fibrous tumour and haemangiopericytoma: evolution of a concept. Histopathology 48:63-74, 2006.**
48. Alston SR, Francel PC, Jane JA Jr. Solitary fibrous tumor of the spinal cord. Am J Surg Pathol 21:477-483, 1997.
49. Tihan T, Viglione M, Rosenblum MK, et al. Solitary fibrous tumors in the central nervous system. A clinicopathologic review of 18 cases and comparison to meningeal hemangiopericytomas. Arch Pathol Lab Med 127:432-439, 2003.
50. **Fletcher CDM, Unni KK, Mertens FE. Pathology and genetics of tumours of soft tissue and bone. In World Health Organization Classification of Tumours. Lyon: IARC Press, 2002.**
51. Nappi O, Ritter JH, Pettinato G, et al. Hemangiopericytoma: histopathological pattern or clinicopathologic entity? Semin Diagn Pathol 12:221-232, 1995.
52. Mena H, Ribas JL, Pezeshkpour GH, et al. Hemangiopericytoma of the central nervous system: a review of 94 cases. Hum Pathol 22:84-91, 1991.
53. Moran CA, Rush W, Mena H. Primary spinal paragangliomas: a clinicopathological and immunohistochemical study of 30 cases. Histopathology 31:167-173, 1997.
54. Bagley CA, Gokaslan ZL. Cauda equina syndrome caused by primary and metastatic neoplasms. Neurosurg Focus 16:e3, 2004.
55. Sonneland PR, Scheithauer BW, LeChago J, et al. Paraganglioma of the cauda equina region. Clinicopathologic study of 31 cases with special reference to immunocytology and ultrastructure. Cancer 58:1720-1735, 1986.
56. Lima J, Feijao T, Ferreira da Silva A, et al. High frequency of germline succinate dehydrogenase mutations in sporadic cervical paragangliomas in northern Spain: mitochondrial succinate dehydrogenase structure-function relationships and clinical-pathological correlations. J Clin Endocrinol Metab 92:4853-4864, 2007.
57. **Masuoka J, Brandner S, Paulus W, et al. Germline SDHD mutation in paraganglioma of the spinal cord. Oncogene 20:5084-5086, 2001.**
58. Sundgren P, Annertz M, Englund E, et al. Paragangliomas of the spinal canal. Neuroradiology 41:788-794, 1999.
59. Strommer KN, Brandner S, Sarioglu AC, et al. Symptomatic cerebellar metastasis and late local recurrence of a cauda equina paraganglioma. Case report. J Neurosurg 83:166-169, 1995.
60. Choudhary KK, Bhytani A, Agarwal R, et al. Extradural myxopapillary ependymoma with sacral osteolysis—a case report. Indian J Pathol Microbiol 45:363-365, 2002.
61. Wippold FJ II, Smirniotopoulos JG, Moran CJ, et al. MR imaging of myxopapillary ependymoma: findings and value to determine extent of tumor and its relation to intraspinal structures. AJR Am J Roentgenol 165:1263-1267, 1995.
62. Wisoff HS, Suzuki Y, Llena JF, et al. Extramedullary hemangioblastoma of the spinal cord. Case report. J Neurosurg 48:461-464, 1978.
63. Toyoda H, Seki M, Nakamura H, et al. Intradural extramedullary hemangioblastoma differentiated by MR images in the cervical spine: a case report and review of the literature. J Spinal Disord Tech 17:343-347, 2004.
64. Neumann HP, Eggert HR, Scheremet R, et al. Central nervous system lesions in von Hippel-Lindau syndrome. J Neurol Neurosurg Psychiatry 55:898-901, 1992.
65. Ramachandran R, Lee HS, Matthews B, et al. Intradural extramedullary leptomeningeal hemangioblastomatosis and paraneoplastic limbic encephalitis diagnosed at autopsy: an unlikely pair. Arch Pathol Lab Med 132:104-108, 2008.
66. Waldmann TA, Levin EH, Baldwin M. The association of polycythemia with a cerebellar hemangioblastoma. The production of an erythropoiesis stimulating factor by the tumor. Am J Med 31:318-324, 1961.
67. Ho KL. Ultrastructure of cerebellar capillary hemangioblastoma. II. Mast cells and angiogenesis. Acta Neuropathol 64:308-318, 1984.

68. Hoang MP, Amirkhan RH. Inhibin alpha distinguishes hemangioblastoma from clear cell renal cell carcinoma. Am J Surg Pathol 27:1152-1156, 2003.
69. Becker I, Paulus W, Roggendorf W, et al. Immunohistologic analysis of neuron-specific enolase and neuropeptides in stromal cells of cerebellar hemangioblastomas. Acta Histochem 38:151-155, 1990.
70. Kepes JJ, Rengachary SS, Lee SH. Astrocytes in hemangioblastomas of the central nervous system and their relationship to stromal cells. Acta Neuropathol 47:99-104, 1979.
71. Stratmann R, Krieg M, Haas R, et al. Putative control of angiogenesis in hemangioblastomas by the von Hippel-Lindau tumor suppressor gene. J Neuropathol Exp Neurol 56:1242-1252, 1997.
72. Wizigmann-Voos S, Plate KH. Pathology, genetics and cell biology of hemangioblastomas. Histol Histopathol 11:1049-1061, 1996.
73. Lee JY, Dong SM, Park WS, et al. Loss of heterozygosity and somatic mutations of the VHL tumor suppressor gene in sporadic cerebellar hemangioblastomas. Cancer Res 58:504-508, 1998.
74. **Catapano D, Muscarella LA, Guarnieri V, et al. Hemangioblastomas of central nervous system: molecular genetic analysis and clinical management. Neurosurgery 56:1215-1221; discussion 1221, 2005.**
75. Altinoz MA, Santaguida C, Guiot MC, et al. Spinal hemangioblastoma containing metastatic renal cell carcinoma in von Hippel-Lindau disease. Case report and review of the literature. J Neurosurg Spine 3:495-500, 2005.

Section III

Operative Techniques

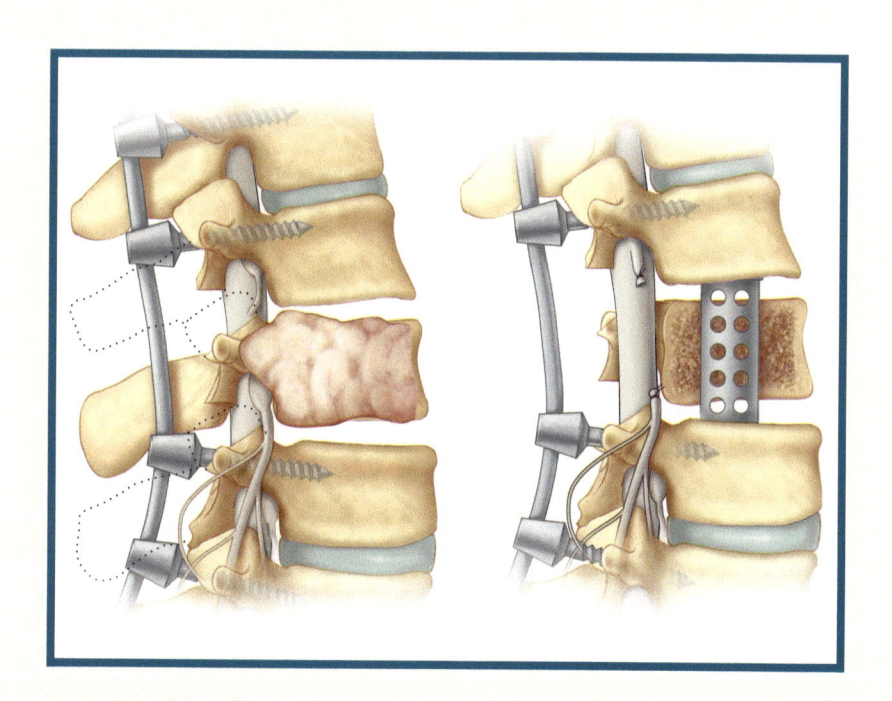

Chapter 24

Approaches to Percutaneous Image-Guided Spine Biopsy

Bihong T. Chen, Mike Y. Chen,
Julie A. Ressler, Chi-Shing Zee

The approaches to percutaneous biopsy of the spine have evolved significantly over the years since it was first performed blindly in the 1930s.[1,2] Conventional radiographs were used as image guidance for spine biopsy in the 1940s. This has been replaced in today's practice by fluoroscopy, CT, MRI, and real-time CT fluoroscopic guidance.[3-8] Advances in image-guided techniques have made percutaneous spine biopsies more accurate, with improved diagnostic yield and fewer complications, compared with open biopsies. Percutaneous biopsy of the spine with the use of fluoroscopy or CT guidance has replaced open biopsy whenever feasible to obtain a histologic diagnosis to guide management of spine lesions.

In this chapter we will discuss the various image-guided techniques available, the reasoning behind the choice among these techniques, the tips and tricks of the trade for spine biopsy, and the variety of techniques in the different spine segments, including the cervical, thoracic, and lumbar spine and the sacrum.

INDICATIONS AND CONTRAINDICATIONS

Spine biopsy is indicated when the differential diagnosis between a neoplastic or inflammatory lesion is difficult or when the blood culture is negative in the presence of spondylodiscitis (Box 24-1). Spine biopsy is also performed when the radiologic diagnosis is confusing. However, even with a classic radiologic appearance and clinical presentation of osteomyelitis, the offending microorganism may need to be isolated to implement optimal antibiotic therapy. Patients with potential primary neoplasms of the spine require a biopsy to confirm the diagnosis and develop the subsequent treatment plan based on a multidisciplinary approach. Even with what clearly appears to be metastatic disease, some patients may have a second primary cancer in the spine that must be identified before a treatment regimen is initiated. At our institution, which is a comprehensive cancer center, patients may have more than one primary cancer and require treatment that can be quite different, depending on the cause (Box 24-1).

The main contraindications are uncorrectable coagulopathy and inaccessibility for percutaneous spine biopsy[9,10] (Box 24-2).

Box 24-1 **Indications for Performing a Percutaneous Spine Biopsy**

- To differentiate between tumor and infection
- To confirm metastasis in patients with known cancer or to determine the diagnosis in patients with an unknown primary tumor
- To evaluate primary bone lesions
- To determine whether a vertebral body fracture resulted from benign or pathologic processes
- To confirm discitis and osteomyelitis and obtain samples to isolate organisms
- To assess spinal or paraspinal soft tissue masses
- To guide treatment of facet joint synovial cysts

Box 24-2 **Contraindications for Percutaneous Spine Biopsy**

- Severe uncorrectable coagulopathy
- Inaccessibility of percutaneously available trajectories used in image-guided biopsies

PREOPERATIVE EVALUATION

Patients should be thoroughly counseled regarding the risks and benefits of the biopsy procedure. They should also be advised of the possible complications of bleeding, infection, injury to the nerve roots, and inadvertent puncture of the thecal sac and spinal cord, which can result in neurologic deficits. In addition, pneumohemothorax can also occur in lower cervical and thoracic spine biopsies. There is also a possibility of insufficient tissue sampling, which renders the biopsy nondiagnostic.

Before the biopsy is performed, the patient should be carefully evaluated with a combination of clinical history, physical examination, and imaging studies. Any coagulopathy should be corrected. Blood-thinning medications, such as aspirin and warfarin (Coumadin), should be discontinued 1 week before the procedure. Patients should also be carefully examined with regard to back pain. Patients who have radiologic or clinical evidence of cord compression may have to be monitored more closely after the procedure. A multidisciplinary approach that includes referring physicians, pathologists, and radiologists is essential to ensure safe needle placement and adequate sampling. Routine preprocedure laboratory studies, such as complete blood cell examination with platelet count, a basic metabolic panel, and coagulation profile, including prothrombin time, partial thromboplastin time, and international normalized ratio (INR), should be obtained. All of the patient's radiologic studies, such as plain radiographs and CT, MRI, positron emission tomography–computed tomography (PET-CT), and nuclear medicine scans, including bone and gallium scans, should be reviewed carefully. MRI scans of the spine can depict anatomic details, especially the soft tissue extension, and can also demonstrate the enhancing parts of the lesion after injection of a contrast medium, which should be targeted for biopsy. PET-CT studies can be helpful to guide the biopsy needle into the PET-positive portion of the lesion to increase diagnostic yield, especially in large, partially necrotic lesions. Biopsy specimens should be obtained of the most superficial and the largest lesions. The lytic component of the spine lesion should always be sampled first when a mixed lytic and sclerotic lesion is encountered. Biopsies should be performed on both soft tissue masses and the bone lesion, if there is an adjacent soft tissue component in the spine bone lesion.[8,9]

TECHNIQUE

For a fluoroscopic-guided spine biopsy, the patient is usually placed in the prone position, and the area of interest for biopsy is prepared and draped in the usual sterile fashion (Fig. 24-1). The needle entry site is then identified with a radiopaque object, such as a needle or clamp, and marked on the skin. A local anesthetic, such as 2% lidocaine, is used to anesthetize the biopsy tract up to the periosteum with a 22-gauge spinal needle. Biopsies can be performed either transpedicularly or extrapedicularly. The C-arm can be adjusted until the pedicle is ovoid in shape, with clear cortical borders, and is in the center of the field of view. This happens when the x-ray beam is projecting down the long axis of the pedicle in an en face view.

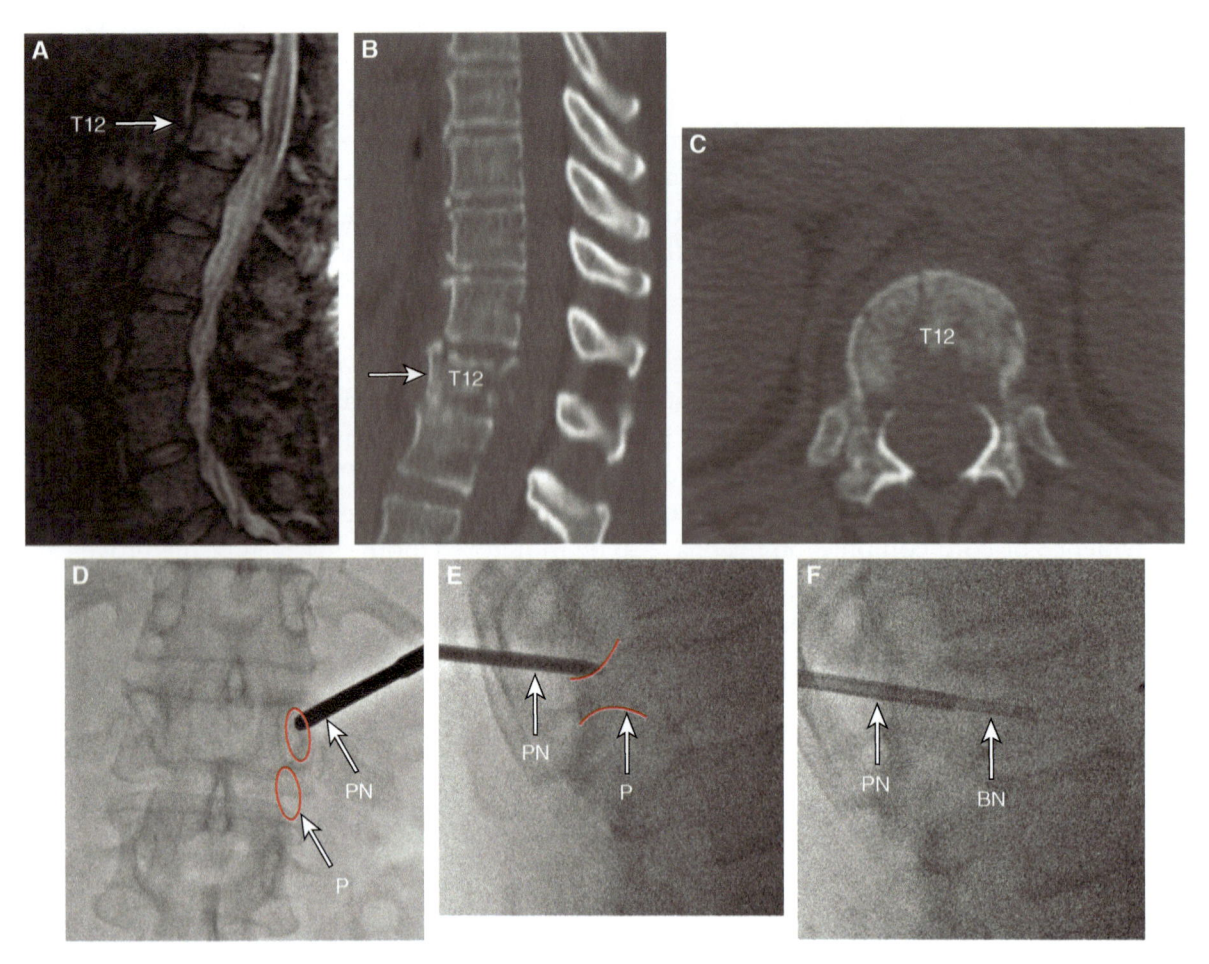

Fig. 24-1 Fluoroscopic-guided thoracic spine biopsy specimen. **A,** An MRI of the spine shows a compression fracture of T12 with retropulsion on the thecal sac. **B,** Sagittal and **C,** axial CT images of the thoracic spine demonstrate gross destruction of the T12 vertebral body with posterior cortical erosion. **D-F,** Radiographic images demonstrate fluoroscopic-guided biopsy findings obtained through a transpedicular approach at the right T12 pedicle. The pathologic diagnosis is metastatic breast cancer. (*BN,* Biopsy needle; *P,* pedicle; *PN,* penetration needle.)

As an alternative, the biopsy can be performed by a transpedicular approach from a midline posterior view in which the spinous processes lie exactly in between the pedicles. Frequent oblique, anteroposterior, and 90-degree tangential lateral views of the vertebral body should also be obtained to ensure proper positioning of the needle. This biopsy technique is similar to that used during percutaneous kyphoplasty or vertebroplasty.[11,12]

For a CT-guided spine biopsy, the patient is usually placed in the prone position (Fig. 24-2). The radiologist identifies the area of interest through evaluation of preprocedure imaging studies. Preliminary axial CT images of the biopsy area are then obtained. The radiologist selects the appropriate slice number and coordinates. A radiopaque grid or a BB pellet is then taped to the skin site corresponding to the line marked by the CT scanner's laser localizer. A subsequent CT scan confirms the appropriate skin entry site and trajectory. The skin site is prepared and draped in sterile fashion. A local anesthetic, such as 2% lidocaine, is used to anesthetize the biopsy tract up to the periosteum with a 22-gauge spine needle. The biopsy needle is advanced step by step, with frequent acquisition of axial CT scans or CT fluoroscopy of the biopsy area for needle adjustment and proper placement.[13,14]

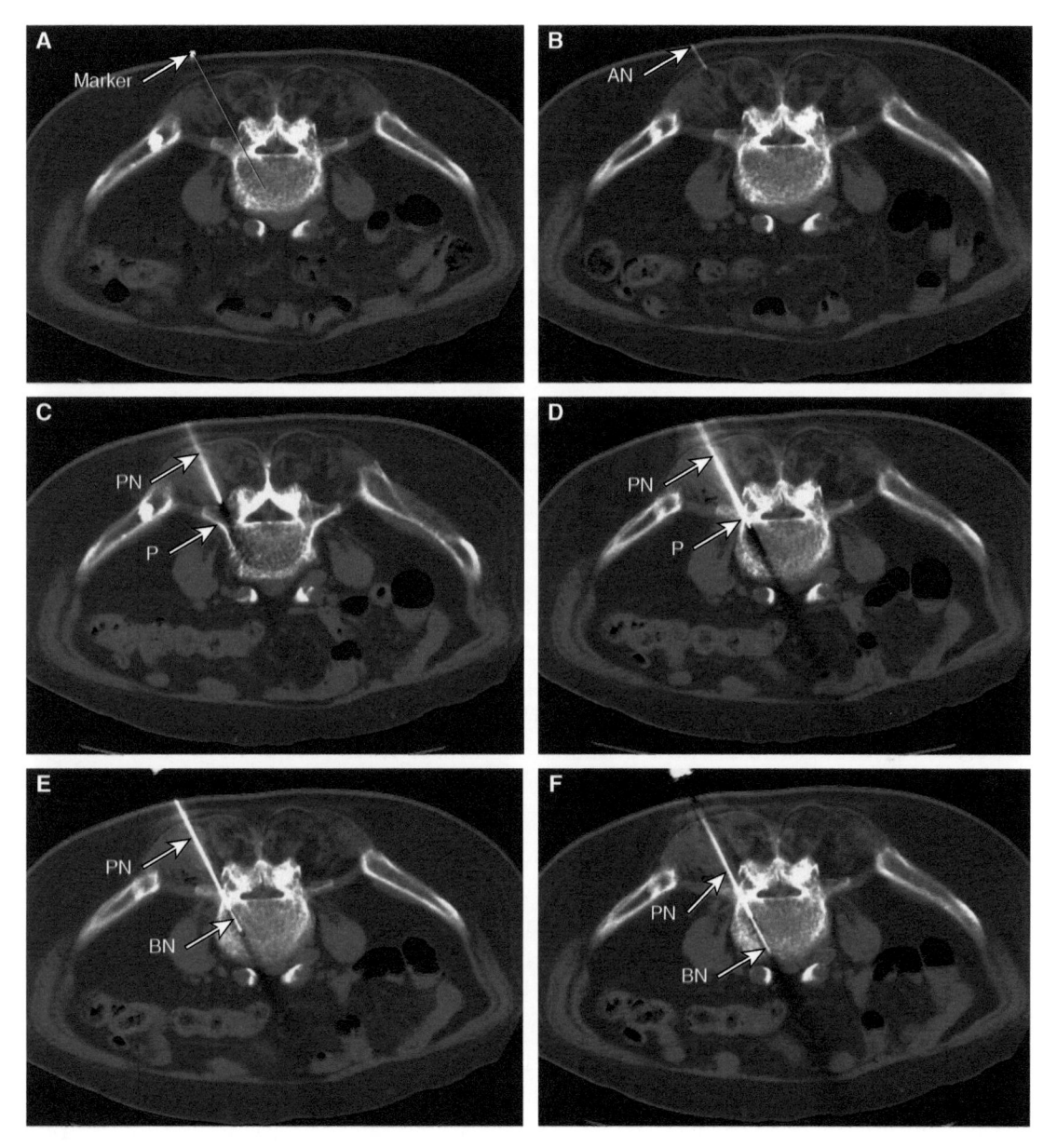

Fig. 24-2 CT-guided biopsy technique. **A,** Axial CT scan with a radiopaque marker on the skin surface to confirm the skin entry site and the trajectory of the biopsy needle. The line in this image indicates the trajectory of the needle. **B,** The *arrow* points to the local anesthetic needle *(AN)* used for injection of 2% buffered lidocaine solution. **C,** The penetration needle *(PN)* of the coaxial biopsy set is at the outer cortex of the pedicle *(P)*. **D,** The penetration needle is advanced through the pedicle. **E,** The biopsy needle *(BN)* is placed coaxially into the penetration needle *(PN)*, and the first core biopsy specimen is obtained. **F,** Then the second core biopsy specimen is obtained.

Various types of image-guided techniques have been used, such as fluoroscopy and CT, MRI, and ultrasound imaging studies. CT is superior to fluoroscopy with cross-sectional capability and soft tissue detail, which makes it more commonly used in clinical practice. CT guidance allows detailed trajectory planning to avoid passage through critical structures, such as the lungs and pleura, thus decreasing the risk of complications. CT also permits direct visualization of both bone and soft tissue, with precise location of the needle tip, especially in small lesions of the spine. However, most CT scans do not have real-time fluoroscopy, which makes the procedure time longer, because the radiologist needs to step out of the CT room and wait each time any positioning image has to be obtained. CT fluoroscopy, when available, shortens the procedure time. There is also concern about more ionizing radiation with CT-guided biopsy procedures.

On the other hand, biopsies performed under real-time fluoroscopy are less time-consuming, less expensive, and allow real-time visualization of needle placement. However, inability to visualize soft tissue details, such as epidural spread of tumor or soft tissue infection, limits the popularity of these biopsies among radiologists.[8]

MRI guidance allows stereotactic targeting and localization techniques for near real-time interventional procedures. Other advantages include greater soft tissue contrast, multiplanar imaging capability, and no ionizing radiation to the patient and physician. However, MRI-guided biopsy with MRI-compatible nonmagnetic titanium needles is both expensive and time consuming and therefore is not widely available at present.

There are reports of ultrasound-guided biopsies of the spine.[15] Ultrasound-guided biopsy is advantageous because it includes real-time monitoring, is quick and inexpensive, and avoids the use of ionizing radiation. However, such biopsies require a radiologist with advanced expertise in the ultrasonic anatomy of the spine and surrounding structures. Although ultrasound-guided biopsies are rarely performed, they may be useful in selected cases, once indications have been further clarified.

Two main types of percutaneous biopsies are performed in the spinal column: the fine-needle aspiration biopsy (FNAB) and the core needle biopsy.[10,12] FNAB is the process of obtaining a sample of cells and bits of tissue for examination by applying suction through a fine needle attached to a syringe. FNAB is frequently used for disc aspiration. Core needle biopsy involves extracting cylindrical samples of tissue with the use of a large, hollow needle. There are a number of biopsy needles available commercially. Chiba (Cook Medical, Bloomington, IN), Franseen (Meditech, Westwood, MA), and Turner (Cook Medical) needles have frequently been used for aspiration. The core needles commonly used include the Ackermann (Tieman, Long Island, NY), Bonopty (RADI Medical Systems, Uppsala, Sweden), Geremia Needle Biopsy System (Cook Medical), Jamshidi (Kormed Co., Minneapolis, MN), and Ostycut (Bard Biopsy Systems, Tempe, AZ). The choice of a biopsy needle depends largely on the experience and personal preference of the radiologist performing the procedure.

CERVICAL SPINE BIOPSY

Percutaneous cervical biopsy is challenging because of potential complications from inadvertent injury of the spinal cord or vascular structures. As a result, fewer cervical spine biopsies have been performed percutaneously. However, in experienced hands, this procedure can be performed safely with either fluoroscopic or CT guidance. Adequate surgical and neurosurgical support must be available, because compromise of the airway or hemorrhage into the spinal canal may require urgent surgical intervention.[16-18]

Prebiopsy Evaluation

Images from preprocedure studies, such as cervical spine radiographs, CT scans, MRI of the spine, radionuclide bone scans, or PET-CT scans, should be carefully studied. The goal of evaluation is to determine whether the cervical spine lesion is accessible by percutaneous biopsy and, if so, what is the best approach. More easily accessible lesions might be present, as shown in the imaging studies. Radiologists are required to correlate all imaging studies with the clinical indications for biopsy and to decide where and how to approach the lesion with available percutaneous biopsy techniques.

The three commonly used approaches for image-guided cervical biopsy are anterolateral, posterolateral, and anterior transoral (Fig. 24-3).

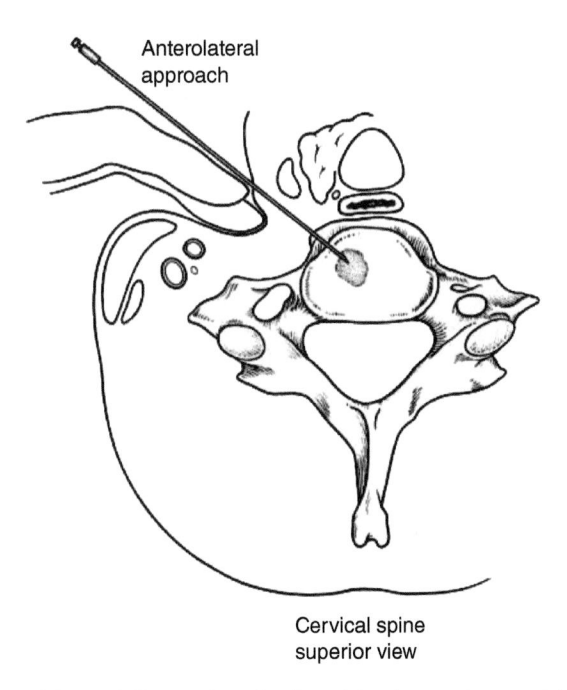

Fig. 24-3 Cervical spine biopsy. The patient is placed in the supine position with the neck in extension with a pillow or bolster underneath the neck. Under C-arm fluoroscopic guidance or CT control, the needle is inserted between the carotid sheath and the esophagus and trachea into the vertebral body. (From Tehranzadeh J, Tao C, Browning CA. Percutaneous needle biopsy of the spine. Acta Radiol 48:860-868, 2007.)

The anterolateral approach is appropriate for lesions located within the vertebral bodies from C2 to C7.[17,18] The patient is placed in the supine position, and the needle is advanced between the pharynx and the carotid artery. It is helpful to manually retract the great vessels laterally, as shown in Figs. 24-3 and 24-4.

For the posterolateral approach, the patient is usually placed in the prone position. The thecal sac and vertebral artery are carefully avoided, especially at the C1-2 level. Because the vertebral artery courses along the upper (cranial) surface of the C1 lamina, it is possible to safely perform a biopsy of the lateral masses of C1 by angling the needle caudal to the lamina (Fig. 24-5).

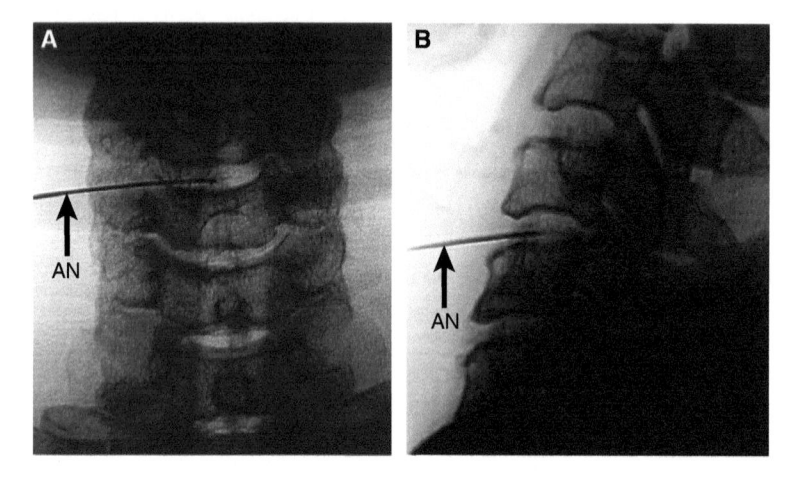

Fig. 24-4 **A** and **B,** Fluoroscopic-guided cervical disc aspiration at the C4-5 level. The aspiration needle *(AN)* is inserted into the disc space at the C4-5 level.

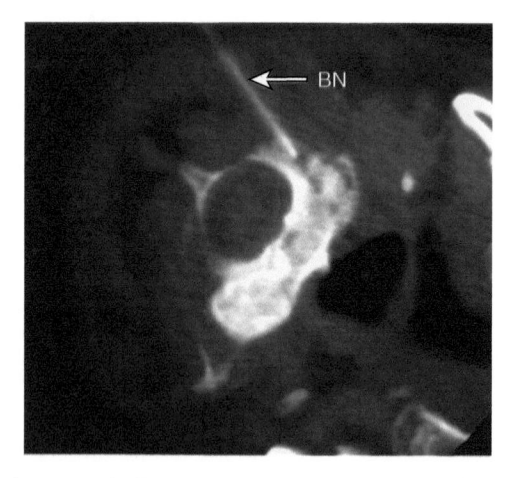

Fig. 24-5 Posterior lateral approach for CT-guided cervical spine biopsy. A biopsy needle *(BN)* is inserted into the sclerotic bone lesion in the cervical spine under CT guidance.

An anterior transoral approach is recommended when the lesion is located at the first three cervical levels to avoid important surrounding anatomic structures.[19] The transoral approach is a more complicated procedure with a higher risk of infection. Fig. 24-6 shows a destructive bone lesion at the dens and C2, where a biopsy was performed transorally.

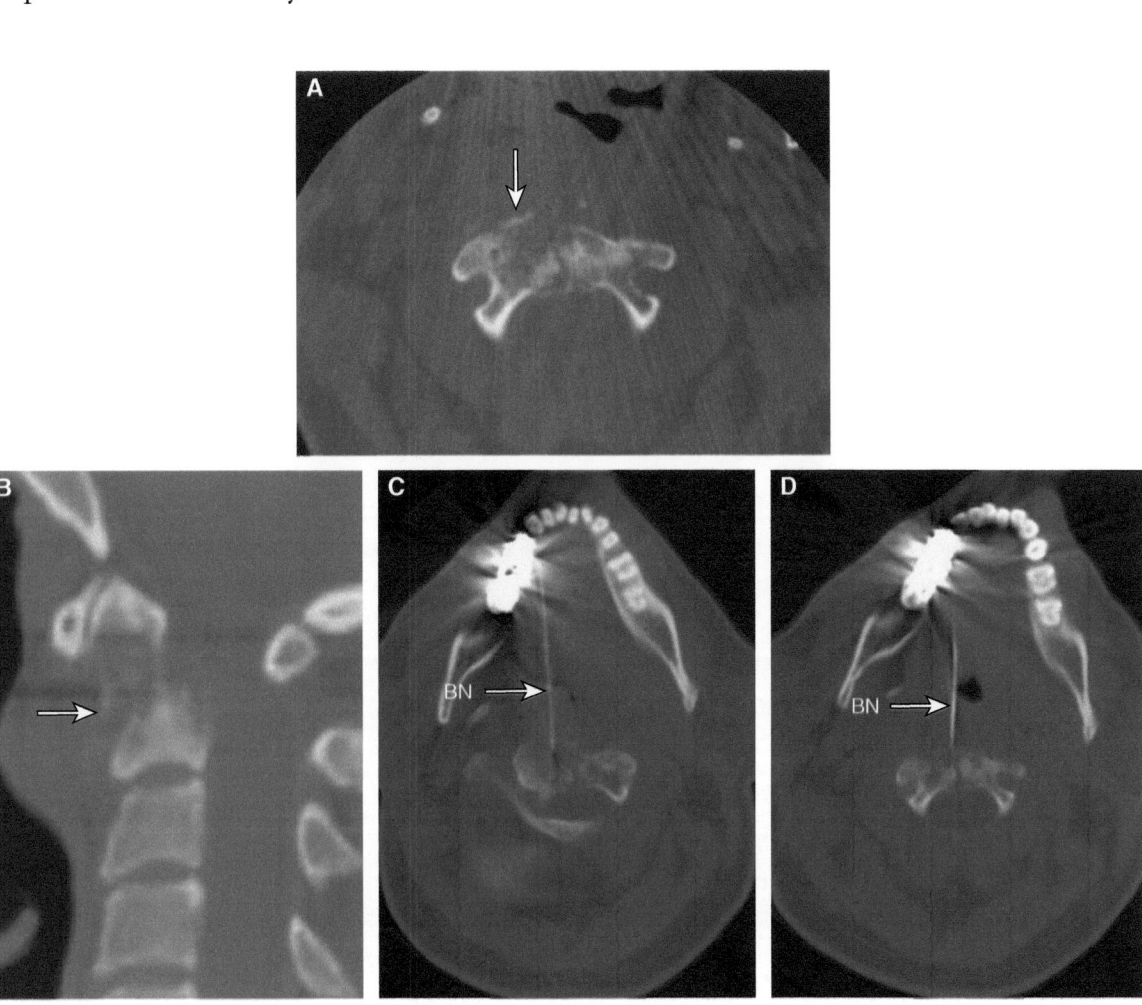

Fig. 24-6 CT-guided transoral biopsy of the upper cervical spine. Both **A,** axial and **B,** sagittal reformations of the upper cervical CT scan show a destructive bone lesion at the dens and C2 *(arrow),* where the lesion is to be biopsied, with anterior displacement of the dens over C2. **C** and **D,** Biopsy needle is advanced into the vertebral lesion transorally. The pathologic diagnosis was a chordoma. (*BN,* Biopsy needle.)

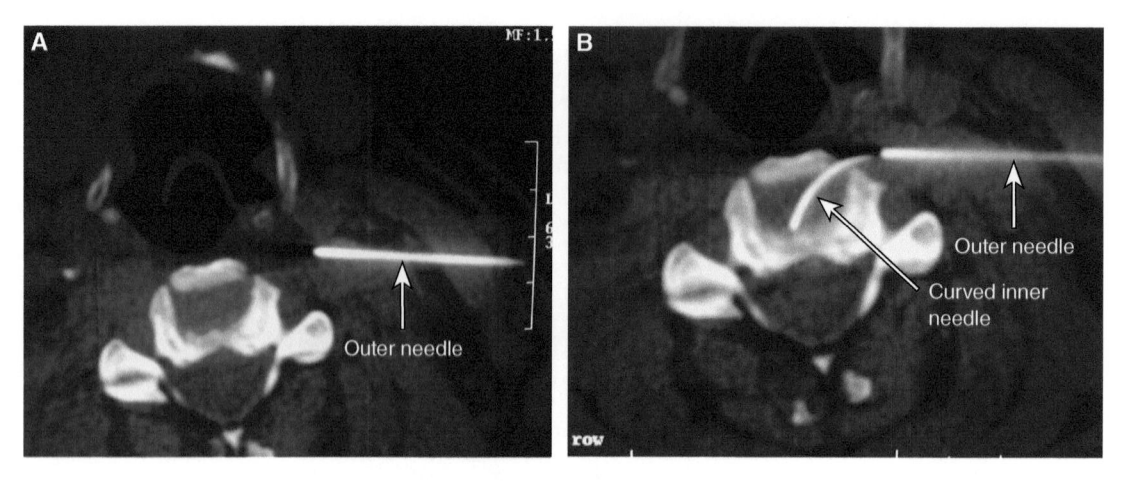

Fig. 24-7 New technique for performing CT-guided cervical spine disc aspiration/discography. This technique uses an anterolateral approach and coaxial needles with a curved inner needle. **A,** The introducer needle (outer needle) tip (21-gauge) is placed at the anterolateral aspect of the disc space; **B,** the 25-gauge curved inner needle is then placed coaxially into the disc space.

We have developed a novel technique for CT-guided cervical spine disc aspiration/discography (Fig. 24-7). This technique uses an anterolateral approach and coaxial needles with a curved inner needle. The introducer needle tip (21-gauge) is placed at the anterolateral aspect of the disc space, followed by placement of the 25-gauge curved needle into the disc space. This new technique, which uses a coaxial curved needle under CT guidance, may be a good alternative to the conventional technique for performing cervical disc aspiration or discography.

THORACIC SPINE BIOPSY

Various approaches have been used for image-guided biopsy of the thoracic spine, such as the transpedicular, posterior lateral, intercostal, and transforaminal discal approaches, as shown in Fig. 24-8.

Transpedicular Approach

Fig. 24-9 demonstrates the transpedicular approach for biopsy of the thoracic spine to confirm osteomyelitis at T9.[20-23] Advantages of percutaneous CT-guided transpedicular biopsy include the following:
1. A short needle tract.
2. The transverse process and the mammillary process join at an acute angle, which helps guide the needle tip perpendicularly toward the pedicle and through the thin cortex at the point of entry.

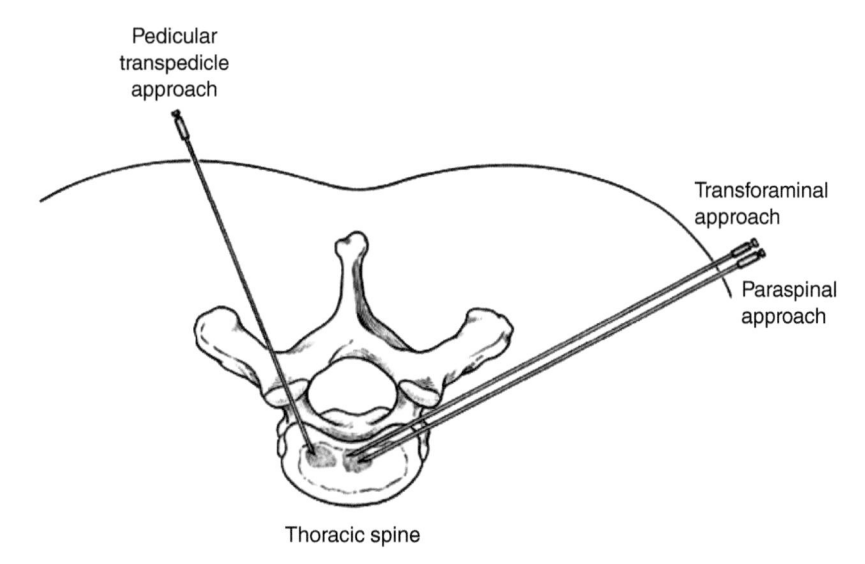

Fig. 24-8 Thoracic spine biopsy. The patient is placed in the prone position. The needle is inserted, aiming for the pedicle for the transpedicular approach, and lateral to the pedicle for the transforaminal or paraspinal approach. (From Tehranzadeh J, Tao C, Browning CA. Percutaneous needle biopsy of the spine. Acta Radiol 48:860-868, 2007.)

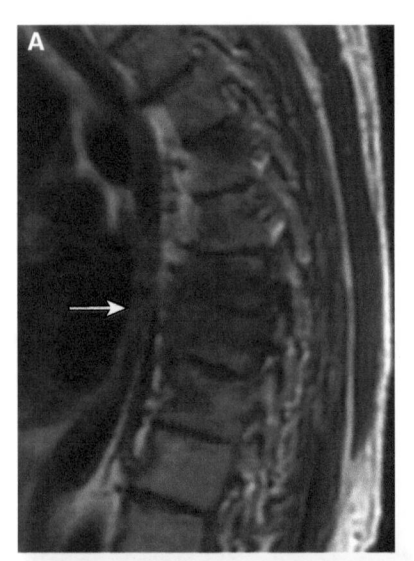

Fig. 24-9 CT-guided transpedicular biopsy of the thoracic spine at T9. T1-weighted fat-suppressed **A,** axial and **B,** sagittal MRI scans of the thoracic spine after contrast-enhanced imaging showing spondylodiscitis, which was confirmed, **C,** with a CT-guided biopsy. (*BN,* Biopsy needle.)

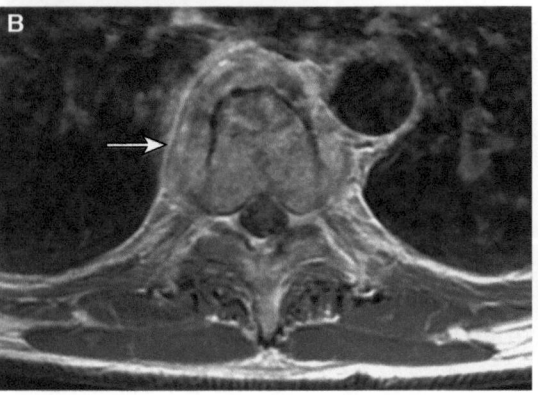

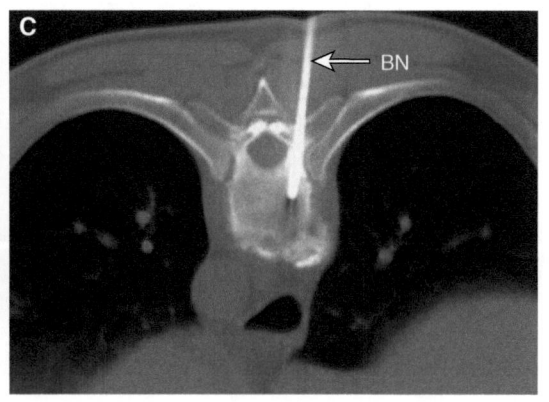

Transcostovertebral Approach

With the patient in the prone or lateral position, after local anesthesia is achieved, the penetration needle of the biopsy set is advanced under CT guidance between the anterior part of the transverse process of the vertebra and the posterior part of the neck of the rib. The lateral side of the vertebral body is approached through the costovertebral joint (transcostovertebral joint approach).[24]

Fig. 24-10 demonstrates a CT-guided biopsy of the thoracic spine through a transcostovertebral approach for spondylodiscitis and psoas abscess. A biopsy of T11 was performed through this approach. A biopsy and aspiration of the right psoas abscess were also performed. This patient was immunocompromised, and *Clostridium perfringens* was the pathogen isolated. This study shows the importance of obtaining specimens from both bone and soft tissue when infection is suspected.

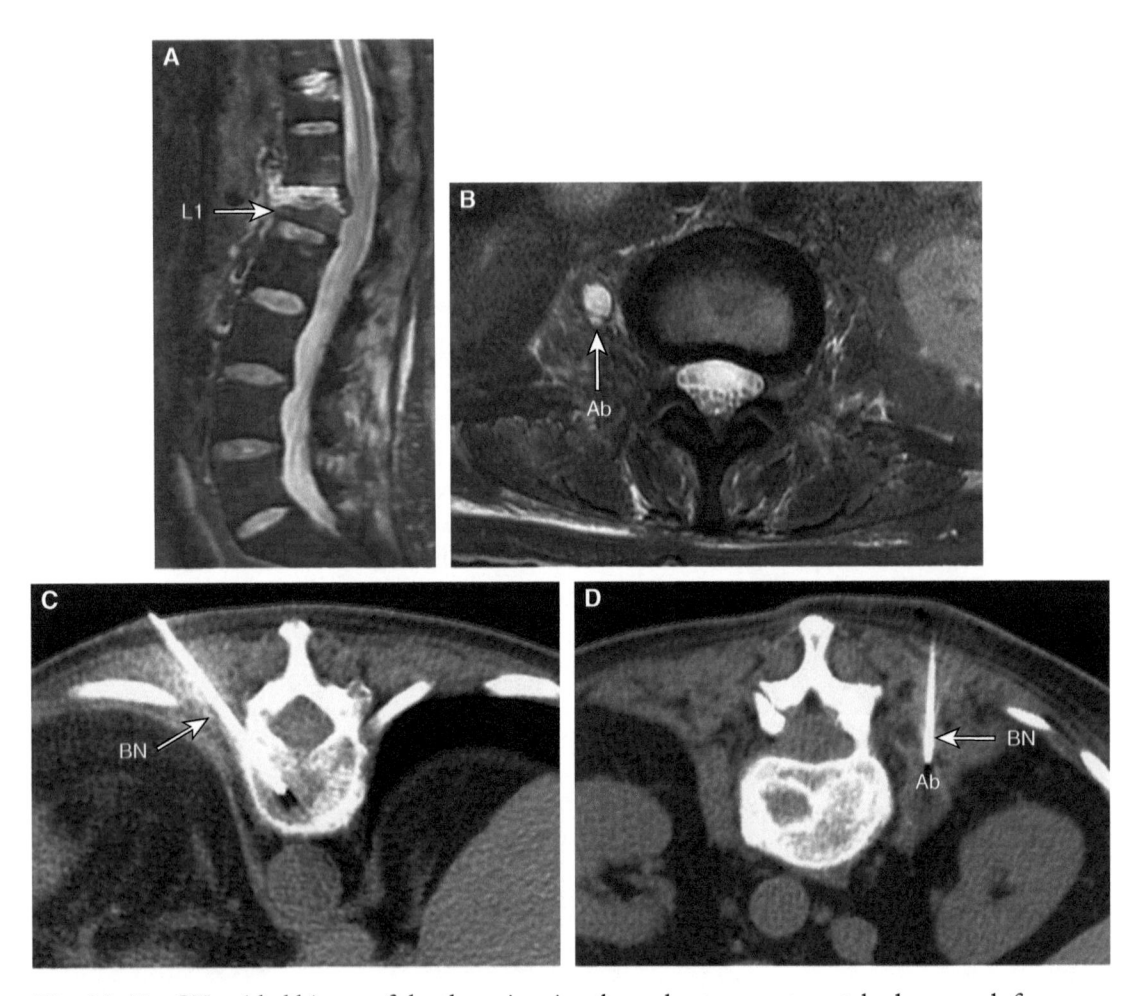

Fig. 24-10 CT-guided biopsy of the thoracic spine through a transcostovertebral approach for spondylodiscitis and psoas abscess. **A,** Sagittal and **B,** axial T3-weighted images of the thoracolumbar spine demonstrate compression fractures of T11 and L1, with abnormal disc signals noted at T10-T11 and T12-L1 levels. Right psoas abscess is also noted. (*Ab,* Abscess.) **C,** T11 was biopsied using a transcostovertebral approach. **D,** Biopsy of the right psoas abscess was also performed. The pathogen isolated was *Clostridium perfringens*.

The transcostovertebral approach does not need any angulation of the needle; it is performed quickly and easily, and avoids any risk of pleural puncture. It is well tolerated because of the distance from intercostal nerves. Because of the anatomic relationship between the costovertebral joint and the intervertebral disc, both disc and bone biopsies are easy to perform. Fig. 24-11 demonstrates CT-guided biopsy of the thoracic spine through a transcostovertebral approach for metastatic disease. A biopsy of T7 was performed with this approach. The pathologic diagnosis was metastatic breast cancer.

The intercostal approach uses posteromedial insertion anterior to the head of the rib and costovertebral joint of the intercostal space. It is helpful for paravertebral soft tissue masses or vertebral body masses. However, it has the added risk of lung puncture and intercostal vascular injury.

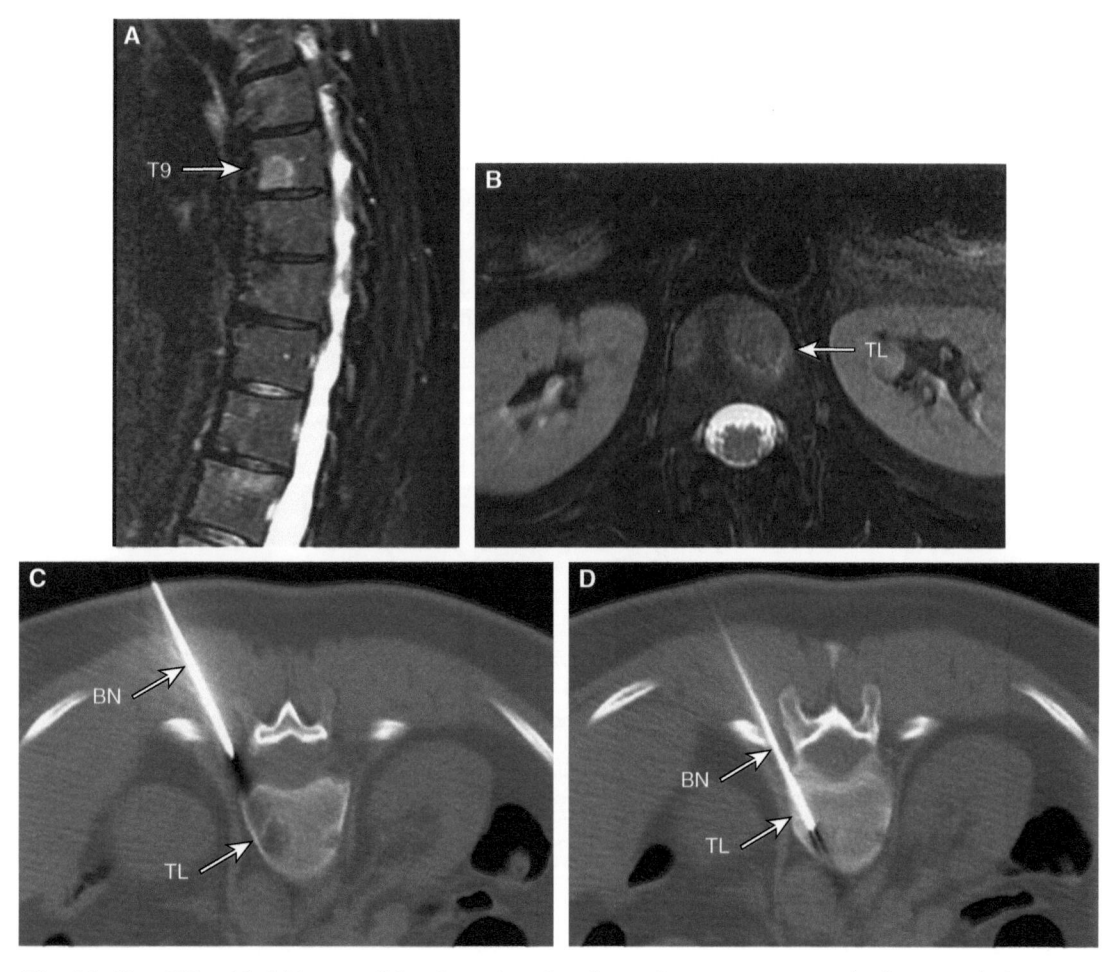

Fig. 24-11 CT-guided biopsy of the thoracic spine through a transcostovertebral approach for metastatic disease. **A,** MRI sagittal short-T1 inversion-recovery (STIR) sequence and **B,** an axial T2 fat-suppressed image demonstrate bone metastasis in the thoracic spine. (*TL,* Target lesion for biopsy.) **C** and **D,** Biopsy of T7 was performed through a transcostovertebral approach. The pathologic diagnosis was metastatic breast cancer.

A transforaminal discal approach is safe and effective for accessing vertebral body lesions in the thoracolumbar spine. The entire vertebral body, except for the extreme superomedial aspect, can be sampled, thereby decreasing the risk of pleural puncture resulting from its entry position with central vertebral body access. However, this is a complex pathway that requires more images and prebiopsy calculations, which lengthens the total procedure time.[25]

LUMBAR SPINE BIOPSY

The most commonly used image-guided approaches for lumbar spine biopsy are transpedicular and posterolateral extrapedicular (Fig. 24-12). A transpedicular approach is used if a lesion is within the pedicle or central vertebral bodies and provides safe passageway to the vertebral body. Described as the *bull's-eye* or *en face* approach, it has been commonly used for treatment of compression fractures with vertebroplasty. Both transpedicular and posterolateral extrapedicular methods for lumbar spine biopsy are similar to thoracic spine biopsy, as described earlier. Fig. 24-12 illustrates the various approaches for image-guided lumbar spine biopsy.

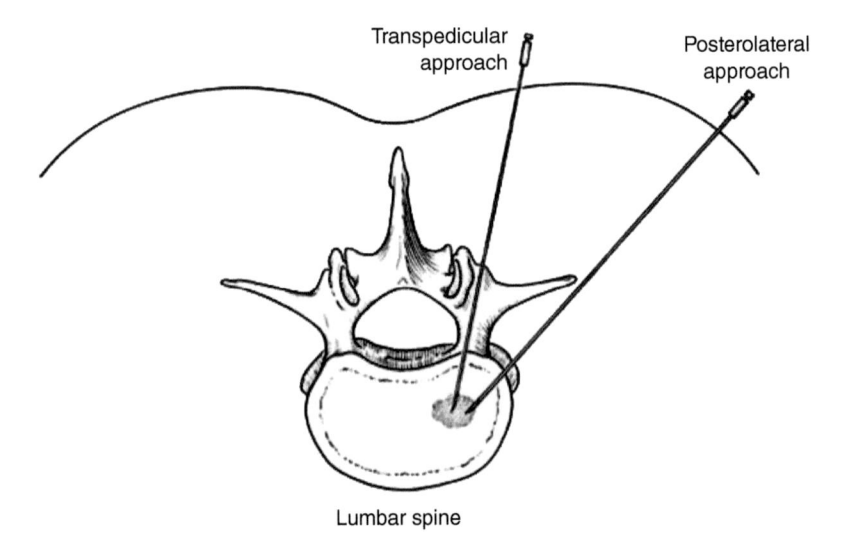

Fig. 24-12 Lumbar spine biopsy. The patient is placed in the prone position. The needle is inserted, aiming for the pedicle with the transpedicular approach and lateral to the pedicle for the paraspinal approach. (From Tehranzadeh J, Tao C, Browning CA. Percutaneous needle biopsy of the spine. Acta Radiol 48:860-868, 2007.)

There are a few important points to keep in mind during spine biopsy procedures. The size of the biopsy needle matters. Patients who have an unsuccessful biopsy or fine needle aspiration with a small needle may be rebiopsied with a larger trocar needle to establish the diagnosis. When biopsies of sclerotic lesions are performed, negative biopsy results should be viewed with caution because of the high rate of false-negative findings for sclerotic lesions. It has been shown in the literature that lytic, mixed lytic, and sclerotic lesions have a higher accuracy rate, compared with sclerotic lesions.[26] Therefore false-negative biopsy results in sclerotic bone lesions may require a repeat percutaneous biopsy or open biopsy to confirm the diagnosis. With malignant tumors there is always concern about disseminating malignant cells through the trocar. Transpedicular access might be advantageous and is noncontaminating. With this method the soft tissue components, such as the retroperitoneum, pleura, peritoneal cavities, and spinal canal, are not traversed. In addition, the biopsy tract can be resected if surgery is contemplated in the future. This also fits the principles of open biopsy of tumors, which dictate that the biopsy be performed through as few compartments as possible and along a resectable tract for the future definitive surgery.[27,28]

Whenever possible, it is important to obtain a percutaneous biopsy to isolate an organism in spine infections before initiating antibiotic treatment. It is often difficult to isolate causative pathogens in blood cultures and biopsy specimen because patients frequently have been started on empiric antimicrobial therapy for *Staphylococcus aureus,* which is responsible for 76% of all spine infections. Nevertheless, percutaneous biopsy specimens should still be obtained in an attempt to isolate *Staphylococcus* and the 20% of cases in which another organism is involved. A biopsy of bone and soft tissue spine lesions is recommended if it is an inflammatory or infectious process. The literature has shown that the growth rate of microorganisms falls from 40% overall to 25% if patients are already on antibiotics. Biopsy of soft tissue and bone components of the infectious spine lesion may increase the diagnostic yield. Fluoroscopic or CT-guided percutaneous needle aspiration is an accurate method for identifying active bacterial disc space infections but is less reliable for identifying fungal infections. There are reports that percutaneous endoscopic discectomy and drainage is a better alternative to CT-guided biopsy for diagnosis of early-stage infectious spondylodiscitis.[29-34]

Fig. 24-13 demonstrates CT-guided biopsy and disc aspiration of the lumbar spine through a transpedicular approach for infection. Both MRI and CT scans of the lumbar spine show spondylodiscitis of L4 and L5. Disc aspiration was performed at L4-5, and 1 ml of cloudy material was obtained. A biopsy of the L5 vertebral body was performed through a transpedicular approach. No organism was isolated, which may be attributed to the fact that the patient had been treated with antibiotics for a few weeks before the biopsy.

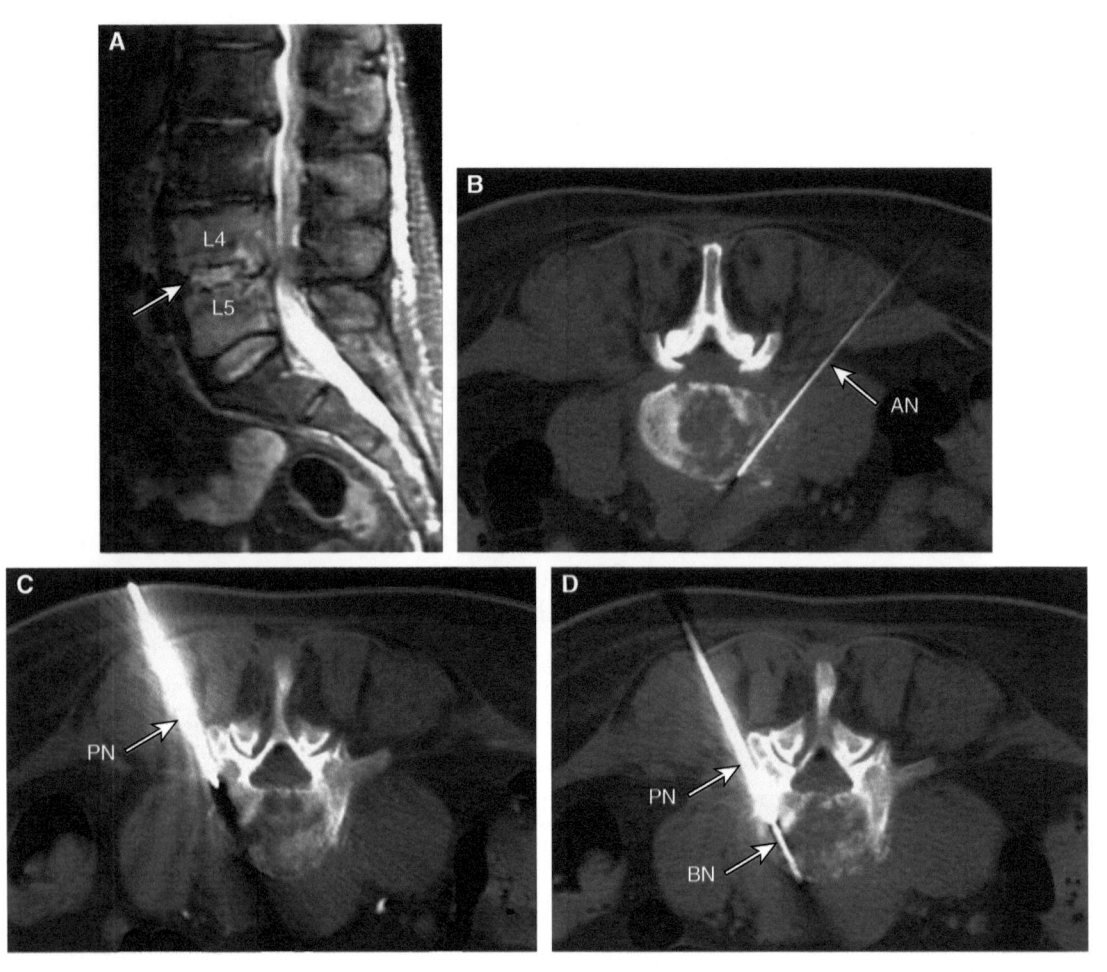

Fig. 24-13 CT-guided biopsy and disc aspiration of the lumbar spine through a transpedicular approach for infection. **A,** Sagittal T2-weighted MRI images of the lumbar spine show spondylodiscitis of L4 and L5. **B,** CT axial image at L4-5 shows disc aspiration; 1 ml of cloudy material was obtained. (*AN,* Aspiration needle.) **C** and **D,** Biopsy of the L5 vertebral body was performed through a transpedicular approach. No organism was isolated, and the patient had been on antibiotics before the biopsy. (*BN,* Biopsy needle; *PN,* penetration needle.)

Prebiopsy images should be studied in detail by the radiologist before biopsy. The same principles of biopsy, in general, also apply to percutaneous spine biopsy. It is important to include the periphery of the lesion in the biopsy if radiographic imaging shows a tumor with central necrosis. The patient's PET-CT scan should be checked, if available, to plan a relevant trajectory for biopsy of the PET-avid portion of the lesion. It is also helpful to perform a biopsy of the lesion if it is infiltrative or malignant. In systemic malignant disease (Hodgkin's and non-Hodgkin's lymphoma and myeloma), the histologic diagnosis is often based on results of immunohistochemical staining, which might require more tissue samples. The biopsy success rate is higher in malignant lesions, primary and secondary, and lower in inflammatory lesions, especially those that are chronic. The highest accuracy rates are obtained in primary and secondary malignant lesions. Most false-negative results are found in cervical lesions and in benign, pseudotumoral, inflammatory, and systemic pathologies.[35,36]

See Fig. 24-16, which demonstrates how to approach the L5-S1 level for disc aspiration. The patient is placed in the prone position. The image intensifier is significantly angulated craniocaudally toward the patient's head. This maneuver is used to optimally visualize the opening of the L5-S1 triangle, which is bordered by the inferior endplate of L5, the lateral margin of the S1 superior articular process, and the iliac crest.

Procedures for Sacral Biopsy

There are three commonly used methods for image-guided sacral biopsy. They are the dorsal approach, the direct anterior approach, and transrectal ultrasound image guidance.

Puncture using a dorsal approach is the most straightforward method, as shown in Fig. 24-14. However, bowel perforation is a major risk factor. A direct anterior approach is used for presacral space lesions and the anterior body. Low-lying pelvic lesions can be approached with transrectal ultrasound image guidance, but approaching masses that lie higher in the pelvis are logistically more difficult and may require laparotomy through the abdomen (Fig. 24-15).

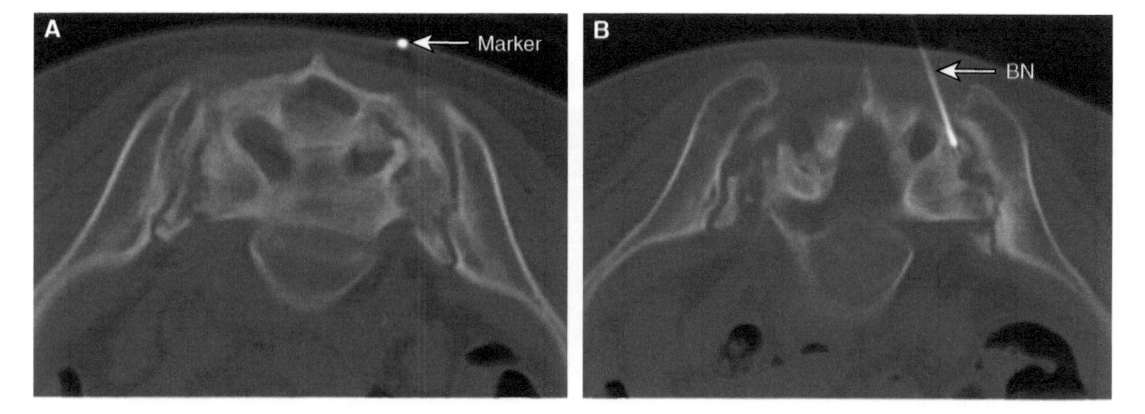

Fig. 24-14 CT-guided sacral biopsy. **A,** Axial CT images of the sacrum with a radiopaque marker on the skin surface to confirm the trajectory and needle path. **B,** Biopsy needle *(BN)* in the right sacral fracture.

428 Section III ▪ Operative Techniques

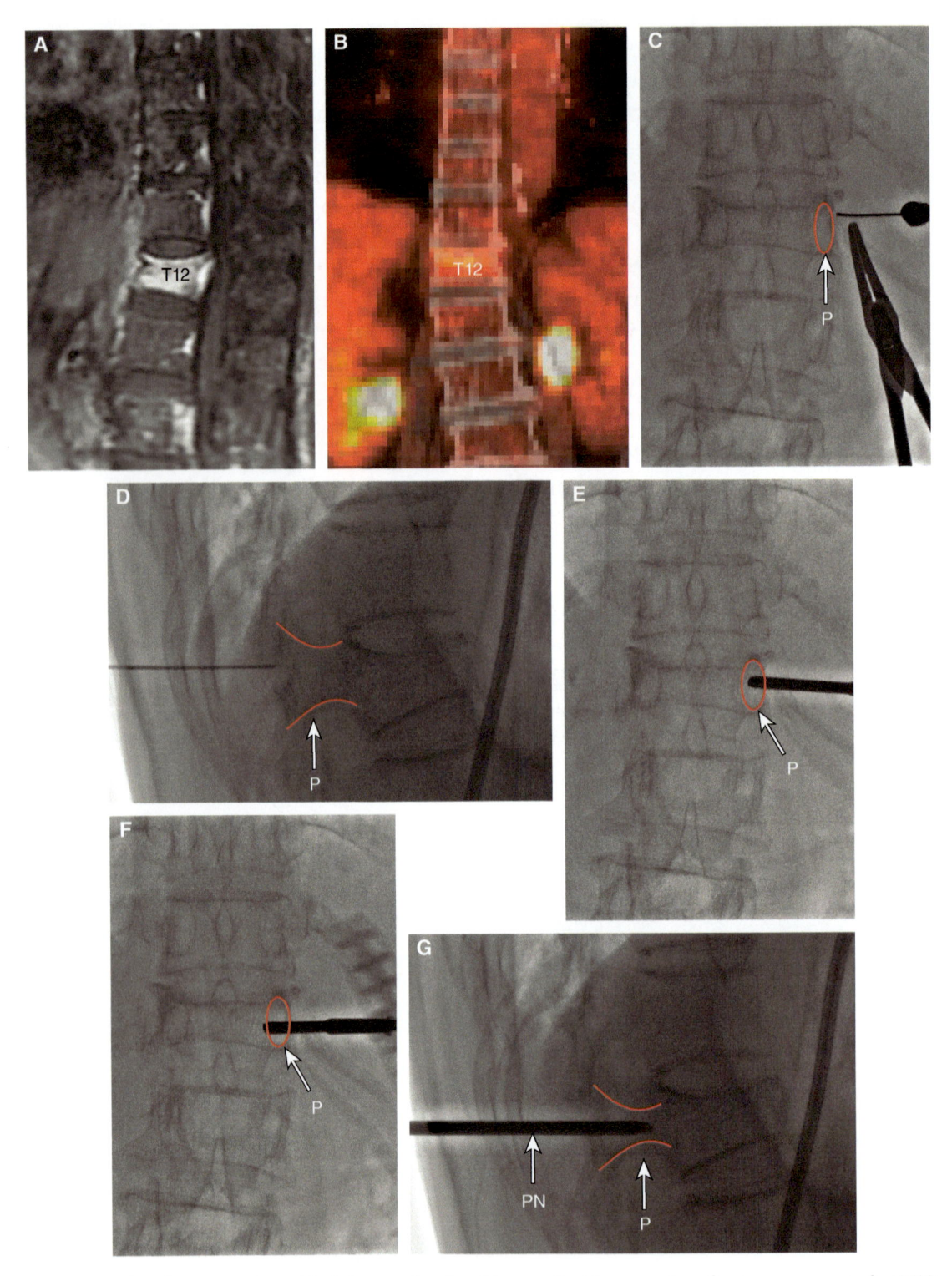

Fig. 24-15 Fluoroscopic-guided thoracolumbar biopsy. **A,** Compression fractures are noted at T12 and L2. **B,** PET-CT shows abnormal fluorodeoxyglucose activity at T12 and L2. **C-G,** Fluoroscopic-guided biopsy of T12 and L2 during vertebroplasty through a transpedicular approach. The pathologic diagnosis was lymphoma. (*P,* Pedicle; *PN,* penetration needle.)

COMPLICATIONS OF PERCUTANEOUS SPINE BIOPSY

The complication rate for percutaneous image-guided biopsy is relatively low (less than 1% to 3%). However, complications do occur, especially in the cervical and thoracic spine, because of the proximity of critical organs, such as the major blood vessels, lungs, pleura, esophagus, and mediastinum. Extrapedicular biopsies have less chance of neural complications but more risk of hematomas (by injuring the segmental vessels) or pneumothorax. Transpedicular biopsies may result in pedicular fractures. Acute complications that occur during or immediately after the procedure include anaphylactic allergic reactions to medication or contrast medium. Pneumothorax can occur with low cervical or thoracic biopsies. Neural injury of the spinal cord and nerve roots can result in foot drop, transient paresis, transient paraplegia, and paraplegia. Nerve injury can be caused by nerve root injury during biopsy or anesthesia. Bleeding near the needle puncture site may occur, which can manifest as an immediate complication. Postprocedure late complications that have been reported from percutaneous bone biopsies include infection, vascular puncture, and death. There are reports of other possible complications, such as aortic punctures, psoas punctures with associated psoas hematomas, biopsy of the incorrect level (especially when the patient has a transitional vertebral body or only 11 ribs), and spread of tumor along the biopsy tract. Tumor spread is a risk with any invasive procedure, and it is imperative to select a biopsy path that, if needed, can be entirely resected during the operative approach. Transient quadriparesis resulting from acute compression of the anterior spinal artery during cervical spine biopsy has been reported.[37]

To avoid possible complications from percutaneous spine biopsy, the clinician should first consider using a needle with a smaller inner diameter to obtain the biopsy specimen because of the higher complication rate associated with large-bore needles. However, in sclerotic lesions, where obtaining an adequate sample can be difficult, the use of a needle with a larger inner diameter might be necessary.[35,36]

Two major technical limitations of vertebral biopsy are crushing and insufficient sample size. In necrotic, sclerotic, or cystic lesions, it is difficult to retrieve an adequate specimen, despite repeated attempts. Another reason for a nondiagnostic biopsy may occur with biopsy of infectious spondylitis in patients who are already receiving broad-spectrum antibiotics. Improper handling of the specimen and failure to perform microbiologic testing also contribute to nondiagnosis.[37]

SIGNATURE CASES
FLUOROSCOPIC-GUIDED APPROACH FOR PERCUTANEOUS BIOPSY OF THE THORACOLUMBAR SPINE

A 59-year-old woman had a history of Hodgkin's lymphoma with progressive back pain. The imaging workup included MRI of the thoracolumbar spine and a PET-CT scan. These studies showed compression fractures of T12 and L2, with abnormal signal intensity, on MRI and corresponding intense fluorodeoxyglucose activity on PET-CT scans. The findings were consistent with pathologic fractures of T12 and L2 from lymphoma. The patient was referred to the interventional radiology service for percutaneous vertebroplasty. Percutaneous biopsy samples with a core specimen through 11-gauge bone biopsy needles were obtained at T12 and L2 during the vertebroplasty procedure. The pathologic diagnosis was lymphoma. Fig. 24-16 shows the results of imaging with the fluoroscopic-guided approach for percutaneous biopsy of the thoracolumbar spine.

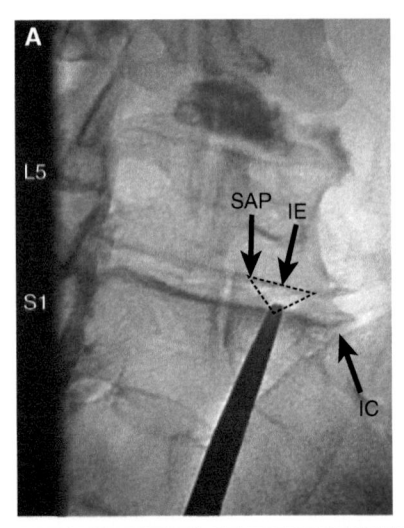

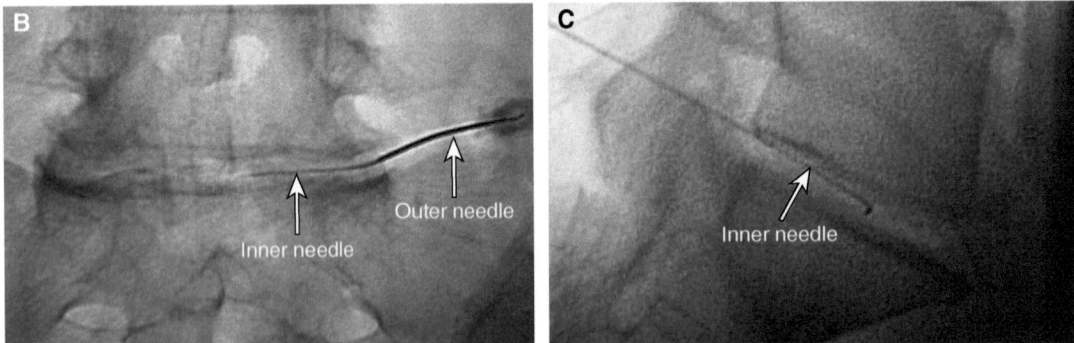

Fig. 24-16 Technique for approaching the L5-S1 level for disc aspiration. The C-arm is rotated into a posterior oblique position and angulated toward the patient's head until, **A**, the clear space bordered by the inferior endplate of L5 *(IE)*, the superior articular process of S1 *(SAP)*, and the iliac crest *(IC)* are visualized for needle positioning, as shown. **B** and **C**, Then the outer needle is placed at the periphery of the L5-S1 disc, with subsequent placement of an inner needle coaxially into the disc space.

FLUOROSCOPIC-GUIDED LUMBAR SPINE BIOPSY

A 43-year-old man was seen in the emergency department with fever and low back pain. Laboratory testing demonstrated an elevated white blood cell count and erythrocyte sedimentation rate. Plain radiographs of the lumbar spine showed severe erosion in the inferior endplate of L4 and the superior endplate of L5 (Fig. 24-17, *A*). There was also narrowing of the disc space at this level. MRI scans of the lumbar spine (Fig. 24-17, *B* and *C*) were obtained, which demonstrated the typical findings of discitis, with abnormal signal and corresponding contrast enhancement at the L4-5 disc level and adjacent vertebral bodies of L4 and L5. The findings were consistent with spondylodiscitis. The patient was then admitted to the hospital, and intravenous antibiotic drug treatment was initiated immediately. Within 24 hours of admission, fluoroscopic-guided disc aspiration was performed at the L4-5 level (Fig. 24-17, *D* through *F*). A total of 2 ml of pus was aspirated and sent for culture and sensitivity testing. The causative organism was confirmed as *S. aureus* in this intravenous drug abuser.

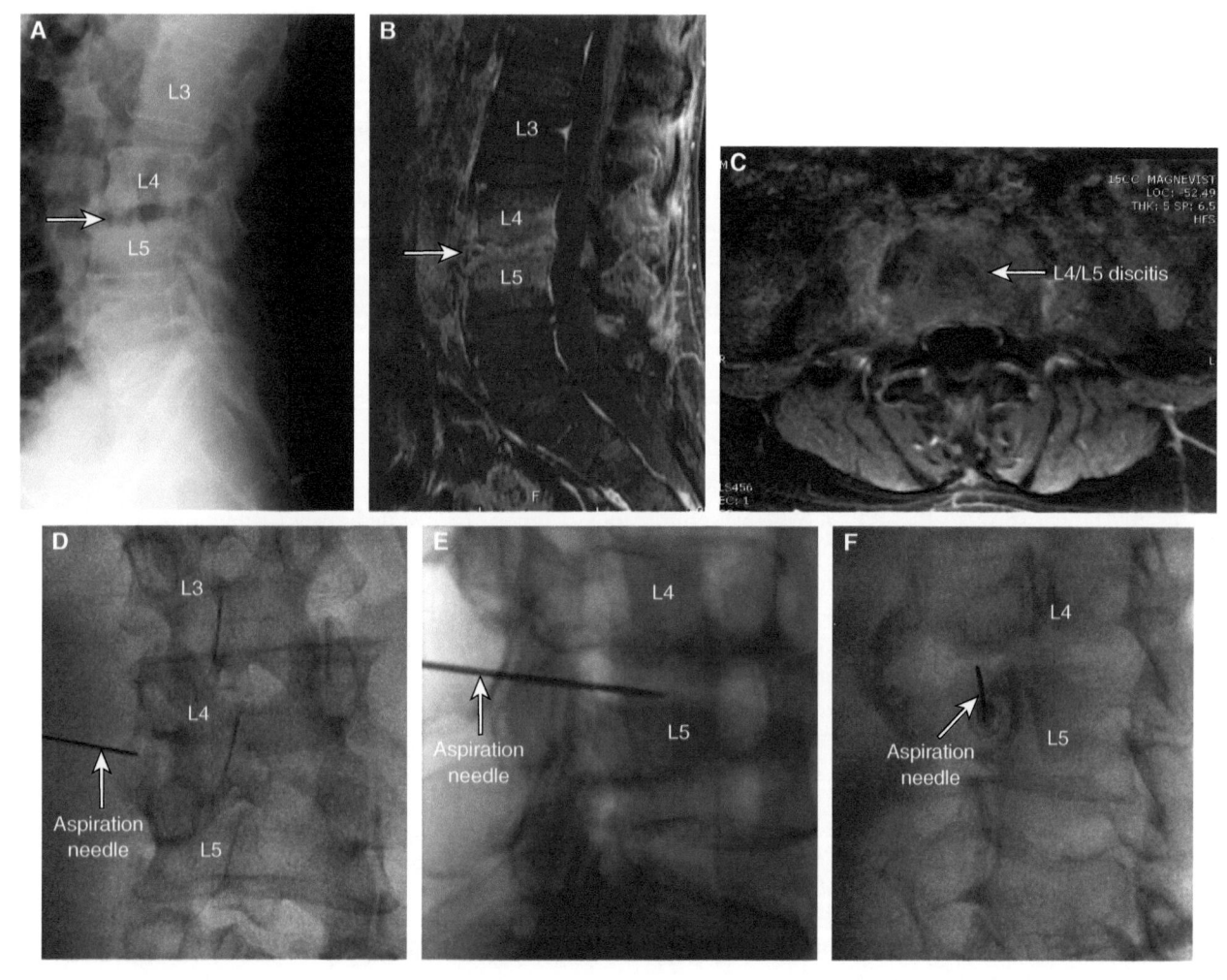

Fig. 24-17 Fluoroscopic-guided disc aspiration at the L4-5 level. **A,** Discitis was noted at L4-5 on a plain radiograph. **B** and **C,** on T1-weighted postgadolinium fat-suppressed sagittal and axial images. **D-F,** Fluoroscopic-guided disc aspiration at L4-5 was performed. The causative organism was *S. aureus*.

CONCLUSION

Percutaneous image-guided biopsy has been widely used for diagnostic purposes in various pathologic conditions of the spine, especially tumors and infections. It has the distinct advantage of being safe and efficient, with precise localization and biopsy of the intended target tissue. Core biopsy specimens are preferred over FNAB, whenever possible, for diagnosis of tumors, especially lymphomas. Careful preoperative planning, attention to details, meticulous image guidance, and direct communication with referring clinicians are prudent measures for a successful biopsy.

TIPS FROM THE MASTERS

- Carefully review all clinical information and results of imaging studies before the biopsy procedure.
- Plan the biopsy trajectory and mode of image guidance ahead of time. For example, use CT imaging rather than fluoroscopic guidance if the target lesion is too close to critical neurovascular structures. CT cross-sectional imaging, with or without intravenous or intrathecal contrast, can help to minimize the risk of injury.
- Obtain large core biopsy specimens rather than FNAB samples to increase the diagnostic yield, whenever feasible.
- Know your limitations. When in doubt, check with a neurosurgeon. There may be times when an open surgical biopsy is indicated for selected clinical scenarios.
- Biopsies of almost anything can be performed.

References (With Key References in Boldface)

1. Ball R. Needle (aspiration) biopsy. J Tenn Med Assoc 27:203-206, 1934.
2. Robertson RC, Ball RP. Destructive spine lesions: diagnosis by needle biopsy. J Bone Joint Surg 17:749-758, 1935.
3. Ackermann W. Vertebral trephine biopsy. Ann Surg 143:373-385, 1956.
4. Ackermann W. Application of the trephine for bone biopsy: results in 635 cases. JAMA 184:11-17, 1963.
5. Ottolenghi C. Diagnosis of orthopaedic lesions by aspiration biopsy: results of 1061 punctures. J Bone Joint Surg Am 37:443-464, 1955.
6. Craig FS. Vertebral-body biopsy. J Bone Joint Surg 38:93-102, 1956.
7. Adapon B, Legada BJ, Lim E, et al. CT guided closed biopsy of the spine. J Comput Assist Tomogr 5:73-78, 1981.
8. **Czervionke L, Fenton D. Percutaneous spine biopsy. In Fenton DS, Czervionke LF, eds. Image-Guided Spine Intervention. Philadelphia: Elsevier-Saunders, 2003.**
9. Kornblum MB, Wesolowski DP, Fischgrund JS, et al. Computed tomography-guided biopsy of the spine—a review of 103 patients. Spine 23:81-85, 1998.
10. **Tehranzadeh J, Tao C, Browning CA. Percutaneous needle biopsy of the spine. Acta Radiol 48:860-868, 2007.**
11. Siffert RS, Arkin AM. Trephine biopsy of bone with special reference to the lumbar vertebral bodies. J Bone Joint Surg 31:146-149, 1949.

12. Jamshidi K, Windschitl H, Swaim W. A new biopsy needle for bone marrow. Scand J Haematol 8:69-71, 1971.
13. Brugieres P, Revel MP, Dumas JL, et al. Apport de la biopsie vertebrale percutanee sous controle tomodensitometrique: a propos de 89 cas. J Neuroradiol 18:351-359, 1991.
14. Sartoris DJ, Resnick D. Computed tomography of the spine: an update and review. Crit Rev Diagn Imaging 27:271-296, 1987.
15. Gupta S, Takhtani D, Gulati M, et al. Sonographically guided fine-needle aspiration biopsy of lytic lesions of the spine: technique and indications. J Clin Ultrasound 27:123-129, 1999.
16. Brugieres P, Gaston A, Voisin MC, et al. CT-guided percutaneous biopsy of the cervical spine: a series of 12 cases. Neuroradiology 34:358-360, 1992.
17. Tampieri D, Weill A, Melanson D, et al. Percutaneous aspiration biopsy in cervical spine lytic lesions: indications and technique. Neuroradiology 33:43-47, 1991.
18. Kattapuram S, Rosenthal D. Percutaneous biopsy of the cervical spine using CT guidance. Am J Roentgenol 149:539-541, 1987.
19. Evarts CM. Diagnostic techniques: closed biopsy of bone. Clin Orthop Relat Res 107:100-111, 1975.
20. Alexander AH. Thoracolumbar needle biopsy. Orthopedics 11:1473-1477, 1988.
21. Renfrew D, Whitten C, Wiese J, et al. CT-guided percutaneous transpedicular biopsy of the spine. Radiology 180:574-576, 1991.
22. Ashizawa R, Ohtsuka K, Kamimura M, et al. Percutaneous transpedicular biopsy of thoracic and lumbar vertebrae—method and diagnostic validity. Surg Neurol 52:545-551, 1999.
23. Donaldson WF, Johnson DW. Percutaneous biopsy of the thoracic spine. Neurosurg Clin North Am 7:135-144, 1996.
24. Brugieres P, Gaston A, Heran F, et al. Percutaneous biopsies of the thoracic spine under CT guidance: transcostovertebral approach. J Comput Assist Tomogr 14:446-448, 1990.
25. Sucu HK, Bezircioglu H, Cicek C, et al. Computerized tomography-guided percutaneous transforaminodiscal biopsy sampling of vertebral body lesions. J Neurosurg 99:51-55, 2003.
26. **Sucu HK, Cicek C, Rezanko T, et al. Percutaneous computed-tomography-guided biopsy of the spine: 229 procedures. Joint Bone Spine 73:532-537, 2006.**
27. Lis E, Bilsky MH, Pisinski L, et al. Percutaneous CT-guided biopsy of osseous lesion of the spine in patients with known or suspected malignancy. Am J Neuroradiol 25:1583-1588, 2004.
28. Yaffe D, Greenberg G, Leitner J, et al. CT-guided percutaneous biopsy of thoracic and lumbar spine: a new coaxial technique. Am J Neuroradiol 24:2111-2113, 2003.
29. Caudron A, Grados F, Boubrit Y, et al. Discitis due to Clostridium perfringens. Joint Bone Spine 75:232-234, 2008.
30. **Chew FS, Kline MJ. Diagnostic yield of CT-guided percutaneous aspiration procedures in suspected spontaneous infectious diskitis. Radiology 218:211-214, 2001.**
31. Fouquet B, Goupille P, Gobert F, et al. Infectious discitis diagnostic contribution of laboratory tests and percutaneous discovertebral biopsy. Rev Rhum Engl Ed 63:24-29, 1996.
32. Yang SC, Fu TS, Chen LH, et al. Identifying pathogens of spondylodiscitis percutaneous endoscopy or CT-guided biopsy. Clin Orthop Relat Res 466:3086-3092, 2008.
33. Yang SC, Fu TS, Chen LH, et al. Percutaneous endoscopic discectomy and drainage for infectious spondylitis. Int Orthop 31:367-373, 2007.
34. Rankine JJ, Barron DA, Robinson P, et al. Therapeutic impact of percutaneous spinal biopsy in spinal infection. Postgrad Med J 80:607-609, 2004.
35. Rimondi E, Staals EL, Errani C, et al. Percutaneous CT-guided biopsy of the spine: results of 430 biopsies. Eur Spine J 17:975-981, 2008.
36. Nourbakhsh A, Grady JJ, Garges KJ. Percutaneous spine biopsy: a meta-analysis. J Bone Joint Surg Am 90:1722-1725, 2008.
37. Olscamp A, Rollins J, Tao SS, et al. Complications of CT-guided biopsy of the spine and sacrum. Orthopedics 20:1149-1152, 1997.

Chapter 25

Embolization and Test Occlusion

James K. Tatum, Van Halbach

Vascular tumors of the spinal axis can be particularly challenging during surgical resections because of their propensity to hemorrhage, which can result in extensive perioperative blood loss. Preoperative embolization may be used as an adjuvant therapy to minimize perioperative hemorrhage and facilitate resection, particularly when corpectomy or complete surgical resection is planned. Estimated perioperative blood loss has been reported to reach 15 liters in rare instances.[1] Such substantial blood loss can be life-threatening and complicate surgical resection, frequently leading to early termination of the operation without complete removal of the tumor.[1-5] In cases where surgical resection is impossible without incurring a high mortality rate or intolerable morbidity, serial palliative embolizations have been advocated by some as a realistic alternative measure.[6-8] In this chapter we will focus on basic understanding, the benefits and limitations, and the safety profile of adjuvant preoperative transarterial embolization of vascular spine tumors. We will also touch briefly on percutaneous techniques that have been reported and the future direction of embolization of spine tumors.

INDICATIONS AND CONTRAINDICATIONS

Preoperative embolization of vascular spine tumors should be considered in all patients before resection and must be weighed against relative contraindications. Patients should be screened for the following: history of allergic reactions to contrast material, renal disease, collagen vascular disease, and coagulopathies. If there is a history of allergy to contrast material, and the benefit of preoperative embolization outweighs the risk of a potential allergic reaction, the patient should be premedicated before angiography. Our standard pretreatment regimen consists of an H_1 blocker (diphenhydramine, 50 mg), an H_2 blocker (cimetidine, 300 mg), and steroids (prednisone, 50 mg) administered before the procedure. The specific protocol is shown in Table 25-1.

Table 25-1 Pretreatment Protocol for Iodine Contrast Allergy

Medication	Dose	Route	Administration (time before examination)
Benadryl (diphenhydramine)	50 mg	PO, IM, IV	1 hr
Tagamet (cimetidine)	300 mg	PO	1 hr
Prednisone	50 mg	PO	13, 7, and 1 hr
Medrol* (methylprednisone)	32 mg	PO	12 and 1 hr
Hydrocortisone*	200 mg	IV	13, 7, and 1 hr

*Alternatives to prednisone.

Table 25-2 Pretreatment Protocol for Patients With Renal Insufficiency Requiring Iodinated Contrast

Medication	Dose	Route	Administration (time before examination)
Sodium bicarbonate 154 mEq/1 L D5W	3 ml/kg over 1 hr; then 1 ml/kg over 6 hr	IV	Start 1 hr before contrast injection
Mucomyst (N-acetylcysteine)	600 mg	PO	Give day before and day of examination; twice a day
Hydration 0.9% saline solution	100 ml/hr	IV	6-12 hr to 6-12 hr after

RENAL FUNCTION

An assessment of renal function should also be performed in all high-risk patients. The term *high-risk* can be arbitrary; at our institution this group includes patients 70 years of age or older, patients with diabetes mellitus, and patients with known renal disease. Screening is based on the estimated glomerular filtration rate calculated according to the Modification of Diet in Renal Disease (MDRD) formula.[9] We use an absolute threshold of 60 ml/min to determine renal insufficiency. It has been demonstrated that patients with renal insufficiency should be regarded as being at risk for contrast-induced nephrotoxicity. In this population of patients there are controversial interventions that may be performed, but these have not shown conclusive benefits in larger studies (Table 25-2).

When a patient with renal insufficiency is encountered at our institution, we perform two separate interventions. First, we administer 600 mg of Mucomyst (N-acetylcysteine; Bristol-Myers Squibb, Princeton, NJ) twice daily for 2 days starting on the day before angiography. Second, we begin a sodium bicarbonate drip 1 hour before angiography and continue the drip for a total of 7 hours. The solution consists of 154 mEq of sodium bicarbonate prepared in 1 L of 5% dextrose in water by the pharmacy. It is infused at a rate of 3 ml/kg over a 1-hour period, and the rate is then decreased to 1 ml/kg/hr for the remaining 6 hours. It should be noted that these measures have shown variable benefits as nephroprotective agents.[10]

BEFORE ANGIOGRAPHY
NONINVASIVE IMAGING

It is helpful and recommended to perform precontrast and postcontrast magnetic resonance imaging (MRI) and computed tomography (CT) of the spine before angiography (Fig. 25-1, *A* and *B*). MRI scans will assist in evaluating the level of the tumor, its intradural or extradural location, and its relationship to the spinal cord and adjacent soft tissues. CT scans are invaluable for evaluation of the cortex, bone density, and detection of fractures. CT or MRI scans may also be used for evaluation of the size and ectasia of the aorta. This additional information is useful in planning angiography and embolization, because it assists the angiographer in locating the level of the tumor quickly during the procedure and typically correlates well with the extent of the tumor blush (Fig. 25-1, *C* through *F*) before embolization.

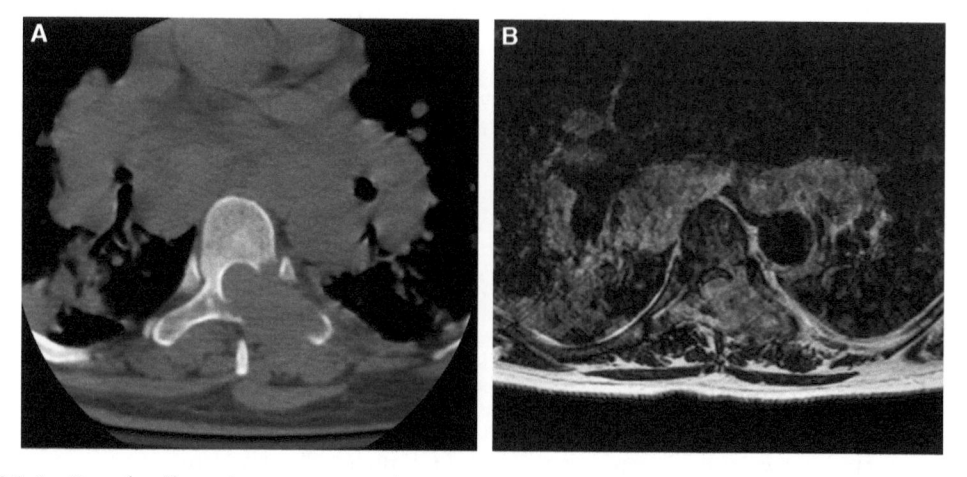

Fig. 25-1 Renal cell carcinoma metastasis to T7. **A,** Noncontrast CT scan demonstrates destructive lesion of the left transverse process of T7 invading the spinal canal and paraspinal soft tissues. Notice the mediastinal adenopathy. **B,** T2 axial MRI scan of the thoracic T7 level reveals a left transverse process mass compressing the spinal cord and extending into the surrounding paraspinal soft tissues.

Continued

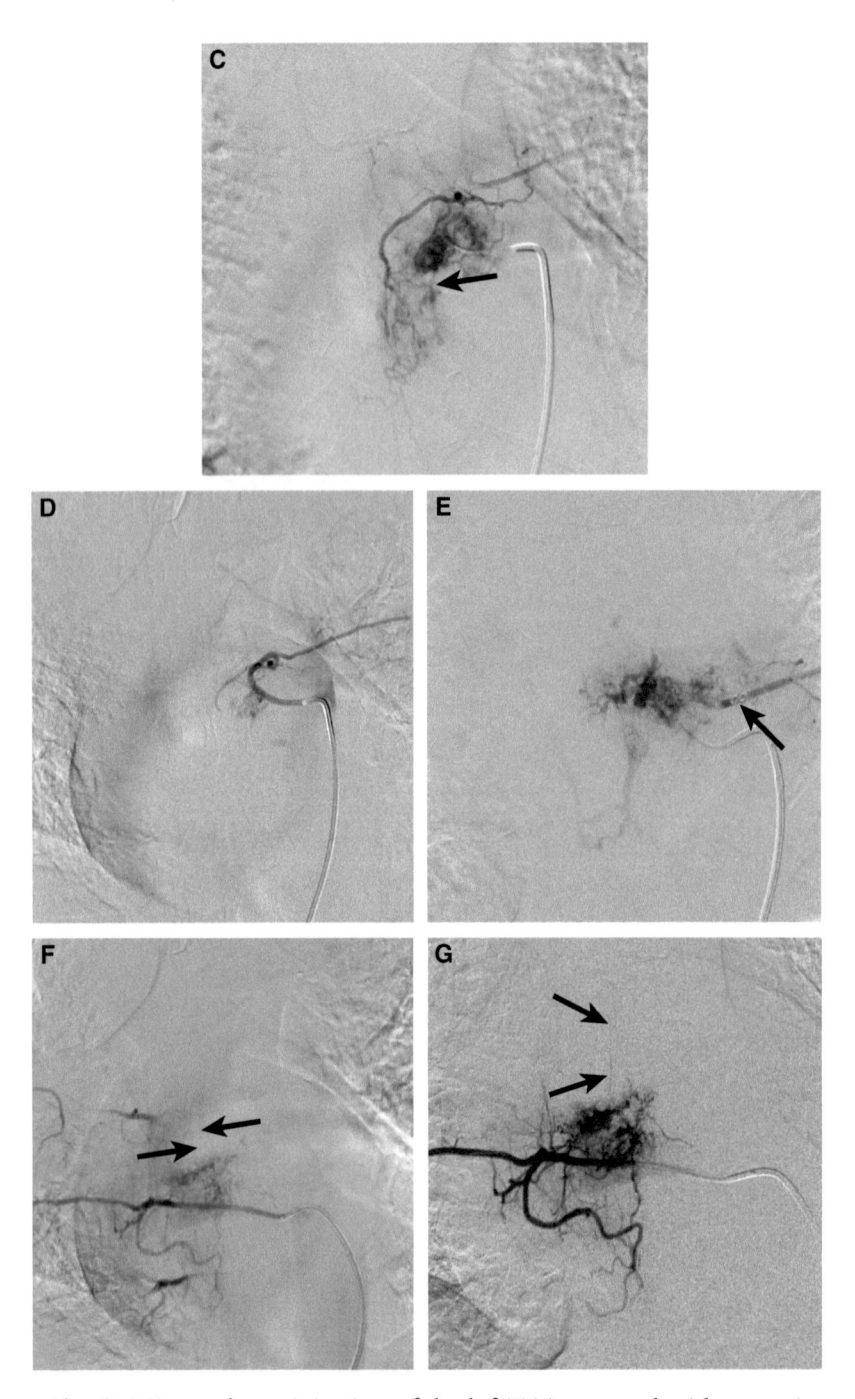

Fig. 25-1, cont'd **C,** Microcatheter injection of the left T6 intercostal with extensive tumor blush and intratumoral shunting into adjacent veins *(arrow).* **D,** Postembolization demonstration of minimal residual tumor blush. **E,** Microcatheter injection of the left T7 intercostal reveals tumor blush demonstrating supply from two adjacent levels. The coil had been placed in the left T7 intercostal *(arrow).* **F,** Injection of the right T7 intercostal reveals tumor blush. Note the subtle opacification of a vertically oriented vessel *(arrows).* **G,** Microcatheter injection of the right T7 intercostal opacifies the subtle right posterior lateral spinal artery *(arrows).* This intercostal was not embolized with PVA particles.

EQUIPMENT

Spinal angiography and embolization should be performed in an angiography suite with a dedicated biplane system. Performing such procedures in the operating room setting will likely result in frustration because of the limitations of the equipment. A dedicated biplane system is equipped with a small focal spot (<3 mm), facilitating a view of 300 to 400 micron blood vessels. Such high spatial resolution will aid in defining dangerous arterial anastomoses of the spine, preventing inadvertent embolization of the arterial supply to the spinal cord (Fig. 25-1, G).

ANESTHESIA AND ADJUNCTIVE MEASURES

We almost always use general anesthesia for angiography and embolization of the spine. General anesthesia eliminates two factors that may result in misguided embolization of the normal spinal cord supply: respiratory motion and patient movement. Apnea eliminates respiratory motion temporarily during injection of contrast material in patients who are paralyzed. Patients who are not paralyzed should be deeply anesthetized to prevent overbreathing of the ventilator.

In addition, bowel motion can be quite problematic in the evaluation and embolization of tumors in the lower thoracic and lumbar spine regions. This may be temporarily remedied by administration of 1 mg of glucagon. Glucagon should not be used in all patients. It is absolutely contraindicated in anyone who harbors a pheochromocytoma, because it may stimulate release of catecholamines and result in a hypertensive crisis.[11,12] In addition, patients with diabetes may have elevated glucose levels after the administration of glucagon, reflecting a relative contraindication in these patients.

An alternative approach that may be undertaken by an interventional neuroradiologist is to perform targeted diagnostic spinal angiography with the patient awake, permitting the use of clinical provocative testing.

PROVOCATIVE TESTING

Provocative testing, in experienced hands, can provide critical feedback regarding supply to the anterior and posterior spinal cord.[13-17] Provocative testing of the spinal cord is akin to the Wada test for speech localization before temporal lobe surgery.[17] It is performed by injecting amytal and lidocaine while the patient is awake. If there is a loss of motor function or if paresthesias develop after injection into the target vessel, embolization should be avoided for fear of spinal cord ischemic injury.

Provocative testing is carried out by injection of 1 ml of amytal (sodium amobarbital), 25 mg/ml, into the target vessel by means of a 1 ml syringe. The patient's neurologic status is monitored for signs of change over 5 to 10 minutes. If no response is elicited, 1 ml of 1% lidocaine without preservatives or epinephrine is injected into the target vessel. It should be noted that these medications must not come in contact with each other, and the catheter should always be flushed with saline solution between injections. When mixed, these medications will form a precipitate that could cause inadvertent embolization and catheter occlusion.

Provocative testing may be performed with the patient under general anesthesia. In such cases one must rely solely on neurophysiologic monitoring as feedback. Neurophysiologic monitoring is executed by monitoring somatosensory evoked potentials (SEPs) or motor evoked potentials (MEPs), or both. The choice of anesthetic can influence SEP and MEP signals, so close coordination between the anesthesiologist and the neurophysiologist is essential. Niimi et al[13] elicited SEPs by stimulating the right and left posterior tibial nerves at the ankle and the median nerves at the wrists with 40 mA, 0.2 msec duration, 4.3 Hz repetition rate, and recorded through corkscrew-type electrodes in the patient's scalp over the primary sensory cortex. MEPs were conducted by transcranial stimulation of the motor cortex by means of corkscrew-type electrodes. Short trains of 5 to 7 square-wave stimuli of 500 µsec duration and 4 msec interstimulus intervals were applied at a 1 Hz repetition rate through electrodes at C1 and C2 scalp sites with the use of the International 10-20 EEG system. Muscle responses were recorded with needle electrodes in the bilateral anterior tibialis, toe abductor, and thenar muscles. Neurophysiologic monitoring was reported to be useful in preventing embolization of the normal spinal cord supply. Of note, there is increased recovery time to baseline SEPs and MEPs after repeated injections.[15] This may limit the repetition of provocative testing.

In some studies provocative testing has been shown to be useful when employed as an adjunct to anatomic evaluation. It rarely produces false-negative results. False-negative results may occur in the setting of high-flow vascular spine lesions. This has been seen in our practice in cases where an arteriovenous malformation or perimedullary fistula acts as a sump, causing blood to flow into a feeding pedicle, thus preventing the pharmacologic agent from reaching normal neural tissue. As the shunt (sump) is shut down during embolization, perfusion to the normal tissue begins to increase, and the provocative testing becomes positive. This was reported in a study by Touho et al.[16]

More commonly, provocative testing suffers from false-positive results, as in the case discussed by Niimi et al.[13] In this case a false-positive result was suspected and led to waking the patient from general anesthesia. The patient was tested clinically, and the clinical examination was unremarkable. The targeted vessel was embolized uneventfully. This illustrates an excellent point regarding neurophysiologic monitoring. It is dependent on a sufficient electrical signal and correct interpretation of that signal. In our own clinical practice we have found monitoring to be heavily dependent on the technician's abilities to exclude erroneous data that may lead to false-positive results.

Our current general consensus is angiographic evaluation under general anesthesia, with the imaging quality that may be achieved from the latest dedicated biplane neuroangiography systems, is sufficient to eliminate inadvertent embolization of the spinal cord supply. Moreover, angiographic data tend to echo physiologic data, as demonstrated in the article by Sala et al.[14] For this reason we have abandoned the use of neurophysiologic monitoring in cases of spinal embolization.

CATHETERS

We will not go into significant detail about the catheters used in spinal angiography and embolization, because it is beyond the scope of this chapter. Generally a 5 Fr diagnostic catheter is used both for angiography and as a guide catheter for embolization (Fig. 25-2). There are a plethora of choices for diagnostic catheters. The choice is dictated by anatomy and personal preference. Therefore one may need to use a different diagnostic catheter for the thoracic aorta than would be used for the abdominal aorta in the same patient. If a diagnostic catheter from the manufacturer is not satisfactory for a patient's particular vascular anatomy, steam shaping the catheter to satisfy the anatomy may be of benefit.

Much like diagnostic catheters, there are many choices of microcatheters. In their most basic form there are two types of microcatheters. The first is an over-the-wire microcatheter. This type of catheter depends on the use of a guidewire for vessel selection. The second type is a flow-directed microcatheter. Flow-directed microcatheters rely on increased relative blood flow to carry the catheter to its target. Over-the-wire microcatheters are typically used for most spine tumor embolizations.

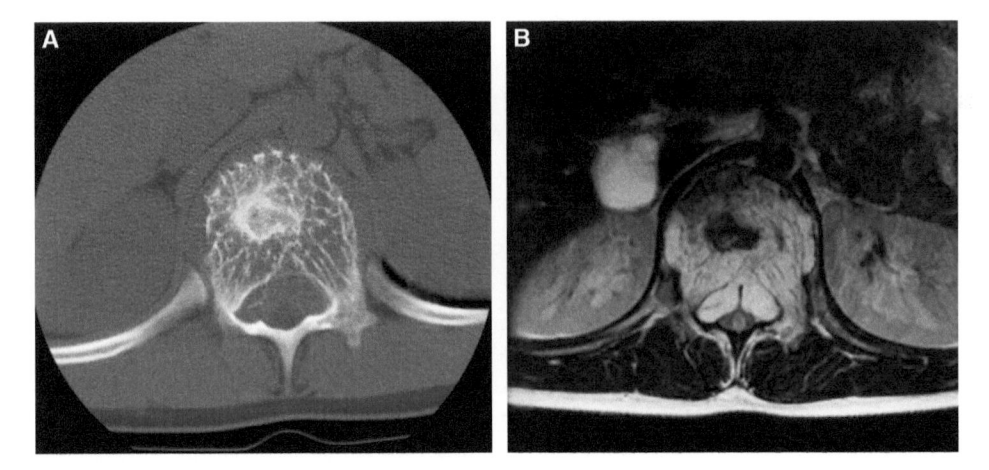

Fig. 25-2 T12 hemangioma. **A,** Noncontrast CT scan demonstrates typical findings with prominent osseous septa and rarefaction of interposed bone. The vertebra is collapsed. The posterior cortex is disrupted with displaced spicules in the spinal canal and the right lamina is remodeled. These findings suggest extension into the spinal canal, which was confirmed by MRI. **B,** T2 axial image reveals involvement of the spinal canal.

Continued

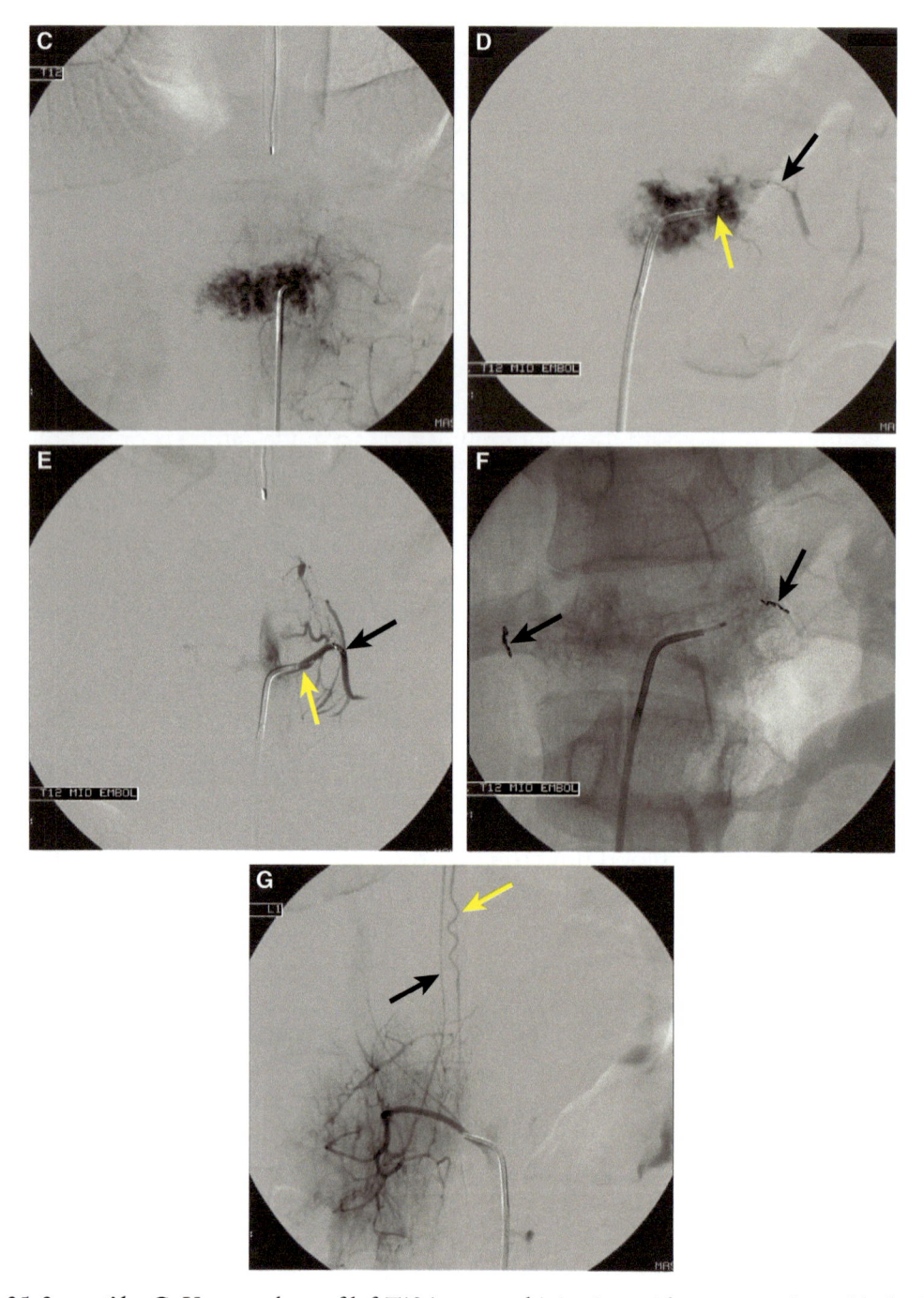

Fig. 25-2, cont'd **C,** Venous phase of left T12 intercostal injection with very prominent blush. **D,** A 5 Fr Cobra-2 diagnostic catheter used as a guide for the microcatheter. Microcatheter *(yellow arrow)* injection after deployment of fibered coil *(black arrow)* in left T12 intercostal artery to protect the tissues supplied distally by the intercostal artery. No dangerous spinal supply is present. **E,** Post-PVA embolization injection through microcatheter *(yellow arrow)* revealing absence of tumor blush. Coil is seen in intercostal *(black arrow)*. **F,** Left anterior oblique projection. The T12 vertebral body is collapsed. Pushable fibered coils in bilateral T12 intercostal arteries *(arrows)*. Microcatheter through diagnostic catheter in left T12 intercostal. **G,** Injection of the right L1 lumbar artery with opacification of the artery of Adamkiewicz *(black and yellow arrows)*. This is important to identify when it resides in close proximity to the level of the tumor so the collateral supply may be disrupted with a coil or carefully observed during embolization to ensure there is no opacification of the intervertebral connection.

ANGIOGRAPHIC PROTOCOL

A complete diagnostic angiogram of the spine is not necessary when tumor embolization is being considered. Cross-sectional imaging has usually already been performed, and targeted therapy is being considered for a particular level of the spine. A more focal angiogram is appropriate in most cases and should begin with selection of the vessels suspected of supplying the lesion first. The protocol followed varies with the level of the tumor (Table 25-3).

Table 25-3 Target Vessels Based on Tumor Levels

Cervical Spine	Thoracic/Lumbar Spine	Sacrum
1. Vertebral arteries 2. Thyrocervical trunk 3. Costocervical trunk 4. External carotid arteries (high cervical lesion) 5. Supreme intercostals (lower cervical lesion)	1. Supreme intercostals (high thoracic spine) 2. Thyrocervical trunk (high thoracic spine) 3. Intercostal/lumbar arteries at level of lesion and two levels above and below lesion	1. Lower lumbar arteries 2. Iliolumbar arteries 3. Median sacral artery 4. Internal iliac arteries

It is of utmost importance that vertebral bodies be counted before angiography is begun and that this system remains unchanged throughout the procedure. We typically employ radiopaque tape applied to the patient along the spine to aid in counting vertebral bodies during angiography. For pediatric patients the use of low fluoroscopic rates, energy and, when appropriate, shielding reduces the dose of radiation and should be used.

A quality intercostal or lumbar artery injection should result in a visible blush of the ipsilateral half of the vertebra. This is important to prevent underinjection of the vessel and unopacification of a posterior spinal or anterior spinal artery (see Fig. 25-1). Most of the time two acquisitions per second are sufficient. Filming should be carried out to include the venous phase. By convention the intercostal or lumbar artery is named according to the rib that it passes beneath or the transverse process that it passes adjacent to on the anteroposterior projection. Any vessel that is not completely seen, and is of importance, should be assessed in its entirety (Fig. 25-3).

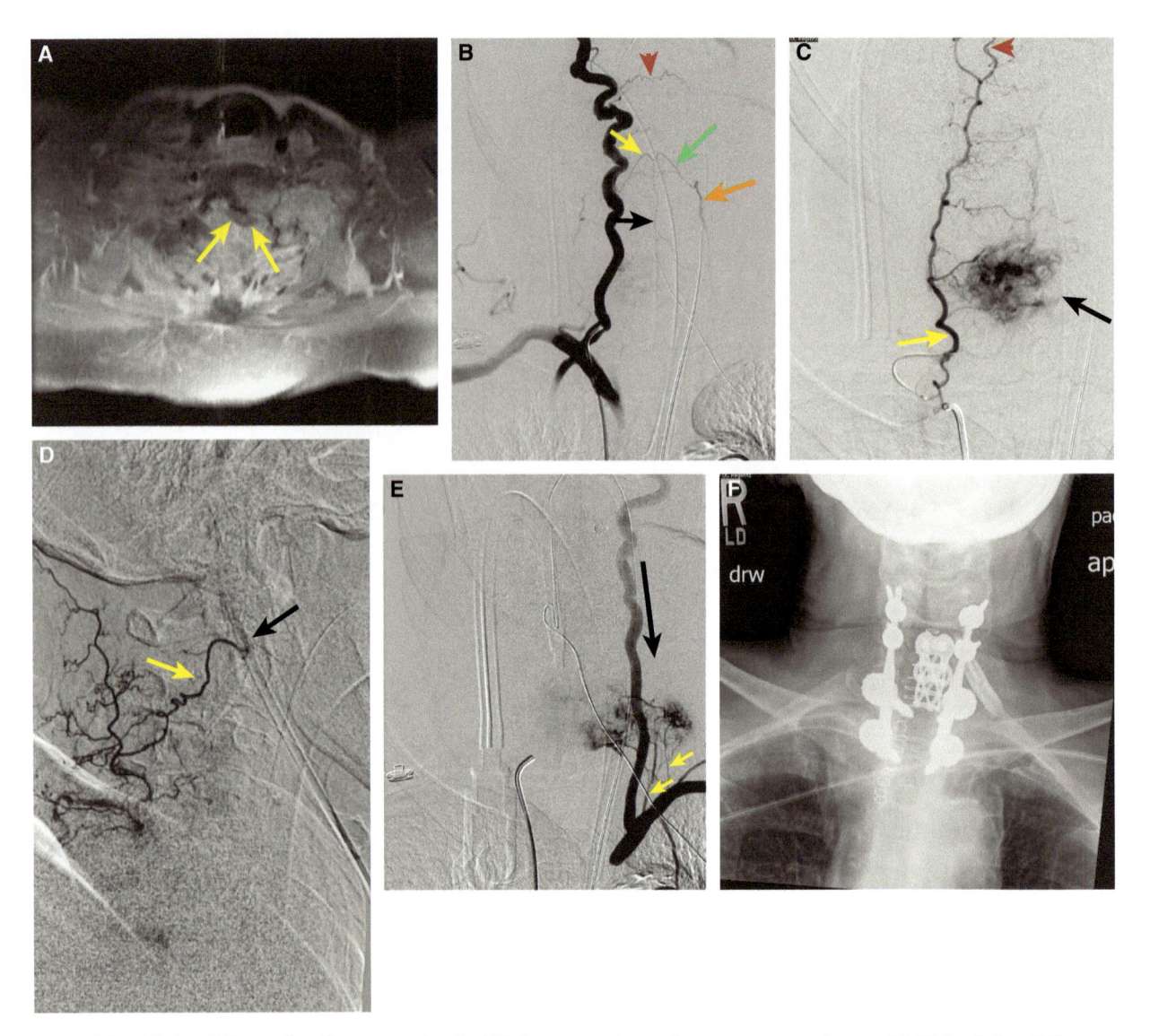

Fig. 25-3 C7 renal cell metastasis. **A,** T1 fat saturation after contrast-enhanced MRI of the C7 level demonstrating large vascular spinal metastasis. There is cord compression *(arrows)* near the mass. **B,** Right vertebral artery injection. Cervical radiculomedullary artery, right *(yellow arrow)* and left *(green arrow)*. Anterior spinal artery *(black arrow)*. Opacification of contralateral vertebral artery *(orange arrow)* across the midline through radiculomedullary arteries. Odontoid arcade *(red arrowhead)*. **C,** Right deep cervical injection *(yellow arrow)* demonstrates extensive tumor blush from the vascular metastasis *(black arrow)*. Distal vessel not included *(red arrowhead)*. **D,** Further evaluation of right deep cervical vessel more distal to image **B** *(yellow arrow)* reveals a dangerous anastomosis with the vertebral artery *(black arrow)*. This must be protected before embolization. **E,** Delayed filming reveals subclavian steal with retrograde flow *(black arrow)* down the left vertebral artery and tumor blush from thyrocervical branches *(yellow arrows)*. This illustrates the importance of delayed filming after the injection. **F,** Postoperative cervical anteroposterior radiograph demonstrates spinal instrumentation in place from anterior and posterior fusion with interbody cage construct.

EVALUATION OF TUMORS IN THE CERVICAL SPINE

The cervical spine differs from other levels in that it requires evaluation of bilateral thyrocervical trunks, costocervical trunks, vertebral arteries, and external carotid arteries or supreme intercostal arteries, depending on the level of the tumor. Because there is a varying supply to the cervical spinal cord, it is absolutely critical to have a clear understanding of vascular anatomy so that inadvertent embolization of normal spinal cord tissue is avoided. One should keep in mind that the vertebral artery branches supplying the spinal cord at this level may differ in appearance from their counterparts in the thoracic and lumbar spine. Unlike in the thoracic and lumbar spine, they do not necessarily make the characteristic "hairpin" loop but ascend slightly before reaching the cord (see Figs. 25-3 and 25-4). They may appear more flattened angiographically on the anteroposterior projection and should not be overlooked as insignificant muscular or vertebral branches. An artery slightly larger than other radiculomedullary branches may be seen in the lower cervical levels during injection of the vertebral, deep cervical, or ascending cervical arteries, and it is a significant contributor to the cervical cord supply. This artery is referred to as the *artery of cervical enlargement* and is most often found at the C4 to C8 levels. It must be avoided during embolization to prevent possible cord infarction.[18]

Because of the close proximity of the vertebral body in the cervical spine to the vertebral artery, large cervical spine tumors often invade the foramina transversarium and encase the vertebral artery. Therefore complete tumor resection must address management of the vertebral artery, including vertebral artery sacrifice.

Several pieces of data are required before vertebral artery occlusion is performed. The vertebral arteries should be evaluated for caliber, patency, and supply to the spinal cord, and the collateral supply to the posterior circulation should be studied. When the vertebral artery to be occluded is nondominant or codominant, the contralateral vertebral artery is patent without stenosis, and the vertebral artery to be occluded provides the nondominant supply to the spinal cord, then the vertebral artery may be occluded most of the time with reasonable safety. Fig. 25-4 shows a C4 chordoma treated with gross total resection after right vertebral artery endovascular occlusion. Other circumstances may warrant additional evaluation with temporary balloon test occlusion (BTO).

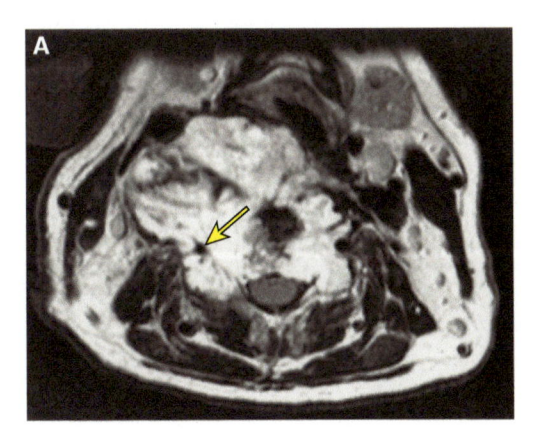

Fig. 25-4 C4 chordoma treated with radical resection after right vertebral artery endovascular occlusion. **A,** The mass invades the paraspinal soft tissues, both transverse processes, and encases the right vertebral artery *(arrow)*.

Continued

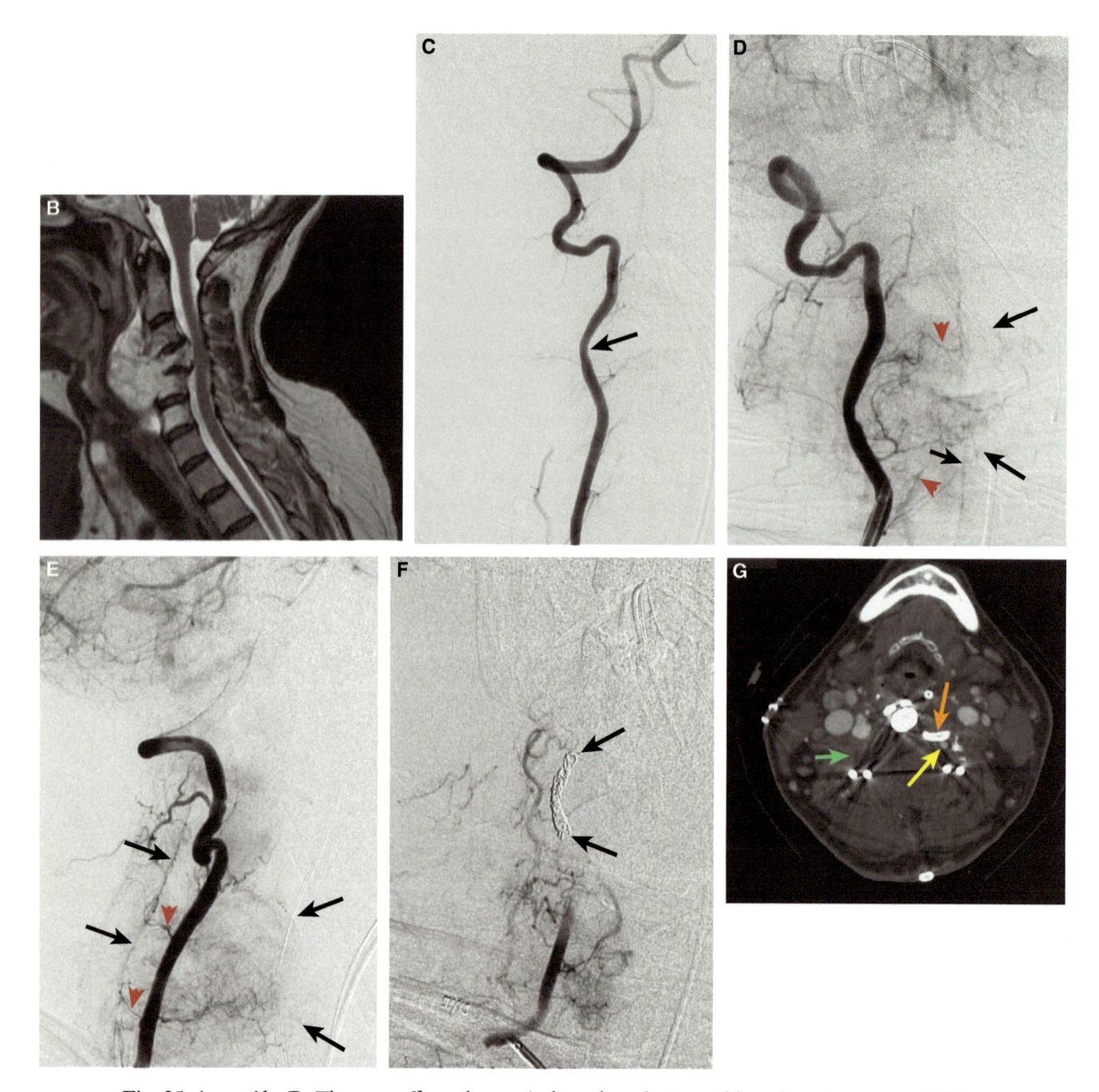

Fig. 25-4, cont'd **B,** The mass effaces the cervical canal producing mild cord impingement. **C,** Vertebral artery injection shows displacement laterally *(arrow)* from mass effect. **D,** Vertebral artery injection in late arterial phase reveals a tumor blush *(black arrows)*. Radiculomedullary branches *(red arrowheads)* are partially masked by tumor blush and should not be mistaken for muscular branches. **E,** Anterior spinal artery *(black arrows)*, radiculomedullary arteries *(red arrowheads)*. **F,** After coil embolization of the right vertebral artery at the site of the tumor, above the spinal artery *(arrows)*. The right vertebral artery was resected along with the tumor at surgery. **G,** Postoperative CT scan demonstrates patency of the left vertebral artery *(yellow arrow)* with absence of the right vertebral artery *(green arrow)*. No residual tumor is seen with construct and posterior rods in place. A surgical drain is noted just anterior to the left vertebral artery *(orange arrow)*.

Balloon Test Occlusion

BTO was first described by Serbinenko[19] in 1974. BTO is most often performed in the internal carotid artery to evaluate the ischemic tolerance of the anterior circulation to permanent occlusion. Although there are many studies describing the stratification of patients on the basis of the BTO, the data are mostly defined by retrospective small case series that use a variety of protocols. The data do suggest a slight advantage in stratification over abrupt occlusion of the internal carotid artery. Before BTO, abrupt internal carotid artery occlusion was associated with a cumulative stroke rate of 26% and a mortality rate of 12%.[20] Some studies suggest a reduction in these numbers with the use of BTO.[20-24] Other studies have suggested no outcome advantage for BTO.[25] Studies have illustrated that approximately 9% to 10% of patients undergoing BTO with only clinical evaluation will fail the test.[24,26] If adjunctive testing is performed, the percentage increases and is variable depending on the type of adjunctive testing used. An example is the use of the hypotensive challenge, which has been reported to increase the failure rate of BTO to 21%.[24] This adjunctive testing, in theory, should detect patients with minimal cerebral blood flow reserve that is inadequate to meet increasing demand in suboptimal physiologic conditions. This outcome advantage remains to be proved in larger controlled trials.

The complication rate is reasonably low in experienced hands. In the largest series to date, Mathis et al[27] described 500 patients who underwent BTO. In their series, eight patients (1.6%) developed asymptomatic complications, including dissection, pseudoaneurysm, and embolus. Eight patients developed a neurologic deficit (1.6%), and in two patients (0.4%) the deficit was permanent. The data were complicated by the use of xenon CT perfusion imaging during BTO, which subjected patients to risk of carotid injury when they were transferred from the angiography table to the CT scanner. Newer imaging modalities, such as flat-panel CT perfusion, that are performed on the angiography table will alleviate this added risk. Smaller studies without the use of CT perfusion have reported similar complication rates.[24,28]

Unfortunately, the predictive value of BTO for posterior circulation ischemia is less well defined. Case reports within small case series provide limited data on its application. If we extrapolate from anterior circulation data, BTO may be of benefit in situations where there is concern about inciting ischemic events in the posterior fossa after vertebral artery sacrifice. In addition, there may be a theoretical risk of spinal cord ischemia after vertebral artery occlusion based on extrapolated data from case reports of cord infarcts in the setting of spontaneous vertebral artery dissection. BTO and careful analysis of major spinal arterial supply could potentially circumvent such a risk.[29,30]

A neurologic examination should be performed before beginning BTO of the vertebral artery, focusing on signs manifested by posterior fossa ischemia. Patients should undergo anticoagulation with heparin to target an activated clotting time that is twice the baseline value. The balloon should be inflated to the level targeted for permanent occlusion. This minimizes the collateral supply from segmental vessels perfusing the vertebral artery distal to the balloon and parallels postocclusion physiology. The balloon remains inflated for 15 minutes. Once the balloon is inflated, a timer is started. The neurologic examination is repeated, again focusing on signs of posterior fossa ischemia. This examination is repeated every 2 to 5 minutes until the balloon is deflated. Any change during the neurologic examination representing a new deficit warrants abrupt termination of the examination, and the balloon should be immediately deflated.

After the balloon has been inflated for 15 minutes, the anesthesiologist is asked to lower the blood pressure by 10% of the patient's mean arterial pressure. Induced hypotension simulates a hemodynamic challenge. This may be encountered at the time of surgical resection for a number of reasons, including general anesthesia, hyperventilation, or perioperative hemorrhage, with a drop in hematocrit. In addition, this is important because patients are recumbent during this examination, and perfusion pressure may drop when they are erect, dehydrated, or develop bacteremia.[31]

There are a limited number of balloons that may be chosen for test occlusion. The balloons currently available are made of silicone or latex material. During inflation of the balloon, one should proceed with caution. Overdilatation or movement of the balloon during inflation may result in severe vasospasm or dissection. Therefore this procedure should be performed by an experienced interventional radiologist to minimize complications. The balloons with a central lumen are mounted on stiff catheters, and we do not recommend navigating these balloons above the C2 level in the cervical vertebral artery or using them in tortuous anatomy because this can lead to arterial injury (see Fig. 25-3). If a high cervical occlusion is needed or the vertebral artery is extremely tortuous or atherosclerotic, a low-profile, softer, silicone, low-compliance balloon, without a central lumen, such as the HyperGlide Occlusion Balloon System (Covidien, Plymouth, MN), should be chosen. This type of balloon does not have a central lumen and may be slightly more prone to thrombus formation, so a shorter test occlusion period (10 minutes) is preferred.

As an adjunctive measure of tolerance to permanent occlusion, we routinely monitor back pressure during test occlusion of the anterior circulation. Similarly, back pressures may be monitored with the central lumen balloons used in the proximal vertebral artery. Back pressures are measured with an arterial transducer by connecting the transducer to the lumen of the balloon catheter. The lumen of the balloon catheter should be perfused with a constant pressurized saline drip containing 3 units of heparin/ml when not acquiring measurements. Back pressure measurements are compared with systemic pressures by means of a transducer connected to the femoral arterial sheath. For the anterior circulation we use a 50/50 rule as a general guide in our clinical practice. If back pressure is at least 50 mm Hg and more than 50% of the mean arterial pressure, then the vessel may be safe to occlude. Although no evidence exists for use of back pressure measurements in the vertebral artery, we find them reassuring, when available, in appropriate cases.

After 25 minutes of total occlusion time using a central lumen balloon, the balloon is deflated and removed. A branch occlusion angiogram should be obtained to ensure that there are no distal embolic occlusions. Assuming similar hemodynamic conditions exist, in comparison with the anterior circulation, this may improve stratification of patients who will tolerate vertebral occlusion.

EVALUATION OF TUMORS IN THE THORACIC AND LUMBAR SPINE

As in the cervical spine, it is extremely important to count the level of the vertebrae starting from T1, when possible. Targeted angiography should be performed to select out the intercostal or lumbar arteries at the level being considered for embolization first. This allows the surgeon to make a rapid determination of the vascularity of the tumor and evaluate the local angioarchitecture for the feasibility of embolization. In cases where there is a high thoracic tumor at T1 or T2, the supreme intercostal arteries and the thyrocervical trunk should be injected. At thoracolumbar levels, two levels above and below the tumor should be evaluated, ensuring that the supply to an anterior spinal artery (ASA) or posterolateral spinal artery (PLSA) at adjacent levels is identified, if present (see Fig. 25-1, *C* and *E*, and Fig. 25-2, *G*). Identifying the cord supply originating from adjacent levels is important. As the supply to the tumor is being brought to stasis during embolization, collateral perfusion may develop, sending embolic material through intervertebral anastomoses to the ASA or PLSA at adjacent levels. This could result in cord infarction.

Additional considerations should be taken when evaluating lower lumbar and sacral tumors for embolization. There is some variation in the origin of the lower lumbar arteries. A common trunk may be found at the L3-4 levels. The L5 lumbar arteries typically arise from the iliac vessels, if present. Moreover, injection of the internal iliac arteries and the median sacral artery is important in evaluating the lumbosacral or pelvic tumor supply.

EMBOLIZATION TECHNIQUE

The patient should be placed under general anesthesia in the supine position on the angiography table. A baseline activated clotting time is measured. After limited diagnostic spinal angiography to confirm the presence of a vascular spine tumor that can be safely embolized, the patient undergoes anticoagulation by means of a bolus of heparin based on the patient's weight in kilograms. We generally administer 70 units/kg as a bolus. A 5 Fr Cobra catheter or suitable diagnostic catheter is advanced into the targeted vessel. The catheter is double flushed and connected to a continuous flush of heparinized saline solution by means of a rotating hemostatic valve. A microcatheter is chosen based on the type of embolization that is to be performed. Similarly, a guidewire is chosen to complement the microcatheter.

A roadmap is obtained through the diagnostic catheter, which acts as a guide catheter in this scenario. The microcatheter is then advanced over the guidewire distally into the pedicle supplying the tumor. The guidewire is then removed. A blank roadmap is then obtained. A small test injection using a 1 ml syringe and 100% contrast material is performed under the blank roadmap to ensure adequate runoff. Digital subtraction angiography is then performed by hand through the microcatheter using a 1 ml syringe with 100% contrast material. This injection is very important because arteries that may not have been seen on the more global injection with the diagnostic catheter, because of either a sump pump effect from other vessels or overlying vessel opacification, suddenly become quite apparent (see Fig. 25-1). It is most important to look for spinal arteries and collateral vessels at adjacent levels that may give rise to the spinal cord supply (see Fig. 25-2). After confirming that there are no crucial vessels, the tumor may be embolized with caution. Before embolization, we recommend placing a pushable fibered coil or detachable coil into the intercostal or lumbar artery distal to the origin of the branches supplying the tumor to protect normal tissues from embolic material and redirect the flow (see Fig. 25-2). This may be used as a radiographic marker at surgery when confirming the surgical level.

The embolic agent of choice is prepared before beginning embolization. In each case embolization is carried out in a slightly different manner depending on the agent chosen. In all cases a blank roadmap is obtained before embolization. Because we use polyvinyl alcohol (PVA) for tumor embolization, we will focus on its use for now and explore the other agents in brief detail later. When using PVA it is important to use 100% contrast material as a solution for the particles to ensure that the mixture is clearly visible during injection. It is equally important to adequately mix the solution before aspirating it into the syringe to ensure that it remains suspended. Injection is then carried out in a pulsatile manner through the microcatheter using a 1 ml syringe with small excursions that vary depending on the flow. Periodically the syringe is flushed with 100% contrast material to prevent clogging of the microcatheter with PVA particles. The microcatheter should be flushed more frequently with larger particles. The procedure should be stopped after stasis is achieved or if reflux occurs. Minimal reflux may be controlled if the angiographer adjusts the injection to less frequent, smaller injections with a longer linear rise. After achieving stasis within the vessels directly supplying the tumor, the catheter is cleared with 1 ml of contrast material or saline solution. It should be noted that saline solution has a much lower resistance and, if not prepared for this difference, the catheter may be rapidly injected, flushing particles from the target vessel. The microcatheter is then removed from the guide/diagnostic catheter. Postembolization digital subtraction angiography is performed by hand to assess the embolization result. Other vessels may be targeted in a similar manner. This approach will work well for most spine tumors involving vertebrae.

There are a small number of tumors that require a different technique because of their pial supply. Hemangioblastomas are an example of an intramedullary extremely vascular tumor that may benefit from preoperative embolization. These tumors, when found in the spinal cord, are routinely supplied by a PLSA or ASA. Although it has been reported, we suggest not proceeding with embolization of the ASA supply because of the increased risk of clinically significant cord infarction. Unless superselective within the tumor, the goal should be subtotal devascularization with preservation of the ASA supply distal to the tumor. It is important to achieve as distal a catheter position as possible to prevent embolization of normal branches more proximally. Equally important is the choice of PVA particle size. The use of particles that are too small may result in occlusion of normal sulcocommissural arteries.[32]

Embolization Material

Once a complete evaluation of the targeted tumor has been performed and angioarchitecture is completely understood, embolization of the tumor can proceed. Several different embolic agents can be used for transarterial tumor embolization. The choice of embolic agent is largely dictated by the time to surgery after embolization, anatomy and, less important, tumor type. PVA (Boston Scientific, Natick, MA), Embosphere Microspheres (BioSphere Medical, Rockland, MA), polyethylene alcohol (Onyx; Micro Therapeutics, Irvine, CA), or N-butyl cyanoacrylate (N-BCA; Cordis, Miami, FL) are the most commonly used agents today for transarterial embolization.

In our practice we perform preoperative tumor embolization of the spinal axis with PVA particles. There are currently no data to suggest an outcome advantage for the use of N-BCA or Onyx rather than PVA. Moreover, PVA has a cost advantage over the other two agents. It is compatible in all catheters, and it is only limited by the size of the lumen of the catheter chosen. Particles that are 150 to 250 and 250 to 355 microns are typically used in our practice and are compatible with all over-the-wire microcatheters.

Polyvinyl Alcohol

PVA particles have been around for many years and are still heavily used in embolization of the spine and in head and neck tumors. The particles come in a variety of sizes, ranging from 45 to 150 to 1100 to 1180 microns. For most spinal axis tumors 150 to 250 and 250 to 355 micron particles are chosen. In general, smaller particles will penetrate deeper within tumor vessels, but there is an increased risk of ischemia in normal tissue. This can occur during the course of embolization as stasis is achieved within the target vessel and reflux occurs. Use of larger particles will not eliminate inadvertent embolization and is not a substitute for careful angiographic assessment. The central artery is typically 100 to 200 microns, the posterior lateral spinal arteries 100 to 400 microns, and the anterior radicular and anterior spinal arteries 200 to 800 microns. Therefore the use of particles that are 250 to 355 microns cannot prevent embolization of the ASA.

N-Butyl Cyanoacrylate

N-BCA may be used for transarterial embolization or percutaneous embolization. We will focus on transarterial embolization at this time. The advantage proposed for using N-BCA rather than PVA particles is the radiopacity of N-BCA when it is admixed with Ethiodol. PVA is radiolucent and, once admixed with contrast material, must be periodically agitated to remain suspended in solution. N-BCA has a lower risk of recannulization, as opposed to PVA, which is not permanent. The disadvantages to using N-BCA include its propensity for reflux in small-caliber vessels, particularly when the mixture of Ethiodol and N-BCA is not optimal, as well as its variable entrance along with the possibility of proximal occlusion. Moreover, in unfamiliar hands there is a high risk of catheter retainment.

Onyx

Onyx is ethylene vinyl alcohol copolymer dissolved in dimethyl sulfoxide (DMSO). It has been approved by the U.S. FDA for use in arteriovenous malformations; however, it has been used off label in recent case series for preoperative embolization of spine tumors and head and neck tumors. In one series of 10 patients in which Onyx was used for preoperative embolization, it was favored over N-BCA for its increased penetrance and the requirement of fewer arterial feeder catheterizations.[33] Onyx has been reported to penetrate vessels as small as 40 microns.[34] It is a permanent agent, which makes it more appealing than PVA particles when complete tumor resection is unlikely. A disadvantage to using Onyx is its requirement of a compatible microcatheter. The catheters are reinforced to withstand higher injection pressures and therefore are stiffer than similar noncompatible microcatheters. This may prevent distal catheterization and facilitate perforations from excessive force on the arterial wall around bends.

COMPLICATIONS

Most complications from spine tumor embolization can be prevented by diligently searching for the spinal arterial supply and avoiding dangerous anastomoses. It may be difficult to identify spinal arteries that are superimposed over a vascular tumor or because of patient movement in patients who are awake and uncooperative. Finstein et al[35] reported paraplegia in a 64-year-old patient who underwent preoperative transarterial embolization of a giant cell tumor involving the T12 and L1 vertebrae with the use of PVA particles. The patient was not placed under general anesthesia and complained of bilateral spasms of the gastrocnemius and soleus muscles during embolization. After completion of the procedure, the patient reported numbness in the legs. On examination he had loss of sphincter tone, saddle anesthesia, and loss of motor and sensory function below T12. The suspected cause was failure to identify the anterior spinal artery at the level of embolization or at an adjacent level, which resulted in inadvertent embolization of the predominant supply to the spinal cord causing cord infarction and paralysis. This case illustrates the need for careful observation before and during embolization to avoid occlusion of spinal arteries or critical anastomotic branches with embolic material. Adequate training in a neurointerventional fellowship program, as well as experience, is recommended to avoid such catastrophic complications.

FUTURE DIRECTIONS

Percutaneous embolization of vascular spine tumors with the use of N-BCA has been reported.[36] As compared with the transarterial technique, the authors suggested that embolization occurs at the level of the capillary bed, as opposed to more proximal arteriole occlusion, yielding superior devascularization of the tumor.[37] The lack of dependence on arterial access to the tumor is advantageous in some cases where arterial access is difficult or limited. However, these investigators tempered their discussion with the possible risk of inadvertent embolization of a spinal artery. Lethal complications have been reported with other agents used in a similar manner in the high cervical spine, and therefore more experience is needed along with outcome studies to prove its advantages over current techniques and agents.[38]

CONCLUSION

Transarterial embolization of spine tumors can be extremely useful in minimizing perioperative blood loss and facilitating complete en bloc resection. The risk of spinal embolization is small in experienced hands and should be considered in cases where planned resection of vascular spine tumors is to be performed.

TIPS FROM THE MASTERS

- A good-quality angiogram to define vascular anatomy is essential. This may be facilitated with general anesthesia and acquisition during apnea.
- Blush of the ipsilateral vertebral body should be seen at all levels in high-quality angiographic spinal injections.
- Anterior spinal arteries (ASA) and posterolateral spinal arteries (PLSA) should be defined before surgical resection or embolization.
- No embolization should be carried out if the ASA or PLSA are present at the level of target embolization. There are very few exceptions to this rule.
- Sodium amytal or 1% preservative-free lidocaine can be used for provocative testing in awake patients or in concert with somatosensory evoked potentials and motor evoked potentials in patients under general anesthesia.
- Experienced physicians with proper training should perform these procedures to limit complications.

References (With Key References in Boldface)

1. Gellad FE, Sadato N, Numaguchi Y, et al. Vascular metastatic lesions of the spine: preoperative embolization. Radiology 176:683-686, 1990.
2. **Berkefeld J, Scale D, Kirchner J, et al. Hypervascular spinal tumors: influence of the embolization technique on perioperative hemorrhage. AJNR Am J Neuroradiol 20:757-763, 1999.**
3. Guzman R, Dubach-Schwizer S, Heini P, et al. Preoperative transarterial embolization of vertebral metastases. Eur Spine J 14:263-268, 2005.
4. **Manke C, Bretschneider T, Lenhart M, et al. Spinal metastases from renal cell carcinoma: effect of preoperative particle embolization on intraoperative blood loss. AJNR Am J Neuroradiol 22:997-1003, 2001.**
5. **Shi HB, Suh DC, Lee HK, et al. Preoperative transarterial embolization of spinal tumor: embolization techniques and results. AJNR Am J Neuroradiol 20:2009-2015, 1999.**
6. Kuether TA, Nesbit GM, Barnwell SL. Embolization as treatment for spinal cord compression from renal cell carcinoma: case report. Neurosurgery 39:1260-1262; discussion 1262-1263, 1996.

7. Hosalkar HS, Jones KJ, King JJ, et al. Serial arterial embolization for large sacral giant-cell tumors: mid- to long-term results. Spine (Phila Pa 1976) 32:1107-1115, 2007.
8. Lin PP, Guzel VB, Moura MF, et al. Long-term follow-up of patients with giant cell tumor of the sacrum treated with selective arterial embolization. Cancer 95:1317-1325, 2002.
9. Levey AS, Bosch JP, Lewis JB, et al. A more accurate method to estimate glomerular filtration rate from serum creatinine: a new prediction equation. Modification of Diet in Renal Disease Study Group. Ann Intern Med 130:461-470, 1999.
10. Merten GJ, Burgess WP, Gray LV, et al. Prevention of contrast-induced nephropathy with sodium bicarbonate: a randomized controlled trial. JAMA 291:2328-2334, 2004.
11. Minamori Y, Yammoto M, Tanaka A, et al. Hazard of glucagon test in diabetic patients. Hypertensive crisis in asymptomatic pheochromocytoma. Diabetes Care 15:1437-1438, 1992.
12. van Lennep JR, Romijn JA, Harinck HI. Multi-organ failure after a glucagon test. Lancet 369:798, 2007.
13. Niimi Y, Sala F, Deletis V, et al. Neurophysiologic monitoring and pharmacologic provocative testing for embolization of spinal cord arteriovenous malformations. AJNR Am J Neuroradiol 25:1131-1138, 2004.
14. Sala F, Niimi Y, Krzan MJ, et al. Embolization of a spinal arteriovenous malformation: correlation between motor evoked potentials and angiographic findings: technical case report. Neurosurgery 45:932-937; discussion 937-938, 1999.
15. **Berenstein A, Young W, Ransohoff J, et al. Somatosensory evoked potentials during spinal angiography and therapeutic transvascular embolization. J Neurosurg 60:777-785, 1984.**
16. Touho H, Karasawa J, Ohnishi H, et al. Intravascular treatment of spinal arteriovenous malformations using a microcatheter—with special reference to serial xylocaine tests and intravascular pressure monitoring. Surg Neurol 42:148-156, 1994.
17. Doppman JL, Girton M, Oldfield EH. Spinal Wada test. Radiology 161:319-321, 1986.
18. Thron AK. Vascular Anatomy of the Spinal Cord. New York: Springer-Verlag, 1988.
19. Serbinenko FA. Balloon catheterization and occlusion of major cerebral vessels. J Neurosurg 41:125-145, 1974.
20. Linskey ME, Jungreis CA, Yonas H, et al. Stroke risk after abrupt internal carotid artery sacrifice: accuracy of preoperative assessment with balloon test occlusion and stable xenon-enhanced CT. AJNR Am J Neuroradiol 15:829-843, 1994.
21. Fox AJ, Vinuela F, Pelz DM, et al. Use of detachable balloons for proximal artery occlusion in the treatment of unclippable cerebral aneurysms. J Neurosurg 66:40-46, 1987.
22. Higashida RT, Halbach VV, Dowd C, et al. Endovascular detachable balloon embolization therapy of cavernous carotid artery aneurysms: results in 87 cases. J Neurosurg 72:857-863, 1990.
23. Gonzalez CF, Moret J. Balloon occlusion of the carotid artery prior to surgery for neck tumors. AJNR Am J Neuroradiol 11:649-652, 1990.
24. Standard SC, Ahuja A, Guterman LR, et al. Balloon test occlusion of the internal carotid artery with hypotensive challenge. AJNR Am J Neuroradiol 16:1453-1458, 1995.
25. Eckard DA, Purdy PD, Bonte FJ. Temporary balloon occlusion of the carotid artery combined with brain blood flow imaging as a test to predict tolerance prior to permanent carotid sacrifice. AJNR Am J Neuroradiol 13:1565-1569, 1992.
26. Michel E, Liu H, Remley KB, et al. Perfusion MR neuroimaging in patients undergoing balloon test occlusion of the internal carotid artery. AJNR Am J Neuroradiol 22:1590-1596, 2001.
27. Mathis JM, Barr JD, Jungreis CA, et al. Temporary balloon test occlusion of the internal carotid artery: experience in 500 cases. AJNR Am J Neuroradiol 16:749-754, 1995.
28. Barr JD. Temporary and permanent occlusion of cerebral arteries: indications and techniques. Neurosurg Clin N Am 11:27-38, vii-viii, 2000.
29. Bergqvist CA, Goldberg HI, Thorarensen O, et al. Posterior cervical spinal cord infarction following vertebral artery dissection. Neurology 48:1112-1115, 1997.
30. Laufs H, Weidauer S, Heller C, et al. Hemi-spinal cord infarction due to vertebral artery dissection in congenital afibrinogenemia. Neurology 63:1522-1523, 2004.

31. Abud DG, Spelle L, Piotin M, et al. Venous phase timing during balloon test occlusion as a criterion for permanent internal carotid artery sacrifice. AJNR Am J Neuroradiol 26:2602-2609, 2005.
32. **Biondi A, Ricciardi GK, Faillot T, et al. Hemangioblastomas of the lower spinal region: report of four cases with preoperative embolization and review of the literature. AJNR Am J Neuroradiol 26:936-945, 2005.**
33. Gore P, Theodore N, Brasiliense L, et al. The utility of onyx for preoperative embolization of cranial and spinal tumors. Neurosurgery 62:1204-1211; discussion 1211-1212, 2008.
34. Gobin YP, Murayama Y, Milanese K, et al. Head and neck hypervascular lesions: embolization with ethylene vinyl alcohol copolymer—laboratory evaluation in swine and clinical evaluation in humans. Radiology 221:309-317, 2001.
35. Finstein JL, Chin KR, Alvandi F, et al. Postembolization paralysis in a man with a thoracolumbar giant cell tumor. Clin Orthop Relat Res 453:335-340, 2006.
36. Liebig T, Henkes H, Kirsch M, et al. Preoperative devascularization of a circumferential osteogenic metastasis to the upper cervical spine by direct percutaneous needle puncture: a technical note. Neuroradiology 47:674-679, 2005.
37. Schirmer CM, Malek AM, Kwan ES, et al. Preoperative embolization of hypervascular spinal metastases using percutaneous direct injection with n-butyl cyanoacrylate: technical case report. Neurosurgery 59:E431-E432; author reply E432, 2006.
38. Peraud A, Drake JM, Armstrong D, et al. Fatal ethibloc embolization of vertebrobasilar system following percutaneous injection into aneurysmal bone cyst of the second cervical vertebra. AJNR Am J Neuroradiol 25:1116-1120, 2004.

Chapter 26

Intramedullary Spinal Cord Tumors

Yoon Ha, Keung Nyun Kim, Do Heum Yoon,
Brian J. Jian, Andrew T. Parsa, Christopher P. Ames

The average annual incidence of primary spinal cord tumors is approximately 1.3 per 100,000 persons, which represents roughly 2% to 4% of all neoplasms of the central nervous system (CNS).[1,2] Primary spinal cord tumors are anatomically separable into two broad categories: intramedullary and extramedullary. Intramedullary glial tumors are composed predominantly of infiltrative astrocytomas and ependymomas. In a recent large retrospective analysis of intramedullary spinal cord tumors at a single institution, ependymomas were the most common tumors (54%), followed by astrocytomas (21%), hemangioblastomas (12%), and miscellaneous tumors (14%).[3]

The purpose of intramedullary tumor surgery is to achieve complete removal of an intramedullary tumor without causing damage to the spinal cord. Improvements in diagnostic testing, development of new operative tools, and technical advances in intraoperative electrophysiologic monitoring have largely contributed to recent improvements in surgical results.[4,5]

The surgical strategy is determined by analyzing the preoperative imaging data regarding the presence of a cleavage plane between the tumor and the normal spinal cord.[6] It is essential to define the extent of the solid portion of the tumor to determine the length of the laminectomy.[7] It is also essential to localize the lesion within the spinal cord with regard to its lateralization and depth. Even though recent advances in surgical techniques for treating intramedullary tumors have improved surgical outcomes and long-term tumor control, selection of surgical principles and management plans are critically important and require skilled and experienced surgeons with a multimodal team approach.[6-12]

Surgical resection of intramedullary spine tumors is often difficult, because ongoing pathologic conditions distort the normal anatomy. In the case of spinal ependymomas, gross total resection of the tumor is possible, given the typical clean surgical planes. However, resection requires a midline myelotomy to avoid injury to the posterior columns. Locating the midline for performing the myelotomy to access the tumor margin is often difficult because of the distorted anatomy. Anatomic landmarks may be misleading in patients with intramedullary spinal cord tumors because of edema, cord expansion and rotation, local reactive gliosis/fibrosis, or neovascularization. An erroneously placed midline myelotomy places the posterior columns at risk for significant postoperative disability.

This chapter will cover the most recent issues surrounding the treatment of intramedullary spinal cord tumors, including intraoperative neurophysiologic monitoring and relevant anatomy and surgical techniques.

TYPES OF TUMORS AND MANAGEMENT STRATEGIES
EPENDYMOMA

Intramedullary ependymomas are the most common spinal cord tumors in adults, representing 34.5% of all CNS ependymomas and approximately half of all intramedullary tumors.[7,13] They can appear at any point in life but more frequently occur in the middle adult years. Histopathologic findings reveal two distinct types: classic (World Health Organization [WHO] grades 2 and 3) and myxopapillary (WHO grade 1).[6,14] Classic ependymomas develop from the intramedullary spinal cord.[15] Myxopapillary ependymomas originate from the filum terminale and occur almost exclusively at the conus medullaris.[16]

Approximately 50% of spinal cord ependymomas are encountered in the cervical spine. Thoracic (14%), lumbar (34%), and conus (14%) lesions are seen less frequently.[10,12,17] Magnetic resonance imaging (MRI) shows a focal expansion of the spinal cord and high signal intensity on T2-weighted images and slight hypointensity on T1-weighted images, with heterogeneous contrast enhancement.[15,18,19] These tumors can also be accompanied by cystic degenerations, hemorrhage, and syrinx. Treatment outcome and prognosis are excellent when tumors can be completely removed; in these cases there is a low risk of recurrence.[3,6,8,10]

The use of microsurgery in the treatment of intramedullary ependymomas has played a significant role in recent years.[6,9,17] Surgery is considered the most effective treatment modality for this encapsulated tumor with well-defined margins.[6,7,9,20] Microsurgical removal alone could achieve long-term tumor control or cure with preservation of neurologic function.[6,9,17]

The most important step during surgical removal is finding the plane between the tumor and the spinal cord. This interface can only be accurately exposed through a meticulous myelotomy, which extends over the entire craniocaudal ends of the tumor. The presence of a syrinx around the tumor may sometimes improve the chances of a gross total resection. Preoperative functional neurologic status is the most important and significant predictor of postoperative functional outcomes.[3,10,21] Patients with profound and long-standing neurologic deterioration rarely achieve significant neurologic improvement, even after technically successful surgical removal.[22,23] Surgical morbidity is also increased in patients with more significant preoperative neurologic deficits.

Somatosensory deficits usually occur in the immediate postoperative period after the results of posterior midline myelotomy are known.[23,24] Traction of the posterior column and transient edema because of microtrauma or vascular insult may cause this postoperative sensory deficit. In general, most patients have resolution of their deficits within a few months' time, although they may not return to their preoperative neurologic status.[22]

Myxopapillary ependymomas are a specific tumor variant of spinal cord ependymomas that occur most commonly in the lumbosacral region. The optimal management for these tumors has been controversial, because their rate of recurrence appears to be higher than that of typical intramedullary spinal ependymomas.[21] In a study by Bagley et al,[25] a total of 1013 patients who underwent surgery for spinal cord tumors were retrospectively analyzed. Of these patients, 52 had a final pathologic diagnosis of myxopapillary ependymoma. Overall, pediatric patients had a much more aggressive clinical course, with a much higher rate of local recurrence and dissemination of the tumor compared with adults (64% versus 32%).[25] The median time to disease recurrence was 88 months for the entire group. The overall survival after 11.5 years of follow-up was 94%. No clear benefit was demonstrated for adjuvant chemotherapy and/or radiation therapy. Consequently aggressive surgical resection is still recommended. In a study by Jeibmann et al,[9] patients were retrospectively analyzed with a mean follow-up of 42 months. The 5-year recurrence-free survival rates were 86% for patients harboring ependymomas, 100% for patients with transitional tumors, and 77% for patients with myxopapillary ependymomas.

SUBEPENDYMOMA

Intramedullary subependymomas are benign, well-demarcated tumors.[26,27] The cell of origin of these tumors is still uncertain. They may originate from cells of the subependymal plate or residual periventricular matrix, and histopathologic findings suggest that they may certainly be a variant of ependymoma. MRI scans show variable intensity on T1-weighted and T2-weighted images, with varying degrees of enhancement.[26,28,29] The most common finding on MRI is homogeneous isointensity or hypointensity on T1-weighted images and slight hyperintensity on T2-weighted images without contrast enhancement. The absence of contrast enhancement may diminish the ability to distinguish subependymomas from other more common intramedullary tumors, with significant enhancement by contrast agents.

During surgery, subependymomas usually have less vasculature and are well circumscribed by the gliotic plane that separates these tumors from the surrounding normal spinal cord. Under these surgical conditions, surgeons are able to remove tumors completely with the use of standard microsurgical instrument and techniques. Because these tumors have benign and noninvasive characteristics, adjuvant radiation therapy or chemotherapy is not required.

ASTROCYTOMA

Intramedullary astrocytomas are the second most common of these tumors, representing approximately 20% of intramedullary tumors.[30,31]

Histopathologic grading is the most important prognostic factor.[30-32] Most of these tumors (75%) are low-grade (WHO grade 2) fibrillary astrocytomas, with a 5-year survival rate of more than 70%.[6,12] The less common high-grade (WHO grades 3 and 4) tumors, anaplastic astrocytomas and glioblastomas, have a poor prognosis and low survival rates.[12,33]

MRI scans show fusiform enlargement of the spinal cord and occasionally cystic degeneration.[6,34] Diffuse edema and syrinx formation are infrequently associated with tumor mass.[6,35] Typically the tumor shows hypointensity on T1-weighted images and hyperintensity on T2-weighted images with contrast enhancement. In case of differential diagnosis with demyelinating disease or vascular malformation is required, repeated MRI follow up or angiography should be required.

Because most spinal cord astrocytomas are infiltrative and are associated with indistinct boundaries with the surrounding normal spinal cord, total removal of these tumors is rarely achieved, and the role of surgery is often limited to safe surgical resection or biopsy only.[6,30,31,36,37] Histologic tumor grading and preoperative functional status are the two most important prognostic variables after surgery.[12,14,30,38]

Because of the high rate of local and remote recurrences in high-grade astrocytomas, postoperative radiation therapy is usually required.[6,33] Postoperative spinal or craniospinal radiation for these types of tumors should also be required. Most series suggest that radiation therapy can improve both the rate of local tumor control and overall survival.[14] In one retrospective study of 57 patients with spinal cord astrocytomas, postoperative radiation therapy prolonged progression-free survival but not overall survival in those with low-grade astrocytomas.[39]

Chemotherapy is indicated for patients with high-grade astrocytomas that continue to progress after surgery and radiation therapy.[40,41] Previous reports concerning the role of temozolomide (TMZ)–based chemotherapy in astrocytomas are very limited.[42-45] In one study of 22 adults with low-grade spinal cord gliomas treated with TMZ, four patients showed a partial response and 12 had stable disease.[42] In another study of six patients with high-grade gliomas treated with several different TMZ schedules, two patients remained stable or showed radiographic improvement, and two patients showed no response to TMZ and eventually died.[44]

HEMANGIOBLASTOMA

Hemangioblastomas are rare vascular tumors and the third most common type of intramedullary spinal cord tumor.[46] Hemangioblastomas develop in one of two ways: as a spontaneous solitary tumor or as hereditary or sporadic von Hippel–Lindau (VHL) syndrome.[47] Approximately 10% to 30% of intramedullary hemangioblastomas are associated with VHL syndrome. VHL is an autosomal dominant genetic condition in which hemangioblastomas are found in the cerebellum, spinal cord, kidney, and retina. These hemangioblastomas are associated with several pathologic conditions: retinal hemangioma, renal cell carcinoma, and pheochromocytoma. VHL is caused by a mutation in the von Hippel–Lindau tumor suppressor gene on chromosome 3p25.3. Whether these tumors are solitary or associated with VHL, their histopathologic characteristics are identical. Most hemangioblastomas occur in the posterior part of the spinal cord, which causes the progressive sensory deficits that are a presenting symptom. The MRI findings show uniform, homogeneous enhancing nodules with high vascularity.[48,49] Cysts, syrinxes, and peritumoral edema are often associated findings. Tumor hypervascularity often indicates the presence of hemangioblastoma rather than ependymoma.

Hemangioblastomas are well-circumscribed and benign tumors and, as such, complete surgical resection is the primary treatment, providing excellent long-term tumor control.[36,46,50] Tumor hypervascularity increases the risk of excessive intraoperative bleeding, resulting in incomplete surgical resection. However, in contrast to hemangioblastomas of the posterior fossa, preoperative embolization may not be recommended because of the high risk of complications associated with spinal angiography and embolization procedures. In contrast to other types of intramedullary tumors, intratumoral decompression should not be carried out before interrupting the arterial supply. To reduce the risk of massive intraoperative bleeding, circumferential dissection outside of the tumor is critical. It is also important to preserve draining veins until the arterial supply has been interrupted to avoid spinal cord injuries resulting from acute swelling of the tumor itself.

GANGLIOGLIOMA

Gangliogliomas are rare CNS tumors that usually develop in the brain and infrequently arise from the spinal cord. Gangliogliomas are slow-growing glial-neuronal tumors, but they occasionally exhibit rapidly progressing characteristics.[51] On MRI scans, gangliogliomas show hypointensity on T1-weighted images and varied signal characteristics on T2-weighted images with contrast enhancement. Secondary changes caused by long-term tumor growth include scoliosis, bone erosion, and scalloping.

Total surgical resection is the mainstay of treatment for spinal cord gangliogliomas. Excellent long-term survival and minimal morbidity can be achieved by means of total or near-total tumor removal.[51]

The role of adjuvant radiation therapy is controversial. Most investigators do not recommend postoperative radiation therapy; although it may be required in the presence of recurrence or progression.

Lymphoma

Primary CNS lymphoma rarely presents as an isolated spinal cord intramedullary tumor.[52] On MRI, the most common finding is a solid and homogeneously enhanced mass that is hyperintense on T2-weighted images, without associated syringomyelia. When patients are diagnosed on the basis of histopathologic findings, a careful investigation of the brain and spinal cord should follow to identify other sites of CNS disease. Because CNS lymphoma is a diffuse infiltrative disease that most often affects the entire craniospinal neuraxis, the role of surgery is limited to biopsy alone.[53] As for other types of CNS lymphoma, chemotherapy including high-dose methotrexate is considered to be the principal treatment.

Melanoma

Melanomas can arise in and be limited to the intramedullary spinal cord region, or they may be secondary to systemic melanoma.[54,55] Reports in the literature of primary intraspinal melanomas are very rare. The clinical presentation is similar to that of other intramedullary tumors, but melanomas often progress more rapidly than other common benign intramedullary tumors.

MRI shows high signal intensity on T1-weighted images and hypointensity on T2-weighted images with contrast enhancement.[56] Intratumoral hemorrhage is commonly found at presentation.

Because complete resection is rarely achievable, the role of surgery is limited to biopsy or decompression alone. Most patients should be required to undergo postoperative radiation therapy.[54,55] Chemotherapy for systemic melanoma could be administered as an adjuvant treatment.

Other Rare Intramedullary Tumors

Other rare primary intramedullary spinal cord tumors include germinoma, primitive neuroectodermal tumor, paraganglioglioma, teratoma, dermoid cyst, epidermoid cyst, and lipoma.[6] The surgical treatment strategies are similar to those for other intramedullary tumors.

ANATOMY AND NEUROPHYSIOLOGIC MONITORING

The cross-sectional anatomy of the spinal cord consists of three funiculi: one posterior and two anterolateral in location. The attachments of the dentate ligaments to the cord define the anterior (ventral) and posterior (dorsal) halves of the spinal cord. The ascending posterior nerves emanating from the dorsal horn gray matter of the spinal cord carry the sensory fibers encoding position, tactile (deep touch), and vibratory axons. They run directly to the ipsilateral half of the posterior funiculi or columns and ascend in the posterior portion of the cord. Given the requisite dorsal approach to spinal cord tumors, the nerves at highest risk for injury during surgical resection are the dorsal funiculi, which carry proprioceptive information. Consequently, temporary deficits in arm and limb position sense can be expected. It is hoped that a pure midline myelotomy might be used to avoid any permanent damage to the fibers.

The remaining sensory fibers encoding pain (sharp, dull), temperature, and light touch cross to the contralateral anterolateral funiculus. These fibers then ascend as anterolateral spinothalamic tracts. These tracts are located anterior to the dentate ligaments. In acute central cord injuries and in the case of damage to this central region during surgical resection of intramedullary tumors, the more centrally located cervical axons of the spinothalamic tract are disrupted. Similar to damage to the dorsal columns, postoperative patients demonstrate altered pain and temperature sensations. These sensory symptoms often go unnoticed by the patient, which is likely the result of many factors, including a concurrent alteration in sensation due to diminished proprioceptive sense.

Motor symptoms are caused by damage to the descending corticospinal or pyramidal tract in the posterior portion of the anterolateral funiculus. Acute disruptions may evoke a flaccid paralysis or weakness that ultimately progresses to spasticity. In both acute and chronic disruptions, motor symptoms are ipsilateral to the pathologic findings. Chronic disruption along this anatomic course causes upper motor neuron or long tract findings that include a segmental level of paralysis or weakness, muscle atrophy, hyperactive deep tendon reflexes, spasticity, a disturbance of fine motor movements, and a pathologic extensor response of the toe to plantar stimulation. Lower motor neuron deficits can originate from the anterior horn cell, nerve root, and any point along the peripheral nerve. The clinical picture may overlap with long tract signs, but its distinguishing features include absence of deep tendon reflexes, decreased tone, fasciculations, and absence of a pathologic extensor response of the toes. Within the descending motor tract, the cervical or arm axons are more centrally located, exiting through the ventral gray matter and ventral nerve roots first. This is the anatomic basis of central cord syndrome, which leaves the arms weaker than the legs when injury to the cervical cord causes edema in a central to peripheral direction.[8,57,58]

In recent years, with improvements in neurophysiologic monitoring, clinicians are beginning to determine whether finely mapped surgical midline myelotomies can reduce the risk of permanent neurodeficits during surgical resection of intramedullary lesions. In a study by Yanni et al,[5] two patients with syringomyelia and five patients with tumors had the dorsal funiculi mapped to determine the anatomic midline. In two of these patients, the midline was identified anatomically. In another two patients, the posterior columns were preserved only on one side. All other patients had intact posterior column function postoperatively.[5]

SURGICAL TECHNIQUES

The operative approach to intramedullary tumors is based on a midline posterior approach. The patient is placed prone on bolsters, freeing the thorax and abdomen from any pressure. This is the most widely used position for all tumor locations. In this position immobilization can be achieved with a three-point head fixation to prevent inadvertent cervical flexion and pressure sores on the face if the tumor is located in the cervical portion. When motor evoked and somatosensory evoked potential monitoring is established, and electrode placement should be checked at this stage of the procedure.

A midline incision is made, centered at the level of the lesion but extending above and below it, cutting across the raphe and allowing symmetrical retraction of muscular masses. Bone removal should provide sufficient access to the solid portion of the tumor. As a rule, exposure of one additional vertebra above and below the tumor is recommended. Laminectomy or laminotomy is performed. Laminectomy should be carried out gently and patiently with the removal of small pieces of bone, avoiding any damage to the adjacent spinal cord. Laminectomy is often performed for only one- or two-level exposure or for thoracic level exposure. But laminoplastic laminotomy or laminectomy with posterior instrumented fusion should be considered for long level exposure, especially in the cervical or cervicothoracic junction in young patients. In rare cases, option of unilateral laminectomy, especially with smaller eccentric tumors and junctional regions could be selected.

Opening of the dura can be performed with or without the microscope, making the incision carefully so as not to violate the arachnoid membrane. Dural suspension by simple traction sutures is sufficient (Fig. 26-1, *A*). The arachnoid mater is opened separately, when possible, with microscissors, particularly when one intends to close it

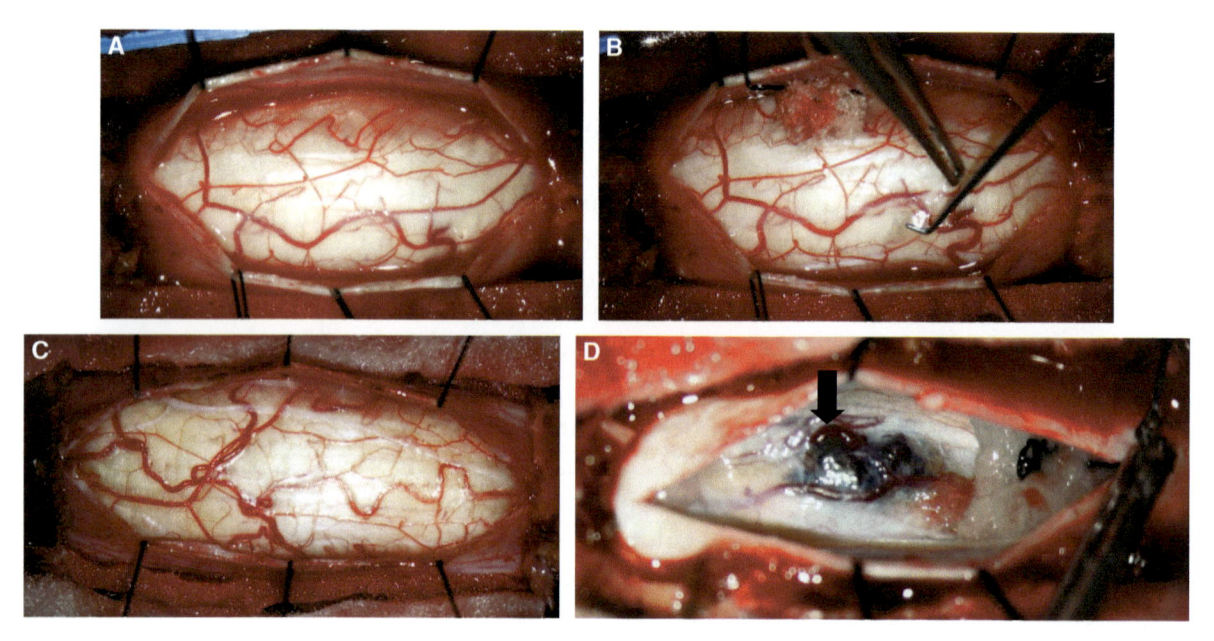

Fig. 26-1 Intraoperative photograph displaying intradural steps before myelotomy. **A,** Dural incision should be performed carefully so as not to violate the arachnoid membrane. Dural suspension by simple traction sutures is sufficient. **B,** Arachnoid is opened with a fine dissector with microscissors. **C,** The spinal cord is then visible, enlarged and swollen, smooth and tense, more or less vascularized. **D,** The spinal cord is sometimes discolored because of previous tumor bleeding (*arrow* indicates engorged tumor vessel and intratumoral bleeding).

(Fig. 26-1, *B*). The spinal cord is then seen, enlarged and swollen, smooth and tense, more or less vascularized, and sometimes discolored because of previous tumor bleeding (Fig. 26-1, *C* and *D*). Gentle evaluation of its firmness will confirm the location of solid and cystic areas.

High-powered microscopic magnification will allow localization of the dorsal median sulcus, which appears as a distinct median raphe, over which runs the tortuous posterior spinal vein (Fig. 26-2, *A*). Occasionally, small veins exiting from the sulcus may also help to establish the midline (Fig. 26-2, *B*). Midline crossing vessels in the pia are cauterized and divided. The dorsal midline can be estimated by noting the midpoint between the dorsal nerve root entry zones, but this may prove impossible because of the asymmetrical distortion of the cord or the adherence of the posterior columns. In such instances the midline is identified above and below this region, and then the two lines may join on the surface of the lesion site (Fig. 26-2, *C*).

Midline myelotomy is performed. During the myelotomy the spinal cord is not incised but opened by spreading the dorsal columns apart. The midline surgical approach is an absolute rule, with one exception—that is, when the lesion is located in one dorsal column and is apparent on the surface without any cortical "mantle." Dissection of

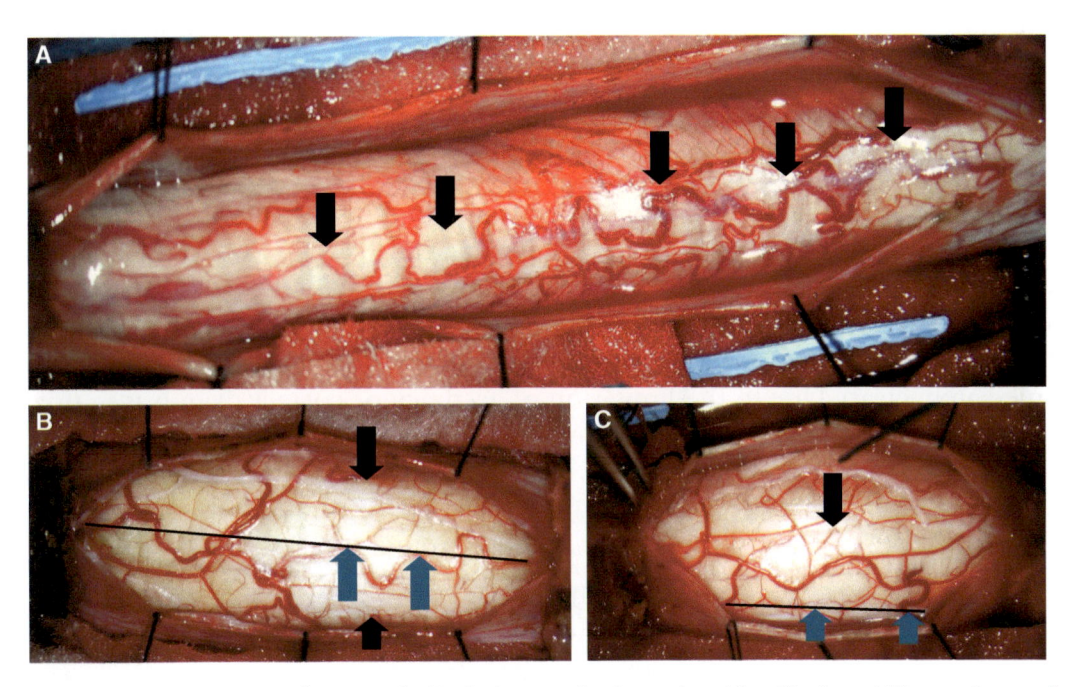

Fig. 26-2 Intraoperative photograph displaying methods used to identify the midline and steps for midline myelotomy. **A,** Identification of median sulcus. Under high-power magnification, median sulcus is identified, over which the very tortuous posterior spinal vein runs. It is not always in the real midline (*arrows* indicate the median sulcus and overlying spinal veins). **B,** The midline between the two dorsal root entry zones can be identified by a line of veins emerging from the dorsal raphe (*black arrows* indicate dorsal root entry zone; *blue arrows* indicate an imaginary line contiguous to the point of veins emerging from the dorsal raphe). **C,** In cases of asymmetrical expansion and distortion of the cord, visual midline determination may be impossible and can be located by a line of veins emerging from the dorsal raphe *(blue arrows)*. *Black arrow* indicates the dorsal root entry zone, which is rotated by asymmetrical tumor location within the spinal cord.

the dorsal column is performed with the finest surgical instruments (microdissectors, microforceps, microscissors, and cottonoids moistened with saline solution at 37° C) (Fig. 26-2, *D* and *E*). Vessels of various sizes that run vertically over the dorsal columns are dissected and mobilized laterally to expose the posterior sulcus, sacrificing the smallest number of vessel branches, bridging the two columns, and trying to spare all of the finest arterial or venous vessels in the sulcocommissural region. The dorsal columns are carefully retracted and opened gently and progressively over the entire length of the solid portion of the tumor. This maneuver is continued to expose the rostral and caudal cysts, if present. The opening of the spinal cord must allow exposure of the poles of the lesion and evaluation of the cyst walls but should not extend further than this. Pial traction suturing improves surgical exposure and reduces the severity of repeated trauma due to dissection. At the same time it exerts a continuous traction effect that alters the monitored evoked potentials. This is not surprising when one uses pial suspension sutures with as much tension. This can be accomplished with the use of a 6-0 suture without tension to hold the median pia mater and the dura mater close together rather than suspension with sutures and weights at the ends of the sutures.

The technique of tumor removal is determined on the basis of the surgical objective, tumor size, and gross and histologic characteristics of the tumor. If no plane is apparent between the tumor and surrounding spinal cord, it is likely that an infiltrative tumor is present. A biopsy specimen is obtained to establish a histologic diagnosis. If an infiltrating or malignant astrocytoma is identified and is consistent with the intraoperative findings, additional tumor removal is not warranted.

The first surgical maneuver consists of exposing a sufficient portion of the tumor to perform a biopsy with forceps and scissors, without coagulation. This is followed by immediate frozen-section histologic analysis, while careful hemostasis is carried out before proceeding with the operation. This examination sometimes provides the surgeon with no information at all. More often, however, it provides a great deal of information (e.g., when the limits between the tumor and the spinal cord are not immediately clear). Due to the limitation of accuracy of correct diagnosis in frozen section, the surgeon makes the ultimate decision with regard to not only the results from frozen section, but also gross findings, MRI and clinical characteristics of tumor.

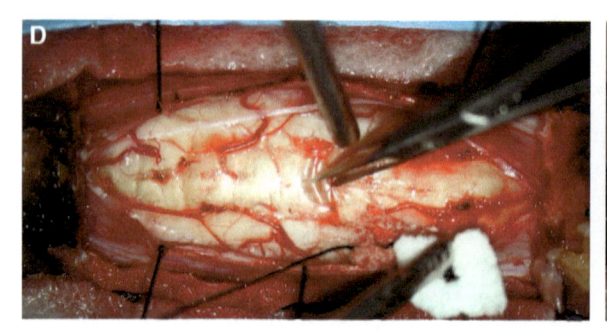

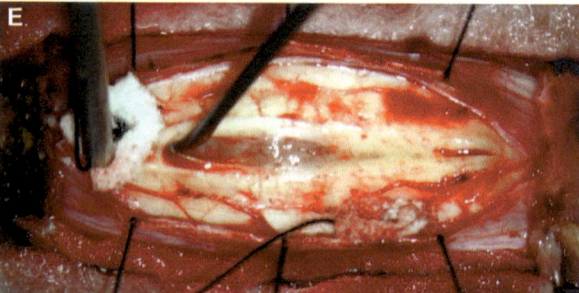

Fig. 26-2, cont'd **D,** Midline myelotomy with microscissors. **E,** Dissection of entire length of tumor with microdissector.

At the same time, the discovery of a cleavage plane (Fig. 26-3, *A*) is crucial. Ependymomas usually appear with a smooth reddish-gray glistening tumor surface that is sharply demarcated from the surrounding spinal cord. Various blood vessels can be seen crossing the tumor surface, distinguishing tumors from astrocytomas, which rarely display such surface characteristics.

Locating the cleavage plane makes tumor removal possible. If the cleavage plane is not found, the decision as to whether to remove the tumor must be deferred (Fig. 26-3, *B*).

However, in both cases the surgeon begins by reducing the tumor volume with the use of the Cavitron Ultrasonic Surgical Aspirator (Covidien, Boulder, CO), after setting the suction and vibratory force to a suitably low level (Fig. 26-3, *C*). Intratumoral resection is performed from inside to outside, and this is sometimes facilitated by the presence of a cyst or an intratumoral hematoma. After strict control of hemostasis, dissection can be started. There is a risk of arterial injury on the anterior side, especially in the thoracic region, the vascular territories of which are extremely precarious. Dissection is continued laterally on the side on which resection proves easier. If there is a capsule or if the tumor is not too friable, it can be grasped, allowing visualization of the correct cleavage plane (Fig. 26-3, *D*), which must be respected. Once it has been slightly re-

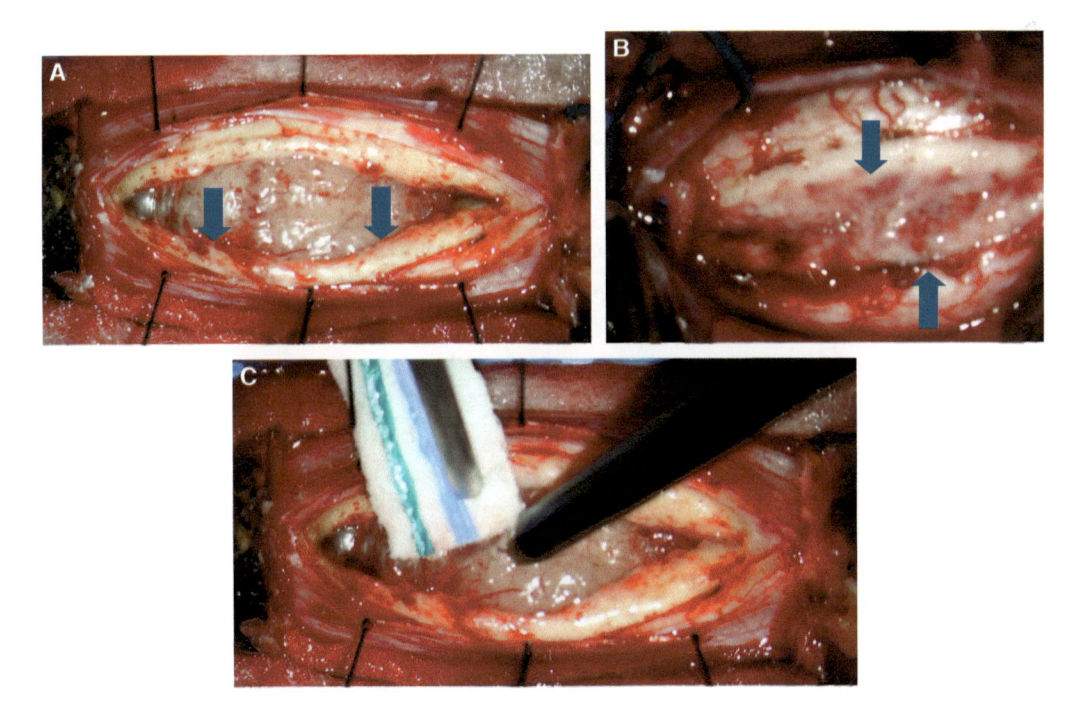

Fig. 26-3 Intraoperative photographs and postoperative x-ray displaying the procedure for removal of tumor with less traumatic methods. **A,** Identify cleavage plane. Ependymomas usually appear with a smooth reddish-gray glistening tumor surface that is sharply demarcated from the surrounding spinal cord (*blue arrows* indicate cleavage plane). **B,** Astrocytoma has a less clear cleavage line between the tumor and surrounding normal spinal cord. Total removal is rarely achieved, and the role of surgery is often limited to safe surgical resection or biopsy only (*blue arrows* indicate indistinct tumor margin). **C,** Reducing the volume of the tumor with the use of the Cavitron Ultrasonic Surgical Aspirator.

tracted, the spinal cord separates itself almost spontaneously from the sulcocommissural vessels, which diminish in size as the procedure progresses along the dorsal column.

The absence of a cleavage plane, particularly if the intraoperative appearance is suggestive of an infiltrating tumor, malignant or not, will prompt the surgeon to be cautious and avoid continuing tumor removal at all costs, because it may be both dangerous and useless.

The last difficulty lies in the vascular pedicle or pedicles that supply the tumor and are connected to the anterior spinal artery (Fig. 26-3, *E*). The danger here is real, as some tumors are large enough to separate and even cleave the spinal cord, resulting in true diastematomyelia and exposing the anterior spinal artery to all kinds of risks. Ignorance of this can lead to catastrophic operative results. In fact, when removal is macroscopically complete, there is no more bleeding. In view of the small size of the cord vessels, which stop bleeding spontaneously, it is unusual to have to coagulate an area outside the tumor. When tumor removal is complete, we inspect the wall of the cyst or cysts adjacent to the tumor bed. When the normal spinal cord tissue can be seen through a transparent cyst wall, the operation can be completed, because the cyst wall is similar to that seen in syringomyelic cavities and does not contain tumors (Fig. 26-3, *F*). If the wall of the cyst is thick, it should be removed along with the tumor and considered an intratumoral cyst; intraoperative histologic examination can help in making this decision.

After tumor removal, the dorsal columns are released from pial traction and brought back together with caution. Whenever possible, the cord is approximated with 6-0 pial sutures, and the arachnoid may be partially reconstituted if it was preserved on opening. The dura is closed in a watertight fashion and without tension. If required, a duraplasty is performed with fascia or lyophilized dura (Fig. 26-3, *G*). In addition to pial suture, there are few methods to prevent tethered cord. Gore-Tex durograft is beneficial to have less postoperative adhesion. Prevention of postlaminectomy focal kyphosis is important to protect posterior displacement of the spinal cord. Cutting the dentate ligaments so that the cord reconforms reestablishes CSF flow. If laminotomy has been performed, the bone is returned to its place, taking care to avoid compressing the spinal cord with internal fixation (Fig. 26-3, *H* and *I*). Depending on the situation, a nonsuction drain is inserted into the subfascial or subcutaneous space.

Postoperatively, early mobilization is encouraged to prevent complications of long-term bed rest, such as deep venous thrombosis and pneumonia. Patients at high risk for thromboembolic complications are usually managed with subcutaneous heparin. Orthostatic hypotension may occasionally occur after the removal of upper thoracic and cervical intramedullary neoplasms. This is usually a self-limiting problem that can be managed with liberalization of fluids and further gradual mobilization. Complications related to wound dehiscence, infection, and cerebrospinal fluid leaks are much more common in patients who have undergone prior surgery and/or radiation therapy. Early and aggressive management with physical and occupational therapy will optimize functional recovery.

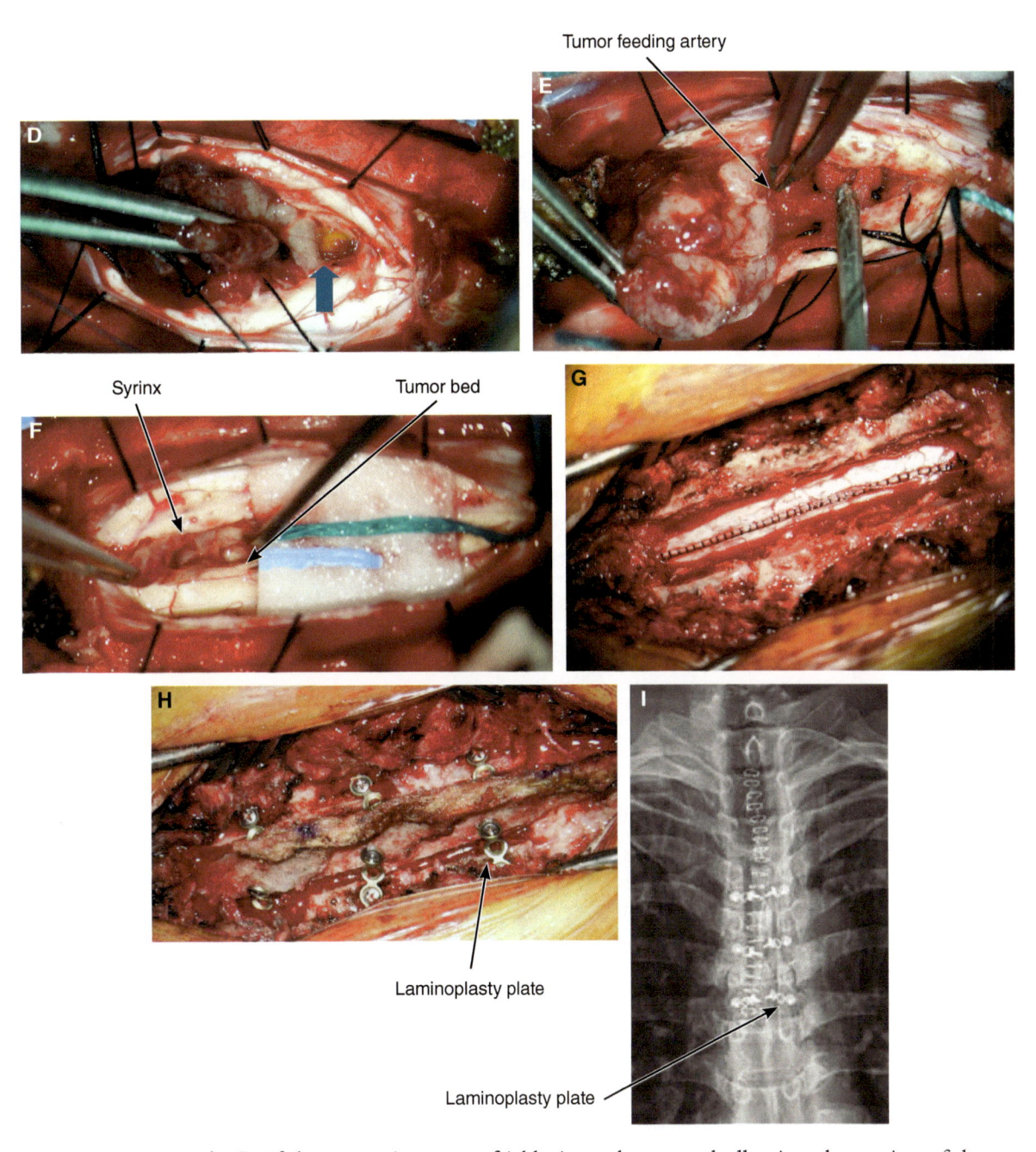

Fig. 26-3, cont'd **D,** If the tumor is not too friable, it can be grasped, allowing observation of the correct cleavage plane (*blue arrow*: identification of the rostral end of the tumor and cleavage plane by gentle traction). **E,** The vascular pedicles are connected to the anterior spinal artery, which should not be injured, and the vessel is cut and coagulated as close to the tumor as possible. **F,** When tumor removal is complete, the wall of the cyst or cysts adjacent to the tumor bed is inspected. When normal spinal cord tissue can be seen through a transparent cyst wall, the operation can be completed. **G,** The dura is closed in a watertight fashion and without tension; if necessary, a duraplasty is performed with fascia or lyophilized dura. **H** and **I,** If laminotomy has been performed, the bone is returned to its place, being careful to avoid compressing the spinal cord, with internal fixation.

CONCLUSION

Intramedullary spinal cord tumors have varying histopathologic types. The most common forms are astrocytomas and ependymomas. Patients with tumors who have progressive neurologic decline should undergo surgical resection or biopsy. The preoperative neurologic status of the patient is the most important variable in determining the postoperative functional outcome. To reduce the surgical risk, neuromonitoring and careful microsurgical dissection are mandatory. Adjuvant radiation therapy and chemotherapy are considered for high-grade astrocytomas or other rare malignant tumors.

TIPS FROM THE MASTERS

- The primary goal of intramedullary tumor surgery is to achieve complete removal of an intramedullary tumor without causing damage to the spinal cord.
- The preoperative neurologic status of the patient is the most important variable in determining the postoperative functional outcome.
- Intraoperative electrophysiologic monitoring have largely contributed to recent improvements in surgical results.
- It is essential to define the extent of the solid portion of the tumor to determine the length of the laminectomy.
- In ependymoma surgery, the most important step during surgical removal is finding the cleavage plane between the tumor and the spinal cord.
- Because most spinal cord astrocytomas are infiltrative and are associated with indistinct boundaries with the surrounding normal spinal cord, total removal of these tumors is rarely achieved, and biopsy and decompression are considered the primary goals of surgery.
- Identification of the dorsal midline spinal cord is critically important to avoid inadvertent posterior column injury. Techniques to identify the midline include identification of the small vein exiting from the sulcus, finding the imaginary midline between both sides of the dorsal root entry zone and making an imaginary line from the midline above and below lesion.
- The preoperative neurologic status of the patient is the most important variable in determining the postoperative functional outcome.

References (With Key References in Boldface)

1. Fogelholm R, Uutela T, Murros K. Epidemiology of central nervous system neoplasms. A regional survey in Central Finland. Acta Neurol Scand 69:129-136, 1984.
2. **Stein BM, McCormick PC. Intramedullary neoplasms and vascular malformations. Clin Neurosurg 39:361-387, 1992.**
3. Karikari IO, Nimjee SM, Hodges TR, et al. Impact of tumor histology on resectability and neurological outcome in primary intramedullary spinal cord tumors: a single-center experience with 102 patients. Neurosurgery 68:188-197; discussion 197, 2011.
4. Morota N, Deletis V, Constantini S, et al. The role of motor evoked potentials during surgery for intramedullary spinal cord tumors. Neurosurgery 41:1327-1336, 1997.
5. Yanni DS, Ulkatan S, Deletis V, et al. Utility of neurophysiological monitoring using dorsal column mapping in intramedullary spinal cord surgery. J Neurosurg Spine 12:623-628, 2010.

6. **Chamberlain MC, Tredway TL. Adult primary intradural spinal cord tumors: a review. Curr Neurol Neurosci Rep 11:320-328, 2011.**
7. Schwartz TH, McCormick PC. Intramedullary ependymomas: clinical presentation, surgical treatment strategies and prognosis. J Neurooncol 47:211-218, 2000.
8. Dvorak MF, Fisher CG, Hoekema J, et al. Factors predicting motor recovery and functional outcome after traumatic central cord syndrome: a long-term follow-up. Spine (Phila Pa 1976) 30:2303-2311, 2005.
9. Jeibmann A, Egensperger R, Kuchelmeister K, et al. Extent of surgical resection but not myxopapillary versus classical histopathological subtype affects prognosis in lumbo-sacral ependymomas. Histopathology 54:260-262, 2009.
10. Joaquim AF, Santos MJ, Tedeschi H. Surgical management of intramedullary spinal ependymomas. Arq Neuropsiquiatr 67:284-289, 2009.
11. **Lee J, Parsa AT, Ames CP, et al. Clinical management of intramedullary spinal ependymomas in adults. Neurosurg Clin N Am 17:21-27, 2006.**
12. Raco A, Esposito V, Lenzi J, et al. Long-term follow-up of intramedullary spinal cord tumors: a series of 202 cases. Neurosurgery 56:972-981; discussion 972-981, 2005.
13. Mork SJ, Loken A. Ependymoma: a follow-up study of 101 cases. Cancer 40:907-915, 1977.
14. Isaacson S. Radiation therapy and the management of intramedullary spinal cord tumors. J Neurooncol 47:231-238, 2000.
15. Kahan H, Sklar EM, Post MJ, et al. MR characteristics of histopathologic subtypes of spinal ependymoma. AJNR Am J Neuroradiol 17:143-150, 1996.
16. Yamada CY, Whitman GJ, Chew FS. Myxopapillary ependymoma of the filum terminale. AJR Am J Roentgenol 168:366, 1997.
17. Kaner T, Sasani M, Oktenoglu T, et al. Clinical analysis of 21 cases of spinal cord ependymoma: positive clinical results of gross total resection. J Korean Neurosurg Soc 47:102-106, 2010.
18. Moelleken SM, Seeger LL, Eckardt JJ, et al. Myxopapillary ependymoma with extensive sacral destruction: CT and MR findings. J Comput Assist Tomogr 16:164-166, 1992.
19. Wagle WA, Jaufman B, Mincy JE. Intradural extramedullary ependymoma: MR-pathologic correlation. J Comput Assist Tomogr 12:705-707, 1988.
20. Ohata K, Takami T, Gotou T, et al. Surgical outcome of intramedullary spinal cord ependymoma. Acta Neurochir (Wien) 141:341-346; discussion 346-347, 1999.
21. **Bostrom A, von Lehe M, Hartmann W, et al. Surgery for spinal cord ependymomas: outcome and prognostic factors. Neurosurgery 68:302-308; discussion 309, 2011.**
22. Hoshimaru M, Koyama T, Hashimoto N, et al. Results of microsurgical treatment for intramedullary spinal cord ependymomas: analysis of 36 cases. Neurosurgery 44:264-269, 1999.
23. Epstein FJ, Farmer JP, Freed D. Adult intramedullary spinal cord ependymomas: the result of surgery in 38 patients. J Neurosurg 79:204-209, 1993.
24. McCormick PC, Torres R, Post KD, et al. Intramedullary ependymoma of the spinal cord. J Neurosurg 72:523-532, 1990.
25. Bagley CA, Wilson S, Kothbauer KF, et al. Long term outcomes following surgical resection of myxopapillary ependymomas. Neurosurg Rev 32:321-334; discussion 334, 2009.
26. Jallo GI, Zagzag D, Epstein F. Intramedullary subependymoma of the spinal cord. Neurosurgery 38:251-257, 1996.
27. Matsumura A, Nose T, Hori A. Intramedullary subependymoma of the spinal cord. Neurosurgery 39:879, 1996.
28. Jang WY, Lee JK, Lee JH, et al. Intramedullary subependymoma of the thoracic spinal cord. J Clin Neurosci 16:851-853, 2009.
29. Yadav RK, Agarwal S, Saini J, et al. Imaging appearance of subependymoma: a rare tumor of the cord. Indian J Cancer 45:33-35, 2008.
30. Houten JK, Cooper PR. Spinal cord astrocytomas: presentation, management and outcome. J Neurooncol 47:219-224, 2000.
31. Roonprapunt C, Houten JK. Spinal cord astrocytomas: presentation, management, and outcome. Neurosurg Clin N Am 17:29-36, 2006.
32. Santi M, Mena H, Wong K, et al. Spinal cord malignant astrocytomas. Clinicopathologic features in 36 cases. Cancer 98:554-561, 2003.

33. Rodrigues GB, Waldron JN, Wong CS, et al. A retrospective analysis of 52 cases of spinal cord glioma managed with radiation therapy. Int J Radiat Oncol Biol Phys 48:837-842, 2000.
34. Abdi S, Lenthall RK. Haemorrhage within an intramedullary astrocytoma presenting with a mild clinical course and a fluid-fluid level on MRI. Br J Radiol 77:691-693, 2004.
35. Abel TJ, Chowdhary A, Thapa M, et al. Spinal cord pilocytic astrocytoma with leptomeningeal dissemination to the brain. Case report and review of the literature. J Neurosurg 105:508-514, 2006.
36. Cristante L, Herrmann HD. Surgical management of intramedullary spinal cord tumors: functional outcome and sources of morbidity. Neurosurgery 35:69-74; discussion 74-76, 1994.
37. Merchant TE, Zhu Y, Thompson SJ, et al. Preliminary results from a Phase II trial of conformal radiation therapy for pediatric patients with localised low-grade astrocytoma and ependymoma. Int J Radiat Oncol Biol Phys 52:325-332, 2002.
38. **Minehan KJ, Brown PD, Scheithauer BW, et al. Prognosis and treatment of spinal cord astrocytoma. Int J Radiat Oncol Biol Phys 73:727-733, 2009.**
39. Abdel-Wahab M, Etuk B, Palermo J, et al. Spinal cord gliomas: a multi-institutional retrospective analysis. Int J Radiat Oncol Biol Phys 64:1060-1071, 2006.
40. Balmaceda C. Chemotherapy for intramedullary spinal cord tumors. J Neurooncol 47:293-307, 2000.
41. Foreman NK, Hay TC, Handler M. Chemotherapy for spinal cord astrocytoma. Med Pediatr Oncol 30:311-312, 1998.
42. Chamberlain MC. Temozolomide for recurrent low-grade spinal cord gliomas in adults. Cancer 113:1019-1024, 2008.
43. Chamoun RB, Alaraj AM, Al Kutoubi AO, et al. Role of temozolomide in spinal cord low grade astrocytomas: results in two paediatric patients. Acta Neurochir (Wien) 148:175-179; discussion 180, 2006.
44. **Kim WH, Yoon SH, Kim CY, et al. Temozolomide for malignant primary spinal cord glioma: an experience of six cases and a literature review. J Neurooncol 101:247-254, 2011.**
45. Tseng HM, Kuo LT, Lien HC, et al. Prolonged survival of a patient with cervical intramedullary glioblastoma multiforme treated with total resection, radiation therapy, and temozolomide. Anticancer Drugs 21:963-967, 2010.
46. Cristante L, Herrmann HD. Surgical management of intramedullary hemangioblastoma of the spinal cord. Acta Neurochir (Wien) 141:333-339; discussion 339-340, 1999.
47. Lonser RR, Weil RJ, Wanebo JE, et al. Surgical management of spinal cord hemangioblastomas in patients with von Hippel-Lindau disease. J Neurosurg 98:106-116, 2003.
48. Colombo N, Kucharczyk W, Brant-Zawadzki M, et al. Magnetic resonance imaging of spinal cord hemangioblastoma. Acta Radiol Suppl 369:734-737, 1986.
49. Rebner M, Gebarski SS. Magnetic resonance imaging of spinal-cord hemangioblastoma. AJNR Am J Neuroradiol 6:287-289, 1985.
50. Lee DK, Choe WJ, Chung CK, et al. Spinal cord hemangioblastoma: surgical strategy and clinical outcome. J Neurooncol 61:27-34, 2003.
51. Jallo GI, Freed D, Epstein FJ. Spinal cord gangliogliomas: a review of 56 patients. J Neurooncol 68:71-77, 2004.
52. Machiya T, Yoshita M, Iwasa K, et al. Primary spinal intramedullary lymphoma mimicking ependymoma. Neurology 68:872, 2007.
53. Abrey LE, Yahalom J, DeAngelis LM. Treatment for primary CNS lymphoma: the next step. J Clin Oncol 18:3144-3150, 2000.
54. Salame K, Merimsky O, Yosipov J, et al. Primary intramedullary spinal melanoma: diagnostic and treatment problems. J Neurooncol 36:79-83, 1998.
55. Yamasaki T, Kikuchi H, Yamashita J, et al. Primary spinal intramedullary malignant melanoma: case report. Neurosurgery 25:117-121, 1989.
56. Farrokh D, Fransen P, Faverly D. MR findings of a primary intramedullary malignant melanoma: case report and literature review. AJNR Am J Neuroradiol 22:1864-1866, 2001.
57. Maroon JC, Abla AA, Wilberger JI, et al. Central cord syndrome. Clin Neurosurg 37:612-621, 1991.
58. Nowak DD, Lee JK, Gelb DE, et al. Central cord syndrome. J Am Acad Orthop Surg 17:756-765, 2009.

Chapter 27

Surgical Management of Nerve Sheath Tumors

Matthew C. Tate, Nicholas M. Barbaro,
Pierre Reynald Theodore, Christopher P. Ames

*A*ggressive microsurgical resection remains the optimal treatment option for intradural extramedullary (IDEM) tumors.[1,2] Recent improvements in surgical techniques have enabled improved control and clinical benefit while allowing for minimal morbidity. In this chapter we will discuss the pertinent clinical features of IDEM tumors as well as modern surgical approaches for resection of IDEM tumors, with a particular emphasis on strategies for aggressive resection of paraspinal tumors because of their complex management and recent advances in surgical technique.

CLINICAL FEATURES

Approximately 10% to 15% of all central nervous system tumors are spine tumors, and two thirds of these intraspinal tumors are IDEM tumors.[3-5] Among IDEM tumors, nerve sheath tumors (NSTs) and meningiomas account for most IDEM tumors. Less common IDEM tumors include paragangliomas, neurenteric cysts, and metastases.[1] In recently published series, the NST/meningioma ratio was 2:1.[4,6] The age distribution among patients with IDEM tumors is bimodal, with one peak occurring at age 40 (primarily NSTs) and a second peak occurring at age 70 (primarily meningiomas).[6] Meningiomas are more common among women, whereas NSTs are more common in men.[1,6] Distribution along the spinal axis depends on tumor type. NSTs are relatively evenly distributed along the spinal axis, whereas meningiomas are primarily localized to the cervical and thoracic spine.[6,7] Tumor size is also a function of location: thoracic tumors are smaller than cervical lesions, and all other regions are intermediate.[1] Four percent of patients have multiple tumors, all of which are schwannomas.[6] Fifteen percent to 44% of NSTs are paraspinal, a finding more common in patients with neurofibromatosis.[7,8] Patients with neurofibromatosis also have a higher incidence of multiple tumors and malignancy and typically present earlier than those with other IDEM tumor subtypes.[7]

The age at presentation for meningiomas was higher than that for NSTs (58 versus 45 years).[6] NSTs present most commonly with localized pain or radiculopathy, whereas meningiomas more often cause myelopathy, which is likely a function of an increased incidence of thoracic tumors.[6,9] The average duration of symptoms at the time of diagnosis among all IDEM tumors is 11 months, with schwannomas having a longer duration than meningiomas (15 versus 8 months).[4,6] Among patients with NSTs, pain, not necessarily radicular, is the most common presenting symptom and is seen in 60% of all NSTs.[7] The frequency of pain as a function of spinal axis level is 95%, 75%, and 30% for lumbar, thoracic, and cervical tumors, respectively. Other common presenting symptoms of NSTs are motor dysfunction (24% overall, 43% of cervical spine tumors, 18% of thoracic tumors), sensory deficits (14% overall), scoliosis (5%), and spasticity (5%, only observed in C1-2 NSTs).[7,10] Only 2% of patients were neurologically intact at the time of diagnosis.

General indications for surgery include intractable pain or paresthesias, weakness, myelopathy, and spinal cord compression. The goal of surgery is maximal resection, which has been shown to decrease recurrence rates.[1] Another important consideration is maintenance of spinal stability and shape. In a recent series, 72% of patients were treated through a posterior approach; the remainder were equally divided between lateral and anterior approaches.[7] Recent series reported gross total resection in 84% to 90% of patients, whereas 10% to 16% underwent subtotal resection, as determined by residual disease on postoperative MRI imaging.[1,7] Among those with subtotal resections, most had paravertebral intraforaminal and extraforaminal extension, and none of these was located in the thoracic spine. In 5% to 6% of patients their IDEM tumors recur, despite apparent complete resection on immediate postoperative imaging.[6,7] Spinal instrumentation was reported to be employed in 13% of NST resections.[7]

Intraoperative monitoring is a useful adjunct in IDEM surgery for evaluating the integrity of the major spinal cord pathways.[11] In particular, somatosensory evoked responses and motor evoked responses can be used continuously throughout the procedure to be sure that there has not been excessive manipulation of the spinal cord. In addition, if it is desirable to attempt resection of the lesion while sparing as much motor function as possible, the use of electrical stimulation and electromyographic (EMG) monitoring of appropriate muscles can be useful. This is typically used for cervical roots that innervate the upper extremities or lumbar roots. Most schwannomas involve primarily the dorsal roots, so ventral motor fascicles can be spared in most cases. The use of microsurgical techniques with neurophysiologic monitoring can allow gross total resections to be performed with minimal motor deficits, if any, in most cases. It should also be noted that in cases where nerve root sacrifice is essential for gross total resection, a series reported by Kim et al[12] demonstrated a milder morbidity profile than predicted. Only 23% of patients with sacrificed roots had a clinically referable neurologic deficit, and none of the deficits were complete.

Complications of IDEM surgery included cerebrospinal fluid leak (7.5%), new neurologic deficit (6%), vertebral artery injury (1.5%), postlaminectomy kyphosis (1.5%), and deep venous thrombosis (1.5%).[7] A recent study evaluated functional outcomes (modified Odom criteria[13]) and demonstrated a 94% excellent or good result and only 1.5% poor outcomes at 1 month postoperatively.[6] Overall, patients in that study had additional, although small, improvements at subsequent follow-up examinations. Another study reported functional outcome (Frankel scale[14]) after NST resection. Forty-four percent of patients improved by one grade and 12% improved two grades, whereas 39% were unchanged and 5% worsened neurologically.[7] This is consistent with results of other studies demonstrating early, sustained postoperative improvement.[4] The extent of resection (total versus subtotal) has been shown to predict clinical improvement in patients with IDEM tumors.[1] However, all patients with surgical morbidity in one series had undergone complete resections, indicating that aggressive resection may impart some additional surgical risk. This may be particularly important in the thoracic spine, where morbidity has been reported to be higher than at other levels.[1] The patient's sex, tumor size, and histologic type (schwannoma versus meningioma) were not found to be predictors of outcome.

SURGICAL APPROACHES AND CONSIDERATIONS

The goals of surgical treatment of IDEM tumors are to maximize resection of the tumor mass while maintaining the stability of the vertebral column. This often requires combined or multiple approaches. In this section we will discuss the basic principles of surgical resection of IDEM tumors as a function of location along the spinal axis (Table 27-1).

CERVICAL AND UPPER THORACIC SPINE (T1-3)

The preferred approaches for most IDEM tumors of the cervical levels are (1) midline, posterior through a standard laminectomy/facetectomy, or (2) the direct anterior approach. For anterior C1-2 tumors, a far-lateral transcondylar approach or suboccipital craniectomy may be used.[10] A recently published classification scheme offers a systematic approach to the selection of a surgical approach based on tumor location[15]

Table 27-1 Recommended Surgical Approach for Each Type of Tumor

PUTH Classification	Tumor Location	Involved Section	Approach
Type 1	Intraspinal, lateral to the cord (intraextradural)	A	Posterior
Type 2	Posterior to the cord	I, II, III ± A	Posterior
Type 3	Intraforaminal or extraforaminal; intraextraspinal	B, C ± A	Posterior ± facetectomy or anterolateral
Type 4	Anterior to the cord and/or far-extraforaminal	IV, V, and/or section D	Anterior or anterolateral
Type 5	Posterior and lateral	Type 2 + 3	Posterior ± facetectomy
Type 6	Anterior and lateral	Type 3 + 4	Anterior or anterolateral
Type 7	Anterior, posterior, and lateral	Type 1 + 2 + 3 + 4	Combined

From Jiang L, Lv Y, Liu XG, et al. Results of surgical treatment of cervical dumbbell tumors: surgical approach and development of an anatomic classification system. Spine 34:1307-1314, 2009.
PUTH, Peking University Third Hospital.

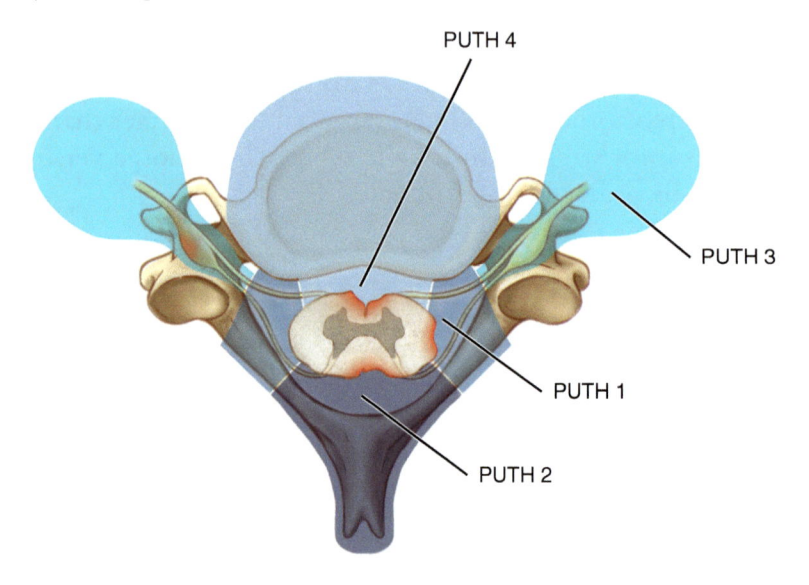

Fig. 27-1 Peking University Third Hospital *(PUTH)* classification scheme based on tumor location. (Adapted from Jiang L, Lv Y, Liu XG, et al. Results of surgical treatment of cervical dumbbell tumors: surgical approach and development of an anatomic classification system.[15])

(Fig. 27-1). For lesions involving multiple levels or resulting in structural compromise, instrumentation and fusion may be required. For the subaxial spine, this generally involves lateral mass screw fixation for C3 through C6 and lateral mass or pedicle screw fixation at C7. For those cases involving C1 and C2, occipital-cervical fusion may be necessary, depending on the extent of bony erosion and joint involvement.

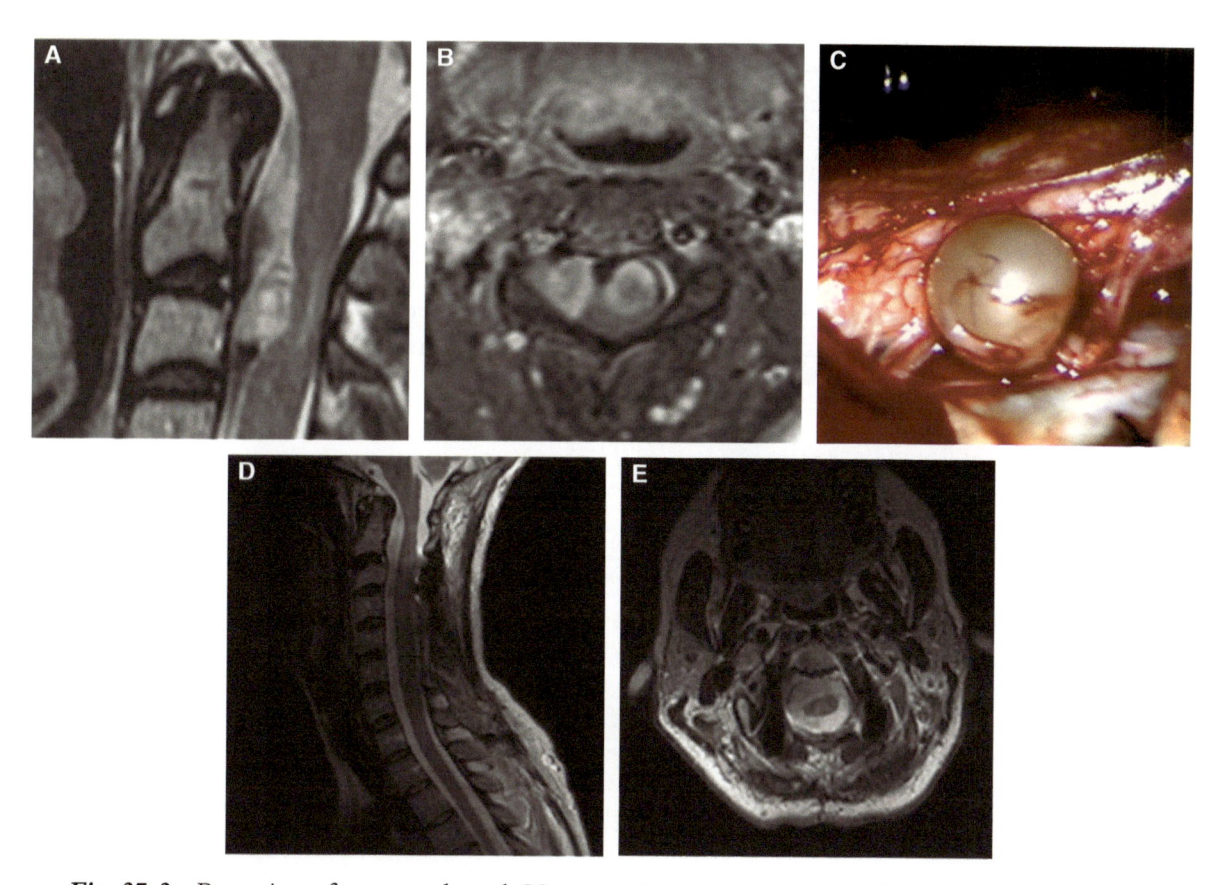

Fig. 27-2 Resection of an anterolateral C2 tumor. **A,** Preoperative sagittal and **B,** axial MRI scans of a C2 nerve sheath tumor. **C,** The tumor was resected through a posterolateral approach, which provides access, as shown in the intraoperative photograph. **D** and **E,** A gross total resection was achieved, as shown in the postoperative MRI scans.

C1-2 tumors represent a challenging subset of cervical NSTs, given the distinctive anatomy at those levels. Tumors at C1-2 are often larger than those in the subaxial spine, presumably because of the increased mean diameter of the bony canal, which results in delayed symptom onset.[10] Surgical access for posterior, anterolateral, or posterolateral lesions is through a standard posterior laminectomy. Debulking of the lateral portion of the tumor during this approach allows improved visualization of the spinal cord–tumor interface. Sectioning of the posterior nerve roots and dentate ligament also improves visualization of the spinal cord–tumor interface in anterolateral tumors accessed through the posterior approach.[16,17] An operating microscope and neurophysiologic monitoring aid in decreasing cord manipulation. For optimal access to anterolateral lesions, a laminectomy and partial facetectomy are a reasonable option (Fig. 27-2), but care must be taken to maintain more than two thirds of the ipsilateral joint surface.[18] In patients with C1 tumors anterior to the spinal cord, a far-lateral transcondylar approach is typically preferred.[10] We favor a two-stage approach for C2 nerve sheath tumors that cross the vertebral artery into the area posterior to the carotid sheath. The lesions are first approached posteriorly and resected up to the capsule at the vertebral artery. A second-stage anterior lateral approach is then used to deliver the lesions from behind the carotid sheath (Fig. 27-3).

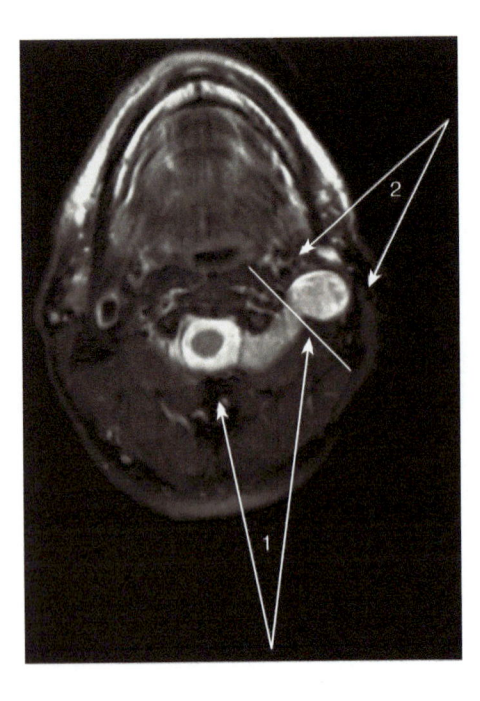

Fig. 27-3 Combined approach to C2 tumor. Axial T2 MRI scan demonstrates a C2 schwannoma crossing the vertebral artery. The lesions are first approached posteriorly *(1)* and resected up to the capsule at the vertebral artery. A second-stage anterolateral approach is then used to deliver the lesions from behind the carotid sheath *(2)*.

Fig. 27-4 Posterior approach to the vertebral artery. This spine model demonstrates the position of the vertebral artery relative to the pedicle and the nerve root, as seen in a standard posterior approach. (*P*, pedicle.)

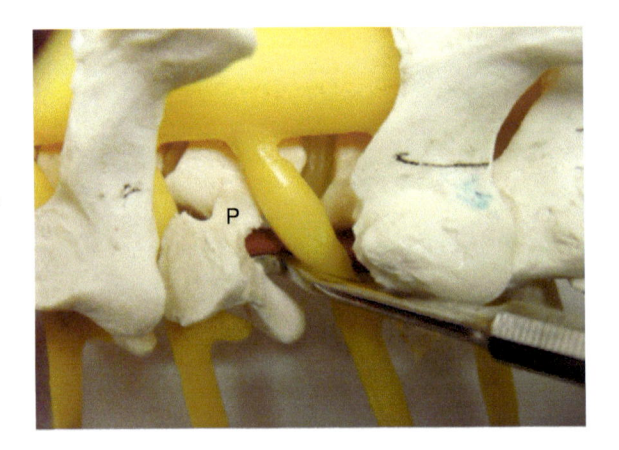

An important consideration in the surgical management of cervical IDEM tumors is the relationship of the vertebral artery to the tumor mass. Proximal and distal control should be attempted before tumor resection for patients in whom the vertebral artery is adherent to and displaced by the tumor capsule, as is most commonly seen with cervical NSTs. The vertebral artery and its branches can then be dissected from the tumor and transposed, if necessary. From a posterior approach, the vertebral artery can be identified by following the nerve root laterally to the edge of the vertebral body, and resection of the pedicle may be necessary (Figs. 27-4 and 27-5). This view of the vertebral artery during a posterior approach is particularly useful for en bloc resection of malignant paraspinal NSTs where a broader exposure is needed. Anterior approaches for spondylectomy or en bloc procedures for sarcomatous NSTs also require identification and often lateral mobilization or sacrifice of the vertebral artery. The vertebral artery can be found directly under the transverse process at the levels of C6 and above and can be mobilized laterally, if necessary (Fig. 27-6).

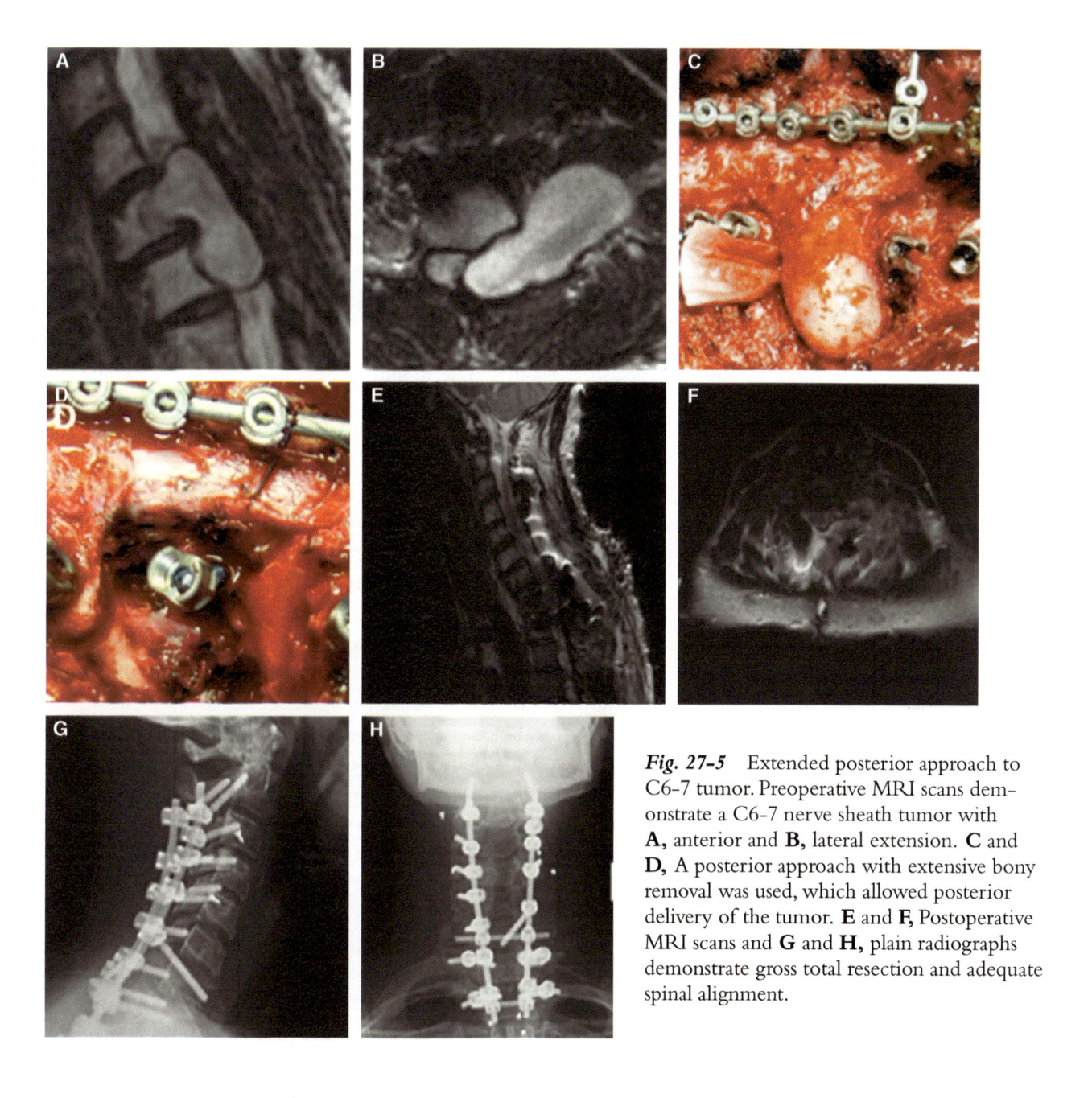

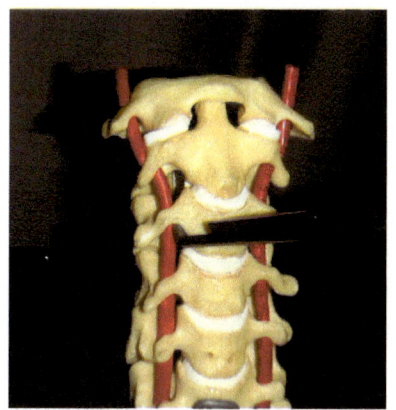

Fig. 27-5 Extended posterior approach to C6-7 tumor. Preoperative MRI scans demonstrate a C6-7 nerve sheath tumor with **A,** anterior and **B,** lateral extension. **C** and **D,** A posterior approach with extensive bony removal was used, which allowed posterior delivery of the tumor. **E** and **F,** Postoperative MRI scans and **G** and **H,** plain radiographs demonstrate gross total resection and adequate spinal alignment.

Fig. 27-6 Anterior approach to the vertebral artery. This spine model shows the vertebral artery posterior to the transverse process, as seen from an anterior cervical approach.

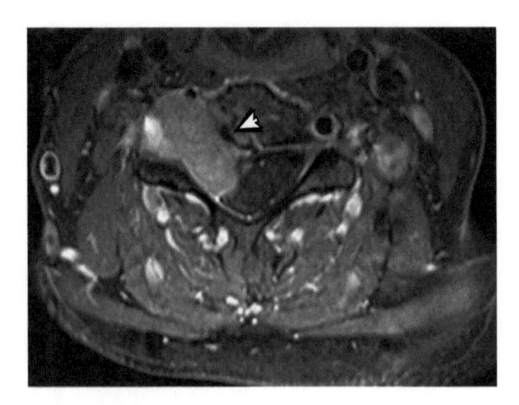

Fig. 27-7 Vertebral artery injury. Axial MRI scan of a nerve sheath tumor demonstrating vertebral artery injury occurring during surgical resection. *Arrowhead* shows the course of the vertebral artery relative to the tumor.

One particular concern during more aggressive anterior approaches is the sympathetic chain. Although postoperative Horner's syndrome is rare, it is important to understand the relationship of the sympathetic chain. Techniques that can decrease the risk of injury to the sympathetic chain are stripping rather than sectioning muscle and placing retractor blades under the longus colli muscle. The sympathetic chain courses, on average, 11 mm lateral to the medial longus colli border. For large paraspinal NSTs, a combination of the two approaches is often needed. In our recent series of large (greater than 2.5 cm) combined intradural and paraspinal NSTs, 2 of 23 patients had intraoperative injury to the vertebral artery. Both cases involved malignant NSTs that had significant vertebral body erosion (Fig. 27-7). Bleeding was controlled in both cases with light packing. Postoperative angiography demonstrated a patent artery in one patient and an occluded artery in the other. Neither patient experienced any significant clinical sequelae from the vertebral artery injury.

In addition to the previously mentioned approaches to the cervical spine, the posterior subscapular technique allows access to the lower brachial plexus and upper thoracic nerve roots (C7-T3) while avoiding the morbidity of anterior approaches to this region.[8] However, most neurosurgeons are less familiar with this technique. An excellent review of the technique was recently published.[8] Briefly, the patient is placed prone with the ipsilateral arm abducted and flexed at the shoulder. A curved incision is made with its center between the thoracic spinous processes and the medial scapula. The muscles connecting the spine to the scapula (trapezius, rhomboid, levator scapulae) are sectioned, and the ends are marked for later reapproximation. A retractor is placed between the scapula and thoracic spinous processes. The first rib is resected to a margin of 5 cm lateral to the rib transverse process junction. The supraclavicular space is opened, and the lower trunk is isolated from the subclavian vessels. This approach is particularly useful for large lesions that extend intraforaminally. The combined posterior foraminotomy, facetectomy, or laminectomy can allow access to both intraspinal and extraspinal tumor, thereby obviating the need for a two-stage procedure. For lesions that are not accessible from a combined posterior midline and subscapular approach, other approaches should be considered.

For midline ventral intradural cervical lesions, especially those that span more than one vertebral segment, we prefer the cervical transpedicular technique, which we developed at the University of California, San Francisco.[19] (For details and case examples, see Chapter 23.) As an alternative, a vertebrectomy can be performed through an anterior cervical approach, followed by anterior fusion and instrumentation.

MIDDLE AND LOWER THORACIC SPINE

The major approaches to this region of the spine are thoracotomy, thoracoscopy, costotransversectomy, transpedicular, or a combination thereof.

Thoracotomy

The traditional method for addressing IDEM tumors with a significant intrathoracic component has been a combined posterior and open thoracotomy approach. True anterior approaches are limited by the inherent morbidity, particularly in patients with comorbid conditions. Most significantly, there is a high risk of cerebrospinal fluid fistula, given the negative intrathoracic pressure during inspiration. Morbidity associated with rib resection and parietal pleura disruption includes intercostal neuralgia and postthoracotomy syndromes. Many neurosurgeons are transitioning to less-invasive techniques for anterior approaches to the thoracic spine, often referred to as *mini-open* thoracotomy. Advantages include a smaller surgical wound, decreased surgical morbidity and, with experience, the ability to perform these transthoracic procedures without the need for assistance from a cardiothoracic surgeon. Disadvantages include a steep learning curve for the neurosurgeon and a diminished operative view. Innovations in video-assisted thoracoscopic surgery (VATS), with selective single-lung ventilation through a dual-lumen endotracheal tube, facilitate exposure and have helped to reduce surgical complications from these more restricted approaches.

Thoracoscopic Approach

The thoracoscopic approach involves placing the patient in a lateral decubitus position. In the midaxillary line, two to three intervertebral spaces below the vertebral l level of interest, a 10 mm camera port is placed. The "working incision" is centered over the vertebrae of interest, as determined by fluoroscopic imaging or direct visualization. One or two additional ports are placed, typically 1.5 cm, to permit suction/irrigation and lung retraction. After medial retraction of the lung and downward retraction of the diaphragm, if needed, the parietal pleura overlying the tumor and vertebral levels is incised, exposing the intercostal segmental arteries and veins. Bipolar cautery is used to ablate segmental vessels, which can be large and associated with brisk bleeding before tumor resection (Fig. 27-8).

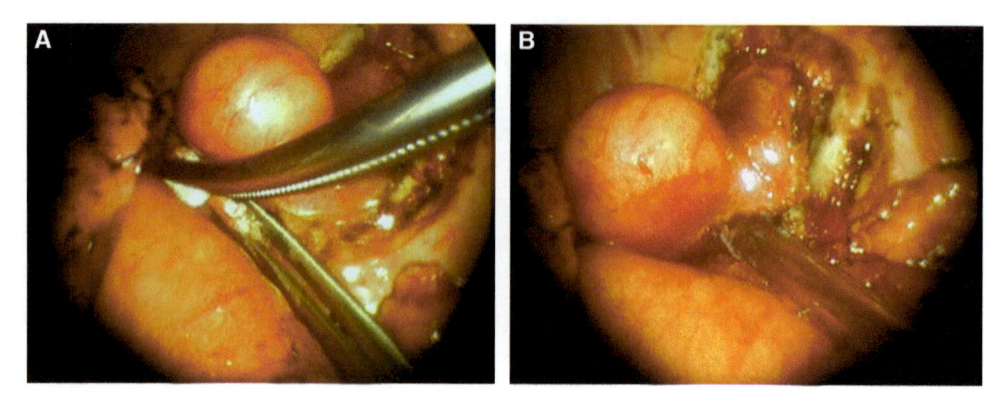

Fig. 27-8 VATS for paraspinal tumor resection. Intraoperative photographs of resection of left thoracic paraspinal ganglioneuroma arising from the sympathetic trunk. The tumor was identified adjacent to **A,** the descending aorta and dissected free from **B,** the fifth rib head.

An additional advantage of the trajectory of these min-open approaches is the minimal bony removal necessary to access the tumor; thus instrumentation is typically not needed. For lesions without a significant foraminal or canal component, single-stage anterior surgery is often sufficient. Small and cystic lesions can be removed thoracoscopically. For lesions with significant medial foraminal involvement, a posterior approach is often performed first to section the nerve root and disconnect the lesion from the spinal canal. The larger portion of the lesion is then delivered from the chest cavity with a mini-open thoracotomy or thoracoscopically.

For patients with dumbbell tumors in this region or primarily intraspinal pathology, a midline posterior incision is used. From this approach it is important to fully visualize the proximal affected nerve roots and their course through the foramina. As with cervical lesions, the use of the operating microscope and neurophysiologic monitoring can reduce the incidence of spinal cord deficits.

Costotransversectomy and Transpedicular Approach
Another surgical option for patients with paraspinal IDEM tumors is costotransversectomy combined with pedicular resection, which allows a posterior-lateral exposure and a more ventral view. Multiple variations of this approach exist, primarily depending on the size of the tumor and the potential for instrumentation. Classically, this involves making a T-shaped or a J-shaped incision, with the transverse portion at the level of tumor involvement. Muscle dissection is performed to expose the transverse process, lamina, facet, and ribs. In practice, we perform a midline incision and increase the length of the incision as needed to facilitate soft tissue retraction and ventral visualization. A subperiosteal circumferential dissection along the rib is followed to the costotransverse joint, which is opened sharply. Eventually the transverse process, medial rib, rib head, and costovertebral ligament are removed, thereby providing a posterolateral view of the spinal canal Next, the canal is opened through laminectomy, facetectomy, and pediculectomy, thereby exposing the lateral spinal cord and allowing visualization of the entire anterior-posterior extent of the vertebral body. For lesions

with a significant midline component or vertebral body erosion, we favor the transpedicular technique.

LUMBAR SPINE

Spine tumors involving the lumbar segments are typically accessed through either a transabdominal anterior, midline posterior, or retroperitoneal approach.

Midline Posterior Approach

Midline posterior approaches are often used for intradural and combined lesions. For combined lesions with large foraminal components, complete facet removal is often necessary to fully visualize the paraspinal area. Instrumented posterior spine fusion is often employed in these cases to address the instability resulting from the complete pars resection.

Retroperitoneal Approach

The retroperitoneal approach is typically the route of choice for anterior paraspinal tumors, either through a paramedian or lateral incision, because of the decreased risk of bowel obstructions/adhesions or retrograde ejaculation as compared with transabdominal approaches (Fig. 27-9). Transperitoneal approaches are used more commonly for malignant nerve sheath tumors and sarcomas where adjacent structure involvement is more common and lymph node biopsy is necessary. In terms of external landmarks, the umbilicus and superior iliac crest overlie the L3-4 and L4-5 levels, respectively. L5-S1 is at the midpoint between the umbilicus and pubic symphysis.[8] A lateral incision is usually optimal for retroperitoneal access of the upper lumbar spine, typically L1-L4. The patient is placed in the lateral decubitus position with the left side up for improved access of the left L4-5 space and easier retraction of the spleen (versus the liver) on the left side. An incision is made extending from the final rib to the iliac crest. Dissection is carried down to the transversus abdominis, which is incised for visualization of the retroperitoneal space. As with the paramedian approach, the peritoneum is swept medially along with the abdominal contents by blunt dissection. The psoas muscle is identified and separated from its attachment to the vertebral bodies, thereby exposing the anterior spine.

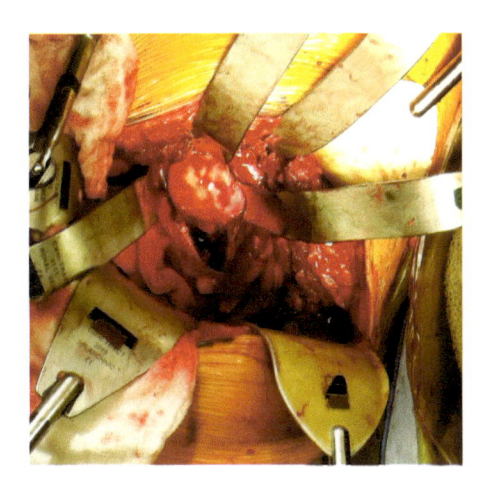

Fig. 27-9 Intraoperative photograph of resection of an L3-4 schwannoma through a retroperitoneal approach.

Paramedian Approach

For the paramedian approach, which is optimal for lower lumbar access, the patient is placed in the supine position, and an incision is made from 5 cm above the umbilicus to 5 mm superior to the pubic symphysis. The dissection is carried down to the posterior rectus sheath, which is incised to expose the retroperitoneal space. Intraabdominal contents are retracted medially, revealing the psoas muscle, taking care to avoid injury to the ureter or genitofemoral nerve. The aorta and inferior vena cava bifurcations are at the L4-5 and L5 levels, respectively. These vessels are mobilized to provide anterior access to the vertebral levels of interest, which may require ligation of lumbar segmental vessels or iliolumbar veins in the case of inferior vena cava manipulation.

SIGNATURE CASE

A 38-year-old woman with a history of neurofibromatosis type I initially presented with progressive lower extremity weakness. MRI demonstrated a right lateral C2 nerve sheath tumor (Fig. 27-10). The patient was taken to the operating room for resection through a posterolateral approach. Postoperative imaging confirmed a gross total resection. The patient's lower extremity strength was stable at the time of discharge.

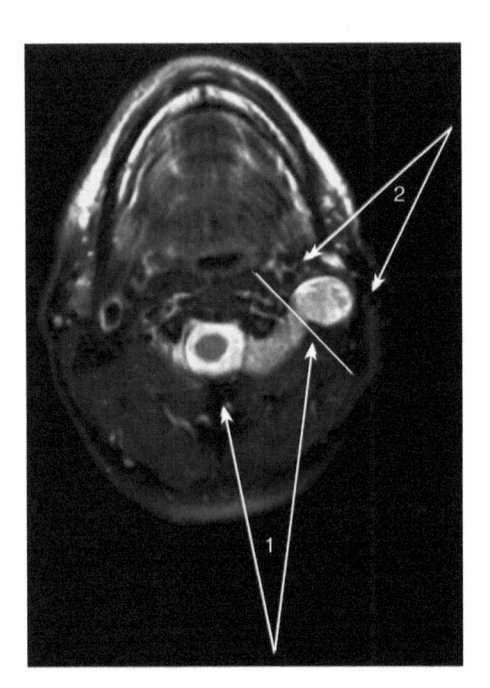

Fig. 27-10 Combined approach to C2 tumor. Axial T2 MRI scan demonstrates a C2 schwannoma crossing the vertebral artery. The lesions are first approached posteriorly *(1)* and resected up to the capsule at the vertebral artery. A second-stage anterolateral approach is then used to deliver the lesions from behind the carotid sheath *(2)*.

CONCLUSION

Aggressive surgical resection remains the mainstay of therapy for intradural, extramedullary spinal cord tumors. Recent advances allowing for improved extent of resection while minimizing morbidity include vertebral artery exposure/manipulation, thoracoscopic assistance, and improved intraoperative neurophysiology. Finally, staged procedures involving colleagues in otolaryngology, thoracic surgery, and vascular surgery provide new avenues for en bloc IDEM tumor resection.

BAILOUT TECHNIQUES

Usually, in patients with intradural extramedullary tumors, a complete resection is possible. In recurrent intradural tumors, such as higher-grade meningiomas, or in patients who have had prior radiation therapy, it is not always possible to separate the tumor from the pial plane or vertebral artery. In these cases the tumor is internally debulked to decrease the effect of the mass on the spinal cord, and postoperative radiosurgery is used.

For ventral tumors, wide transpedicular exposure can be of tremendous benefit for directly visualizing the spinal cord plane. Neuromonitoring can be quite helpful in patients with intradural tumors but becomes less reliable for combined intradural extradural lesions with brachial plexus or retroperitoneal peripheral nerve extension. In these cases we use nerve root stimulation during resection.

Occasionally, vertebral artery injury may occur in more malignant lesions in the cervical spine with extradural extension. Usually, persistent Surgicel tamponade will stop the bleeding, but occasionally, additional bone resection may be required to locate the site of injury. Postoperative angiography is then performed to evaluate for dissection.

TIPS FROM THE MASTERS

- For cervical tumors with a component anterior to the cord, a two-stage approach with posterior resection up to the vertebral artery followed by anterolateral removal is effective.
- Monitoring of somatosensory and motor evoked potentials during resection are helpful adjuncts to ensure that excessive cord manipulation has not occurred.
- Particularly for cases of en bloc tumor removal, adequate visualization of the vertebral artery proximal and distal to the intended resection margins is essential.
- Vertebral artery injury during tumor resection can often be successfully treated with a combination of a hemostatic agent and direct pressure.

References (With Key References in Boldface)

1. **Prevedello DM, Koerbel A, Tatsui CE, et al. [Prognostic factors in the treatment of the intradural extramedullary tumors: a study of 44 cases]. Arq Neuropsiquiatr 61:241-247, 2003.**
2. Wilkins RH, Rengachary SS. Neurosurgery. New York: McGraw-Hill, 1985.
3. Ropper AH, Adams RD, Victor M, et al. Adams and Victor's Principles of Neurology, 9th ed. New York: McGraw-Hill, 2009.
4. Hufana V, Tan JS, Tan KK. Microsurgical treatment for spinal tumours. Singapore Med J 46:74-77, 2005.
5. Porchet F, Sajadi A, Villemure JG. [Spinal tumors: clinical aspects, classification and surgical treatment] Praxis (Bern 1994) 92:1897-1905, 2003.
6. Stawicki SP, Guarnaschelli JJ. Intradural extramedullary spinal cord tumors: a retrospective study of tumor types, locations, and surgical outcomes. The Internet Journal of Neurosurgery, vol 4, No. 2, 2007.
7. **el-Mahdy W, Kane PJ, Powell MP, et al. Spinal intradural tumours: Part I—Extramedullary. Br J Neurosurg 13:550-557, 1999.**
8. **Cherqui A, Kim DH, Kim SH, et al. Surgical approaches to paraspinal nerve sheath tumors. Neurosurg Focus 22:E9, 2007.**
9. **Cohen-Gadol AA, Zikel OM, Koch CA, et al. Spinal meningiomas in patients younger than 50 years of age: a 21-year experience. J Neurosurg 98(3 Suppl):258-263, 2003.**
10. **Krishnan P, Behari S, Banerji D, et al. Surgical approach to C1-C2 nerve sheath tumors. Neurol India 52:319-324, 2004.**
11. Gonzalez AA, Jeyanandarajan D, Hansen C, et al. Intraoperative neurophysiological monitoring during spine surgery: a review. Neurosurg Focus 27:E6, 2009.
12. Kim P, Ebersold MJ, Onofrio BM, et al. Surgery of spinal nerve schwannoma. Risk of neurological deficit after resection of involved root. J Neurosurg 71:810-814, 1989.
13. Odom GL, Finney W, Woodhall B. Cervical disk lesions. J Am Med Assoc 166:23-28, 1958.
14. Frankel HL, Hancock DO, Hyslop G, et al. The value of postural reduction in the initial management of closed injuries of the spine with paraplegia and tetraplegia. I. Paraplegia 7:179-192, 1969.
15. **Jiang L, Lv Y, Liu XG, et al. Results of surgical treatment of cervical dumbbell tumors: surgical approach and development of an anatomic classification system. Spine 34:1307-1314, 2009.**
16. Bucci MN, McGillicuddy JE, Taren JA, et al. Management of anteriorly located C1-C2 neurofibromata. Surg Neurol 33:15-18, 1990.
17. Tubbs RS, Salter G, Grabb PA, et al. The denticulate ligament: anatomy and functional significance. J Neurosurg 94(2 Suppl):271-275, 2001.
18. Bartolomei JC, Crockard HA. Bilateral posterolateral approach to mirror-image C-2 neurofibromas. Report of four cases. J Neurosurg 94(2 Suppl):292-298, 2001.
19. Ames CP, Wang VY, Deviren V, et al. Posterior transpedicular corpectomy and reconstruction of the axial vertebra for metastatic tumor. J Neurosurg Spine 10:111-116, 2009.

Chapter 28

T-Saw Laminoplasty

Yoshiyasu Fujimaki, Hideki Murakami,
Norio Kawahara, Katsuro Tomita

The resection of a large dumbbell tumor in the cervical spine has several concerns, including preservation of the nerve root, management of the vertebral artery, and maintaining spinal stability. Injury to the vertebral artery during total resection of a cervical dumbbell schwannoma can be a serious complication. A recapping T-saw laminoplasty and dissection off the surface of these encapsulated tumors allows single-stage posterior resection of the dumbbell schwannoma.[1] We report three cases of cervical dumbbell-type schwannoma compressing the vertebral artery. We used the posterior approach, with total tumor removal without laceration of the vertebral artery and spinal instability.

EQUIPMENT

The T-saw is a device for cutting bone. It has a number of advantages over the conventional Gigli saw devised by Gigli in 1894.[2] The T-saw is made of stainless steel microcable with a diameter of 0.36 mm or 0.54 mm. The surface of the T-saw is smooth and safe for soft tissue. The T-saw is thin and flexible, and it can be introduced safely into a confined space, such as the epidural space or the intervertebral foramen, with the use of an epidural catheter (T-saw catheter) or a specially made T-saw guide, and can cut the lamina or the pedicle or the spinous process sharply. It is possible to cut the lamina safely without injuring the dura and to obtain a good view of the operative field. The cut is so thin that bone loss may be negligible. As a result, the replaced laminae after the intraspinal operation are likely to remain in their primary position and be stable. The recapping T-saw laminoplasty makes it possible to achieve exact matching when replacing the lamina or when reapproximating after cutting. The posterior approach with the recapping T-saw laminoplasty permits a wide view of the spinal cord and the nerve root. Tumor dissection was safely performed.

SURGICAL APPROACH

Various surgical approaches for cervical dumbbell tumors have been described, with their respective advantages, disadvantages, and limitations in the exposed area. The choice depends on the surgeon's degree of familiarity. The standard anterior approach is usually insufficient for total tumor resection. Although the anterolateral approach[3-5] provides excellent exposure and control of the vertebral artery, intraspinal access is limited, and most surgeons are unfamiliar with this approach. Tumor removal by a lateral approach poses a risk of injuring the vertebral artery.

Most surgeons are familiar with the single posterior approach. The hemilaminectomy combined with the facetectomy has a great advantage for excising the dumbbell tumor, because most tumors are located unilaterally in the spinal canal. This approach can minimize bone removal and preserve spinal stability.[6] In the experimental study by Cusick et al,[7] isolated unilateral facetectomy resulted in an average loss of strength of 31.6% in response to a constant flexion/compression load, as compared with an intact motion segment. A posterior approach that uses the recapping T-saw laminoplasty provides as wide a view as unilateral facetectomy. Spinal stability is not affected. Reconstruction with spinal instrumentation is not necessary.

MANAGEMENT OF THE VERTEBRAL ARTERY

In the middle and lower cervical area, the brachial plexus roots are immediately posterior to the artery. The vertebral artery is surrounded by a venous plexus and is thin walled, so it can easily be injured. The vertebral artery is consistently displaced anteromedially by dumbbell schwannomas of the cervical spine. The vertebral artery has a well-defined plane separating it from the tumor capsule.[8] The tumor can be removed safely with an intrafascicular tumor dissection *enucleation* resection.

If there is a residual tumor component anterior to the vertebral artery after the posterior approach, we would remove the anterior tumor component at a second-stage anterior approach. Because residual tumor is far from the vertebral artery and nerve root, it can be removed easily and safely.

TECHNIQUE
POSITION AND EXPOSURE

The patient should be placed in the prone position, with the neck in a neutral position. The neck is maintained in a slightly fixed position with a Mayfield head clamp. A standard midline incision is performed. A bilateral muscle dissection is performed.

The muscle dissection continues laterally to expose the entire facet joint at the affected level.

RECAPPING T-SAW LAMINOPLASTY

The T-saw is inserted into a thin polyethylene tube, and the saw and tube are passed under the lamina from caudal to cranial.[9] A reciprocating motion divides the lamina at its lateral margin, just medial to the facet joints on the other side of the tumor. On the tumor side, the lamina with the lateral mass can be removed after removing the pedicle (Fig. 28-1). The pedicle on the tumor side can be removed easily with a high-speed air drill because the pedicle is eroded (Fig. 28-2). Two laminae were excised, as shown in Figs. 28-6 and 28-7. Three laminae were excised, as shown in Fig. 28-8.

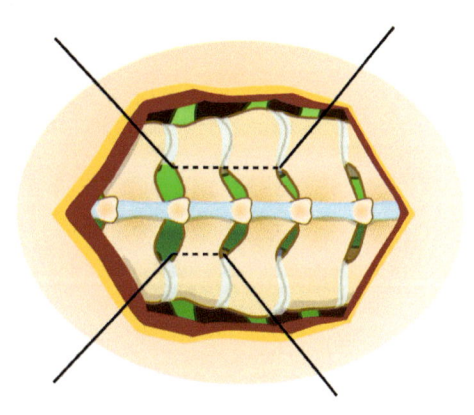

Fig. 28-1 The T-saw is passed under the lamina. A reciprocating motion divides the lamina at its lateral margin, just medial to the facet joints on the other side of the tumor. On the tumor side, the lamina with the lateral mass can be removed after removing the pedicle.

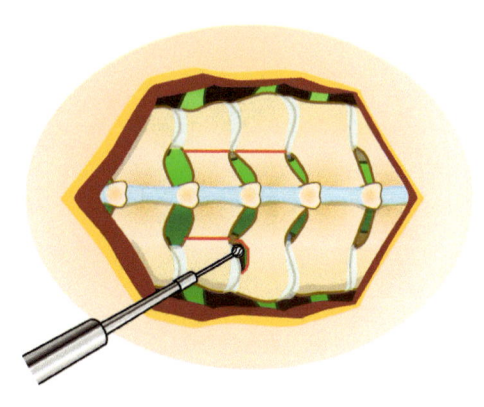

Fig. 28-2 The pedicle on the tumor side can be easily removed with a high-speed air drill because the pedicle is erosive.

TUMOR REMOVAL

We recommend introducing the operating microscope at this point. The dura mater is opened and tacking sutures are placed. The intraspinal tumor component is removed first. Removal of the foraminal and extraforaminal tumor components depends on their size and relationship to the nerve root and nerve root sleeve. The tumor is followed distally along the lateral margin of the root. The tumor capsule is opened along the nerve root (Fig. 28-3). The vertebral artery is separated from the tumor capsule by a thin layer of periosteum and perivertebral veins. Therefore an intrafascicular tumor dissection and "enucleation" resection is performed safely. We suture the extraspinal tumor component. We mobilize the tumor from its capsule gradually and pull out the extraspinal tumor. We excised the extraspinal tumor totally in three cases (Fig. 28-4).

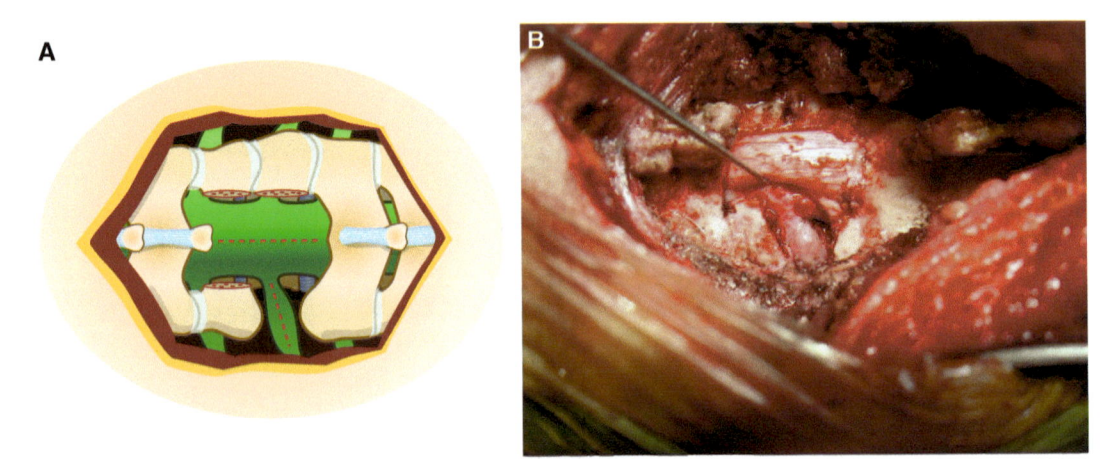

Fig. 28-3 **A** and **B**, The dura mater is opened, and tacking sutures are placed. The intraspinal tumor component is removed first. The tumor capsule is opened along the nerve root.

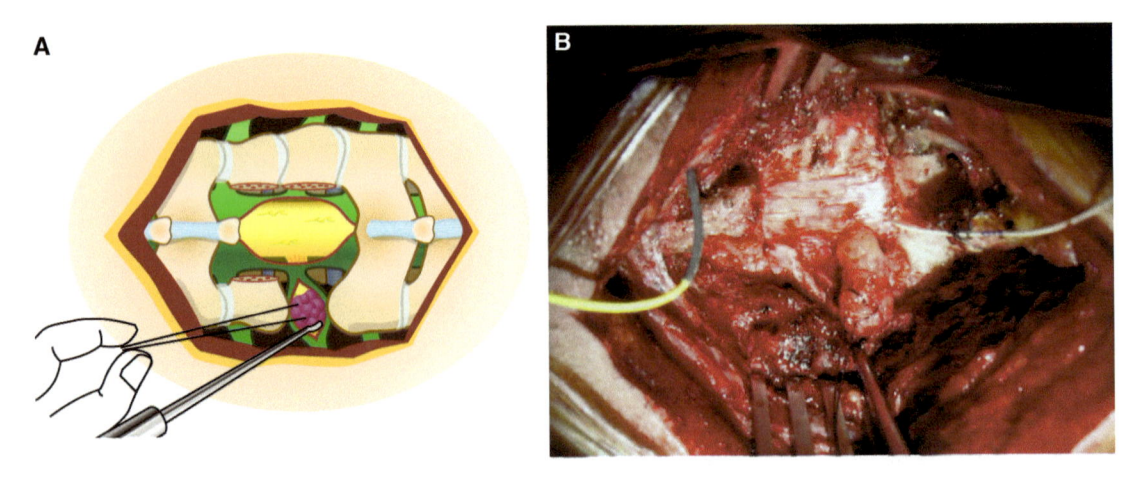

Fig. 28-4 **A** and **B**, The tumor from the tumor capsule is abraded gradually, and the extraspinal tumor is pulled out.

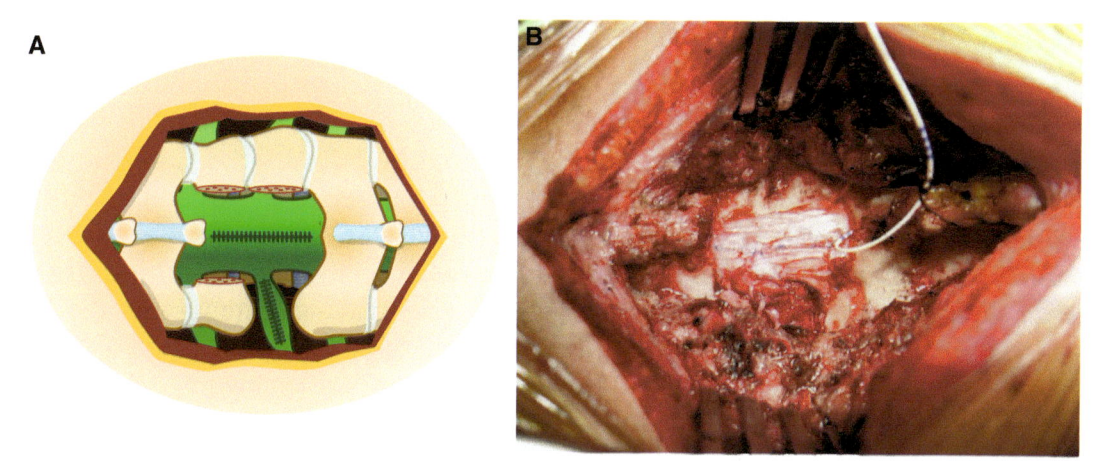

Fig. 28-5 **A** and **B,** After the tumor resection is completed, the dural tube and tumor capsule are constructed with interrupted or running sutures so that they are watertight.

Blood flow of the vertebral artery was confirmed with Doppler ultrasound imaging. After the tumor resection was completed, the dural tube and tumor capsule were constructed to be watertight with interrupted or running sutures (Fig. 28-5). We routinely use spinal cord evoked potential monitoring and compound muscle action potentials during spinal cord surgery. In case 3, the bone defect of C4 and C5 vertebrae were filled with α-tricalcium phosphate.

RECONSTRUCTION OF THE POSTERIOR ARCH

After the tumor resection, the posterior arches are reconstructed. The excised two or three laminae can be restored to their exact original anatomic position, because the amount of bone lost with the T-saw cut is negligible. They are secured with sutures passed through the holes fashioned with a 1.0 mm diameter burr and/or a bone clamp.

OUTCOMES WITH EVALUATION OF RESULTS

Intraoperative inspection, as well as computed tomography (CT) and magnetic resonance imaging (MRI), confirmed an apparently total tumor resection without sacrifice of the nerve root or laceration of the vertebral artery in all three cases. Although extraspinal tumor extended up to 4 cm from the lateral dural margin in case 3, we were able to resect the extraspinal tumor completely. In all three patients there was apparent involvement of the periosteal sheath but no invasion of the vessel wall itself.

In the following case, follow-up was 6 years (Fig. 28-6), 8 years (Fig. 28-7), and 7 years (Fig. 28-8). All patients had normalization of the initial signs and symptoms at their follow-up evaluations. There were no embolic or ischemic complications. Postoperatively none of the patients had any radicular deficits or recurrences. Delayed spinal instability has not developed in any of the three cases.

SIGNATURE CASES

A 53-year-old woman had numbness in the left upper extremities and causalgia of the right lower extremity consistent with C6 Brown-Séquard syndrome for 6 months. She had a bilateral fine motor disturbance in her fingers during the last 3 months. On neurologic examination she had mild weakness of the left biceps and wrist extensors. Left oblique radiographs of the cervical spine showed a large intervertebral foramen (foraminal enlargement) between C4 and C5 on the left side. On MRI the tumor showed low intensity on the T1-weighted image and high intensity on the T2-weighted image. The tumor appeared to be dumbbell shaped on gadolinium-DTPA–enhanced T1-weighted images. On magnetic resonance arteriography (MRA) the left vertebral artery was displaced anteriorly (Fig. 28-6).

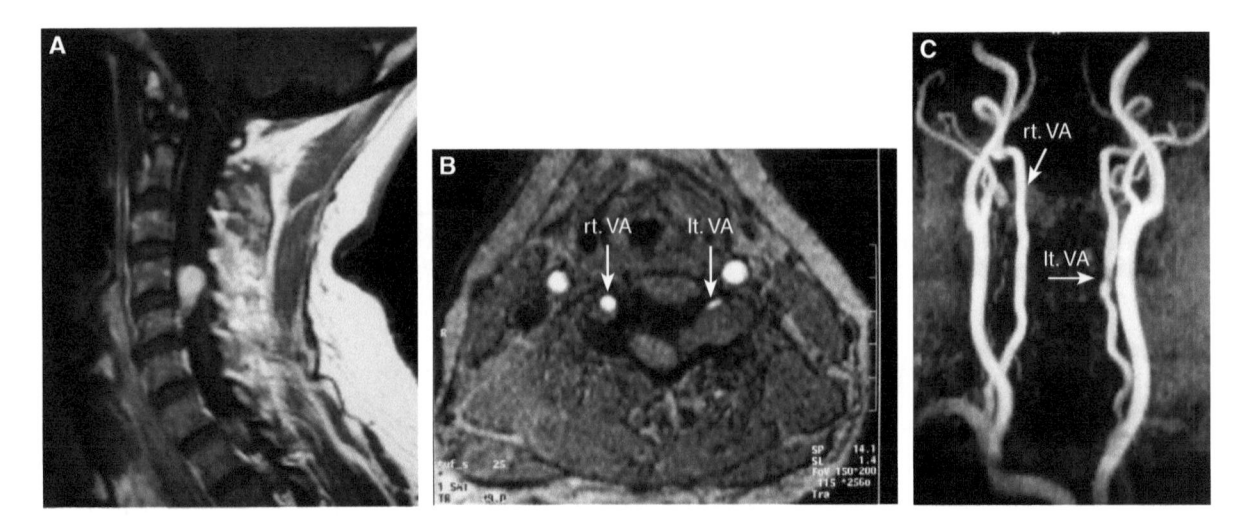

Fig. 28-6 **A,** Sagittal and **B,** axial T1-weighted gadolinium-enhanced MRI scans demonstrating a dumbbell schwannoma at C4/5. **C,** MRA demonstrates occlusion of the left vertebral artery by tumor.

A 49-year-old man had numbness of the right hand for 4 months. On neurologic examination there was no muscle weakness or evidence of myelopathy. A right oblique radiograph of the cervical spine showed a large intervertebral foramen between C3 and C4 on the right side. CT scans revealed a lesion involving C4. On MRI the tumor showed low intensity on the T1-weighted image and high intensity on the T2-weighted image. The MRI scan showed a dumbbell-shaped tumor on gadolinium-DTPA–enhanced T1-weighted images. MRA showed that the right vertebral was occluded (Fig. 28-7).

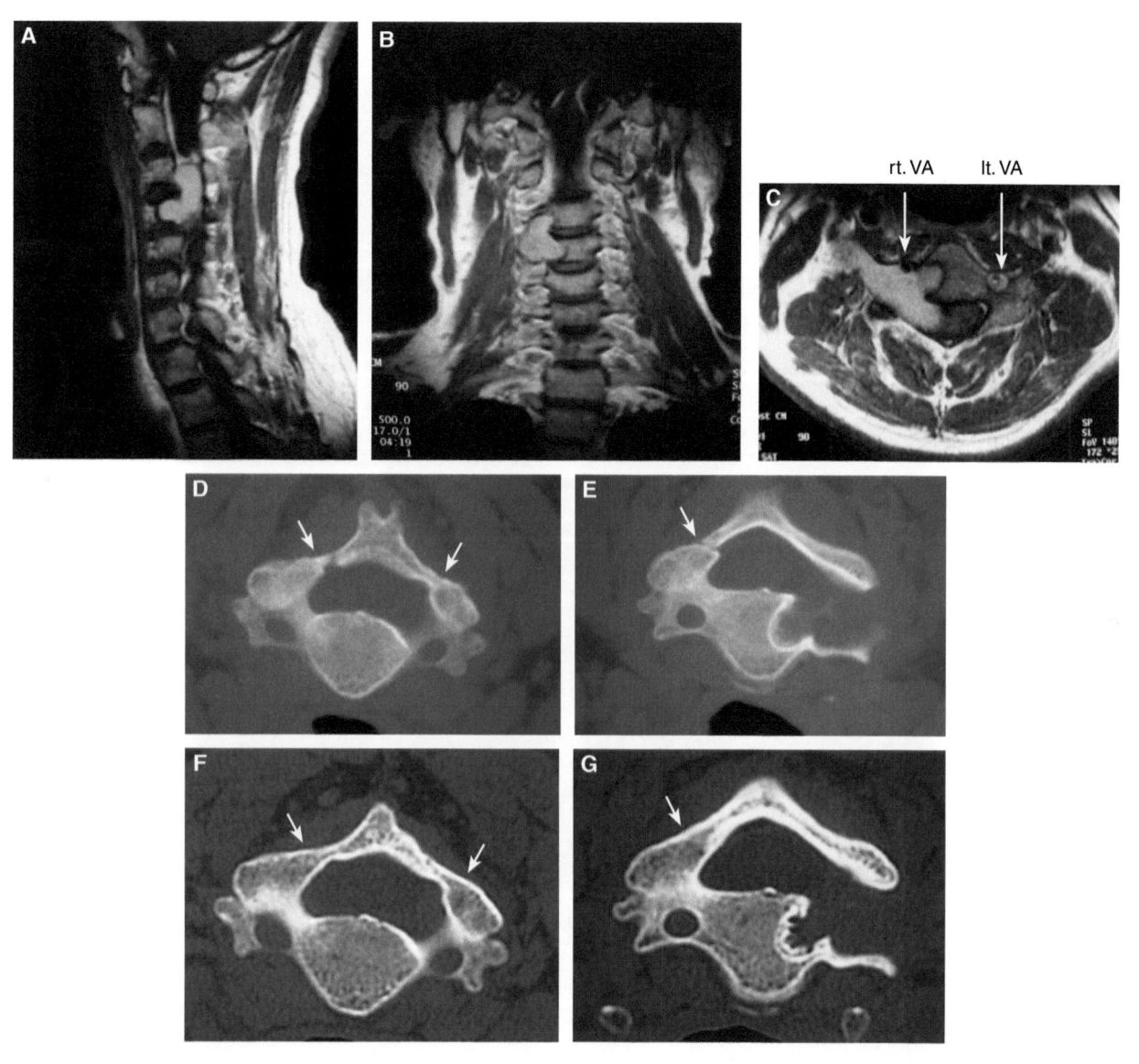

Fig. 28-7 **A,** Sagittal, **B,** coronal, and **C,** axial T1-weighted gadolinium-enhanced MRI scans demonstrating a dumbbell schwannoma eroding the C4 vertebra. **D** and **E,** Postoperative (3 months) CT scans show negligible bone loss when the T-saw is used. **F** and **G,** Postoperative (12 months) CT scans showing bony union of the lamina.

A 55-year-old man had numbness of the left hand for 12 months. On neurologic examination there was no muscle weakness or evidence of myelopathy. Left oblique radiographs of the cervical spine showed a large intervertebral foramen between C3 and C4, C4 and C5, C5 and C6 on the left side. CT scans revealed a lesion involving C4 and C5. On MRI the tumor showed low intensity on the T1-weighted image and high intensity on the T2-weighted image. MRI scans showed a dumbbell-shaped tumor on gadolinium-DTPA–enhanced T1-weighted image. MRA showed that the right vertebral artery was occluded and displaced anteriorly. We obtained a preoperative vertebral artery arteriogram, which demonstrated occlusion of the left vertebral artery. Balloon test occlusion of the involved vessel was performed before surgery (Fig. 28-8).

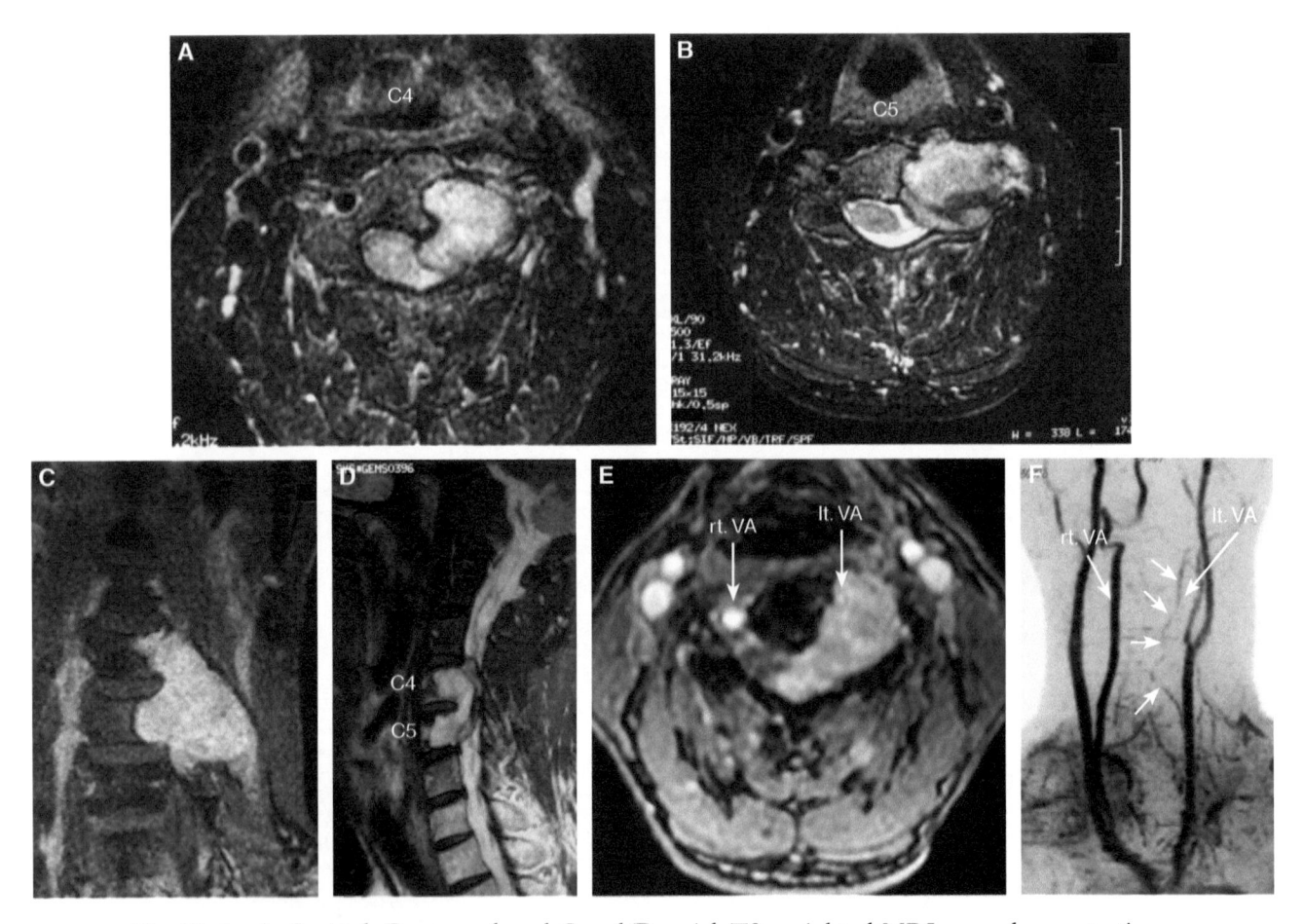

Fig. 28-8 **A,** Sagittal, **B,** coronal, and **C** and **D,** axial T2-weighted MRI scans demonstrating a dumbbell schwannoma eroding the C4 and C5 vertebrae. **E,** Axial T1-weighted gadolinium-enhanced MRI scan demonstrating a dumbbell schwannoma at the C4 level compressing the left vertebral artery. **F,** Vertebral arteriogram showing distortion and occlusion of the left vertebral artery. Balloon test occlusion was performed before surgery.

CONCLUSION

Recapping T-saw laminoplasty provides a wide view and anatomic reconstruction. Tumor can be removed safely with an intrafascicular tumor dissection and *enucleation* resection. These are effective for cervical dumbbell-type schwannomas compressing the vertebral artery.

TIPS FROM THE MASTERS

- The posterior approach with the recapping T-saw laminoplasty permits a wide view of the spinal cord and the nerve root.
- Since spinal stability is not affected in the recapping T-saw laminoplasty, reconstruction with spinal instrumentation is not necessary.
- The tumor can be removed safely with an intrafascicular tumor dissection and *enucleation* resection.

References (With Key References in Boldface)

1. **Kawahara N, Tomita K, Shinya Y, et al. Recapping T-saw laminoplasty for spinal cord tumors. Spine 24:1363-1370, 1999.**
2. Gigli L. Über ein neues Instrument sum Durchtrennen der Knochen, die Drahtsäge. Zentralbl Chir 21:409-411, 1894.
3. George B, Lot G. Neurinomas of the first two cervical nerve roots: a series of 42 cases. J Neurosurg 82:917-923, 1995.
4. Hakuba A, Komiyama M, Tsujimoto T, et al. Transuncodiscal approach to dumbbell tumors of the cervical spinal canal. J Neurosurg 61:1100-1106, 1984.
5. Sen C, Eisenberg M, Casden AM, et al. Management of the vertebral artery in excision of extradural tumors of the cervical spine. Neurosurgery 36:106-115, 1995.
6. Ozawa H, Kokubun S, Aizawa T, et al. Spinal dumbbell tumors: an analysis of a series of 118 cases. J Neurosurg Spine 7:587-593, 2007.
7. Cusick JF, Yoganandan N, Pintar F, et al. Biomechanics of cervical spine facetectomy and fixation technique. Spine 13:808-812, 1988.
8. McCormick PC. Surgical management of dumbbell tumors of the cervical spine. Neurosurgery 38:294-300, 1996.
9. **Tomita K, Kawahara N. The threadwire saw (T-saw): a new device for cutting bone. J Bone Joint Surg [Am] 78:1915-1917, 1996.**

Chapter 29

Paramedian Transpedicular Approach for Ventral Intradural Extramedullary Tumors of the Cervical and Cervicothoracic Spine

Frank L. Acosta, Jr., Christopher P. Ames

*I*ntraoperative spinal cord monitoring for cervical spinal cord tumors can be unreliable.[1-4] Ultimately the only certain way to prevent new or worsening neurologic deficits after intradural spine surgery is to avoid manipulation of the cord. Although not possible for intramedullary spinal cord tumors, this is possible for certain types of large ventral intradural extramedullary tumors of the spinal canal.

Dorsal intradural extramedullary spinal cord tumors of the cervical and upper thoracic spinal canal can be accessed after standard midline laminectomy or laminoplasty and partial facetectomy and, if not adherent to the spinal cord, they may be removed without cord manipulation. Similarly, thoracic laterally situated lesions may be directly exposed by means of posterolateral approaches, including costotransversectomy, lateral extracavitary, and lateral extrapleural-parascapular exposures.[5-8] However, ventral and ventrolaterally located lesions in the cervical and cervicothoracic spinal canal present several obstacles to safe and effective surgical management.[9-12] In most cases there is no single approach that provides adequate surgical exposure across multiple levels of this region. Two main approaches have been described to access the ventral cervical and cervicothoracic spinal canal: (1) anterior cervical or transthoracic approaches, and (2) posterolateral approaches. Recent advances in spinal instrumentation and reconstruction, however, now allow spine surgeons to sacrifice a significant amount of bone from the vertebral canal to achieve a much wider and more direct approach with minimal or no neural manipulation. This has been a common theme of skull base surgery for many years: remove the bone rather than retract neural elements. Here we demonstrate the possible advantages of taking a *spine-based* approach for resecting intradural extramedullary spinal cord tumors of the ventral cervical and cervicothoracic spinal canal. Specifically, we describe the use of a paramedian cervical transpedicular, thoracic parascapular approach with partial dorsal corpectomy, wide eccentric dural opening, and immediate posterior spinal reconstruction for the resection of ventral intradural extramedullary spinal cord tumors of the cervical and cervicothoracic spine. This technique is a modification of traditional thoracic, posterolateral, extracavitary, and transpedicular approaches. Combined with angulation of the operating table, removal of the posterior and posterolateral elements, and occasionally the dorsal vertebral body, this approach provides excellent exposure of the ventralmost thecal sac and creates a potential space into which certain intradural extramedullary spinal cord tumors can be delivered without spinal cord retraction or rotation.

INDICATIONS AND CONTRAINDICATIONS
INDICATIONS
- Ventral intradural extramedullary tumors of the cervical and/or cervicothoracic spine
- Ventral extradural tumors of the cervical and cervicothoracic spine (dural opening unnecessary)
- Multilevel ventral cervical/cervicothoracic tumors

CONTRAINDICATIONS
- Tumors requiring en bloc resection from an anterior approach (chordoma)
- Ventral intramedullary tumors

PREOPERATIVE EVALUATION
A complete history is obtained and a physical examination is performed in all patients. Any relevant history of cancer, prior spinal instrumentation, bleeding disorders, or osteoporosis should be noted. All patients should undergo diagnostic MRI and CT imaging, with sagittal and coronal reconstructions demonstrating an intradural extramedullary spinal cord tumor of the anterior cervical and/or cervicothoracic spinal canal. CT scans are also useful for assessing the anatomy of the C2 pedicles to plan instrumentation.

CLINICAL DECISION-MAKING

For small, purely ventral extramedullary one- or two-level lesions situated in the intradural space immediately behind the vertebral body, an anterior corpectomy approach may allow the fusion of fewer operative levels, but the dural repair can be quite difficult. For all other intradural extramedullary ventral lesions, especially multilevel lesions with some lateral component, we recommend the transpedicular approach described herein.

TECHNIQUE

All patients are monitored with somatosensory evoked potentials and transcranial motor evoked potentials throughout the procedure. The patient's head is secured in a Mayfield pin fixation device, and the patient is then placed in the prone position on uneven chest rolls so that he or she is angled away from the surgeon at approximately 45 degrees, with the surgeon standing on the side with the larger chest roll. The patient is heavily padded and taped, because significant rotation of the operating table is required during the procedure. The table is rotated so that the patient's back and neck are level with the floor for exposure, bone removal, and instrumentation. The table is subsequently rotated back to 45 degrees for tumor resection. Although certain variations of the posterolateral approach to the ventral cervical and upper thoracic cord require both a midline and a transverse incision, we use a 2 cm paramedian incision on the side of approach from at least three levels above and below the target level or levels. The paraspinous muscles and ligaments are dissected free, and the soft tissue dissection is carried at least 2 cm lateral to the edges of the lateral masses in the cervical spine and lateral enough to expose 4 to 6 cm of rib in the thoracic spine on the side of approach, which is determined by tumor location relative to the midline. Fish hook retractors on the Leyla bar (Leyla Retractor System; Integra, Plainsboro, NJ) are used to pull the skin and soft tissues ventrally on the side of the exposure to enlarge the visualization corridor.[13]

Contralateral spinal instrumentation is placed first. Pedicle screws or bicortical lateral mass screws are placed at each level on the opposite side of the planned paramedian transpedicular approach before decompression. Fixation is extended at least two levels above and below the location where the pediculectomies or costotransversectomies are to be performed. A stabilizing rod is placed on the side contralateral to the pedicle removal before any decompression. This is especially important when the integrity of the anterior column is compromised, which could cause intraoperative spinal instability. Moreover, dural tack-up sutures can be secured to this stabilizing rod during tumor resection.

Wide laminectomies are performed to at least one level above and below the planned dural opening, allowing spinal cord decompression and identification of a normal dural plane without tumor involvement. Subsequently, unilateral facetectomies and pedicle resection to the floor of the spinal canal are performed on the side selected for the lateral approach with the use of a high-speed drill and Lempert rongeurs. The pediculectomy permits improved visualization of the ventral spinal canal, as well as increased working room for nerve root mobilization. At this stage of the procedure, the entire nerve root sleeves and dorsal root ganglions can be clearly seen, but access to the ventral spinal canal would require significant spinal cord retraction (Fig. 29-1).

VERTEBRAL ARTERY MOBILIZATION AND EXPOSURE OF THE VENTRAL SPINAL CANAL

In the cervical spine it is sometimes necessary to dissect and mobilize the vertebral artery from the foramen transversarium. This step enhances exposure of the ventral cervical spinal cord and allows for safe retraction of the vertebral artery during tumor resection or later instrumentation. First, the nerve root immediately below the level of interest is gently retracted inferiorly. The venous plexus around the vertebral artery is usually then easily seen. Removal of the lateral posterior bony strut of the transverse foramen affords more mobilization of the underlying vertebral artery laterally. With gentle retraction of the vertebral artery, Kerrison rongeurs are again used to complete the anterior transverse process resection that forms the anterior margin of the foramen transversarium, providing access to the lateral vertebral body (Fig. 29-2, *A*). This step is only used when wide control and mobilization are needed for very large lesions. With gentle ventral retraction of the vertebral artery and nerve roots, a dorsal partial corpectomy can be accomplished using a high-speed drill to enhance exposure of the ventral spinal canal (Fig. 29-2, *B* and *C*). Removal of the dorsal 20% to 25% of the vertebral body creates an anterior working space into which tumor can be delivered away from the spinal cord. The removal of the dorsal body and posterior portion of intervening discs also creates a secondary site for bone fusion into which autograft may be placed after tumor resection.

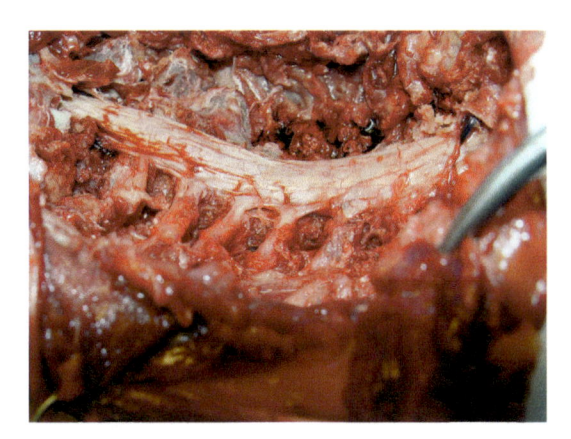

Fig. 29-1 Cadaveric dissection after midline incision and right-sided facetectomy and pediculectomy across both the cervical and cervicothoracic spine. Note that although the entire dorsal thecal sac and ipsilateral nerve roots are visible, the ventral spinal canal remains inaccessible.

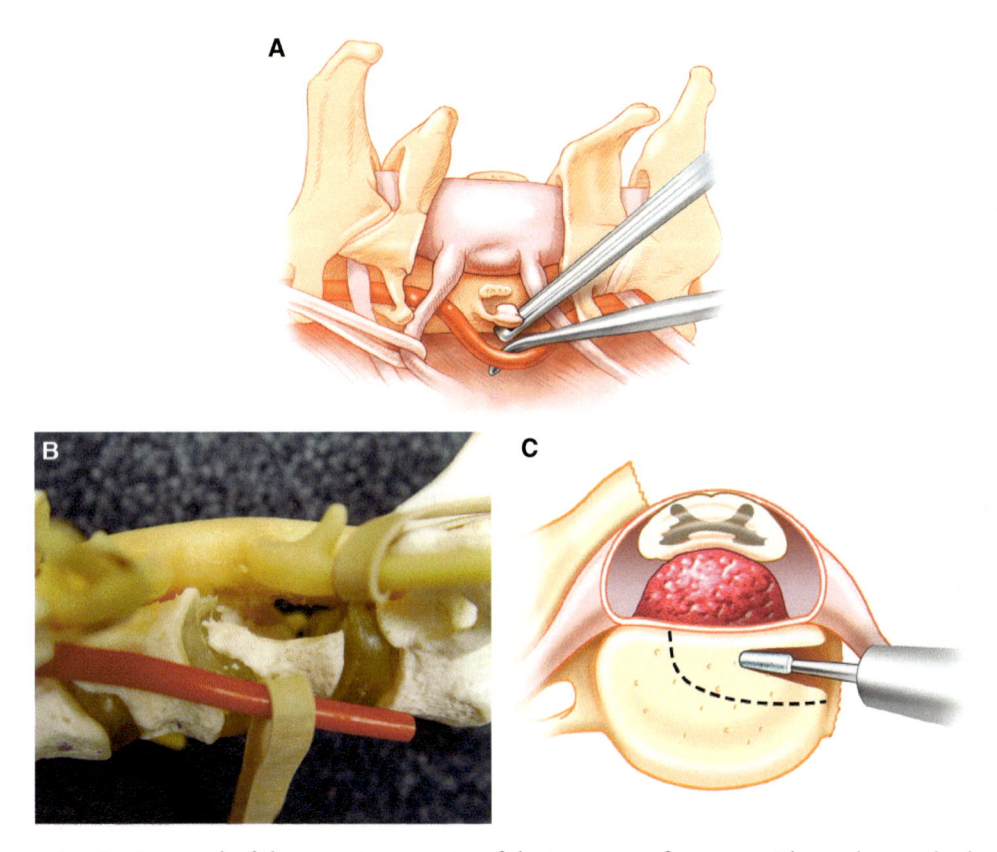

Fig. 29-2 **A,** Removal of the anterior margin of the transverse foramen with gentle vertebral artery retraction. **B,** Sawbone model. **C,** Partial dorsal corpectomy performed with a pneumatic drill after resection of the anterior bone of the transverse foramen with gentle lateral retraction of the vertebral artery. Dorsalmost cortical bone adjacent to the thecal sac may be removed with Lempert or upbiting pituitary rongeurs.

TUMOR RESECTION

Extra-large fish hook retractors are placed over the lateral soft tissue and secured to a Leyla bar. The tissue is then retracted as ventrally as possible by means of rubber bands and the retractor arm to establish the pure lateral line of sight. After the bone work is complete, the posterior, lateral, and ventral thecal sac is exposed, and extradural tumor, if present, can be dissected. The operating microscope is brought into the field, and the dura is then opened through a longitudinal eccentric H-shaped incision at the midpoint between the nerve root sleeve and the dorsal midline. A transverse incision directed toward the ventral midline is then used to create dural flaps for further exposure of the cord and intradural tumor. These lateral flaps are easily closed and allow a dural flap that is completely flush with the level of the vertebral body. The dural flaps on the contralateral side may be secured with dural tack-up sutures to the previously placed rod for further exposure (Fig. 29-3, *A*). The operating table is then rotated 45 degrees away from the surgeon, allowing direct vision of the ventral spinal cord and intradural space (Fig. 29-3, *B* and *C*). With gentle retraction of the ventral dura, the tumor can be delivered into the pediculectomy and corpectomy defect without manipulation of the cord itself (Fig. 29-3, *D* and *E*). Previous pedicle removal allows significant nerve root retraction superiorly and inferiorly. The tumor is then resected by means of a combination of bipolar cautery, suction, and Rhoton dissectors. A watertight dural closure is then achieved by use of a dural patch graft, if necessary. Specifically, the ventralmost dura is closed from the inside out, whereas the lateral and posterior dura is closed in the standard fashion from the outside in.

RECONSTRUCTION

After dural closure, ipsilateral lateral mass or pedicle screws are placed two levels above and below the exposed segment. Artificial pedicles are then created at the levels requiring pediculectomy with the use of a standard lateral mass screw inserted directly into the vertebral body[14] (Fig. 29-4). A final lateral mass/pedicle screw-rod construct is created, followed by thorough decortication of the remaining facet joints, and transverse processes and bone graft placement for fusion. The ipsilateral area of bone removal for tumor resection does not leave any lateral bone for fusion; however, autograft can be packed into the lateral disc space after discectomy for a lateral disc fusion. Moreover, most of the autograft has been placed on the contralateral side from exposure. A standard cervical rod, rod-extended, or tapered rod can be secured to the lateral mass/pedicle screws to cross the cervicothoracic junction.

Chapter 29 ▪ *Paramedian Transpedicular Approach for Ventral Intradural Extramedullary Tumors of the Cervical and Cervicothoracic Spine*

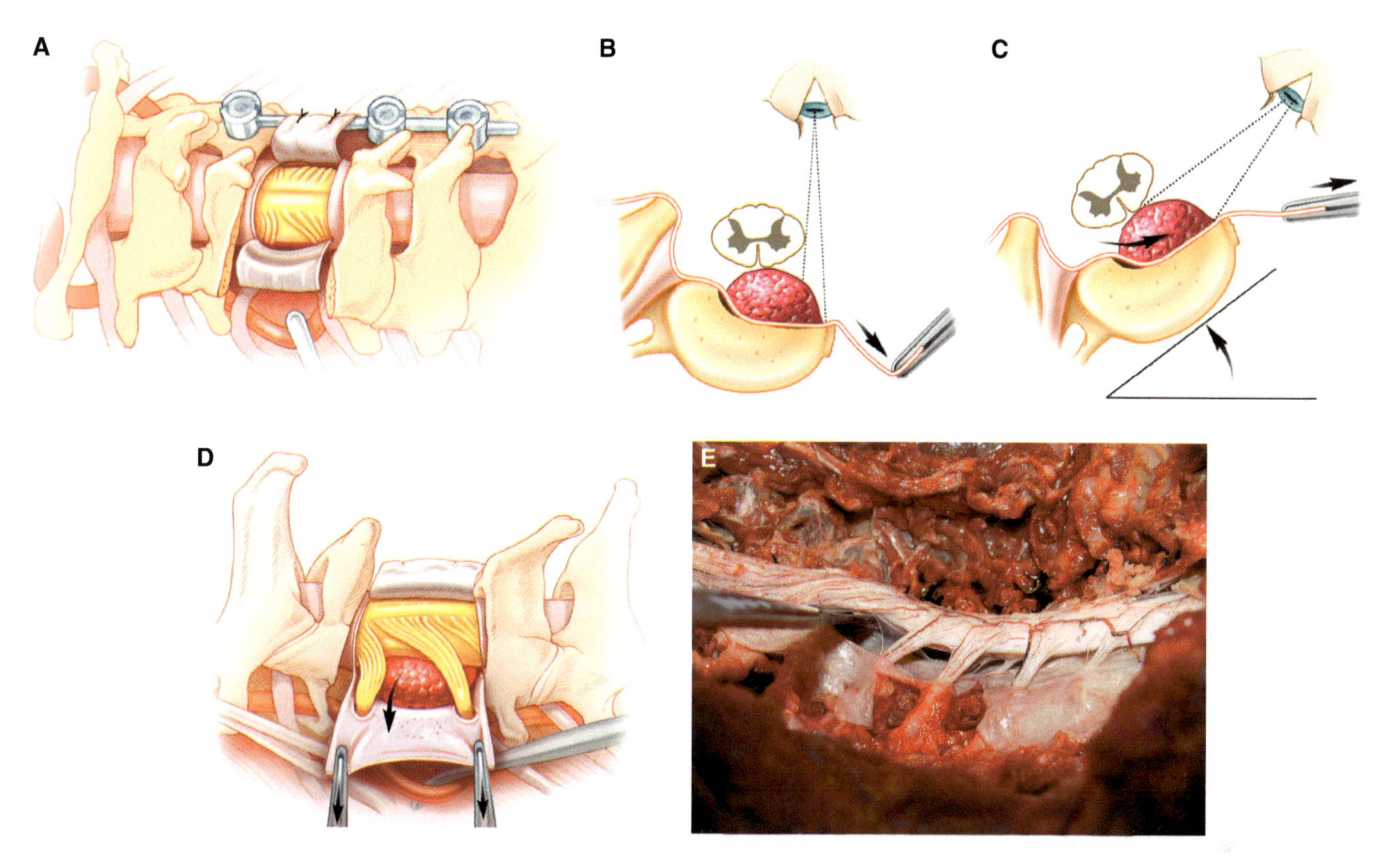

Fig. 29-3 **A,** Dural H-shaped flap. **B** and **C,** Rotating the operating room table 45 degrees permits a direct view of the ventral spinal cord and intradural space. Ventral tumor exposure is enhanced with a modified paramedian transpedicular approach, partial corpectomy, and patient rotation. **D,** Gentle downward retraction of the dural flap allows tumor delivery into the previously created corpectomy defect. **E,** Cadaveric dissection after partial corpectomy and dural H-flap demonstrating an unobstructed view across the ventral spinal canal.

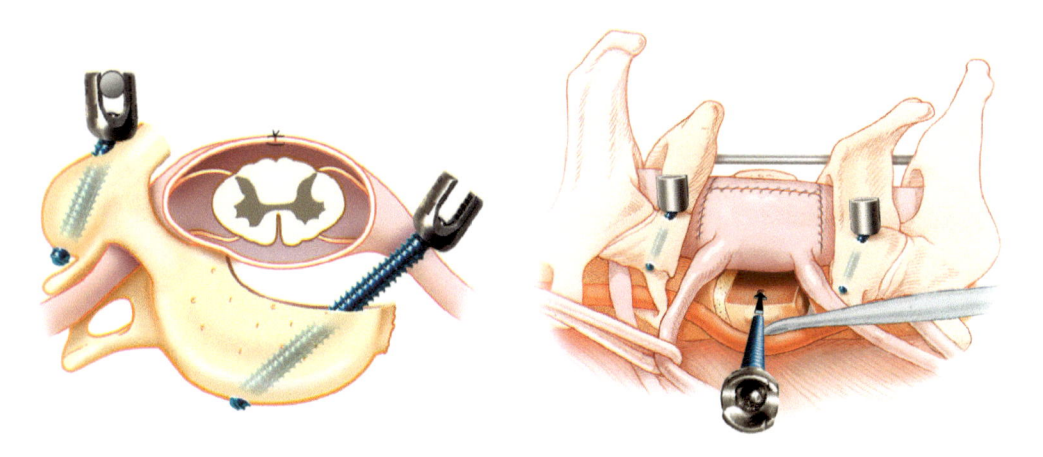

Fig. 29-4 Placement of standard lateral mass screws directly into the cervical vertebral body after pediculectomy to create artificial cervical pedicles.

POSTOPERATIVE CARE

Patients are immobilized in a rigid collar after surgery and are monitored in the intensive care unit for 1 or 2 days. Immediate plain radiographs are obtained to document proper instrumentation position. MRI is also performed before discharge to evaluate tumor resection.

OUTCOMES WITH EVALUATION OF RESULTS

We previously published our results with this technique in 14 patients with intradural extramedullary spinal canal tumors involving multiple levels of the anterior cervical and cervicothoracic spine (Box 29-1). Nine patients had tumors that extended across the cervicothoracic junction, and five had tumors limited to the cervical spine. All patients had pain and/or radiculomyelopathy, which were attributed to a ventral intradural extramedullary spinal cord tumor of the cervical or cervicothoracic spine. Lesions extended across an average of 3.5 levels (range 2 to 7) from C2 to T3.

Box 29-1 Patient Characteristics

Total number of patients	14
Mean age (yr)	39.6 (range 20-62)
Sex	
Number of males	4 (29%)
Number of females	10 (71%)
Presenting symptoms	
Number of patients with radiculomyelopathy	5 (36%)
Number of patients with radiculomyelopathy and pain	9 (64%)
Mean length of hospital stay (days)	9 (range 6-22)
Tumor location	
Cervical	5 (2.2)
Cervicothoracic	9 (4.2)
Mean operative time (hr)	7.6 (range 5-15)
Mean follow-up (mo)	14.6 (range 5-30)

Surgical, radiographic, and clinical data are presented in Table 29-1. The average follow-up period was 14.6 months. Pathologic findings included meningioma in seven patients, schwannoma in three, neurofibroma in one, leptomeningeal pilocytic astrocytoma in one, and exophytic ependymoma in one. Gross total resection was achieved in all cases, and none of the patients required additional surgery through an anterior approach for residual tumor. Mean operative time was 7.6 hours. No manipulation of the spinal cord was necessary, and no changes were observed in the transcranial motor evoked potentials or somatosensory evoked potentials in any of the patients.

Table 29-1 Clinical Outcomes

Case No.	Age (yr)/Sex	Pathology	Location	Intraoperative TcMEP/ SSEP Signal	Preoperative/ Postoperative VAS (change)	Preoperative/ Postoperative NDI (change)	Follow-up (mo)
1	44/M	Schwannoma	C7-T2	No change	4/2 (2)	13/6 (7)	30
2	20/F	Meningioma	C5-T3	No change	8/4 (4)	25/15 (10)	20
3	29/M	Meningioma	C6-T1	No change	7/3 (4)	16/9 (7)	7
4	35/F	Schwannoma	C5-T1	No change	6/3 (3)	17/12 (5)	5
5	37/F	Meningioma	C2-4	No change	3/2 (1)	12/6 (6)	22
6	25/F	Schwannoma	C2-T2	No change	8/5 (3)	24/14 (10)	18
7	54/M	Neurofibroma	C3-T1	No change	8/3 (5)	27/21 (6)	22
8	58/M	Meningioma	C2-4	No change	7/4 (3)	18/12 (6)	10
9	35/F	Ependymoma	C3-5	No change	4/2 (2)	15/4 (11)	5
10	36/F	Meningioma	C5-T1	No change	5/3 (2)	12/5 (7)	18
11	27/F	Pilocytic astrocytoma	C2-T1	No change	4/2 (2)	13/7 (6)	14
12	37/F	Neurofibroma	C1-T1	No change	4/2 (2)	15/12 (3)	8
13	56/F	Meningioma	C2-4	No change	3/2 (1)	12/5 (7)	12
14	62/F	Meningioma	C3-6	No change	7/4 (3)	16/10 (6)	14
AVERAGE	39.6				5.6/2.9 (2.7)	16.8/9.9 (6.9)	14.6

F, Female; *M*, male; *NDI*, neck disability index; *SSEP*, somatosensory evoked potential; *TcMEP*, transcranial motor evoked potential; *VAS*, visual analog scale.

SIGNATURE CASES

A 25-year-old woman with a history of a cervical mass after laminectomy and biopsy 2 years earlier was seen with new right upper and lower extremity weakness and neck pain. The previous biopsy had only revealed evidence of an epidural hematoma. Physical examination was significant for the following strength measurements: 2/5 for grip strength and 4/5 for lower extremity strength. MRI showed evidence of an extensive, multilevel partially intramedullary, partially extramedullary, intradural extramedullary tumor of the cervical and cervicothoracic spine (Fig. 29-5, *A* and *B*). The patient was taken to the operating room and underwent a paramedian transpedicular approach for access to the ventral spinal canal (Fig. 29-5, *C*). Immediate spinal reconstruction was performed (Fig. 29-5, *D* and *E*). Pathologic findings were consistent with pilocytic astrocytoma.

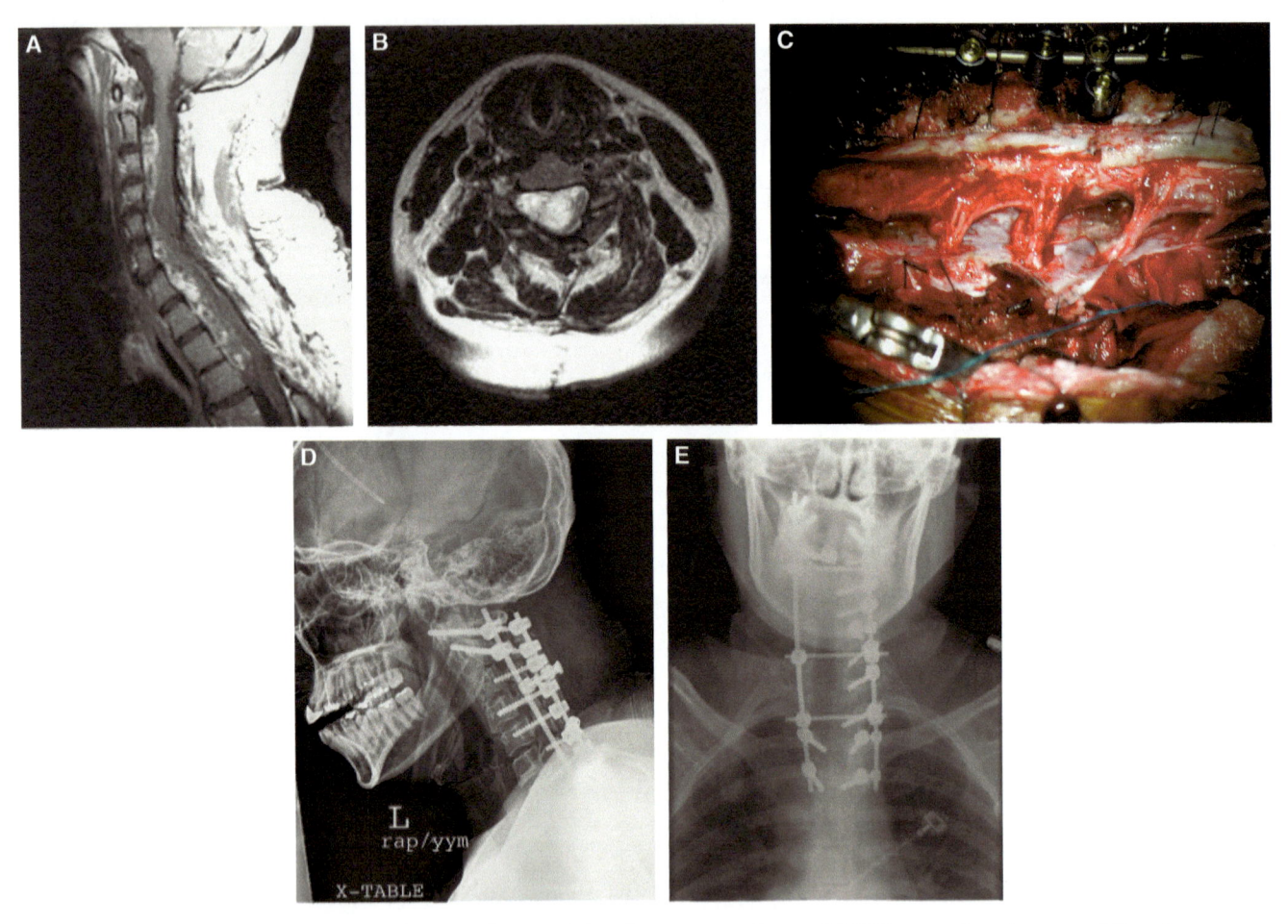

Fig. 29-5 **A,** Sagittal and **B,** axial T1-weighted contrast-enhanced MRI scans showing a multilevel ventral intradural extramedullary mass of the cervical and cervicothoracic spine. **C,** Intraoperative photograph showing a direct view of the ventral cervicothoracic spinal canal. **D** and **E,** Postoperative radiographs demonstrating spinal reconstruction after a paramedian transpedicular approach.

A 38-year-old mother of two with a history of neurofibromatosis-1 (NF1) was first seen with progressive lower extremity weakness. MRI showed a ventral intradural extramedullary mass at the C2-3 level (Fig. 29-6, *A* and *B*). She underwent a C2-3 paramedian transpedicular approach for resection of this mass (Fig. 29-6, *C*). Reconstruction was performed with artificial pedicle screws at C2 and C3 (Fig. 29-6, *D*).

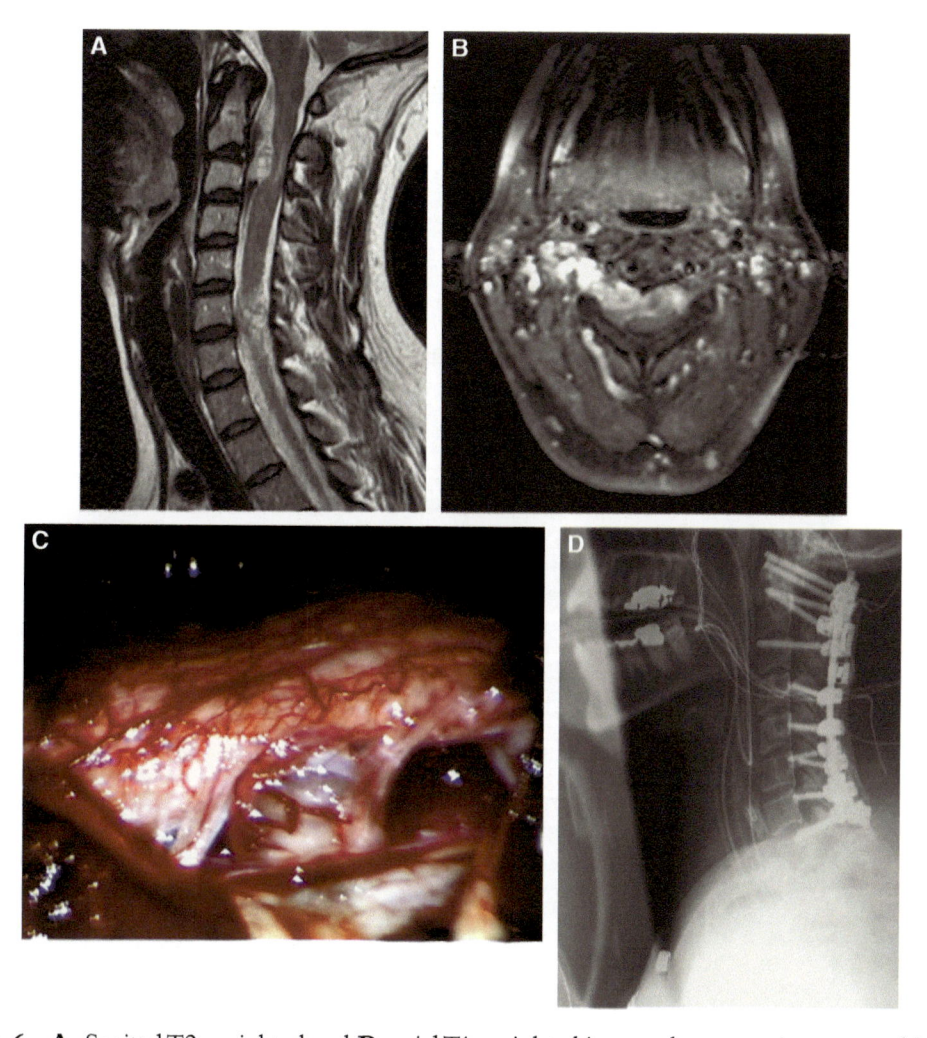

Fig. 29-6 **A,** Sagittal T2-weighted and **B,** axial T1-weighted images demonstrating a ventral intradural extramedullary mass at C2-3 with cord compression. **C,** Intraoperative photograph demonstrating access to the ventral canal. A direct view of the ventral mass is obtained. **D,** Lateral plain radiograph demonstrating spinal reconstruction with artificial pedicle screws at C2 and C3.

A 35-year-old woman was first seen with signs of myelopathy from a ventral intradural extramedullary mass at C4-5 (Fig. 29-7, *A* and *B*). A paramedian transpedicular approach was used, with reconstruction through artificial pedicle screws at C4-5 (Fig. 29-7, *C* and *D*). Pathologic findings were consistent with exophytic ependymoma.

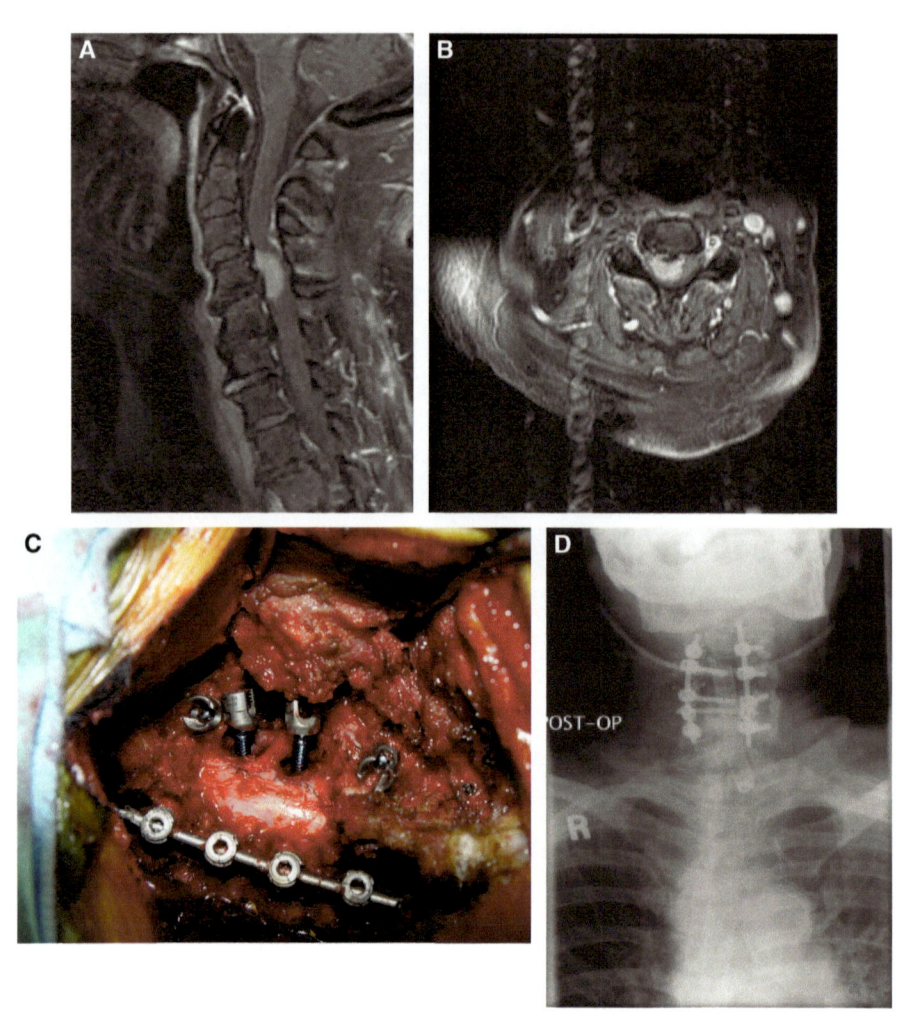

Fig. 29-7 **A,** Sagittal and **B,** axial T1-weighted MRI scans showing a ventral intradural extramedullary mass at C4-5. **C,** Intraoperative photograph and **D,** postoperative plain radiograph demonstrating C4-5 artificial pedicle screws for spinal reconstruction.

CONCLUSION

The paramedian transpedicular approach we describe in this chapter is a variation of traditional thoracic posterolateral transpedicular extracavitary approaches and offers direct access to lesions of the ventral cervicothoracic spinal canal. This approach avoids the morbidity of anterior transcervical, transoral, or transthoracic procedures while providing a view of the entire ventral cervicothoracic canal. We find this approach useful for resection of intradural tumors extending across the cervicothoracic junction. Potential complications with our approach include nerve root avulsion, cerebrospinal fluid leakage, postoperative spinal deformity or fusion failure, and cerebrospinal fluid–pleural fistula. We recommend our technique for resecting ventral intradural lesions spanning the cervicothoracic junction and multilevel intradural lesions of the ventral cervical spine. Postoperative instability is prevented by immediate posterior spinal reconstruction performed by means of lateral mass, artificial pedicle, and pedicle screw-rod fixation.

BAILOUT TECHNIQUE

In the event that artificial pedicle screws cannot be placed, the fusion levels may be extended as needed. As an alternative, the surgeon may decide to perform an anterior cervical fusion and plating as needed.

TIPS FROM THE MASTERS

- The paramedian transpedicular approach is a variation of traditional thoracic posterolateral transpedicular extracavitary approaches.
- It is useful for resection of ventral intradural extramedullary tumors that extend across the cervicothoracic junction.
- Postoperative instability is prevented by immediate posterior spinal reconstruction performed by means of lateral mass, artificial pedicle, and pedicle screw-rod fixation.

References (With Key References in Boldface)

1. Leung YL, Grevitt M, Henderson L, et al. Cord monitoring changes and segmental vessel ligation in the "at risk" cord during anterior spinal deformity surgery. Spine 30:1870-1874, 2005.
2. Morota N, Deletis V, Constantini S, et al. The role of motor evoked potentials during surgery for intramedullary spinal cord tumors. Neurosurgery 41:1327-1336, 1997.
3. Quinones-Hinojosa A, Lyon R, Ames CP, et al. Neuromonitoring during surgery for metastatic tumors to the spine: intraoperative interpretation and management strategies. Neurosurg Clin N Am 15:537-547, 2004.
4. Quinones-Hinojosa A, Lyon R, Zada G, et al. Changes in transcranial motor evoked potentials during intramedullary spinal cord tumor resection correlate with postoperative motor function. Neurosurgery 56:982-993; discussion 993, 2005.
5. Hernigou P, Duparc F. Lateral exposure of the cervicothoracic spine for anterior decompression and osteosynthesis. Neurosurgery 35:1121-1124; discussion 1124-1125, 1994.
6. McCormick PC, Post KD, Stein BM. Intraduralextramedullary tumors in adults. Neurosurg Clin N Am 1:591-608, 1990.
7. McCormick PC, Stein BM. Intramedullary tumors in adults. Neurosurg Clin N Am 1:609-630, 1990.

8. Steck JC, Dietze DD, Fessler RG. Posterolateral approach to intradural extramedullary thoracic tumors. J Neurosurg 81:202-205, 1994.
9. Gambardella G, Gervasio O, Zaccone C. Approaches and surgical results in the treatment of ventral thoracic meningiomas. Review of our experience with a postero-lateral combined transpedicular-transarticular approach. Acta Neurochir (Wien) 145:385-392; discussion 392, 2003.
10. Kraus DH, Huo J, Burt M. Surgical access to tumors of the cervicothoracic junction. Head Neck 17:131-136, 1995.
11. Kurz LT, Pursel SE, Herkowitz HN. Modified anterior approach to the cervicothoracic junction. Spine 16:S542-S547, 1991.
12. Marchesi DG, Boos N, Aebi M. Surgical treatment of tumors of the cervical spine and first two thoracic vertebrae. J Spinal Disord 6:489-496, 1993.
13. **Acosta FL Jr, Aryan HE, Chi J, et al. Modified paramedian transpedicular approach and spinal reconstruction for intradural tumors of the cervical and cervicothoracic spine: clinical experience. Spine 32:E203-E210, 2007.**
14. **Acosta FL Jr, Ames CP. Artificial pedicle screw reconstruction of the cervical spine after lateral paramedian transpedicular approach for lesions of the ventral cervical spinal canal. Neurosurgery 57:281-285; discussion 285, 2005.**

Chapter 30

Combined Far-Lateral Approaches and Reconstruction for Tumors of the Craniocervical Junction

Brendan D. Killory, Peter Nakaji, Robert F. Spetzler

Compared with the standard posterior midline approach to the craniocervical junction or the retrosigmoid approach to the cerebellopontine angle, the approaches to lesions located lateral or anterior to the medulla are considerably more complex. In the former approaches, the trajectory is straightforward and landmarks are plentiful. In contrast, the far-lateral approach requires "seeing ahead" through layers of muscle and bone, and dissection can feel somewhat blind. Furthermore, the anatomy of this region is more difficult because of the location of the sigmoid sinus, the vertebral artery, and the veil formed by the lower cranial nerves.

The trajectory that this approach offers, however, can provide surgeons with invaluable advantages for addressing pathology in this region. The same trajectory is not available with the midline posterior approach or through a traditional retrosigmoid approach. The far-lateral approach was first described by Heros[1] for the treatment of vertebral and vertebrobasilar aneurysms, and it is now frequently used to treat tumors of the foramen magnum and jugular foramen region as well. Familiarity with the nuances of this technique gives neurosurgeons an option for accessing vascular, neoplastic, degenerative, and inflammatory pathologies at the craniocervical junction, many of which lie lateral or anterior to the brainstem.

INDICATIONS AND CONTRAINDICATIONS

The most common indication for a far-lateral approach is a lesion located anterior or lateral to the brainstem or uppermost spinal cord that cannot be approached directly from a direct posterior approach. If the brainstem is deflected by the tumor to one side, the ipsilateral far-lateral approach is preferable. Foramen magnum meningioma is the classic lesion that grows in this fashion (Fig. 30-1). Other common lesions in this category include tumors of the ninth, tenth, or eleventh cranial nerve complex; vertebral artery aneurysms; clival meningiomas; and chordomas. If a tumor creates a corridor that allows it to be accessed from a purely posterior approach, then the simpler posterior approach is preferable. Extradural lesions, which are entirely anterior to the brainstem (i.e., in the clivus), should be considered for an endonasal, transpalatal, or transoral approach rather than a far-lateral approach. For lesions that are higher up (i.e., midclival or located at the level of the middle third of the basilar artery), a transpetrosal approach may be necessary. In all cases, radiosurgical or endovascular options should be considered, where appropriate, in the treatment plan.

Contraindications to the far-lateral approach include the presence of an anomalous vertebral artery or sigmoid sinus that precludes adequate exposure from this direction. In fact, such findings are rare. In these cases, the vertebral artery can be mobilized. If the dominant vertebral artery is on the same side as the lesion, caution should be exercised, because sacrifice of this artery could be catastrophic. However, the vertebral artery is quite sturdy and, if exposed in an orderly fashion, it should not be at undue risk. The presence of a dominant or sole sigmoid sinus on the exposure side creates a similar concern. The risk to the sigmoid sinus is somewhat greater than the risk to the vertebral artery. However, this risk does not present an absolute contraindication to accessing pathology in this region through a far-lateral approach.

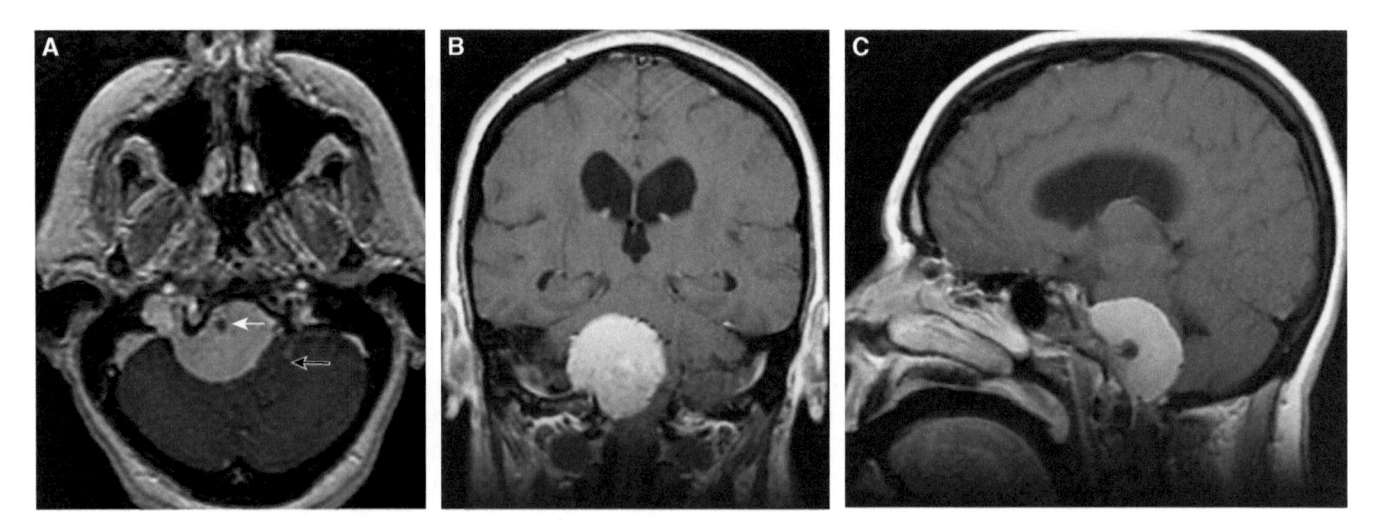

Fig. 30-1 **A,** T1-weighted axial, **B,** coronal, and **C,** sagittal scans enhanced with gadolinium show a typical foramen magnum meningioma. The tumor is biased to the right, displacing the brainstem *(A, white arrow)* and encasing the right vertebral artery *(A, black arrow)*. A midline approach would be obstructed by thinned-out lower cranial nerves that are highly susceptible to injury with manipulation. (Used with permission from Barrow Neurological Institute.)

PREOPERATIVE EVALUATION

Physical Examination

All patients undergoing this procedure should undergo standard physical and neurologic examinations. Particular attention should be paid to the lower cranial nerves (VII-XII), which are most often involved in pathologies addressed by this approach and are most susceptible to injury during surgery. The presence of hoarseness or swallowing problems may indicate preexisting weakness of the ninth or tenth cranial nerve. In these instances, laryngoscopy performed in the office by an otolaryngologist may help document the weakness. Weakness of these nerves on the side contralateral to the planned approach should raise particular concern, because weakness on the approach side may necessitate a tracheostomy and gastrostomy. Atrophy of the tongue usually indicates involvement of the twelfth cranial nerve.

Attention should be paid to the patient's cervical range of motion, because appropriate positioning is the key to an optimal exposure. The better a patient can rotate, flex, and laterally bend his or her neck, the better the surgical access will be.

Diagnostic Studies

Routine preoperative studies should be obtained (complete blood cell count, basic metabolic panel, coagulation profile, electrocardiogram), and more extensive testing should be individualized based on medical comorbidity. Formal audiographic assessment and direct laryngoscopy should be considered for patients with involvement of cranial nerves VIII, IX, and X.

Radiologic Studies

Gadolinium-enhanced and unenhanced magnetic resonance imaging (MRI) is usually the best modality to delineate pathology. Magnetic resonance angiography can be used to define vascular structures. Computed tomography (CT) often best delineates bony involvement and is helpful for surgical planning to determine when fusion may be needed. CT angiography is particularly useful to define the course of the vertebral artery, to identify anatomic variants of the vertebral artery, and to determine whether the bony anatomy will support safe fusion.

CT venography or magnetic resonance venography is important to determine whether the venous sinuses are patent bilaterally. If a single dominant sinus is present on the approach side, great caution must be exerted because damage to the sinus can result in catastrophic intracranial venous hypertension.

If the occipitocervical or C1-2 articulations are involved, flexion-extension radiographs may show instability that necessitates fixation or fusion. This finding also may be evident during surgery.

Table 30-1 Posterior Approaches to Brainstem and Upper Cervical Spinal Cord

Approach	Regions Accessed	Pathologies Addressed
Midline suboccipital	Posterior-inferior brainstem, foramina of Luschka	Distal PICA aneurysms, vascular/neoplastic/infectious/inflammatory processes of dorsolateral foramen magnum
Retrosigmoid	Dorsolateral pons/midbrain CPA	Intra-axial and extra-axial tumors, vascular/neoplastic/infectious/inflammatory processes of CPA
Far-lateral	Anterolateral cervicomedullary junction and lower pons	Vertebral artery aneurysms neoplastic/vascular/degenerative/infectious/inflammatory processes of ventrolateral foramen magnum
Transpetrous	Anterior pons, clivus	Basilar trunk aneurysms, vascular/neoplastic/infectious inflammatory processes of clivus and anterior ventral pons

CPA, Cerebellopontine angle; *PICA,* posterior inferior cerebellar artery.

CLINICAL DECISION-MAKING
TREATMENT DECISIONS

Surgical approaches to the posterior fossa should be chosen by assessing the trajectory needed to resect a given lesion (Table 30-1). If the optimal trajectory is below the level of the pons, above the cervical cord, directed inferior to superior toward the lesion, and extends laterally, as opposed to posteriorly, then a far-lateral approach is preferable. If a lesion can be approached at the level of the pons or lies predominantly in the cerebellopontine angle, it should be accessed typically from a retrosigmoid approach. If a lesion is at the level of the pons and is entirely anterior to the brainstem, some type of transpetrosal approach may be necessary. Lower lesions, which are located in the posterior 180 degrees of the brainstem or in the foramen of Luschka bilaterally, are best approached through a suboccipital midline approach (Fig. 30-2).

CHOICE OF TECHNIQUE

Once the far-lateral approach has been selected, the degree of bony removal must be tailored to the lesion. As a general rule, the further anteriorly and medially that the pathology being addressed is located, the more extensive the removal of the occipital bone and condyle must be to avoid retracting the brainstem and lower cranial nerves. Exceptions are large tumors with a lateral extension, where the lesion itself creates a surgical corridor.

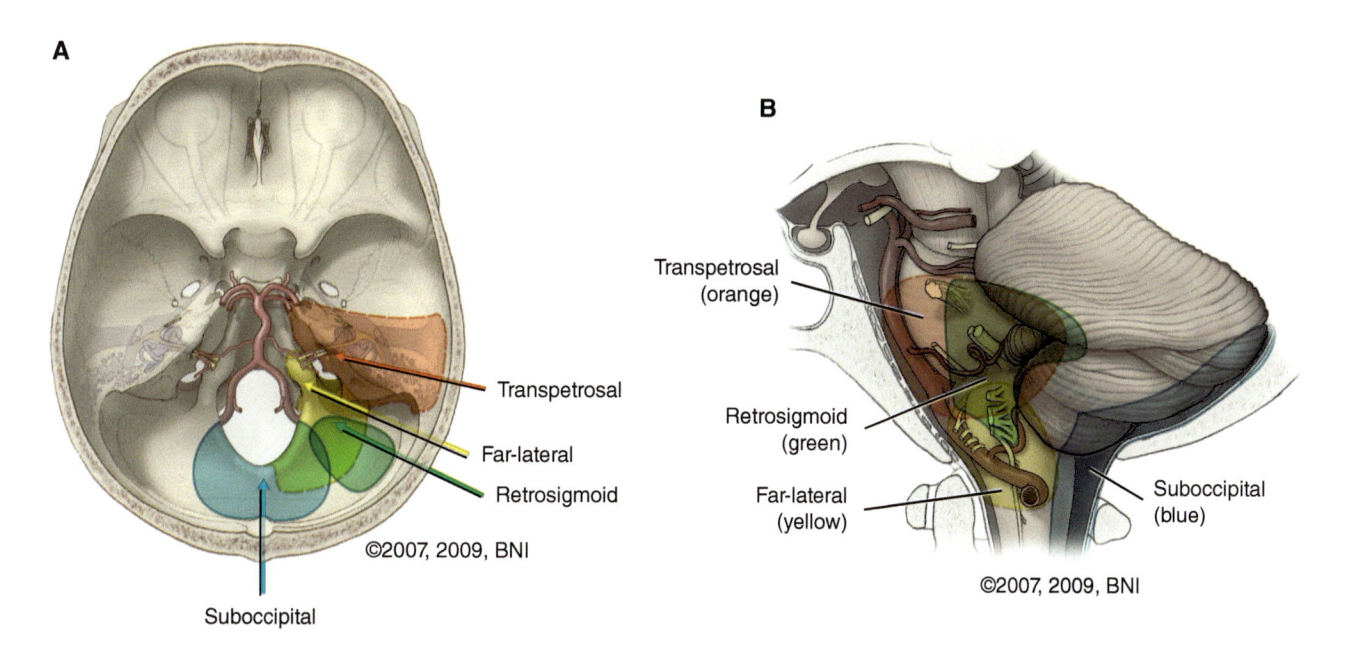

Fig. 30-2 **A,** Superior and **B,** lateral views of the skull base show exposures accessed by various posterior approaches to the brainstem and upper cervical cord. (Used with permission from Barrow Neurological Institute.)

TECHNIQUE

POSITIONING AND SETUP

Although patients can be positioned prone or supine with a large "bump" sandbag or equivalent placed under the shoulder ipsilateral to the lesion, we favor a modified park bench position, with the patient lying on his or her side with the lesion side up, turned slightly prone (Fig. 30-3). The operating table is extended rostrally with a plexiglass board, and the dependent arm is padded and secured to the Mayfield stand. An axillary roll should be used, and both somatosensory evoked potentials and pulse oximetry should be used throughout the operation to monitor this limb. Additional monitoring is tailored to the specifics of the operation but usually includes complete somatosensory evoked potentials, cranial nerves VII to XI, often cranial nerve XII, and sometimes motor evoked potentials.

Exact positioning of the patient is necessary to achieve all of the advantages of the far-lateral approach. The patient's head is positioned with the mastoid at the highest point with three key maneuvers. First the head is flexed, bringing the chin toward the chest to open the space between the axis and foramen magnum and to facilitate superior visualization. Next the head is rotated away from the lesion and bent laterally toward the opposite shoulder, further opening the space between the ipsilateral atlas and foramen magnum, and bringing the entry point to the bone uppermost in the surgical field. The exposure can be augmented by taping the ipsilateral arm caudally

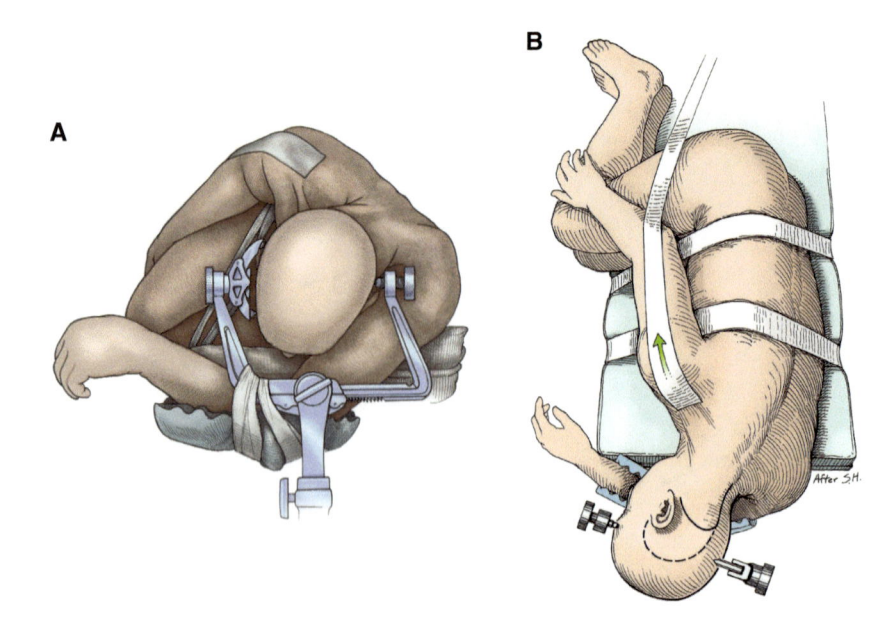

Fig. 30-3 **A,** Modified park bench position. Patient lies on his or her side, with the lesion side up, turned slightly prone. The operating table is extended rostrally with a plexiglass board, and the dependent arm is padded and secured to a Mayfield stand. An axillary roll should be used. A pillow is positioned between the patient's knees. (From Barrow Neurological Institute.) **B,** Patient should be secured firmly with tape over the hips and upper thorax. (Modified from Baldwin HZ, Miller CG, van Loveren HR, et al. The far lateral/combined supra- and infratentorial approach. A human cadaveric prosection model for routes of access to the petroclival region and ventral brain stem. J Neurosurg 81:60-68, 1994. Used with permission from Journal of Neurosurgery.)

and inferiorly. If the arm is taped, evoked potentials should be monitored to confirm that the brachial plexus is not being stretched unacceptably. The working direction is upward into the craniocervical junction. Therefore the microscope must be set up to allow visualization without affecting the patient. For a left-sided approach, the observer should be on the right; for a right-sided approach, the observer should be on the left. In most operating microscopes, an attached still camera will be in the way for this approach and therefore must be removed.

After the patient is positioned, the image guidance frame should be positioned on the side contralateral and caudal to the surgical field. We have found image guidance to be helpful in maintaining orientation during exposure, especially when a paramedian incision is used where the vertebral artery can be encountered suddenly during the transmuscular exposure. Image guidance also can help identify the location of the sigmoid sinus, allowing it to be exposed more rapidly.

Skin Incision and Bony Exposure

There are two basic techniques for exposing the soft tissue during a far-lateral approach (Fig. 30-4)[9]. The first uses a "hockey-stick" incision, which is formed by a midline incision beginning at the level of the second or third cervical spinous process. The incision proceeds above the nuchal line and then curves over to the ipsilateral mastoid.

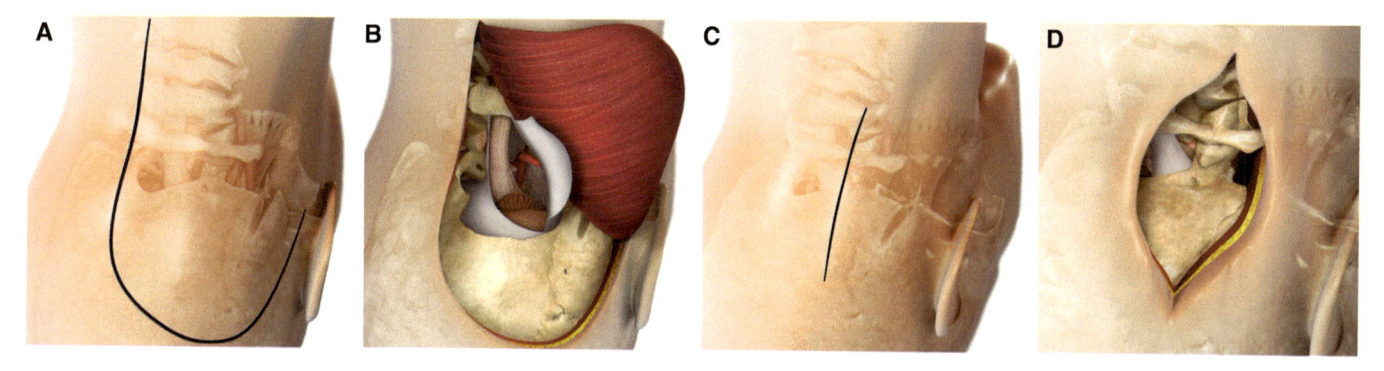

Fig. 30-4 Two basic variants of skin incision. **A,** Hockey-stick incision and **B,** corresponding flap maintain the surgeon's orientation to midline, but the incision is long, extensive muscle mobilization is needed, and the large flap can potentially obscure the surgical view. **C,** Paramedian incision avoids these issues but is directly over the **D,** vertebral artery. (Used with permission from Barrow Neurological Institute.)

A muscular cuff can be left at the superior insertion of the suboccipital muscles to facilitate closure. The incision extends down to the midline of the axis and atlas, and the myocutaneous flap is reflected off the occipital bone and the laminae of C1 and C2 laterally and inferiorly with sharp technique.

Although its course is variable, the vertebral artery can usually be identified in the sulcus arteriosus of the axis. The vessel may even contact the occipital bone.[2] The advantage of this technique is that it is easier to identify the landmarks, which remain recognizable throughout the approach and, consequently, protect the vertebral artery and dura more reliably. If the occipital artery is needed for bypass, this technique allows it to be saved and then dissected from within the flap. The disadvantage of the approach is that the extensive muscle elevation creates a large myocutaneous flap that may itself obstruct the viewing and working angles.

The second technique involves a paramedian incision with a muscle-splitting trajectory directed at the lateral foramen magnum and occipital condyle. In addition to frequently palpating the spinous and transverse processes of the atlas and axis, respectively, we have found image guidance to be invaluable in maintaining the surgeon's orientation with this approach, especially early in the surgeon's experience. Monopolar electrocauterization must not be used in the deeper muscle layers, because the vertebral artery is quite variable and the vessel can be injured inadvertently. Splitting these fibers with Metzenbaum scissors allows a more controlled encounter with the vessel.

The horizontal portion of the vertebral artery lies within the suboccipital triangle. This triangle is formed by the major and minor rectus capitis muscles medially, by the superior oblique muscle superiorly, and by the inferior oblique muscle inferiorly. The artery is covered with a venous plexus. Bleeding from this structure can be controlled with judicious bipolar cauterization or with application of a variety of hemostatic agents. Care must be taken not to damage any branches of the vertebral artery, inasmuch as extradural origins of the posterior inferior cerebellar artery (PICA) and the posterior spinal artery have been described.[2]

The bony exposure should extend medially to the midline and laterally to the sigmoid sinus and proximal transverse process of the axis. We have found fish hook retractors to be superior to self-retaining retractors; the former tend to flatten the edges of the incision, whereas the latter elevates them. The benefits of this paramedian incision include a relatively shorter incision with less muscle elevation and, consequently, less lateral retraction of tissue that can potentially obstruct the surgical corridor. The disadvantage of this technique is that it is easier for the surgeon to become disoriented. Consequently the potential for injury to the vertebral artery is increased. Directing a more medial trajectory, aiming toward the midline rather than coming down on the occipital condyle directly, can ameliorate this risk to some degree.

BONE REMOVAL AND DURAL OPENING

Bony removal includes the inferior retrosigmoid bone down to the foramen magnum, as well as the ipsilateral lamina of C1. The actual extent of bone removal must be tailored to the lesion in question. Typically the limits of maximal exposure are the transverse sinus superiorly; the sigmoid sinus, hypoglossal canal, and vertebral artery laterally; the foramen magnum and beyond it the arch of C1 inferiorly; and the midline (or a bit contralateral to the midline) medially. Rarely does a lesion require this full exposure. After the entire course of the vertebral artery, from the vertebral foramen of the transverse process of the axis to its entrance through the dura, is exposed and protected, we start with a C1 hemilaminectomy (Fig. 30-5, *A*). The high-speed drill and footplate are ideal for this purpose, but bone rongeurs can also be used. Bone removal should extend from the midline to the lateral mass and can be extended to skeletonize and mobilize the vertebral artery in its foramen.

Next a high-speed drill and footplate are used to turn a small craniotomy upward from the foramen magnum (Fig. 30-5, *B*). If the lip of the foramen magnum is particularly thick, it may help to thin the planned extent of the craniotomy with the burr before the craniotomy is turned. The craniotomy should extend from the midline to as lateral as possible at the foramen magnum. If indicated, the craniotomy can extend superiorly to the transverse-sigmoid junction, and the entire course of the sigmoid sinus can be skeletonized. When such an "extended" craniotomy is required, an additional burr hole should be drilled at the transverse-sigmoid sinus, and image guidance should be used to map the sigmoid anatomy.

The surgeon must next decide how much of the occipital condyle to remove (Fig. 30-5, *C*). The extent of bony removal is determined by the geometry of the pathology being addressed. For ventrolateral tumors, little drilling is necessary, because the tumor itself creates an operative corridor. For vertebrobasilar aneurysms or other lesions that have not themselves retracted the brainstem for the surgeon, removing the posterior third of the condyle usually suffices. We recommend using the diamond burr and microscopic magnification for drilling. The hypoglossal canal runs anteriorly and laterally along its course from proximal to distal and can be identified by a transition from spongy bone to its cortical canal.

Condylar emissary veins are frequently encountered running from the condylar fossa, which lies immediately posterolateral to the condyle, to the sigmoid sinus. Bleeding from these vessels can easily be controlled with bone wax, packing, or both. After the condyle has been drilled, further exposure can be obtained by drilling the jugular tubercle either extradurally or intradurally (Fig. 30-5, *D*).

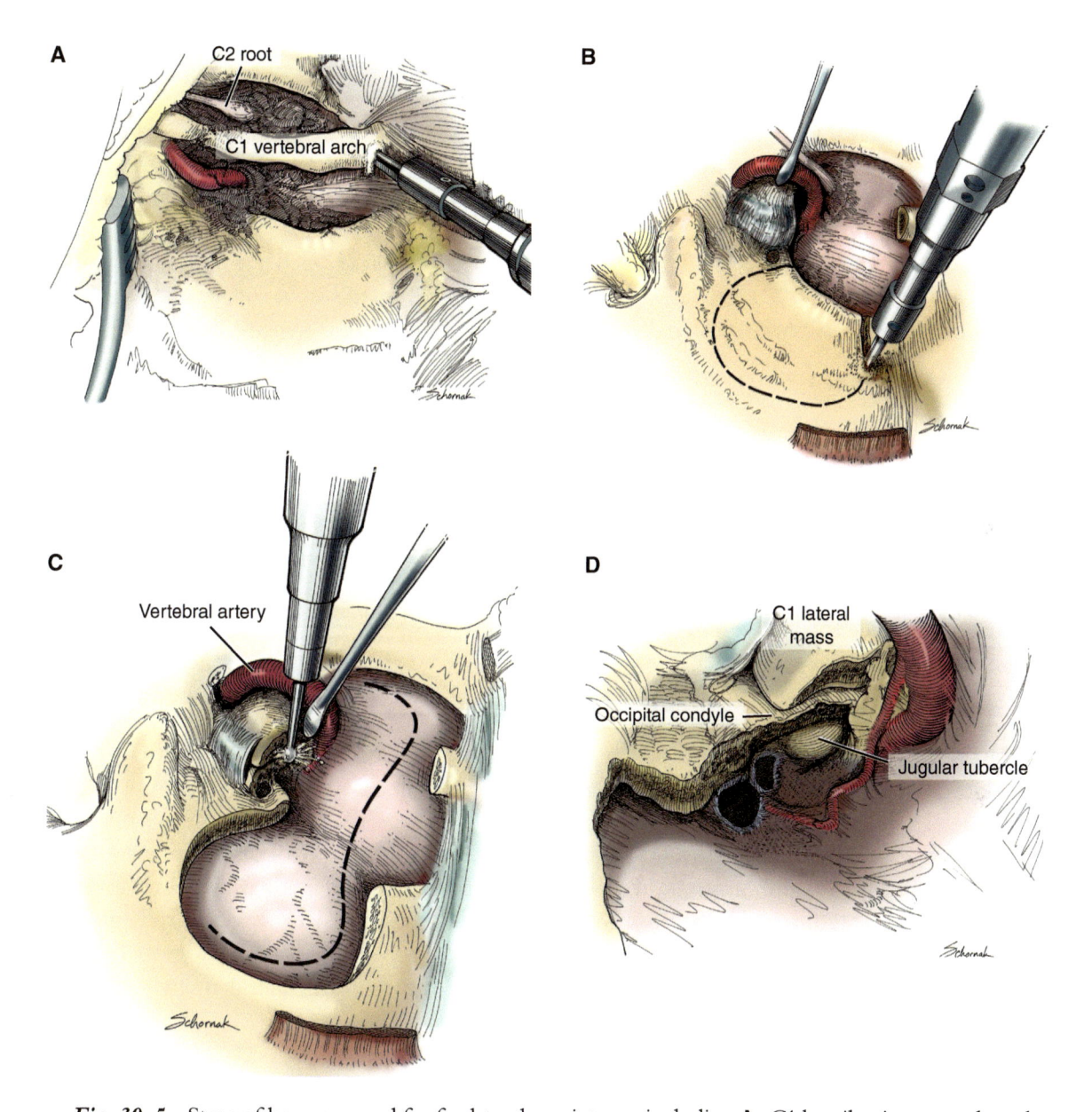

Fig. 30-5 Steps of bony removal for far-lateral craniotomy, including **A**, C1 hemilaminectomy, lateral suboccipital craniotomy, and condylectomy; **B**, small craniotomy upward from the foramen magnum; and **C**, drilling of the occipital condyle and **D**, jugular tubercle, both tailored to the patient's anatomy and the lesion's geometry. Note that the vertebral artery is identified and protected throughout the procedure. (Modified from Baldwin HZ, Miller CG, van Loveren HR, et al. The far lateral/combined supra- and infratentorial approach. A human cadaveric prosection model for routes of access to the petroclival region and ventral brain stem. J Neurosurg 81:60-68, 1994. Used with permission from Journal of Neurosurgery.)

Continued

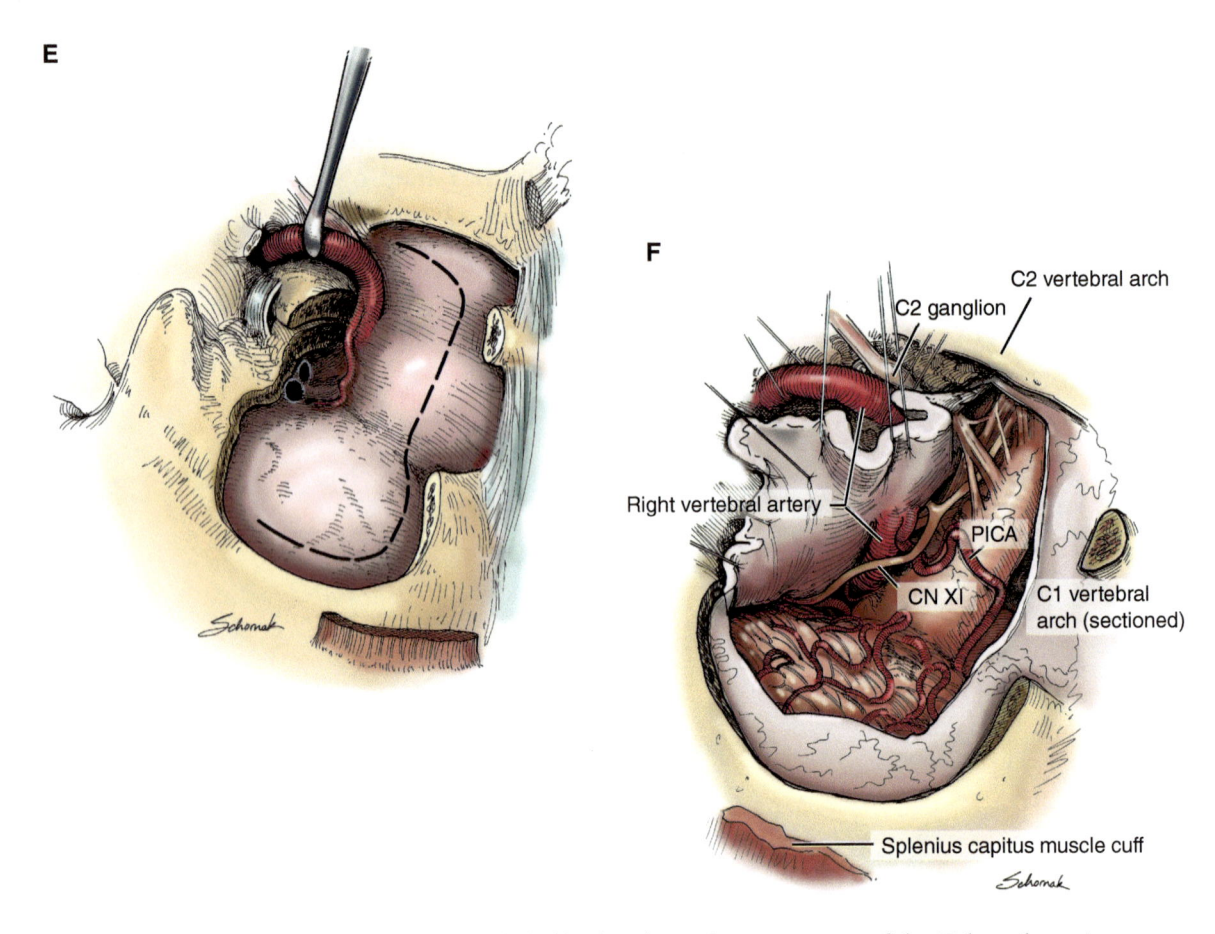

Fig. 30-5, cont'd **E,** Dural opening *(dashed line)* with resultant exposure of the **F,** lateral cervicomedullary junction. Note that the vertebral artery is mobilized with the dural flap.

A curvilinear dural incision should be made to create a flap with its base flush along the lateral aspect of the craniotomy (Fig. 30-5, *E* and *F*).

Removal of the occipital condyle rarely destabilizes the atlantooccipital joint and requires fusion. Vishteh et al[3] studied the biomechanics in cadavers and determined that statistically significant hypermobility is created after a 50% condylectomy. Major biomechanical changes resulted from a 75% condylectomy. These investigators recommended considering fusion if more than half of the condyle is resected.

Bejjani et al[4] reviewed their series of 27 transcondylar far-lateral craniotomies and reported that one third of their patients required a fusion. These investigators were extremely aggressive with their condylectomies, and all patients who ultimately required fusion had more than 70% of their condyles resected. In our experience, short of resecting ventral extradural lesions, as described by al-Mefty et al,[5] it is rarely necessary to drill more than one third of the condyle, and instrumentation can generally be avoided.

CLOSURE

A watertight dural closure, either with or without a dural graft, should be attempted. One benefit of a craniotomy over a craniectomy is that the bone can be replaced with miniplates, adding another layer of closure to prevent cerebrospinal fluid (CSF) leakage. If the mastoid is opened extensively, fat can be used to fill the gap. If possible, the posterior arch of the atlas can be replaced. However, this option may not be available if bone removal has been extensive. The suboccipital muscles should be reapproximated, and careful attention should be paid to closing the deep cervical fascia, which is the most crucial layer in preventing a CSF leak. If a hockey-stick incision was used, this attention should extend to reattaching the muscular cuff. The dermis and skin should be closed in the standard fashion.

OUTCOMES WITH EVALUATION OF RESULTS

As with many surgical approaches, no comparative series documents the superiority of the far-lateral approach compared with its alternatives. D'Ambrosio et al[6] reported that they achieved good outcomes in more than 90% (1 or 2 on the Glasgow Outcome Scale) of patients treated for ruptured proximal PICA aneurysms with a far-lateral technique similar to that described earlier in this chapter. Their outcomes for these challenging lesions were comparable to those of patients treated surgically for ruptured posterior communicating artery aneurysms, a patient population traditionally considered to respond well to surgery. In their review of the literature, these investigators noted that the incidence of lower cranial nerve palsies for these lesions was 20% to 66%. The highest incidence was in a series of patients who did not undergo a C1 hemilaminectomy.[7] This finding underscores the importance of this technique in exposing the anterolateral brainstem.

SIGNATURE CASES
FORAMEN MAGNUM MENINGIOMA

A typical lesion appropriate for a far-lateral approach in a 63-year-old woman is seen on sagittal (Fig. 30-6, *A*) and axial (Fig. 30-6, *B*) gadolinium-enhanced T1-weighted MRI scans. The amount of bony removal necessary to remove the tumor is shown in this montage of the foramen magnum and the ring of C1 (Fig. 30-6, *C*). The final appearance of the tumor removal achieved is seen on these 4-year postoperative sagittal and axial MRI scans (Fig. 30-6, *D* and *E*).

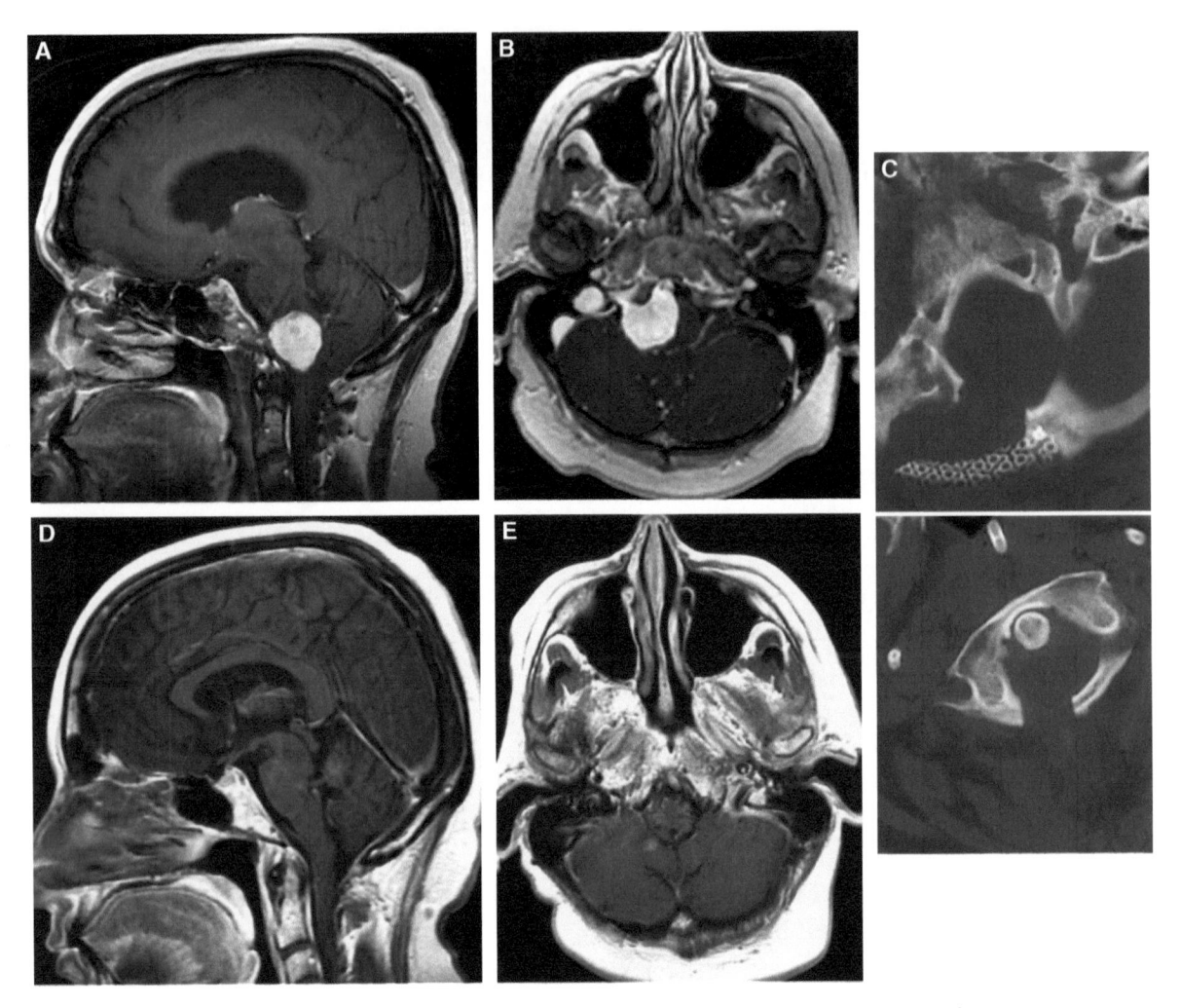

Fig. 30-6 **A,** Gadolinium-enhanced T1-weighted sagittal and **B,** axial MRI scans demonstrating a foramen magnum meningioma. Postoperative imaging demonstrates bony removal on **C,** axial CT image and complete tumor removal on enhanced **D,** sagittal and **E,** axial T1-weighted MRI scans. (Used with permission from Barrow Neurological Institute.)

A small tumor located anterior to the brainstem requires a far-lateral approach even more so than a larger tumor, because the tumor itself does not move the brainstem enough to the side to create a path to reach it (Fig. 30-7, A and B). By approaching from the side, access anterior to the brainstem can be obtained that will allow safe removal of the tumor (Fig. 30-7, C and D). The location of the skin incision can be seen on the postoperative axial MRI scan (see *arrow* in Fig. 30-7, D).

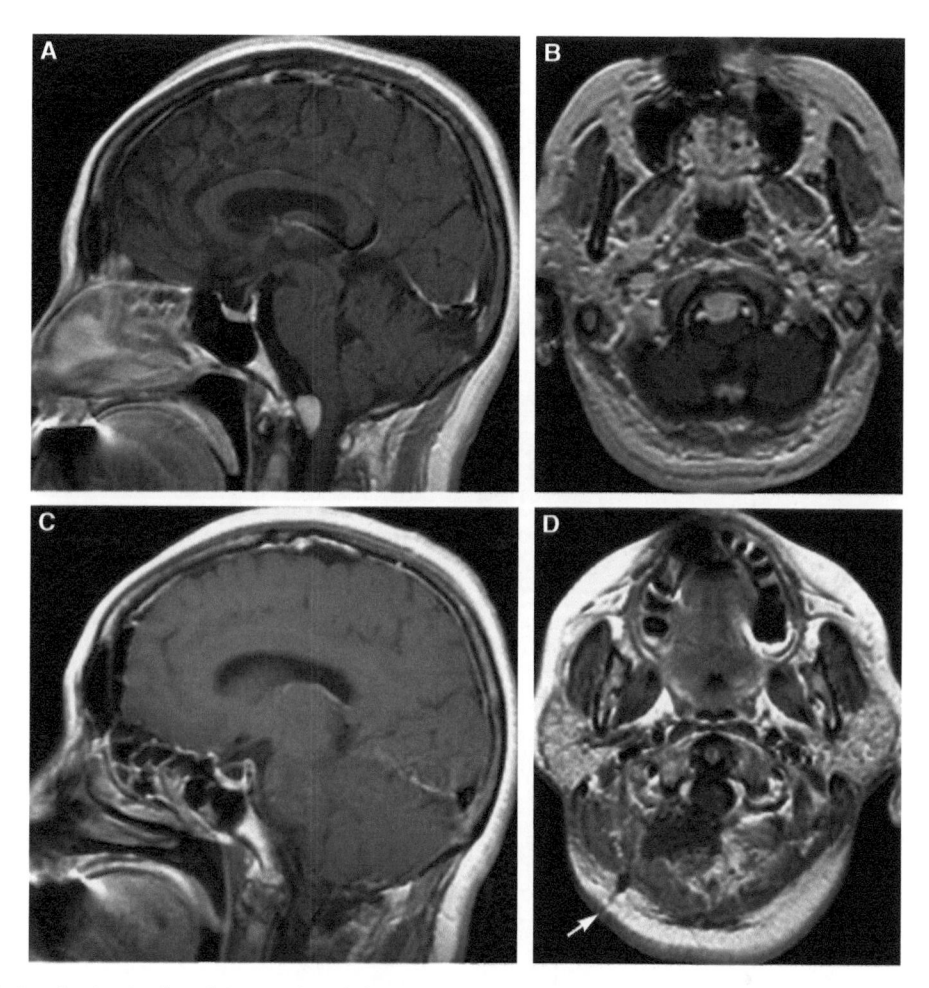

Fig. 30-7 **A,** Sagittal and **B,** axial gadolinium-enhanced T1-weighted MRI scans show a small foramen magnum meningioma ventral to the brainstem. Postoperative **C,** sagittal and **D,** axial gadolinium-enhanced T1-weighted MRIs confirm gross total removal of the tumor. *Arrow* in D indicates location of skin incision. (Used with permission from Barrow Neurological Institute.)

In this case the tumor has displaced the brainstem so much that a posterior approach would almost be possible, as seen in this axial T1-weighted gadolinium-enhanced MRI scan (Fig. 30-8, *A*). Therefore the bony removal does not have to be as extensive. As shown in the axial CT bone window views, the craniotomy extended only to the condyle and lateral mass of C1 (Fig. 30-8, *B* and *C*). In this case the arch of C1 was not replaced, and the bone at the level of the foramen magnum was left off, with no obvious clinical consequence. Postoperative axial T1-weighted MRI scans enhanced with gadolinium confirmed complete tumor removal (Fig. 30-8, *D*).

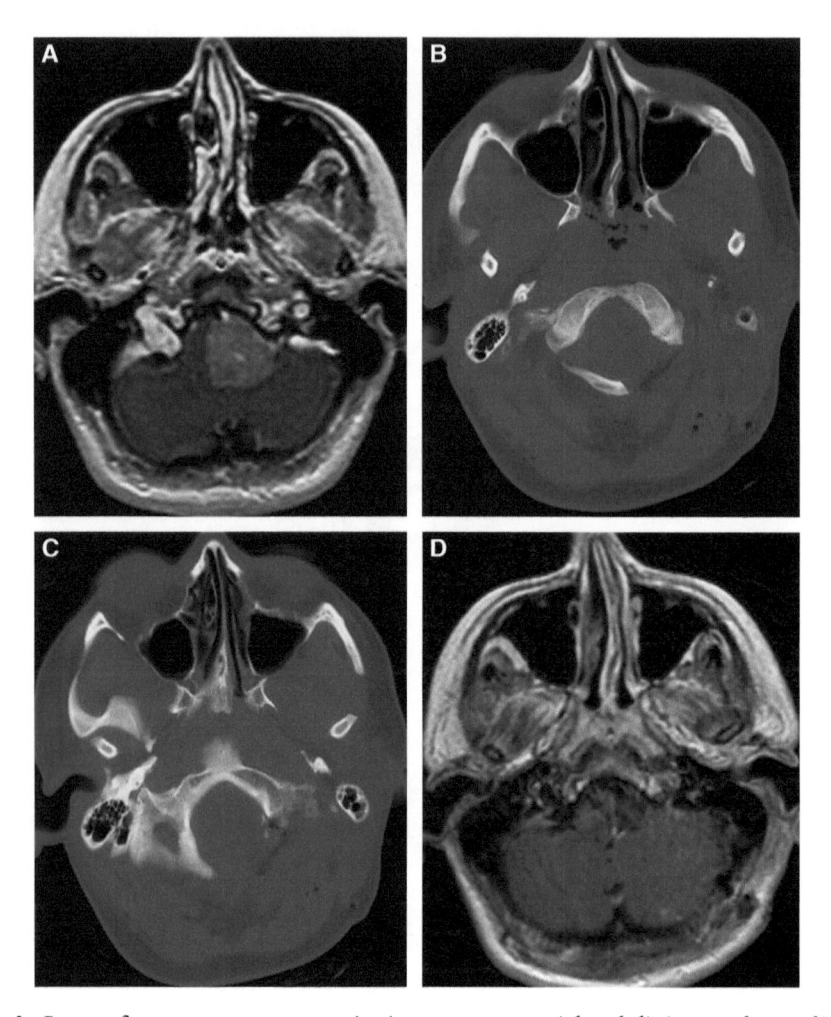

Fig. 30-8 **A,** Larger foramen magnum meningioma seen on axial gadolinium-enhanced T1-weighted MRI. The lesion displaces the brainstem, and axial CT imaging demonstrates that a less extensive bony removal of the **B,** axis and **C,** foramen magnum is required to achieve complete tumor removal, as confirmed on **D,** gadolinium-enhanced T1-weighted axial MRI scan. (Used with permission from Barrow Neurological Institute.)

JUGULAR FORAMEN SCHWANNOMA

A 38-year-old woman presented with gait instability and headache. The tumor was located below the cerebellopontine angle (Fig. 30-9, *A* and *B*) and could be reached alternatively through a retrosigmoid approach. However, the angle under the cerebellum is better accessed from below. The far-lateral approach affords this trajectory and improves access to the jugular tubercle, which needs to be drilled to improve exposure of the tumor in the jugular foramen. The extensive bony removal, which included the posterior third of the condyle, is shown in Fig. 30-9, *C*. The tumor had excellent margins and was removed completely, while sparing cranial nerves IX, X, and XI (Fig. 30-9, *D* and *E*). Reconstruction included placement of an abdominal fat graft and a titanium plate. At a 20-month follow-up, the cosmetic result was excellent.

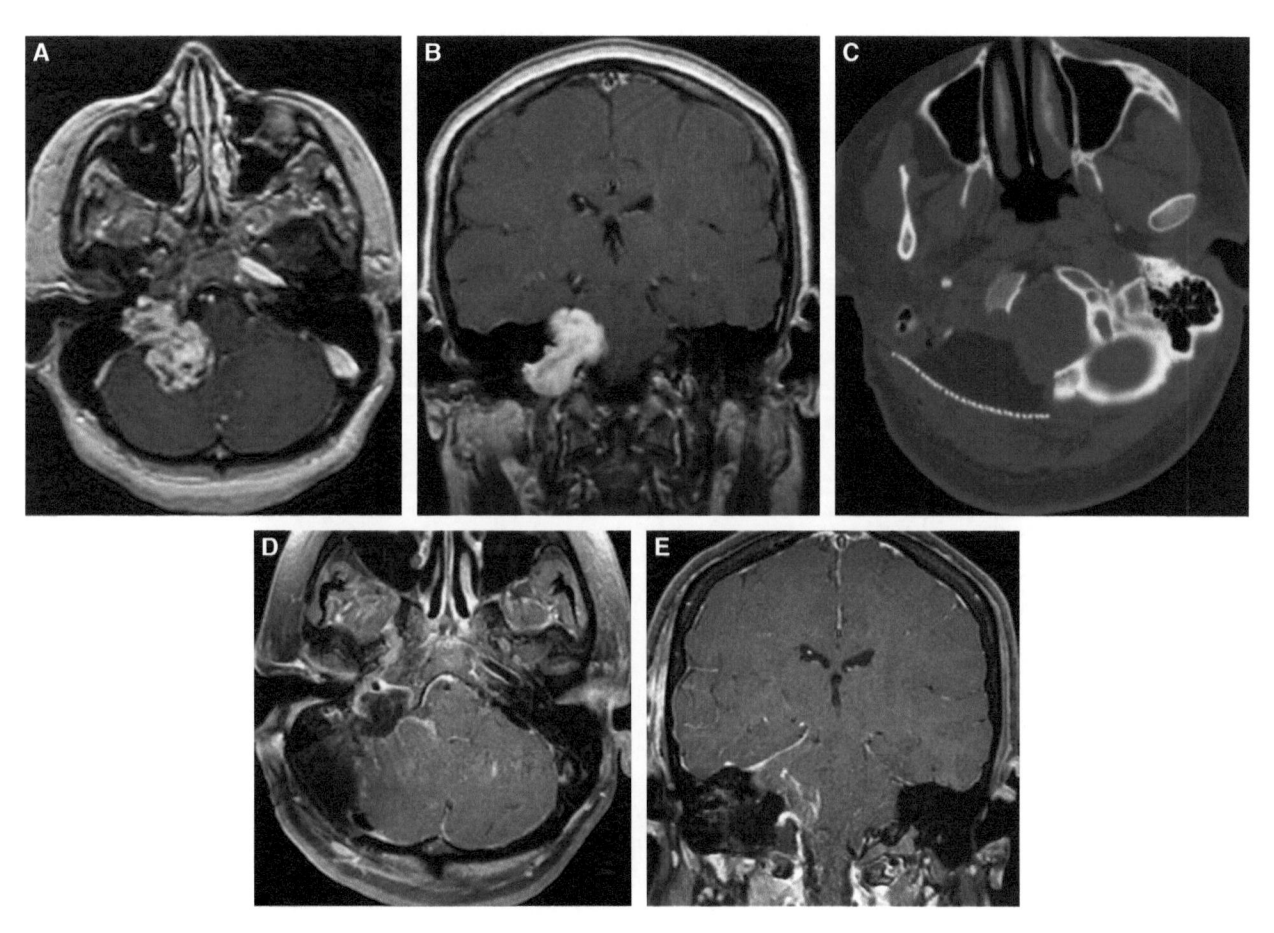

Fig. 30-9 **A,** Axial and **B,** coronal gadolinium-enhanced T1-weighted MRI scans showing a jugular foramen schwannoma. **C,** Postoperative axial CT scan demonstrates the extensive bony removal, including the posterior occipital condyle and jugular tubercle, that was necessary to achieve gross total removal of the tumor, which was confirmed on gadolinium-enhanced T1-weighted **D,** axial and **E,** coronal MRI scans. (Used with permission from Barrow Neurological Institute.)

CLIVAL CHORDOMA

This tumor arises from the clivus and extends far to both sides, as shown on T1-weighted gadolinium-enhanced axial (Fig. 30-10, *A*) and sagittal (Fig. 30-10, *B*) MRI scans. No single trajectory affords an optimal view of the tumor. The brainstem is located posteriorly and to the right. A left far-lateral approach allows the bulk of the tumor to be removed, as shown in axial (Fig. 30-10, *C*) and sagittal (Fig. 30-10, *D*) MRI scans. The residual can be accessed through a contralateral approach or, as in this case, addressed with adjuvant radiosurgery.

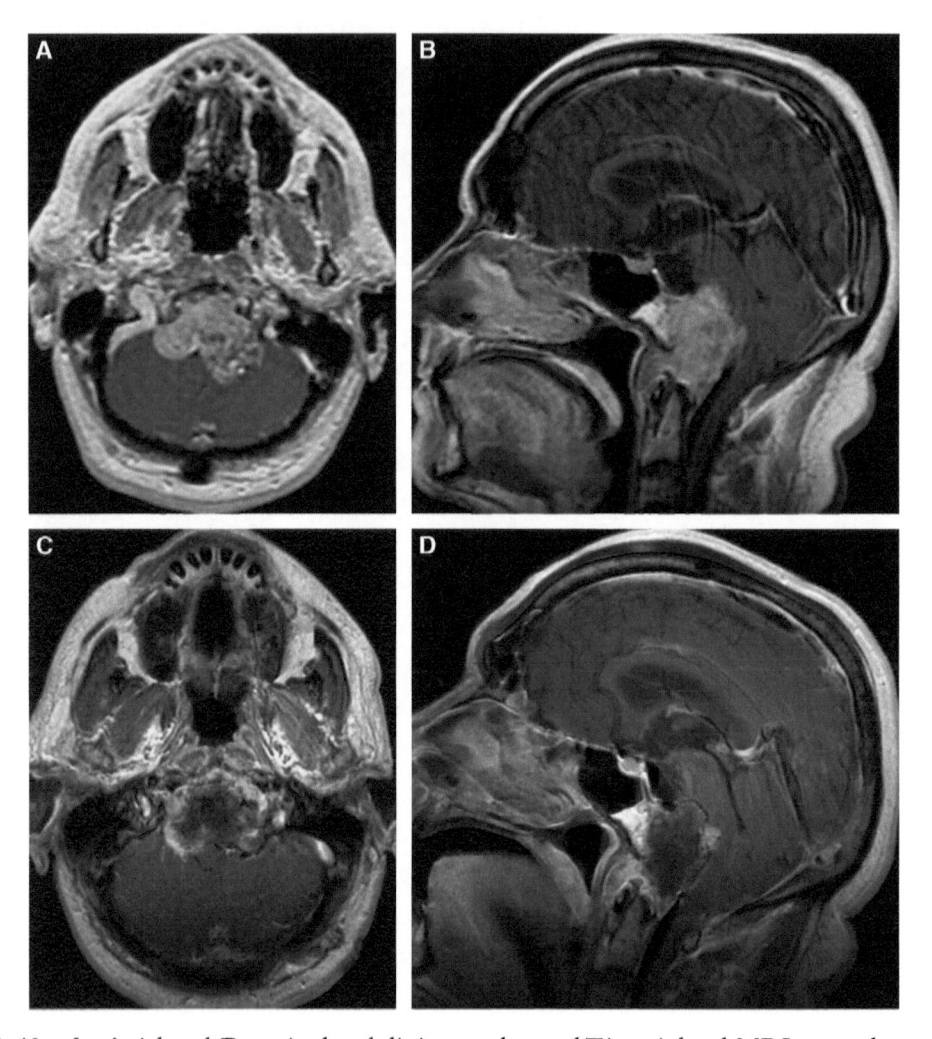

Fig. 30-10 **A,** Axial and **B,** sagittal gadolinium-enhanced T1-weighted MRI scans show a clival chordoma with posterior displacement of the brainstem. A left far-lateral approach was used to aggressively debulk the tumor, as seen on postoperative gadolinium-enhanced T1-weighted **C,** axial and **D,** sagittal MRI scans. (Used with permission from Barrow Neurological Institute.)

CONCLUSION

The far-lateral approach is a valuable tool in the neurosurgeon's armamentarium. It is particularly valuable when approaching lesions at the base of the skull or at the craniocervical junction, especially when they are best approached from below or located anterior to the brainstem. It provides valuable access to targets lateral or anterior to the cervicomedullary junction. Adherence to strict anatomic principles will help surgeons to overcome potential disorientation in this area and to work safely around the vertebral artery. Neurosurgeons should not hesitate to use this approach for the improved access and decreased neural element manipulation that it affords.

BAILOUT TECHNIQUES

VASCULAR INJURIES

If the vertebral artery is damaged during the operation and cannot be repaired primarily, there are multiple rescue strategies. A diminutive vessel can be sacrificed as long as the contralateral vertebral artery feeds the ipsilateral PICA. An end-to-side occipital-to-vertebral artery bypass can be performed. The occipital artery is most easily identified distally at the nuchal line and can be dissected proximally until adequate length is available to mobilize it for the bypass. The calibers of the occipital artery and the PICA are usually well matched. If the injury involves the PICA, a side-to-side PICA-to-PICA bypass can be performed near the foramen of Magendie. The craniotomy must be expanded to expose the contralateral foramen magnum. Both vessels must be dissected free of their arachnoid membrane to expose and mobilize them for the midline bypass.

DURAL CLOSURE

If the patient refuses an allograft dural substitute, periosteum is an excellent option. It can be harvested from the occipital bone, above the nuchal line, either by extending the incision rostrally or by undermining the scalp, as described by Stevens et al.[8] Another option is a tensor fascia lata graft, which can be harvested from the lateral thigh. D'Ambryosio et al[6] advocate securing an abdominal fat graft over the durotomy site to further reduce the risk of CSF leakage. Finally, several days of continuous postoperative CSF drainage through a lumbar drain is an option, especially in previously irradiated or operated surgical sites.

TIPS FROM THE MASTERS

- The far lateral approach should be reserved for patients whose lesions lie anterior or anterolateral to the brainstem. If the tumor is purely lateral, it may create enough space that a simpler midline approach will suffice.
- Preoperative evaluation of the vertebral arteries is essential so that collateral vasculature is known in case one of the vessels needs to be purposely sacrificed or is inadvertently damaged.
- In many cases, the upper part of the condyle can be removed without damaging its articular surface, thus preserving stability at the occiput-C1 joint.
- In cases where a bypass could be required, a hockey-stick incision should be used, because it saves the occipital artery to serve as a possible donor vessel.

References (With Key References in Boldface)

1. Heros RC. Lateral suboccipital approach for vertebral and vertebrobasilar artery lesions. J Neurosurg 64:559-562, 1986.
2. **Rhoton AL Jr. The far-lateral approach and its transcondylar, supracondylar, and paracondylar extensions. Neurosurgery 47(3Suppl):S195-S209, 2000.**
3. Vishteh AG, Crawford NR, Melton MS, et al. Stability of the craniovertebral junction after unilateral occipital condyle resection: a biomechanical study. J Neurosurg 90:91-98, 1999.
4. Bejjani GK, Sekhar LN, Riedel CJ. Occipitocervical fusion following the extreme lateral transcondylar approach. Surg Neurol 54:109-115, 2000.
5. **al-Mefty O, Borba LA, Aoki N, et al. The transcondylar approach to extradural nonneoplastic lesions of the craniovertebral junction. J Neurosurg 84:1-6, 1996.**
6. D'Ambrosio AL, Kreiter KT, Bush CA, et al. Far lateral suboccipital approach for the treatment of proximal posteroinferior cerebellar artery aneurysms: surgical results and long-term outcome. Neurosurgery 55:39-50, 2004.
7. Horowitz M, Kopitnik T, Landreneau F, et al. Posteroinferior cerebellar artery aneurysms: surgical results for 38 patients. Neurosurgery 43:1026-1032, 1998.
8. Stevens EA, Powers AK, Sweasey TA, et al. Simplified harvest of autologous pericranium for duraplasty in Chiari malformation Type I. Technical note. J Neurosurg Spine 11:80-83, 2009.
9. **Lanzino G, Paolini S, Spetzler RF. Far-lateral approach to the craniocervical junction. Neurosurgery 57:367-371, 2005.**

Chapter 31

Transoral and Transglossal Approach or Transmandibular Circumglossal Approach to the Cervical Spine

Ted H. Leem, Ivan Homer El-Sayed

Anterior approaches to the cervical spine have been used for many years to address a variety of pathologic conditions. Traditionally these approaches have been open, regardless of the pathologic condition to be treated. With the recent development of newer technologies and instrumentation, minimally invasive approaches to the cervical spine have become widely accepted. These techniques allow for a tailored approach to the cervical spine while minimizing morbidity. Thus they have become part of the standard repository for cervical spine surgery. This is of paramount importance as the population ages and the number of cervical spine procedures increases. In addition, the role of multidisciplinary surgical teams involving spine surgeons and otolaryngologists (head and neck surgeons) in complex cases and revision surgery is emerging. Several approaches have been described for accessing the craniocervical junction and anterior spine, including transmaxillary with a LeFort I approach, transcervical, and transoral.[1-4] The transoral approach has gained wide acceptance, but few guidelines exist concerning its use. The transoral approach can be used as part of a sequential approach, depending on the patient's anatomy and the amount of access needed. Anatomic variations may occur in the form of an elongated palate and uvula, a large tongue, a short or long mandibular ramus or mandibular body, and the presence or absence of teeth. At times a tracheostomy can be performed to provide an additional few centimeters of access and also to stabilize the airway.

A sequential approach can be used to address lesions of the upper anterior spine transorally. Increasing exposure can be achieved by retracting the palate, splitting the soft palate, removing a portion of the posterior hard palate, performing a midline glossotomy without mandibulotomy, and performing a midline mandibulotomy.[5] Recently a variation of the transoral approach has been described that uses an endonasal and endonasal/endoral approach.[6-8]

The lower neck can be approached transcervically to provide access down to the T1 level. When a few segments are addressed, the exposure is relatively simple. However, exposing multiple segments requires mobilization of additional structures in the neck, with a greater potential for secondary injury. The proximity of the great vessels, cranial nerves, esophagus and pharyngeal constrictors, and laryngeal structures creates potential for significant postoperative morbidity, which should be discussed with the patient preoperatively. In extreme cases the entire cervical spine can be exposed by using a combination of transcervical approaches with a mandibulotomy. Enlisting the help of a surgeon who is an expert in this anatomy, such as an otolaryngologist, can aid in the dissection and postoperative management. This chapter will discuss the transoral and transcervical approaches to the cervical spine.

INDICATIONS AND CONTRAINDICATIONS

Transoral and transcervical techniques are indicated whenever access to the craniovertebral junction and/or anterior cervical spine is required. Each approach can be tailored to the pathology, dictating which technique or techniques should be used. The craniocervical junction involving the clivus, odontoid process, ring of C1, and body of C2 may be affected by trauma, congenital malformations, inflammatory lesions, and a variety of benign or malignant tumors requiring biopsy or decompression. The common factor in many lesions of the craniocervical junction is upper cord compression requiring decompression. The lower spine can be approached for biopsy, tumor extirpation, or rigid fixation. When pathology overlapping the upper and lower spine exists, the approaches can be tailored to extend a transoral approach inferiorly or a transcervical approach superiorly, depending on the nature of the procedure being undertaken.

Transoral approaches are indicated for high lesions involving the odontoid process, C1 arch, and extending potentially into the body of C2. The transoral approach is well suited for lesions of the odontoid process with basilar impression or rheumatoid pannus. Depending on the pathology and surgical plan, transoral/transpharyngeal approaches can provide access to the lower cervical spine down to C4, which lies approximately posterior to the base of the tongue. There is, of course, overlap of access provided by a given technique, and approach selection is dictated by the planned surgical procedure. For instance, a biopsy or resection of lesions in the C2, C3, or C4 vertebrae of the spine can be performed transorally, whereas rigid fixation of these discs is best performed without oral contamination through a transcervical approach. However, accessing the C2 vertebra through a transcervical approach may create difficulty with application of the screws because of obstruction by the mandible.

Relative contraindications to the open transoral/transpharyngeal approach include the need to apply rigid fixation of the spine. Contamination of the implants may occur when they are exposed to the oral flora. Furthermore, a midline split of the pharynx with the use of a transpharyngeal approach can present problems with wound healing over the plate. When appropriate, traction and posterior fixation may avoid the need for additional work anteriorly.

The transcervical approach can provide a wide axis from C2 to T1, depending on the patient's anatomy. Preoperative assessment with radiographic imaging and correlation with anatomic landmarks can help to assess these lesions. Relative contraindications to a transcervical approach are few when patients are appropriately selected for biopsy, reduction, or fixation.

PREOPERATIVE EVALUATION

A preoperative examination and complete history determine the indications for surgery of the anterior spine. In addition to the overall health of these patients and their suitability for surgery, there are several factors that should be explored during preoperative planning. The physical examination should be thorough and include a neurologic assessment and evaluation of the degree of mouth opening and neck mobility. Evaluation by an otolaryngologist, along with a speech therapist for laryngeal examination, may also be warranted when a significant potential for speech and swallowing morbidity exists or when there is a history of prior surgery in the neck, such as a thyroidectomy, or a prior spine approach. In patients who report that they have had permanent or temporary hoarseness after a previous surgery, the possibility of vocal cord paresis should be considered. Furthermore, injury to the superior laryngeal nerve around the level of C3 can result in anesthesia of the supraglottis, with subtle dysphagia that can complicate postoperative recovery. Laryngeal sensation testing can be performed by an otolaryngologist when indicated. Radiographic studies include CT, MRI, plain radiography, and angiography in selected cases. The use of intraoperative computer-assisted navigation and intraoperative imaging (fluoroscopy, CT, MRI) can be useful.

Approaches to the cervical spine will depend on the spinal level and patient anatomy. The craniocervical junction and upper spine can be addressed through transoral approaches, whereas the middle and lower cervical spinal levels are addressed through transcervical approaches. Spinal level can be correlated with external anatomy. For instance, the hyoid bone estimates the C3 body, the laryngeal thyroid cartilage correlates with the C4 vertebrae, and the cricoid ring overlies C6. The bodies of C2 and C1 lie deep to the ramus of the mandible.

Because of associated comorbid conditions, such as trismus and inability to extend or flex the neck, airway management should be considered. Difficult intubations may be handled with fiberoptic oral intubation. Any necessary neurophysiologic monitoring should be arranged for at this time. Vigilance at this juncture will ensure the best outcome while avoiding complications.

CLINICAL DECISION-MAKING
TRANSORAL APPROACH

The preoperative assessment and the nature of the lesion will determine the best approach. For lesions selected for a transoral approach, physical examination and radiographic assessment are vital. The images should be evaluated to determine how high above the palate the odontoid lesion extends. It is notable that inflammatory rheumatoid pannus, one of the major conditions requiring surgery of the odontoid process, is associated with arthritic fixation of the temporomandibular joint, with resultant trismus or restricted opening of the mouth. As a result of this trismus, access to the oral cavity may be limited. In patients who can open their mouths adequately, the length of the palate is assessed, the height of the posterior tongue is identified, and the level of the palate with respect to the lesion is confirmed. Externally the ramus of the mandible can be correlated with the lesion, on the basis of imaging, to estimate where the lesion lies. A prior transoral approach with a palatal split portends a worse outcome, with respect to dysphagia and velopharyngeal insufficiency.

Fig. 31-1 is an algorithm for an approach to the cervical spine.

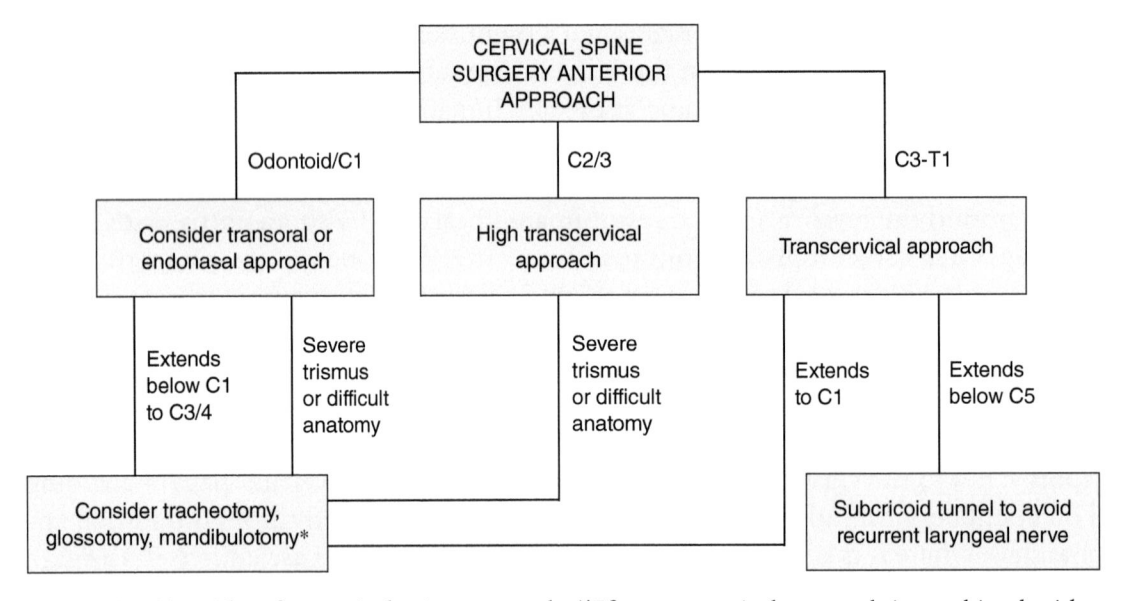

Fig. 31-1 Algorithm for cervical spine approach. (*If a transcervical approach is combined with a mandibulotomy, a circumglosssal approach is used to join the pharyngeal incision with the lateral palate incision. When a midline tongue split is used, the posterior pharyngeal wall must be incised directly over the spine.)

TRANSCERVICAL APPROACH

The transcervical approach is best suited for lesions of the middle and lower spine. Patients who are undergoing revision spine surgery pose a difficult problem. In cases of revision surgery, the exposure usually needs to be greater than that used in the initial surgery. There is always the concern that scarring and fibrosis can impede the dissection and increase injury to important neural structures, such as the recurrent laryngeal nerve. If a preexisting vocal cord paresis is present, it is usually wiser to approach the spine from the ipsilateral side. This will avoid the bilateral vocal fold paralysis that can occur with injury to the contralateral side. If a superior laryngeal nerve injury is identified with functional bilateral vocal folds, then the decision becomes more difficult. Bilateral superior laryngeal nerve injury can result in complete anesthesia of the larynx and unexpected dysphagia and aspiration. However, a combined superior and inferior laryngeal nerve deficit can also be devastating, especially in elderly patients. In our experience this situation is handled on a case-by-case basis, depending on the extent of the lesion and prior surgery, the patient's age and health, and the nature of the existing deficit. The superior laryngeal nerve is often located in the center of the surgical field and is at great risk for a stretch injury when the larynx is mobilized, whereas the recurrent laryngeal nerve is typically preserved. The selection-of-side approach merits some consideration for the lower spine. The right nerve is reportedly at greater risk of injury from stretching. This risk is greatly increased when there is a nonrecurrent laryngeal nerve, which can occur on the right side as the nerve emanates directly off of the vagus nerve. A nonrecurrent laryngeal nerve occurs in approximately 1% of the population and is almost always associated with a retroesophageal subclavian artery, which may be identifiable on preoperative imaging.[9] A nonrecurrent laryngeal nerve can be found by tracing the course of the vagus nerve when it is suspected.[10]

Initially a transoral approach to C1 and the odontoid process can be accomplished with retraction of the soft palate. More cranial exposure can be obtained by splitting the soft and hard palate or by using a combined endoscopic technique. More caudal access can be obtained by a transglossal or a combined transglossal/transmandibular approach. If more inferior access is necessary after the palate is split, a tracheotomy can be performed because removing the endotracheal tube from the oral cavity allows more working room. Splitting the tongue in the midline can provide another few centimeters of inferior extension down to the level of the larynx. Depending on the preoperative assessment, consent should be obtained as indicated.

TECHNIQUES
TRANSORAL-TRANSPHARYNGEAL APPROACH

This is the most direct route to the upper cervical spine and affords exposure from the clivus to the upper cervical vertebrae. Perioperative antibiotics are administered and should cover normal oral flora. We routinely use a combination of cephalexin and metronidazole or clindamycin. If a dural resection is expected, a lumbar drain is placed at this time. The head is positioned with as much extension as permitted, with neurophysiologic monitoring of the spinal cord. Care is taken to rinse and suction out the decontaminant to avoid aspiration. In addition, perioperative dexamethasone is used

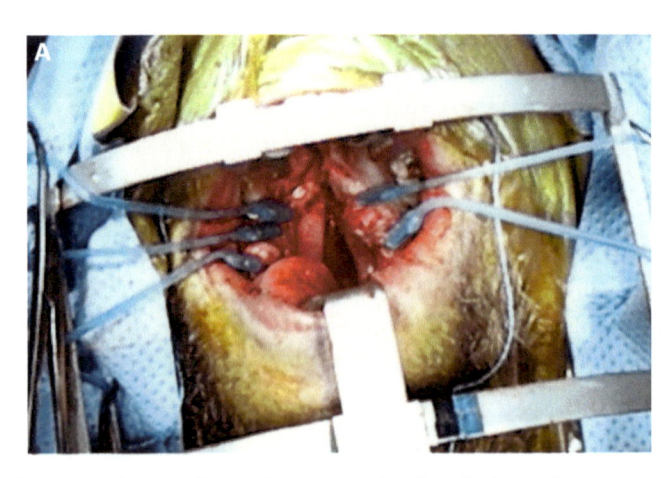

Fig. 31-2 Transoral approach. **A,** The oral retractor is placed. A tracheotomy can be performed to remove the endotracheal tube from the oral cavity; this will provide about 1 cm more exposure with the retractor in the oral cavity.

to prevent edema. General anesthesia is induced in patients who are orally intubated. The need for fiberoptic intubation or the use of newer video laryngoscopes should be anticipated preoperatively. The endotracheal tube should be taped to the lower lip in the midline or, as an alternative, sutured to the mental crease. A tracheostomy is performed at this time, if the need is anticipated postoperatively. However, this is less common.[4] Next the head is fixed, and the oral cavity is rinsed with either chlorhexidine mouthwash or another antiseptic regimen of choice. Finally, the face and neck are prepared in sterile fashion, followed by standard draping procedures. Exposure of the nasopharynx and oropharynx is achieved with a Dingman (V. Mueller Surgical Instruments, Cleveland, OH) or Crockard (Codman, Raynham, MA) mouth retractor. These allow the tongue and endotracheal tube to be simultaneously depressed and make it possible to secure lateral retractors (Fig. 31-2, *A*). If a palatal split can be avoided, the soft palate is retracted with two red rubber catheters brought through the nasal cavity and out through the mouth. These are secured with Kelly clamps over gauze rolls on the oral retractor to prevent pressure ulcers on the skin or nose. The oropharynx can then be evaluated to determine whether the exposure is adequate. For more cranial exposure, the uvula can be pulled into the nasopharynx/nasal cavity by suturing it to a red rubber catheter that has been placed through the nasal cavity.

TRANSPALATAL APPROACH

A transpalatal approach is often needed for greater exposure. An incision is made starting lateral to the uvula and is brought immediately to the midline raphe and continued posteriorly to the hard palate (Fig. 31-2, *B*). Midline incisions in the uvula will usually result in necrosis of the uvula and should be avoided. If more exposure is needed, the muscular attachments medially are freed from the hard palate laterally. Care is taken to keep the muscular attachments of the tensor veli palatini on the pterygoid hamulus. To allow lateral retraction of the palate, the hard palate is incised. A curvilinear incision is brought from the soft palate to within 5 mm of the incisors. This incision has been described as a C-shaped flap, sacrificing the greater palatine vessels and nerve on one

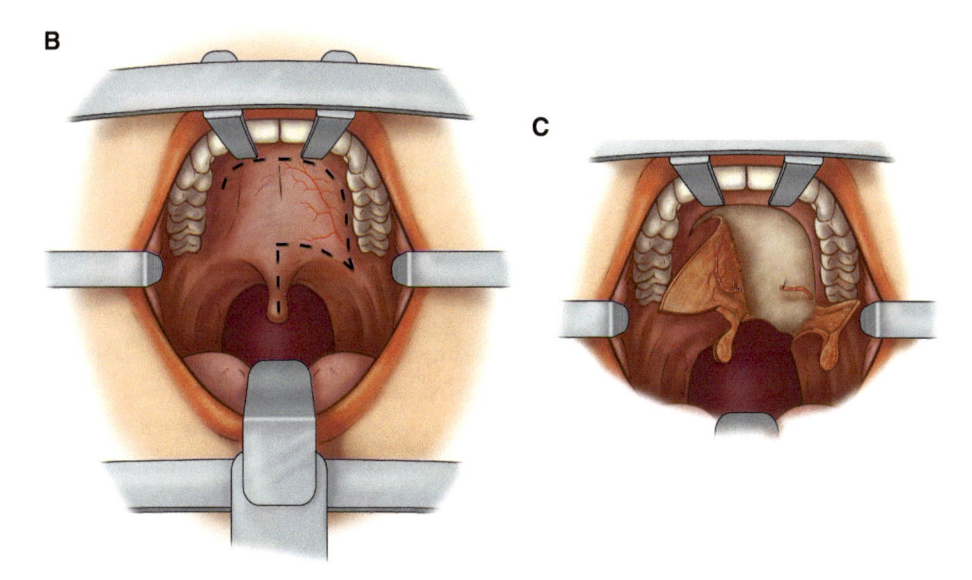

Fig. 31-2, cont'd **B,** The mucosa and deep tissue of the palate are incised in the midline raphe of the soft palate. The uvula is usually left intact and brought to one side, because dividing it can result in necrosis. **C,** On the hard palate, the mucosa can be incised in the midline or with a C shape to one side to aid retraction. The neurovascular bundle is often transected in that case. An attempt should be made to keep the tensor veli palatini attachments to the pterygoid hamulus intact to decrease velopharyngeal incompetence. Sutures or self-retaining retraction hooks retract the palate. This provides access to the posterior pharyngeal wall.

side (Fig. 31-2, *C*), but we often keep these pedicles intact bilaterally.[3] The dense mucosa on the hard palate is elevated with a Freer elevator to allow retraction of the soft palate laterally. If more exposure is needed superiorly, the posterior edge of the hard palate can be resected with a drill or rongeur. In general, removal of a small amount of bone should allow access. However, removal of the hard palate bone can increase postoperative dysfunction, with increased velopharyngeal insufficiency.

Maxillotomy Approach

When even greater exposure is required than what the hard palate resection affords, the maxillotomy technique is the desired approach. Once the patient is prepared and draped, access to the maxilla is achieved by a transfacial Weber-Fergusson incision. The skin is incised along the nasofacial groove, and the incision is carried around the nasal ala to the philtrum, then down the midline to split the lip. Next the incision is extended down to bone and laterally in the gingivobuccal sulcus. Alternatively, a midface degloving incison can be used. A sublabial incision is made bilaterally. All of the soft tissue, including the periostium, is elevated superiorly and laterally; the surgeon identifies and preserves the infraorbital neurovascular bundle. In the nose, an incision is made through the nasal mucosca onto the palate. This soft tissue is elevated medially and laterally. Posteriorly, an incision is made to separate the soft palate from the hard palate unilaterally. At this point, the bone cuts can be made with either a gigli saw or powered instrumentation. It is helpful to preplate the bone cuts to allow easy reconstruction at the end of the procedure. The anterior cut goes through the hard palate on the nasal side, with preservation of the hard palate mucosa. The superior cut extends from the superior aspect of the piriform aperature laterally through the pterygoid plates. At this point, the maxilla can be swung inferiorally and medially. It should be pedicled on the hard palate, nasal mucosa, and soft palate. The internal maxillary artery and its branches may need to be controlled.[4]

Next the posterior pharyngeal incision is made by incising the mucosa in the midline plane and splitting the prevertebral muscles. The incision is carried up to the clivus and can be joined with a horizontal T incision superiorly. U-shaped flaps along the posterior pharynx wall have also been recommended. However, in our experience, U-shaped flaps create a large denervated portion of pharynx that prevents sphincteric contraction and potentially worsening velopharyngeal insufficiency. Therefore we convert to a midline incision that would keep the pharyngeal constrictors innervated bilaterally. The tendinous fibers of the prevertebral muscle are detached with a Bovie cautery and deflected laterally, exposing the C1 ring, clivus, and odontoid process (Fig. 31-3). Retraction of the oropharyngeal flaps is achieved with rigid retractors or heavy silk suture material. If additional inferior exposure is necessary, the endotracheal tube can be removed and a tracheotomy placed. If further inferior exposure is necessary, the tongue can be divided.

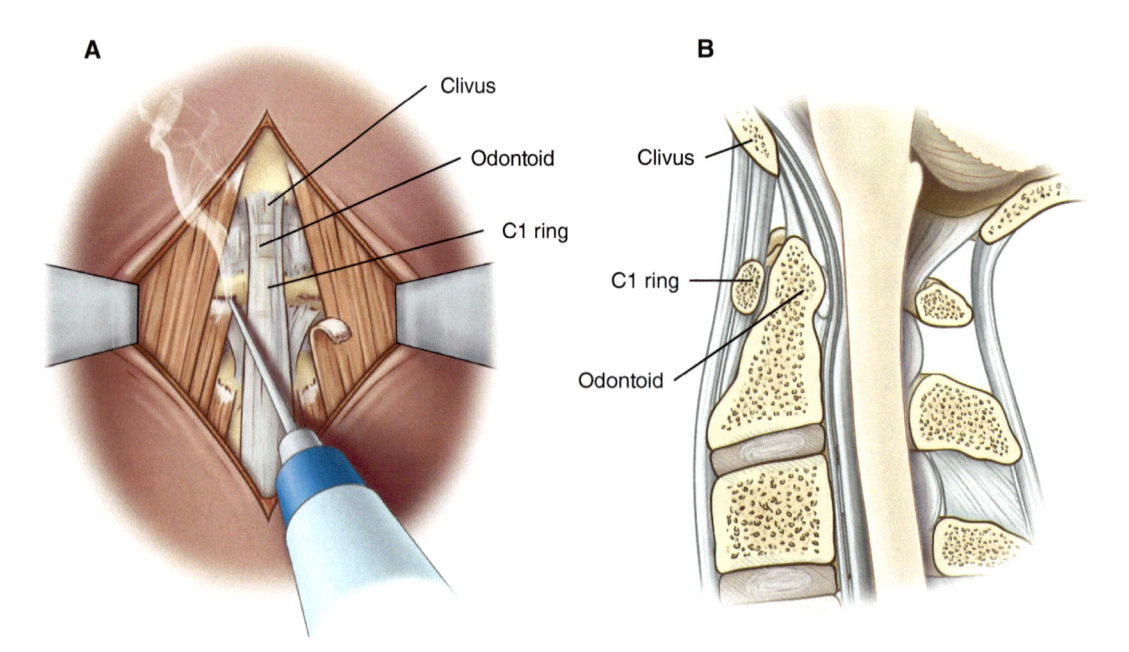

Fig. 31-3 **A,** The craniovertebral junction can be addressed through a direct incision through the posterior pharyngeal wall. A midline incision is made and the prevertebral muscles are divided down to prevertebral fascia. The muscular insertions are divided and the tissue elevated laterally. The fascia can then be divided, exposing the ring of C1 overlying the odontoid. **B,** The relationship of the clivus, odontoid, and ring of C1 is shown.

Once the goal of the procedure has been achieved, hemostasis is obtained and the wound is copiously irrigated. The pharyngeal incision is closed in two layers. The muscle layers are reapproximated with interrupted 3-0 sutures. The flaps are closed with interrupted 3-0 absorbing sutures and the use of a tapered needle. The soft palate is similarly closed in three layers consisting of the nasopharyngeal mucosa, palatal musculature, and oropharyngeal mucosa. A nasogastric feeding tube is placed and sutured to the nasal septum. If necessary, the cervical spine is immobilized at this point. Next appropriate airway management ensues, depending on the level of edema. Postoperative neurologic and airway monitoring occurs in the intensive care unit.

TRANSGLOSSAL APPROACH

When more caudal exposure is needed, a transglossal modification can be employed. A temporary tracheostomy is routinely performed under these circumstances because of expected postoperative edema. The soft tissues of the floor of mouth are divided in the midline and extended through the relatively avascular midline raphe of the tongue, using a needle point electrocautery tip on a low setting at 12 to 15 watts. The tongue is split down the midline raphe to the floor of the mouth and the epiglottic space fascia. The tongue is retracted with heavy 0 silk sutures. At this point the epiglottis is identifiable, and the pharynx should be exposed to C4. At the end of the procedure, hemostasis is obtained, and the tongue is reapproximated with 3-0 absorbable sutures in both the muscular and mucosal layers. The floor of the mouth is similarly closed. If exposure is limited, a midline mandibulotomy can be performed for superior or inferior exposure.

TRANSMANDIBULAR-TRANSGLOSSAL APPROACH

A transmandibular approach is used for large tumors. A transmandibular-transglossal approach affords the widest bilateral-lateral exposure of the cranial base, anterior foramen transversarium of C2, and C1 lateral masses. The approach to the posterior oropharynx and spine can be through a midline glossotomy as outlined previously, or circumglossal. The skin of the lip is marked down the midline, from the vermilion border to the mentum, into the submental skin. The incision can be modified into a stairstep Z pattern from the vermilion border to the labiomental crease and, circumferentially around the mentum back to the midline at the inferior aspect of the chin to break up the scar. However, if this modification is used, care must be taken to avoid the mental nerve as the incision is carried through the subcutaneous tissue and skived toward the midline. Care should be taken to avoid inadvertent injury to Wharton's ducts, which can be seen just lateral to the lingual frenulum. The cervical incision is U shaped and begins at the mastoid tip, extends inferiorly into a skin crease on the neck, and then joins the incision for the chin and lip. After injecting it with local anesthetic with epinephrine, the incision is made sharply and carried down through the platysma muscle. At this point subplatysmal myocutaneous flaps are raised sharply, with care to avoid injury to the marginal branch of the facial nerve by elevating this flap immediately deep to the muscle. The nerve will be in the investing fascia of the submandibular gland. On the face the incision is carried through the subcutaneous tissue to the mentum. The vermilion border is either tattooed with methylene blue on either side of the incision or scored with the back edge of a scalpel to aid in reapproximation. The lip is split, and the incision is brought to 5 to 10 mm of the gingivolabial sulcus. Next horizontal limbs are extended and carried down through the mentalis muscle to expose bone. The soft tissue is elevated, revealing the inferior border of the mentum. Extending this too far laterally will place the mental nerves at risk. The osteotomy is then planned in a linear or stairstep fashion, avoiding the midline to protect the central incisors. A miniplate is preplated and then saved for later use. The osteotomy is then made with a sagittal saw. Some surgeons prefer to make the osteotomy through the socket of an extracted tooth.

The circumglossal approach differs in that the soft tissue on the floor of the mouth is divided in the lingual gutter, and the tongue is retracted rather than split. Extensions of the incision can be carried onto the anterior tonsil pillar and the soft and hard palate as necessary. Care is taken to identify the hypoglossal and lingual nerves and keep them intact as they drape across the surgical field. The anterior tonsil pillar is incised, and the superior constrictors are elevated laterally in a contralateral direction to expose the longus colli muscles. The longus muscles are split down the midline, and the spine is exposed. The soft tissue and bone are retracted with hooks and/or retractors as necessary. At the end of the procedure, hemostasis is obtained and the wound is copiously irrigated. The soft tissues are reapproximated with absorbable sutures in layers when feasible. The mandible is repositioned and fixed with the previously applied miniplate. The facial incision is closed with 6-0 nylon interrupted sutures. Finally, after a suction drain is placed, the neck is closed in layers consisting of at least the platysma muscle and the skin. A nasogastric feeding tube is placed and sutured to the nasal septum. If necessary, the cervical spine is then immobilized. Postoperative neurologic and airway monitoring occurs in the intensive care unit.

Transnasal Approach

The transnasal technique was introduced within the past decade, and its application to the craniovertebral junction and the skull base is continually expanding. It can be used alone or in conjunction with the transoral approaches outlined previously. The importance of surgical expertise and proper equipment cannot be underestimated. Preoperative imaging by means of both CT and MRI is of paramount importance. In addition, surgical navigation is used in all cases. Perioperative antibiotics are also used in all cases.

After induction of general anesthesia, a lumbar drain may be placed at the discretion of the surgeons. Next the nose is packed with pledgets containing either oxymetazoline, Neo-Synephrine, or 4% cocaine. The face is then prepared and draped accordingly.

The navigation system is then applied in sterile fashion. The procedure begins with endoscopy of each nasal cavity, paying particular attention to any anatomic variants that could cause difficulties with access, such as septal deviation, concha bullosa (pneumatized middle turbinate), or polypoid sinusitis. If these are present, they are addressed at this time. The middle turbinates are either outfractured or one is resected for exposure. At this point preparations are made for reconstructing the defect. The nasoseptal flap based on the posterior septal artery is preferred and will be described. Harvesting the nasoseptal flap begins with two horizontal incisions and needle-tip electrocautery—one along the nasal floor extending to the choana and the other 1.0 to 1.5 cm below the base of the skull.

The anterior incision is placed 1.5 cm posterior to the caudal nasal septum and connects the two horizontal incisions. Posterolaterally the inferior incision is carried up the posterior septum to where it transitions onto the sphenoid rostrum. The mucoperichondrial flap is raised with a Cottle, Freer, or suction elevator off of the septum and the sphenoid rostrum. It is then tucked into the maxillary antrum or nasopharynx for protection while the procedure continues. At that point the posterior septum is resected to increase the angle of exposure from either nasal cavity. This can be accomplished with backbiting instruments or a drill. Next bilateral sphenoidotomies are performed, and the remaining sphenoid rostrum is taken down. This should provide access to the upper clivus. The rest of the clivus is exposed by elevating the mucosa and muscle of the nasopharynx. The clivus is now ready to be drilled to gain access to the tumor. Reconstruction begins with a Duragen inlay graft, which is carefully placed so that it lies flush with the underlying surface. Some investigators advocate using a fat graft next, which is taken from the subcutaneous tissue of the abdomen in a sterile manner. The nasoseptal flap is then positioned as an onlay graft to cover the bony defect. A dural sealant is used to reinforce the flap followed by Gelfoam. Last, a Foley catheter is placed, and the balloon is inflated to support the reconstruction along with nasal packs. A nasogastric feeding tube is placed and sutured to the nasal septum. If necessary, the cervical spine is immobilized at this point. Next appropriate airway management ensues, depending on the level of edema. Postoperative neurologic and airway monitoring occurs in the intensive care unit.

TRANSCERVICAL APPROACH

After induction of anesthesia with an orotracheal tube, the patient's neck is placed into slight extension with a shoulder roll. A horizontal incision is marked in a natural skin crease, according to the level of surgery. The thyrohyoid membrane serves as a landmark for the upper cervical vertebrae, the middle of the thyroid cartilage for the middle cervical vertebrae, and the cricoid cartilage and clavicles for the lower vertebrae. Typically the length of the incision extends from the midline to the sternocleidomastoid muscle. The incision is then injected with lidocaine with epinephrine, and the patient is prepared and draped using sterile technique. The incision is made

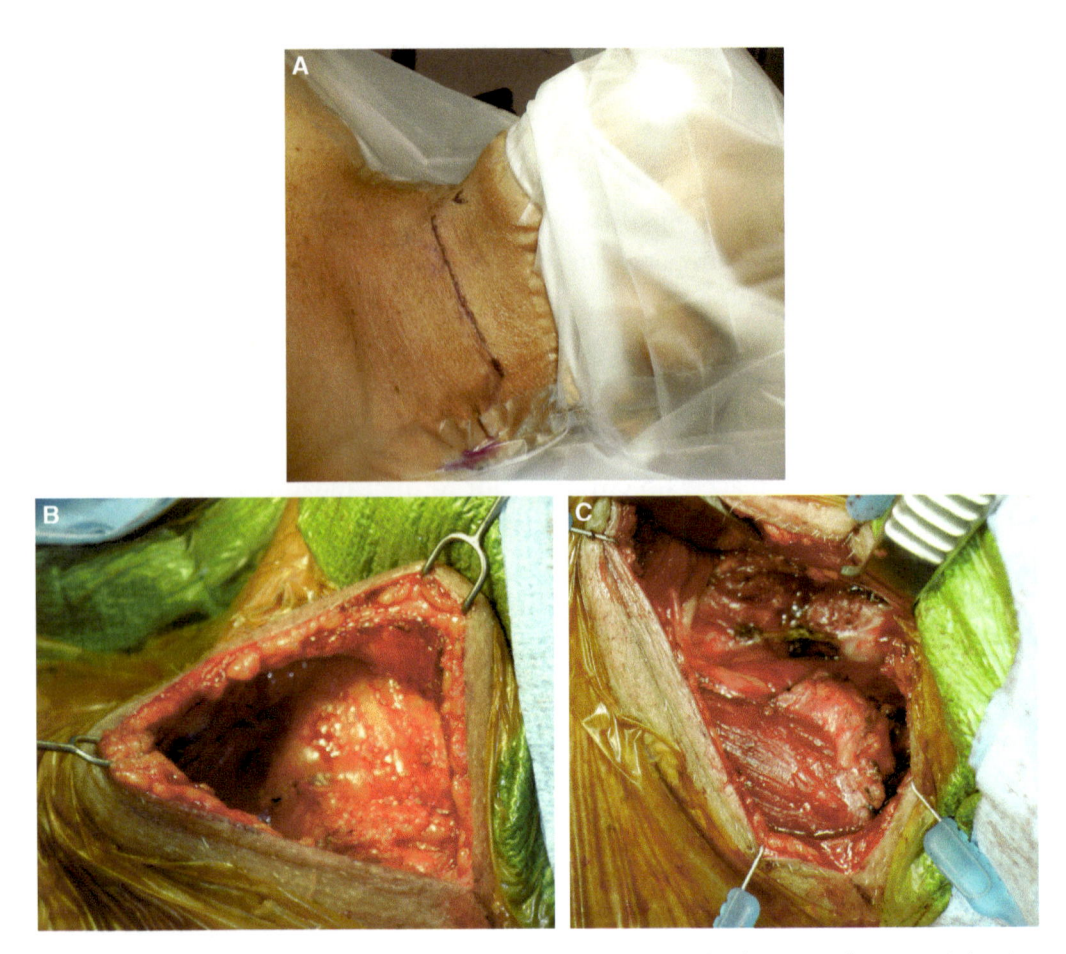

Fig. 31-4 Transcervical approach. **A,** Planned skin incision in the horizontal crease. A horizontal skin incision is favored over a vertical incision for improved healing and cosmesis. The incision is centered over the target zone but kept at least two fingerbreadths above the clavicle or below the mandible. Inferiorly, there is nothing gained by a lower incision, and superiorly, the incision is kept low to avoid the marginal branch of the facial nerve. **B,** Subplatysmal flaps are elevated as high as the mandibular body and as low as the clavicle. The drapes are purposely kept off the skin and placed at the level of the mandible and clavicle to avoid tethering retraction. **C,** The laryngopharynx is retracted off of the spine revealing multiple disc levels. Sternocleidomastoid muscles and great vessels are retracted laterally from the spine.

sharply and taken down through the platysma muscle. Next subplatysmal myocutaneous flaps are elevated. Once the flaps are elevated, they are retracted for adequate exposure (Fig. 31-4).

For superior exposure, the fascia overlying the submandibular gland is incised along the inferior border of the gland. The deep surface of the gland is elevated and retracted superiorly to expose the digastric muscle and twelfth cranial nerve (Fig. 31-5). The fascia between the anterior border of the sternocleidomastoid and strap muscles is opened both superiorly and inferiorly. The internal jugular vein and carotid sheath are identified, and blunt dissection is used to gain access to the prevertebral fascia between the carotid sheath and the aerodigestive tract. The superior laryngeal nerve courses medially to the carotid and enters the thyrohyoid membrane and should be

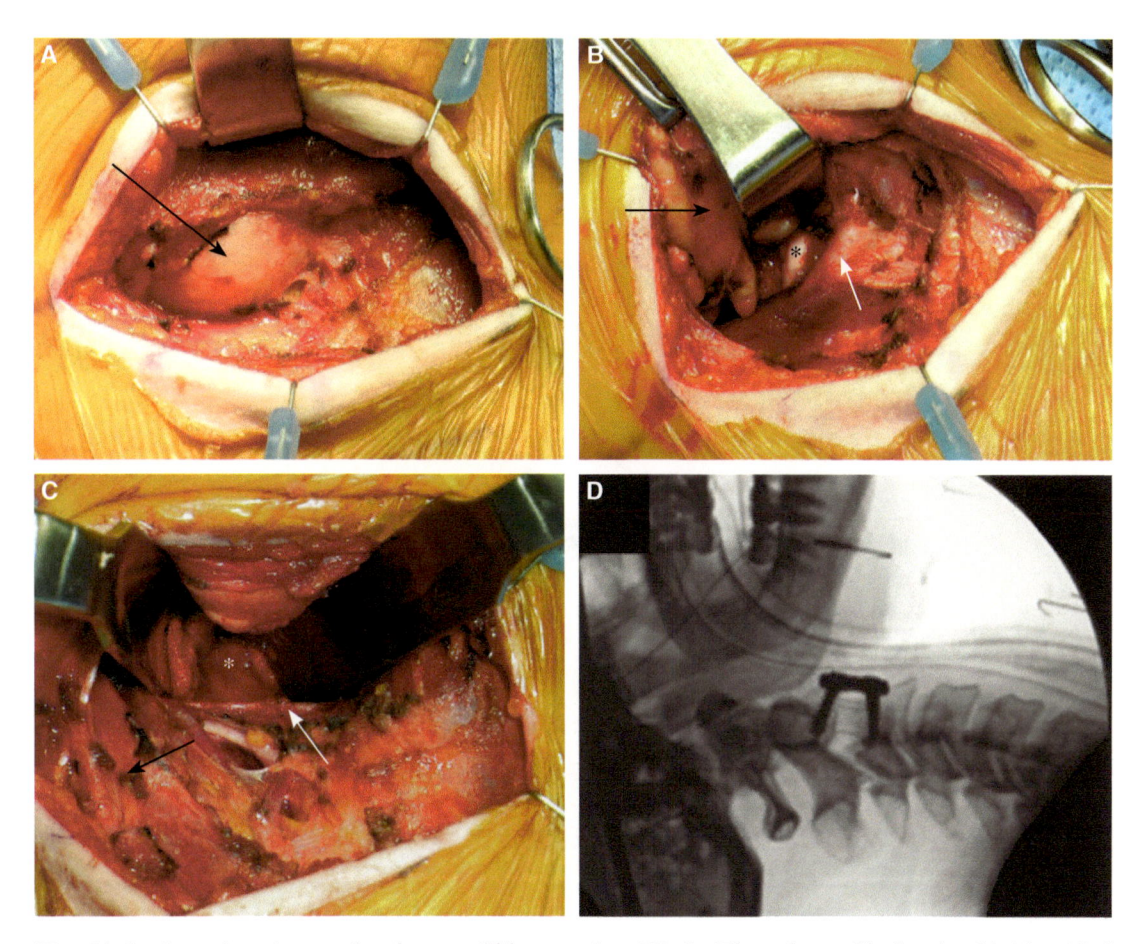

Fig. 31-5 Superior view under the mandible exposing C2. **A,** The submandibular gland is identified and retracted superiorly. **B,** The submandibular gland is retracted *(black arrow)* and cranial nerve 12 is identified *(black asterisk)* above the digastric muscle *(white arrow)*. **C,** The digastric muscle is divided and the submandibular gland is retracted superiorly. The tissue plane medial to the great vessels (internal jugular vein demonstrated by *black arrow*) is dissected down to the prevertebral fascia of the spine *(asterisk)*. The tissue plane is created inferior to cranial nerve twelve. In this manner the C2 vertebrae can be reached. A plane above and below the superior thyroid neurovascular bundle can be made *(white arrow)* for inferior extension as needed. **D,** Placement of the plate fusing C2 and C3 is shown.

preserved. If needed, these can be dissected free and gently retracted. Identification of the esophagus may be aided by palpation of an esophageal temperature probe or an orogastric tube.

For lesions involving the C5 to T1 spine, the position of the recurrent laryngeal nerve must be considered. It emerges from the mediastinum in the tracheoesophageal groove and enters the cricothyroid joint (Fig. 31-6). The cricothyroid joint may be palpated, and the prevertebral fascia can be entered superior to the joint. The nerve may be identified and protected. As an alternative, the tissue between the carotid sheath and the trachea can be tunneled under to avoid injury to the recurrent laryngeal nerve. The prevertebral fascia is exposed further by retracting the laryngopharynx medially. Once this is completed, the endotracheal tube cuff pressure should be tested to avoid excess compression on the intralaryngeal segment of the recurrent laryngeal nerve.

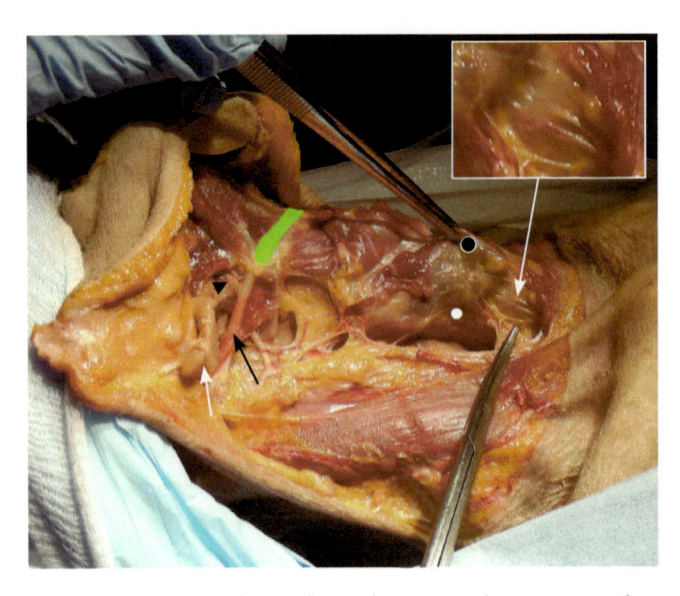

Fig. 31-6 Critical structures in the neck. Cadaver dissection demonstrates key anatomic structures. The submandibular gland is retracted *(small white arrow)* off the digastric muscle *(black arrow)*. The cranial nerve twelve runs over the carotid artery and deep to the nerve toward the tongue musculature *(black arrowhead)*. The hyoid bone is shaded green and demonstrates the attachment of the digastric tendon. The laryngopharyngeal complex has been elevated off the spine. The thyroid gland is retracted off the trachea *(black dot)*. The esophagus and tracheal esophageal groove can be appreciated *(white dot)*. The inset demonstrates the recurrent laryngeal nerve running in the tracheoesophageal groove to enter the larynx on the inferior surface of the cricoid cartilage.

fascia is then incised in the midline, and the longus colli muscles are dissected free. Confirmation of the correct level is obtained by localizing a spinal needle with a lateral radiograph. At the end of the procedure, the wound is irrigated and hemostasis is obtained. The wound is closed in layers.

Combined Transmandibular-Transcervical Approach

The transcervical approach is followed with the skin incision extending posteriorly over the sternocleidomastoid muscle. The superior flap is elevated up to the mandibular body and joined to meet a midline lip split. The mandibulotomy is completed, and a circumglossal approach is used to push the tongue to the contralateral side. Inferiorly the plane of the superior constrictor muscles is contiguous with the pharynx, overlying the spine, the larynx, and trachea, all of which are retracted.

OUTCOMES WITH EVALUATION OF RESULTS

These approaches afford excellent exposure to the cervical spine, successful surgical outcomes, and acceptable complications. However, dysphonia and dysphagia are common after these procedures. Tervonen et al[11] reported speech and swallowing difficulties in 60% and 69% of patients, respectively, in the immediate postoperative period. In addition, recurrent laryngeal nerve paralysis was noted in 12% of patients. However, most cases of symptomatic dysphonia and dysphagia had resolved by 3 months, but a persistent recurrent laryngeal nerve paralysis rate of 3% was observed. In a study with a mean follow-up period of 7.2 years, Yue et al[12] reported a persistent dysphonia rate of 18.9% and a dysphagia rate of 35.1%. More recently results of a prospective study evaluating the incidence of and risk factors for dysphagia were reported over a 2-year period. Lee et al[13] found that the prevalence of dysphagia at 1, 2, 6, 12, and 24 months was 54.0%, 33.6%, 18.6%, 15.2%, and 13.6%, respectively. Risk factors included female sex, greater than two-level surgery, and revision surgery. The dysphagia can be attributed to edema, esophageal injury, and injury to the hypoglossal nerve, recurrent laryngeal nerve, superior laryngeal nerve, and the nerves of the pharyngeal plexus.[13] Similarly, causes of dysphonia can be multifactorial. They can range from intubation-related changes (i.e., laryngeal edema, vocal fold granuloma, and vocal fold trauma) to physiologic alterations, such as laryngopharyngeal reflux.[14] However, the most studied cause is recurrent laryngeal nerve injury from direct trauma, such as ligation or stretch injury. There is debate regarding which side is best for approaching the cervical spine to reduce recurrent laryngeal nerve injury. Some believe that the handedness of the surgeon should determine the side—that is, right-handed surgeons should approach from the right, and vice versa. Others think that the remote possibility of having a nonrecurrent laryngeal nerve on the right should prompt a left-sided approach. In an effort to determine which operative side is safest for reducing recurrent laryngeal nerve injury, a retrospective review of more than 400 patients was carried out by Kilburg et al.[15] They found that the relative rate of recurrent laryngeal nerve injury was not significantly different between right- and left-sided approaches (1.8% versus 2.1%) or between one- and two-level operations.

Another mechanism of injury has been proposed as a cause of recurrent laryngeal nerve paresis/paralysis. Two studies have evaluated the amount of intralaryngeal pressure placed on the recurrent laryngeal nerve by the cuff of the endotracheal tube after retractors are placed. In the first study, when the cuff was deflated and reinflated to a pressure of 15 mm Hg, a decrease in recurrent laryngeal nerve paralysis was observed.[16] Another group evaluated this prospectively, using 20 mm Hg as their pressure limit, and found no difference in recurrent laryngeal nerve injury.[17] Clearly this is not completely understood, as evidenced by the persistent low rate of recurrent laryngeal nerve injury reported. However, knowledge of the recurrent laryngeal nerve anatomy, minimizing retraction, and adjusting cuff pressures may all help reduce recurrent laryngeal nerve injuries.

Last, infectious complications can range from wound infection to meningitis.[18] Fortunately these rates are low. Lee et al[13] reported a wound infection rate of 3.1%, a meningitis rate of 3.1%, and a sepsis rate of 2.1% in 132 operations. Similarly, only two wound infections and one case of meningitis were reported in 53 procedures by Mouchaty et al.[19] Overall, morbidity and complication rates are low, and careful planning and cautious tissue handling should help maintain these low rates.

SIGNATURE CASES
Endonasal and Transoral Approach

A patient with a history of Chiari malformation and basilar impression by the odontoid process had previously undergone an odontoidectomy through a transoral approach, with a palatal split, at another institution (Fig. 31-7). The patient developed recurrent symptoms, and a residual odontoid process and body of C2 were seen on preoperative images. The lesion was noted to extend approximately 1.5 cm over a line drawn along the nasal cavity floor and palate (palatal line) and reside high in the nasopharynx. This case was managed with an endonasal and transoral approach with the use of a red rubber catheter to retract the soft palate. In this manner a palatal split was avoided.

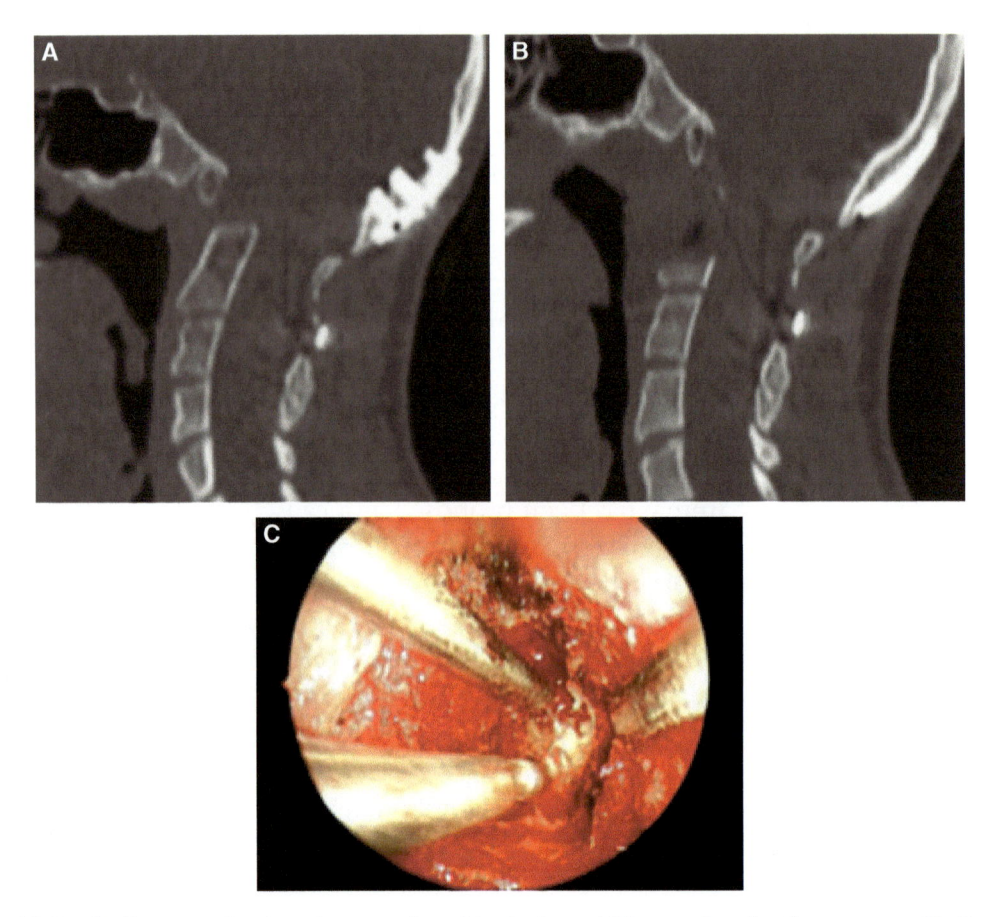

Fig. 31-7 **A,** Preoperative imaging reveals residual odontoid bone after the first surgery. **B,** Postoperative imaging reveals resection of the offending segment of bone, and the patient had resolution of symptoms. **C,** A midline incision was used over the posterior pharyngeal mucosa, and the lesion was resected with a high-speed endoscopic drill and rongeurs.

MIDLINE GLOSSOTOMY

A 49-year-old with a history of polysubstance abuse, hepatitis C, and liver cirrhosis and esophageal varicosities presented with a 1-year history of chronic neck pain and 4 days of acute onset of severe neck pain (Fig. 31-8). Imaging revealed a destructive lesion at C2-3 with a kyphotic deformity. Indications for surgery were instability with kyphosis at C2-3 and spinal stenosis with spinal cord compression. The first stage was performed as a transoral completion corpectomy, placement of an allograft bone strut, and anterior plating from C2 to C4. In the second stage, a posterior cervical laminectomy and fusion of C1 through C5 were performed. During the transoral approach, the patient had a limited oral opening with 4 cm distance between incisors. A tonsil retractor exposed the soft palate, which was divided. However, the inferior exposure was limited, and a tracheotomy was performed. This provided an additional 1.5 cm inferior exposure, and the oral endotracheal tube was removed. More access was needed, and a midline glossotomy was performed. This allowed exposure of the epiglottis and down to the C5 body, avoiding the need for a mandibulotomy.

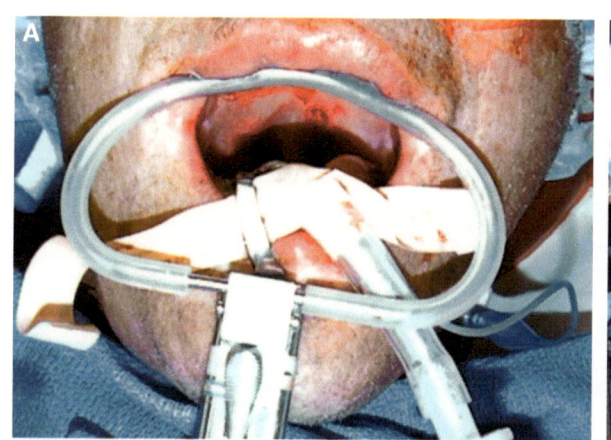

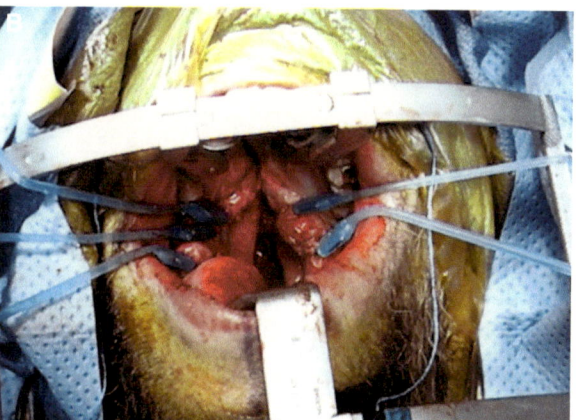

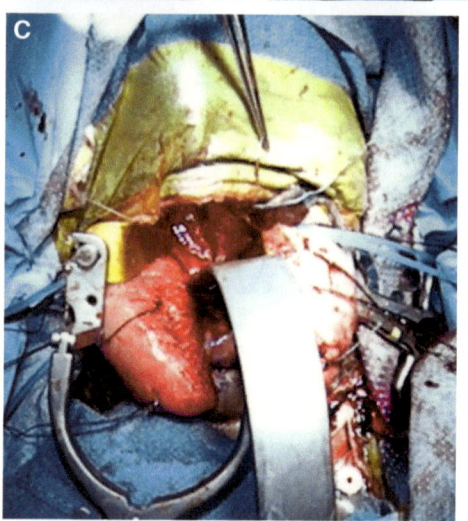

Fig. 31-8 **A,** Transoral retraction before tracheotomy with limited superior exposure. **B,** After tracheotomy, the endotracheal tube is removed. A palatal split provides access to the superior target. A glossotomy can be performed without a mandibulotomy to provide a few more centimeters of exposure. The mandible can be divided in conjunction with a glossotomy, or a circumglossal approach can be used. **C,** The tongue is split down the midline, with the retractor on the preepiglottic fat and the floor of the mouth, improving the inferior view.

Transcervical-Transmandibular Exposure From C1 to C7

A 65-year-old man had a history of prior multilevel fusion levels for treatment of tumor and degenerative disease (Fig. 31-9). The patient required revision surgery, with removal of the hardware and the diseased disc, and placement of a cage from C1 to C7. A transmandibular circumglossal approach was combined with a transcervical approach to provide adequate access.

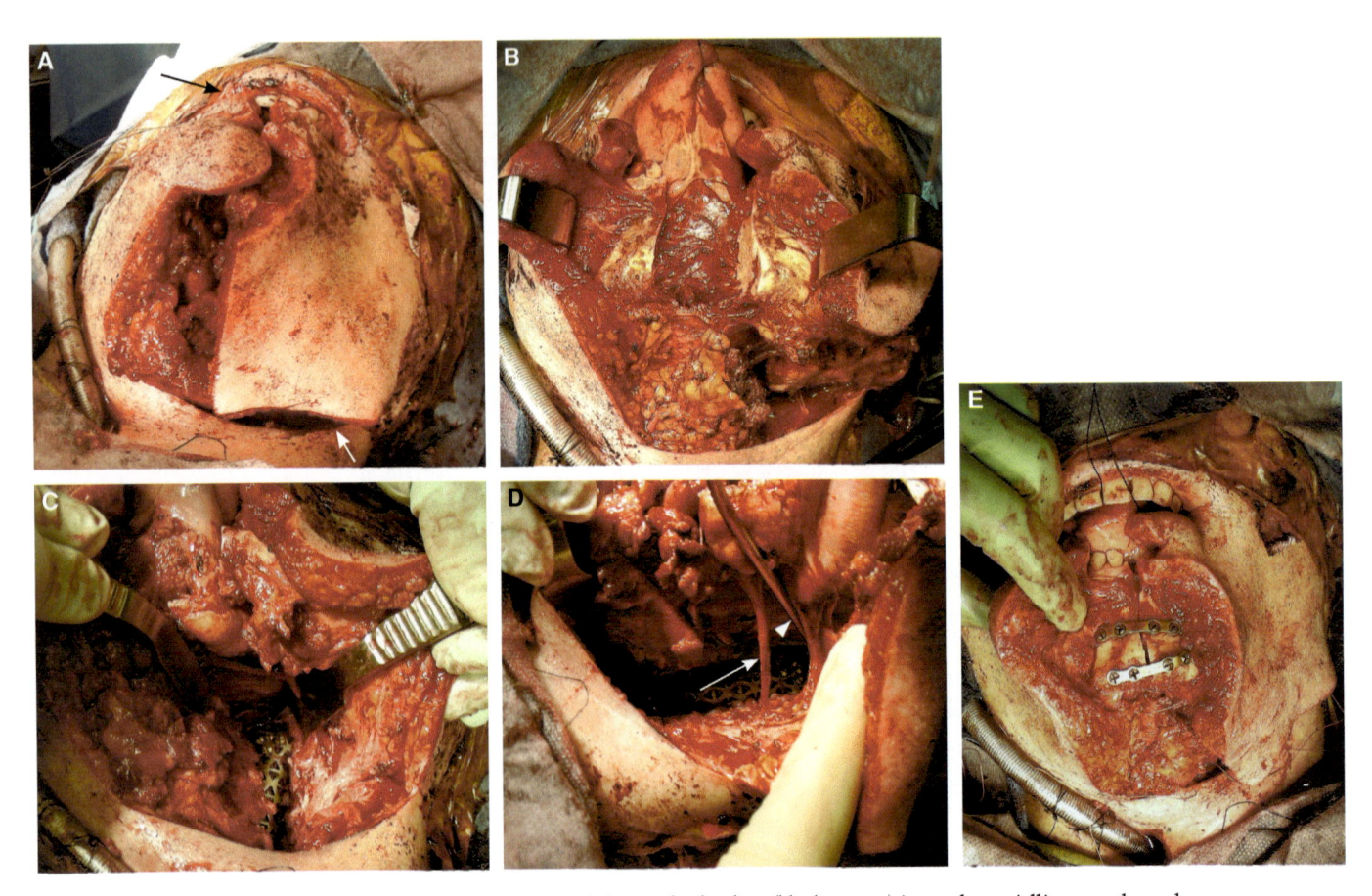

Fig. 31-9 **A,** Skin incisions are carried through the lip *(black arrow)* into the midline neck and are joined with a horizontal neck incision *(white arrow).* **B,** Midline mandibulotomy is performed with preplating of the mandible. **C,** Transcervical exposure with subplatysmal flap elevated to the mandible and clavicle. If a transcervical approach is combined with a mandibulotomy, a circumglossal approach is used to join the pharyngeal incision with the lateral palate incision. When a midline tongue split is used, the posterior pharyngeal wall must be incised directly over the spine. **D,** Critical structures are preserved, including the superior laryngeal nerve *(arrow)* and hypoglossal nerve *(arrowhead).* **E,** The mandible is plated with low-profile mandibular reconstruction plates, with two fixating screws on either side of the incision.

CONCLUSION

Advances in surgical anatomy techniques and instruments, along with the emergence of multidisciplinary surgical teams, has allowed for growth in the field of comprehensive spine surgery. Contemporary spine surgeons should be familiar with basic and extended approaches to the craniovertebral junction and cervical spine. In many cases a stepwise approach can be taken that will allow for a tailored approach to these areas and the given pathology. In complicated procedures, advanced techniques such as surgical navigation or use of complementary surgical teams can be of great benefit. Because these procedures are quite successful, attention should be given to the avoidance of complications.

BAILOUT TECHNIQUES

In the case of revision surgery, a preoperative endoscopy and evaluation of vocal cord fixation can be performed. For planned surgery of the C5-7 region, if the vocal fold function is intactbilaterally and the larynx sensation is intact, then the approach can be performed via the contralateral side. If there is evidence of superior laryngeal nerve or recurrent laryngeal nerve injury, the ipsilateral side should be used. During revision surgery where scar tissue is present, it is helpful to perform a horizontal skin incision in a skin crease and raise subplatysmal flaps. Elevating beyond the scar tissue plane to normal tissue aids in identification of the correct tissue plane.

To avoid injury to the marginal nerve, the superficial layer of the deep cervical fascia is incised at the inferior border of the submandibular gland and the gland is retracted superiorly off the posterior belly of the digastric.

Recurrent laryngeal injury is a signficant event. The recurrent nerve runs in the fascia between the carotid artery and tracheal esophageal grove. To reduce chance of injury to the recurrent laryngeal nerve, a subcricoid tunnel can be created. Below the level of the cricoid ring, the fascia between the carotid fascia and tracheal esophageal groove is left intact. The prevertebral fascia is identified just above the level of the cricoid ring and the constrictor muscles and esophagus are then elevated off the prevertebral fascia creating a tunnel deep to the deep layer of the cervical fascia below the level of the cricoid. The recurrent laryngeal nerve is within this fascia which serves to protect the nerve if retractors are placed. The authors have tunneled to the level of T1 on multiple occasions using this technique.

TRANSORAL APPROACH

To gain more access superiorly after a palatal split, a rongeur can be used posteriorly in the hard palate to increase the superior angle of view. In patients with significant trismus and limited opening of the oral cavity, a tracheotomy can allow more working room. An endoscope placed transorally can aid in visualization for decompression or biopsies to avoid a mandibulotomy. A mandibulotomy can be avoided at times by performing a midline tongue split and retracting the tongue laterally.

Continued

TRANSCERVICAL APPROACH

During revision procedures or in patients who have had prior neck surgery, identification of the recurrent laryngeal nerve can be challenging due to scar. In these cases, avoidance of the nerve may be safer. The recurrent laryngeal nerve travels in the fascia of the tracheoesophageal groove. By remaining below that fascia, inferior to the level of the cricoid ring, the nerve can be avoided. Rarely, perforation of the pharynx or esophagus occurs and should be closed with the tissue inverted into the lumen using 3.0 sutures in an interrupted fashion.

TIPS FROM THE MASTERS

- Postoperative dysphagia is common, and patients should be counseled about this possibility preoperatively. Increasing the extent of exposure increases the risk of dysphagia and velopharyngeal incompetence (escape of air and food into the nose with speech and swallowing). A midline pharyngeal incision may reduce trauma to the posterior pharynx. Significant tissue reduction at the level of the nasopharynx may prevent closure of the velopharynx and result in unavoidable velopharyngeal insufficiency.
- In complicated and revision cases, preoperative laryngeal, speech, and swallowing evaluations by means of fiberoptic examination can be useful.
- A stepwise approach during transoral and extended approaches will minimize morbidity.
- The use of endoscopic assistance may obviate the need for palatal splitting, which increases the risk of velopharyngeal incompetence and fistula formation.
- For multilevel surgery, an extended horizontal incision in a skin crease provides better access and cosmesis than an oblique incision along the sternocleidomastoid muscle.
- Translocation and, rarely, resection of the submandibular gland will aid in transcervical exposure of the upper cervical spine.
- Preservation of the superior laryngeal nerve will help with postoperative dysphagia and aspiration.
- The recurrent laryngeal nerve travels in the tracheoesophageal groove and can usually be avoided by staying deep to the tissue plane, connecting the carotid fascia with the trachea and the esophagus inferior to the level of the cricoid ring. Tunneling under this tissue usually provides adequate exposure to C7 or T1.
- Rarely, a nonrecurrent laryngeal nerve is encountered on the right. This is associated with a retroesophageal subclavian artery, which may be identified on preoperative imaging.
- The choice of side for a revision transcervical approach should be tailored to whether there is existing cranial nerve dysfunction. If the recurrent nerve is functional, either side can be used, but dissecting the contralateral side may aide in preservation of the nerve. If the recurrent nerve is nonfunctional, an approach from the ipsilateral side is indicated.

- If a pharyngeal/esophageal perforation is identified at the time of surgery, a primary watertight two-layer closure should be performed, with inversion of the constrictors into the lumen. Methylene blue can be insufflated into the oral cavity to ensure that the closure is watertight. Nasogastric tube feeding should be implemented for 7 days in nonirradiated patients and 14 days in irradiated patients before feeding is attempted.

References (With Key References in Boldface)

1. **Menezes AH. Surgical approaches: postoperative care and complications "transoral-transpalatopharyngeal approach to the craniocervical junction." Childs Nerv Syst 24:1187-1193, 2008.**
2. **Lu J, Ebraheim NA, Nadim Y, et al. Anterior approach to the cervical spine: surgical anatomy. Orthopedics 23:841-845, 2000.**
3. Crumley RL, Gutin PH. Surgical access for clivus chordoma. The University of California, San Francisco, experience. Arch Otolaryngol Head Neck Surg 115:295-300, 1989.
4. **Cocke EW, Robertson JH, Robertson JT, et al. The extended maxillotomy and subtotal maxillectomy for excision of skull base tumors. Arch Otolaryngol Head Neck Surg 116:92-104, 1990.**
5. **Kingdom TT, Nockels RP, Kaplan MJ. Transoral-transpharyngeal approach to the craniocervical junction. Otolaryngol Head Neck Surg 113:393-400, 1995.**
6. Logroscino CA, Casula S, Rigante M, et al. Transmandible approach for the treatment of upper cervical spine metastatic tumors. Orthopedics 27:1100-1103, 2004.
7. **Kassam AB, Snyderman C, Gardner P, et al. The expanded endonasal approach: a fully endoscopic transnasal approach and resection of the odontoid process: technical case report. Neurosurgery 57(1 Suppl):E213; discussion E213, 2005.**
8. **Messina A, Bruno MC, Decq P, et al. Pure endoscopic endonasal odontoidectomy: anatomical study. Neurosurg Rev 30:189-194; discussion 194, 2007.**
9. Nayak JV, Gardner PA, Vescan AD, et al. Experience with the expanded endonasal approach for resection of the odontoid process in rheumatoid disease. Am J Rhinol 21:601-606, 2007.
10. Hermans R, Dewandel P, Debruyne F, et al. Arteria lusoria identified on preoperative CT and nonrecurrent inferior laryngeal nerve during thyroidectomy: a retrospective study. Head Neck 25:113-117, 2003.
11. Tervonen H, Niemelä M, Lauri ER, et al. Dysphonia and dysphagia after anterior cervical decompression. J Neurosurg Spine 7:124-130, 2007.
12. **Yue WM, Brodner W, Highland TR. Persistent swallowing and voice problems after anterior cervical discectomy and fusion with allograft and plating: a 5- to 11-year follow-up study. Eur Spine J 14:677-682, 2005.**
13. **Lee MJ, Bazaz R, Furey CG, et al. Risk factors for dysphagia after anterior cervical spine surgery: a two-year prospective cohort study. Spine J 7:141-147, 2007.**
14. Daniels AH, Riew KD, Yoo JU, et al. Adverse events associated with anterior cervical spine surgery. J Am Acad Orthop Surg 16:729-738, 2008.
15. Kilburg C, Sullivan HG, Mathiason MA. Effect of approach side during anterior cervical discectomy and fusion on the incidence of recurrent laryngeal nerve injury. J Neurosurg Spine 4:273-277, 2006.
16. Kriskovich MD, Apfelbaum RI, Haller JR. Vocal fold paralysis after anterior cervical spine surgery: incidence, mechanism, and prevention of injury. Laryngoscope 110:1467-1473, 2000.

17. Audu P, Artz G, Scheid S, et al. Recurrent laryngeal nerve palsy after anterior cervical spine surgery: the impact of endotracheal tube cuff deflation, reinflation, and pressure adjustment. Anesthesiology 105:898-901, 2006.
18. Choi D, Melcher R, Harms J, et al. Outcome of 132 operations in 97 patients with chordomas of the craniocervical junction and upper cervical spine. Neurosurgery 66:59-65, 2010.
19. Mouchaty H, Perrini P, Conti R, et al. Craniovertebral junction lesions: our experience with the transoral surgical approach. Eur Spine J 18(Suppl 1):13-19, 2009.

Chapter 32

Vertebral Artery Sacrifice and Mobilization

Bernard George, Michaël Bruneau, Damien Bresson

*F*or modern surgical approaches to complicated pathology of the cervical spine, a complete understanding of vertebral artery mobilization techniques and/or sacrifice is invaluable. This holds true for surgical complications as well.

Decisions regarding vertebral artery sacrifice are made on the basis of two very different circumstances.[1] In one instance, the vertebral artery sacrifice is planned, with the goal of achieving a better oncologic resection. In the other, the vertebral artery has been inadvertently injured with no possibility of repair. The second case is clearly more hazardous because, in general, the consequences of vertebral artery occlusion have not been evaluated preoperatively. Whenever possible, rather than sacrificing the vertebral artery, it is preferable to preserve the vertebral artery by alternative means. Vertebral artery mobilization allows preservation of the vertebral artery, as well as new or expanded corridors to the cervical spine and spinal cord. One of these means is control and mobilization of the vertebral artery so that it does not obstruct the operative field. Precise preoperative planning is therefore necessary to be prepared for any problems relating to the vertebral artery during cervical spine surgery.

CLINICAL DECISION-MAKING

Some surgical techniques can be problematic for the vertebral artery. Although this is an infrequent occurrence, we strongly recommend that the surgical team be prepared for any inadvertent vertebral artery injury and become familiar with the strategies for control, repair, or occlusion. This applies specifically to oncologic surgery in and around the vertebral artery. In theory, any surgery involving the cervical spine or any tumor near or including the lateral part of the cervical vertebral bodies places the vertebral artery at risk. This means that for any tumor in close proximity to the vertebral artery, consideration should be given to preoperative imaging, and possibly angiography, if the artery is encased[2-4] (Figs. 32-1 and 32-2).

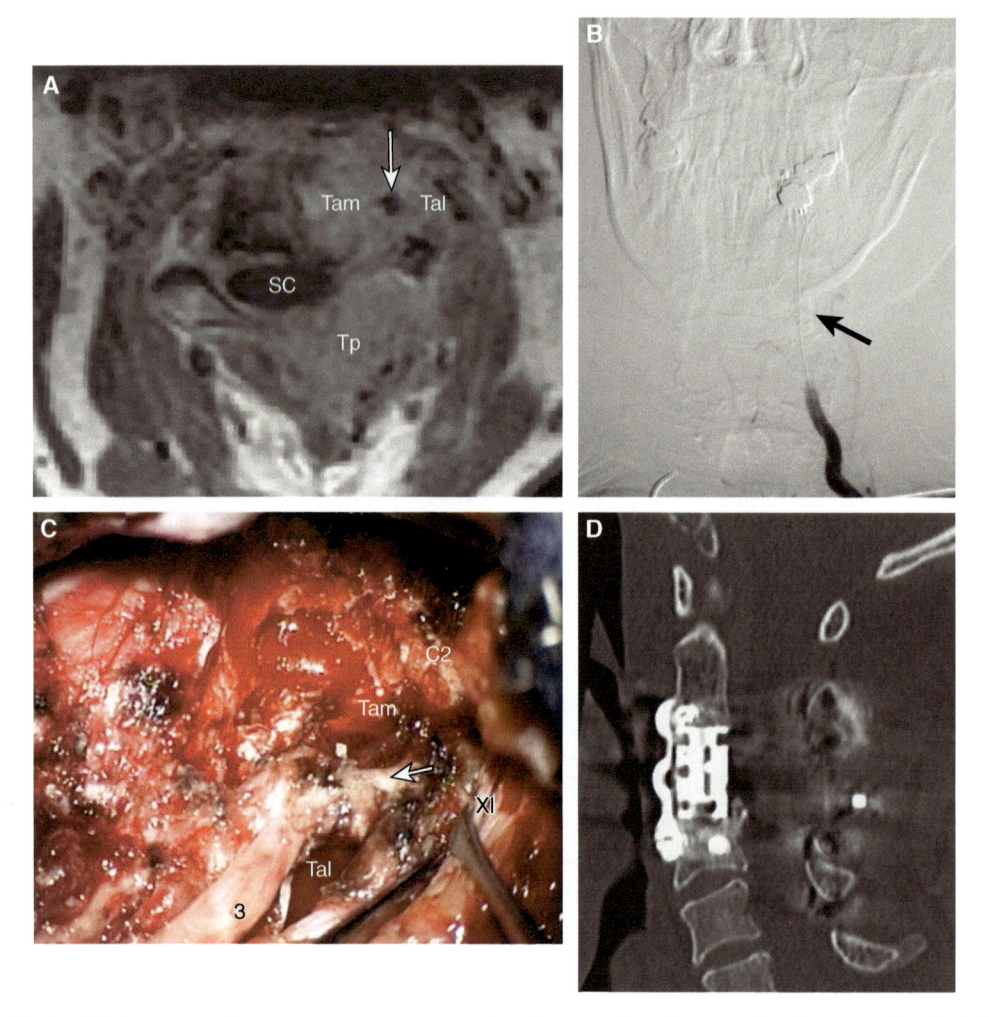

Fig. 32-1 C3 hypernephroma metastases completely encasing the vertebral artery. **A,** Axial T1-weighted MRI with gadolinium enhancement. Left vertebral artery *(arrow)* is completely embedded within the tumor. The lesion will be resected in two operations. The anterior parts (anteromedial and anterolateral to the vertebral artery) of the tumor will be resected through an anterolateral approach, and the posterior part through a posterior lateral approach. The lesion has already destroyed the anterior and posterior parts of the vertebra. **B,** Balloon test occlusion *(arrow)* has been performed and well tolerated. **C,** Operative view during anterolateral approach. The vertebral artery has been dissected from the tumor. Anteromedial and anterolateral portions of the lesion have been resected. **D,** Postoperative CT scan after complete tumor resection and C3 vertebral reconstruction with an expandable cage. Notice the posterior opening. (*C2,* Axis; *SC,* spinal cord; *Tam,* tumor–anteromedial component; *Tal,* tumor–anterolateral component; *Tp,* tumor–posterior component; *XI,* accessory nerve; *3,* C3 nerve root.) (From Université Libre de Bruxelles, Hôpital Erasme.)

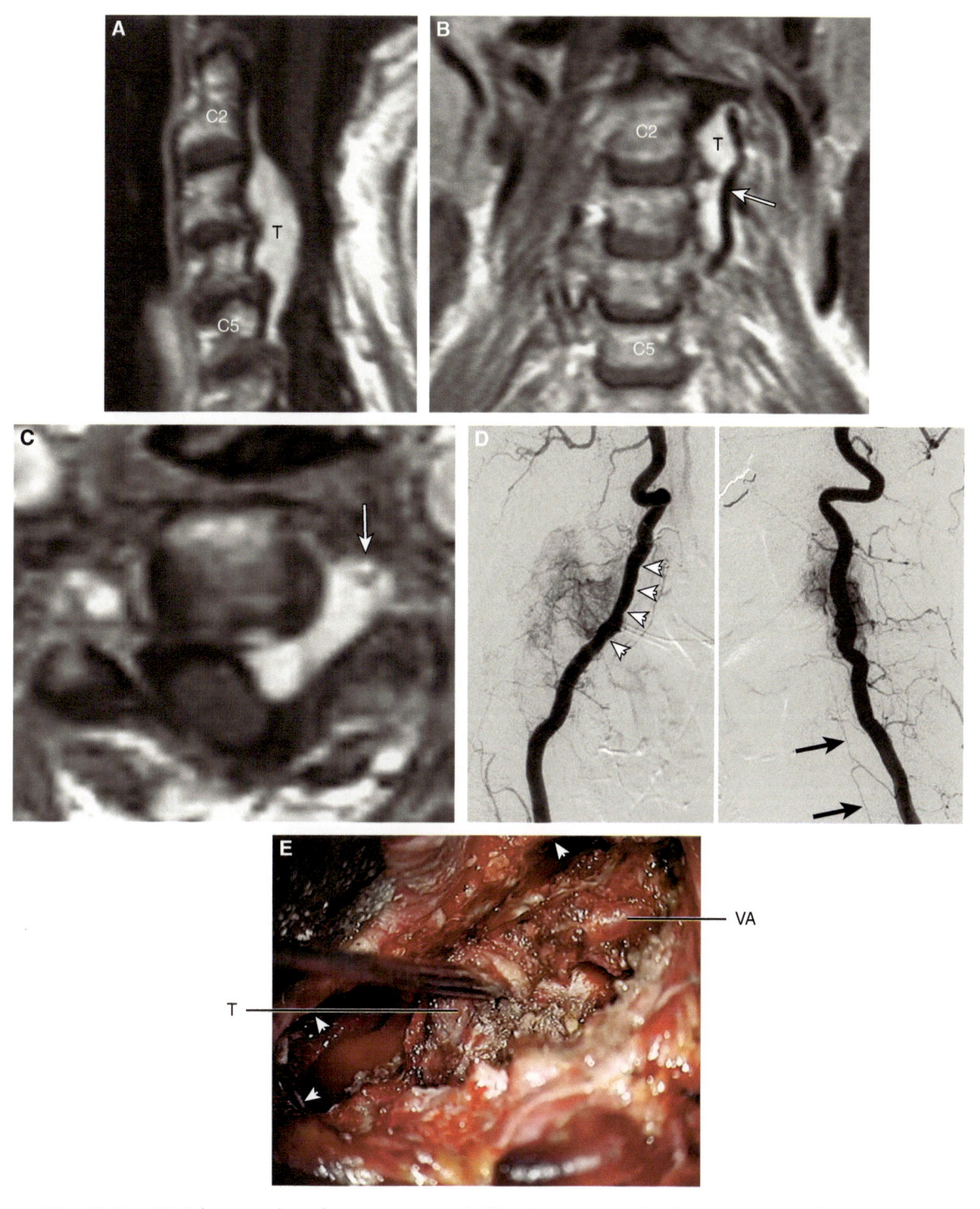

Fig. 32-2 C2-5 low-grade soft tissue sarcoma infiltrating the vertebral artery periosteal sheath. Preoperative **A,** sagittal, **B,** coronal, and **C,** axial T1-weighted MRI scans with gadolinium enhancement. The tumor extends through the intervertebral foramen from the intradural compartment toward the vertebral artery *(arrow),* which is displaced. **D,** Left vertebral artery angiogram. *Left,* Arterial wall appears irregular with several constricted areas *(arrowheads),* leading to suspected wall infiltration. *Right,* Anterior spinal artery *(arrows)* originates at C6-7 level. **E,** Operative view after C2-5 oblique corpectomy (delineated by *arrowheads*) and dissection of the vertebral artery. Adventitial layer of the vertebral artery is seen, whereas tumor remnants are observed infiltrating the periosteal sheath of the artery. (*T,* Tumor; *VA,* vertebral artery.) (From Université Libre de Bruxelles, Hôpital Erasme.)

Continued

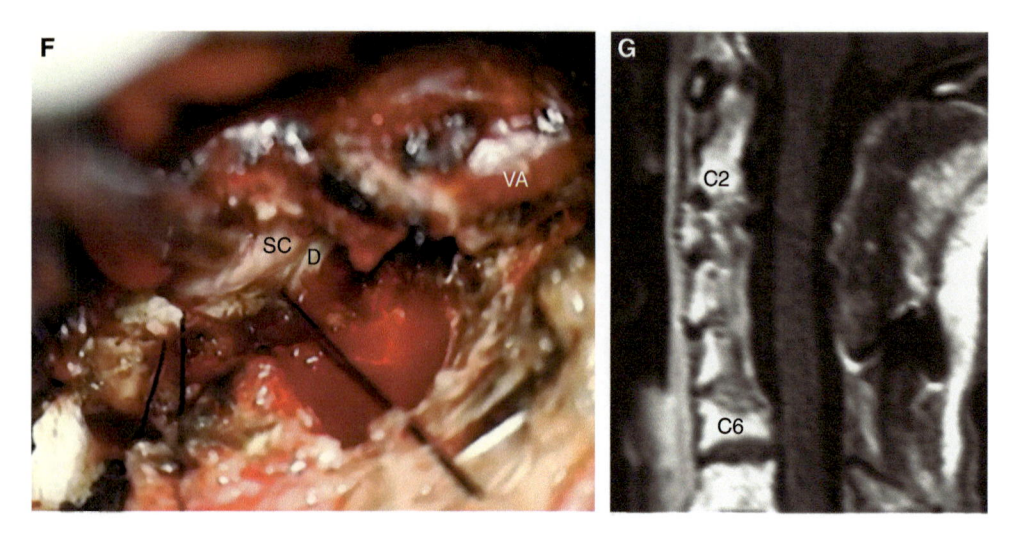

Fig. 32-2, cont'd **F,** Operative view at completion of tumor resection. The intradural component has been resected through an opening in the dura mater *(D)*, releasing the spinal cord *(SC)* compression. (*VA,* Vertebal artery). **G,** Postoperative sagittal MRI scan.

In posterior approaches, vertebral artery injury is most frequently attributed to an errant lateral mass or pedicle screw placement. In these cases the screw should be left in place, which often resolves the profuse bleeding. Subsequently angiography must be performed to check for pseudoaneurysm or vertebral artery occlusion.

With any lateral approach to the cervical spine, including the craniocervical junction, the vertebral artery is, of necessity, encountered as part of the surgical corridor and should be evaluated preoperatively by means of angiography and balloon test occlusion.[5-9] Release of extrinsic intermittent compression of the vertebral artery is another example in which the vertebral artery is at risk of injury. A lateral approach is useful to decompress the spinal cord and the cervical nerve roots through an oblique corpectomy. Even during routine anterior cervical discectomies, the vertebral artery can be injured during drilling of the uncovertebral processes and lateral osteophytes. In cervicothoracic surgery, the vertebral artery may be encountered in supraclavicular brachial plexus approaches and during removal of superior sulcus (Pancoast) tumors. At the level of the craniocervical junction, an anterolateral approach (extreme lateral approach) is used to reach bony and extradural lesions of the anterior and lateral wall (Fig. 32-3). Conversely, the posterolateral approach provides access to intradural and anteriorly located lesions (foramen magnum tumors).

SURGERY WITHOUT VERTEBRAL ARTERY EXPOSURE

A major component of clinical decision-making in surgical approaches that place the vertebral artery at risk is anticipating when vascular and bony abnormalities may increase the risk of injury. Redundancy of the vertebral artery, vertebral artery loops, or an abnormal level of entry into the transverse canal significantly increase the risk of injury to the vertebral artery.[11-16] In anterior procedures the landmarks can be lost,

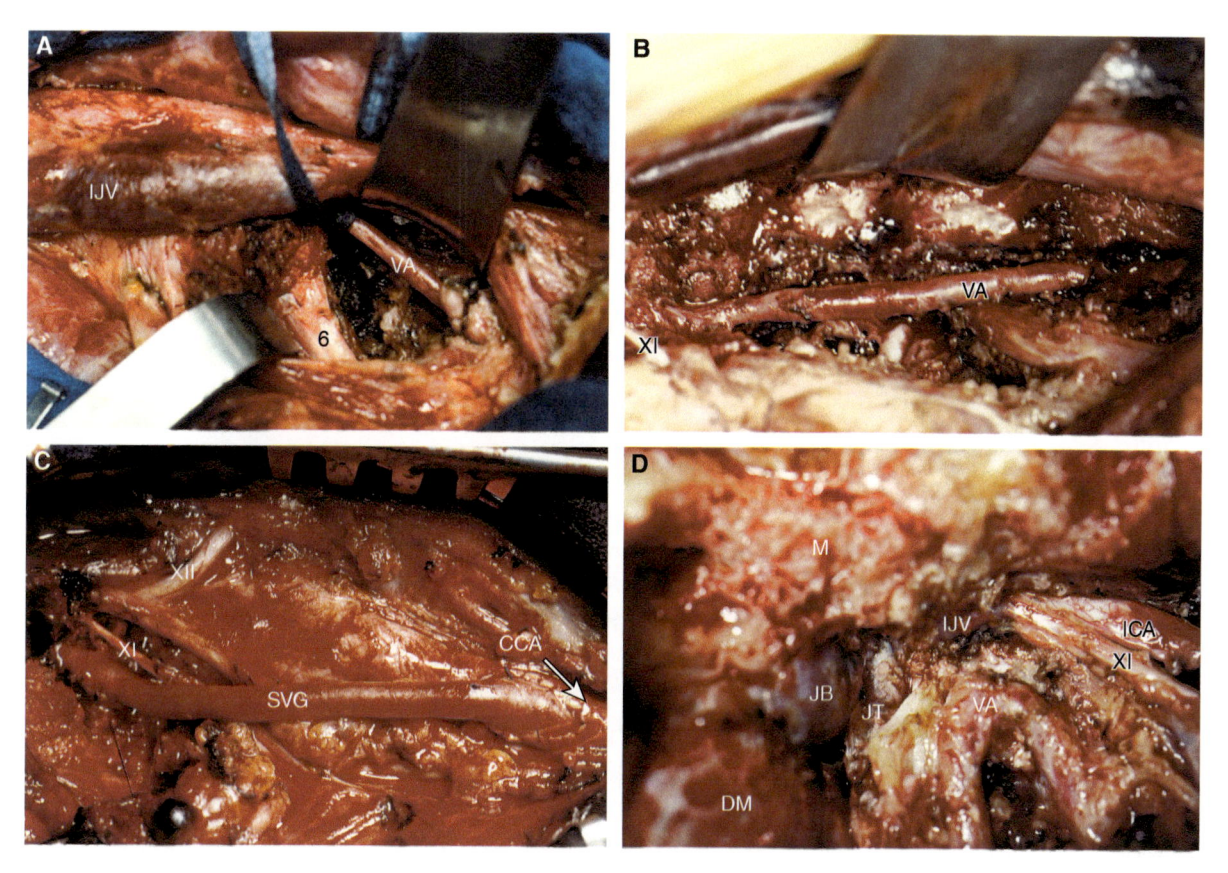

Fig. 32-3 Surgical exposure of the vertebral artery at different levels. **A,** Proximal (V1) segment. (*IJV,* Internal jugular vein; *C6,* C6 cervical nerve root; *VA,* vertebral artery.) **B,** Transversary (V2) segment. (*VA,* Vertebral artery; *XI,* accessory nerve.) **C,** Carotid to vertebral artery bypass with saphenous vein graft performed in a case where the vertebral artery occlusion test was not tolerated. (*CCA,* Common carotid artery; *SVG,* saphenous vein graft; *XI,* accessory nerve; *XII,* hypoglossal nerve.) **D,** Distal (V3) segment. (*M,* Mastoid; *DM,* dura mater of the cerebellum; *JB,* jugular bulb; *JT,* jugular tubercle; *IJV,* internal jugular vein; *ICA,* internal carotid artery; *XI,* accessory nerve; *VA,* vertebral artery.) (From Hôpital Lariboisière.)

and maneuvers such as drilling or screwing may be inadequate.[17-20] In these situations it may be difficult to solve the problem of vertebral artery injury. Very often the procedure ends with compressive packing or blind coagulation, with the end result being vertebral artery occlusion. With posterior procedures the vertebral artery injury is, in most cases, the result of screw misplacement. In these cases the best option is to leave the screw in place.

Factors Increasing the Risk of Vertebral Artery Injury

Vertebral Artery Anomalies

Some anomalies in the course of the vertebral artery place the vertebral artery at much greater risk of injury, such as redundant vertebral artery loops or an abnormal level of entry into the transverse canal.[21] In the case of a redundant vertebral artery, the vertebral artery does not run straight in the transverse canal but instead runs out of it more superficially into the muscles.[21] This is seen, in particular, at the C1-2 level and above the C1 level.[21] In the case of loops the vertebral artery encroaches medially on the vertebral body (or bodies) or the intervertebral foramen.[21] When the vertebral artery enters the transverse canal at the C5, C4, or even the C3 level, rather than at the typical C6 level, it runs in front of the anterior part of the transverse process and behind the muscles (longus colli muscle).[21] Therefore it is no longer protected by bone, and mobilization of the longus colli may lead to vertebral artery injury.[21] Posterior transarticular C1-2 screw placement may be dangerous and is contraindicated in the presence of a high-riding vertebral artery that blocks passage of the screw.[21]

Bone Anomalies

Very occasionally the anterior branch of the transverse process may be absent, thereby rendering the vertebral artery unprotected by bone. If the surgeon is unaware of this anomaly, it can lead to inadvertent injury to the vertebral artery. We have observed this anomaly in only one case out of more than 1300 vertebral artery exposures.

Recurrence and Radiation Therapy

In patients presenting with recurrent pathology and in those who have undergone radiation therapy, fibrotic scarring and adhesions make the dissection more tedious.

SACRIFICE OF THE VERTEBRAL ARTERY

Vertebral artery sacrifice is often well tolerated in patients with normal posterior circulation anatomy. However, in salvage reoperations or postradiation settings, it can be complicated and hazardous. It is of paramount importance that the surgeon be cognizant of the course of the vertebral artery and its correlation with both the ipsilateral and contralateral sides; this is accomplished with preoperative magnetic resonance imaging (MRI) and computed tomographic (CT) angiography.[14] Sacrifice of the vertebral artery may be a simple procedure under quiet conditions, or it may be more difficult and hazardous when used as salvage treatment. In fact on MRI scans, and even on CT scans, it is rather simple to identify the vertebral artery and to get an idea of the size and course of both the ipsilateral and contralateral vertebral artery.[14] In these cases a risk of injury can be anticipated. In some cases an abnormal level of entry of the vertebral artery into the transverse process canal (above C6), a vertebral artery loop, or a lack of the anterior aspect of the transverse process are easily recognizable conditions where the vertebral artery is at risk of injury. The only major branch that cannot be identified on angiographic CT or MRI scans is the anterior radiculomedullary artery.

Deliberate occlusion of one vertebral artery is best performed after balloon test occlusion (BTO) demonstrating a good contralateral supply and good clinical tolerance. BTO must be done each time the vertebral artery to be occluded is dominant or of a substantive caliber. There is a general assumption that small and minor (larger contralateral vertebral artery) vertebral arteries can be occluded with no clinical consequences. However, this is not always true. In the case of an atretic vertebral artery that does not connect with the contralateral vertebral artery and ends at the posterior inferior cerebellar artery, the result of its occlusion may be a cerebellar infarction because of a lack of collateral supply. Conversely, interruption of a large and dominant vertebral artery may be well tolerated, especially if this is performed proximally, because of a collateral network through muscular branches from the external carotid artery, ascending cervical artery, and deep cervical artery, which may be sufficiently developed to compensate for the vertebral artery occlusion.

In the literature there are only a few reports of vertebral artery injuries, most likely because they remain unrecognized and therefore unpublished.[11-16,22-24] We have encountered vertebral artery injury in five patients out of 1300 vertebral artery exposures over a 30-year period. In three cases the vertebral artery injury occurred during exposure of the vertebral artery. In one case the vertebral artery was small, and it entered the transverse canal at the C4 level and was coagulated. In another two cases, the vertebral artery ruptured while it was being separated from a schwannoma. One small vertebral artery was ligated, and the other was repaired with sutures after proximal and distal clamping. In two other patients a delayed rupture was observed 8 hours and 10 days after surgery, respectively. The first patient had a recurrent and irradiated chordoma. The second patient had an osteoid osteoma removed with no problem but developed a late infection of the wound. Both patients were treated with ligation. In only one case were any consequences of these injuries noted. One of the patients with a schwannoma and vertebral artery ligation had some gait disturbances, which improved over the following weeks. These were the result of two small infarctions in the cerebellar vermis, as seen on MRI.

Conversely, we deliberately occluded eight vertebral arteries. In all of them the decision was made to sacrifice the artery to achieve a radical resection of a malignant tumor. BTO was performed in five of them to assess their tolerance to occlusion. One patient was unable to tolerate occlusion and underwent a saphenous vein bypass between the common carotid artery and the distal vertebral artery. In the other patients only ligation was performed. In three patients no BTO was carried out. Two of these patients had a small vertebral artery that was occluded without consequence. The third patient, a 6-year-old boy, required bypass on both sides to resect a huge osteoblastoma involving both vertebral arteries. In the literature there are four large studies of inadvertent vertebral artery injury during anterior cervical spine surgery.[9,25] The incidence of vertebral artery injury varies from 0.18% to 0.3% and 0.8%.[17,21,25,26] Among reported cases, only two patients had brain stem ischemic infarcts, including one who died. In fact, consequences of vertebral artery occlusion are usually rare because of compensation by the opposite vertebral artery, the circle of Willis, and the muscular collateral network connecting the vertebral artery with the external carotid arteries and the cervical branches of the subclavian artery. Ischemic complications after vertebral artery occlusion, regardless of the cause (traumatic or surgical), are reported at rates varying from 0% to 33%.*

The potential complication of sacrificing a vertebral artery giving rise to the anterior radiculomedullary artery has never been reported. However, occlusion of this branch may lead to severe ischemic lesions with tetraplegia. This branch always originates below C3. Therefore sacrifice or mobilization of the lower part of the vertebral artery should be studied in advance by means of angiography.

Exposure and Mobilization

As previously mentioned, the best way to avoid the unexpected need for sacrifice of the vertebral artery is sometimes to mobilize the vertebral artery out of the working place. Obviously this means perfect control of the vertebral artery. This is accomplished through a lateral approach, which provides the best exposure of the vertebral artery. The lateral approach is similar, with some modifications, regardless of the level of exposure.

The lateral approach is now well known, as it has been described in several articles[4-8] (Fig. 32-4). Briefly, the patient is placed in the supine position, with the head slightly extended and rotated toward the opposite side. The skin incision follows the medial edge of the sternocleidomastoid muscle at the appropriate level. For the upper or lower part of the cervical spine, the sternocleidomastoid muscle is detached from the mastoid process or the sternum, respectively. The plane between the internal jugular vein and the sternocleidomastoid muscle is then opened, and the vasculonervous elements with the esophagus and trachea are retracted all together without any dissection. The prevertebral aponeurosis is incised longitudinally, medial to the sympathetic trunk, which is retracted laterally (Fig. 32-4, *A*). The prevertebral (longus colli) muscle is divided along the lateral aspect of the chosen vertebral bodies and along the transverse processes (Fig. 32-4, *B*). The anterior aspect of the transverse processes is then subperiosteally exposed to preserve the periosteal sheath surrounding the vertebral artery and its venous plexus. The transverse foramina are then opened, and the vertebral artery is exposed to the desired length (Fig. 32-4, *C*). The general principle is to open the transverse foramina at the level of the lesion, including the ones above and below.

---

*References 10, 18, 19, 23, 27-30.

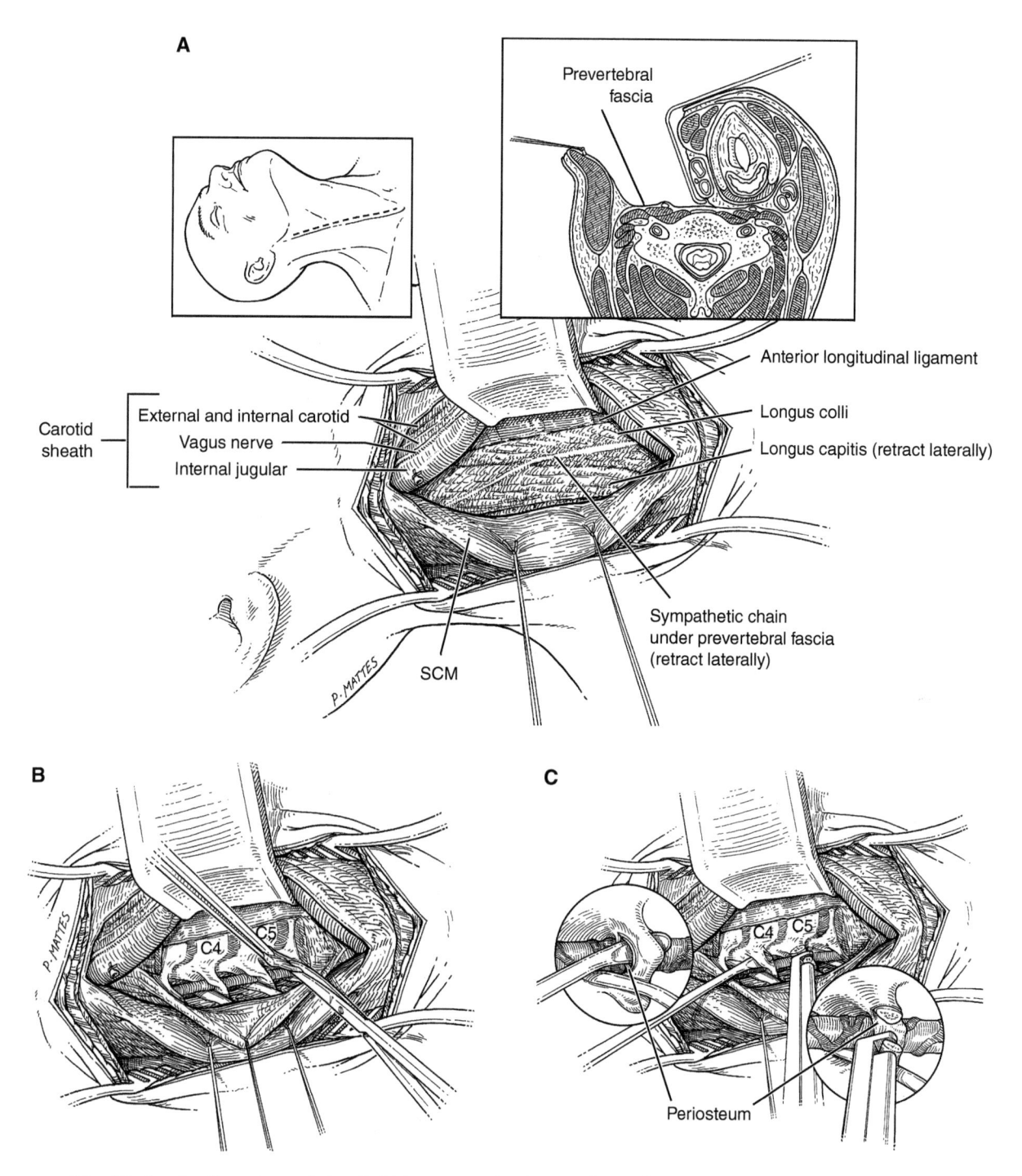

Fig. 32-4 A, Opening of the field between the internal jugular vein and the sternocleidomastoid muscle *(SCM)*. Inset *(left)*, positioning and skin incision; inset *(right)*, axial view of the opening. **B,** Exposure of the lateral aspect of the vertebral bodies (C4 and C5) and corresponding transverse processes; the sympathetic chain is laterally retracted by stitches. **C,** Opening of the transverse canal by resection of the anterior branch of the transverse process after the bone is split from the periosteum surrounding the vertebral artery (see insets).

Continued

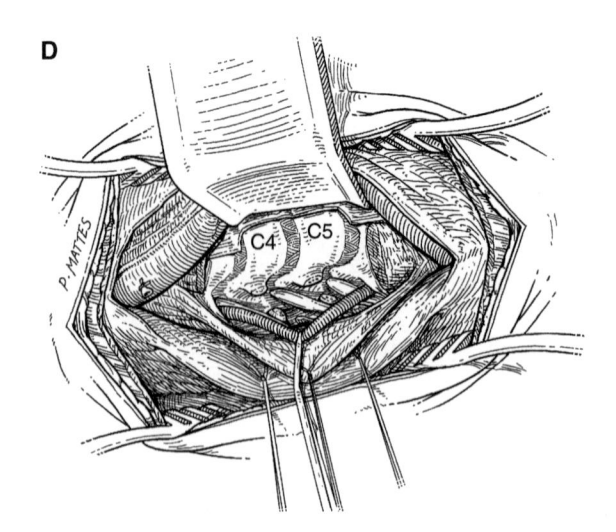

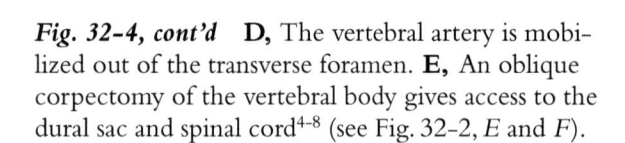

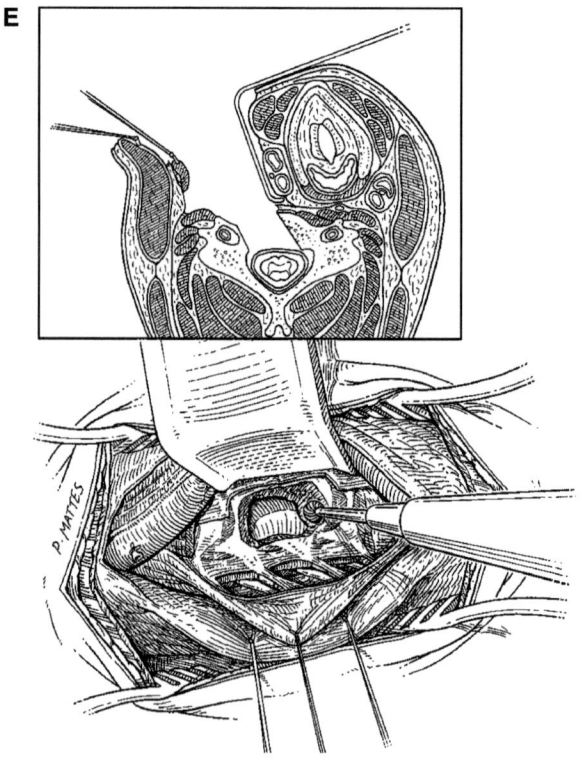

Fig. 32-4, cont'd **D,** The vertebral artery is mobilized out of the transverse foramen. **E,** An oblique corpectomy of the vertebral body gives access to the dural sac and spinal cord[4-8] (see Fig. 32-2, *E* and *F*).

Working subperiosteally, the vertebral artery can be fully controlled all around its circumference. At the level of the vertebral bodies, the subperiosteal dissection separates the vertebral artery from the bone. At the level of the intervertebral foramen, the vertebral artery must be separated from the sheath of the cervical nerve root or roots (Fig. 32-4, *D* and *E*). Often the nerve sheath and the vertebral artery periosteal sheath are adherent. However, it is always possible to find a plane between the two. It may be useful to divide the longus capitis muscle to gain access to the cervical nerve roots. In the presence of tumor, especially neurinoma, the vertebral artery is more or less compressed, and it is generally easier to identify after the tumor has been debulked lateral and anterior to the vertebral artery. In some cases the periosteal sheath of the vertebral artery is ruptured or even invaded. This cannot be detected on preoperative examination and is the reason why control of the vertebral artery must begin above and below the level of the lesion.

Still more difficult is mobilization of the vertebral artery in reoperations, when fibrous scar tissue makes the plane disappear. As a rule the vertebral artery must be controlled out of fibrosis above and below before progressing toward the scar tissue. In two situations (reoperation with fibrous tissue and tumor severely compressing or encasing the vertebral artery), BTO must be considered before surgery to be prepared for any difficulties that may arise during vertebral artery exposure.

VERTEBRAL ARTERY TRANSPOSITION

Transposition corresponds to mobilization of the V3 segment (C2 to foramen magnum) out of the transverse foramen of the atlas. This is a more complex technique because of the complex anatomy of this segment, which changes according to head position. Because the head is usually rotated (toward the opposite side), the two parts of the VA-3 segment (C1-2 and above C1) are stretched on both sides of the posterior arch of the atlas (Fig. 32-5). The sternocleidomastoid muscle is detached from the mastoid process, and the field is opened between the sternocleidomastoid muscle and the internal jugular vein. The accessory nerve (cranial nerve XI) crosses the field and must be dissected free and is then usually retracted anteromedially. The transverse process of the atlas is identified 15 mm below the tip of the mastoid. All of the little muscles inserting on it are divided flush to it (levator scapulae, inferior and superior oblique, and rectus capitis muscles) until the two parts of the vertebral artery come into view. The C1-2 part is crossed anteriorly by the second cervical nerve root, which often must be divided. Then the tip of the transverse foramen of the atlas is resected, and the transverse foramen is unroofed. Again this must be done with preservation of the vertebral artery periosteal sheath. Care must be taken to resect the bone in the concavity of the vertebral artery loop at the level of the transverse foramen, so that pulling the vertebral artery out of the transverse foramen does not result in the tearing of it. This transposition can be extended to the junction between the V2 and V3 segments by opening the transverse foramen of C2.

Transposition of the V3 segment gives access to the lateral wall of the craniocervical junction, including the C1-2 joint and the C0 (occipital condyle)-C1 joint. It also leads to the jugular tubercle, which is the inferolateral wall of the jugular foramen.[31]

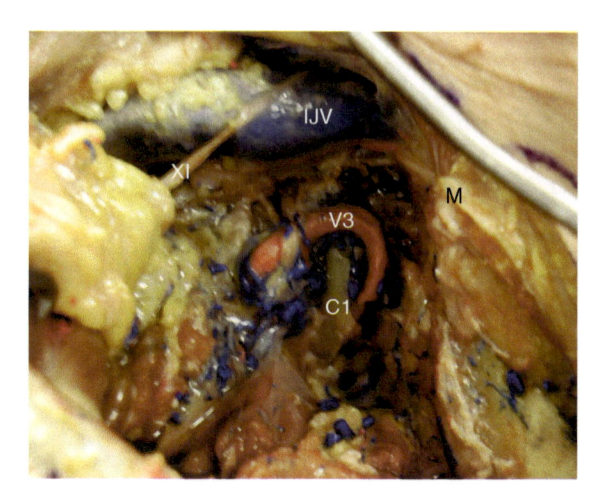

Fig. 32-5 Exposure of the vertebral artery V3 segment on a cadaveric dissection. (*C1,* Posterior arch of atlas; *IJV,* internal jugular vein; *M,* mastoid process; *XI,* accessory nerve.) (From Hôpital Lariboisière.)

BAILOUT TECHNIQUES

- In case of no vertebral artery control, packing is the best option (with post operative angiographic control.)
- In case of vertebral artery exposure and of dominant vertebral artery, direct repair or bypass (from the carotid artery) has to be done.

TIPS FROM THE MASTERS

- The ability to locate and mobilize the vertebral artery from an anterior, anterior lateral, and posterior approach is a vital skill for dealing with complex cervical spine tumors and deformities.
- CT angiography can be very helpful to rule out rare anatomic variations in treatment planning.
- Malignant disease is more likely to invade the vertebral artery, and therefore the risk is high in cases of intraoperative injury.
- Proximal and distal control, as is the case with all types of vascular surgery, is critical in high-risk patients.

References (With Key References in Boldface)

1. **George B, Cornelius JF, Bruneau M. Complications of surgery around the vertebral artery and their management. In George B, Bruneau M, Spetzler RF, eds. Pathology and Surgery Around the Vertebral Artery. New York: Springer, 2012.**
2. Lot G, George B. Cervical neuromas with extradural components: surgical management in a series of 57 patients. Neurosurgery 41:813-820; discussion 820-822, 1997.
3. George B, Laurian C. Impairment of vertebral artery flow caused by extrinsic lesions. Neurosurgery 24:206-214, 1989.
4. **George B, Carpentier A. Compression of and by the vertebral artery. In Spetzler RF, ed. Operative Techniques in Neurosurgery. Philadelphia: WB Saunders, 2001, pp 202-218.**
5. Bruneau M, Cornelius JF, George B. Anterolateral approach to the V1 segment of the vertebral artery. Neurosurgery 58:ONS-215-219; discussion ONS-219, 2006.
6. **George B. Extracranial vertebral artery anatomy and surgery. In Pickard JD, Akalan N, Di Rocco C, et al, eds. Advances and Technical Standards in Neurosurgery. New York: Springer-Verlag, 2002, pp 179-216.**
7. Bruneau M, Cornelius JF, George B. Anterolateral approach to the V2 segment of the vertebral artery. Neurosurgery 57:262-267; discussion 267, 2005.
8. Bruneau M, Cornelius JF, George B. Antero-lateral approach to the V3 segment of the vertebral artery. Neurosurgery 58:ONS29-35; discussion ONS35, 2006.
9. Lot G, George B. Cervical neuromas with extradural components: surgical management in a series of 57 patients. Neurosurgery 41:813-820; discussion 820-822, 1997.
10. **George B, Blanquet A, Alves O. Surgical exposure of the vertebral artery. In Septzler RF, ed. Operative Techniques in Neurosurgery. Philadelphia: WB Saunders, 2001, pp 182-194.**

11. Schweighofer F, Passler JM, Wildburger R, et al. Interbody fusion of the lower cervical spine: a dangerous surgical method? Langenbecks Arch Chir 377:295-299, 1992.
12. Pfeifer BA, Freidberg SR, Jewell ER. Repair of injured vertebral artery in anterior cervical procedures. Spine 19:1471-1474, 1994.
13. de los Reyes RA, Moser FG, Sachs DP, et al. Direct repair of an extracranial vertebral artery pseudoaneurysm: case report and review of the literature. Neurosurgery 26:528-533, 1990.
14. Cosgrove GR, Theron J. Vertebral arteriovenous fistula following anterior cervical spine surgery. Report of two cases. J Neurosurg 66:297-299, 1987.
15. Cloward RB. Complications of anterior cervical disc operation and their treatment Surgery 69:175-182, 1971.
16. Cloward RB. New method of diagnosis and treatment of cervical disc disease. Clin Neurosurg 8:93-132, 1962.
17. Neo M, Fujibayashi S, Miyata M, et al. Vertebral artery injury during cervical spine surgery: a survey of more than 5600 operations. Spine 33:779-785, 2008.
18. **Wright NM, Lauryssen C. Vertebral artery injury in C1-C2 transarticular screw fixation: results of a survey of the AANS/CNS section on disorders of the spine and peripheral nerves. American Association of Neurological Surgeons/Congress of Neurological Surgeons. J Neurosurg 88:634-640, 1998.**
19. Madawi AA, Casey AT, Solanki GA, et al. Radiological and anatomical evaluation of the atlantoaxial transarticular screw fixation technique. J Neurosurg 86:961-968, 1997.
20. Paramore CG, Dickman CA, Sonntag VK. The anatomical suitability of the C1-2 complex for transarticular screw fixation. J Neurosurg 85:221-224, 1996.
21. Burke JP, Gerszten PC, Welch WC. Iatrogenic vertebral artery injury during anterior cervical spine surgery. Spine J 5:508-514; discussion 514, 2005.
22. Daentzer D, Deinsberger W, Boker DK. Vertebral artery complications in anterior approaches to the cervical spine: report of two cases and review of literature. Surg Neurol 59:300-309; discussion 309, 2003.
23. Weinberg PE, Flom RA. Traumatic vertebral arteriovenous fistula. Surg Neurol 1:162-167, 1973.
24. **Bertalanffy H, Eggert HR. Complications of anterior cervical discectomy without fusion in 450 consecutive patients. Acta Neurochir (Wien) 99:41-50, 1989.**
25. Golfinos JG, Dickman CA, Zabramski JM, et al. Repair of vertebral artery injury during anterior cervical decompression. Spine 19:2552-2556, 1994.
26. Smith MD, Emery SE, Dudley A, et al. Vertebral artery injury during anterior decompression of the cervical spine. A retrospective review of ten patients. J Bone Joint Surg Br 75:410-415, 1993.
27. Higashida RT, Halbach VV, Tsai FY, et al. Interventional neurovascular treatment of traumatic carotid and vertebral artery lesions: results in 234 cases. AJR Am J Roentgenol 153:577-582, 1989.
28. **Bruneau M, Cornelius JF, Marneffe V, et al. Anatomical variations of the V2 segment of the vertebral artery. Neurosurgery 59:ONS20-24; discussion ONS24, 2006.**
29. Taneichi H, Suda K, Kajino T, et al. Traumatically induced vertebral artery occlusion associated with cervical spine injuries: prospective study using magnetic resonance angiography. Spine 30:1955-1962, 2005.
30. Steinberg GD, Drake GG, Peerless SJ. Deliberate basilar or vertebral artery occlusion in the treatment of intracranial aneurysms. Immediate results and long-term outcome in 201 patients. J Neurosurg 79:161-173, 1993.
31. **Bruneau M, George B. The juxtacondylar approach to the jugular foramen. Neurosurgery 62:75-78; discussion 80-81, 2008.**

Chapter 33

Pancoast Tumors

Matthias Setzer, Lary A. Robinson, Frank D. Vrionis

Pancoast tumors are primary carcinomas arising from the apex of the lung; they are usually located in the superior pulmonary sulcus. They are named after Henry Kunrath Pancoast (1875 to 1939), a radiologist at the University of Pennsylvania in Philadelphia, first described the radiologic features that now bear his name.[1-3] Because the term *superior pulmonary sulcus* is not clearly defined anatomically, some authors dismiss the term *superior sulcus tumors,* which has gained widespread use, nevertheless, in the literature.[4] Pancoast tumors may extend in three directions: anteriorly, invading major blood vessels, such as the subclavian artery; superiorly, primarily invading the brachial plexus; and medially, invading the stellate ganglion or vertebral bodies.[5]

Due to their position in the apex of the lung, with invasion of the lower part of the brachial plexus, ribs, vertebrae, subclavian vessels, and/or stellate ganglion, Pancoast tumors cause characteristic symptoms, such as arm, shoulder, or scapular pain, radicular pain and muscle weakness in the distributions of the C8, T1, and T2 nerve roots; and Horner (ptosis, miosis, and anhidrosis) syndrome, when the sympathetic chain is involved.[6] This symptom complex is also called *Pancoast syndrome*. However, the first patient with this syndrome was described 90 years earlier by the British surgeon, Edwin Hare,[7] in 1838. Pancoast[2] initially believed the tumor to be extrapulmonary in origin and erroneously described these tumors as derived from epithelial remnants of the fifth branchial cleft. J.W. Tobías,[6] from Buenos Aires, Argentina, later described the syndrome independently in 1932 and correctly assigned these tumors to the bronchopulmonary compartment. Therefore some authors refer to this symptom complex as *Pancoast-Tobías syndrome*.

Although superior sulcus primary lung-tumors are the most common cause of Pancoast-Tobías syndrome, there are a variety of rarer pathologic conditions that can cause this syndrome.[8] In most cases Pancoast tumors are non–small cell bronchogenic carcinomas, most commonly squamous cell (52%), followed by adenocarcinomas (23%) and large cell carcinomas (20%). Only about 5% of Pancoast tumors are of small cell origin. Pancoast tumors invading the mediastinal pleura, chest wall, and spine have been considered unresectable, and the remaining therapeutic options have been radiation therapy, alone or in combination with chemotherapy, but the overall prognosis is poor.[9] However, the introduction of newer diagnostic, medical, and surgical therapies has led to an improvement in the overall prognosis. Recent progress in spinal instrumentation, with the development of reliable hardware and wider acceptance of total spondylectomy, make more radical surgical modalities feasible.[10] An incomplete resection is considered a poor prognostic factor, and recent studies have focused on exploring the use of extended operations to achieve complete resection of Pancoast tumors invading the spine.[11,12] The aim of the present chapter is to introduce some current concepts regarding the surgical management of locally advanced Pancoast tumors with spine involvement.

EPIDEMIOLOGY

Non–small cell lung cancer (NSCLC) is the most common histologic entity among Pancoast tumors. Lung cancer is the most common cancer worldwide, with an incidence of 1.35 million new cases per year, and an annual mortality of 1.18 million deaths, with the highest rates in industrial countries in North America and Europe.[13,14] Lung cancer is the second most commonly occurring form of cancer in most Western countries, and it is the leading cancer-related cause of death.[15] The incidence of lung cancer is highest in current or former smokers greater than 50 years of age. Although the mortality rate for lung cancer in men is declining in the United States, the rate has been increasing in women over the past few decades and is only recently beginning to stabilize.[15] However, Pancoast tumors account for only 3% to 5% of all NSCLCs, or approximately 7000 cases per year in the United States.

CLASSIFICATION OF PANCOAST TUMORS
The Tumor-Node-Metastasis System

As with other types of lung cancer, Pancoast tumors are classified according to the tumor, lymph node, metastasis (TNM) system of the American Joint Committee on Cancer and the International Union Against Cancer. Because of their peripheral location and the frequent involvement of the chest wall, most Pancoast tumors are classified as T3 tumors, typically invading easily resectable areas of the chest wall or superficially extending into the mediastinum. Further invasion of the brachial plexus, mediastinal structures, or the vertebral bodies classifies the tumor as a T4 tumor, which is less readily resectable. Table 33-1[16] provides an overview of the new seventh revision of the TNM descriptors for staging NSCLC developed by the International Association for the Study of Lung Cancer (IASLC) and adopted by the International Union Against Cancer. Table 33-2[16] lists the revised staging system. Therefore, based on this staging classification, Pancoast tumors are either stage IIb or stage IIIa in the absence of nodal or distant metastasis.

Table 33-1 Seventh Revision of Tumor-Node-Metastasis (TNM) Descriptors for Non–Small Cell Lung Cancer

Tumor (T)

- T1a Tumor ≤2 cm in diameter, with no visceral pleural or lobar bronchial involvement
- T1b Tumor 2.1-3.0 cm in diameter, with no visceral pleural or lobar bronchial involvement
- T2a Tumor 3.1-5.0 cm in diameter; visceral pleural involvement or involvement of main bronchus >2 cm from the carina
- T2b Tumor 5.1-7.0 cm in diameter, visceral pleural involvement or >2 cm from the carina
- T3   Tumor >7.0 cm in diameter; 2 tumor nodules in the same lobe; direct extension to visceral pleura, phrenic nerve, or chest wall; involvement of C8/T1, or pericardial invasion
- T4   Tumor nodules in different lobes of the same lung or direct extension into mediastinal structures and organs, carina, trachea, recurrent laryngeal nerve, brachial plexus, vertebrae, or major extrapulmonary vessels pericardial invasion

Node (N)

- N0 No lymph node involvement
- N1 Involvement of peribronchial or ipsilateral hilar lymph nodes
- N2 Involvement of ipsilateral mediastinal lymph nodes
- N3 Contralateral mediastinal/hilar lymph nodes; any supraclavicular or scalene lymph node involvement

Metastasis (M)

- M0   No distant metastases
- M1a Malignant pleural effusion or tumor involvement of contralateral lung
- M1b Any distant metastases

Adapted from Detterbeck FC, Boffa DJ, Tanoue LT. The new lung cancer staging system. Chest 136:260-271, 2009.

Table 33-2 Seventh Revision Stage Groupings for Non–Small Cell Lung Cancer

Grouping	TNM Staging
Occult carcinoma	TX N0 M0
Stage 0	Tis N0 M0
Stage IA	T1a N0 M0
	T1b N0 M0
Stage IB	T2a N0 M0
Stage IIA	T1a N1 M0
	T1b N1 M0
	T2a N1 M0
	T2b N0 M0
Stage IIB	T2b N1 M0
	T3 N0 M0
Stage IIIA	T1a N2 M0
	T1b N2 M0
	T2a N2 M0
	T2b N2 M0
	T3 N1 M0
	T3 N2 M0
	T4 N0 or N1 M0
Stage IIIB	Any T N3 M0
	T4 N2 M0
Stage IV	Any T Any N M1a or M1b

Adapted from Detterbeck FC, Boffa DJ, Tanoue LT. The new lung cancer staging system. Chest 136:260-271, 2009.

SURGICAL CLASSIFICATION

Although the TNM staging system helps in general decision-making, with regard to surgical treatment versus nonoperative therapy, it does not help in determining the extent of vertebral body resection, the operative approach, and whether instrumentation is needed. Therefore spine surgeons dealing with this disease have developed a classification of vertebral involvement to facilitate surgical planning.[17,18]

TYPE A TUMORS

The tumor involves the transverse process and extends to but not beyond the neuroforamina. The tumor may be attached to the vertebral body, but there is no infiltration of the vertebral body.

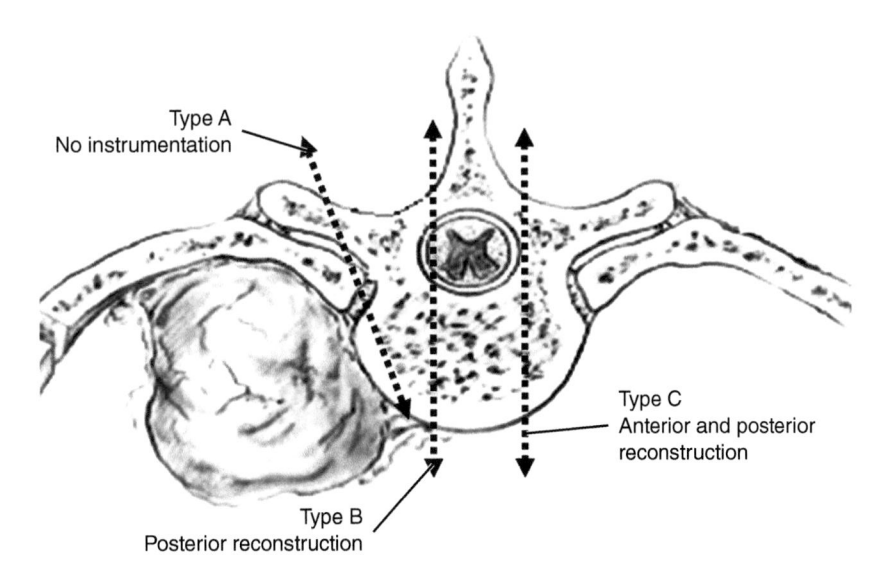

Fig. 33-1 Diagram illustrating assessment of resectability. The need for spinal stabilization depends on the degree of tumor extension to the vertebral body and ipsilateral or contralateral pedicle. Extension of the tumor to the vertebral body or pedicle is an indication for partial or total vertebrectomy. (From Jain S, Sommers E, Setzer M, et al. Posterior midline approach for single-stage en bloc resection and circumferential spinal stabilization for locally advanced Pancoast tumors. Technical note. J Neurosurg Spine 9:71-82, 2008.)

TYPE B TUMORS

These tumors extend beyond the neural foramina into the epidural space and may cause cord compression and involvement of one or more roots. The vertebral body is infiltrated or destroyed, but no more than one third of the vertebral body is affected. These tumors require one or more vertebral body resections.

TYPE C TUMORS

Tumors with vertebral body involvement of more than one third in one or more levels are classified as type C. In addition to vertebral body involvement, nerve root and/or cord compression are also found (Fig. 33-1).

SURGICAL ANATOMY

The lower trunk of the brachial plexus consists of the ventral rami of the C8 and T1 (and occasionally T2) roots (Fig. 33-2). It is seen posterior to the subclavian artery. It emerges above the first rib between the anterior and middle scalene muscles. The subclavian vein is anterior to the subclavian artery, separated by the anterior scalene muscle. Medially and anterior to the vertebral bodies are the esophagus, trachea, recurrent laryngeal nerve, and thoracic duct *(left)*. The recurrent laryngeal nerve curves around the subclavian artery *(right)* or the aortic arch *(left)*. It can be seen during right-sided approaches. The vertebral artery arises from the posterior aspect of the proximal subclavian artery and courses upward toward the transverse foramen of C6.

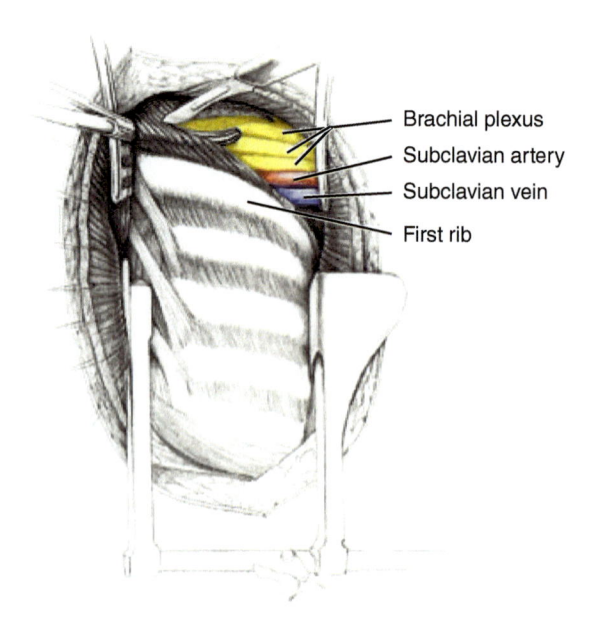

Fig. 33-2 Anatomic view of the inferior trunk of the brachial plexus as seen from a posterior approach. After sectioning of the scalene attachments to the first rib, the C8 and T1 nerve roots are seen. Anterior to them is the subclavian artery and further anterior is the subclavian vein. (From Atlas of Peripheral Nerve Surgery, Kline DG, Hudson AR, Kim DH, Chapter 6, Copyright WB Saunders [2001].)

The phrenic nerve courses on the anterior surface of the anterior scalene muscle and then descends between the subclavian artery and vein. The cervicothoracic (stellate) ganglion is formed by a fusion of the lower two cervical and first thoracic ganglia and lies anterior to the neck of the first rib and lateral to the lateral border of the longus colli muscle. All of these anatomic structures in the superior mediastinum and thoracic outlet can be exposed and involved by Pancoast tumors.

CLINICAL FEATURES
PRESENTATION

Pancoast tumors are closely related to structures surrounding the superior sulcus, including the lower brachial plexus, the first, second, and third ribs, and the vertebrae with the overlying parietal pleura and endothoracic fascia, the subclavian vessels, and the stellate ganglion.[1,19] Because of these anatomic relationships, Pancoast tumors can cause a variety of symptoms, such as pain in the shoulder or scapular area; radicular pain and sensory deficits, as well as muscle weakness in the distributions of the C8, T1, and T2 nerve roots.[19] The pain may radiate up to the head and neck or down to the medial scapula, axilla, and anterior chest.[1] Because the lower trunk of the brachial plexus is usually involved, the pain often radiates down to the ipsilateral arm along the ulnar nerve distribution. Shoulder pain is the most common initial symptom and may imitate frequent degenerative shoulder problems, such as osteoarthritis and bursitis.[1] This pain is often attributed to benign degenerative conditions, and as a result the correct diagnosis of Pancoast tumor is often delayed for some months, as reported in many series.[20,21] A typical presentation of a Pancoast tumor is Horner syndrome, which occurs in 14% to 83% of patients and consists of ipsilateral ptosis, meiosis, and anhidrosis, which are caused by destruction of the paravertebral sympathetic chain or the inferior stellate ganglion.[1,19,21,22] Irritation of the sympathetic chain before the development of Horner syndrome is thought to be responsible for ipsilateral flushing and hyperhidrosis of the face.[21] Involvement of the C8 and T1 nerve roots is responsible for weakness and atrophy of the hand, as well as pain and paresthesias along the distribution of the ulnar nerve at the medial aspect of the arm, forearm, and fourth and fifth digits.[1,19]

Advanced tumor growth through the intervertebral foramina into the spinal canal may lead to epidural spinal cord compression with subsequent paraplegia in up to 25% of patients.[1,23] Another early sign of Pancoast syndrome is involvement of the T2 nerve root and the intercostobrachial nerve, which results in pain, paresthesia, and decreased sensation in the axilla and the medial aspect of the upper arm.[24] Less common manifestations of Pancoast tumors may also involve the phrenic and recurrent laryngeal nerves,[23,25] as well as compression of structures such as the subclavian vessels or the superior vena cava (SVC syndrome), resulting in dyspnea, hoarseness, or vascular obstructive symptoms.[23] Pulmonary complaints, such as cough, hemoptysis, and dyspnea, which are common in later stages of the disease, are usually absent in the early stages because of the peripheral location of the tumor, with pain as the initial symptom.[9]

THERAPEUTIC MANAGEMENT
PATIENT SELECTION AND DECISION-MAKING

The management of Pancoast tumors has changed significantly over the past decades. Before the introduction of radiation treatment in 1954[26] and the first successful removal of a Pancoast tumor with postoperative adjuvant radiation,[27] this cancer was uniformly fatal.[9] Subsequently Shaw et al,[28] in 1961, published the first clinical series that used preoperative neoadjuvant radiation, demonstrating improved tumor resectability and long-term survival.[29,30] Neoadjuvant radiation and surgical resection then became the standard method for management of Pancoast tumors, with reported 5-year survival rates ranging from 27% to 46% for tumor stages up to IIB.[31,32] The following prognostic factors predicting a poor prognosis have been identified: direct extension of the tumor into the vertebral bodies, great vessels, brachial plexus, and neck base; involvement of mediastinal lymph nodes; and incomplete resection with positive margins.[20,33-38] Therefore the surgical treatment of locally advanced Pancoast tumors continues to be controversial, with many surgeons arguing that tumors with involvement of the trachea, esophagus, or great vessels cannot or should not be resected completely.[33]

However, the fact that survival is associated with a complete resection has triggered the search for new treatment modalities. With the introduction of modern spine reconstruction techniques, some recently published series have stressed the benefit of complete resection of locally advanced tumors with vertebral and subsequent spine reconstruction.* There are two major strategies in the treatment of tumors invading

---

*References 11, 12, 17, 31, 39-41.

the spine: (1) circumferential spinal cord decompression with subsequent spine reconstruction, and (2) radical en bloc resection of the tumor and subsequent spine reconstruction. Although the first strategy involves an intralesional resection and is thus palliative, the second strategy is intended to be curative. In particular, it is necessary to resect the tumor en bloc, without violating the tumor borders, particularly with the histologic proof of tumor-free margins.[31,41] In certain cases, where the tumor is in the epidural space, a true en bloc resection is impossible. In those cases, the resection is termed *en bloc with planned transgression* and may include the involved dura.[42,43]

In general, the following criteria are considered when deciding in favor of or against Pancoast tumor resection with spine involvement: (1) histologic diagnosis, (2) whether the tumor is attached to the vertebral column, as evidenced by radiographic findings, (3) the presence or absence of mediastinal nodal involvement, and (4) the presence or absence of distant metastasis.[41,44]

Usually patients with locally advanced NSCLC of the superior sulcus, without mediastinal lymph node involvement and without distant metastases, are considered appropriate candidates for surgical therapy.

If the decision to proceed with surgery is made, the appropriate approach must be selected. This selection is usually made on the basis of MRI and CT studies of the chest. MRI is important to reveal or rule out tumor growth through the neuroforamina into the spinal canal, with resulting spinal cord compression (Fig. 33-3). With MRI and CT scans, it should be possible to assign the tumor to one of three spine tumor types (see pp. 568-569) to make the appropriate decision concerning the need for vertebral body resection and, if this is necessary, how much of the vertebral body must be resected (partial versus complete vertebrectomy). Also, if spinal stabilization is necessary, which approach is most appropriate and should it be a staged surgical procedure?

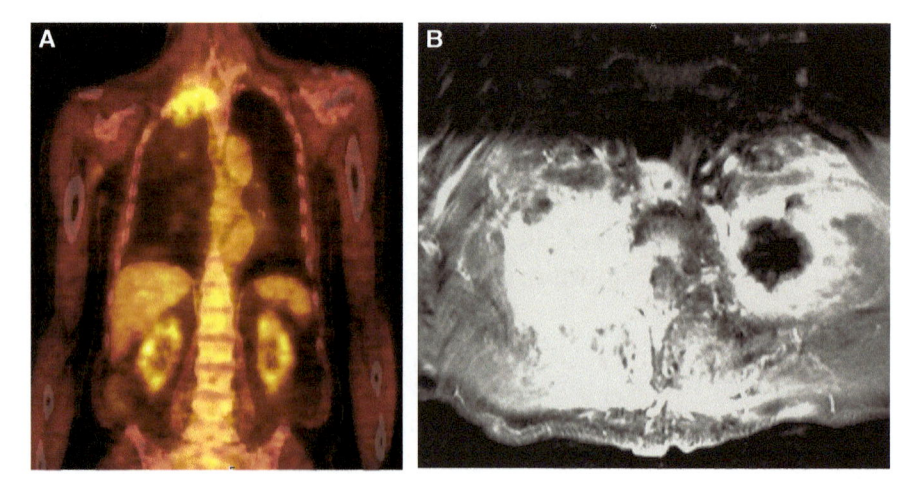

Fig. 33-3 Typical Pancoast tumor (type C) with spine involvement. **A,** PET scan and **B,** axial T1 MRI sequence with contrast enhancement showing a right-sided tumor with involvement of the lateral vertebral body.

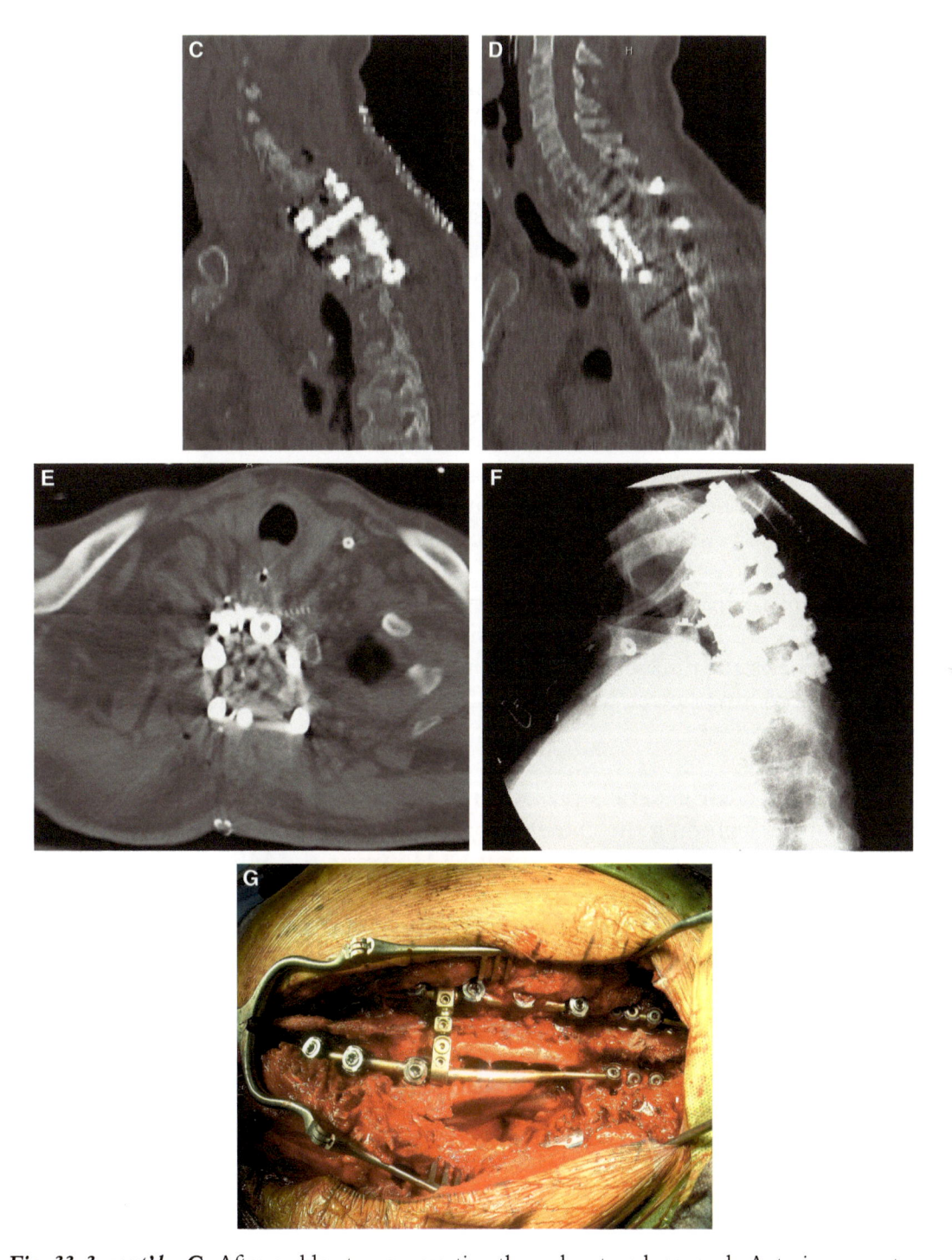

Fig. 33-3, cont'd **C,** After en bloc tumor resection through a staged approach. Anterior reconstruction with cage and vertebral body screws (sagittal CT reconstruction). **D,** A cross-link connector is placed to connect the anterior rod to the posterior instrumentation. **E** and **F,** Additional views of the construct. **G,** Intraoperative image after resection of a type C Pancoast tumor (anterior and posterior reconstruction).

PREOPERATIVE STAGING EVALUATION

The initial evaluation should include a thorough physical examination, including a detailed neurologic examination, CT scans of the chest with three-dimensional reconstructions, MRI of the thorax, including the brachial plexus and thoracic inlet, fusion positron emission tomographic (PET)/CT scans, MRI of the brain, pulmonary function tests, standard laboratory tests, and possibly a cardiac evaluation depending on risk factors. Use of standard CT scanning with intravenous contrast material to evaluate the mediastinum for lymph node metastases is limited by substantial false-positive and false-negative results, with pooled estimates of 51% sensitivity and 85% specificity. Newer generation fusion PET/CT scans have greatly improved the accuracy of staging the mediastinum, with 74% sensitivity and 85% specificity.[45] With equivocal lymph node enlargement (≥1.5 cm diameter nodes in short axis), whether the PET findings are positive or negative, surgeons generally recommend an invasive assessment of the mediastinum with sampling of lymph nodes before a curative surgical approach is attempted.[25,32] Current techniques for mediastinal lymph node sampling include endobronchial ultrasound-guided needle biopsy, transesophageal endoscopic ultrasound-guided needle biopsy, or the more invasive mediastinoscopy.[46-50] As the presence of distant metastases is also of paramount importance in the selection of patients with Pancoast tumors, a thorough search for distant metastatic spread should begin with an analysis of the patient's history, physical examination findings, and blood test results. The PET/CT scan plays a critical role in searching for common sites of extracranial metastatic disease. Because of the elevated incidence of brain metastasis in locally advanced lung cancer, MRI scans of the brain are recommended to complete the metastatic workup.

CT scans of the chest generally provide information concerning the extent of the Pancoast tumor, including the extent of parenchymal disease along with chest wall and mediastinal lymph node involvement.[1,51] However, the MRI scans are superior to CT scans in terms of imaging tumor extension to the brachial plexus, subclavian vessels, vertebral bodies, and the spinal canal.[52-55] With the accuracy of CT and MRI scans, only rarely is venous or arterial angiography needed, in suspicious cases, to determine whether subclavian vessels are invaded by tumor. Because knowledge about any spinal canal involvement is crucial to planning surgery of locally invasive Pancoast tumors with apparent spine involvement, we recommend preoperative MRI of the thoracic inlet, brachial plexus, and cervical and upper thoracic spine, with three-plane reconstruction in all cases.

TUMOR DIAGNOSIS

Cytologic analysis of expectorated sputum generally yields a malignant diagnosis in 11% to 20% where the tumor is located centrally.[20,21,56,57] Fiberoptic bronchoscopy, with transbronchial biopsy and lavage with cytologic analysis, may increase the diagnostic accuracy to 30% or 40%, even in peripheral tumors.[20,56,58]

However, most Pancoast tumors are peripheral, and the most sensitive procedure for the diagnosis is a percutaneous transthoracic needle biopsy, usually performed with CT guidance through a posterior or, occasionally, a cervical approach.[57,59,60] Direct needle biopsy of the tumor yields a positive diagnosis in at least 95% of cases.[20,32,57,59] Very rarely is a more invasive option, such as thoracoscopy, needed to make a diagnosis.

PREOPERATIVE RADIATION THERAPY AND CHEMOTHERAPY

The potential benefits of preoperative radiation therapy, first promoted by Shaw et al,[28] include a decrease in the size of the tumor, with improved resectability and a reduction in the number of viable cells, which theoretically prevents dissemination of the tumor during surgery.[61] In addition, the pathologist may determine, by examining the specimen, whether the irradiation had a significant effect on the tumor, which frequently affects the overall prognosis. The disadvantages of radiation therapy include difficulty in determining "true" margins during surgery, because the tumor is frequently smaller, and postradiation scarring limits useful tactile surgical feedback. In addition, complications such as infection, cerebrospinal fluid leakage, pseudarthrosis, and hardware failure increase with preoperative irradiation. Other disadvantages of preoperative radiation therapy include symptomatic debilitation of patients before they undergo a major surgical procedure and potential wound-healing problems where the surgical incision (superior-posterior extent) is located in the radiation field. The recent addition of chemotherapy to preoperative radiation therapy is motivated by the rationale of improving resection rates and preventing or treating occult systemic disease.[38,61-65] This approach has proved beneficial as preoperative neoadjuvant therapy in the treatment of high-grade sarcomas, but the optimum neoadjuvant regimen for Pancoast tumors remains to be determined. The only major published, multiinstitutional phase II trial of combined preoperative induction chemotherapy and radiation therapy in Pancoast tumors (Intergroup Trial 0160) showed a 92% complete resection rate and a significantly improved survival rate compared with historical control trials of preoperative radiation therapy alone followed by surgery.[66] Other approaches recently reported include high-dose three-dimensional radiation therapy, with doses ranging from 50 to 70 Gy, that were integrated into trimodality therapy by Kwong et al.[63] These investigators recommended performing restaging mediastinoscopy after induction therapy with chemotherapy and radiation therapy and, if the nodes are positive, surgical options are reassessed in terms of palliation of local symptoms rather than curative surgery. Despite the widespread use of preoperative chemotherapy and radiation therapy for Pancoast tumors, there are no randomized trials supporting this treatment, and the paucity of cases with this presentation will likely limit completion of randomized studies. The role of stereotactic radiosurgery in Pancoast tumors has not yet been explored, but the difficulty in precise radiographic delineation of tumor margins and the proximity to major vascular and nerve structures will likely limit its usefulness in this setting. Despite the popularity of induction chemotherapy and radiation therapy, the usual recommended dose of induction radiation therapy is only

45 Gy, which is minimally cytotoxic for lung cancer. If there are positive margins at the subsequent surgical resection, then adding 20 Gy of postoperative radiation therapy, which is split-course radiation, will have little additional effect. An empiric approach now favored by a number of major cancer centers, including our own, is for induction doublet chemotherapy alone followed 3 to 5 weeks later by resection, and then full-dose postoperative radiation therapy (65 to 70 Gy), a dose that is much more cytotoxic and will likely cover any close or positive margins. With this approach, we and others have not found resectability to be impaired, and the patients are in much better shape coming to surgery after chemotherapy alone versus concurrent chemotherapy and radiation therapy. Although this approach has not yet been validated in clinical trials, we suspect that local recurrence rates will be lower than the reported 33% local recurrence rate for induction chemotherapy and radiation therapy.

ANESTHETIC CONSIDERATIONS

The preoperative anesthetic workup includes the following standard pulmonary function tests: forced vital capacity (FVC), maximum breathing capacity (MBC), and forced expiratory volume in 1 second (FEV_1). Patients with FVC and FEV_1 of less than 70% and MBC of less than 60% are at higher risk for postoperative pulmonary complications and may need extended postoperative respiratory therapy. When indicated by appropriate risk factors, a cardiac workup, including a cardiac stress test, is necessary. Nevertheless, in experienced centers that commonly treat Pancoast tumors surgically, these major surgical procedures proceed smoothly with low morbidity and mortality. Routine double-lumen endotracheal intubation for the thoracotomy is necessary to deflate the lung for adequate exposure. As with other thoracotomies, the following are recommended: peripheral venous access, urinary catheter, arterial line, and ECG. If a vertebral body resection is anticipated, neurophysiologic monitoring (motor evoked potentials and somatosensory evoked potentials) is highly recommended.

SURGICAL APPROACHES

Different surgical approaches have been described for invasive Pancoast tumors with spine involvement that require vertebral body resection.[11,12,67-70] Recent studies of surgical case series have shown that the use of extended operations to achieve complete resection of locally advanced Pancoast tumors that invade the subclavian vessels or spinal column is feasible.[11,12,17,41] The surgical goal is to resect the upper lobe with the involved ribs and transverse processes and all involved structures, such as the lower trunk of the brachial plexus (T1 nerve root), the stellate ganglion, and spinal elements, in an en bloc fashion to obtain negative margins.[41,70] These tumors are usually resected in two stages because instrumentation and spinal stabilization are required. In certain studies a single lateral approach was used for both resection and instrumentation placement, but it is technically demanding to perform dorsal spinal fixation and maintain proper alignment with the patient in a lateral position. In the event that instrumentation is not necessary (no vertebral body involvement—only chest wall involvement), single-stage surgery through a posterolateral thoracotomy (classic Shaw-Paulson approach[28]) typically suffices.[61,71] For greater exposure DeMeester et al[67] proposed an extended posterolateral approach to the paraspinal muscles, expanding the length of the thoracotomy to perform an oblique osteotomy through the transverse process up to the vertebral body, with ligature of the root outside the foramen. One alternative approach that is favored occasionally is the anterior transcervical approach popularized by Dartevelle et al.[72-74] This method allows better exposure of the extreme anterior apex of the lung and cervically based structures (brachial plexus and subclavian vessels). The incision parallels the lower sternocleidomastoid muscle and courses over the manubrium and then turns laterally below the involved clavicle. Grunenwald and Spaggiari[75] developed a transmanubrial technique that involves a manubrial L-shaped transection and first costal cartilage resection. Dartevelle,[76] Fadel et al,[77] and Grunenwald et al[70] developed techniques that combine a transcervical or transmanubrial and a posterior midline approach.[76,77]

Perhaps the most versatile and popular of the anterior approaches is the trapdoor approach described by Nazzaro et al,[78] in 1994. This is a combination of the anterolateral cervical approach, partial median sternotomy, and anterolateral thoracotomy, and it is the most suitable intervention for gaining access not only to the T1-4 vertebral bodies anteriorly but also to the entire ventral cervical column and the midthoracic and upper thoracic spine. The main indication is an anteriorly located tumor, resulting in spinal cord compression, or a tumor mass with kyphotic angulation and/or involvement of the esophagus or the subclavian artery (Fig. 33-4). Although the anterior weight-bearing spinal column can be effectively reconstructed with the use of polymethylmethacrylate, bone graft, or mesh after the removal of a vertebra, the placement of adequate anterior instrumentation is difficult to achieve. Although anterior cervical plate and screw constructs can be used for fixation of this region in the absence of severe kyphotic angulation, additional posterior instrumentation is usually recommended for patients who have significant spinal deformity or multilevel involvement.[79]

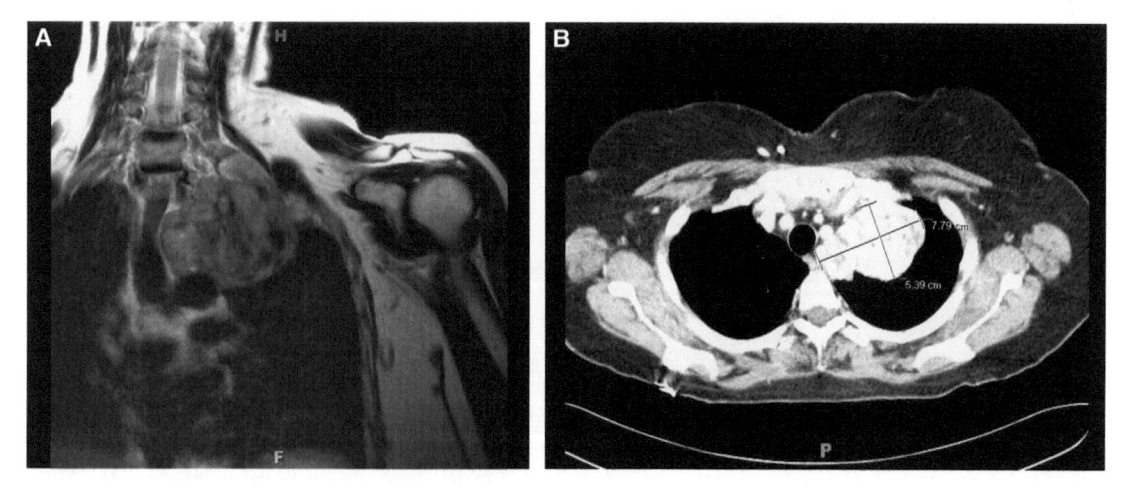

Fig. 33-4 Anteriorly located Pancoast tumor that is best accessed through a trapdoor type of approach. **A,** Coronal MRI and **B,** axial CT scan.

Whenever possible, a lobectomy is favored for the pulmonary resection (lower recurrence rates than with apical segmentectomy).[28,80] However, in these anterior apical approaches, an apical segmentectomy may be substituted, especially for small tumors, with an anticipated good outcome.[28,80] However, most described surgical methods involve at least two stages (type B and type C tumors). Typically spinal stabilization is performed through a posterior approach (first stage) followed by a posterolateral or trapdoor thoracotomy for definitive resection (second stage). Our group recently showed that a single-stage posterior approach is feasible in selected patients and can lead to a good outcome in patients with Pancoast tumors who require spinal stabilization and en bloc resection.[18] The merits of this single-stage posterior approach include a wide exposure that allows aggressive removal of tumor involving multiple columns of the spine. This approach offers one-stage definitive resection, spinal stabilization (anterior, posterior, or both), and simultaneous chest wall and lobectomy resection. This type of surgery is well tolerated when performed in experienced centers and eliminates the need for patients to undergo a two-stage operation.[18] The choice of approach depends on several factors, including the medical and neurologic status of the patient; the nature, location, and extent of the tumor; the need for spinal stabilization; and the experience of the surgeons and anesthesiologists. In general, three types of spine tumor involvement are identified. For selection of the appropriate approach, Pancoast tumors with spine involvement are classified according to the extent of vertebral involvement (see "Surgical Classification," pp. 568-569).

In type A tumors, only the chest wall, including the ribs and transverse processes, is involved, and there is no need for instrumentation. Therefore type A tumors can be approached and resected by a single-stage posterolateral thoracotomy (Fig. 33-5).

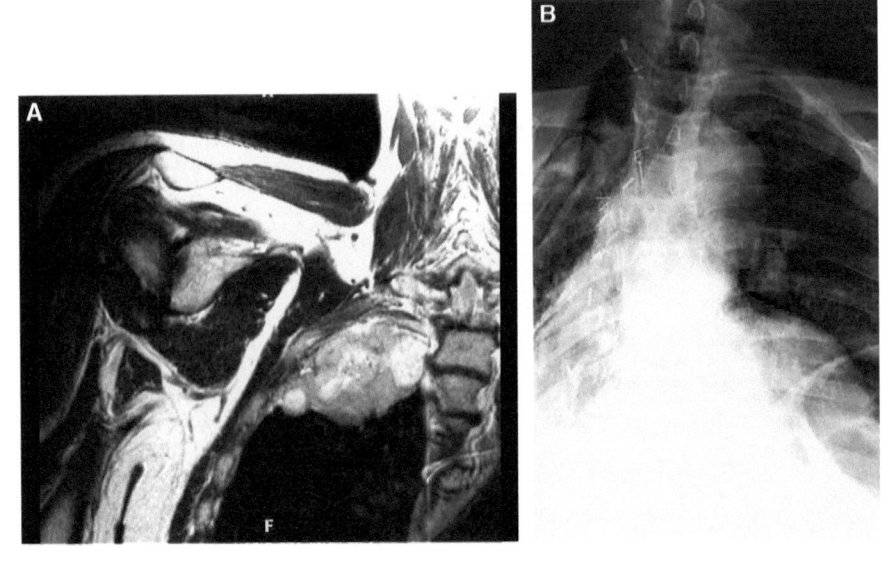

Fig. 33-5 **A,** Type A Pancoast tumor with chest wall but no vertebral body involvement. **B,** After en bloc resection without instrumentation, the patient developed a compensatory scoliotic deformity without kyphosis.

In type B tumors there is infiltration of part of the vertebral body, but it is confined to one side. In such cases all that is required is osteotomy through the medial wall of the involved pedicle obliquely, then incision through the vertebral body (partial vertebrectomy), combined with posterior instrumentation and fusion. It is not necessary to perform an anterior reconstruction because at least 50% of the vertebral body remains intact. This can be achieved by means of an initial posterior midline approach with posterior instrumentation followed later by a definitive resection in a second-stage posterolateral thoracotomy.

In type C the tumor crosses over the midline, involving more than 50% of the vertebral body, necessitating anterior reconstruction with a cage, allograft, or polymethylmethacrylate and additional posterior instrumentation in a second stage. In such cases bilateral nerve root clipping is carried out, and the osteotomy is performed from the opposite side (total vertebrectomy). This is also carried out as a two-stage surgical approach, with a posterolateral thoracotomy and a posterior midline approach. As mentioned previously, in selected cases it is possible to achieve an en bloc resection with circumferential stabilization in a single stage through a posterior midline approach.[18] An anterior trapdoor approach is employed when the tumor invades the subclavian artery, esophagus, sternum, and anterior mediastinum. This surgical technique provides excellent exposure in highly selected cases.

SURGICAL TECHNIQUES
RESECTION OF TYPE A TUMORS BY A SINGLE-STAGE POSTEROLATERAL THORACOTOMY

The patient is placed in a lateral decubitus position with the arm extended upward (see Fig. 33-5). A posterolateral thoracotomy is then performed, typically between the fourth and fifth ribs. A lobectomy is then performed to disconnect the tumor from the remaining lung. The hilar vessels are then ligated. At the hilar reflection, the bronchus to the upper lobe is stapled and divided. Frozen-section biopsy specimens of mediastinal nodes are obtained and analyzed. Provided that the nodes are negative, the initial thoracotomy incision is then curved cranially, parallel to the spine. The trapezius and rhomboid attachments to the spine are divided at the midline, and this allows the scapula to be elevated from the chest wall. The transverse processes are identified. The lateral aspect of the facet joints is identified. An osteotome is then used to cut the involved transverse processes in line with the lateral aspect of the facet joints above and below. The osteotome then enters the costovertebral articulation. With the use of a Cobb elevator, the proximal rib is disconnected from the spine. This places the exiting nerve root below under tension. The nerve root is identified just outside the foramen, double clipped, and cut. At the T1 level the nerve root courses upward and diagonally across the first rib, and it is possible, in rare cases, to preserve the T1 nerve while removing the proximal T1 rib. Subsequently, through the thoracotomy defect, the tumor attachment to the upper ribs is defined. Cuts are made 1 to 2 cm lateral and inferior to the tumor attachment to disconnect the chest wall involvement laterally and inferiorly. The first rib is then approached first superiorly. The middle scalene attachment to the rib is severed, and that allows identification of the C8 nerve root proximally and the subclavian artery and then the vein distally. The junction of the C8 and T1 nerve roots is identified. With the vessels and C8 nerve root in view, the first rib is cut laterally. At this point the entire tumor becomes mobile and is pushed inferiorly into the thoracotomy defect. Remaining pleural attachments and the stellate ganglion (if involved) are ligated at this stage. The tumor specimen is delivered en bloc and is marked for margins. Additional frozen-section biopsy specimens of soft tissue are obtained. Clips may be placed in the periphery of the resection to help with the planning of additional radiation. Chest tubes are placed. For resections below the third intercostal space, it is useful to close the defect with mesh to prevent future scapular entrapment. If there is concern about a leak of lymphatic fluid at the end of the case in the right pleural cavity, the thoracic duct is easily ligated at the level of the inferior pulmonary vein to prevent a later chylothorax, with no expected side effects from the ligation.

RESECTION OF TYPE B AND C TUMORS BY A POSTERIOR MIDLINE APPROACH AND SECOND-STAGE POSTEROLATERAL THORACOTOMY

For tumors that involve the vertebral column, a posterior midline approach can be used as a first stage followed by a second-stage posterolateral thoracotomy. During the first stage the dorsal spinal elements are exposed. The correct level is verified (typically the first identifiable transverse process is the one at T2). Instrumentation is then placed with the use of lateral mass screws in the low cervical spine and thoracic pedicle screws at the uninvolved side and approximately two levels below the lesion. The pedicles are smaller at T4 and T5 (4 to 5 mm) and largest at T1 and T2 (7.1 mm). Significant medial angulation is used at T1 and T2 (30 to 45 degrees). The in-out-in technique is typically employed for the pedicles caudal to T2, using a Lenke-type pedicle finder. A rod (preferably transitional) may be placed on the uninvolved side. A laminectomy and medial facetectomy (on the tumor side) are performed. The medial pedicle wall is identified, as well as the exiting nerve roots T1-T4. The nerves are then temporarily clipped using aneurysm clips and monitoring of motor evoked potentials (MEPs) and somatosensory evoked potentials (SSEPs) is performed. If there is no change, the nerves are double clipped and cut. The epidural veins are coagulated, and a small cutting burr is used to perform osteotomies medial to the pedicle (type B tumors). The osteotomies are then completed with the aid of an osteotome that is marked with regard to the anticipated depth of the vertebral body. A C7 pedicle screw can be placed on the tumor side after the laminectomy (average diameter 5.2 mm). The second rod is then secured, and the wound is closed. The second stage involves a posterolateral thoracotomy, as described previously, with the difference being no further osteotomies are performed at the transverse processes because they have already been performed medial to the pedicles. For type C tumors the staged approach is the same as that described for type B tumors, with the exception that a laminectomy (facetectomy) is also performed contralateral to the lesion, and both side nerve roots are sacrificed. The osteotomies are then performed medial to the contralateral pedicle. For type C tumors an anterior reconstruction using a mesh (or expandable) cage is recommended to achieve fusion, because these patients are typically long-term survivors or are even considered cured. In certain cases the entire surgery can be performed through a posterior approach alone, as previously described.[18] Other instrumentation options for the cervicothoracic junction include hooks, long 3.5 or long 4.5 mm rods, or end-to-end connectors (wedding band). No superiority of any one system over another has been established.[81]

INTRAOPERATIVE MONITORING
SPINAL CORD MONITORING

Although a radical resection is the ultimate goal for Pancoast tumors, vertebrectomy and reconstruction of the spine may cause neurologic deficits as a result of direct injury to the spinal cord, aggressive tumor resection with interruption and cutting of nerve roots, and a decrease in spinal cord perfusion pressure caused by a decrease in the mean arterial pressure or an increase in intradural pressure resulting from spinal cord edema, or by a combination of the two. Even if the aggressiveness of the tumor resection is related to patient survival, we believe it should not go beyond a point where it causes expected and severe neurologic damage that leaves the patient severely disabled and dramatically reduces the quality of the patient's remaining life. Therefore we believe that avoiding severe neurologic damage is of paramount importance. Intraoperative neurophysiologic monitoring helps to achieve this goal by revealing the integrity of the spinal cord physiology and alerting the surgeon to any deterioration before irreversible neural injury has occurred. SSEP monitoring assesses the sensory pathways through the posterior column, whereas MEPs assess the descending motor pathways, especially in cases where the spinal cord is compromised by a pathologic process.[82-86] Electrophysiologic monitoring has become a commonly used procedure in intramedullary and spine tumor surgery.[83,84,87-89] Motor and sensory pathways can be affected independently both preoperatively and postoperatively. Therefore MEPs can be present when SSEPs are absent and vice versa.[84,90] Several studies have shown that postoperative motor deficits can occur even in the case of stable SSEPs.[90-92] Because there is no correlation between SSEPs and postoperative motor function, it is necessary to monitor both MEPs and SSEPs.[84,93] SSEPs are influenced by several factors, such as stability and depth of aesthesia, temperature, and blood flow autoregulation of the spinal cord. Thus it is imperative to keep the mean arterial pressure between 60 and 70 mm Hg, the temperature within normal range, the end-tidal CO_2 and fluid volumes at normal levels and the hemoglobin above 7 g/dl.[94-97] For spinal cord monitoring, SSEPs usually are recorded after tibial and median nerve stimulation. Recordings of SSEPs can be affected in their latencies and/or their amplitudes. A decrease of 50% or more and/or a 10% or 2 msec increase in latency are indicators of spinal cord damage, given that the aforementioned factors are within normal limits.[92] These changes correlate with a new postoperative sensory pathway–related deficit if they persist and do not reverse after intraoperative corrective measures.[98]

MEPs can be recorded in peripheral nerves (compound nerve action potential), in muscles (compound muscle action potential), and from the epidural or subdural space of the spinal cord after transcranial electrical or magnetic stimulation of the motor cortex. Epidural spinal cord stimulation can also be performed at the level above the affected one.[82,87] Many inhalational anesthetics substantially affect cortical function and suppress both SSEPs and MEPs,[99,100] whereas transcranial magnetic MEPs seem to be more susceptible to anesthesia-induced artifacts than transcranial electrical MEPs.[101] A complete motor blockade with muscle relaxants will inhibit a muscle response and the recording of both cranial and spinal cord induced MEPs. Therefore it is necessary to control the use of muscle relaxants.[102,103] A permanent decrease in the MEP amplitude of more than 50% or an increase in the response threshold of 100 volts indicates spinal cord damage and correlates well with neurologic outcome.

SPINAL NERVE ROOT MONITORING

Pancoast tumors with nerve root or plexus involvement are obvious. Because it is sometimes unavoidable to resect nerve roots to achieve a radical tumor resection, some spine surgeons argue that spinal nerve root monitoring is needless. Injury of spinal nerve roots can damage neural tissue in the following two ways: (1) direct lesion of motor or sensory fibers within the nerve root and (2) damage or occlusion of the medullary branches of the spinal segmental arteries. Sensory and motor spinal nerve root fibers can be monitored with the use of upper or lower limb or dermatomal SSEPs and the use of continuous electromyographic (EMG) recording.[104-106] The vascular situation can be checked by temporary clipping of the spinal nerve root and careful monitoring of SSEPs and MEPs for approximately 5 minutes. If no changes in SSEPs or MEPs are seen, then in our experience the nerve root can be cut without further sequelae for the spinal cord.[84]

At our institutions neurophysiologic monitoring is performed routinely in spine surgery; however, whether neurophysiologic monitoring is a standard procedure that should be performed in every complex spine procedure remains controversial, especially in spine tumor surgery. Among published series on the surgical treatment of locally advanced Pancoast tumors, the routine use of neurophysiologic monitoring was mentioned in only one.[18]

POSTOPERATIVE MANAGEMENT

Postoperatively patients are transferred to the intensive care unit and remain there for at least 1 day. A regular deep venous thrombosis (DVT) prophylaxis with low molecular heparin and graduated compression stockings or intermittent pneumatic compression is begun postoperatively. For postoperative pain management usually intravenous narcotics (hydromorphone) via a patient-controlled anesthesia (PCA) pump, plus an intravenous nonsteroidal antiinflammatory drug (ketorolac) and intravenous acetaminophen are used for the first few days and then switched to a parenteral or oral schedule. After thoracotomy, the chest drains stay in place until there is no leak and the drainage is minimal. Before chest drains are removed, some surgeons recommend clamping them for 24 hours. Extension and ventilation of the lungs is monitored by regular chest radiography. CT of the chest is necessary only if there are problems and/or complications. Arterial blood gases and constant pulse oximetry should be monitored during the patient's stay in the intensive care unit. Urinary and central venous catheters should remain in place until the patient is mobile and can be transferred to the regular ward. After thoracotomy, a chest physiotherapy and incentive spirometry are ineffective and are not used. Frequent ambulation, vigorous coughing/deep breathing, and inhaled bronchodilators along with good pain control are the most effective means to maintain good pulmonary toilet. After posterior midline approaches, the wound drain is removed after 24 hours. Patient mobilization is begun on postoperative day 1. We do not use braces or orthoses on a regular basis; however, they are recommended by some surgeons.[41] Regular postoperative follow-up is necessary and should include MRI and CT scans/radiographs for early detection of tumor recurrence and complications.

COMPLICATIONS

Pancoast tumor surgery has expected side effects related to the need for an en bloc resection and the frequent sacrifice of the T1 nerve root and stellate ganglion. Although T1 is not the dominant root innervating the intrinsic muscles of the hand (C8), its sacrifice leads to hand weakness. However, patients typically can continue to use their hands for daily activities but not for heavy labor. Horner syndrome presents mainly as an aesthetic-related issue rather than a functional issue. Some atrophy of the muscles, along with prominence of the posterior hardware, can also be expected. Ipsilateral shoulder misuse because of pain issues can occur, and early physical therapy is instrumental in the patient's recovery. Pulmonary complications (pneumothorax, atelectasis, chylothorax, and pneumonia) can arise and should be treated with aggressive pulmonary toilet and appropriate interventions. Patients with type A tumors who undergo chest wall resection only, over time, develop a compensatory scoliosis that is typically nondisabling (see Fig. 33-5, *B*). As with any surgery, appropriate planning will prevent most complications. Preoperatively it is imperative to assess the number of vertebrae involved, the extent of osteotomies, and the relationship of the tumor to the subclavian vessels (Fig. 33-6, *A* and *B*). Furthermore, the extent and type of

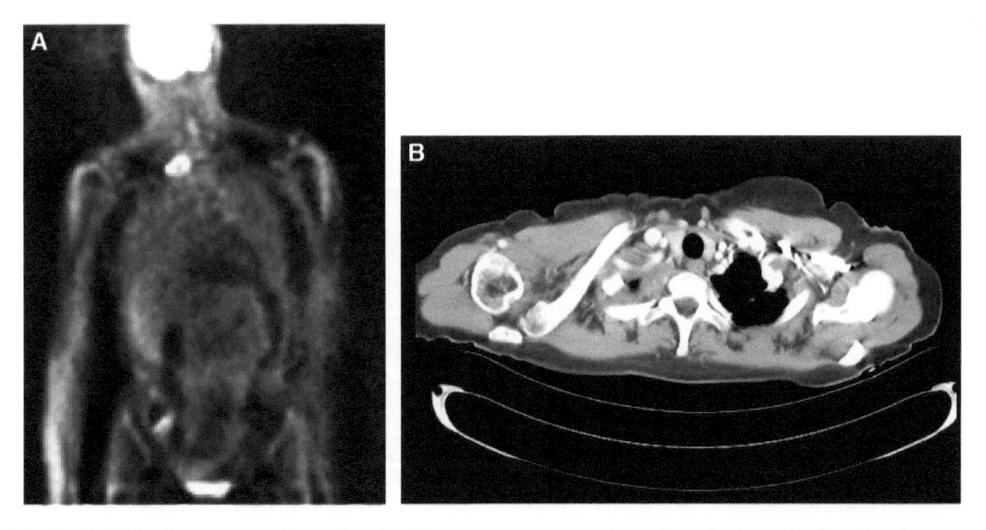

Fig. 33-6 Subclavian artery thrombosis after surgery necessitated replacing the involved segment of the artery with a Gore-Tex vascular graft (W.L. Gore, Newark, DE). **A,** Coronal preoperative MRI and **B,** axial CT scan of the thorax showing that the tumor is in close relationship to the subclavian artery.

Continued

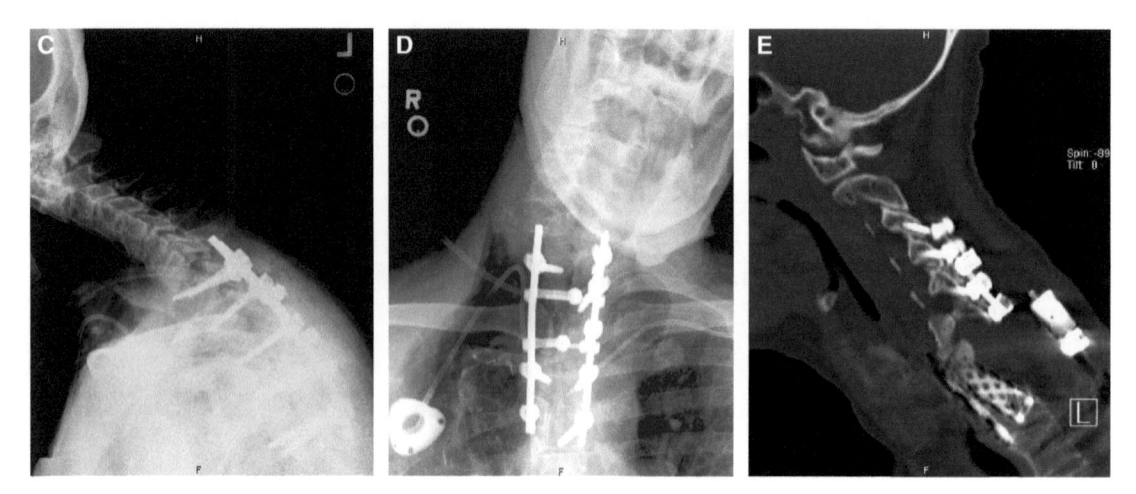

Fig. 33-6, cont'd **C** and **D,** Junctional kyphosis at the cervicothoracic junction after resection of a Pancoast tumor requiring further revision and extension of the instrumentation to the cervical spine. **E,** Rod breakage at the rod transition 1 year after surgery, the result of pseudarthrosis.

instrumentation must be determined. Hardware failure can occur including the following: junctional kyphosis/scoliosis, rod breakage (typically at transition points), and pulling out of screws or hooks. Late failures are usually the result of pseudarthrosis and require revision of the fusion.

Complications included three junctional revisions (Fig. 33-6, *C* and *D*) and one subclavian artery thrombosis. All complications occurred in the instrumentation group. A similar group of 30 patients also underwent palliative surgery for cervicothoracic tumors. In this group 90% of patients underwent instrumentation, and there were four hardware-related complications, including two instances of rod breakage (Fig. 33-6, *E*), one case of junctional kyphosis, and one misplaced screw.

Among reported series on surgical treatment of locally advanced Pancoast tumors, mortality rates ranged from 0% to 5% and complication rates ranged from 28% to 52%. The most frequent complications in these series were the result of pulmonary issues, such as prolonged intubation for respiratory failure, pneumonia, and atelectasis.

The most frequent instrumentation-related complications included hardware failure in combination with or without tumor progression.[11,12,17,39,44] Other complications that should be mentioned in the patient consent form are DVT, pulmonary embolism, excessive blood loss, wound dehiscence/infection (especially in combination with postoperative radiation), injury of nerve roots, spinal cord, and dura with neurologic deficits, and cerebrospinal fluid (CSF) leakage. If there is a CSF leak within the thoracic cavity, treatment may be difficult because of negative intrathoracic pressure. In our experience this problem usually requires a surgical repair with a multilayered patch or even a vascularized graft.

SURGICAL RESULTS

In our series of 30 patients with Pancoast tumors, an en bloc resection was performed in 25 of them. Several surgical series on locally advanced Pancoast tumors could prove that an en bloc resection with tumor-free margins results in prolonged survival and an increased median time to recurrence. The rates of complete tumor resections ranged from 56% to 79% versus 21% to 44% for incomplete resections.[11,12,17,39,70] Some investigators found a significant difference in median survival times between complete and incomplete resection groups.[39] Two-year survival rates ranged from 47% to 54%, and 5-year survival rates from 14% to 27%.[11,17,70] Recurrence rates were reported to range from 41% to 59%.[11,17]

CONCLUSION

En bloc resection with tumor-free margins improves survival in patients with locally advanced Pancoast tumors with vertebral involvement. However, surgical resection of these tumors, which involve the cervicothoracic junction, is technically demanding and is associated with considerable morbidity. In addition, it is essential that these types of operations be performed by a multidisciplinary team and be reserved for carefully selected patients.

BAILOUT TECHNIQUES

- If the temporary clipping of the spinal nerve root shows a significant change (decrease of amplitude, increase in latency) of MEPs or SSEPs, a decision has to be made between permanent neurologic deficits, with possible reduction of quality of life and the limitation of aggressiveness of tumor resection with possible shorter survival time.
- If significant changes of MEPs or SSEPs occur suddenly that cannot be attributed to a surgical step, technical problems should be ruled out first. Mean arterial pressure should be maintained above 80 mm Hg in these cases.
- Treating unstable conditions at the cervicothoracic junction is challenging because of the sharp transition between the flexible lordotic cervical spine and the more rigid kyphotic thoracic spine. Therefore the construct needs to be long and stable enough to accommodate the flexibility changes at this site.
- Instead of lateral mass screws above C6, pedicle screws can be used if cervical pedicles are large enough. In this case preoperative CT angiography and intraoperative navigation is recommended.

References (With Key References in Boldface)

1. Arcasoy SM, Jett JR. Superior pulmonary sulcus tumors and Pancoast's syndrome. N Engl J Med 7:1370-1376, 1997.
2. Pancoast HK. Importance of careful roentgen-ray investigations of apical chest tumors. JAMA 83:1407-1411, 1924.
3. Pancoast HK. Superior pulmonary sulcus tumor: tumor characterized by pain, Horner's syndrome, destruction of bone and atrophy of hand muscles. JAMA 99:1391-1396, 1932.
4. Davis GA, Knight S. Pancoast tumor resection with preservation of brachial plexus and hand function. Neurosurg Focus 22:E15, 2007.
5. Pitz CC, de la Riviere AB, van Swieten HA, et al. Surgical treatment of Pancoast tumours. Eur J Cardiothorac Surg 26:202-208, 2004.
6. Tobías JW. Sindrome ápico-costo-vertebral doloroso por tumor apexiano: su valor diagnóstico en el cáncer primitivo pulmonar. Rev Med Latino Am 17:1522-1556, 1932.
7. Hare ES. Tumor involving certain nerves. Lond Med Gaz 1:16-18, 1838.
8. Arcasoy SM, Bajwa MK, Jett JR. Non-Hodgkin's lymphoma presenting as Pancoast's syndrome. Respir Med 91:571-573, 1997.
9. Attar S, Krasna MJ, Sonett JR, et al. Superior sulcus (Pancoast) tumor: experience with 105 patients. Ann Thorac Surg 66:193-198, 1998.
10. Komagata M, Nishiyama M, Imakiire A, et al. Total spondylectomy for en bloc resection of lung cancer invading the chest wall and thoracic spine. Case report. J Neurosurg 100:353-357, 2004.
11. Gandhi S, Walsh GL, Komaki R, et al. A multidisciplinary surgical approach to superior sulcus tumors with vertebral invasion. Ann Thorac Surg 68:1778-1784, 1999.
12. York JE, Walsh GL, Lang FF, et al. Combined chest wall resection with vertebrectomy and spinal reconstruction for the treatment of Pancoast tumors. J Neurosurg 91:74-80, 1999.
13. Ferlay J, Autier P, Boniol M, et al. Estimates of the cancer incidence and mortality in Europe in 2006. Ann Oncol 18:581-592, 2007.
14. Weir HK, Thun MJ, Hankey BF, et al. Annual report to the nation on the status of cancer, 1975-2000, featuring the uses of surveillance data for cancer prevention and control. J Natl Cancer Inst 95:1276-1299, 2003.
15. Jemal A, Thun MJ, Ries LA, et al. Annual report to the nation on the status of cancer, 1975-2005, featuring trends in lung cancer, tobacco use, and tobacco control. J Natl Cancer Inst 100:1672-1694, 2008.
16. Detterbeck FC, Boffa DJ, Tanoue LT. The new lung cancer staging system. Chest 136:260-271, 2009.
17. Bolton WD, Rice DC, Goodyear A, et al. Superior sulcus tumors with vertebral body involvement: a multimodality approach. J Thorac Cardiovasc Surg 137:1379-1387, 2009.
18. Jain S, Sommers E, Setzer M, et al. Posterior midline approach for single-stage en bloc resection and circumferential spinal stabilization for locally advanced Pancoast tumors. Technical note. J Neurosurg Spine 9:71-82, 2008.
19. Komaki R, Roh J, Cox JD, et al. Superior sulcus tumors: results of irradiation of 36 patients. Cancer 48:1563-1568, 1981.
20. Anderson TM, Moy PM, Holmes EC. Factors affecting survival in superior sulcus tumors. J Clin Oncol 4:1598-1603, 1986.
21. Hepper NG, Herskovic T, Witten DM, et al. Thoracic inlet tumors. Ann Intern Med 64:979-989, 1966.
22. Sundaresan N, Hilaris BS, Martini N. The combined neurosurgical-thoracic management of superior sulcus tumors. J Clin Oncol 5:1739-1745, 1987.
23. Attar S, Miller JE, Satterfield J, et al. Pancoast's tumor: irradiation or surgery? Ann Thorac Surg 28:578-586, 1979.
24. Marangoni C, Lacerenza M, Formaglio F, et al. Sensory disorder of the chest as presenting symptom of lung cancer. J Neurol Neurosurg Psychiatry 56:1033-1034, 1993.

25. Stanford W, Barnes RP, Tucker AR. Influence of staging in superior sulcus (Pancoast) tumors of the lung. Ann Thorac Surg 29:406-409, 1980.
26. Haas LL, Harvey RA, Langer SS. Radiation management of otherwise hopeless thoracic neoplasms. JAMA 154:323-326, 1954.
27. Chardack WM, MacCallum JD. Pancoast syndrome due to bronchiogenic carcinoma: successful surgical removal and postoperative irradiation; a case report. J Thorac Surg 25:402-412, 1953.
28. Shaw RR, Paulson DL, Kee JL. Treatment of superior sulcus tumor by irradiation followed by resection. Ann Surg 154:29-40, 1961.
29. Ginsberg RJ, Martini N, Zaman M, et al. Influence of surgical resection and brachytherapy in the management of superior sulcus tumor. Ann Thorac Surg 57:1440-1445, 1994.
30. Hilaris BS, Martini N, Wong GY, et al. Treatment of superior sulcus tumor (Pancoast tumor). Surg Clin North Am 67:965-977, 1987.
31. Rusch VW, Parekh KR, Leon L, et al. Factors determining outcome after surgical resection of T3 and T4 lung cancers of the superior sulcus. J Thorac Cardiovasc Surg 119:1147-1153, 2000.
32. Wright CD, Moncure AC, Shepard JA, et al. Superior sulcus lung tumors. Results of combined treatment (irradiation and radical resection). J Thorac Cardiovasc Surg 94:69-74, 1987.
33. Muscolino G, Valente M, Andreani S. Pancoast tumours: clinical assessment and long-term results of combined radiosurgical treatment. Thorax 52:284-286, 1997.
34. Okubo K, Wada H, Fukuse T, et al. Treatment of Pancoast tumors. Combined irradiation and radical resection. Thorac Cardiovasc Surg 43:284-286, 1995.
35. Pisters KM, Ginsberg RJ, Giroux DJ, et al. Induction chemotherapy before surgery for early-stage lung cancer: a novel approach. Bimodality Lung Oncology Team. J Thorac Cardiovasc Surg 119:429-439, 2000.
36. Rosell R, Gomez-Codina J, Camps C, et al. A randomized trial comparing preoperative chemotherapy plus surgery with surgery alone in patients with non-small-cell lung cancer. N Engl J Med 330:153-158, 1994.
37. Roth JA, Fossella F, Komaki R, et al. A randomized trial comparing perioperative chemotherapy and surgery with surgery alone in resectable stage IIIA non-small-cell lung cancer. J Natl Cancer Inst 86:673-680, 1994.
38. Rusch VW, Albain KS, Crowley JJ, et al. Neoadjuvant therapy: a novel and effective treatment for stage IIIb non-small cell lung cancer. Southwest Oncology Group. Ann Thorac Surg 58:290-294, 1994.
39. Bilsky MH, Vitaz TW, Boland PJ, et al. Surgical treatment of superior sulcus tumors with spinal and brachial plexus involvement. J Neurosurg 97:301-309, 2002.
40. Kent MS, Bilsky MH, Rusch VW. Resection of superior sulcus tumors (posterior approach). Thorac Surg Clin 14:217-228, 2004.
41. **Mazel C, Grunenwald D, Laudrin P, et al. Radical excision in the management of thoracic and cervicothoracic tumors involving the spine: results in a series of 36 cases. Spine (Phila Pa 1976) 28:782-792, 2003.**
42. Boriani S, Bandiera S, Donthineni R, et al. Morbidity of en bloc resections in the spine. Eur Spine J 19:231-241, 2010.
43. Li H, Gasbarrini A, Cappuccio M, et al. Outcome of excisional surgeries for the patients with spinal metastases. Eur Spine J 18:1423-1430, 2009.
44. **Mazel C, Balabaud L, Bennis S, et al. Cervical and thoracic spine tumor management: surgical indications, techniques, and outcomes. Orthop Clin North Am 40:75-vii, 2009.**
45. Silvestri GA, Gould MK, Margolis ML, et al. Noninvasive staging of non-small cell lung cancer: ACCP evidenced-based clinical practice guidelines, 2nd ed. Chest 132:178S-201S, 2007.
46. Eckardt J, Petersen HO, Hakami-Kermani A, et al. Endobronchial ultrasound-guided transbronchial needle aspiration of undiagnosed intrathoracic lesions. Interact Cardiovasc Thorac Surg 9:232-235, 2009.
47. Ernst A, Eberhardt R, Krasnik M, et al. Efficacy of endobronchial ultrasound-guided transbronchial needle aspiration of hilar lymph nodes for diagnosing and staging cancer. J Thorac Oncol 4:947-950, 2009.

48. Rintoul RC, Tournoy KG, El DH, et al. EBUS-TBNA for the clarification of PET positive intrathoracic lymph nodes—an international multi-centre experience. J Thorac Oncol 4:44-48, 2009.
49. Tournoy KG, De RF, Vanwalleghem LR, et al. Endoscopic ultrasound reduces surgical mediastinal staging in lung cancer: a randomized trial. Am J Respir Crit Care Med 177:531-535, 2008.
50. Tournoy KG, Rintoul RC, van Meerbeeck JP, et al. EBUS-TBNA for the diagnosis of central parenchymal lung lesions not visible at routine bronchoscopy. Lung Cancer 63:45-49, 2009.
51. Webb WR, Jeffrey RB, Godwin JD. Thoracic computed tomography in superior sulcus tumors. J Comput Assist Tomogr 5:361-365, 1981.
52. Gefter WB. Magnetic resonance imaging in the evaluation of lung cancer. Semin Roentgenol 25:73-84, 1990.
53. Takasugi JE, Rapoport S, Shaw C. Superior sulcus tumors: the role of imaging. J Thorac Imaging 4:41-48, 1989.
54. Webb WR, Gatsonis C, Zerhouni EA, et al. CT and MR imaging in staging non-small cell bronchogenic carcinoma: report of the Radiologic Diagnostic Oncology Group. Radiology 178:705-713, 1991.
55. Webb WR, Sostman HD. MR imaging of thoracic disease: clinical uses. Radiology 182:621-630, 1992.
56. Maxfield RA, Aranda CP. The role of fiberoptic bronchoscopy and transbronchial biopsy in the diagnosis of Pancoast's tumor. N Y State J Med 87:326-329, 1987.
57. Walls WJ, Thornbury JR, Naylor B. Pulmonary needle aspiration biopsy in the diagnosis of Pancoast tumors. Radiology 111:99-102, 1974.
58. Miller JI, Mansour KA, Hatcher CR Jr. Carcinoma of the superior pulmonary sulcus. Ann Thorac Surg 28:44-47, 1979.
59. Paulson DL, Weed TE, Rian RL. Cervical approach for percutaneous needle biopsy of Pancoast tumors. Ann Thorac Surg 39:586-587, 1985.
60. Yang PC, Lee LN, Luh KT, et al. Ultrasonography of Pancoast tumor. Chest 94:124-128, 1988.
61. Paulson DL, Shaw RR, Kee JL, et al. Combined preoperative irradiation and resection for bronchogenic carcinoma. J Thorac Cardiovasc Surg 44:281-294, 1962.
62. Barnes JB, Johnson SB, Dahiya RS, et al. Concomitant weekly cisplatin and thoracic radiotherapy for Pancoast tumors of the lung: pilot experience of the San Antonio Cancer Institute. Am J Clin Oncol 25:90-92, 2002.
63. Kwong KF, Edelman MJ, Suntharalingam M, et al. High-dose radiotherapy in trimodality treatment of Pancoast tumors results in high pathologic complete response rates and excellent long-term survival. J Thorac Cardiovasc Surg 129:1250-1257, 2005.
64. Martinez-Monge R, Herreros J, Aristu JJ, et al. Combined treatment in superior sulcus tumors. Am J Clin Oncol 17:317-322, 1994.
65. Wright CD, Menard MT, Wain JC, et al. Induction chemoradiation compared with induction radiation for lung cancer involving the superior sulcus. Ann Thorac Surg 73:1541-1544, 2002.
66. Rusch VW, Giroux DJ, Kraut MJ, et al. Induction chemoradiation and surgical resection for non-small cell lung carcinomas of the superior sulcus: initial results of Southwest Oncology Group Trial 9416 (Intergroup Trial 0160). J Thorac Cardiovasc Surg 121:472-483, 2001.
67. DeMeester TR, Albertucci M, Dawson PJ, et al. Management of tumor adherent to the vertebral column. J Thorac Cardiovasc Surg 97:373-378, 1989.
68. **Grunenwald D, Mazel C, Baldeyrou P, et al. En bloc resection of lung cancer invading the spine. Ann Thorac Surg 61:1878-1879, 1996.**
69. **Grunenwald D, Mazel C, Girard P, et al. Total vertebrectomy for en bloc resection of lung cancer invading the spine. Ann Thorac Surg 61:723-725, 1996.**
70. **Grunenwald DH, Mazel C, Girard P, et al. Radical en bloc resection for lung cancer invading the spine. J Thorac Cardiovasc Surg 123:271-279, 2002.**
71. Shaw RR. New approaches to treatment of bronchogenic carcinoma. Med Bull (Ann Arbor) 27:231-238, 1961.
72. Dartevelle P, Levasseur P, Rojas-Miranda A, et al. [Combined cervical and thoracic approach to the removal of tumours responsible for the Pancoast and Tobias syndrome (author's translation)] Nouv Presse Med 10:1051-1054, 1981.

73. Dartevelle P, Levasseur P, Rojas-Miranda A, et al. [Value of the combined cervical and thoracic approach in the surgery of Pancoast and Tobias's syndrome of tumoral origin] Chirurgie 109:399-403, 1983.
74. Dartevelle PG, Chapelier AR, Macchiarini P, et al. Anterior transcervical-thoracic approach for radical resection of lung tumors invading the thoracic inlet. J Thorac Cardiovasc Surg 105:1025-1034, 1993.
75. Grunenwald D, Spaggiari L. Transmanubrial osteomuscular sparing approach for apical chest tumors. Ann Thorac Surg 63:563-566, 1997.
76. Dartevelle PG. Herbert Sloan Lecture. Extended operations for the treatment of lung cancer. Ann Thorac Surg 63:12-19, 1997.
77. Fadel E, Missenard G, Chapelier A, et al. En bloc resection of non-small cell lung cancer invading the thoracic inlet and intervertebral foramina. J Thorac Cardiovasc Surg 123:676-685, 2002.
78. Nazzaro JM, Arbit E, Burt M. "Trap door" exposure of the cervicothoracic junction. Technical note. J Neurosurg 80:338-341, 1994.
79. Gokaslan ZL, Walsh GL. "Trap door" exposure of the cervicothoracic junction. In Rengachary SS, ed. Neurosurgical Operative Color Atlas, vol VIII. Lebanon, NH: AANS Publications, 1999, pp 253-260.
80. Jones DR, Detterbeck FC. Pancoast tumors of the lung. Curr Opin Pulm Med 4:191-197, 1998.
81. Eleraky MA, Setzer M, Baaj AA, et al. Biomechanical comparison of posterior cervicothoracic instrumentation techniques after one level laminectomy and facetectomy. J Neurosurg Spine 13:622-629, 2010.
82. Deletis V. Intraoperative monitoring of the functional integrity of the motor pathways. Adv Neurol 63:201-214, 1993.
83. Deutsch H, Arginteanu M, Manhart K, et al. Somatosensory evoked potential monitoring in anterior thoracic vertebrectomy. J Neurosurg 92:155-161, 2000.
84. Eleraky MA, Setzer M, Papanastassiou ID, et al. Role of motor-evoked potential monitoring in conjunction with temporary clipping of spinal nerve roots in posterior thoracic spine tumor surgery. Spine J 10:396-403, 2010.
85. Ibanez V, Fischer G, Mauguiere F. Dorsal horn and dorsal column dysfunction in intramedullary cervical cord tumours. A somatosensory evoked potential study. Brain 115(Pt 4):1209-1234, 1992.
86. Koyanagi I, Iwasaki Y, Isu T, et al. Spinal cord evoked potential monitoring after spinal cord stimulation during surgery of spinal cord tumors. Neurosurgery 33:451-459, 1993.
87. Kothbauer K, Deletis V, Epstein FJ. Intraoperative spinal cord monitoring for intramedullary surgery: an essential adjunct. Pediatr Neurosurg 26:247-254, 1997.
88. Lang EW, Chesnut RM, Beutler AS, et al. The utility of motor-evoked potential monitoring during intramedullary surgery. Anesth Analg 83:1337-1341, 1996.
89. Morota N, Deletis V, Constantini S, et al. The role of motor evoked potentials during surgery for intramedullary spinal cord tumors. Neurosurgery 41:1327-1336, 1997.
90. Lesser RP, Raudzens P, Luders H, et al. Postoperative neurological deficits may occur despite unchanged intraoperative somatosensory evoked potentials. Ann Neurol 19:22-25, 1986.
91. Ginsburg HH, Shetter AG, Raudzens PA. Postoperative paraplegia with preserved intraoperative somatosensory evoked potentials. Case report. J Neurosurg 63:296-300, 1985.
92. Nuwer MR, Dawson EG, Carlson LG, et al. Somatosensory evoked potential spinal cord monitoring reduces neurologic deficits after scoliosis surgery: results of a large multicenter survey. Electroencephalogr Clin Neurophysiol 96:6-11, 1995.
93. Kelleher MO, Tan G, Sarjeant R, et al. Predictive value of intraoperative neurophysiological monitoring during cervical spine surgery: a prospective analysis of 1055 consecutive patients. J Neurosurg Spine 8:215-221, 2008.
94. Markand ON, Warren C, Mallik GS, et al. Effects of hypothermia on short latency somatosensory evoked potentials in humans. Electroencephalogr Clin Neurophysiol 77:416-424, 1990.
95. Markand ON, Warren C, Mallik GS, et al. Temperature-dependent hysteresis in somatosensory and auditory evoked potentials. Electroencephalogr Clin Neurophysiol 77:425-435, 1990.
96. Noonan KJ, Walker T, Feinberg JR, et al. Factors related to false- versus true-positive neuromonitoring changes in adolescent idiopathic scoliosis surgery. Spine (Phila Pa 1976) 27:825-830, 2002.

97. Owen JH. The application of intraoperative monitoring during surgery for spinal deformity. Spine (Phila Pa 1976) 24:2649-2662, 1999.
98. Stevens WR, Glazer PA, Kelley SD, et al. Ophthalmic complications after spinal surgery. Spine (Phila Pa 1976) 22:1319-1324, 1997.
99. Sloan TB. Evoked potential monitoring. Int Anesthesiol Clin 34:109-136, 1996.
100. Sloan TB, Koht A. Depression of cortical somatosensory evoked potentials by nitrous oxide. Br J Anaesth 57:849-852, 1985.
101. Sloan TB. Anesthetic effects on electrophysiologic recordings. J Clin Neurophysiol 15:217-226, 1998.
102. Jellinek D, Jewkes D, Symon L. Noninvasive intraoperative monitoring of motor evoked potentials under propofol anesthesia: effects of spinal surgery on the amplitude and latency of motor evoked potentials. Neurosurgery 29:551-557, 1991.
103. Lang EW, Beutler AS, Chesnut RM, et al. Myogenic motor-evoked potential monitoring using partial neuromuscular blockade in surgery of the spine. Spine (Phila Pa 1976) 21:1676-1686, 1996.
104. Hormes JT, Chappuis JL. Monitoring of lumbosacral nerve roots during spinal instrumentation. Spine (Phila Pa 1976) 18:2059-2062, 1993.
105. Padberg AM, Bridwell KH. Spinal cord monitoring: current state of the art. Orthop Clin North Am 30:407-33, viii, 1999.
106. Shinomiya K, Fuchioka M, Matsuoka T, et al. Intraoperative monitoring for tethered spinal cord syndrome. Spine (Phila Pa 1976) 16:1290-1294, 1991.

Chapter 34

Advanced Thoracic Approaches to the Spine

Eric B. Jelin, Pierre Reynald Theodore

A variety of pathologic conditions involve the thoracic spine and may require surgical intervention. These conditions include metastatic neoplasms, congenital malformations, degenerative diseases, chronic infections, primary bone tumors, and primary soft tissue tumors. Although metastases, which represent the most frequently encountered pathology, are increasingly managed nonoperatively in patients with intractable pain and/or spinal cord compression, occasionally thoracic surgeons are asked to participate in anterior approaches, particularly for lesions adjacent to the aorta, reoperative procedures, and some lesions at the cervicothoracic junction.

The cornerstone of safe access to the spine is communication between the surgical teams responsible for each part of the procedure. The type of incision and the extent of sternal division or rib resection are determined by the spine level being treated, encompassing spine oncologic principles, and the anticipated reconstructive needs of the spine surgeon. By developing a clear and well-reasoned surgical plan, errors that may complicate challenging cases can often be avoided. Close attention to preoperative evaluation and intraoperative anatomic findings can assist the thoracic surgeon in providing consistent reliable approaches to the thoracic spine.

In this chapter, access to the cervicothoracic junction and the entire thoracic spine will be covered. Approaches will be described based on the level of instrumentation required, with an emphasis on anterior approaches to the spine in which the assistance of a thoracic surgeon is often required. Technical pitfalls and anatomic landmarks will be considered along with complications of thoracotomy.

INDICATIONS AND CONTRAINDICATIONS

The first accounts of spinal access surgery were reported by Hodgson and Stock,[1] in the mid-twentieth century, for treatment of tuberculous disease of the spine. Although indications for accessing the spine have largely shifted from infectious diseases to neoplastic and degenerative diseases, the basic operative approaches to the thoracic spine remain unchanged.

Approaches to the thoracic spine are divided between posterior (translaminar or transpedicular) and anterior approaches, such as median sternotomy or median sternectomy, high axillary thoracotomy, posterolateral thoracotomy, and thoracoabdominal approaches. The global approach of posterior versus anterior is dictated by the operating spine surgeon and is influenced by the surgeon's level of experience, the presence of bulky neoplastic disease of the spine, previous operations, and the requirement for a coincident procedure (chest wall resection and pulmonary resection). Experience at major spine centers suggests a decrease in anterior approaches to the spine, with growing enthusiasm for posterior transpedicular approaches. However, anterior transsternal or transthoracic approaches remain the mainstay of operative therapy for superior sulcus tumors, some lesions of the cervicothoracic junction, large masses, and masses abutting major vascular structures or invading the chest wall.

Thoracic incisions and exposures are associated with significant disability and risk of complications, including chronic pain, neurapraxia resulting from retractor placement, recurrent laryngeal nerve injury, hemorrhage, myocardial infarction, pneumonia, sternal disunion, and lung herniation. Given these risks, it is incumbent on both spine surgeons and access surgeons to choose an approach that yields adequate exposure for uncompromised visualization and instrumentation, while minimizing complications and disabilities. In patients with unilateral recurrent laryngeal nerve injuries, every effort should be made to avoid contralateral injuries resulting in mandatory tracheostomy. Videoscopic techniques are being used with increasing frequency in thoracic spine surgery to help minimize complications from invasion into the thorax.

Careful orchestration of the operation can prevent needless delays during exchanges between teams, minimizing the time spent with an open wound and the attendant increased risk of infection. By communicating with the neurosurgical team and understanding the neurosurgical operation, the access surgeon can, for example, harvest autologous tissue for bone grafting (morcelated rib) at the same time that ideal exposure to the thoracic spine is provided. Close communication among colleagues from different disciplines is particularly important during thoracic spine surgery for metastatic cancer, a multidisciplinary undertaking involving medical oncology, radiation oncology, thoracic surgery, and rehabilitative medicine.

PREOPERATIVE EVALUATION

The preoperative evaluation of patients before intrathoracic procedures is extensive. Because all operations represent a balance of risks and benefits, careful risk stratification before the intervention is important. The morbidity of a thoracotomy should not be underestimated by practitioners. Rates of significant complications from thoracotomy alone range from 10% to 50%.[2] Patients with pulmonary compromise, coagulopathy, widely metastatic tumor burden, or general debilitation are at high risk for major adverse events after operations that violate the thoracic cage.

Along with a thorough physical examination, an initial screening assessment should include spirometric pulmonary function testing. Patients are at high risk for postoperative respiratory failure if their predicted postoperative forced expiratory volume in the first second (FEV_1) is less than 0.8 L. Although often impractical in patients with spine disorders, exercise testing demonstrating a mixed venous oxygen (MVO_2) value of less than 10 to 15 ml/kg/min or predicting a postoperative MVO_2 value of less than 10 ml/kg/min identifies a patient at very high risk for complications and mortality[3] (Box 34-1). Patients with pulmonary hypertension or right ventricular dysfunction often tolerate single-lung ventilation poorly.

ACCESS TO THE CERVICOTHORACIC JUNCTION

The cervicothoracic junction provides unique access challenges because of the high density of critical structures within a relatively compact region. In addition, because of the normal kyphosis of the high thoracic spine, the junction can be at the deepest recess of a cramped cervical incision, complicating exposure, lighting, and dutiful assistance.

Box 34-1 Factors That Identify Low-Risk and High-Risk Patients

Low-Risk Patients	High-Risk Patients
FEV_1 >2 L	PCO_2 >45
MVV >50% predicted	PO_2 <50
Predicted postoperative FEV_1 >0.8 L and 40% predicted	Predicted postoperative FEV_1 <0.7 L and/or 40% predicted
Absence of cardiac disease	Age >70 yr
	Poor exercise performance

From Reilly JJ Jr. Evidence-based preoperative evaluation of candidates for thoracotomy. Chest 116:474S, 1999.

The cervicothoracic junction is located at the border between regions that can be accessed through a high lateral thoracotomy (T2 to T5) and those that can often be reached through a purely cervical approach (T1 and T2). Traditionally, to avoid median sternotomy, incision of the sternoclavicular joint was performed to permit access to levels T1 to T3.[6] However, sternoclavicular joint disruption is associated with an inordinately high incidence of chronic pain syndrome, immobility of the upper extremities, and pseudarthrosis. A better alternative to complete median sternotomy is the approach known as the *upper sternal split*. The sternum is comprised of three fused congenital bones, with a persistent pseudojoint observed between the manubrium and the body of the sternum (Fig. 34-1) that represents a natural cleavage plane that can be exploited by the access surgeon. The upper sternal split has been undertaken with a good outcome and provides better exposure to the upper thoracic spine with a smaller scar (Fig. 34-2).[7,8]

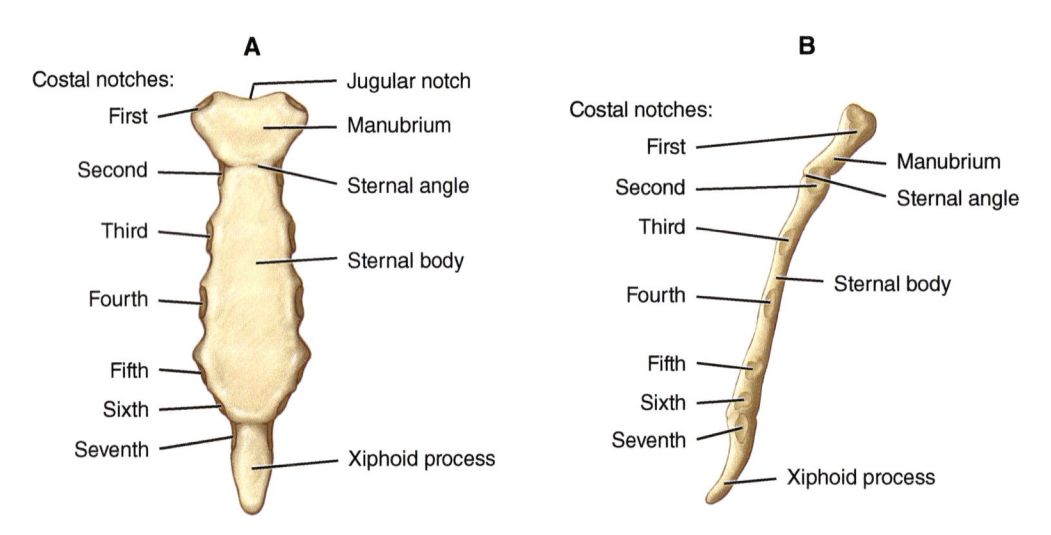

Fig. 34-1 Surface landmarks of the manubrium and sternum. **A,** Anteroposterior and **B,** sagittal views. (Adapted from Gray H. Anatomy of the Human Body, 20th ed. Philadelphia: Lea & Febiger, 1918. *www.bartleby.com*.)

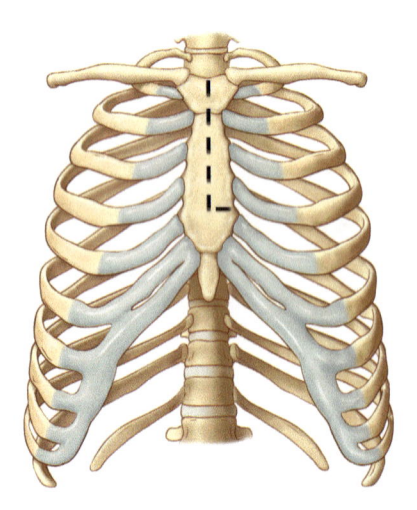

Fig. 34-2 Inverted-T upper sternal split technique. Traditional presternocleidomastoid incision is continued over the upper sternum.

TECHNIQUE
UPPER STERNAL SPLIT

The exposure provided by the upper sternal split, coupled with the low rate of complications compared with clavicular dislocations, makes this the approach of choice for tumors of the cervicothoracic junction.

We begin the upper sternal split with a 3 to 4 inch (7 to 10 cm) incision over the sternum, which can be extended anteriorly to the sternocleidomastoid muscle (Fig. 34-3). Next, subdermal flaps are elevated over the pectoralis major. Taking care to keep the incision in the midline of the sternum, a path is created in the periosteum, by means of electrocautery, from the manubrium to the upper several centimeters of the body of the sternum. At the apex of the sternum, between the sternal heads of the sternocleidomastoid muscles, the tough suprasternal ligament is divided by means of electrocautery, allowing the passage of a finger gently under the sternum to sweep away the loose fascial attachments of the retrosternal space. The oscillating sternal saw, with an inferior safety guard in place, is positioned at the upper border of the sternum facing downward. The manubrium is split up to the angle of Louis at the junction of the second and third chondrosternal junctions.

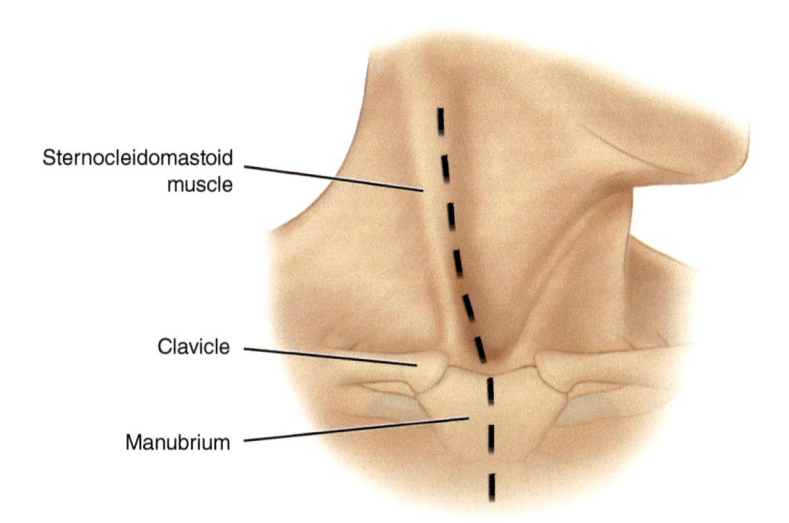

Fig. 34-3 Upper sternal split with a 3 to 4 inch (7 to 10 cm) incision over the sternum, which can be extended anteriorly to the sternocleidomastoid muscle. (Adapted from Luk KD, Cheung KM, Leong JC. Anterior approach to the cervicothoracic junction by unilateral or bilateral manubriotomy. A report of five cases. J Bone Joint Surg Am 84A:1013, 2002.)

Two techniques can be used to achieve lateral extension of the midline sternal division (T-ing off the sternotomy). We prefer to split the sternum bilaterally at the manubriosternal junction to provide improved exposure and ease of sternal reconstruction. Some investigators have described the use of unilateral transverse sternotomy (L-shaped sternotomy). However, this technique is not associated with a better cosmetic or functional result and limits exposure to both sides of the thoracic spine. An oscillating sternal saw can be used to divide the anterior table and cancellous portion of the sternum, and heavy Mayo scissors can be used to divide the posterior table. Care should be taken to avoid the internal mammary artery and vein pedicle lying approximately 2 cm lateral to the sternal borders. The alternative is to place a retractor from the cut edge of the sternum superiorly down to the level of the manubrium, which generally will split along the manubriosternal junction with opening of the retractor. Bone wax is placed against the cut edges of the sternum, and small penetrating vessels along the periosteum are touched with the electrocautery pen. After the manubrium is slightly separated, the first structure generally encountered is the H-shaped thymus gland, which can be removed up to its superior lobes extending into the neck. Removal of the superior horn of the thymus gland facilitates further dissection to the cervicothoracic junction.

The crossing brachiocephalic (innominate) vein is readily visualized. It is important that this vein not be placed under excessive tension from retractor opening, because it can be torn or thrombose under extremes of tension. Once the brachiocephalic vein is dissected free, it is surrounded with a vessel loop and retracted gently in a caudal direction. Damage to the recurrent laryngeal nerve is a cause of significant morbidity and, in the case of bilateral nerve injury, is potentially life-threatening. Thus preservation of the recurrent laryngeal nerve function is critical. Although some investigators advocate isolating and even surrounding the nerve with a vessel loop, we have favored considering the trachea and the esophagus as a unit in combination with the recurrent laryngeal nerve. By mobilizing the trachea and esophagus together and sweeping the carotid artery sheath laterally, we can avoid significant injury to the nerve (Fig. 34-4).

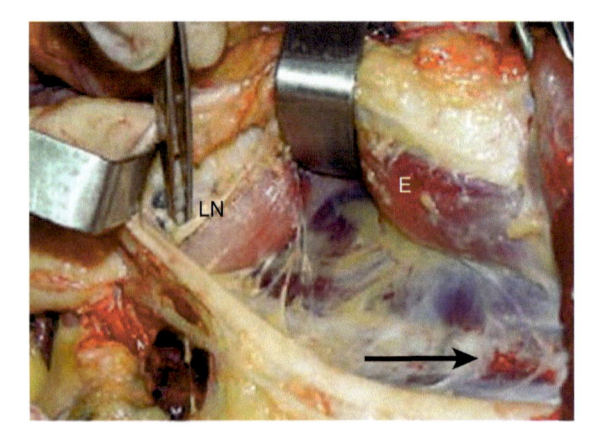

Fig. 34-4 Neck dissection as viewed from the left side of the table with the recurrent laryngeal nerve *(LN)* pulled anteriorly and medially in concert with the esophagus *(E)* and trachea.

Although the left-neck approach is the most straightforward means of mobilizing the esophagus, either side can be approached if there is a specific concern regarding one recurrent laryngeal nerve (known previous unilateral nerve injury) or unilateral predominance of tumor. Once the anterior vertebral ligaments are encountered, deep self-retaining retractors are placed to hold the trachea and esophagus medially. A peanut-sized piece of Kuettner sponge is used to incise the prevertebral fascia to the bone. Precise bipolar electrocautery is used to coagulate any small penetrating fascial vessels that are encountered. Care in applying the lateral retractor used for pushing aside the carotid sheath is required to avoid rupture of carotid atherosclerotic plaques and carotid thrombosis, both of which can lead to stroke.

With adequate hemostasis and retractors in place, the field is returned to the spine surgeon for instrumentation. In most patients, access to the T3-T4 interspace is readily achieved from the exposure as described. Periodically the carotid sheath should be inspected for thrombus or stretch injury.

At the conclusion of the instrumentation of the spine, a flat 7 Fr Jackson-Pratt drain is placed adjacent to the spine and is then brought through the thoracic inlet and through a stab incision at the base of the neck. Typically this drain is removed on postoperative day 2. The sternum should be closed very carefully to avoid the complications of nonunion. After checking for hemostasis along the inferior edge of the sternum and placement of another flat Jackson-Pratt drain in the anterior mediastinum, the edges of the sternum are reapproximated. It is important that the edges are brought evenly together to promote healing. At the T of the sternotomy, either a figure-of-eight sternal wire is placed parallel to the midline incision or a sternal plating system is used to reconnect the sternum to the manubrium. Then either two sternal wires or a second plate is used to reapproximate the manubrium. It is critical that the deep fascial layer overlying the sternum be closely reapproximated and that the suprasternal notch be completely closed to avoid infection in any remaining potential space anterior or superior to the sternum. The dermis is reapproximated with absorbable material, and the skin is typically closed with staples.

Upper sternal split is well tolerated, but a small risk of complications is incurred. Some widening of the mediastinum is to be expected in the postoperative period, but any increase after the initial postoperative radiographs are obtained raises concern about mediastinal hemorrhage, for which the patient must undergo an exploratory reoperation to prevent compromise of venous return and tamponade-like physiology. Hematomas of the anterior mediastinum are generally avoided by placement of a small drain, but significant hematomas associated with widening of the mediastinum on chest radiographs, hypotension, or a drop in hematocrit are managed with exploratory reoperation after correction of coagulopathy.

Sternal osteomyelitis and mediastinitis are feared complications, but fortunately they are uncommon when the internal mammary arteries are preserved. Although some thoracic surgeons have advocated division of the internal mammary arteries, we have not found this to be necessary, as this would place the ischemic sternum at greater risk for infection. Recurrent laryngeal nerve injury can be avoided through knowledge of its anatomy, moving the trachea and the esophagus as a unit, and careful retractor placement. The nerve is considered at greater risk for injury on the right side, given its longer course outside of the tracheoesophageal groove after it "recurs" around the innominate artery. It is critical to confirm that the esophagus is mobilized free of the spine, because transesophageal screw placement can result in swallowing disorders and chronic infection.[9]

Long-term sequelae from upper sternal splits are rare. On occasion, delayed disunion of the sternal plates may occur and require reintervention. In very thin patients, sternal wires may irritate the dermis and subcutaneous tissues and require removal (after a 2-month period of sternal healing).

ANTEROLATERAL THORACOTOMY WITH MEDIAN STERNOTOMY—TRAPDOOR INCISION

Large bulky tumors involving the bodies of the upper thoracic spine, either primarily or from direct extension from lung neoplasms, can be approached by a combination of a median sternotomy and an anterior thoracotomy incision (*trapdoor* or *hemiclamshell*). The division of the sternum and lateral extension of the incision essentially combines the exposure provided through an upper sternal split with that of a high (axillary) thoracotomy, giving unfettered anterior access to the spine from the midcervical vertebrae to the lower thoracic vertebrae (Fig. 34-5). This approach is facilitated by single-lung ventilation, which is accomplished through the use of a Carlin's dual-lumen endotracheal tube. After confirmation of proper placement with a pediatric bronchoscope, the appropriate lung is deflated before incision.

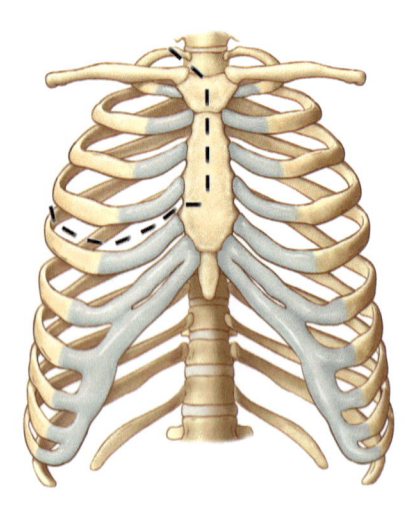

Fig. 34-5 Trapdoor or hemiclamshell incision.

Initially a stack of towels is placed behind the patient's shoulder on the side and in line with the anterior thoracotomy. The operating table is then tilted with the patient level to the ground. This permits the surgeon to perform an initial sternotomy with an anterior oblique view of the spine. The incision is made as described for the upper sternal split, but at the level of the third intercostal space the incision is taken laterally between the third and fourth ribs. The internal mammary artery and vein pedicle are identified and divided between silk ties or clips, and the curvilinear intercostal space is opened with electrocautery, taking care not to reach the sympathetic trunk. By using two Finochietto retractors, the first to distract the sternum and the second to separate the ribs, this approach effectively disarticulates the upper extremity and upper chest wall, exposing the thoracic spine posterior to the pericardium. If either side is suitable, a right-sided approach is preferable, because early division of the azygous vein permits more complete visualization of the thoracic spine lying medial to it (see Fig. 34-4). Conversely, the same approach through the left chest is associated with an obscured view of the spine at level T4 to T6 because of the transverse arch of the aorta. Care should be taken to avoid placing the brachial plexus and subclavian vein under too much distraction stress from the opening of the retractors, which can result in brachial plexus neuralgia or, rarely, subclavian vein injury.

The principal advantage of the trapdoor approach is its exposure for pathology that extends from the cervicothoracic junction to the midthoracic spinal bodies. This region is challenging to reach from the neck alone, and a primary thoracic approach gives poor exposure to the cervical vertebrae because of the confinements of the thoracic outlet. In Pancoast-type tumors arising from lung parenchyma, this anterior approach coupled with thoracotomy permits anatomic pulmonary resection, reconstruction of major vascular structures as required, and spine instrumentation in a one-stage procedure.[10] Closure of the trapdoor incision is performed first by reapproximation of the ribs with braided heavy absorbable Vicryl sutures (Covidien, Boulder, CO) and then reapproximation of the serratus anterior muscle and pectoralis major muscle with heavy Vicryl sutures. The sternum is closed in the same manner as described previously. Two chest tubes are placed: the first one overlaying the dome of the diaphragm and the second one directed to the apex of the chest to permit adequate drainage of blood and air in the postoperative period. The lung is reinflated before the chest is closed.

Complications of the combined anterolateral thoracotomy with median sternotomy include the following: sternotomy disunion or infection, injury to the brachial plexus, hemothorax, chronic thoracotomy pain syndrome from injury to the intercostal nerves, and empyema. The functional results are typically good, with minimal long-term disability in upper extremity function stemming from the approach alone.

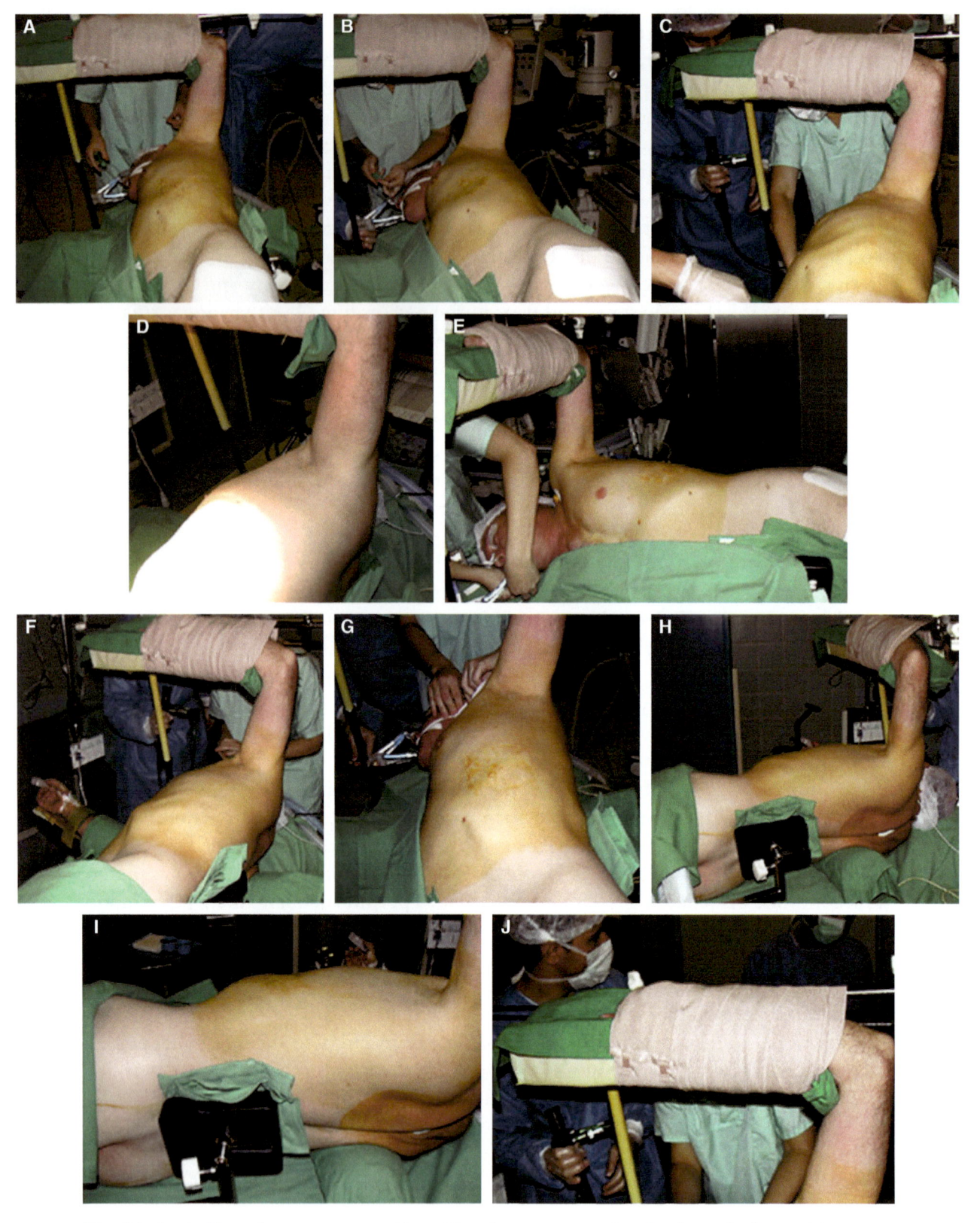

Fig. 34-6 Axillary thoracotomy position. The chest must stay in a horizontal plane with an arm placed at right angles to this plane, but without any tension to avoid stretching the brachial plexus. (From Dürrleman N, Massard G. Axillary thoracotomy. Multimedia Manual Cardio-Thoracic Surgery doi:10.1510/mmcts.2006.001834. Copyright 2006 European Association for Cardio-Thoracic Surgery, with permission from the European Association for Cardio-Thoracic Surgery.)

Axillary Thoracotomy

The high muscle-sparing lateral thoracotomy provides superb exposure to levels T2 to T6 with acceptable morbidity. The patient is placed in the lateral decubitus position with the upper extremity extended from a support device to provide ready access to the axilla (Fig. 34-6). The incision begins at the lateral border of the pectoralis major muscle lateral to the nipple in male patients and proceeds posteriorly over the latissimus dorsi. The latissimus dorsi is spared through posterior mobilization, whereas the pectoralis major and serratus anterior are displaced anteriorly, providing access to the third or fourth intercostal space. After the intercostal muscle is divided, a small (Tuffier) retractor is placed to open the thoracotomy. As described previously, the right-sided approach is favored to avoid the aortic arch. If autologous osseous tissue is requested, the third or fourth rib can be removed in the subperiosteal plane to avoid injuring the intercostal neurovascular bundle and improve visualization. A dual-lumen endotracheal tube with single-lung ventilation is required. The lung is grasped with an atraumatic grasping clamp (Fig. 34-7) and pulled anteriorly and inferiorly. The azygous vein is surrounded by a right-angle clamp and divided with a 30 mm vascular articulating stapler. The lung is reflected medially away from the spine and the parietal pleura is incised, giving access to the periosteum of the vertebral bodies. Attention should be paid to the thoracic duct, which should be ligated if it is seen. The axillary thoracotomy is very well tolerated, even in elderly patients, and provides access to vertebral levels T2 to T5. Disability is minimized by sparing the latissimus dorsi and pectoralis muscles.

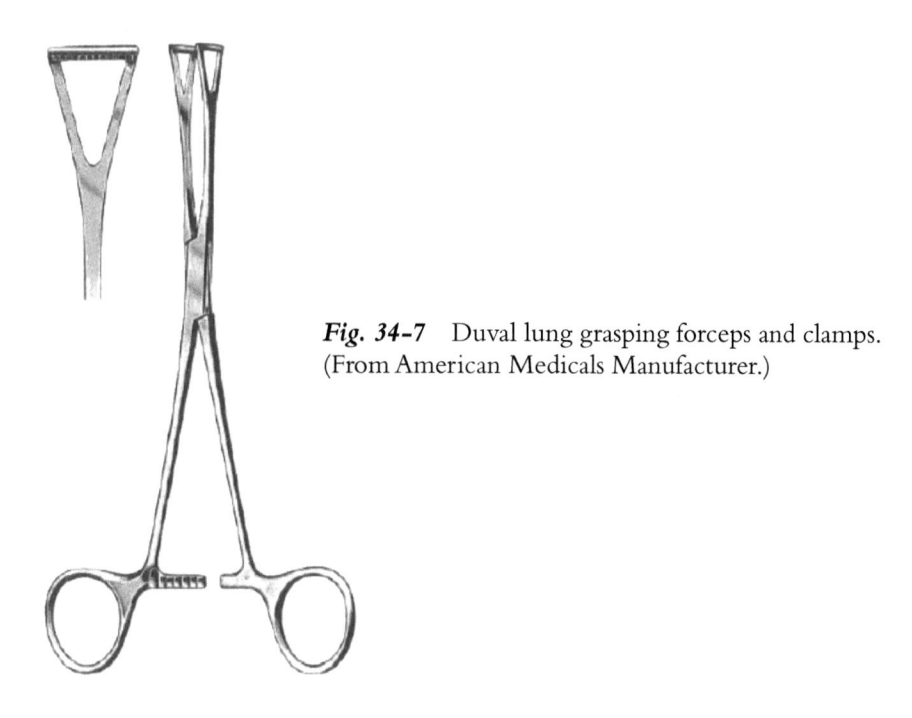

Fig. 34-7 Duval lung grasping forceps and clamps. (From American Medicals Manufacturer.)

Classic Posterolateral Thoracotomy

The most common approach to the anterior thoracic spine is by posterolateral thoracotomy. The patient is placed in the lateral decubitus position so that the tip of the scapula is centered and the plane of the scapula is horizontal. Proper positioning of the patient is important for ease of exposure and to avoid inadvertent pressure injuries to the anesthetized patient. Once the patient is placed in the lateral position, it is imperative that the dependent extremity be padded to avoid ulnar nerve injury; it is also essential that a soft pad be placed under the patient in the axilla to minimize stretching of the brachial plexus (see Fig. 34-6). Somatosensory evoked potential monitors are placed before positioning to confirm that lateral positioning or intraoperative spinal manipulations are not impairing nerve conduction.

The incision is shifted slightly posteriorly, relative to that used for pulmonary pathology, to provide easier access to the spine. The incision begins between the scapula and the spinous processes and runs parallel to the spine before aligning with the path of the ribs at the fifth, seventh, or ninth intercostal space, depending on the vertebral level of interest. Soft tissue flaps are raised above the latissimus dorsi, and the muscle is divided in its entirety. The cut ends of the latissimus dorsi are mobilized 3 to 4 cm to permit easier closure at the conclusion of the operation. The obliquely running fibers of the serratus anterior muscle are mobilized without division and distracted medially. This allows the surgeon to access the subscapular plane, which can be entered bluntly. The ribs are counted, and the proper interspace is entered. The intercostal muscles are divided with electrocautery, and care is taken when entering the pleural space to avoid thermal or mechanical injury to the underlying lung. The ribs are distracted slightly, and the intercostal muscles along with the endothoracic fascia are divided from the inside out. If an autograft is required, a rib is resected in the subperiosteal plane and morcelated, as directed by the spine surgeon. With a right-sided low thoracotomy, attention is required to avoid potential injury to the thoracic duct. Evident lymphatic vessels should be ligated, because chylothorax is another risk.

If a thoracolumbar approach with division of the diaphragm is favored, the incision is extended anteriorly across the costal margin (Fig. 34-8). This extension is preferably performed on the left to avoid the liver. The ninth or tenth rib is resected with an incision that crosses the costal margin, exposing the dome of the diaphragm. The diaphragm is divided circumferentially, leaving a 1 to 2 cm rim of diaphragm attached to the lateral chest wall. The psoas insertion and the bodies of the lumbar vertebrae are visualized, developing the retroperitoneal plane by medial rotation of the abdominal contents. At the time of closure, a nonabsorbable polypropylene suture is used to reassemble the diaphragm.

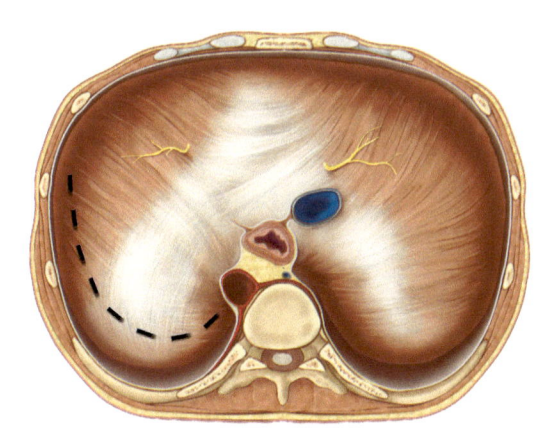

Fig. 34-8 View of the diaphragm from above, demonstrating line of division to preserve phrenic nerve function.

In addition to drains left in the retroperitoneal space, a chest drain should remain to evacuate the small pleural effusions that inevitably result from the manipulation of the diaphragm and retroperitoneum. We routinely place two 28 Fr chest tubes to drain both the posterior costophrenic angle for fluid and the apex of the residual pneumothorax. The apical chest tube can be removed early in the postoperative period once full expansion of the lung has been confirmed. The basilar chest tube remains in place until less than 300 cc/day of chest tube drainage is achieved.

Complications of posterolateral thoracotomy are numerous and include the following: pneumonia, wound infection, chylothorax, persistent pneumothorax, pleural effusion, lung herniation, neuralgia, chronic pain syndromes, and respiratory failure. Pain control can be aided by placement of intercostal nerve blocks with 0.25% bupivicaine injections at the conclusion of the operation, taking care to avoid inadvertent intravascular injection. Early ambulation, incentive spirometry, and prompt removal of chest drains, when appropriate, can reduce pain and complications.

VIDEO-ASSISTED THORACOSCOPIC SURGERY

Recently the use of video-assisted thoracoscopic surgery (VATS) has become widespread in the management of thoracic disease. VATS involves the use of a fiberoptic camera and light source for visualization through small percutaneous portals, offering direct illumination and magnification of the operative field. With the use of VATS, outcomes are improved because rib spreading with traditional retractors is avoided, preventing intercostal nerve injury and reducing postoperative pain.

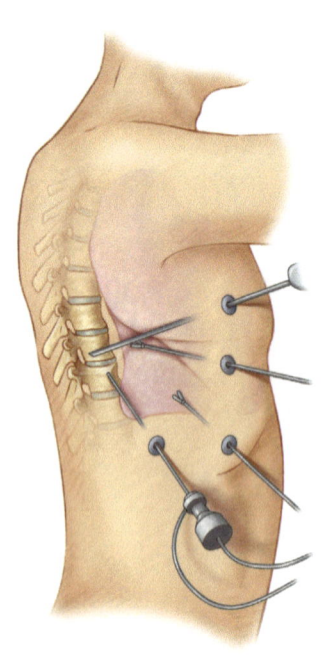

Fig. 34-9 Placement of ports for videoscopic access to the spine.

The first clinical report of thoracoscopic surgery was in 1910, when Jacobaeus[11] used a thoracoscope to diagnose and lyse a tuberculosis lung adhesion. At present, virtually every procedure within the realm of general thoracic surgery can be performed with VATS, and this technique is used frequently for a variety of spine conditions. VATS is probably most beneficial in the treatment of scoliotic deformity, when multiple levels require instrumentation, or in the treatment of intervertebral disc disease, when a minimal access technique can achieve functional results similar to those used in open procedures without the need for thoracotomy.[12,13]

VATS requires selective single-lung ventilation with double-lumen endotracheal intubation to fully collapse the lung to facilitate surgery. (Recently the execution of an anterior thoracoscopic soft tissue release in a patient in the prone position has been examined.[14]) The camera ports are placed in the midaxillary line and the operating ports in the posterior axillary line. Often many levels of port placement are required to permit instrumentation along the thoracic spine (Fig. 34-9).[15]

POSTOPERATIVE CONCERNS

Noncardiac thoracic surgery has been associated with significant risks of major adverse cardiac events in several large retrospective series. Patients more than 70 years of age, and those with a history of recent myocardial infarction, dysrhythmia, heart failure, or known valvular heart disease, are at significant cardiac risk after thoracotomy and require intensive monitoring and sometimes preoperative intervention (revascularization or medical optimization) before spine surgery.[4,5]

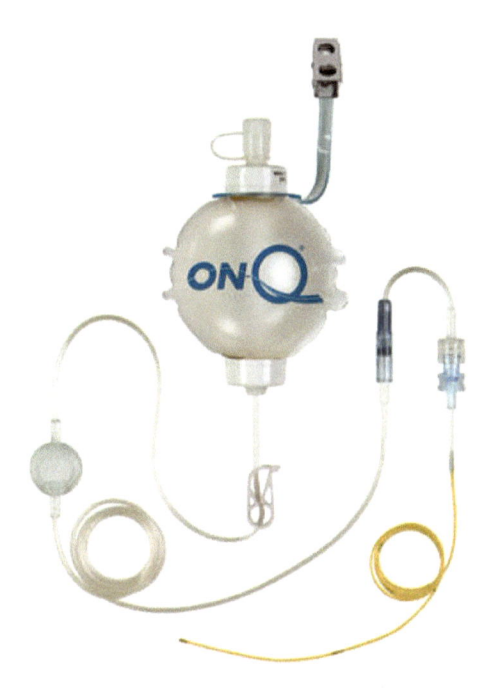

Fig. 34-10 On-Q PainBuster postoperative analgesia system. (From I-Flow, a Kimberly-Clark Healthcare Company, Lake Forest, CA.)

A principal concern in the postoperative period after thoracotomy is pneumonia. Postoperative pain and immobility discourage the patient from taking deep breaths, causing atelectasis. The patient's atelectatic lungs are further impaired by dysfunctional mucociliary clearance, which is known to occur postoperatively. These factors conspire to identify these patients as high risk for nosocomial pneumonia. Early ambulation, as appropriate, and pain control with intercostal analgesics (Fig. 34-10) or systemic narcotics can help reduce the risks of hypoventilation, atelectasis, and pneumonia.

CONCLUSION

Surgical interventions involving the thoracic spine are common and increasing in number. A variety of distinct incisions provide optimized access from the cervicothoracic junction to the thoracolumbar spine. The capacity of the spine surgeon to restore function, limit disability, and reduce pain must be weighed against the morbidity associated with thoracic cavity access. Preoperative evaluative tools can aid in risk stratification of patients with spine disorders, who frequently have major comorbidity. With proper preoperative evaluation, intraoperative precision, and attentive postoperative care, the significant risk of complications from median sternotomy, thoracotomy, and cervicothoracic incisions can be reduced. Communication among surgical teams promotes better outcomes through reduced operative times and incisions that provide optimal visualization.

TIPS FROM THE MASTERS

- Posterior thoracic transpedicular approaches have decreased the need for many of the anterior thoracic approaches for tumor surgery.
- In cases of anterior organ or vessel involvement, these approaches are still quite critical for adequate tumor exposure.

References (With Key References in Boldface)

1. Hodgson A, Stock FE. Anterior spinal fusion a preliminary communication on the radical treatment of Pott's disease and Pott's paraplegia. Br J Surg 44: 266, 1956.
2. Darling GE, McBroom R, Perrin R. Modified anterior approach to the cervicothoracic junction. Spine (Phila Pa 1976) 20:1519, 1995.
3. **Reilly JJ Jr. Evidence-based preoperative evaluation of candidates for thoracotomy. Chest 116:474S, 1999.**
4. Detsky AS, Abrams HB, McLaughlin JR, et al. Predicting cardiac complications in patients undergoing non-cardiac surgery. J Gen Intern Med 1:211, 1986.
5. **Goldman L, Caldera DL, Nussbaum SR, et al. Multifactorial index of cardiac risk in noncardiac surgical procedures. N Engl J Med 297:845, 1977.**
6. Pointillart V, Aurouer N, Gangnet N, et al. Anterior approach to the cervicothoracic junction without sternotomy: a report of 37 cases. Spine (Phila Pa 1976) 32:2875, 2007.
7. Wang VY, Chou D. The cervicothoracic junction. Neurosurg Clin N Am 18:365, 2007.
8. Liu YL, Hao YJ, Li T, et al. Trans-upper-sternal approach to the cervicothoracic junction. Clin Orthop Relat Res 467:2018, 2009.
9. Lu DC, Theodore P, Korn WM, et al. Esophageal erosion 9 years after anterior cervical plate implantation. Surg Neurol 69:310, 2008.
10. Lebreton G, Baste JM, Thumerel M, et al. The hemiclamshell approach in thoracic surgery: indications and associated morbidity in 50 patients. Interact Cardiovasc Thorac Surg 9:965-969, 2009.
11. Jacobaeus HC. Ueber die Möglichkeit der Zystoskopie bei Untersuchung seröser Höhlungen anzuwenden. Münch Med Wochenschr 57:2090, 1910.
12. Al-Sayyad MJ, Crawford AH, Wolf RK. Early experiences with video-assisted thoracoscopic surgery: our first 70 cases. Spine (Phila Pa 1976) 29:1945, 2004.
13. **Anand N, Regan JJ. Video-assisted thoracoscopic surgery for thoracic disc disease: classification and outcome study of 100 consecutive cases with a 2-year minimum follow-up period. Spine (Phila Pa 1976) 27:871, 2002.**
14. King AG, Mills TE, Loe WA Jr, et al. Video-assisted thoracoscopic surgery in the prone position. Spine (Phila Pa 1976) 25:2403, 2000.
15. Liu GK, Kit WH. Video assisted thoracoscopic surgery for spinal conditions. Neurol India 53:489, 2005.

Chapter 35

Thoracoscopic Resection and Reconstruction

Frank S. Bishop, Meic H. Schmidt

*M*inimally invasive thoracoscopic spine surgery is an alternative to open thoracotomy for tumor and vertebral body resection, thoracic corpectomy, anterior neural decompression, and anterolateral spine reconstruction. This closed endoscopic approach, alternately referred to as endoscopic-assisted or video-assisted thoracoscopic surgery (VATS), is used to access the anterior thoracic and thoracolumbar spine (T5-L2). The goals of surgery are to resect the tumor and diseased vertebral body, decompress the anterior spinal canal, and restore biomechanical stability with interbody reconstruction augmented with anterolateral plating.

Historically, resection of spine tumors was performed through a posterior approach. Thoracic laminectomy, however, failed to adequately address most tumors located ventrally in the spinal column and increased the risk of spinal cord injury when the lesion was associated with epidural masses.[1-4] Therefore anterior open thoracotomy and thoracoabdominal approaches were developed; these demonstrated improved outcomes by more effectively addressing the goals of tumor resection, neural decompression, and anterior reconstruction.[5,6] Unfortunately these open procedures were associated with high-access morbidity.[7]

Minimally invasive thoracoscopic techniques have been used by thoracic surgeons for many years and have now been adapted for use in spine surgery, beginning with treatment of thoracic disc herniations and traumatic fractures.[8-14] As with other endoscopic procedures, access to the thoracic cavity is achieved by using small chest incisions for access portals, and the surgery is performed with specially designed instruments. By using small thoracoscopic incisions, which minimize chest wall dissection and retraction, postoperative morbidity has been significantly reduced by decreasing blood loss, postoperative pain, pulmonary and shoulder dysfunction, days in the intensive care unit, and overall length of hospital stays.[8,10,15-18] Since its inception, minimally invasive thoracoscopic surgery has improved significantly, with the advancement of endoscopic video technology and the development of instruments and instrumentation systems. These have further expanded the use of the technique for treatment of spine tumors.[15] Many procedures that had previously been performed by open thoracotomy can now be performed safely and effectively with the minimally invasive thoracoscopic approach.

INDICATIONS AND CONTRAINDICATIONS

Surgical treatment for spine tumors is indicated for spinal instability, most cases of neural compression, failure of tumor control with radiation treatment, histologic diagnosis, or intractable pain that is not relieved by more conservative measures.[4,19-22] The thoracoscopic technique is indicated in patients with tumors involving the vertebral body that require resection and reconstruction, with interbody replacement and instrumentation. The endoscopic approach is best suited for tumors limited to one vertebral body and the anterior spinal canal.

Thoracoscopic spine surgery is contraindicated in patients with significant medical diseases that would prohibit surgery and in those with terminal illness. Advanced cardiopulmonary disease severe enough to preclude the use of single-lung ventilation, such as severe chronic obstructive pulmonary disease or asthma, is also a contraindication. The presence of significant pleural adhesions, which may occur in patients with a history of trauma, infection, or thoracic surgery, can make the surgery technically challenging. Furthermore, this approach may provide insufficient exposure for extensive tumors with significant posterior column involvement requiring circumferential resection or total spondylectomy. An open thoracotomy or lateral extracavitary approach may be better suited for patients with these conditions.

PREOPERATIVE EVALUATION
HISTORY AND PHYSICAL EXAMINATION

Patients with thoracolumbar tumors may present with a variety of symptoms, including pain, neurologic deficits, spinal malalignment, instability, or with incidental radiographic findings, without clinical symptoms. Pain is the most common presenting symptom and initially may be nonspecific. Furthermore, the extent of tumor involvement may not correlate with the severity of pain or other symptoms. Characteristic tumor pain is chronic and persistent, is present with recumbency and at night, and begins before other neurologic symptoms appear. Localized pain may be caused by vertebral body fracture or destruction, or by mechanical instability, which worsens with weight-bearing or movement. Because the onset of pain is insidious and diffuse, the diagnosis of spine tumors is often delayed until indicated by the presence of a neurologic deficit resulting from tumor compression of the spinal cord or nerve roots. In such cases, patients may report weakness, gait instability, radicular pain, lower extremity numbness or tingling, or bowel and bladder retention or incontinence. Other systemic symptoms, including weight loss, fatigue, and general malaise, may also be present.

The physical examination findings may be grossly normal or may reveal varying degrees of neurologic compromise ranging from subtle weakness and abnormal reflexes to complete paraplegia. These signs can occur as a result of direct spinal cord compression or vascular occlusion and secondary spinal cord ischemia. Local tenderness or muscle spasms may be present, and a mass may be palpable in cases of posterior involvement. Back pain resulting from mechanical instability may be aggravated with flexion-extension maneuvers and axial loading.

RADIOGRAPHIC AND DIAGNOSTIC STUDIES

Radiographic studies are essential for determining the appropriate treatment modality and algorithm. Imaging is carefully reviewed to evaluate the extent of tumor involvement of the vertebral body and bony structures, the degree of osseous destruction, the stability and anatomic alignment of the involved segments, and the amount of neural compression. Initial evaluation is by plain radiography to localize the levels of involvement. Magnetic resonance imaging (MRI) is the primary imaging modality for evaluating the tumor, neural elements, epidural space, and paraspinous soft tissue structures. Computed tomography (CT) is also employed to assess the bony anatomy, differentiate between osteoblastic and osteolytic lesions, and evaluate the vertebral cortical integrity. These imaging modalities offer views in three orthogonal planes, which is important in precisely determining the tumor morphology and local anatomy. In addition, spinal angiography is used for vascular tumors, such as hemangiomas, aneurysmal bone cysts, and renal and thyroid metastases. Preoperative embolization is performed, when necessary, to decrease intraoperative blood loss and facilitate safe aggressive tumor resection.

The preoperative workup for spine tumors also includes appropriate additional radiographic and laboratory studies. In cases of suspected metastasis, a plain chest radiograph, CT images of the chest, abdomen, and pelvis, or a radionuclide bone scan may be useful for identifying the cancer stage. Laboratory tests, including complete blood count, a metabolic panel including liver function tests and coagulation studies, are necessary for routine evaluation. Additional tests may include prostate-specific antigen levels, carcinoembryonic antigen levels, stool occult blood tests, protein electrophoresis of the serum and urine, and urinalysis for Bence Jones proteins. In general, benign tumors are more likely to occur in younger patients or in those with involvement of the posterior elements, whereas malignancy, whether primary or metastatic, tends to occur more often in older patients and in anterior locations.

Thoracoscopic surgery may also require a preoperative evaluation by a pulmonologist, anesthesiologist, or qualified internist to assess pulmonary function and the ability of the patient to undergo general anesthesia with single-lung ventilation. In patients who have a prior lung injury or infection, an evaluation by a cardiothoracic surgeon may be warranted to discuss the patient's ability to undergo thoracoscopic surgery rather than open thoracotomy. When planning the timing of the operation, a cardiothoracic surgeon should be available, with advance knowledge of the patient, if possible, in the event that conversion to an open procedure becomes immediately necessary.

CLINICAL DECISION-MAKING
CHOICE OF TECHNIQUE

The minimally invasive thoracoscopic approach offers several advantages over an open thoracotomy. Current high-definition endoscopic technology provides a view of the surgical field with superb resolution. The small intercostal incisions with the minimally invasive approach do not involve rib resection or retraction, whereas open approaches require a large incision, extensive muscle dissection, and rib resection with significant retraction. With appropriate port placement, multiple levels of the spine may be seen and treated without increasing the surgical exposure. This approach has produced decreases in intraoperative blood loss, perioperative pain, days of mechanical ventilation, and length of hospital stay.[16-18]

The advantages of the approach, however, must be weighed against the disadvantages on a per patient basis. The main drawback of the thoracoscopic approach for most spine surgeons is their lack of familiarity with the technique. Endoscopic surgery requires working in two dimensions at a distance from the surgical site strictly by viewing the video monitors. Learning these new techniques and acquiring these new skills entails overcoming a steep learning curve and an initial investment of time and resources for didactic and practical training before performing the procedure on patients. Operative times can initially increase by several hours before the surgeon and operating room staff become familiar with the approach. Intraoperative complications can be more difficult to address with the endoscopic approach, which may require conversion to an open thoracotomy in difficult cases. An open approach is chosen for patients with contraindications to the thoracoscopic approach and for those with extensive tumors that are difficult to adequately treat with minimally invasive techniques.

PREOPERATIVE PLANNING OF APPROACH, RESECTION, AND RECONSTRUCTION

A thorough understanding of the general regional and individual patient anatomy of the thoracolumbar spine and spinal cord, chest wall and thorax, and the mediastinal structures is essential for these operations to be successful. Imaging studies must be carefully examined preoperatively to determine the side of the surgery and the dimensions of the construct and instrumentation.

The side of surgery is determined based on the location and lateralization of disease in relation to the surrounding anatomy (e.g., the aorta). In general, a left-sided approach is used for the thoracolumbar junction (T11-L2) and disease on the left side. A right-sided approach is preferred for the middle to upper thoracic spine (T3-10). The position of the aorta and vena cava is noted on preoperative imaging when choosing the approach side, as individual anatomy may vary.

The bony anatomy is studied preoperatively to plan the reconstruction. The widths of the vertebral bodies are measured to determine the length of the posterolateral vertebral body screws. The extent of resection, or the distance between the inferior endplate of the cranial level and the superior endplate of the caudal level, is also measured to determine the size of the interbody implant. Finally, the amount of pathologic intrusion into the spinal canal is noted to help determine the extent of bony removal needed for adequate anterior decompression and tumor resection.

TECHNIQUE
ROOM LAYOUT AND INSTRUMENTS

Minimally invasive thoracoscopic surgery requires a high-quality endoscopic camera, which is essential for optimal illumination and visualization. We prefer to use a high-definition 0- to 30-degree angled camera with a high-output xenon light source, which provides the best possible digital resolution and improves the surgeon's ability to operate endoscopically. In the operating room the endoscopic image is projected onto a video monitor in front of the patient. A monitor for the fluoroscope is placed beside the endoscopic video monitor. The surgeon stands directly behind the patient and the operative site, while an assistant who is operating the camera stands to the right of the surgeon. This gives both the surgeon and the camera operator a clear view of the two monitors directly across from them. The third assistant stands in front of the patient for suction, irrigation, and retraction.

Endoscopic instruments are highly specialized and specifically developed for this application. The instruments are designed with nonreflective surfaces for decreased glare, they are of adequate length for safe intrathoracic maneuvering, and they have large handles for ease of use. Endoscopic instrument sets contain many sizes of probes and hooks, curettes, rongeurs, graspers, osteotomes, graft holders, and measurement devices. The surgeon must become familiar with the various instruments and their applications for a smooth and effective operation.

In addition to endoscopic instruments, specialized instrumentation for thoracoscopic spinal reconstruction has been developed. The MACS-TL anterolateral spinal implant (Aesculap, Tüttlingen, Germany) is a rigid fixation plate specifically designed for endoscopic use (Fig. 35-1). It differs from most other thoracolumbar plating systems that have been developed for open surgery. The MACS-TL plating system incorporates

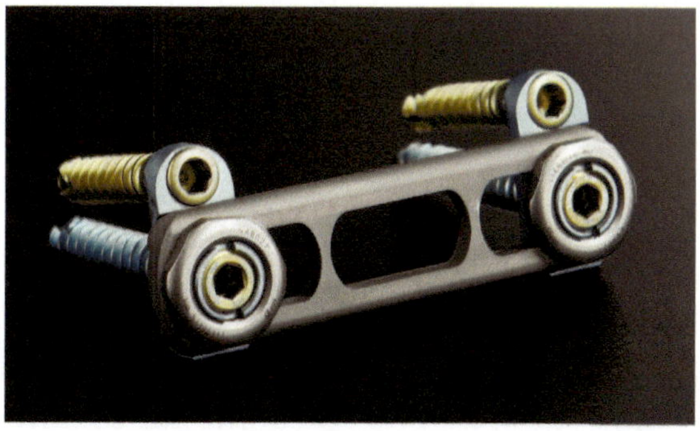

Fig. 35-1 The MACS-TL minimally invasive anterolateral spinal implant is a rigid fixation plate designed for thoracoscopic spinal stabilization.

four fixation screws: two posterior polyaxial vertebral body screws and two anterior stabilizing screws. The screws are placed into the normal vertebral bodies flanking the diseased vertebrae, and a fixation plate is rigidly secured to the screws. The biomechanical properties of the plating system have been characterized in several models of spine trauma, including monosegmental and bisegmental partial and full corpectomy models, with and without posterior ligamentous injury, and its clinical efficacy has been demonstrated in case series.[12,14,15,23-25]

ANESTHESIA AND PATIENT POSITIONING

Thoracoscopic spine surgery is performed while the patient is under general anesthesia. Endotracheal intubation is performed with a double-lumen tube for single-lung ventilation, which provides maximum surgical exposure. A bronchoscope is used before and after final positioning of the endotracheal tube to confirm correct placement. Before the patient is positioned, a Foley catheter, arterial line, and central venous access are placed.

The patient is placed in a lateral decubitus position on a radiolucent operating table, with the side of surgery chosen preoperatively based on a thorough study of the anatomy of the patient. Stabilizing supports secured to the table are placed against the coccyx, sacrum, and sternum, and between the scapulae for four-point stabilization. The legs are slightly flexed, and an inflatable axillary roll is placed. The top-lying arm is supported in a Krause armrest and elevated cranially to prevent intraoperative interference with the thoracoscopic instrumentation. The C-arm fluoroscope is positioned for a lateral view of the spine, and the patient is placed in final position with the spine parallel to the operating table.

LOCALIZATION AND ACCESS

After the patient is positioned optimally, a lateral view of the spine is obtained with the use of the C-arm fluoroscope to determine the relation of the spine and access portals. The lateral image is centered over the affected area, which is often radiographically evident because of bony involvement and changes in alignment, and is projected orthograde onto the chest wall. The involved vertebral bodies are marked on the skin, and the diagram is completed by outlining the intervertebral discs, anterior spinal line, and posterior spinal line (Fig. 35-2, *A*). The four portal access sites are then marked centered on the lesion (Fig. 35-2, *B*). Proper positioning of these portals is essential for optimal working distances, retraction, and imaging with the thoracoscopic camera. The working portal is centered exactly over the lesion and is approximately 3 to 4 cm in length (twice the length of the other access sites) to accommodate insertion of the fusion instrumentation later in the operation. Poor positioning of this portal site can make resection and instrumentation difficult to achieve. Furthermore, the risk of spinal cord and vascular injury may be increased as a result of misdirected instruments sliding on slanted resection surfaces. The access site for the thoracoscopic camera is located two to three intercostal spaces away from the working portal along the axis of the spinal column. The camera portal site is placed in the cranial direction for le-

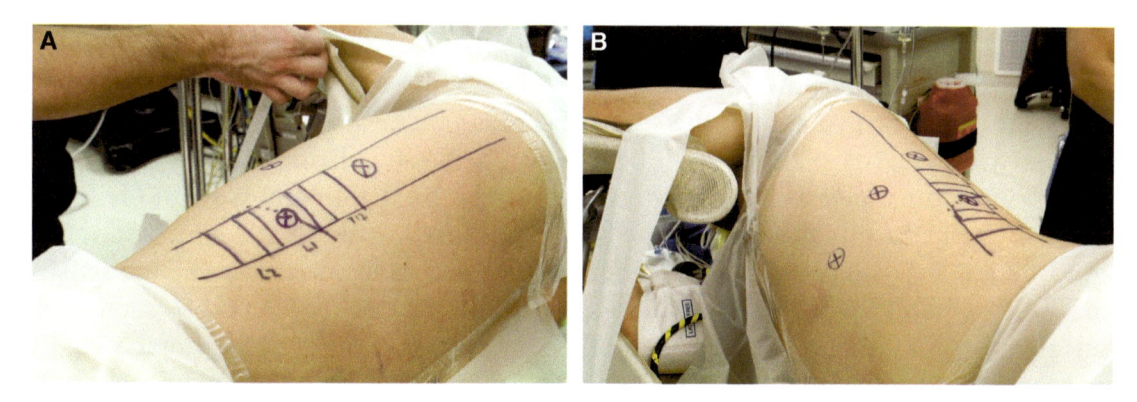

Fig. 35-2 The spine and portal sites are marked on the skin under fluoroscopic guidance. **A,** The involved and adjacent vertebral bodies are marked, then **B,** the four portal access sites are marked, centered on the lesion.

sions at the thoracolumbar junction and in the caudal direction for middle to upper thoracic spine surgery. The portal for suction/irrigation is situated ventrally and in a slightly cranial direction to the working portal. Care must be taken to avoid placing this portal too far from the working portal, which can make suction and irrigation of the surgical bed difficult. The portal for the lung and diaphragm retractor is placed further ventral to the suction/irrigation portal and slightly caudal to the working portal to avoid conflicting with the instruments at the working portal intraoperatively.

After the spinal anatomy is outlined and the portal sites are marked, the entire area of the lateral chest wall is sterilized and draped to prepare for possible conversion to open thoracotomy. Single-lung ventilation is initiated. The portal located in the most cranial direction is opened first to minimize the risk of injury to the diaphragm and underlying organs. After the skin incision is made, the opening is carried down to the rib using a minithoracotomy technique. The subcutaneous tissues and intercostal muscle layers are freed from the rib by means of a blunt dissection technique, without removing any rib, to minimize injury to the underlying lung. After the pleural space is entered, palpation and direct visualization are used to confirm the absence of significant pleural adhesions and ascertain that single-lung ventilation has been achieved. The first trocar is then inserted, and the 30-degree endoscope is used to inspect the thoracic cavity. A similar technique is used to insert the three remaining trocars under direct endoscopic view. The ports for suction/irrigation and retraction are placed next. Because the working portal lies closest to the diaphragm and intraabdominal organs, it is placed last, after the diaphragm has been safely retracted away from the trocar.

EXPOSURE

With the diaphragm retracted and the lung collapsed, the intrathoracic anatomy is inspected. The endoscope is rotated so that the spine is oriented horizontally on the video monitor. The anterior margin of the spine is visualized dorsal to the ventrally situated aorta. The diaphragm is typically attached to the spine between T12 and L1.

The retractor can be manipulated with stretching and relaxing maneuvers to expose the diaphragmatic insertion optimally. When operating at or below the insertion, the diaphragm is incised to expose the spine (Fig. 35-3). The surgeon should make the incision with a Harmonic scalpel (Ethicon Endo-Surgery, Cincinnati, OH), 1 to 2 cm away from and parallel to the insertion site, where the diaphragm is naturally thin. The 1 to 2 cm margin also facilitates closure at the end of the procedure. The incision is made layer by layer and continued along the spine and ribs in a semicircular line. For lesions at L1, a 2 to 3 cm incision typically suffices. The length is increased caudally to 5 cm for exposure of L2. As L3 is approached by means of a thoracoscopic approach, the diaphragm is incised extensively and a mini–open endoscopic–assisted retroperitoneal exposure is used. Retractors are placed through the opening after the diaphragm is split. The peritoneal sac and retroperitoneal fat are mobilized with blunt dissection from the psoas muscle fascia, and then retracted caudally and ventrally to expose the anterior spine.

The prevertebral soft tissue dissection is performed next for exposure of the thoracic vertebral bodies and intervertebral discs. The correct level is identified visually. Endoscopic visualization is often possible by noting a mass under the pleura or a local deformity. Radiographic visualization with fluoroscopy is used for confirmation. The Harmonic scalpel with a hooked tip is used to incise the parietal pleura in line with the spinal axis. Care is taken to avoid damaging the underlying segmental blood vessels, which are located at the midportion of the vertebral body and lie transverse to the direction of the incision. The pleura is dissected bluntly and elevated off of the vertebrae. Once the segmental vessels have been identified, they are carefully ligated with endoclips and divided. The pleura is incised with the Harmonic scalpel along the proximal portion of the ribs of the involved vertebral bodies, as well as the vertebrae one level above and below the lesion. Continuing the exposure in a mediolateral direction and elevating the pleural flap exposes the underlying tumor, lateral vertebral body wall, and intervertebral discs. Wide exposures may be required, depending on the extent of tumor involvement.

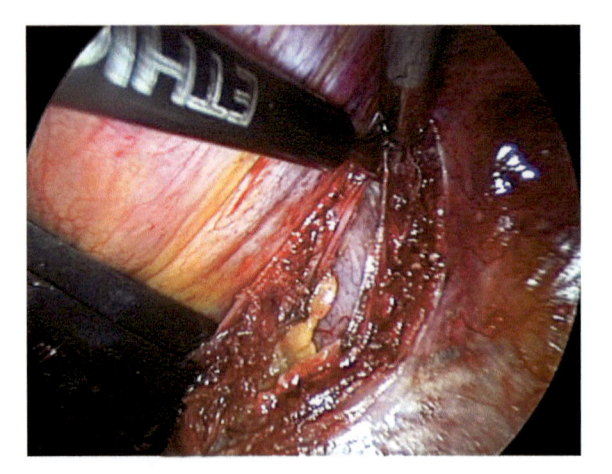

Fig. 35-3 The diaphragm is incised with a Harmonic scalpel when operating at or below the site of insertion. The incision is made approximately 1 to 2 cm away from and parallel to the insertion site, where the diaphragm is naturally thin.

PLACEMENT OF VERTEBRAL BODY SCREWS

Once adequate exposure has been achieved, the surgeon proceeds with placement of the vertebral body screws, which is followed by tumor resection, decompression, alignment correction, and reconstruction. Screws for the MACS-TL endoscopic plating system are placed in the uninvolved vertebral bodies above and below the diseased levels. Attention is first directed to the caudal level, where the first posterior polyaxial screw will be placed. The lower-level screws are placed first because this keeps the surgical field visually free and avoids the need to look over a cranially placed screw. The entry point for the screw is in the upper third of the vertebral body, approximately 10 mm away from the endplate, avoiding the segmental blood vessels located along the midportion of the vertebrae, and approximately 10 mm anterior to the spinal canal (Fig. 35-4, *A*). The radiolucent targeting device loaded with a short Kirschner wire (K-wire) is placed perpendicular to the cortical surface under fluoroscopic guidance. The K-wire will appear on end, and the concentric ring on the device will align when the proper perpendicular position is achieved (Fig. 35-4, *B*). The targeting device is impacted with a mallet, and the K-wire is detached from the instrument once it has been stably inserted into the bone, approximately 25 mm deep (Fig. 35-4, *C*). With

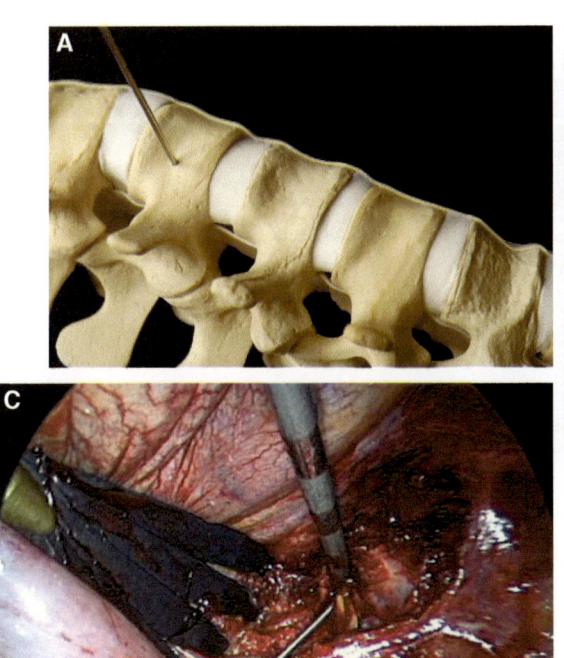

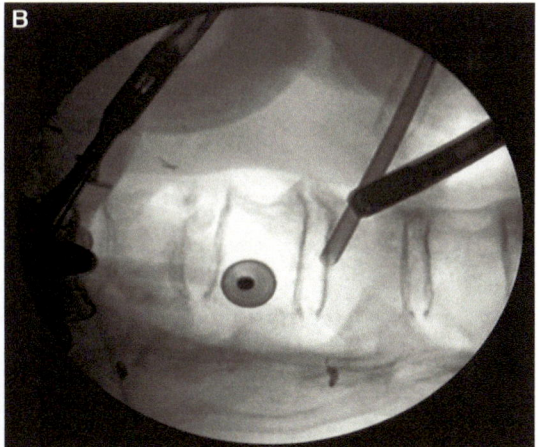

Fig. 35-4 **A,** The entry point for the caudal screw is in the upper third of the vertebral body, approximately 10 mm away from the endplate and 10 mm anterior to the spinal canal, which is demonstrated with a K-wire in a saw bone model. **B,** The radiolucent targeting device loaded with a short K-wire is placed perpendicular to the cortical surface under fluoroscopic guidance. The K-wire will appear on end, and the concentric ring on the device will align when the proper perpendicular position is achieved. **C,** The targeting device is impacted with a mallet, and the K-wire is detached from the instrument once it has been stably inserted into the bone.

Continued

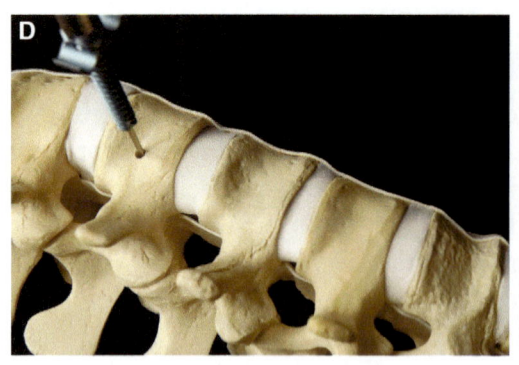

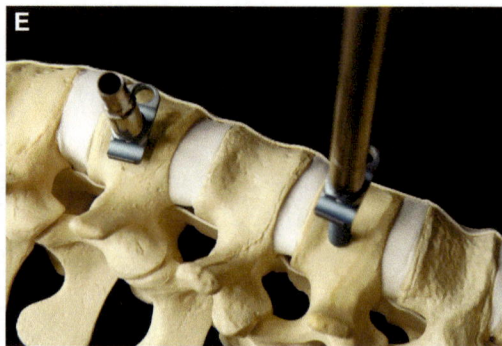

Fig. 35-4, cont'd **D,** The screw clamp assembly is inserted over the K-wire, and the holes for the anterior stabilizing screws are placed ventrally. Placement of the screws into the caudal level is performed first, which keeps the surgical field clear for instrumentation at the cranial level. **E,** The screw clamp assembly is placed into the cranial level in the inferior third of the vertebral body, approximately 10 mm anterior to the spinal canal and 10 mm away from the endplate.

the K-wire in place, the entry point is decorticated with a cannulated awl to prepare for screw insertion.

The MACS-TL screws are attached to a polyaxial clamp before insertion. The screw clamp assembly is inserted over the K-wire while attached to a centralizer tube, with the hole for the anterior stabilizing screw placed ventrally (Fig. 35-4, *D*). As noted earlier, the lengths of the screws are determined preoperatively by measuring the width of the vertebral bodies to be instrumented. After the screw is firmly engaged past the cortical surface with the first few turns of the screwdriver, the K-wire is removed by a clockwise turn of the removal instrument. The screw can then be inserted safely to its full depth without concern for K-wire advancement and the possibility of soft tissue and vascular perforation.

Attention is now turned to the cranially located vertebral body. A similar technique is used to insert the screw in the inferior third of the vertebral body approximately 10 mm anterior to the spinal canal and 10 mm cranial to the inferior endplate (Fig. 35-4, *E*).

TUMOR AND VERTEBRAL BODY RESECTION

Spine tumors can extensively invade the involved vertebral body, pedicles, proximal rib, spinal canal, and surrounding structures. The boundaries of the corpectomy are defined by the intervertebral discs cranially and caudally. The clamps attached to the screw heads are oriented parallel to the endplates, with the holes for the stabilizing screws situated anteriorly. These define the anteromedial and posterolateral borders of an area that includes both the extent of the corpectomy and a safety zone (Fig. 35-5, *A*) that protects critical structures. The resection is performed by keeping instruments within these safe boundaries.

The discectomies are performed endoscopically at the disc spaces above and below the lesion, similar to an open procedure. First, annulectomies are performed with an endoscopic scalpel, and the discs are resected with endoscopic rongeurs. The endplates are prepared by removing any attached cartilage and soft tissue. The tumor and vertebral bodies between the resected disc spaces are removed next by performing a central corpectomy. A rectangular trough is created with osteotomes in the vertebral bodies and extended with curettes, rongeurs, or a high-speed burr (Fig. 35-5, *B*). The anterior, posterior, and contralateral cortices are preserved. Tissue and bone samples are sent for preservation as frozen-section and permanent pathology specimens. The corpectomy cavity is enlarged until normal, vascularized bone can be seen. Intraoperative fluoroscopy is used to confirm the corpectomy depth across the midline.

Decompression of the spinal canal is necessary for tumors extending past the posterior vertebral body wall. To access the anterior spinal canal, the ipsilateral rib head and/or pedicle are identified and removed. The rib head is visualized and followed to the anterolateral spine at its attachment, and the proximal 2 cm are removed with a high-speed drill. The underlying pedicle is now exposed and may be further defined with a blunt hook. Resection is performed with the high-speed drill and endoscopic rongeurs. This maneuver decompresses the neuroforamen and simultaneously allows access to the anterior spinal canal (Fig. 35-5, *C*). Tumor and bone fragments in the epidural space are carefully brought into the corpectomy cavity and removed. The thecal sac overlying the anterior spinal cord can be viewed directly and avoided during this process. The resection is complete when gross tumor is removed, the anterior spinal canal is decompressed, and the corpectomy adequately accommodates the interbody device.

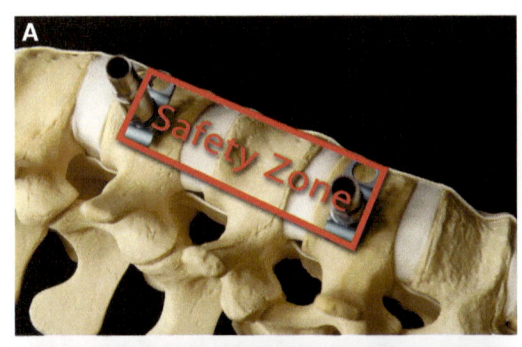

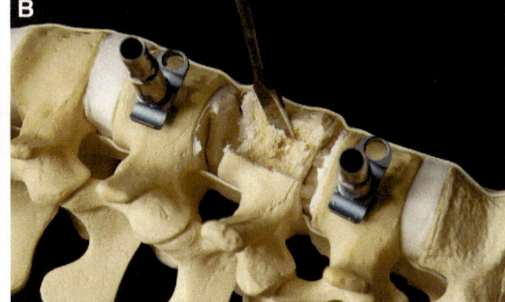

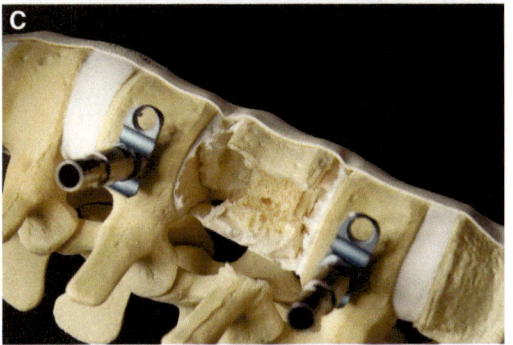

Fig. 35-5 **A,** The borders of the clamps define a safety zone and the extent of corpectomy. The resection is performed within these safe boundaries. **B,** The corpectomy is performed by creating a rectangular trough with osteotomes, curettes, rongeurs, or a high-speed burr. **C,** The rib head and pedicle may be removed for visualization and decompression of the anterior spinal canal.

Endoscopic Vertebral Body Reconstruction and Stabilization

After tumor resection, spinal cord decompression, and corpectomy, an anterolateral vertebral body reconstruction is performed. We prefer to use an expandable titanium cage as the interbody device. The dimensions of the corpectomy cavity are measured with calipers, the working portal is removed, and the expandable cage is inserted through a speculum through the working portal site. Once it has been inserted, the cage is expanded with endoscopic and fluoroscopic visualization, noting its position in the coronal and sagittal planes. Allograft or normal autologous morselized bone may be placed in and around the cage to promote fusion.

Fitting and securing the anterolateral plate completes the reconstruction. The distance between the screw heads is measured, and a suitable plate length is selected by adding 30 mm to the measurement. The plate is dropped over the caudal screw clamp assembly first and then fitted over the cranial assembly (Fig. 35-6, *A*). The screws are left slightly loose to allow angulation of the polyaxial heads while fitting the plate. Fixation nuts are placed and secured over the plates with a torque handle, and the centralizer attached to the polyaxial clamp is removed (Fig. 35-6, *B*).

Final fixation is performed by tightening the construct, inserting the anterior stabilizing screws, and locking the polyaxial screws. First the polyaxial screws are tightened to their final positions, bringing them in direct contact with the vertebral bodies and eliminating the rotational freedom previously preserved for plate placement. The screw guide sleeve is then attached to the polyaxial clamp, and bone is decorticated with the decorticator through the guiding sleeve and anterior hole in the clamp. An

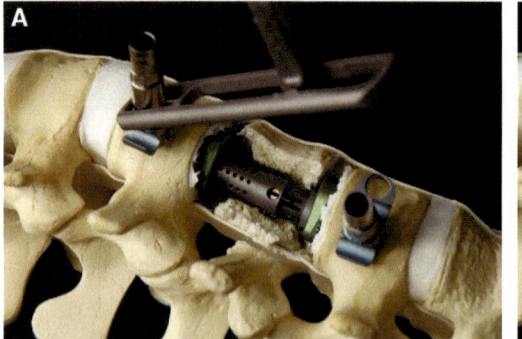

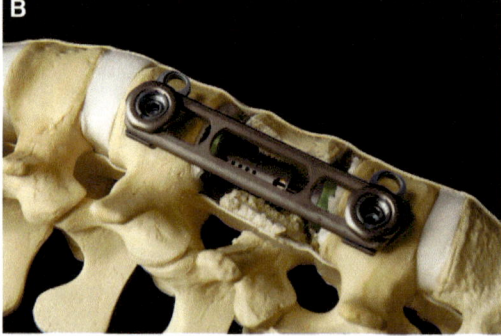

Fig. 35-6 **A,** The plate is placed over the caudal screw clamp assembly and then fitted over the cranial assembly, with the screws left slightly loose to allow angulation of the polyaxial heads. **B,** Fixation nuts are secured on the screw clamp assembly over the plate with a torque handle, and the centralizers attached to the polyaxial clamps are removed after the fixation nuts are secured. The entire assembly is then tightened, bringing the construct in direct contact with the vertebral bodies.

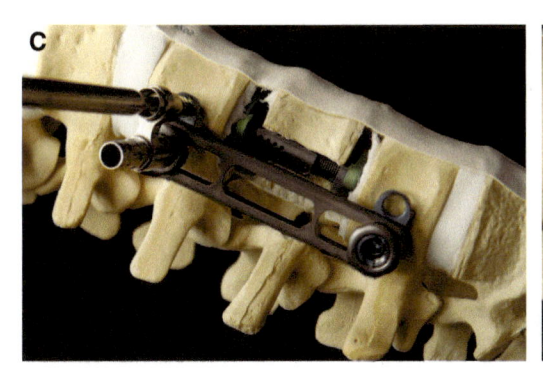

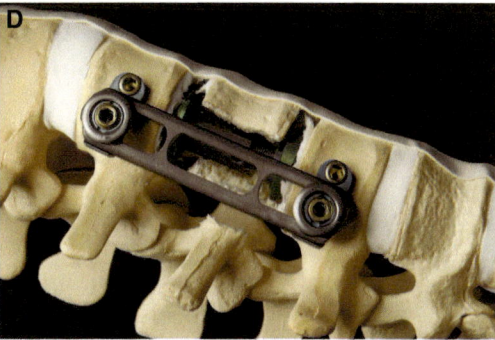

Fig. 35-6, cont'd **C,** Anterior stabilizing screws are placed through the screw guide sleeve after decortication through the anterior hole in the clamp. **D,** Locking screws are inserted over the polyaxial screw head and tightened with a torque wrench, which completes the construct.

appropriate length is selected for the anterior stabilizing screw, which is inserted into the vertebral body with a driver (Fig. 35-6, *C*). The guiding sleeve is then removed. The construct is completed by inserting the yellow locking screw over the polyaxial head and locking it in place with a torque wrench, which converts the polyaxial screw clamp system into a rigid construct. The final position of the construct is verified by means of anteroposterior and lateral fluoroscopic imaging (Fig. 35-6, *D*).

CHEST TUBE PLACEMENT AND CLOSURE

Closure of the operative site begins with reapproximation of the diaphragm. The retractors are rearranged to expose the incision, which is closed with staples or interrupted, absorbable sutures. The thoracic cavity is inspected for hemostasis and irrigated, removing visible blood clots. A 24 Fr chest tube is inserted through the more ventrally located lung/diaphragm retractor portal or the suction/irrigation portal. Placement is performed under endoscopic visualization with the end of the chest tube directed at the apex of the chest cavity. The lung is reinflated and inspected endoscopically to ensure that all lobes are properly inflated. The trocars are removed, and the incisions are closed in multiple layers. The chest tube is secured, and a chest radiograph is obtained immediately to verify lung inflation.

The patient is extubated immediately after surgery. The chest tube is connected to intermittent wall suction initially and advanced to water seal if the chest radiograph demonstrates proper lung inflation on postoperative day 1. Postoperative CT scans and plain radiographs centered on the construct are obtained. Patient mobilization and incentive spirometry training also begin on postoperative day 1. The chest tube is removed once the output decreases below 100 ml/day, and chest radiography continues to demonstrate lung inflation without pneumothorax, typically on postoperative day 2. After removal of the chest tube, a final chest radiograph is used to verify stable lung inflation. Before the patient is discharged from the hospital, plans are made for treatment and follow-up with oncology and radiation oncology services, if needed.

The patient returns to the clinic at 1-, 3-, 6-, 12-, and 24-month intervals for follow-up examination and plain radiographs. The patient is typically allowed to return to work with light activity after 4 weeks and full activity after 3 months.

OUTCOMES AND EVALUATION OF RESULTS
Results

Operative results for the minimally invasive thoracoscopic approach have demonstrated its efficacy and safety and are generally better than those associated with open surgery. Operative times initially increase to an average of 6 hours or more while the surgeon and operating room staff learn the new technique.[8,12,15-18] Incising and reattaching the diaphragm may add an additional 30 minutes to the surgery. The duration of surgery for tumor resection and reconstruction is decreased to 4 hours for the entire procedure after the technique has been mastered.[15] The estimated blood loss has been reported to be 600 ml in thoracoscopic tumor surgery,[15] compared with 1.0 L during open thoracotomy.[7] With care, intraoperative complications such as uncontrollable bleeding, cerebrospinal fluid or chyle leaks, or injuries to the vessels or viscera can largely be avoided.[15] The rate of conversion to an open procedure in skilled hands and with meticulous adherence to surgical technique is 1% or less.[17]

The principal advantages of thoracoscopic surgery are the favorable clinical outcomes. The overall morbidity is low, primarily because of the limited surgical exposure and approach. Although the morbidity rate for all open thoracotomy procedures ranges from 14% to 29.5%,[7,16-18,26] with tumor surgery having a higher incidence than other open procedures, the complication rates for the thoracoscopic procedure range from 0% to 5.4%.[12,15-18] Reported complications include persistent pleural effusion and pneumonia, intercostal neuralgia, shoulder dysfunction, and transient L1 deficit. Furthermore, open thoracotomy for tumor has a reported mortality rate of 8.2%,[7] whereas no deaths have been reported with the thoracoscopic approach.[15,16] Infection rates are low for both thoracotomy and thoracoscopic surgery, approximately 0.5%.[16-18]

Patients have a significant reduction in pain postoperatively with minimally invasive thoracoscopic surgery.[15] Duration and dosages of postoperative analgesic therapy have been reported to decrease by 31% and 42%, respectively.[16-18] Rates of chronic postoperative pain after thoracoscopic surgery range from 4% to 35%, which compares favorably with reported rates of 7% and 55% for open thoracotomy.[18] The median length of stay in the hospital was 7 days (range 4 to 10 days) in a series of patients who underwent thoracoscopic tumor surgery,[15] compared with a median of 9 days (range 4 to 57 days) for patients who underwent open thoracotomy for tumor resection.[7] With the use of the MACS-TL plating system for anterolateral instrumentation, fusion rates of up to 90% have been reported at 1-year radiographic follow-up.[17]

COMPLICATIONS

Significant intraoperative complications are uncommon. Injury to the internal organs and great vessels has been reported but rarely occurs.[10,12,14,15] The most hazardous complications include injury to the aorta or vena cava, which may occur directly when sharp instruments are used with excessive force or indirectly through tearing of the segmental vessels. Intraoperative fluoroscopy is used to gauge the depth of corpectomy and ensure that the opposite cortex, which may be overlain by vascular structures, is not breached. Insufficient exposure and coagulation of the segmental vessels may also result in significant blood loss. The lung parenchyma may sustain local injury, which is typically sufficiently treated with suturing or stapling. The spleen, kidneys, and ureters may be injured through the diaphragm with aggressive diaphragmatic incisions or retraction. When injuries or hemostasis cannot be adequately addressed thoracoscopically, conversion to an open thoracotomy with the assistance of a cardiothoracic surgeon is necessary.

Neural structures are also at risk during thoracoscopic procedures. Overaggressive maneuvers during anterior spinal canal decompression can lead to dural tears or spinal cord injury. Conversely, an inadequate decompression can lead to these same injuries from forced impaction of the interbody device into a smaller corpectomy resection cavity. The risk of wound breakdown and infection is significantly increased with persistent spinal fluid leaks. Every effort should be made to create a watertight dural closure if a defect is discovered intraoperatively. If a defect is discovered postoperatively, the chest tube should be kept on no more than 20 cm H_2O suction and changed to water seal as soon as possible to prevent formation of a cerebrospinal fluid fistula. Damage to the spinal cord is most likely during the corpectomy, decompression, and reconstruction. The exiting nerve roots may be injured during the exposure with excessive electrocautery.

Early postoperative complications are generally pulmonary and include atelectasis, pleural effusions, persistent pneumothorax, hemothorax, and pneumonia.[16-18] Intrathoracic adhesions may also form over time. Intercostal neuralgia and, rarely, shoulder dysfunction may develop in patients who undergo thoracoscopic procedures, although the incidence is lower than that seen in patients who undergo open thoracotomy. Wound infection, both superficial and deep, and dehiscence are risks associated with any surgery, and the risk can be decreased with proper multilevel closure. Although significant advances have been made in minimally invasive technology, instrumentation failure remains a potential late complication, which may be particularly increased in cancer patients with poor bone quality from tumor burden or treatment. Potential instrumentation complications include hardware loosening, pullout, or fracture, which may be prevented with improved surgical technique and choice of reconstruction. If significant osteoporotic bone is encountered intraoperatively, posterior instrumentation increases construct stability and may be necessary to supplement anterior endoscopic reconstruction.[27]

SIGNATURE CASES

A 61-year-old man with a 1-year history of untreated prostate adenocarcinoma was seen in the emergency department with severe back pain, lower extremity weakness and paresthesias, and difficulty walking, which had worsened over 2 weeks. He denied having bowel and bladder dysfunction. On examination the patient reported severe (8/10) thoracolumbar pain on a visual analog scale. He was nonambulatory with diffuse weakness (4/5) of the bilateral lower extremities, corresponding to a Frankel classification grade C. Thoracic spine imaging demonstrated a T10 pathologic burst fracture with canal compromise of approximately 80% on CT scans, and spinal cord compression and edema on MRI (Fig. 35-7, *A* and *B*). Multiple additional cervical and thoracic spinal metastases, without spinal canal compromise, were also present on MRI.

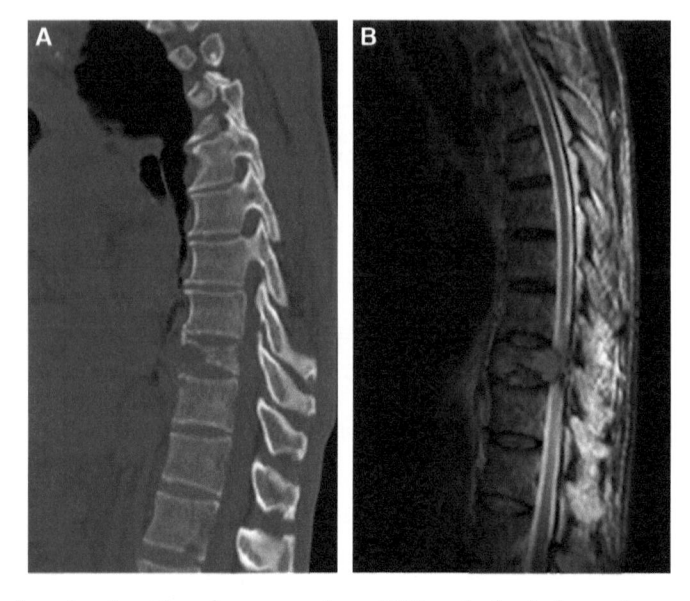

Fig. 35-7 Thoracic spine imaging demonstrating a T10 pathologic burst fracture with canal compromise of approximately 80% on **A,** CT scan and **B,** spinal cord compression with edema on MRI.

The patient underwent a right T10 thoracoscopic corpectomy and reconstruction with a Synex interbody expandable cage (Synthes, West Chester, PA) and T9 to T11 anterolateral instrumentation with the MACS-TL plating system. The postoperative CT scan demonstrated decompression of the spinal cord and reconstruction of the spinal column (Fig. 35-7, C through F). Pathologic examination was consistent with adenocarcinoma. On postoperative day 2 the chest tube was removed. The patient had recovery of lower extremity strength and improvement of back pain. At the time of transfer to the oncology service for spinal radiation treatment on postoperative day 4, the patient was able to walk with a cane. The minithoracotomy incisions were healing well (Fig. 35-7, G). The patient was discharged to home with plans for follow-up treatment with the medical oncology team; however, shortly thereafter, he moved out of state.

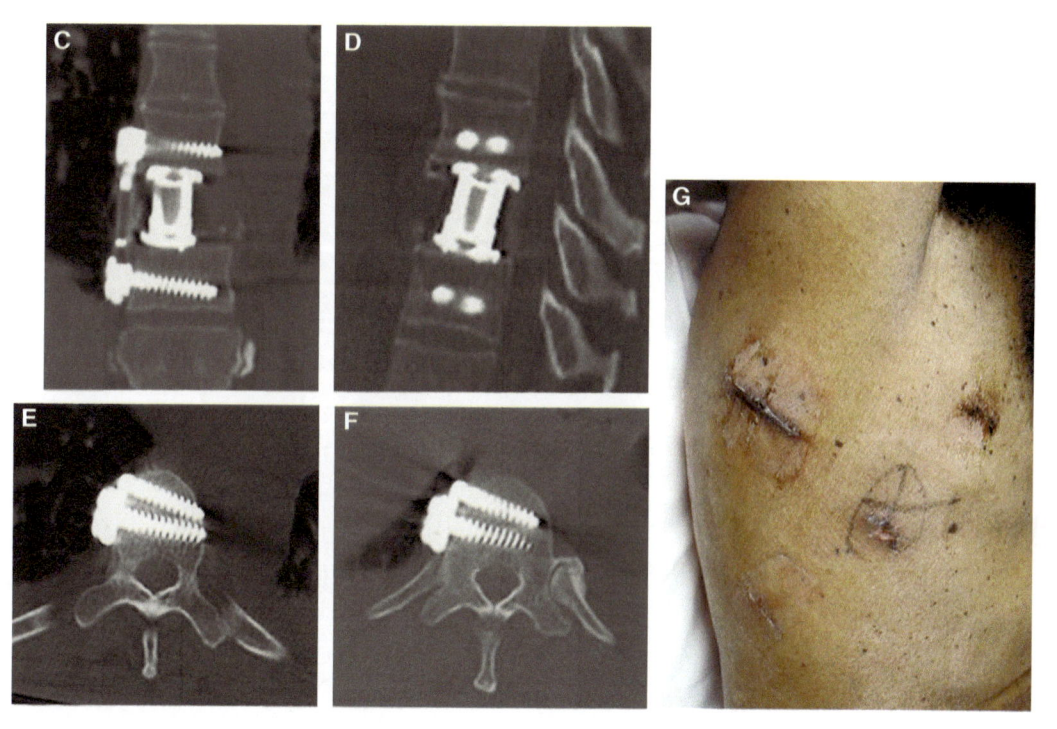

Fig. 35-7, cont'd Postoperative CT scans: **C,** coronal; **D,** sagittal; and **E** and **F,** axial images demonstrating the final construct after right T10 thoracoscopic corpectomy and reconstruction. **G,** Minithoracotomy incisions are seen on postoperative day 4.

A 54-year-old man with a 1-year history of lung cancer initially was seen in the neurosurgery clinic with back pain. He was found to have metastatic spine disease involving multiple levels of the thoracolumbar spine. The other neurologic findings were unremarkable, and he was treated initially with radiation therapy from T11 to L5, which was followed by chemotherapy. He initially had mild improvement of the pain, but the pain worsened several months after treatment, corresponding to a visual analog score of 5/10 despite treatment with narcotic medication. CT imaging of the thoracic spine demonstrated a lytic lesion and pathologic burst fracture of T12 without spinal cord compression on MRI (Fig. 35-8, *A* and *B*).

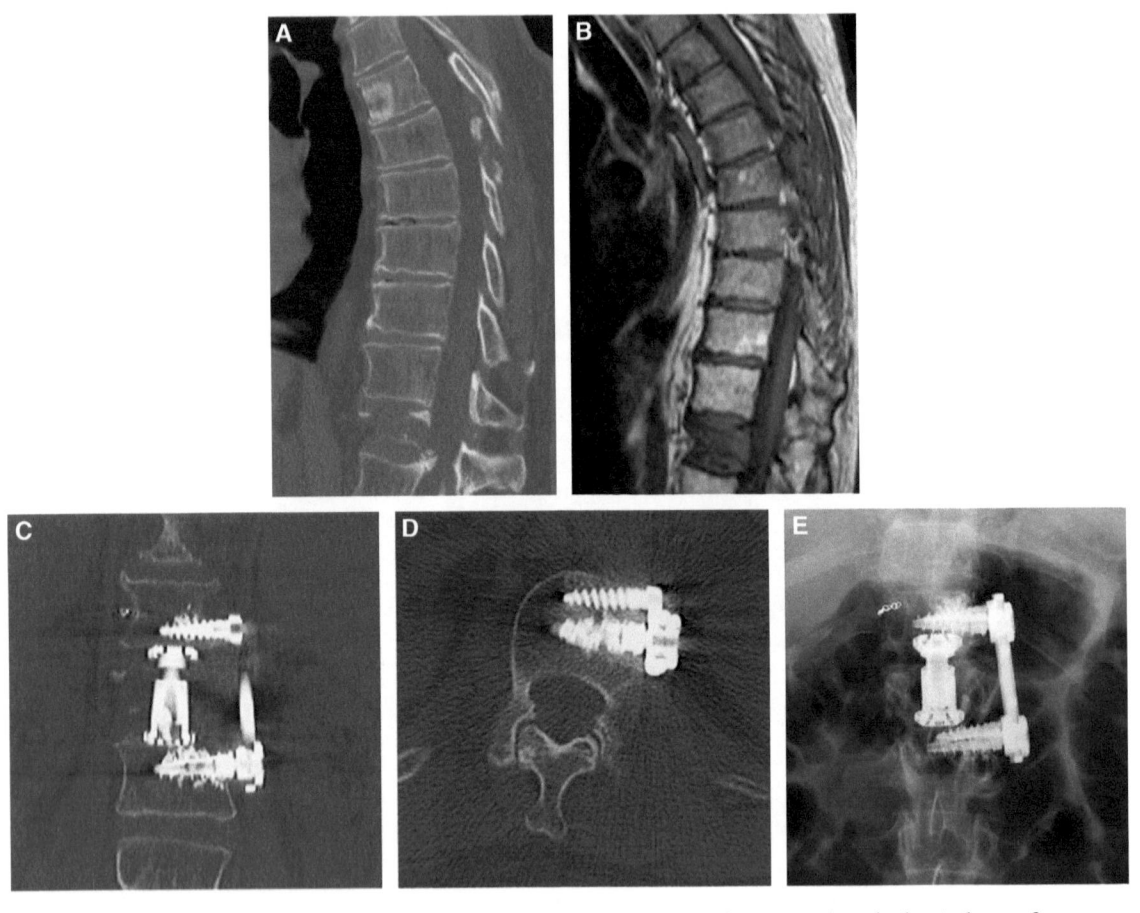

Fig. 35-8 Imaging of the thoracic spine demonstrating a lytic lesion and pathologic burst fracture of T12 on **A,** CT scan and **B,** without spinal cord compression on MRI. Postoperative imaging: **C,** coronal and **D,** axial CT scans and **E,** anteroposterior radiograph demonstrating the final construct after left T12 thoracoscopic corpectomy and reconstruction with cementable polyaxial screw MACS-XL screws. The injected polymethylmethacrylate cement is seen surrounding the screws.

The patient was admitted to the hospital and underwent successful preoperative embolization of the tumor arterial supply. On the second day after admission, he underwent a left T12 thoracoscopic corpectomy and reconstruction with a Synex II expandable cage. Intraoperatively the bone was found to be significantly osteoporotic from his prior treatments. Cementable polyaxial screw MACS-XL screws (Aesculap) were placed into the polyaxial clamps and used in place of the standard MACS-TL screws (Fig. 35-8, *C* through *E*). After the construct was placed and tightened, 1.5 ml of polymethylmethacrylate cement was placed into each screw. Results of pathologic examination were consistent with metastatic poorly differentiated carcinoma.

The patient had improved back pain postoperatively and remained neurologically intact. His chest tube was removed on postoperative day 1. He was discharged to home on postoperative day 3. At his 1-year follow-up visit, the patient showed continued improvement in back pain (visual analog score 3/10) and was taking no narcotic medications. The overall construct remained intact, with mild subsidence of the interbody cage. With continued chemotherapy the patient had stable metastatic disease.

CONCLUSION

Endoscopic technology and surgical techniques have advanced significantly in recent years and continue to be improved and refined. Once rarely used for tumor treatment, minimally invasive thoracoscopic surgery is now one of the standard procedures for resection of thoracolumbar spine tumors of the vertebral body and anterior spinal canal. The development of endoscopic spinal instrumentation has made anterior stabilization and reconstruction possible, in addition to decompression. The thoracoscopic approach is safe and effective and has decreased postoperative morbidity and complication rates when compared with open thoracotomy. With proper patient selection, knowledge of local and patient-specific anatomy, and familiarity with the surgical technique, the surgeon is able to successfully treat a variety of thoracolumbar spine tumors with this minimally invasive endoscopic technique.

BAILOUT TECHNIQUES

- Ease or difficulty of an operation is largely determined during the initial setup. Positioning the patient and accessing portals correctly is extremely important for the successful completion of the remainder of the operation. By using the C-arm fluoroscope, the endplates and edges of the vertebral bodies of interest are inspected to ensure that no overlap is present, which indicates that the patient is positioned with the spine in a true lateral position. This ensures that the instruments and instrumentation are aimed perpendicular to the spine. Incorrect positioning may lead to inaccurate screw placement and potential injury. The portals

Continued

are placed with sufficient distance between them to avoid instrument conflicts during the operation.
- Being mindful of the surrounding anatomy during the exposure decreases the chances of complications and injury. The monopolar electrocautery is used with care when nearing the segmental blood vessels. Unsuccessful identification and ligation of these vessels can lead to significant hemorrhage. Damage to the nerve roots is also possible with electrocautery, which should not be used posterior to the vertebral body. If the surgeon encounters significant bleeding or injury to the internal organs at any point during the operation, conversion to an open thoracotomy with the assistance of a cardiothoracic surgeon is warranted. This transition can be aided by early intervention and preoperative coordination.
- Once the exposure is complete, the corpectomy must be adequately sized for the interbody implant. The clamps attached to the screws act as landmarks to define both a safety zone for operating and the corpectomy borders. During the resection the extent of corpectomy can be seen with the fluoroscope or measured directly by filling the corpectomy bed with irrigation fluid and placing a scaled instrument on the defect floor. This measurement is then compared with preoperative measurements of the vertebral body width and planned corpectomy. Once adequate, the interbody device can be placed into the corpectomy cavity with ease, avoiding the unnecessary force that can damage the dura and spinal cord.
- Endoscopic fusion can be relatively complex compared with other techniques, and thus it is important that each step be performed in the specified order and with attention to technical details. The operation is performed more smoothly if preoperative measurements of the vertebral bodies and screws are available and communicated to the surgical staff. The instrumentation can then be optimally prepared before placement, which decreases lag time and increases operative efficiency.
- For patients with poor bone quality as a result of cancer, radiation, or chemotherapy, cementable screws provide increased fixation strength and spinal stability[28,29] (Fig. 35-9). These hollow screws have been designed with increased thread diam-

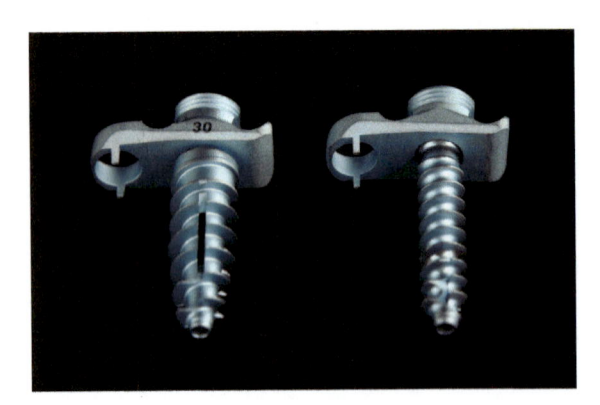

Fig. 35-9 Cementable screws *(left)* have increased thread diameter and pitch compared with standard screws *(right)* to decrease screw pullout. The cementable screws have a hollow core with three longitudinal slits through which 1.5 ml of injectable cement is delivered into the surrounding bone. The cement is injected just before the final step of securing the locking nuts, after the construct is flush against the vertebral bodies and tightened into its final position.

eter and pitch to decrease screw pullout and with three longitudinal slits through which the injectable cement is delivered into the surrounding bone. The screws are inserted into the polyaxial clamps in place of the posterolateral MACS-TL screws, and the same technique is used for implantation. Once the resection and reconstruction have been completed and just before the final step of securing the locking nuts, 1.5 ml of cement is injected through the hollow screw head. After the cement is delivered and allowed to harden, the locking nuts are secured and the construct is complete. It is important to note that the construct must be flush against the bone and in its final position, with all screws and nuts tightened, before the cement is injected. Once the screws are cemented, it is extremely difficult to adjust the construct position.

TIPS FROM THE MASTERS

- Preoperative embolization can limit the blood loss with vascular tumors such as renal cell carcinoma.
- If thoracoscopic surgery is complicated by bleeding or other unexpected difficulties, we recommend early conversion to an open procedure.
- If the bone quality is extremely poor, posterior fixation should be considered.

References (With Key References in Boldface)

1. Grant R, Papadopoulos SM, Greenberg HS. Metastatic epidural spinal cord compression. Neurol Clin 9:825-841, 1991.
2. Grant R, Papadopoulos SM, Sandler HM, et al. Metastatic epidural spinal cord compression: current concepts and treatment. J Neurooncol 19:79-92, 1994.
3. Jacobs WB, Perrin RG. Evaluation and treatment of spinal metastases: an overview. Neurosurg Focus 11:E10, 2001.
4. Klimo P Jr, Kestle JR, Schmidt MH. Treatment of metastatic spinal epidural disease: a review of the literature. Neurosurg Focus 15:E1, 2003.
5. Gokaslan ZL, York JE, Walsh GL, et al. Transthoracic vertebrectomy for metastatic spinal tumors. J Neurosurg 89:599-609, 1998.
6. Schwarzenbach O, Boos N, Aebi M. [Spinal metastases and metastasis-induced pathological fractures of the spine] Unfallchirurg 93:457-466, 1990.
7. Walsh GL, Gokaslan ZL, McCutcheon IE, et al. Anterior approaches to the thoracic spine in patients with cancer: indications and results. Ann Thorac Surg 64:1611-1618, 1997.
8. Amini A, Beisse R, Schmidt MH. Thoracoscopic spine surgery for decompression and stabilization of the anterolateral thoracolumbar spine. Neurosurg Focus 19:E4, 2005.
9. Beisse R. Video-assisted techniques in the management of thoracolumbar fractures. Orthop Clin North Am 38:419-429; abstract vii, 2007.
10. **Beisse R, Muckley T, Schmidt MH, et al. Surgical technique and results of endoscopic anterior spinal canal decompression. J Neurosurg Spine 2:128-136, 2005.**
11. Caputy A, Starr J, Riedel C. Video-assisted endoscopic spinal surgery: thoracoscopic discectomy. Acta Neurochir (Wien) 134:196-199, 1995.

12. Khoo LT, Beisse R, Potulski M. Thoracoscopic-assisted treatment of thoracic and lumbar fractures: a series of 371 consecutive cases. Neurosurgery 51:S104-S117, 2002.
13. McAfee PC, Regan JR, Fedder IL, et al. Anterior thoracic corpectomy for spinal cord decompression performed endoscopically. Surg Laparosc Endosc 5:339-348, 1995.
14. Schultheiss M, Kinzl L, Claes L, et al. Minimally invasive ventral spondylodesis for thoracolumbar fracture treatment: surgical technique and first clinical outcome. Eur Spine J 12:618-624, 2003.
15. Kan P, Schmidt MH. Minimally invasive thoracoscopic approach for anterior decompression and stabilization of metastatic spine disease. Neurosurg Focus 25:E8, 2008.
16. Beisse R. Thoracoscopically assisted anterior approach to thoracolumbar fractures. In Mayer HM, ed. Minimally Invasive Spine Surgery: A Surgical Manual. New York: Springer, 2005, pp 203-214.
17. Beisse R. Thoracoscopic decompression and fixation (MACS-TL). In Kim D, Fessler RG, Regan JJ, eds. Endoscopic Spine Surgery and Instrumentation. New York: Thieme, 2004, pp 180-198.
18. Beisse R. Endoscopic anterior repair in spinal trauma. In Regan JJ, Lieberman IH, eds. Atlas of Minimal Access Spine Surgery, 2nd ed. St Louis: Quality Medical Publishing, 2004, pp 285-320.
19. Heary RF, Bono CM. Metastatic spinal tumors. Neurosurg Focus 11:E1, 2001.
20. Hosono N, Yonenobu K, Fuji T, et al. Orthopaedic management of spinal metastases. Clin Orthop Relat Res:148-159, 1995.
21. Klimo P Jr, Thompson CJ, Kestle JR, et al. A meta-analysis of surgery versus conventional radiotherapy for the treatment of metastatic spinal epidural disease. Neuro Oncol 7:64-76, 2005.
22. Witham TF, Khavkin YA, Gallia GL, et al. Surgery insight: current management of epidural spinal cord compression from metastatic spine disease. Nat Clin Pract Neurol 2:87-94; quiz 116, 2006.
23. Schultheiss M, Hartwig E, Kinzl L, et al. Thoracolumbar fracture stabilization: comparative biomechanical evaluation of a new video-assisted implantable system. Eur Spine J 13:93-100, 2004.
24. Schultheiss M, Hartwig E, Sarkar M, et al. Biomechanical in vitro comparison of different mono- and bisegmental anterior procedures with regard to the strategy for fracture stabilisation using minimally invasive techniques. Eur Spine J 15:82-89, 2006.
25. Schreiber U, Bence T, Grupp T, et al. Is a single anterolateral screw-plate fixation sufficient for the treatment of spinal fractures in the thoracolumbar junction? A biomechanical in vitro investigation. Eur Spine J 14:197-204, 2005.
26. Oskouian RJ Jr, Johnson JP. Vascular complications in anterior thoracolumbar spinal reconstruction. J Neurosurg 96:1-5, 2002.
27. Bishop FS, Samuelson MM, Finn MA, et al. The biomechanical contribution of varying posterior constructs following anterior thoracolumbar corpectomy and reconstruction. J Neurosurg Spine 13:234-239, 2010.
28. Schultheiss M, Claes L, Wilke HJ, et al. Enhanced primary stability through additional cementable cannulated rescue screw for anterior thoracolumbar plate application. J Neurosurg 98:50-55, 2003.
29. Schultheiss M, Hartwig E, Claes L, et al. Influence of screw-cement enhancement on the stability of anterior thoracolumbar fracture stabilization with circumferential instability. Eur Spine J 13:598-604, 2004.

Chapter 36

Sagittal Osteotomy for En Bloc Resection of Lateralized Tumors of the Lumbar Spine

S. Samuel Bederman, Christopher P. Ames, Vedat Deviren

Bone tumors are classified as either benign or malignant, based on their potential for local invasion and distant spread. Malignant tumors can be primary (arising from the local cells) or metastatic. Less than 5% of all tumors of the spinal column are considered primary malignancies, and metastatic disease comprises the vast majority of spinal column tumors.[1]

Some examples of primary malignant tumors of bone include osteosarcoma, chondrosarcoma, fibrosarcoma, angiosarcoma, chordoma, Ewing's sarcoma, lymphoma, and myeloma, and they are often categorized by their matrix histology. Each tumor may have different affinities for differing treatment modalities, namely, chemotherapy, radiation, or surgery. However, most primary malignant tumors of bone require complete surgical resection. Although deaths from benign tumors are rare, mortality rates are highly dependent on the type of tumor, as well as the extent of resection.[2] Intralesional resection carries a fivefold increase in local recurrence rates and a 5-year survival rate of less than 50%, compared with 80% for en bloc excision.[3,4] Enneking[5] established the classification system for tumors affecting the appendicular skeleton and introduced the concept of intracompartmental and extracompartmental disease.

The Weinstein-Boriani-Biagini (WBB) surgical staging system is the most widely used classification system for spine tumors.[6] This classification system (Fig. 36-1) is based on the anatomic location of the tumor as it relates to regions of the vertebrae. Each vertebra is divided into 12 arcs similar to the face of a clock centered on the spinal canal, with the 12 o'clock position at the spinous process and five circumferential layers, labeled from A to E, in a superficial to deep direction. Although adjuvant treatment, such as chemotherapy and radiation therapy, is of paramount importance in treating many malignancies, rates of survival and local recurrence are also highly dependent on the type of surgical resection. Surgical resection can be considered either intralesional or en bloc, based on whether the resection respects the margins of the tumor. Intralesional resections occur when the margin of the resection violates the tumor, whereas en bloc resections are complete resections that leave no detectable tumor behind. Because of the proximity of vital structures, such as nerves and vessels, en bloc resection of bone tumors, although it maintains limb function, is challenging. In the spinal column, en bloc resections present even more difficulties because of the intimate anatomic relationships between the osseous and neural structures.

Most benign tumors that require surgical resection are amenable to intralesional strategies, whereas widely metastatic lesions are often not considered curable. In metastatic disease the surgical goals are mainly palliative, targeting either decompression for nerve or spinal cord compression or stabilization for mechanical pain, instability, or progressive deformity. The goal of surgical treatment for most primary malignancies, to lower the risk of local recurrence and increase the chance of disease-free survival, is complete (en bloc) resection.

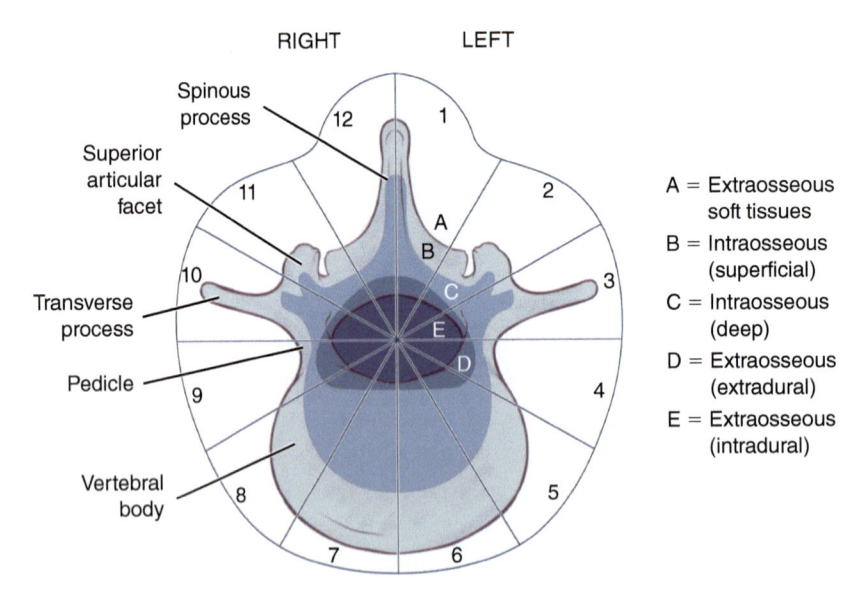

Fig. 36-1 Weinstein-Boriani-Biagini surgical staging system. (Modified from Boriani S, Weinstein J, Biagini R. Primary bone tumors of the spine. Terminology and surgical staging. Spine 22:1036-1044, 1997.)

Many strategies aimed at achieving en bloc resection of spine tumors have been developed, but the specific technique used must be selected on the basis of careful evaluation of the patient, the lesion, and the surrounding anatomy, and is therefore individualized to each patient.[7-14] Sagittal osteotomy for en bloc resection is one strategy that has been developed for lateralized tumors of the thoracic and lumbar spine.

INDICATIONS AND CONTRAINDICATIONS

The indications for sagittal osteotomy for en bloc resection of lateralized spine tumors include the following tumors that require complete negative-margin resection:
- Primary malignancies of the spinal column
- Certain benign aggressive lesions (e.g., giant cell tumors)
- Certain solitary metastatic malignancies (e.g., single renal metastasis)

Contraindications include the following:
- Primary bone tumors with widespread metastases
- Primary bone tumors amenable to adjuvant therapy alone (e.g., myeloma and lymphoma)
- Patients who are deemed medically unfit for major surgery
- Tumor invasion into both pedicles or involving the entire vertebral body (based on the WBB surgical staging system)

PREOPERATIVE EVALUATION

Proper evaluation of patients with spinal column tumors requires careful consideration of the clinical history, physical examination findings, plain radiographs, and advanced cross-sectional imaging. Patients benefit from a multidisciplinary team consisting of surgeons, medical oncologists, radiation oncologists, radiologists, and pathologists.

A thorough clinical history includes a detailed understanding of the extent of the patient's pain and disability, the presence of neurologic symptoms, including lower extremity pain, weakness, and altered sensation, bowel and bladder function, and the patient's relevant medical history. The physical examination should document detailed neurologic findings, including an assessment of rectal tone. Posture, spinal alignment, and the presence of local masses or tenderness should be evaluated in all patients. Furthermore, a general physical examination is necessary to assess both the respiratory system and the lymphatic system for the presence of distant metastases.

Radiologic studies begin with plain radiographs centered on the affected area and radiographs of the entire spine to allow for an overall evaluation of spinal alignment and the presence of other noncontiguous, or skip, lesions. Initial characterization of the lesion based on its location, size, matrix, presence of a soft tissue mass or pathologic fracture, and the reaction between bone and lesion can be ascertained. Further characterization requires cross-sectional imaging, including MRI and/or fine-cut CT.

If the tumor is believed to be aggressive or malignant, a tissue biopsy is required to confirm the diagnosis and establish the tumor grade. Local and systemic staging requires CT and MRI of the entire spine, as well as a CT scan of the chest, total body bone scan, positron emission tomography (PET), and, potentially, bone marrow biopsy, gallium scan, and skeletal surveys. Screening for the presence of occult venous thrombosis should be undertaken, given higher risk factors (e.g., malignancy and decreased ambulation). The chest CT scan should be carefully scrutinized for sarcomatous metastases. Patients who have lung metastases should be referred to a thoracic surgeon to discuss the priority of metastasis resection through a thoracotomy versus primary resection.

After confirmation that the tumor requires surgical resection and satisfies the appropriate indications and contraindications, patients should be properly prepared so that they are in optimal physical condition for surgery, taking into consideration medical and nutritional status, particularly in those patients who have undergone adjuvant chemotherapy.

CLINICAL DECISION-MAKING

Depending on the type of tumor, adjuvant chemotherapy, radiation therapy, and/or the need for preoperative embolization should be considered. Resection of tumors that are highly vascular (e.g., angiosarcomas and solitary renal cell metastasis) benefits from preoperative embolization. The choice of technique for en bloc resection is dependent on the structures involved in the tumor. A detailed understanding of the three-dimensional extent of the tumor is paramount, and an appreciation of the potential margins in a three-dimensional space is required. As mentioned previously, sagittal osteotomy is indicated for lateralized tumors that involve only a single pedicle (Fig. 36-2).

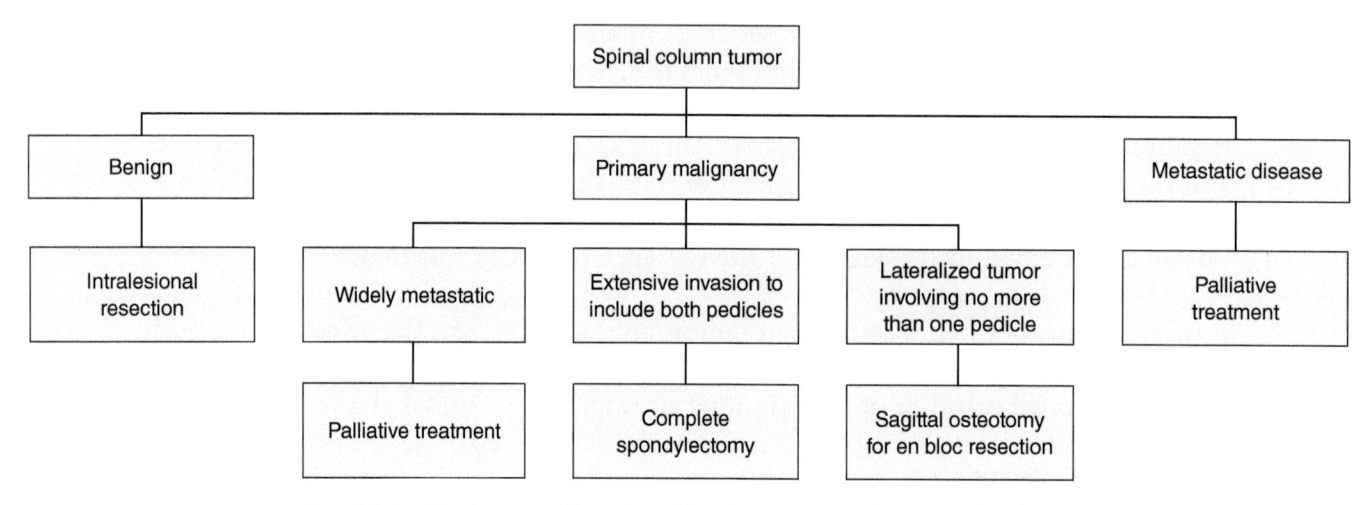

Fig. 36-2 Decision-making algorithm for tumors of the spinal column.

TECHNIQUE

Surgery is performed with patients under general anesthesia. We routinely use electromyography (EMG) and motor and sensory evoked potential neurophysiologic monitoring. Intravenous broad-spectrum antibiotics are administered, and patients are positioned for the anterior (or lateral) approach first. We prefer not to use the Cell Saver intraoperative cell salvage machine in these patients to reduce the remote chance of recirculating blood with microscopic tumor cells.

ANTERIOR APPROACH

A vascular access surgeon can help facilitate the anterior approach, particularly in cases of prior abdominal surgery, anatomic variations, or close proximity of the tumor to the great vessels. The anterior approach consists of discectomies (for fusion) at two disc levels above the resection margin and complete circumferential discectomies/osteotomies at the disc levels at the resection margins.

For lesions at L1 or L2, patients are placed in the decubitus position with the tumor side up. A standard tenth rib thoracoabdominal approach is used to expose two levels above and two levels below the vertebra to be resected. The rib is harvested and used for bone graft.

For lesions at or below L3, patients are placed in the supine position, and a vertical paramedian incision is used along with a standard anterior approach to the lumbar spine. The key to the anterior release is to expose the disc levels above and below the lesion without exposing the vertebral body on the ipsilateral side of the tumor. A circular retractor frame attached to the operative table with deep retractors facilitates the exposure. Intraoperative radiography is used to verify the correct level. The corresponding nerve root on the ipsilateral side of the tumor exiting from the psoas is identified and divided (Fig. 36-3).

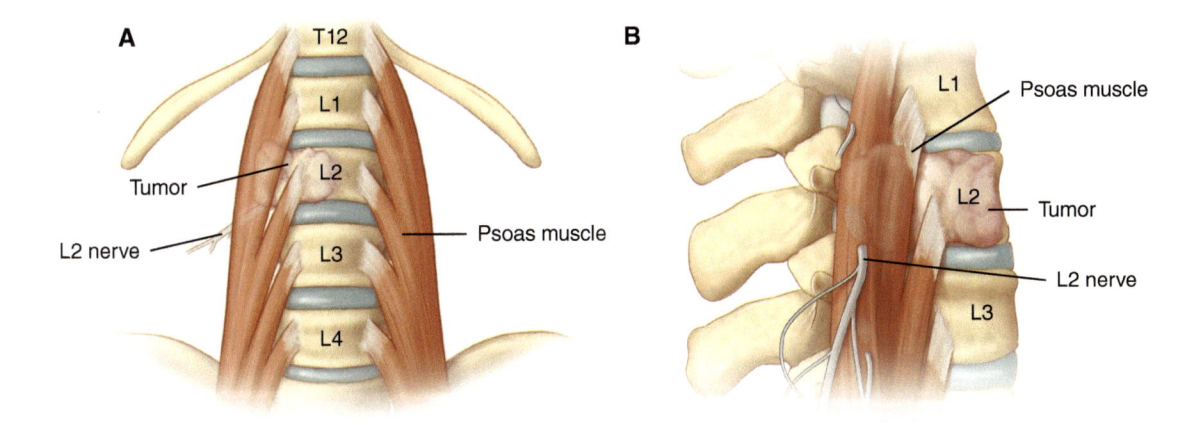

Fig. 36-3 Anterior exposure. **A,** Frontal and **B,** lateral views showing tumor on the right side of the L2 vertebral body beneath the psoas. The distal end of the right L2 nerve is transected after emerging from the psoas.

Continued

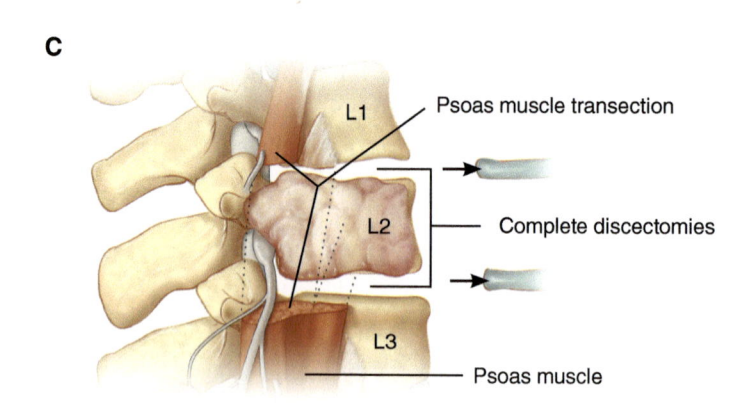

Fig. 36-3, cont'd **C,** Lateral view showing the complete circumferential discectomies and left psoas transection at the level above and below the tumor.

Once the most cephalad and caudad discs are exposed above the resection margin, a complete discectomy and interbody fusion are performed. At the disc spaces adjacent to the level of resection, the entire circumference is transected horizontally, beginning with the overlying psoas muscle on the ipsilateral side, continuing through the disc spaces and anterior and posterior longitudinal ligaments, carried all the way back to the paraspinal muscles to expose the corresponding transverse processes of the levels above and below the lesion. Care is taken not to expose the vertebral body beneath the psoas muscle on the side ipsilateral to the tumor (see Fig. 36-3, C). The anterior margin and two thirds of the superior and inferior margins (anterior and middle column) have now been completed. In addition, interbody fusion has been performed at the levels above and below the resection margin. A rubber mesh is then placed over the anterior margin deep to the vessels to protect them during the osteotomy. The wound is irrigated, and hemostasis is achieved. The wound is then closed in layers, including the diaphragm with chest tube, if necessary, after a complete instrument, sponge, and needle count is confirmed.

POSTERIOR APPROACH

Next the patient is placed prone on a four-poster frame with the legs in extension for a standard posterior approach. An ellipse centered at the biopsy tract is marked so that the medial side is at the midline and an equivalent distance is left laterally. The length of the incision should be adequate to expose two levels above and two levels below the lesion (Fig. 36-4). Intraoperative radiography is used to verify the correct levels preoperatively. It is crucial during the posterior approach to avoid disrupting all soft tissues from the biopsy tract to the pedicle.

The incision is carried down through the skin and subcutaneous tissue. The midline lumbodorsal fascia is incised on the side contralateral to the lesion and dissected from the posterior margins of the spinous processes in the usual manner on that side out to the transverse processes. On the ipsilateral side, at the level of the resection, the fascia and muscle are divided well lateral to the biopsy tract and the tumor margin. At the levels above and below the lesion, the fascia and paraspinal muscles are divided transversely from the vertical muscular interval to the midline, connecting with the transverse resection margins performed anteriorly (Fig. 36-5). A standard medial-to-lateral spinal exposure is carried out two levels above and two levels below the planned resection to expose the laminae, facet capsules, and transverse processes on the side ipsilateral to the tumor (Fig. 36-6).

Fig. 36-4 Posterior skin incision. Posterior longitudinal incision with ellipse centered around the biopsy tract is shown.

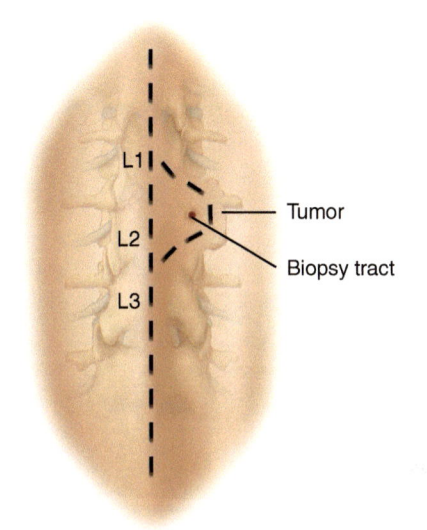

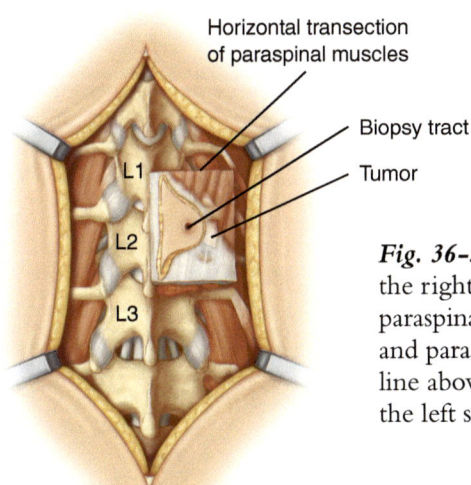

Fig. 36-5 Posterior muscle dissection. Paraspinal muscles cover the right side, and the longitudinal interval through the fascia and paraspinal muscles is lateral to the margin of the tumor. The fascia and paraspinal muscles are transected horizontally back to the midline above and below the disc spaces, respectively. The exposure on the left side is performed in the usual way.

Fig. 36-6 Final posterior exposure. The bone is exposed above and below the level of the resection on the right side, and the myocutaneous cover over the tumor is left intact.

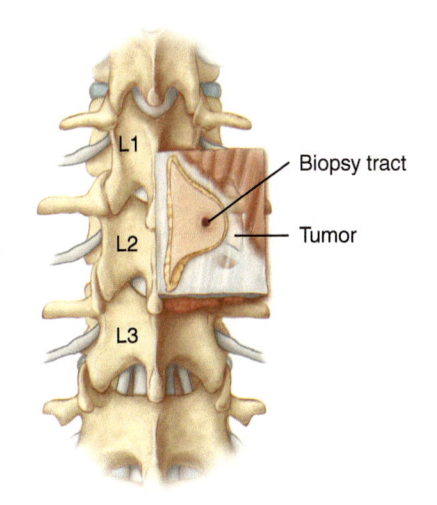

At this stage, pedicle screws are inserted into the pedicles at the two levels cephalad and caudad to the tumor level, and a temporary rod is inserted on the ipsilateral side. The facet joints adjacent to the resection bilaterally are osteotomized. A laminectomy is performed above and below the level of the resection, and the hemilamina on the contralateral side of the tumor is resected. The underlying contralateral pedicle of the vertebra to be resected and the exiting nerve root are exposed (Fig. 36-7). Below the level of the conus, the dura is retracted from the contralateral to the ipsilateral side.

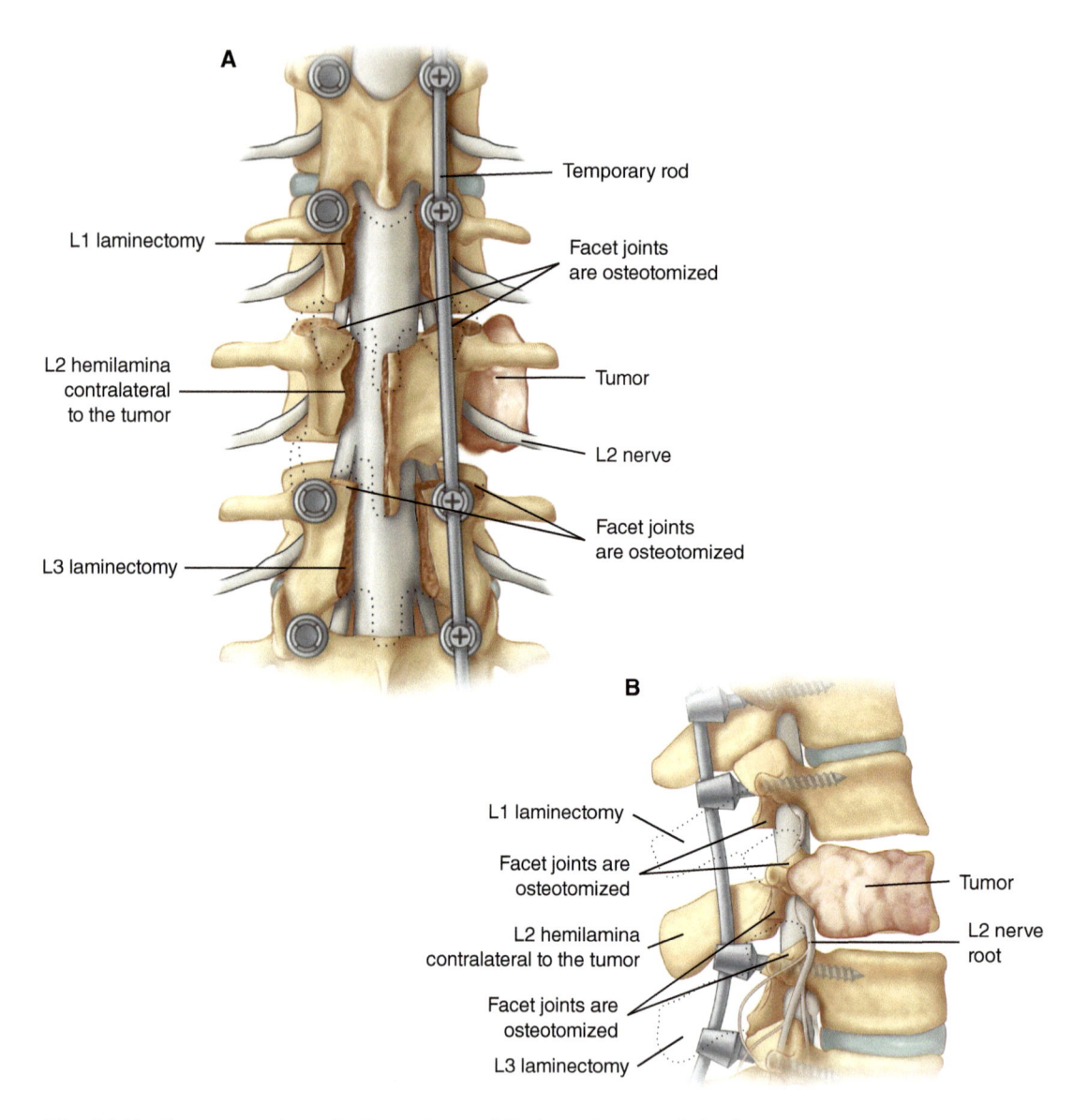

Fig. 36-7 Bone resection. **A,** Posterior and **B,** lateral view of the bone exposure. Laminectomies above and below the resection are carried out, and the hemilamina on the contralateral side of the tumor is resected, isolating the left L2 pedicle and nerve.

Above the conus, the contralateral nerve root can also be sacrificed to facilitate the osteotomy without retraction on the spinal cord. An osteotome is used to osteotomize the vertebral body vertically on the contralateral side, just medial to the pedicle, from a posterior to an anterior direction, as preoperatively planned on the cross-sectional axial scans. The osteotomy is completed from the cephalad to the caudad disc (Fig. 36-8) The exiting nerve root on the ipsilateral side of the tumor is divided as the tumor is mobilized laterally (Fig. 36-9).

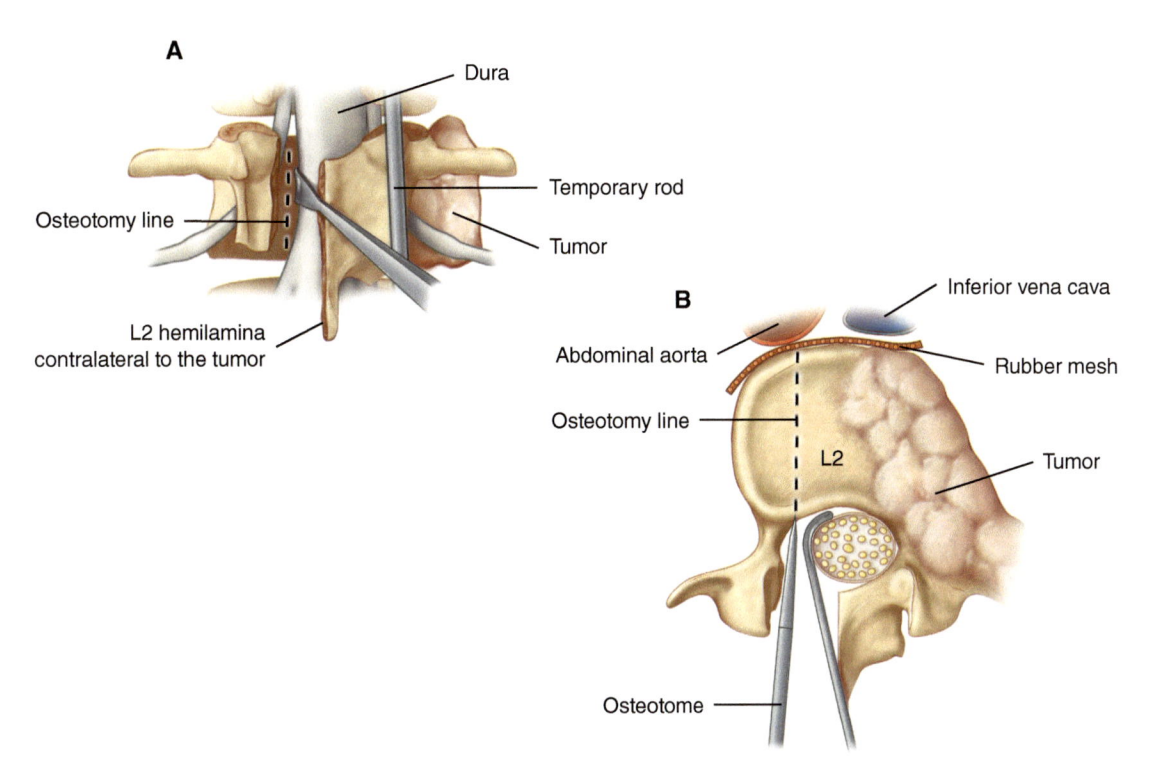

Fig. 36-8 Sagittal osteotomy. **A,** Posterior and **B,** axial views of the dural retraction and osteotomy line. The dura is carefully retracted toward the side of the tumor. The rubber mesh protects the great vessels anteriorly during the osteotomy.

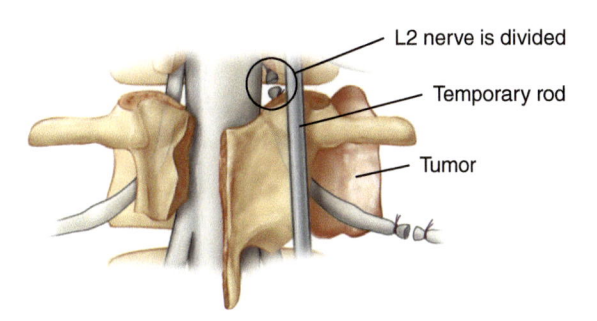

Fig. 36-9 Sacrifice of L2 nerve. The proximal end of the L2 nerve is then identified and ligated at the axilla proximal to its path through the tumor.

After completion of the osteotomy, a temporary rod is placed on the contralateral side, and the ipsilateral rod is removed. The en bloc vertebrectomy is delivered posteriorly on the ipsilateral side to the cauda equina (Fig. 36-10). After the tumor has been resected, the rubber mesh is removed and hemostasis is achieved. The remaining endplates are prepared, and an interbody prosthetic cage or structural allograft with iliac crest autograft or morselized allograft is inserted into the corpectomy site so that it is well seated on the endplates of the vertebrae above and below. The remaining rod is reinserted (Fig. 36-11).

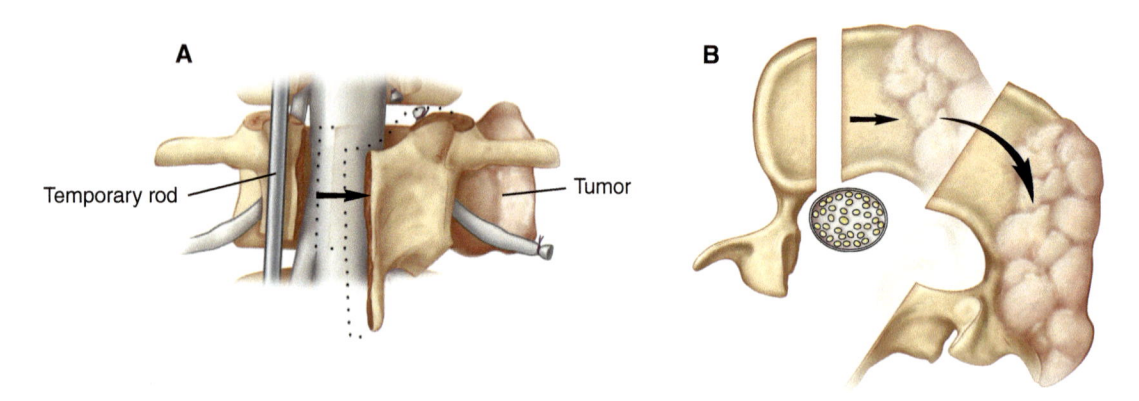

Fig. 36-10 Delivery of the tumor. **A,** Posterior and **B,** axial views showing the direction of tumor delivery from the surgical field.

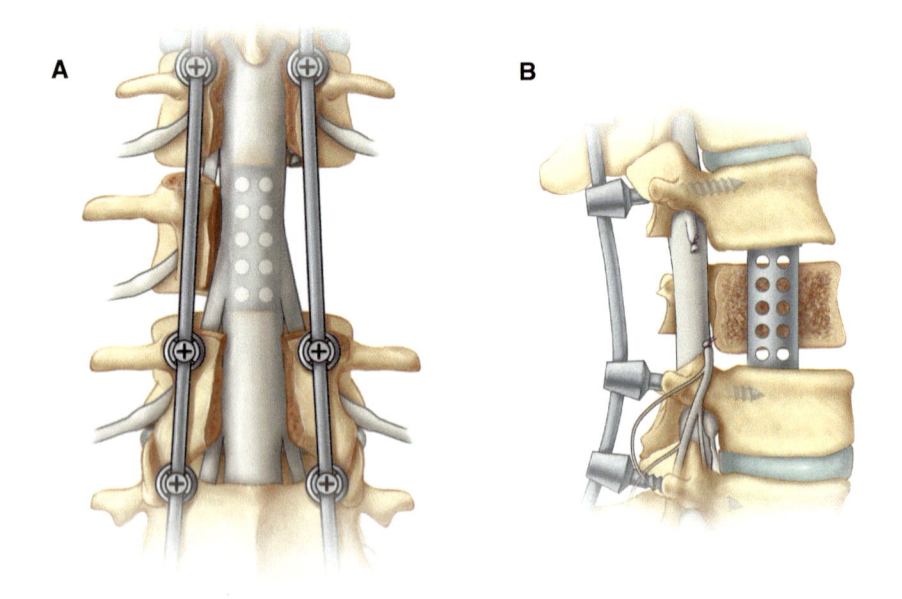

Fig. 36-11 Final reconstruction. **A,** Posterior and **B,** lateral views showing the final construct with interbody prosthetic cage and posterior instrumentation.

The facet joints are prepared for fusion, transverse processes are decorticated, and posterolateral bone grafting is performed. The assistance of a plastic surgeon for possible creation of advancement flaps to cover the defect in the paraspinal musculature is often required. The lumbodorsal fascia is reapproximated over a drain, and the wound is closed in the standard manner.

Postoperatively a soft lumbar corset may be used for comfort. Intravenous antibiotics are continued for 24 hours, and the patient is fully mobilized with restrictions on deep bending and heavy lifting for 3 months.

OUTCOMES WITH EVALUATION OF RESULTS

This novel technique facilitates the removal of lateralized tumors of the spine. Although no long-term studies or clinical series have been published on this specific technique, other reports of en bloc spondylectomy have been published.

Boriani et al[15] reported on a series of 29 patients treated with en bloc resections of the thoracolumbar spine after staging according to the WBB classification system. A wide margin was achieved in 20 patients, a marginal margin in eight patients, and an intralesional margin in one patient. These investigators reported no deaths, one deep infection, and three mechanical failures of the implants requiring additional surgery. Neurologic deficits observed were only related to planned root sacrifice. No local recurrences were found at follow-up evaluation after 6 to 134 months. The investigators concluded that en bloc resection can be safely performed on the basis of the oncologic stage and with careful planning.

Hasegawa et al[10] reported on the outcomes of 13 patients undergoing margin-free spondylectomy with a combined anterior-posterior approach. These investigators found that neurologic status and pain improved in all cases. There were no local recurrences in 11 patients. Two patients with chondrosarcomas were free of disease 14 years and 13 years after surgery, respectively.

A recent systematic review by Yamazaki et al[16] identified eight studies of en bloc resection for primary tumors after excluding small case series and studies incorporating other pathologic conditions (e.g., metastatic disease). The investigators found that the WBB surgical staging system predicted the ability to achieve a wide or marginal resection in 88% of cases and that tumor recurrence was highly correlated with a prior intralesional procedure. A recurrence significantly shortened overall survival, and complications from surgery ranged from 13% to 56%, whereas mortality rates ranged from 0% to 7.7%.

With the development of improved techniques for en bloc resections of primary spine tumors, such as sagittal osteotomy for lateralized tumors, resections can be achieved that balance wide oncologic margins while maintaining more spinal stability, thus, in turn, improving clinical outcomes and reducing complications.

SIGNATURE CASES

A 38-year-old male patient had a history of progressive back pain and was neurologically intact. A lesion was identified at L2, and a transpedicular core biopsy confirmed the diagnosis of angiosarcoma. Cross-sectional imaging, including CT and MRI, demonstrated that the tumor remained predominantly on the right side of L2 (Fig. 36-12, A through C). The tumor crossed the midline of the vertebral body but spared the left lateral body and pedicle. The tumor extended extracompartmentally into the right psoas and paraspinal muscles. On the sagittal MRI (see Fig. 36-13), the tumor remained within the vertical plane of L2 and did not cross the adjacent disc spaces.

The multidisciplinary team recommended en bloc resection along with postoperative radiation therapy. Because the tumor was an angiosarcoma, the lesion was embolized preoperatively. The patient was counseled that the right L2 nerve would need to be sacrificed and that he would likely experience weakness of the right hip flexor and thigh.

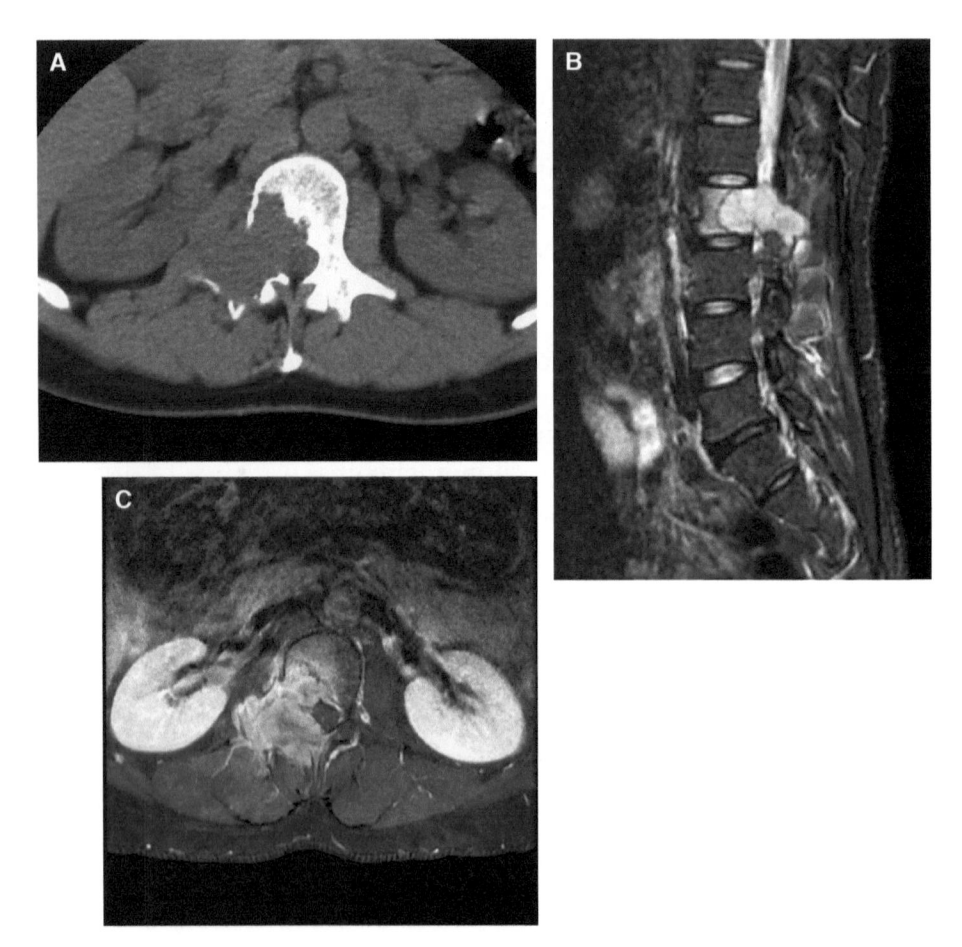

Fig. 36-12 **A,** Axial CT scan of L2 tumor. **B,** Sagittal and **C,** axial T1-weighted MRI of L2 with gadolinium.

The patient underwent a two-stage procedure involving a sagittal osteotomy for en bloc resection (described later in this chapter), first with an anterior approach followed by a posterior approach. The tumor was resected with negative margins (Fig. 36-12, *D* and *E*), and the spine was reconstructed anteriorly and posteriorly (Fig. 36-12, *F* and *G*). The patient tolerated the procedure well and remained disease free at the 6-month follow-up examination.

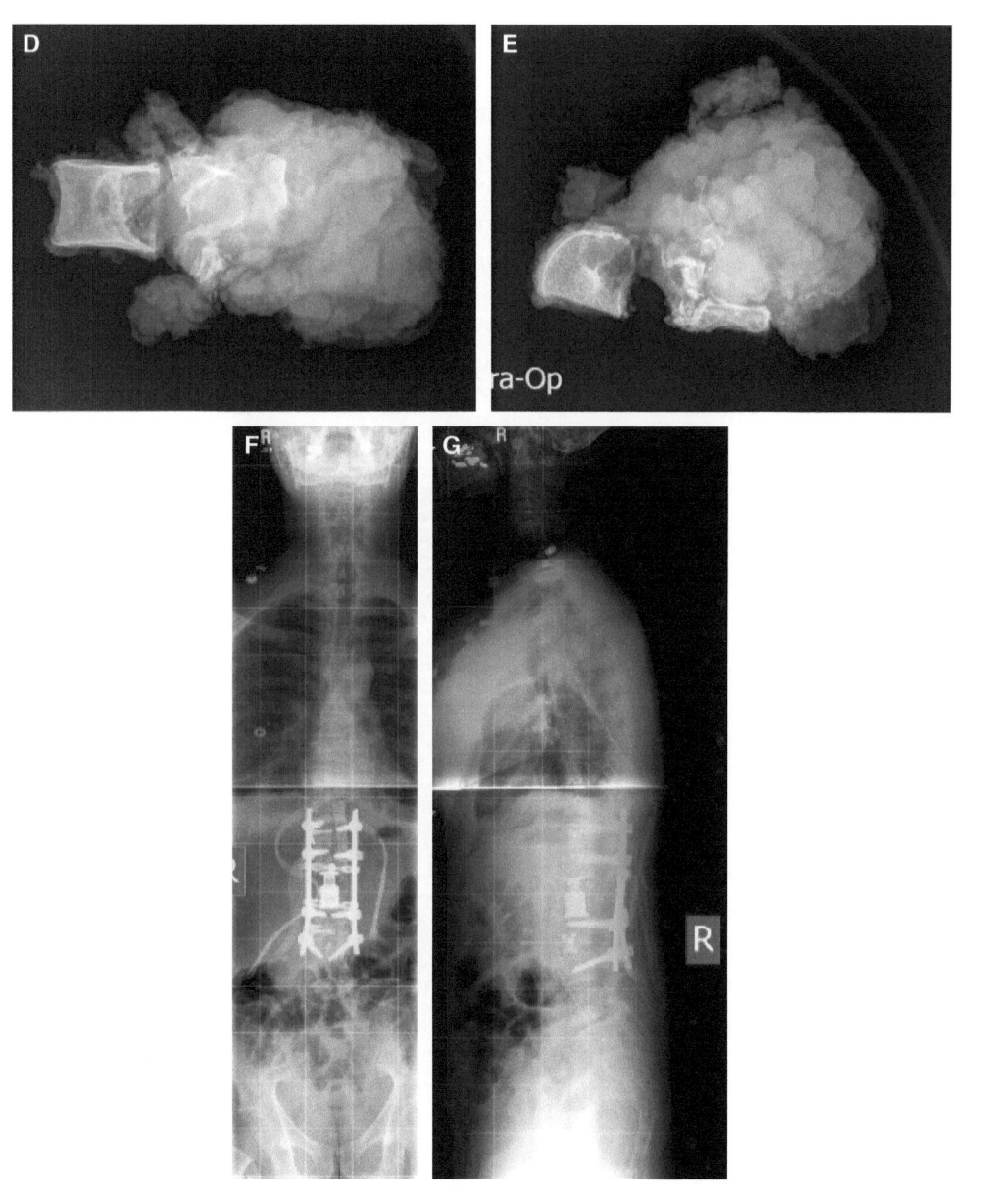

Fig. 36-12, cont'd Intraoperative **D,** lateral and **E,** axial radiographs of resected specimen. **F,** Postoperative anteroposterior and **G,** lateral spine radiographs.

A 71-year-old male patient presented with a history of abdominal pain and cachexia. He was neurologically intact. A large retroperitoneal mass emanating from the left psoas muscle was identified. A core biopsy confirmed the diagnosis of soft tissue sarcoma. MRI demonstrated that the tumor was in the retroperitoneum and was adherent to the left side of the spine from L1 to L4 (Fig. 36-13, *A* through *C*). The multidisciplinary team recommended surgical en bloc resection with left nephrectomy. The patient was counseled that the left L1, L2, and L3 nerves would need to be sacrificed and that he would likely experience weakness of the left hip flexor and thigh.

The patient underwent a two-stage procedure involving a sagittal osteotomy for en bloc resection in reverse order because the tumor was to be delivered from the anterior approach. The surgical plan began first with a posterior approach followed by an anterior approach. From the posterior approach, we performed a laminectomy from T12 to L5 but did not expose the transverse processes on the left L1 to L4. The left L1, L2, and L3 nerve roots were sacrificed from this approach. The T12-L1 and L4-5 discs were incised around the posterolateral corner on the left side. Finally, the dura was retracted from left to right, and an incomplete sagittal osteotomy was begun from the T12-L1 disc to the L4-5 disc in a posterior-to-anterior direction without penetrating through the anterior cortex (Fig. 36-13, *D*). We prepared the right side for facet and intertransverse fusion.

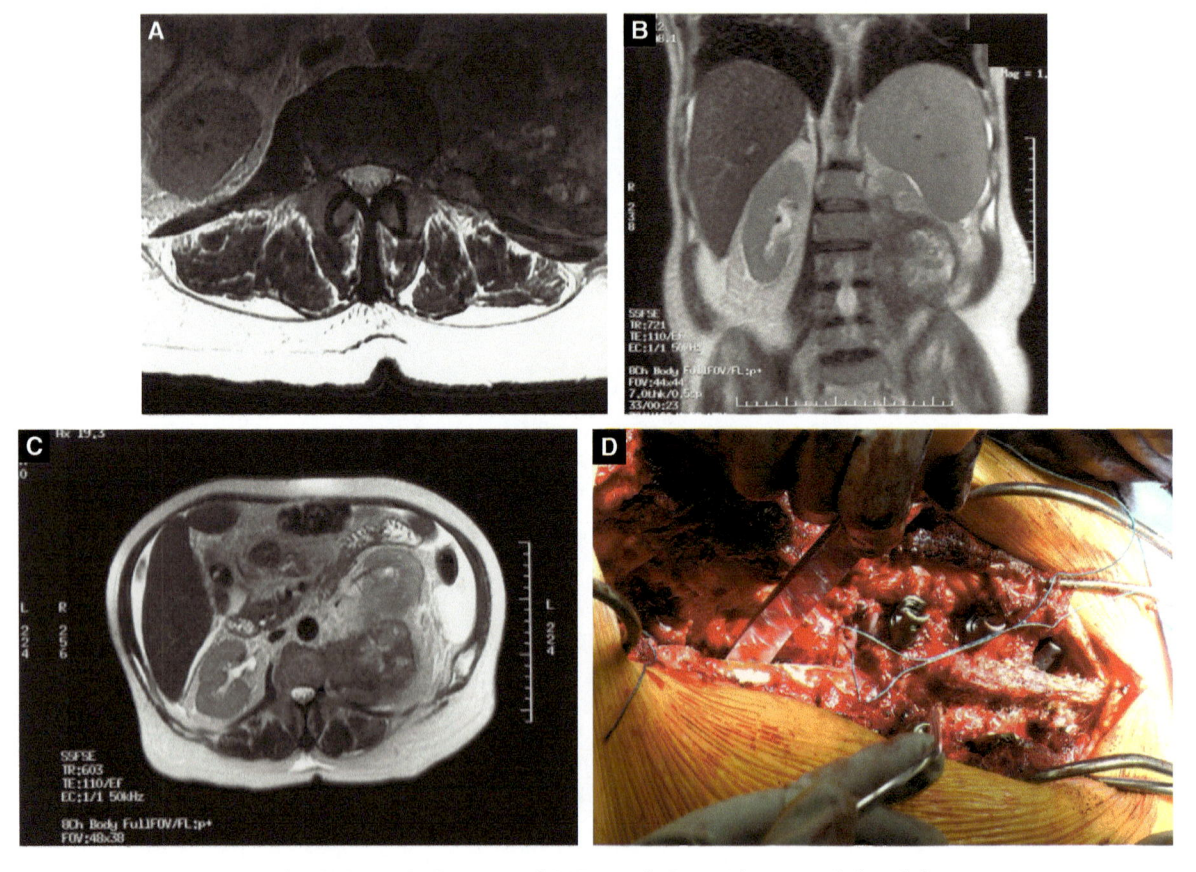

Fig. 36-13 **A,** Axial MRI at L2, **B,** coronal MRI and **C,** axial MRI of the abdomen. **D,** Intraoperative photograph from the posterior approach demonstrating incomplete sagittal osteotomy with dural retraction.

The next day the patient returned to the operating room, where the tumor was approached through a thoracoabdominal retroperitoneal approach. We identified the T12-L1 disc above and the L4-5 disc below. Both discs were incised from the midline all the way back to the posterior corner. The tumor margins were developed medially and laterally. The peripheral nerves emerging from the tumor were sacrificed. Once we identified the anterior spine between the aorta and the tumor, we then performed an osteotomy through L1 to L4 from anterior to posterior to connect with our posterior incomplete osteotomy. The tumor was then removed en bloc with the lateral margin of the spine (Fig. 36-13, *E* and *F*).

A positive margin was identified on the peritoneal wall on the medial surface of the tumor, and we therefore decided against complete discectomies at the resected levels because the patient would need postoperative radiation therapy. The spine was reconstructed with an expandable cage supporting the lateral column from T12 to L5 (Fig. 36-13, *G* and *H*).

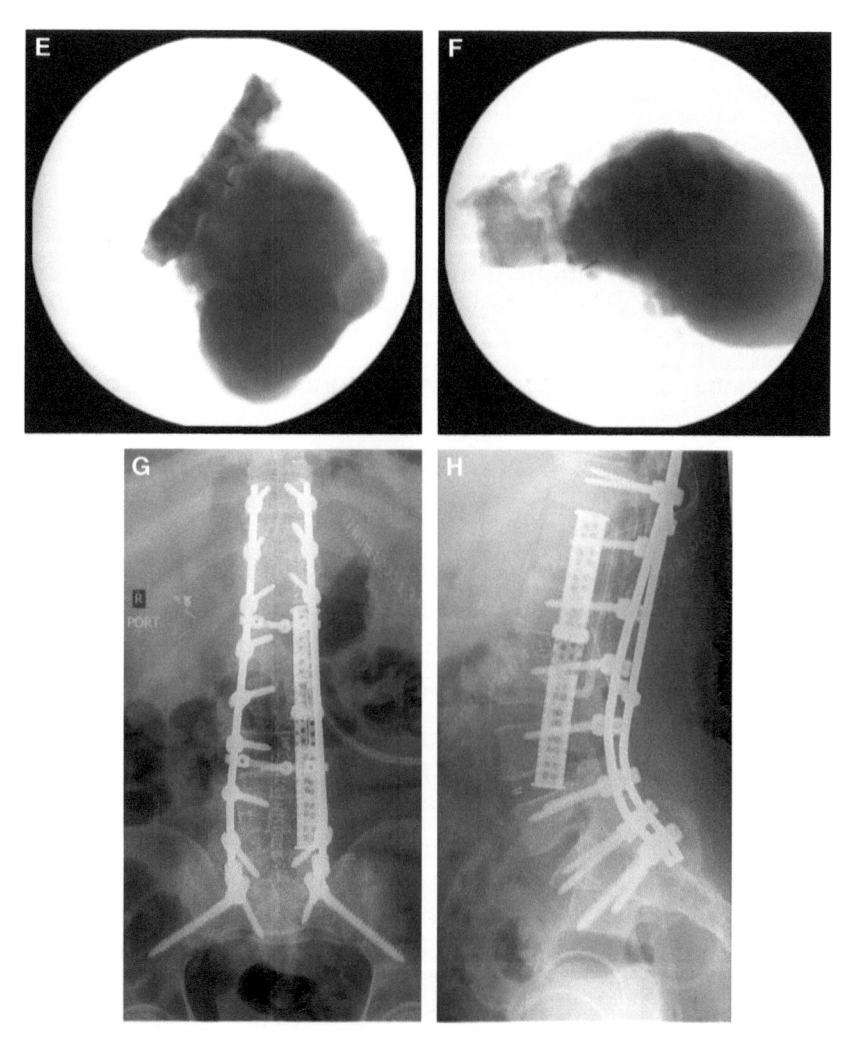

Fig. 36-13, cont'd **E,** Intraoperative anteroposterior and **F,** lateral radiographs of resected specimen. **G,** Postoperative anteroposterior and **H,** lateral spine radiographs.

The patient remained on prolonged ventilatory support and required renal dialysis, tracheostomy, and a percutaneous feeding tube. He died 3 months postoperatively from complications relating to gastrointestinal bleeding.

CONCLUSION

Surgical resection with negative margins for primary malignancies of the musculoskeletal system has been shown to improve survival and lower the rate of local recurrence. A multidisciplinary approach is beneficial in managing these patients. The specific surgical resection technique must be selected based the results of detailed evaluation of the patient and the lesion. With a better understanding of spinal anatomy, stability, and instrumentation techniques, en bloc resections in the spine have become more technically feasible. The sagittal osteotomy technique described in this chapter demonstrates the feasibility of a complete resection with the potential for negative margins in lateralized tumors of the lumbar spine. With close scrutiny of cross-sectional imaging and detailed preoperative planning, a carefully performed sagittal osteotomy for en bloc resection has the potential to improve survival and decrease local recurrence in patients with appropriately selected lateralized tumors of the lumbar spine and offers spine surgeons an alternative surgical option.

BAILOUT TECHNIQUES

- The main pitfall of this technique is inadequate release of the discs above and below in the initial approach, complicating the final resection in the second stage.
- Whether the technique is performed first from an anterior or a posterior approach, it is essential to completely release the disc at the cranial and caudal ends on the side of the resection.
- Sufficient release needs to be performed from the initial approach to facilitate the en bloc removal in the second stage.
- If insufficient release is performed, the lesion may not be excised as planned in the second stage. In this case, to achieve a true en bloc resection, the patient will most likely need to return to the initial positioning to avoid injury to the neurologic structures or violation of the tumor margin.

TIPS FROM THE MASTERS

- Careful review of all imaging studies is essential to ensure that the margins are clear for the sagittal osteotomy.
- Complete circumferential release at the upper and lower margins, including complete discectomies anteriorly and facet osteotomies, is crucial.

References (With Key References in Boldface)

1. Boriani S, Biagini R, De IF, et al. Primary bone tumors of the spine: a survey of the evaluation and treatment at the Istituto Ortopedico Rizzoli. Orthopedics 18:993-1000, 1995.
2. Abdu WA, Provencher M. Primary bone and metastatic tumors of the cervical spine. Spine 23:2767-2777, 1998.
3. Takaishi H, Yabe H, Fujimura Y, et al. The results of surgery on primary malignant tumors of the spine. Arch Orthop Trauma Surg 115:49-52, 1996.
4. Talac R, Yaszemski MJ, Currier BL, et al. Relationship between surgical margins and local recurrence in sarcomas of the spine. Clin Orthop Relat Res 39:127-132, 2002.
5. Enneking WF. Musculoskeletal Tumor Surgery. New York: Churchill Livingstone, 1983.
6. **Boriani S, Weinstein J, Biagini R. Primary bone tumors of the spine. Terminology and surgical staging. Spine 22:1036-1044, 1997.**
7. Biagini R, Boriani S, Andreoli I, et al. Surgical technique: dorsal vertebral hemiresection for bone tumors. Chir Organi Mov 79:331-337, 1994.
8. **Biagini R, Casadei R, Boni F, et al. Spondylectomy (thoracolumbar spine) combined with dural resection for bone tumor: surgical technique. Chir Organi Mov 87:97-101, 2002.**
9. Boriani S, Biagini R, De IF, et al. Lumbar vertebrectomy for the treatment of bone tumors: surgical technique. Chir Organi Mov 79:163-173, 1994.
10. **Hasegawa K, Homma T, Hirano T, et al. Margin-free spondylectomy for extended malignant spine tumors: surgical technique and outcome of 13 cases. Spine 32:142-148, 2007.**
11. Magerl F, Coscia MF. Total posterior vertebrectomy of the thoracic or lumbar spine. Clin Orthop Relat Res 232:62-69, 1988.
12. Stener B. Complete removal of vertebrae for extirpation of tumors. A 20-year experience. Clin Orthop Relat Res 245:72-82, 1989.
13. Sundaresan N, Digiacinto GV, Krol G, et al. Spondylectomy for malignant tumors of the spine. J Clin Oncol 7:1485-1491, 1989.
14. **Tomita K, Kawahara N, Baba H, et al. Total en bloc spondylectomy. A new surgical technique for primary malignant vertebral tumors. Spine 22:324-333, 1997.**
15. Boriani S, Biagini R, De Iure R, et al. En bloc resections of bone tumors of the thoracolumbar spine. A preliminary report on 29 patients. Spine 21:1927-1931, 1996.
16. **Yamazaki T, McLoughlin GS, Patel S, et al. Feasibility and safety of en bloc resection for primary spine tumors: a systematic review by the Spine Oncology Study Group. Spine 34(22 Suppl):S31-S38, 2009.**

Chapter 37

Combined Lateral/Posterior Approach for Large Anterior/Lateral Lesions

Daniel K. Fahim, Laurence D. Rhines

Despite advances in chemotherapy and radiation therapy, surgical resection continues to play an integral role in the management of tumors involving the spine. Even in an era dominated by advances in minimally invasive techniques,[1] clinical circumstances remain in which extended, multistage, open procedures are necessary to achieve optimal oncologic outcomes. The combined posterior/lateral approaches described in this chapter can be used to achieve complete extirpation of tumors involving the spine with extension into the adjacent chest wall and/or paraspinal soft tissues. By providing circumferential access, these tumors can be better visualized and resected by both intralesional and en bloc techniques.

The concept of aggressive surgical resection of spinal neoplasms is not novel. The technique of complete spondylectomy was first described by Stener[2] in 1971 for the resection of a chondrosarcoma of the thoracic spine. Two decades later he published the first clinical case series describing the use of complete spondylectomy for resection of tumors.[3] Subsequently, many other authors have described the use of similar techniques for aggressive benign,[4-7] primary malignant,[5,8-10] and even metastatic spine tumors.[5,11-12] Certainly, in the case of primary malignant bone tumors such as chordoma and chondrosarcoma, the data suggest that the ability to achieve "en bloc" surgical resection with negative margins correlates with improved disease-free survival.[13-14]

Most spine surgeons have more experience with posterior approaches to the spine. Although metastatic disease typically arises in the vertebral body and is frequently amenable to an anterior surgical approach (transthoracic, retroperitoneal), surgeons tend to be more familiar with the posterior approach, which is easier to instrument and better facilitates multilevel resection and stabilization. Techniques for accessing and resecting anteriorly situated tumors from a posterior approach have been reported and are increasingly used. The techniques of transpedicular vertebrectomy, costotransversectomy, and lateral extracavitary approaches have been well described.[15-16] These can be quite effective for the intralesional resection of tumors restricted to the spine with limited extraspinal extension.

However, in circumstances in which the tumor extends beyond the spine, such as into the chest wall or paraspinal soft tissues, a more extensive approach is required to improve access to the tumor. A staged anterior/posterior or posterior/anterior technique can be used for the resection of tumors involving the vertebral body and posterior elements with extraspinal extension, but there are situations in which the simultaneous combination of these approaches (a simultaneous posterior approach combined with a transthoracic or retroperitoneal approach) provides the visualization, access, and protection of vital paraspinal structures necessary to achieve safe and efficacious tumor resection.[17-18] The purpose of this chapter is to describe these combined approaches.

INDICATIONS AND CONTRAINDICATIONS

The principal indication for using the combined approach is the presence of disease that cannot be adequately or optimally addressed by either a posterior or anterolateral approach alone, and when the simultaneous combined posterior and lateral access provides an advantage over staged resection. There are three clinical scenarios that favor this combined approach: (1) superior sulcus tumors (Pancoast tumors) with extension into the chest wall and spine, (2) hypervascular spinal metastases with significant paraspinal extension, and (3) primary spinal tumors involving the lateral aspect of the spine and adjacent chest wall and/or paraspinal tissues where en bloc resection is necessary. These are the situations in which the combined approach is most anatomically advantageous. The ability to simultaneously visualize the posterior, lateral, and anterior limits of the tumor, completely mobilize the adjacent paraspinal structures, and incise the spine while triangulating from both anterior and posterior views improves the surgeon's ability to completely resect these tumors. Obviously, such an aggressive surgical undertaking is reserved for patients whose disease is potentially curable (superior sulcus tumors, primary spinal tumors) or whose metastatic disease is very limited.

In all of these cases, the presence of a neurologic deficit, intractable pain, or spinal instability or the potential to improve survival are indications for surgery. For superior sulcus tumors, patients are screened thoroughly to rule out distant metastatic and unresectable nodal disease, two harbingers of a poor prognosis. In patients without metastases and without nodal disease, a complete tumor resection with negative margins, combined with either neoadjuvant or adjuvant chemoradiation, has been shown to significantly improve survival compared with incomplete resection.[18-19] The combined posterior/lateral approach is extremely useful for ensuring total resection of tumors involving the chest wall and spine.

In metastatic disease, the goal of surgery is palliation. The need for complete tumor removal is confined to cases of solitary (or extremely limited) sites of disease. The role of en bloc resection in cases of solitary spinal metastases remains unclear with respect to the risk/reward balance. With the emergence of spinal stereotactic radiosurgery as an alternative or adjunct to surgery, the need for these aggressive surgical approaches is less clear. Certainly palliative decompression of the spinal cord/nerve roots and effective spinal reconstruction can be performed without a simultaneous combined approach. We reserve this approach for cases of isolated spinal metastasis (no or extremely limited systemic disease) that are hypervascular (notably renal cell carcinoma and thyroid carcinoma), involve anterior and posterior columns of the spine, and have significant extension into the chest wall or paraspinal musculature. For these patients, the combined approach allows maximum tumor devascularization before resection, as well as an improved ability to visualize and remove tumor remnants that can be a source of postoperative hemorrhage or recurrence.

For primary malignant and aggressive benign bone tumors, en bloc surgical resection provides the best chance of local tumor control and a prolonged disease-free survival.[13-14] Patients must be screened thoroughly for any distant metastatic disease that could negate the benefits of an aggressive approach to the primary tumor. For patients with osteosarcoma and Ewing's sarcoma, neoadjuvant chemotherapy is necessary before consideration of any surgery, because this may decrease the likelihood of local recurrence and distant metastasis. Given the need to free these tumors completely from their spinal and paraspinal attachments while avoiding contamination, an extralesional approach is quite helpful, particularly for tumors extending beyond the lateral aspect of the spine into the chest wall or paraspinal musculature.

Finally, in addition to the indications described, patients need to be healthy enough to tolerate these extensive surgeries. In all of these cases, the presence of widespread metastatic disease, limited life expectancy, or severe medical comorbidities preventing the safe administration of general anesthesia are all contraindications.

PREOPERATIVE EVALUATION

Evaluation begins with a careful clinical history. This provides information regarding the patient's cognitive status as well as his or her understanding of the disease and disease burden. It also allows the astute physician to identify patients who may have signs of untreated depression, which is a common malady in patients suffering with cancer. The acute or chronic progression of any neurologic symptoms must be elucidated. Finally, the presence and severity of pain must be investigated. Distinguishing between biologic pain and mechanical instability pain is also helpful in treatment planning.

The physical examination begins when the patient enters the examination room, noting the need for any ambulatory aids or assistance from family members. A sense of the patient's overall health is of fundamental importance. Thorough neurologic examination is essential, including strength testing, sensory examination, and assessment of reflexes. Confirming the dermatomal distribution of any possible radiculopathies is also necessary. When appropriate, a mini-mental status examination should be performed. The Karnofsky performance score should be determined and noted in the medical record.

Diagnostic studies, especially radiographic assessment, play a pivotal role in modern-day preoperative evaluation. In patients with a known malignancy, back pain must be regarded as an indication of metastatic disease until proven otherwise,[20] warranting radiologic workup for an early and accurate diagnosis. This would initially include a contrast-enhanced MRI in the region of pain. Should metastatic disease be discovered, a full radiologic staging workup is indicated to adequately evaluate for additional sites of metastases.

The accurate diagnosis of patients with primary malignancies of the spinal column is usually delayed. These patients most commonly present with pain,[21] and plain radiographs of the spine are obtained. However, there must be approximately 30% to 50% destruction of the trabecular bone in a vertebral body before a lytic lesion can be detected by plain radiographs.[22] Persistence of symptoms frequently leads to further imaging studies and recognition of the pathologic process. Biopsy is performed to establish the histologic diagnosis, which then dictates subsequent steps in the treatment algorithm.

When preparing for any oncologic spine operation, T1-weighted images with and without contrast and T2-weighted images without contrast will be the most helpful. These imaging modalities allow accurate delineation of the extent of the spinal and extraspinal disease as well as the degree of thecal sac or nerve root compression. For operations such as those discussed in this chapter, a CT scan without contrast imaging of all the segments to be included in the planned construct is essential to evaluate for pathologic fractures, integrity of the bone, and the relationship of the tumor to normal bone and paraspinal structures.

Any concern for osteopenia or osteoporosis in the surrounding bone should be assessed by a dual-energy x-ray absorptiometry (DEXA) scan before an instrumentation operation. Finally, any evidence of deformity should be thoroughly evaluated with upright anteroposterior and lateral radiographs to evaluate sagittal and coronal balance. Dynamic flexion-extension and lateral bending radiographs may also be helpful in treatment planning.

As mentioned earlier, a full staging workup is absolutely necessary when considering operative intervention for patients with metastatic disease. It is also appropriate to perform a staging workup when encountering an isolated spinal lesion without a known history of malignancy. This is completed for two reasons: first, the patient may have an undiagnosed primary tumor that has metastasized to the spine; second, primary malignant neoplasms of the spine may metastasize to other organs.

In terms of preoperative planning for the types of operations discussed in this chapter, it is important to evaluate the extent of spinal and extraspinal disease. The operative plan must address the spinal and paraspinal extension of the tumor. This is critical to achieve the surgical objective of complete resection, to appropriately counsel patients regarding the risks of surgery, and to ensure that multidisciplinary surgical expertise is available to assist with the surgical approach and soft tissue reconstruction.

CLINICAL DECISION-MAKING

Proper oncologic terminology must be used when referring to surgical approaches for resection of neoplasms. *Curettage* is the piecemeal resection of a tumor and is by definition, an intralesional procedure. *En bloc resection* involves removing the entire tumor in one piece; the success of such an approach is determined by the subsequent pathologic examination which grades the margin as either intralesional, marginal (along the reactive pseudocapsule around the tumor), or wide (a layer of healthy tissue around the tumor). There is essentially no role for *radical resection* in spinal tumor surgery, as this involves removal of the entire compartment from which the tumor arises (not feasible in the spine).[23] The combined approach may be used to excise a tumor in an intralesional fashion or to perform an en bloc resection.

PANCOAST TUMOR WITH SPINAL INVOLVEMENT

Although superior sulcus tumors account for less than 5% of non–small cell lung cancer (NSCLC) cases,[24] their treatment is difficult because of the frequent extension into surrounding structures. Pancoast[25] first described these apical chest tumors in 1924, and his patients presented with a combination of pain, weakness of the hand muscles, Horner's syndrome, and bone destruction. These tumors commonly involve the adjacent ribs (chest wall) and can also involve the great vessels, trachea, esophagus, brachial plexus, and the spine. When these tumors involve the spine by direct extension in a patient without metastases or nodal disease, surgical resection to negative margins provides a clear survival benefit when combined with neoadjuvant or adjuvant concurrent chemoradiation.[19,26]

If involvement of the spine is minimal, a single-stage thoracotomy (anterior clamshell or posterolateral) approach for resection of the lung mass or ribs and any minor involvement of the vertebral body is appropriate. If involvement of the vertebral body is extensive, requiring complete or near complete resection of the vertebral body, a two-stage procedure (posterior followed by combined lateral/posterior) for optimal resection, reconstruction, and stabilization is warranted. This is described in detail next.

Hypervascular Metastases With Circumferential Spinal Column Involvement and Significant Paraspinal Extension

It is well established that metastatic epidural spinal cord compression frequently requires direct decompressive surgery and spinal stabilization.[27] Most metastases to the spine involve the vertebral body with ventral epidural cord compression, although some extend into the pedicles and further along the posterior elements. As previously mentioned, vertebrectomy, posterior decompression, and anterior/posterior reconstruction and stabilization for metastatic lesions can frequently be performed from a single-stage posterior approach via a transpedicular or lateral extracavitary vertebrectomy.[15,16]

A small subset of metastatic lesions will have more extensive paraspinal involvement involving the chest wall or paraspinal soft tissues. When, in addition to this paraspinal extension, the lesion is also extremely hypervascular, we find that the combined posterior/lateral approach facilitates safe and complete resection. Hypervascular histologies include renal cell carcinoma, thyroid carcinoma, hepatocellular carcinoma, pheochromocytoma, angiosarcoma, hemangioendothelioma, and giant cell tumors. For lesions that are not particularly hypervascular, a staged approach can certainly be used, because the spinal and paraspinal components can be removed from the trajectory of optimal visualization. For hypervascular tumors, however, we find that the simultaneous access to the entire lesion afforded by the combined approach improves our ability to devascularize and visualize the tumor and remove it entirely during one operation, rather than leave a potential source of hemorrhage in the patient between stages. With the combined approach, the surgeon has better access to these larger tumors and thus maintaining hemostasis is easier. This improves respectability and patient safety. Clearly, this aggressive approach should be reserved for patients with a very limited overall disease burden.[28]

Certainly, when addressing a highly vascular metastatic lesion, preoperative embolization is strongly encouraged. Preoperative angiographic embolization should routinely be performed approximately 24 hours before the planned operation. This will significantly reduce intraoperative blood loss.[16,29,30] Occasionally this cannot be accomplished due to aberrant anatomical variations of the spinal vasculature.

Primary Spine Tumors

The staging system initially described by Enneking and colleagues[31-33] for bone tumors of the extremities has been applied to primary spine tumors.[14,34-36] A full discussion of this staging system is addressed in earlier chapters. Of relevance to the discussion of combined approaches to the spine is knowledge of which stages of benign and malignant spine tumors require an en bloc resection which might be facilitated by a combined lateral/posterior approach.

Stage IA, IB, IIA, and IIB malignant tumors of the spine should all be addressed with en bloc resection whenever possible. Surgical resection should aim for widest possible margin around an intact tumor mass.[37] Depending on the specific tumor histology, neoadjuvant or adjuvant chemotherapy and/or radiation may also be necessary. Benign stage II tumors (benign-aggressive) should also be treated with an en bloc resection if this can be achieved with reasonable morbidity. An intralesional excision of these tumors, even when supplemented by radiation, is associated with a high rate of recurrence.[38-39] Benign stage II tumors have a low rate of recurrence with intralesional excision, and therefore this is an acceptable surgical strategy for these tumors.[35]

Determining the appropriate surgical approach when planning for en bloc resection of these primary tumors of the spine depends on its location within the vertebra. The current standard for surgical staging is the Weinstein, Boriani, Biagini (WBB) system.[14,23,36] The WBB system describes the anatomic extent of the tumor by dividing the vertebra into 12 radiating zones and five concentric layers.[23] En bloc resection strategies must aim to open the bony ring of the spine in areas of normal bone, providing a corridor of delivery for the thecal sac, allowing for resection of the diseased bone in one piece. Large tumors involving the vertebra and the adjacent chest wall and/or paraspinal musculature may be optimally approached with a simultaneous combined lateral and posterior approach to the spine.

At MDACC, we strongly espouse a multidisciplinary surgical approach to these complex tumors. All surgical teams that will be involved in the tumor resection and reconstruction should be involved in designing the operative plan. When tumors involve the chest wall or lung, oncologic thoracic surgeons must be involved in the decision-making process. Plastic surgeons should be involved whenever resection of a substantial amount of soft tissue is anticipated—especially for surgical incision planning—to maximize reconstruction options.

Consideration of the combined approach is appropriate whenever the extent of the disease cannot be adequately or optimally addressed by any one approach alone and when simultaneous access to posterior and anterior structures provides improved visualization and safety for en bloc resection.

TECHNIQUE

Historically, at M.D. Anderson Cancer Center, these combined lateral/posterior operations have been performed in a single stage.[17] Even our technique for combined chest wall resection with vertebrectomy and spinal reconstruction for the treatment of Pancoast tumors was performed in a single stage in the lateral position.[18] This required the spinal stabilization to be performed in the lateral position, a particularly challenging task in the cervicothoracic region. These single-stage procedures were quite lengthy, and the stabilization in the lateral position did not always result in optimal spinal alignment. Thus more recently we are using a two-stage operation for many of the patients requiring a combined lateral/posterior approach for the management of their oncologic disease. The first stage is performed with the patient in the prone position and focuses on spinal stabilization and any resection or osteotomy that is more easily achieved with the patient prone. In the second stage the patient is positioned lateral decubitus, with simultaneous access to the posterior and anterolateral aspects of the spine.

The general strategy involves starting with a posterior approach with the patient in the prone position to stabilize the spine and initiate the resection of the tumor. Whether any tumor is actually resected depends on the pathologic entity being treated. In the setting of aggressive benign or primary malignant tumors of the spine, where en bloc resection is of oncologic significance, some osteotomies may be initiated during the posterior approach but no tumor is resected. This allows completion of the resection of the mass in an en bloc fashion from the lateral second-stage approach. Similarly, if the tumor is extremely hypervascular, resection may be reserved for the second stage when the tumor can be more easily devascularized and removed entirely. However, in the setting of metastatic or locally invasive disease (such as a Pancoast tumor involving the vertebral body) where an intralesional resection is acceptable, some tumor resection is begun posteriorly (particularly of that tumor which is more easily accessed in the prone position). The second-stage combined lateral/posterior approach is performed to complete the resection, followed by anterior column reconstruction where appropriate.

Notwithstanding these considerations, we continue to perform the single-stage combined lateral/posterior approach for the resection of highly vascular lesions when the lesion is in the mid to low thoracic spine or upper lumbar spine, because stabilization in these regions can be performed in the lateral position with relative ease, sparing the patient a second procedure.

Spinal cord electrophysiologic monitoring is used in all cases, and the surgeon is kept abreast of any intraoperative changes. Preoperative antibiotics titrated to patient weight are administered before the skin incision is made and are redosed as necessary during the procedure. If there is any evidence of cord compression or effacement on preoperative imaging, 10 mg of dexamethasone is administered intravenously. Throughout the procedure, blood pressure is maintained at a normotensive level tailored to the awake, preoperative baseline of the individual patient. Hypotension may result in ischemia of the spinal cord, especially when the cord is already compressed. All patients are typed and cross-matched for blood transfusion.

RESECTION OF PANCOAST TUMOR WITH SPINE INVOLVEMENT

As stated previously, patients with Pancoast or superior sulcus tumors require extensive preoperative staging. Aggressive resection is reserved for patients with no evidence of metastatic or nodal disease as determined by PET or CT scans and mediastinal lymph node sampling. Moreover, patients with local invasion of the brachial plexus or esophagus are generally excluded from surgical consideration due to the challenges of obtaining negative margins in these cases. Finally, it should be noted that surgical resection constitutes only one part of the treatment for these patients. Chemotherapy and radiation are both used in either the neoadjuvant or adjuvant setting.

For the first stage, the patient is placed prone on chest rolls. The Mayfield clamp is used to secure the head in a neutral position as evaluated both radiographically and by direct visual inspection. A midline posterior incision is made beginning at the lower cervical spine and extending to the midthoracic spine. The number of levels exposed depends on the length of the fixation, which is based on the location and number of vertebral levels to be resected. The uninvolved side of the spine is exposed in the usual subperiosteal manner. Along the involved side of the spine, the dissection is carried out as usual above and below the area of pathology, and the medial portion of the chest wall mass is exposed as it meets the spine. The medial portion of the mass can be resected to allow access to the spine for adequate bony decompression.

Laminectomies can then be performed at the involved levels to expose the thecal sac, and the bony resection can be extended laterally to include all the posterior elements infiltrated by tumor (facets and pedicles). Nerve roots that are encased by tumor are suture-ligated and sharply divided lateral to the ligature (Fig. 37-1). The nerve roots can be ligated at levels below T1 with minimal, if any, neurologic impact. The T1 nerve root may be spared if it is not coursing through the tumor. Ligation of the T1 nerve root will often lead to some degree of hand dysfunction and patients should be counseled appropriately. Ligation of these roots can facilitate the resection of the diseased facets and pedicles allowing a plane of dissection to be created between the involved chest wall and vertebra and the thecal sac. A Silastic sheet may be inserted to demarcate this plane and help identify the location of the dura during the second stage procedure. Once adequate posterior and lateral decompression of the thecal sac is completed, posterior instrumentation can be placed.

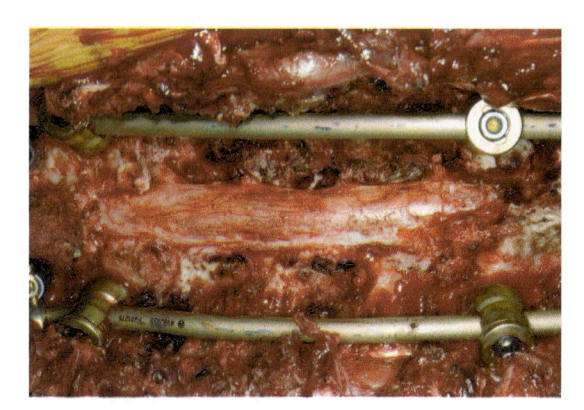

Fig. 37-1 Intraoperative photograph of the posterior approach (stage one) of a Pancoast tumor resection. Laminectomies have been performed, along with suture ligation of the nerve roots along the affected side, with associate facetectomies and partial pediculectomies.

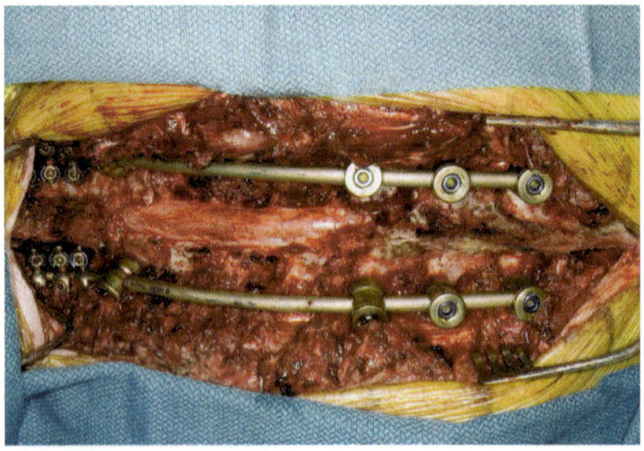

Fig. 37-2 Intraoperative photograph showing the posterior instrumentation and construct, including three levels of thoracic pedicle screw instrumentation below the levels of involvement and extending superiorly to C5 with lateral mass screws.

Pedicle screws are placed in the thoracic spine extending at least two levels below the pathology. In the cervical spine, lateral mass screws or pedicle screws are placed extending up two to three levels above the area of pathology (Fig. 37-2). After instrumentation is complete, copious antibiotic irrigation is used to wash out the wound. The posterior bony surfaces are then decorticated and the rods secured into place. Morselized allograft is then packed along the decorticated bony surfaces and closure is carried out in the usual fashion. The patient is extubated and monitored in the surgical intensive care unit until the second-stage operation.

The second stage of the operation is performed with the patient in the lateral decubitus position, with the affected side up (Fig. 37-3, *A*). The thoracic surgeons begin the operation with a posterolateral thoracotomy incision extended posteriorly to include the previous midline spinal incision which is reopened. The angle at which these incisions are connected is kept as close to ninety degrees as possible so as not to create a thin, poorly vascularized island of tissue. The latissimus dorsi and the serratus anterior muscles are routinely preserved while the trapezius and rhomboid muscles are dissected to allow elevation of the scapula, which is necessary to expose the underlying chest wall. The ribs that are involved by the chest wall tumor are divided lateral to the tumor and a formal thoracotomy is performed at the fourth or fifth interspace (Fig. 37-3, *B*). This provides access into the chest, which facilitates the upper lobectomy and freeing of the tumor from other intrathoracic structures. At this point, the chest wall is resected along with the diseased upper lobe of the lung. With the assistance of the neurosurgeons, the ribs are disarticulated from the spine in sequential fashion beginning inferiorly. The monopolar cautery is used to divide the costotransverse and costovertebral joints, and a Cobb elevator is used to elevate the ribs away from the spine. The neurovascular bundle to each rib is ligated and cut and the pleura is divided, allowing the chest wall to become increasingly free (Fig. 37-3, *C*). One must be mindful of the adjacent T1 and C8 nerve roots while disarticulating the first rib. Once the disarticulation is completed, the diseased chest wall and upper lobe are removed (Fig. 37-3, *D*). This exposes the upper thoracic vertebrae that are involved with tumor.

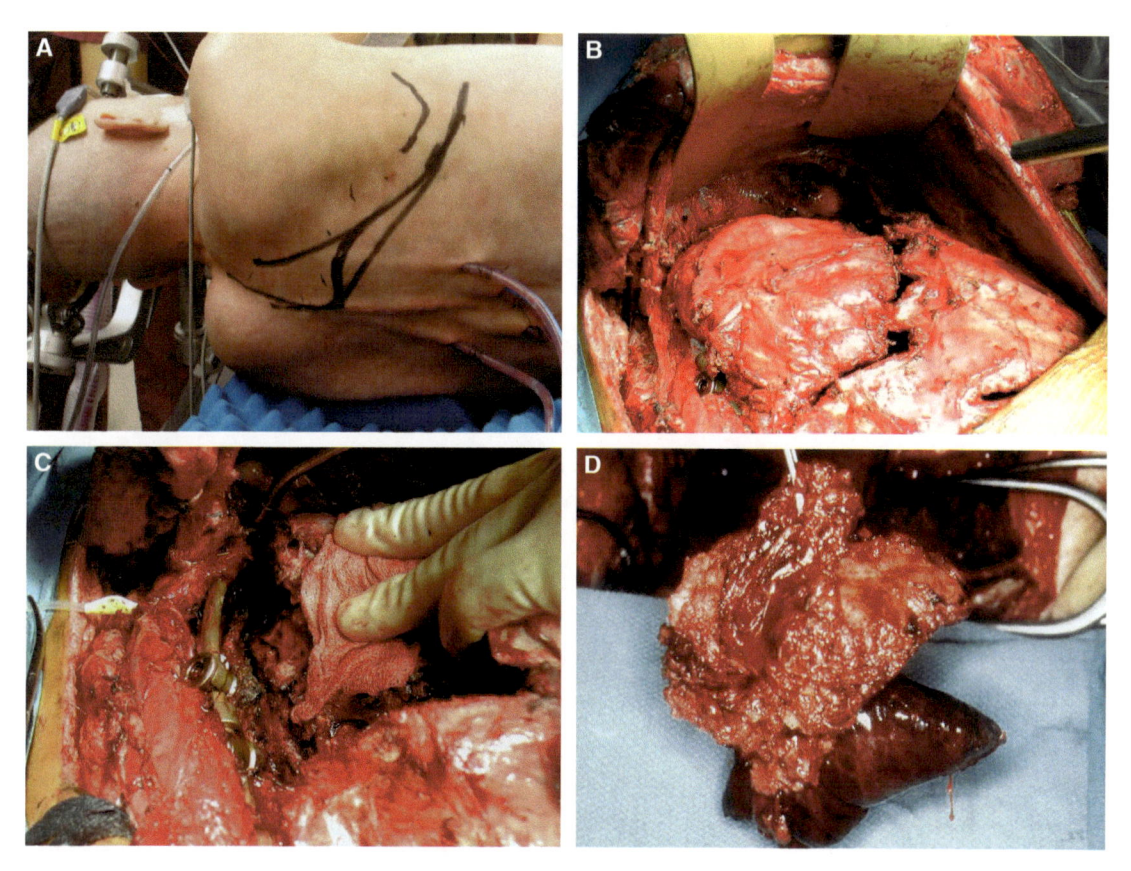

Fig. 37-3 **A,** Positioning for the lateral approach (stage two) for resection of a right-sided Pancoast tumor with spine involvement. The patient is in Mayfield pin fixation to maintain neutral cervicothoracic alignment in both the coronal and sagittal planes. The previous midline incision from the first stage with the associated drains can be observed. This incision will be reopened, along with the posterior thoracotomy incision drawn. **B,** The scapula is being gently retracted anteriorly, and the ribs have been divided lateral to the tumor. **C,** The ribs are carefully disarticulated from the spine at the costovertebral joints to separate the tumor involving the chest (on the right side) from the spine (on the left side). **D,** The pathologic specimen showing the chest wall and upper lobe of the lung.

Removal of the chest wall provides a direct lateral view of the upper thoracic vertebra (Fig. 37-4, *A*). A high-speed drill is used to perform the vertebrectomy of the involved levels (Fig. 37-4, *B*). A helpful tip to prevent ventral dural tears is to place a flat retractor, such as a number 2 Penfield dissector, in front of the silastic sheath during drilling. This serves as additional protection for the thecal sac. Once the involved vertebral bodies are completely resected, the discs above and below are cut at the rostral and caudal attachments respectively with a 15 blade and removed with a combination of pituitaries and curettes. The posterior longitudinal ligament is then sharply divided and resected. There are a variety of options for the anterior column reconstruction including structural allograft, static/expandable cages packed with morselized allograft or methylmethacrylate based on the principles described elsewhere in this chapter (Fig. 37-4, *C*). A chest tube is then placed by the thoracic surgeon, the lung is reinflated, and the thoracotomy is closed in layers. For large chest wall defects, the plastic surgeons may choose to mobilize the latissimus or serratus muscles to cover exposed

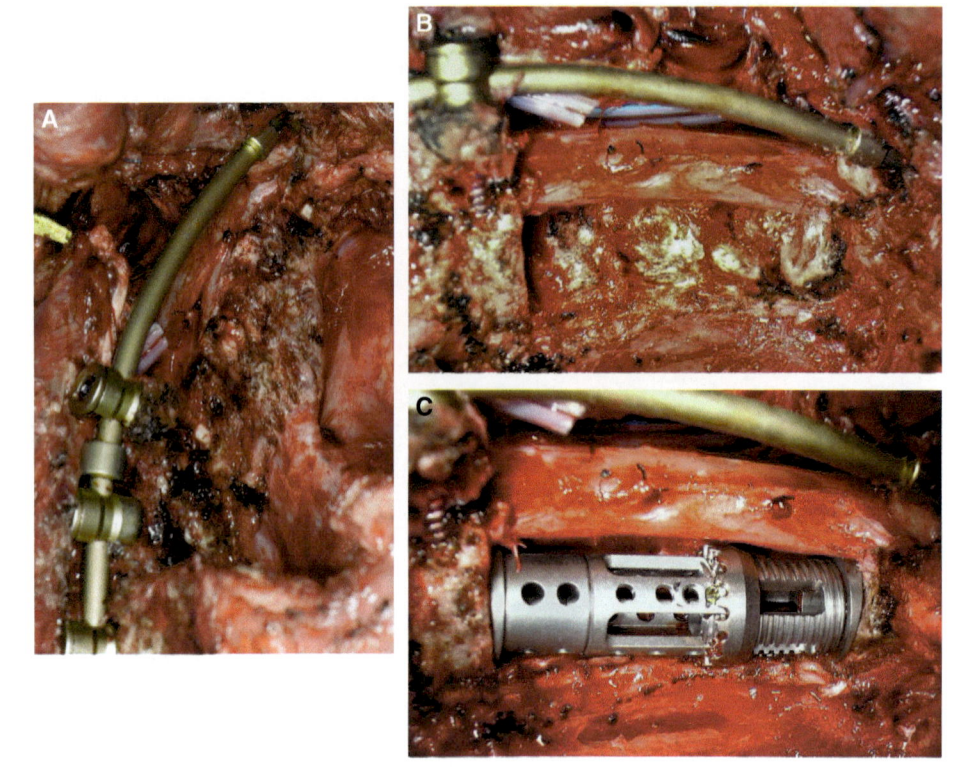

Fig. 37-4 A, Intraoperative view of the lateral aspect of the upper thoracic spine (involved with tumor). The disarticulated surfaces of the costovertebral joints can be seen just anterior to the right-sided rod. The thecal sac and the tip of the drain that was placed at the completion of the first stage of the operation can be seen. **B,** Intraoperative view showing the surgical defect that remains after completion of a three-level vertebrectomy (T2-4). The thecal sac can be clearly seen, along with the suture ligated nerve roots. **C,** The anterior column has now been reconstructed with an expandable titanium cage. This cage spans the three-level vertebrectomy defect, and the superior end is angulated to maintain the normal thoracic kyphosis. The cage will subsequently be filled with morselized allograft.

chest wall or spinal hardware. The patient is extubated and recovers in the surgical intensive care unit.

Resection of Hypervascular Spinal Metastasis with Paraspinal Extension

A single-stage combined lateral/posterior approach may be the most appropriate choice for hypervascular spinal metastasis involving the vertebral body, posterior elements, and paraspinal tissues. This is true whether the metastasis is located in the thoracic or lumbar spine. As discussed previously, the simultaneous access to the lateral and posterior, paraspinal, and spinal components of these tumors can be helpful in controlling bleeding and facilitating complete tumor removal. Anesthesia is induced and the patient is intubated and placed in the lateral decubitus position with the involved side up (Fig. 37-5). A flank incision overlying the level of interest is then planned in consultation with the thoracic or general surgeons. This is carried to the posterior midline, where a connecting incision is planned over the spine, centered over the level of pathology.

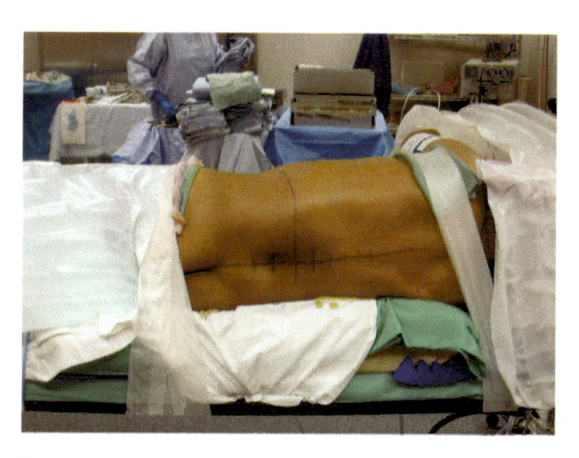

Fig. 37-5 Positioning of a patient for a single-stage combined lateral/posterior approach for a renal cell carcinoma involving the L1 vertebral body. The patient is in the true lateral position on a Jackson table with hips and knees flexed. The posterior midline is clearly marked, along with the flank incision that will allow a retroperitoneal approach for the L1 vertebrectomy.

The approach surgeon (a general surgeon or vascular surgeon for lower lumbar lesions or a thoracic surgeon for upper lumbar or thoracic lesions) generally begins the operation with the flank incision/thoracotomy. Adequate exposure of the superior, inferior, and anterior extent of the tumor and the spine above and below the tumor is necessary for safe resection of the mass. Once adequate exposure is obtained the case is turned over to the neurosurgeons for resection of the tumor. Because the resection of a thoracic spine/chest wall mass is described below, we will describe the appropriate technique for resecting a mass involving the lumbar spine.

Once the retroperitoneal space is exposed, the tumor mass must be clearly delineated. Often the mass is beneath the psoas muscle, which can be mobilized in a medial to lateral direction. If the mass is involving the psoas, the muscle may need to be truncated above and below the tumor. The nerves of the lumbar plexus are in close proximity running in the deep, posterior aspect of the muscle and should be avoided. Patients should be counseled on the risks of lower extremity weakness with these extensive tumors. Finding normal spine above and below the mass is critical for identifying the location of the spine deep to the tumor and for establishing recognizable anatomic landmarks. Once the anterior anatomy is clear, the posterior midline incision is opened. The spine is exposed in the usual subperiosteal fashion on the uninvolved side and on the involved side above and below the affected levels. Where tumor is encountered along the involved side, the dissection is carried out around it. Every effort should be made to stay outside the tumor until the resection is begun, because premature entry into the tumor can lead to prolonged and increased blood loss. The spine is completely exposed two levels above and two levels below the level of pathology. The paraspinal muscles must be elevated off of the tumor mass and a Penrose drain placed around the paraspinal muscle can aid in the lateral retraction so that the spine is well exposed.

With the spine completely exposed, before initiating the tumor resection, we typically place the pedicle screws and stabilize the spine on the uninvolved side with a spinal fixation rod. Not only does this allow completion of this step before tumor bleeding ensues, but also the stabilization helps to maintain the spinal alignment during the subsequent laminectomies, facetectomies, and vertebrectomies. Instrumentation of the pedicles is carried out in standard fashion with fluoroscopic guidance, except that the patient is in the lateral position. A helpful tip for successfully placing instrumentation with patients in this position is to use AP and lateral fluoroscopy at the time of positioning (before skin incision) to ensure that the patient is in the true lateral position, and to adjust the patient as needed.

The laminectomies are performed next. Any posterior or lateral epidural tumor invasion is resected to allow complete posterior and lateral exposure of the thecal sac. If a nerve root in the lumbar spine is encased in tumor and is unsalvageable with meticulous dissection, it may need to be suture ligated and divided sharply. The neurologic ramifications of this should be discussed extensively with the patient before surgery.

Frequently there is tumor involvement along the posterior elements involving the pedicles and facets, and this should be removed at this stage of the operation. Essentially, the tumor is now resected circumferentially around the spine, progressing from posterior to lateral to anterior. In high lumbar lesions with extensive tumor involvement of the psoas muscle, this can be safely resected above the level of the L2 vertebral body. Below this level, resection of the psoas muscle may compromise the lumbar plexus and motor function of the lower extremity. As tumor is resected and the psoas is elevated along the vertebral body, encountered segmental vessels at the level of resections should be cauterized with bipolar cautery and occluded with Weck clips or silk ties before sharp division. The lateral aspects of the vertebral bodies above and below the area of pathology should be exposed to allow adequate visualization for the vertebrectomy and permit lateral plating when indicated.

Attention can now be turned to the vertebrectomy. This can be performed with Leksell rongeurs or a high-speed drill. In general, we maintain a thin cortical shell of bone along the anterior and contralateral aspect of the resected vertebral body to protect adjacent structures. Resection of the posterior wall of the vertebral body is facilitated by direct visualization of the thecal sac afforded by resection of the facet or pedicle. Once the bone is removed, the discs above and below are cut sharply and removed with a combination of Kerrison punches and curettes. Next the posterior longitudinal ligament is dissected free from the thecal sac and resected with sharp division. Once the ventral thecal sac has been completely decompressed, the resected vertebral body can be reconstructed.

There are multiple options for reconstruction of the vertebral body. When there are healthy endplates, an expandable or static cage can be placed. However, when the endplates are irregular, with possible early involvement of tumor or significant osteoporosis, methylmethacrylate reconstruction may be more appropriate (Fig. 37-6). When using methylmethacrylate, we usually employ the chest tube technique first described by Errico and Cooper.[40] After vertebral reconstruction, the posterior stabilization can be completed by placing the ipsilateral rod and set screws.

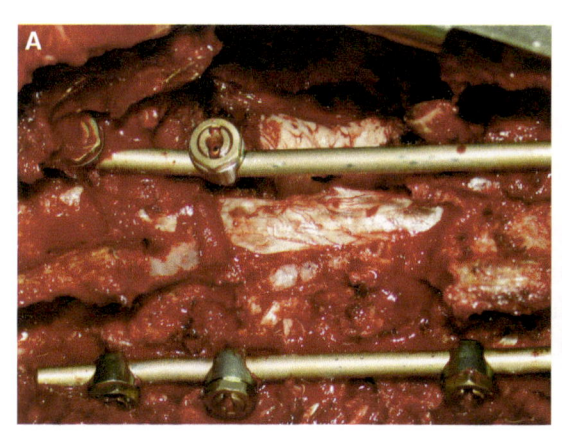

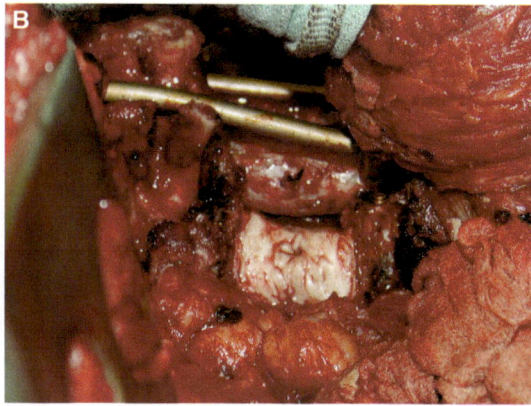

Fig. 37-6 **A,** Posterolateral and **B,** straight lateral intraoperative views during a combined posterior/lateral approach for resection of a hypervascular metastatic lesion. The L1 vertebrectomy has been completed and the vertebral body defect has been reconstructed with polymethylmethacrylate using the chest tube technique. Posterior segmental fixation with pedicle screw instrumentation has been placed.

It is helpful to provide some compression along the reconstructed vertebral body before final tightening of the posterior hardware. The crosslinks can then be placed, followed by morselized allograft for arthrodesis. The posterior incision is closed in the usual fashion while the vascular/thoracic surgeons place a chest tube and close the anterior flank incision. The patient is then extubated and admitted to the surgical intensive care unit for postoperative care.

RESECTION OF A PRIMARY SPINE TUMOR INVOLVING THE CHEST WALL

Surgery is performed in two stages. For the first stage, the patient is placed in the prone position. A midline skin incision is centered over the levels of neoplastic involvement, extending exposure rostrally and caudally to allow instrumented fusion of at least two levels above and two levels below the levels of tumor resection. In general, these tumors tend to involve one side of the posterior elements and chest wall more extensively than the other. On the uninvolved side, the spine can be exposed in the usual subperiosteal manner. On the tumor side, the dissection can be completed in the usual manner until the medial aspect of the facets involved by the tumor are encountered.

Once the medial aspect of the tumor mass comes into view, dissection is carried rostrally and caudally to find uninvolved tissue above and below. Care must be taken to avoid violating the tumor during this dissection, in keeping with sound oncologic principles. The transverse process and medial aspect of the rib are identified at the level above and below the tumor. These will serve as the superior and inferior aspects of the resection margin. In addition to identifying the osseous margins above and below the tumor, the paraspinal muscles may be truncated along the superior and inferior margins, leaving a border of healthy muscle tissue overlying the tumor mass. Once exposure of the spine is completed, posterior instrumented stabilization is done. We use frameless stereotactic navigation for placement of lumbar and thoracic pedicle screws.

The screws are placed on both sides, avoiding the levels on the side of the tumor where the vertebra will be sectioned. Depending on the size of the tumor mass and its medial extent, it may or may not be possible to place the rod on the involved side.

Generous laminectomies are then performed from pedicle to pedicle in the usual manner to allow complete decompression of the involved spinal segments (Fig. 37-7). Next the nerve roots of the involved side are suture-ligated with 2-0 silk ties and cut sharply. This allows unfettered access to the ventral epidural space. The superior articulating facet of the uppermost involved level and the inferior articulating facet of the lowest involved level are removed to free the upper and lower spinal attachments. Finally, a 1 mm cutting burr is used to initiate the sagittal vertebral osteotomy beginning at the disc space above the uppermost involved vertebra and extending down to the disc space below the lowest involved vertebra. This will serve as the "docking point" for the osteotomes during the second stage operation to complete the sagittal osteotomies. Great care must be taken while operating the drill in close proximity to the thecal sac, and an assistant is necessary to protect the dura. As illustrated in Fig. 37-13, frameless stereotactic navigation can be used to determine the location of this trough, which is oriented sagittally along the medial base of the pedicles. The wound is closed in layers in the usual manner. The patient is then extubated and admitted to the surgical intensive care unit for close monitoring until the second stage of the operation.

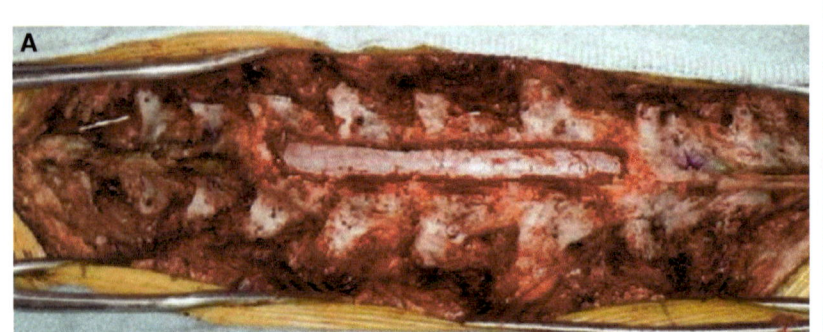

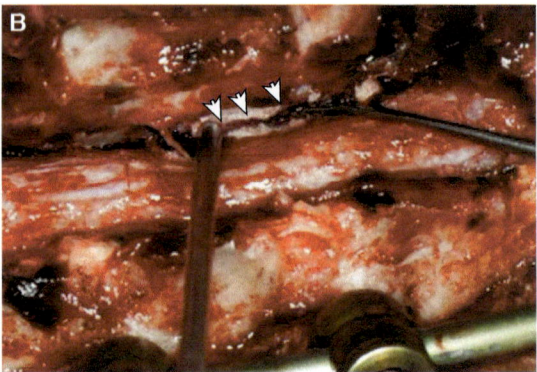

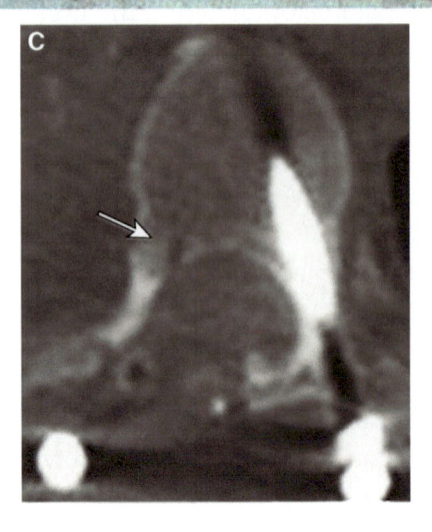

Fig. 37-7 Intraoperative photographs after **A,** complete laminectomies with medial facetectomies from T4 to T7 and **B,** drilling of a sagittal trough *(arrowheads)* along the posterior T6 vertebral body. The 3 mm deep trough was drilled using a 2 mm cutting burr extending from the mid-T4 vertebral body caudally to the T7-8 disc. This trough provides a safe and secure docking point for the osteotome during the sagittal osteotomy in the second-stage procedure. **C,** Axial CT scan between the first and second stages showing the trough *(white arrow)*. (Reprinted with permission from Smitherman SM, Tatsui CD, Rao G, et al. Image-guided multilevel vertebral osteotomies for en bloc resection of giant cell tumor of the thoracic spine: case report and description of operative technique. Eur Spine J 19:1021-1028, 2010.)

The second stage of the operation usually involves a multidisciplinary team comprising plastic surgeons, thoracic surgeons, and spine surgeons. The spine surgeon must be intimately familiar with the work of his or her colleagues as it relates to this approach to effectively lead this multidisciplinary team. The second stage operation begins with the patient in the lateral decubitus position on a bean bag, with the involved side up. First, the previous posterior midline incision is reopened. The plastic surgeons (in coordination with the thoracic surgeons) then make a standard thoracotomy incision that essentially overlies the mass and connects with the posterior midline incision approximately halfway along its rostrocaudal dimension.

The plastic surgeons then mobilize muscle flaps as they deem necessary to accomplish several goals. First, any large defect created by resection of the mass must be filled to avoid postoperative seroma formation. Second, the thecal sac must be separated from the lung if at all possible. Finally, and perhaps most important for the prevention of wound dehiscence, the posterior spinal hardware must be separated from the overlying skin with viable muscle. This is especially vital for patients who are likely to receive adjuvant radiation, which further compromises wound healing. The junction of the spinal and thoracotomy incisions is a notorious location for wound failure, and a tension-free closure is mandatory. The plastic surgeons will frequently use a latissimus dorsi pedicled muscle flap or a trapezius pedicled muscle flap to reconstruct the defects and accomplish the stated goals. In addition, the paraspinous muscles are often mobilized and advanced to cover the hardware in the posterior midline.

After the plastic surgeons have mobilized the appropriate muscle flaps, attention is turned back to completing the en bloc resection of the tumor. The thoracic surgeons define the lateral margin of the tumor resection by cutting the involved ribs lateral to the extent of the tumor (Fig. 37-8). The intercostal neurovascular bundles along the

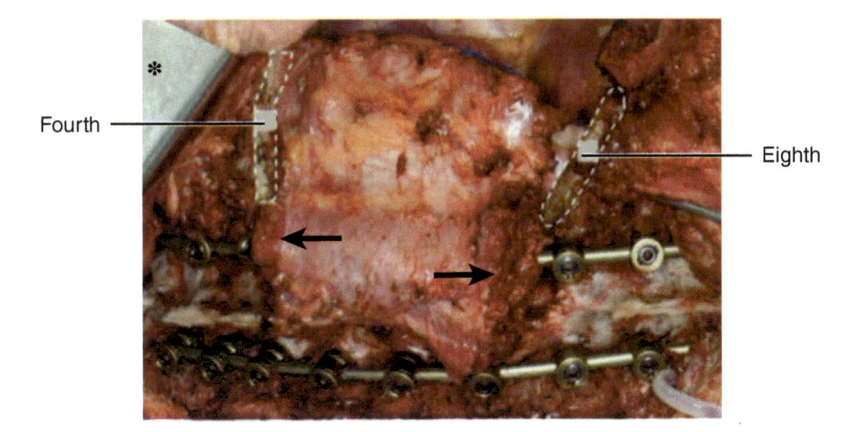

Fig. 37-8 Stage two intraoperative photograph showing preparation for resection of the tumor. The paraspinous muscles *(black arrows)* have been cut and will be removed with the specimen. The ribs have been cut lateral to the mass. The fourth and eighth ribs have been exposed *(dashed white outline)*. There is a retractor under the right scapula *(asterisk)*. (Reprinted with permission from Smitherman SM, Tatsui CD, Rao G, et al. Image-guided multilevel vertebral osteotomies for en bloc resection of giant cell tumor of the thoracic spine: case report and description of operative technique. Eur Spine J 19:1021-1028, 2010.)

involved nerves are individually dissected, suture-ligated with silk ties, and cut sharply. Once the lateral edge of the en bloc resection is defined, the thoracic surgeons are able to address the anterior border of the resection within the chest. Anteriorly, these tumors of the spine and chest wall frequently parasitize the lung for additional blood supply. The involved portion of the lung may be divided with the stapler so that the involved portion can be included with the en bloc resection. Finally, the thoracic surgeons create a safe dissection plane anterior to the spinal column, mobilizing and protecting the vital vascular and digestive structures, depending on the level of the thoracic spine involved. By placing a hand or retractor between the spine and these critical structures, the thoracic surgeon is able to protect these tissues during the subsequent osteotomies.

In preparation for the osteotomies, the frameless stereotactic navigation system is registered and will be used to guide the osteotomes as they create the medial vertebral border of the resection (Fig. 37-9, *A* through *C*). This navigation is based on a new CT obtained after the first stage of the operation. The array may need to be clamped to the spinous process of the inferiormost level of the stabilization (below the hardware) to minimize metal artifact and ensure an accurate registration. After registering, the accuracy of the setup can be checked by placing the pointer probe in the osteotomy groove created during the first surgery and confirming this location on the CT image. Now the tracking probe can be clamped directly to the osteotome so that it can be tracked in real time. This greatly expedites the procedure by precluding the need for constant alternation between the osteotome and a pointer probe to check the accuracy of the trajectory. The osteotome is then seated in the previous osteotomy groove created during the first stage of the procedure. The sagittal osteotomies are carried anteriorly through the involved vertebral bodies, medial to the extent of the tumor. Any remaining attachments of the discs are then cut and the mass is rotated out of the body en bloc (Fig. 37-9, *D* and *E*).

Bone wax is applied to the cut edges of the vertebral bodies to obtain hemostasis. The size of the vertebrectomy defect determines whether or not anterior column reconstruction is warranted. Finally, the posterior bony surfaces are decorticated and the posterior stabilization is completed by placing the missing titanium rod and set screws. Morselized allograft or autograft is then packed along the decorticated surfaces after the placement of one or two crosslinks (depending on the length of the construct).

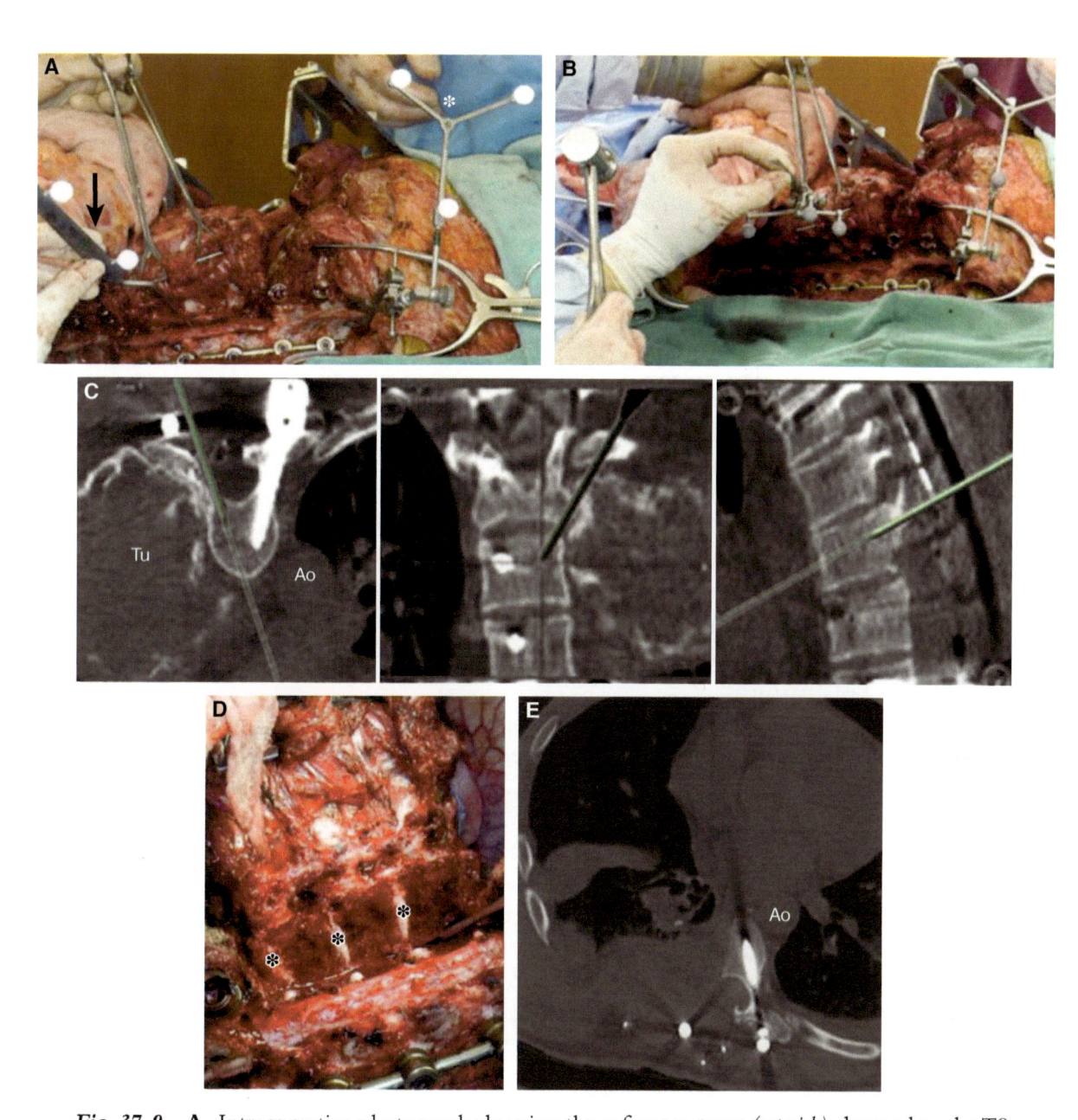

Fig. 37-9 **A,** Intraoperative photograph showing the reference array *(asterisk)* clamped to the T9 spinous process and the pointer probe *(black arrow)* placed into the trough that was drilled in the posterior vertebral body during the first stage of the procedure, verifying accuracy of registration. **B,** A tracking probe is clamped to the osteotome and registered to the navigation system to accurately follow the proposed trajectory. **C,** Intraoperative axial, coronal, and sagittal images demonstrating the path and depth of the osteotomy in real time. **D,** The sagittal osteotomies have been completed. The cut vertebral surfaces along with the T4-5, T5-6, and T6-7 discs are visible *(asterisk)*. **E,** Postoperative axial CT scan at the T7 level. (*Ao,* Aorta; *Tu,* tumor.) (Reprinted with permission from Smitherman SM, Tatsui CD, Rao G, et al. Image-guided multilevel vertebral osteotomies for en bloc resection of giant cell tumor of the thoracic spine: case report and description of operative technique. Eur Spine J 19:1021-1028, 2010.)

A chest tube is placed by the thoracic surgeons, then the plastic surgeons begin filling the resection defect with the muscle flaps mobilized earlier in the case. The muscle flaps are sutured to the prevertebral fascia to separate the neural elements from the lung and to provide an anchor for the muscle filling the resection defect. Posteriorly, the muscle flaps are advanced over the hardware to prevent direct contact between the underlying hardware and the overlying skin. Multiple drains are routinely placed. The closure is then completed in the usual fashion, and after extubation, the patient is taken to the surgical intensive care unit.

OUTCOMES AND EVALUATION OF RESULTS

In appropriately selected patients with metastatic disease to the spine, aggressive surgical resection improves quality of life and may extend survival.[27,41,42] As previously stated, this can frequently be performed through a solitary posterior or anterior approach. However, when a metastatic lesion is hypervascular and has circumferential (anterior and posterior) spinal involvement, the combined approach may be useful to facilitate aggressive surgical resection while optimizing hemostasis. Our experience with this simultaneous combined approach to the thoracic or lumbar spine for metastatic disease shows a mean survival of 22.5 months, with no instances of locally recurrent metastatic disease.[17]

The extent of resection clearly affects local recurrence rates and may have an impact on survival in the management of primary malignant and aggressive benign tumors of the spine. In one study, 5-year survival was 33% in patients who underwent an incomplete excision and 75% in patients who had a complete resection.[23] With regard to chordoma above the sacrum, a retrospective review showed that debulking or palliative surgery was associated with recurrence or progression in 80% of cases (even with radiation), while intralesional resection was associated with 100% recurrence.[13] Only en bloc excision with adjuvant radiation was associated with disease free survival in 100% of patients during the follow-up period (39 to 112 months, mean of 77 months).[13] Boriani's long-term follow-up data[43] (50-year experience) further supports these findings, with 75% recurrence in patients who underwent intralesional resection compared to 33% recurrence in patients who underwent en bloc resection. Similar results were reported for chondrosarcoma of the mobile spine, where the recurrence rate was 8% in patients with en bloc excision and negative histologic margins while the recurrence rate was 100% in patients in intralesional resection (even with radiation). Similarly, survival was 92% in the en bloc resection group, but only 20% in the intralesional resection group at final follow-up.[14] En bloc resection should be attempted whenever possible in these cases.

Pancoast tumors with involvement of the spine have historically been associated with a poor prognosis.[44-47] More recently, however, the combination of neoadjuvant or adjuvant concurrent chemoradiation with aggressive surgical resection has yielded an increasing proportion of long-term survivors among carefully selected patients without distant or nodal disease.[42] Our initial description of combined chest wall resection with vertebrectomy and spinal reconstruction for the treatment of Pancoast tumors showed encouraging short-term follow-up results with regard to ambulatory status and survival.[18,26] Our longer term follow-up shows that negative surgical margins are associated with a 39% 5-year survival, compared with 12% for patients with positive margins[19] (Fig. 37-10). We think the combined approach described is the best way to obtain negative margins when resecting these difficult tumors.

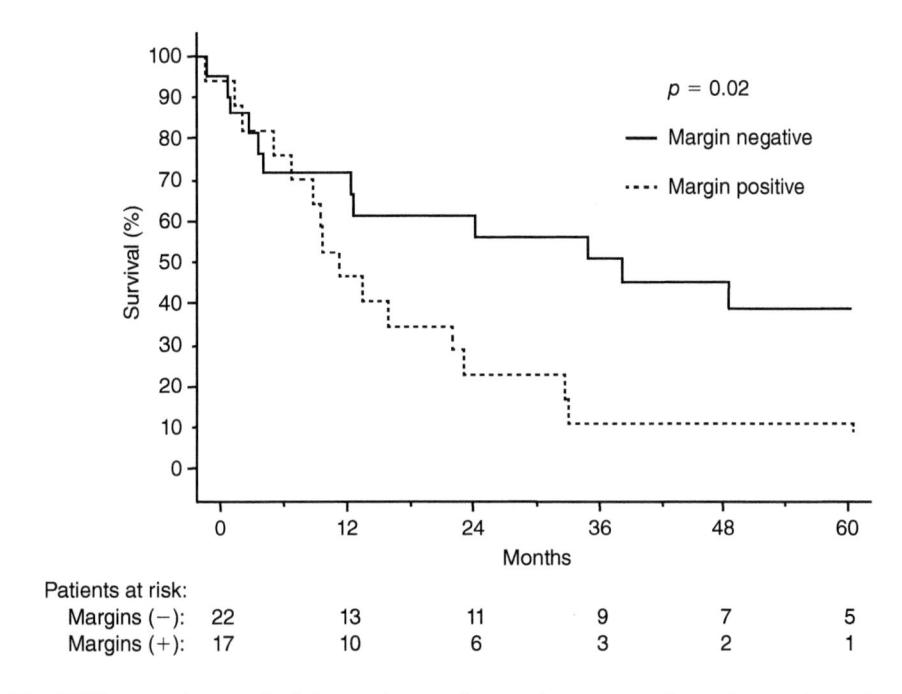

Fig. 37-10 Difference in survival for patients who undergo resection of superior sulcus tumors with negative margins compared with those with positive margins. (From the Journal of Thoracic and Cardiovascular Surgery, Vol 137, Bolton WD, Rice DC, Goodyear A, et al, Superior sulcus tumors with vertebral body involvement: a multimodality approach, pages 1379-1387, Copyright 2009, with permission from Elsevier.)

SIGNATURE CASES

PANCOAST TUMOR WITH UPPER THORACIC SPINE INVOLVEMENT

A 38-year-old woman with an extensive smoking history presented with "lava-like" pain in the right upper ribcage and chest. On physical examination, she was found to have a right Horner's syndrome. Otherwise, the patient had full strength in her bilateral upper and lower extremities without sensory deficits or abnormal reflexes. Her workup revealed a right apical mass involving the right chest wall (Fig. 37-11, *A* and *B*). This tumor involved the second, third, and fourth ribs as well as the lateral aspects of the T2, T3, and T4 vertebrae (Fig. 37-11, *C* through *E*). The staging workup revealed no other sites of disease. The patient elected to undergo resection of this mass.

A two-stage resection of her Pancoast tumor was performed, along with the involved chest wall and vertebral bodies, as detailed in the Technique section above (see Fig. 37-3, *B* through *D*). In this particular case, posterior instrumentation was carried out from C5 to T7, with bilateral laminectomies and right-sided facetectomies from T2-T4 (see Figs. 37-1 and 37-2). A three level vertebrectomy (T2-T4) was undertaken with expandable titanium cage anterior column reconstruction, packed with morselized allograft and demineralized bone matrix (see Fig. 37-4, *B* and *C*). Postoperative three-dimensional CT images show good alignment and reconstruction of the anterior column with posterior segmental instrumentation (Fig. 37-11, *F* and *G*). Negative margins were achieved.

Postoperatively, the patient's right-sided arm and shoulder pain were dramatically improved. She was discharged to home 1 week postoperatively. She received postoperative concurrent chemoradiation. She remained without evidence of disease 3 years after surgery.

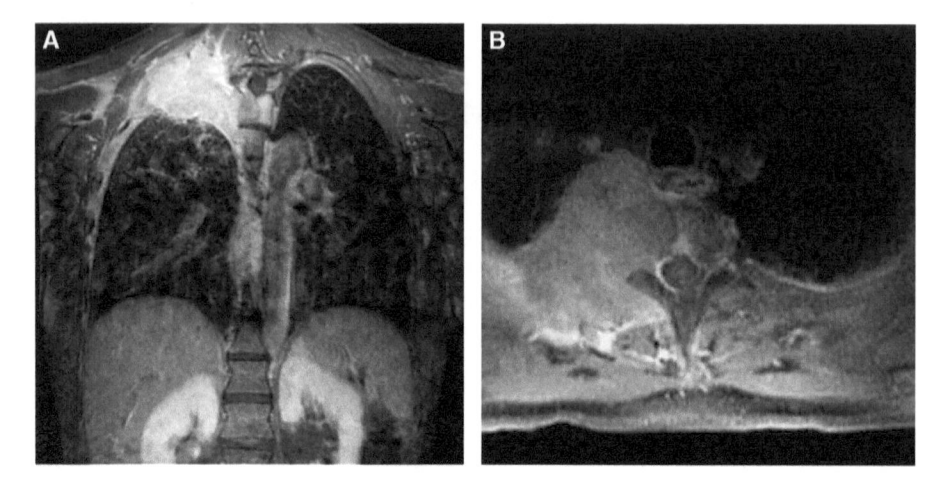

Fig. 37-11 **A**, Coronal and **B**, axial T1-weighted MRI with contrast images showing a right apical lung mass involving the thoracic vertebrae and ribs at T2, T3, and T4.

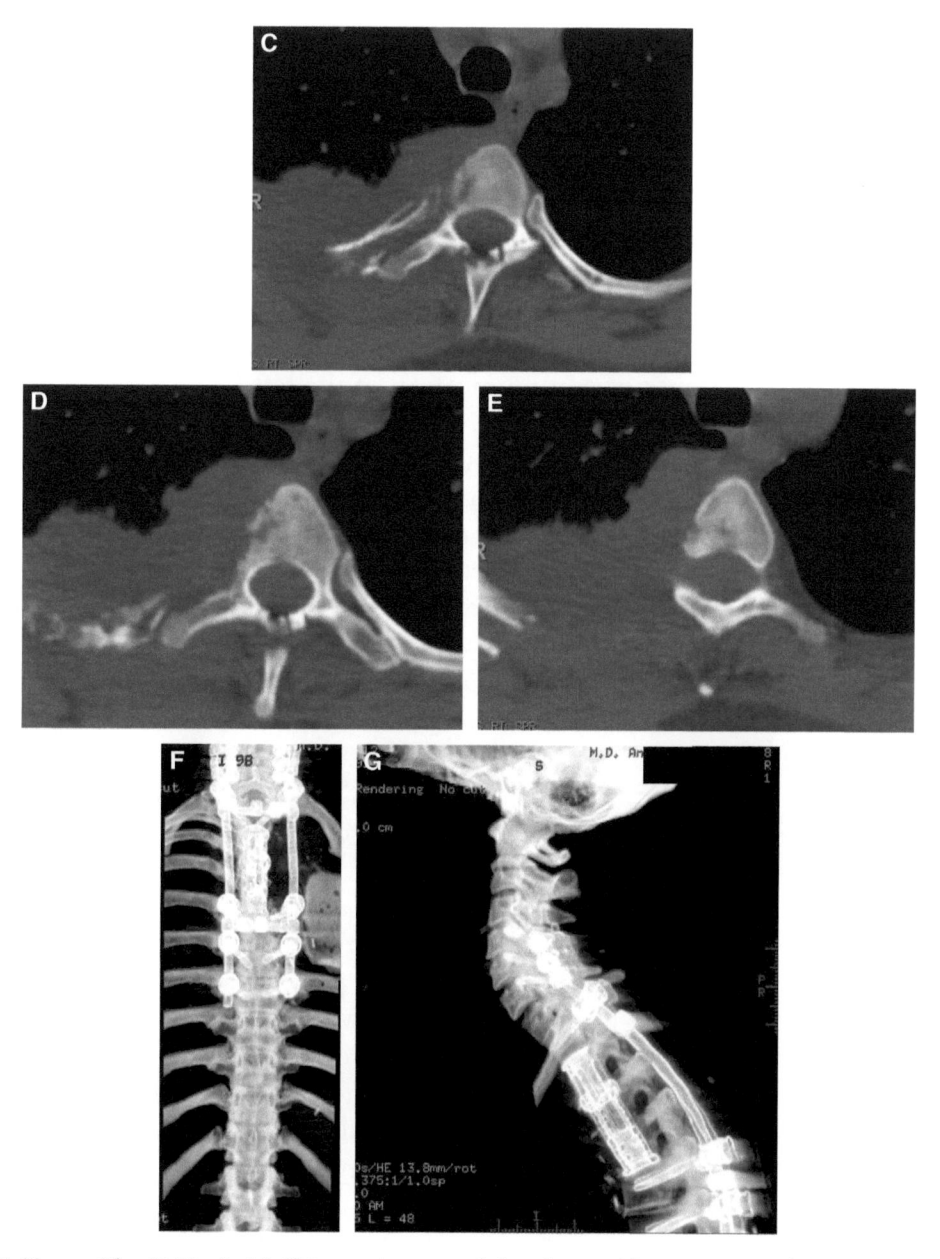

Fig. 37-11, cont'd **C-E,** Axial CT scan images of the chest without contrast show tumor involvement and destruction of the lateral aspects of the vertebral bodies and ribs at the T2, T3, and T4 levels. Postoperative **F,** coronal and **G,** sagittal CT reconstructed images showing anterior column reconstruction with an expandable cage to fill the three-level vertebrectomy defect with posterior segmental instrumentation extending from C5 to T7.

Renal Cell Cancer Metastasis to the L1 Vertebral Body

A 53-year-old man with a history of metastatic renal cell carcinoma presented with significant upper lumbar back pain and radiation into the left hip region. MRI revealed a destructive lesion of the L1 vertebral body with significant canal compromise (Fig. 37-12, *A*). This lesion appeared to be secondarily invading the spine from the psoas muscle with involvement of the left L1 vertebra, pedicle, foramen, and posterior elements (Fig. 37-12, *B*). On examination, he was neurologically intact with normal strength, sensation, and reflexes, as well as normal bowel and bladder function.

Preoperatively, the patient underwent attempted embolization of the mass; however, this was unsuccessful because of communication of the left L1 radicular artery with the artery of Adamkiewickz (Fig. 37-12, *C* and *D*). The patient underwent a single-stage combined anterior/posterior resection and anterior column reconstruction with posterior instrumented fusion, as described in the Technique section. In this case, the L1 vertebral body was resected along with the superiormost portion of the iliopsoas muscle, and the L1 nerve root was sacrificed, because it was completely encased in tumor. The anterior column reconstruction was completed with methylmethacrylate because of the suboptimal consistency and contour of the superior endplate of L2, as observed intraoperatively (see Fig. 37-6). Given the preoperative radiographic appearance of the T12 vertebral body, vertebroplasty was performed intraoperatively before pedicle screw placement (with the patient in the lateral position). The patient's posterior construct spanned from T11 to L3. Postoperatively, the patient recovered in the surgical intensive care unit, then was transferred to the neurosurgery floor on the second postoperative day.

Postoperative imaging showed excellent alignment of the spinal column (Fig. 37-12, *E* and *F*). The patient retained the ability to ambulate postoperatively, although formal neurologic strength testing revealed the expected weakness in the left iliopsoas. By 1 week postoperatively, the patient's pain was significantly decreased compared with his preoperative pain level. He was eventually transferred to a rehabilitation facility. Unfortunately, this patient succumbed to widespread metastatic disease within 1 year of surgery (although he had no evidence of locally recurrent disease).

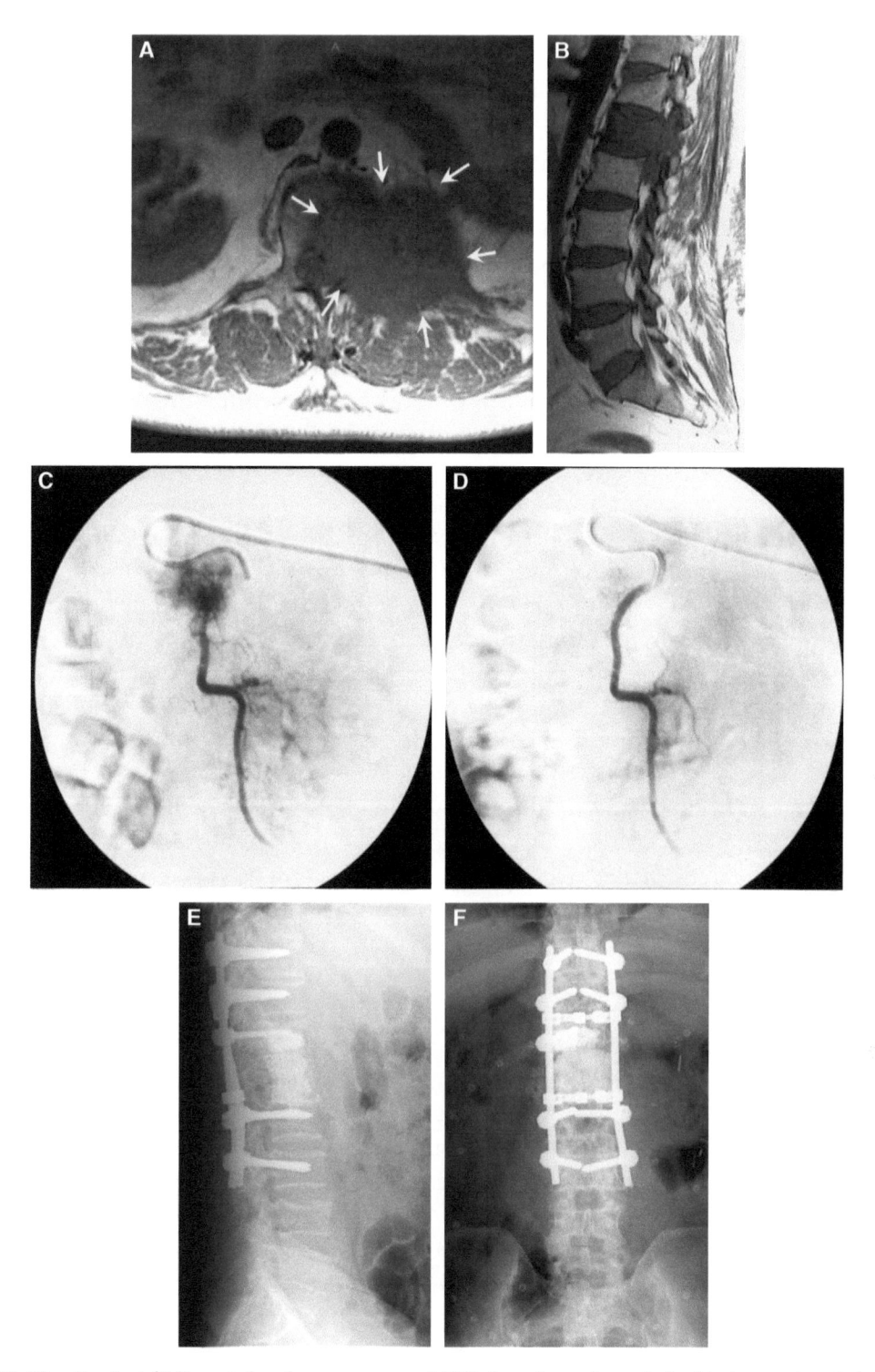

Fig. 37-12 **A,** Axial T1-weighted postcontrast MRI showing a large left-sided mass involving the L1 vertebral body, pedicle, and psoas muscle, with encroachment into the extradural space and compression of the thecal sac. **B,** The mass extended into the L1-2 foramen and posterior elements as well as the extradural space behind the L2 vertebral body. Preoperative angiograms of the spine show **C,** the extensive vascularity of the metastatic renal cell carcinoma lesion, with **D,** an aberrant artery of Adamkiewickz, precluding the possibility of preoperative embolization. Postoperative **E,** lateral and **F,** anteroposterior radiographs showing reconstruction of the L1 vertebral body defect, kyphoplasty at T12, and posterior thoracolumbar segmental instrumentation extending from T10 to L3.

GIANT CELL TUMOR OF THE THORACIC SPINE INVOLVING THE CHEST WALL

A 35-year-old man with a remote history of a motorcycle accident began developing progressive pain and right-sided "bandlike" numbness of the thorax. Chest radiographs and subsequent CT scans demonstrated a right posterior chest wall mass measuring 9 by 9 by 7.5 cm involving the fifth, sixth, and seventh ribs as well as the right anterolateral portion of the fourth through seventh vertebral bodies (Fig. 37-13, *A* through *D*). A CT-guided biopsy revealed histiocytes and giant cells; a diagnosis of giant cell tumor was made. The patient was treated with weekly pegylated interferon injections for 1 year by the sarcoma service. Subsequently he underwent staged monthly endovascular embolizations of the lesion for 4 months. After completing this neoadjuvant treatment and preoperative course, he was referred for definitive surgical resection.

En bloc resection of the mass was planned in two stages. The first stage consisted of posterior instrumented fusion, decompression, and initiation of the sagittal osteotomies. Wide laminectomies were performed from T4 to T7, along with medial facetectomies on the right side (see Fig. 37-7). The right T4 through T7 nerve roots were ligated and cut, allowing for gentle medial retraction of the thecal sac and initiation of the osteotomies. Using imaging guidance, a sagittal trough was created with the pneumatic drill just medial to the pedicles, extending from the middle of T4 to the T7-8 disc. This trough would serve as the docking point for the osteotome during the second stage of the procedure. Image guidance was then used to place posterior instrumentation from T2-T9 on the left with pedicle screws at T2, T3, T4, T8, and T9 on the right. The rods were placed and the wound was closed in layers. A postoperative CT scan confirmed accurate hardware placement and served as the source imaging for frameless stereotactic intraoperative image guidance during the second-stage vertebral osteotomies.

The second stage was performed 2 days later, with the patient placed in the left lateral decubitus position. A right posterolateral thoracotomy incision was made between the fifth and sixth ribs, extending posteriorly to the previous midline incision, which was reopened. The right trapezius, latissimus dorsi, and serratus anterior muscles were mobilized during the exposure to provide sufficient soft tissue coverage during closure. The thoracotomy was augmented by cutting the fifth through seventh ribs lateral to the tumor, and a wedge resection of the right upper and lower lobes was performed, leaving involved portions of the lung attached to the tumor mass. Blunt dissection was then used to free the medial margin of the tumor from the azygous vein, the aorta, and the esophagus, and the anterior aspect of the spine could be palpated

Once the intrathoracic dissection was complete, the right paraspinal muscles were truncated at the fourth and eighth ribs to ensure a negative posterior margin (see Fig. 37-8). Frameless stereotactic navigation was then used to guide the osteotomies from the previously drilled trough to the anterior aspect of the vertebral body (see Fig. 37-9 *A* through *C*), allowing a complete en bloc resection of the mass (Fig. 37-13, *E* through *G*).

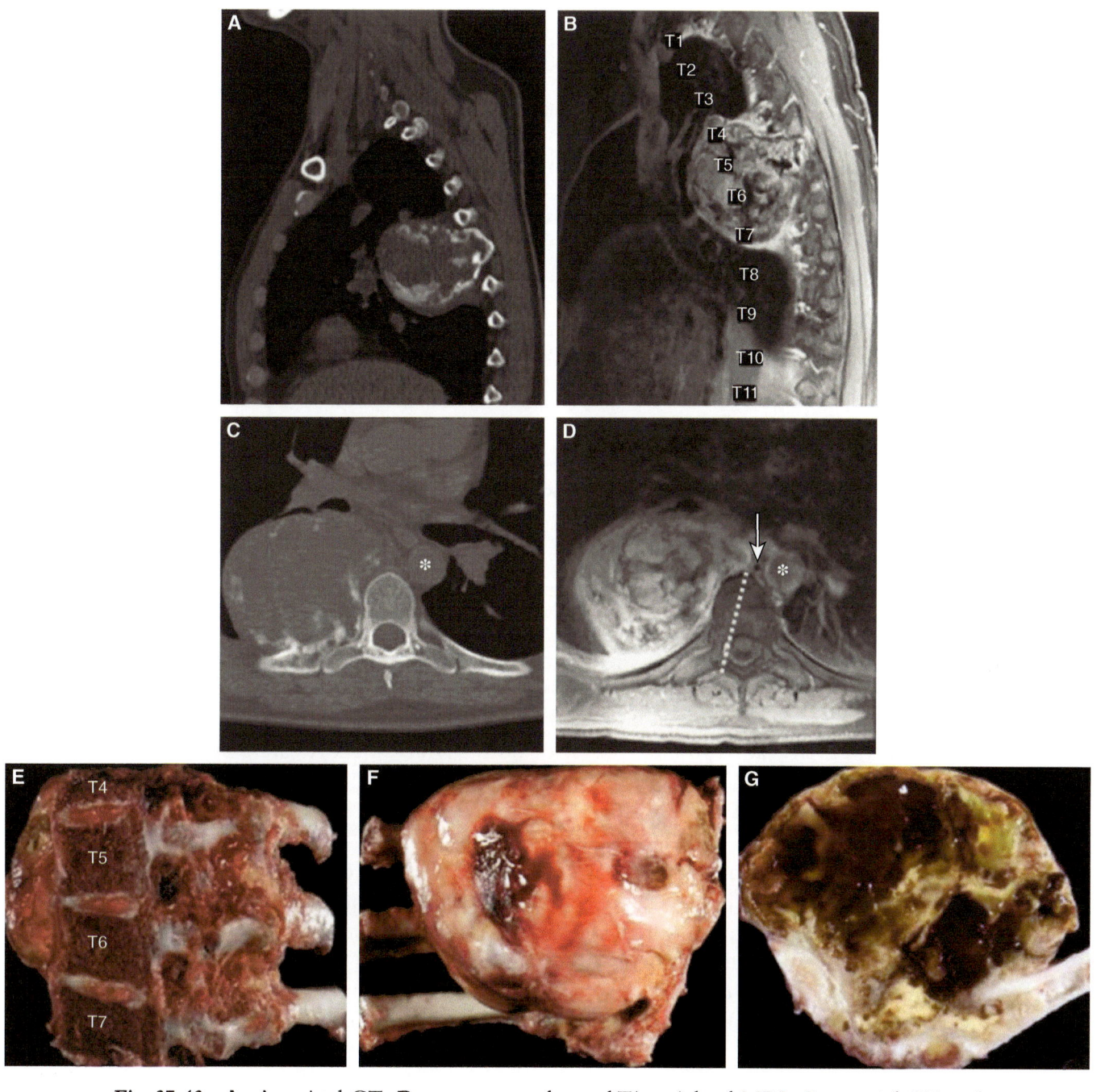

Fig. 37-13 **A,** A sagittal CT; **B,** a contrast-enhanced T1-weighted MRI; **C,** an axial CT; and **D,** contrast-enhanced T1-weighted MRI showing this patient's giant cell tumor involving the right lung, chest wall, and the fourth through seventh thoracic vertebral bodies and ribs. The CT images (**A** and **C**) show evidence of calcifications within the mass. The tumor abuts the aorta *(asterisk)* and the azygous vein *(white arrow)*. *Dashed white line* indicates the planned osteotomy. The gross specimen is shown after en bloc resection; **E,** the medial surface of the specimen, along the sagittal osteotomies; **F,** the ventral surface of the tumor specimen showing the chest wall mass and the resected ribs; and **G,** cross-section cut surface of the specimen revealing its heterogeneous appearance.

Continued

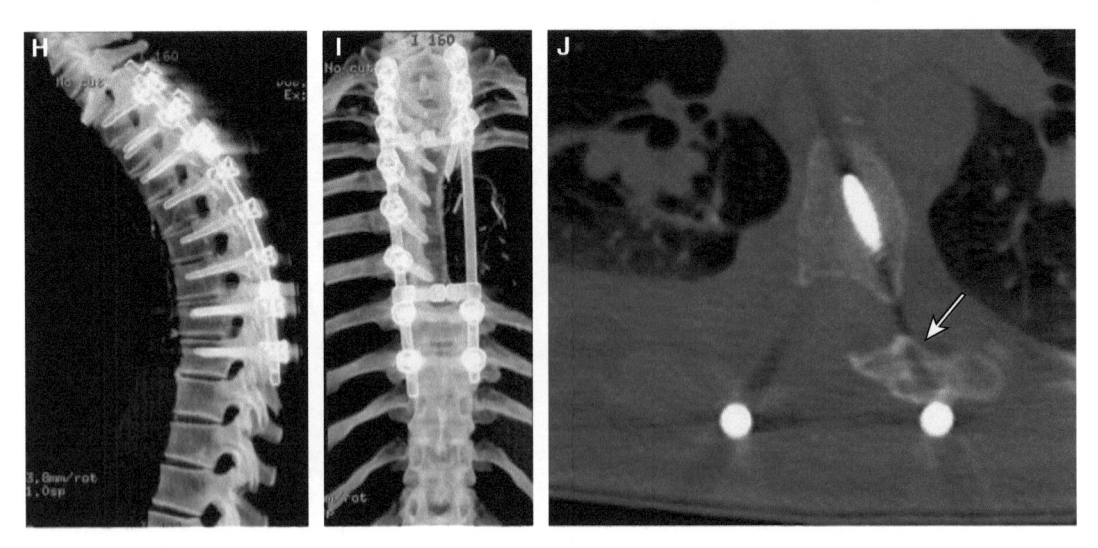

Fig. 37-13, cont'd At 1 year postoperatively, **H**, sagittal and **I**, coronal CT demonstrate that spinal alignment has been maintained, with no evidence of hardware failure. **J**, *Arrow* in axial CT image showing evidence of a posterior fusion mass, suggesting successful arthrodesis. (Reprinted with permission from Smitherman SM, Tatsui CD, Rao G, et al. Image-guided multilevel vertebral osteotomies for en bloc resection of giant cell tumor of the thoracic spine: case report and description of operative technique. Eur Spine J 19:1021-1028, 2010.)

With the help of image guidance, the trajectory of the osteotomes could be precisely determined. The anterior vascular and aerodigestive structures could be protected by placing a hand between these structures and the anterior aspect of the spine. The right-sided rod was then placed and the posterior bony surfaces decorticated and covered with allograft and demineralized bone matrix. Multiple muscle flaps were used to fill the chest wall defect and cover the posterior instrumentation and construct.

Postoperatively, the patient recovered in the surgical intensive care unit for 2 days and was then transferred to the neurosurgery floor. He was neurologically intact, and his right-sided chest wall pain subsided. His spinal alignment is well maintained, with no evidence of hardware failure (Fig. 37-13, *H* through *J*). A CT scan completed 1 year postoperatively revealed continued excellent sagittal and coronal plan alignment and evidence of posterior arthrodesis. The patient remained ambulatory with full strength and no evidence of recurrent disease nearly 3 years after his resection.

CONCLUSION

The combined posterior/lateral approach to the thoracic and lumbar spine is an extensive surgical undertaking that is sometimes necessary for the optimal treatment of patients with neoplastic disease involving the spine. This approach is useful when the pathologic process cannot be adequately addressed by an anterior or posterior approach alone. There are three major categories of spinal neoplastic disease that may benefit from the combined approach: superior sulcus tumors with extension into the spine, hypervascular metastases with extensive spinal and paraspinal involvement, and primary spine tumors extending into the chest wall. Adherence to strict oncologic principles in clinical decision making and thorough preoperative planning will optimize patient outcomes.

TIPS FROM THE MASTERS

- The surgeon must recognize instances in which the combined lateral/posterior approach may provide advantages for spinal resection and reconstruction: Pancoast tumors with spinal involvement, hypervascular spinal metastases with circumferential spinal involvement and paraspinal extension, and primary spinal column tumors with chest wall involvement.
- Patients must undergo appropriate oncologic and surgical staging to determine whether these extensive surgical procedures are warranted and feasible.
- These procedures often extend beyond the spine, and multidisciplinary surgical expertise may provide improved outcomes.
- These patients will often require radiation therapy and chemotherapy as part of their overall therapeutic regimen. These surgical procedures should be coordinated with these other forms of treatment so that the ideal multimodal approach is employed.
- Plan, plan, plan—these are complex surgical procedures. The surgeon must have a conceptual framework for the approach, resection, spinal stabilization/fusion, and soft tissue reconstruction prior to performing the surgery.

References (With Key References in Boldface)

1. Kim DH, O'Toole JE, Ogden AT, et al. Minimally invasive posterolateral thoracic corpectomy: cadaveric feasibility study and report of four clinical cases. Neurosurgery 64:746-753, 2009.
2. **Stener B. Total spondylectomy in chondrosarcoma arising from the seventh thoracic vertebra. J Bone Joint Surg Br 53:288-295, 1971.**
3. Stener B. Complete removal of vertebrae for extirpation of tumors. A 20-year experience. Clin Orthop Relat Res 245:72-82, 1989.
4. Abe E, Sato K, Tazawa H, et al. Total spondylectomy for primary tumor of the thoracolumbar spine. Spinal Cord 38:146-152, 2000.
5. Abe E, Kobayashi T, Murai H, et al. Total spondylectomy for the primary malignant, aggressive benign, and solitary metastatic bone tumors of the thoracolumbar spine. J Spinal Disord 14:237-246, 2001.
6. Faraj AA, O'Dowd J, Webb JK. Osteoblastoma of the vertebral body of the third lumbar vertebra. Eur Spine J 7:249-251, 1998.

7. Laffargue P, Cotten A, Cortet B, et al. [Giant cell tumors of the spine. Report of a case, literature review] Acta Orthop Belg 63:28-34, 1997.
8. Marmor E, Rhines LD, Weinberg JS, et al. Total en bloc lumbar spondylectomy. Case report. J Neurosurg 95(2 Suppl):264-269, 2001.
9. Sundaresan N, Digiacinto GV, Krol G, et al. Spondylectomy for malignant tumors of the spine. J Clin Oncol 7:1485-1491, 1989.
10. Tomita K, Kawahara N, Baba H, et al. Total en bloc spondylectomy. A new surgical technique for primary malignant vertebral tumors. Spine 22:324-333, 1997.
11. Tomita K, Kawahara N, Baba H, et al. Total en bloc spondylectomy for solitary spinal metastases. Int Orthop 18:291-298, 1994.
12. Tomita K, Toribatake Y, Kawahara N, et al. Total en bloc spondylectomy and circumspinal decompression for solitary spinal metastasis. Paraplegia 32:36-46, 1994.
13. Boriani S, Chevalley F, Weinstein JN, et al. Chordoma of the spine above the sacrum. Treatment and outcome in 21 cases. Spine 21:1569-1577, 1996.
14. **Boriani S, De Iure F, Bandiera S, et al. Chondrosarcoma of the mobile spine. Report on 22 cases. Spine 25:804-812, 2000.**
15. Akeyson EW, McCutcheon IE. Single-stage posterior vertebrectomy with anterior and posterior reconstruction via a single posterior approach. J Neurosurg 85:211-220, 1996.
16. Bilsky MH, Boland P, Lis E, et al. Single-stage posterolateral transpedicle approach for spondylectomy, epidural decompression, and circumferential fusion of spinal metastases. Spine 25:2240-2250, 2000.
17. **Fourney DR, Abi-Said D, Rhines LD, et al. Simultaneous anterior-posterior approach to the thoracic and lumbar spine for the radical resection of tumors followed by reconstruction and stabilization. J Neurosurg Spine 94:232-244, 2001.**
18. **York JE, Walsh GL, Lang FF, et al. Combined chest wall resection with vertebrectomy and spinal reconstruction for the treatment of Pancoast tumors. J Neurosurg Spine 91:74-80, 1999.**
19. **Bolton WD, Rice DC, Goodyear A, et al. Superior sulcus tumors with vertebral body involvement: a multimodality approach. J Thorac Cardiovasc Surg 137:1379-1387, 2009.**
20. Vitaz T, Bilsky M. Staging, classification, and oncological approaches for metastatic tumors involving the spine. In Dickman CA, Fehlings MG, Gokaslan ZL, eds. Spinal Cord and Spinal Column Tumors. New York: Thieme, 2005, p 387.
21. Boriani S, Weinstein JN. Oncological classification of vertebral neoplasms. In Dickman CA, Fehlings MG, Gokaslan ZL, eds. Spinal Cord and Spinal Column Tumors. New York: Thieme, 2005, p 24.
22. Scott DL, Pedlow FX, Hecht AC, et al. Primary benign and malignant extradural spine tumors. In Frymoyer JW, Wiesel SW, An HS, et al, eds. The Adult and Pediatric Spine, 3rd ed. Philadelphia: Lippincott Williams & Wilkins, 2004, p 193.
23. **Boriani S, Weinstein JN, Biagini R. Primary bone tumors of the spine. Terminology and surgical staging. Spine 22:1036-1044, 1997.**
24. Komaki R, Roth JA, Walsh GL, et al. Outcome predictors for 143 patients with superior sulcus tumors treated by a multidisciplinary approach at the University of Texas M.D. Anderson Cancer Center. Int J Radiat Oncol Biol Phys 48:347-354, 2000.
25. Pancoast H. Importance of careful roentgen-ray investigations of apical chest tumors. JAMA 83:1407-1411, 1924.
26. Ghandi S, Walsh GL, Komaki R, et al. A multidisciplinary surgical approach to superior sulcus tumors with vertebral invasion. Ann Thorac Surg 68:1778-1784, 1999.
27. **Patchell RA, Tibbs PA, Regine WF, et al. Direct decompressive surgical resection in the treatment of spinal cord compression caused by metastatic cancer: a randomised trial. Lancet 366:643-648, 2005.**
28. Tomita K, Kawahara N, Kobayashi T, et al. Surgical strategy for spinal metastases. Spine 26:298-306, 2001.

29. Olerud C, Jonsson H, Lofberg AM, et al. Embolization of spinal metastases reduces perioperative blood loss: 21 patients operated on for renal cell carcinoma. Acta Orthop Scand 64:9-12, 1993.
30. Sundaresan N, Galicich JH, Bains MS. Vertebral body resection in the treatment of cancer involving the spine. Cancer 53:1393-1396, 1984.
31. Enneking WF, Spanier SS, Goodmann M. A system of surgical staging of musculoskeletal sarcoma. Clin Orthop 153:106-120, 1980.
32. Enneking WF. Musculoskeletal Tumor Surgery. New York: Churchill Livingstone, 1983.
33. **Enneking WF. A system of staging musculoskeletal neoplasms. Clin Orthop 204:9-24, 1986.**
34. Enneking WF. Staging of musculoskeletal neoplasms. In Sundaresan N, Schmidek HH, Schiller AL, et al, eds. Tumors of the Spine: Diagnosis and Clinical Management. Philadelphia: WB Saunders, 1990.
35. Boriani S, Capanna R, Donati D, et al. Osteoblastoma of the spine. Clin Orthop 278:37-45, 1992.
36. Hart RA, Boriani S, Biagini R, et al. A system for surgical staging and management of spine tumors. A clinical outcome study of giant cell tumors of the spine. Spine 22:1773-1782, 1997.
37. **Boriani S, Saravanja D, Yamada Y, Varga PP, Biagini R, Fisher CG. Challenges of local recurrence and cure in low grade malignant tumors of the spine. Spine 34:S48-S57, 2009.**
38. Campanacci L, Boriani S, Giunti A. Giant cell tumors of the spine. In Sundaresan N, Schmidek HH, Schiller AL, et al, eds. Tumors of the Spine: Diagnosis and Clinical Management. Philadelphia: WB Saunders, 1990, pp 163-172.
39. Healey JH, Ghelman B. Osteoid osteoma and osteoblastoma: current concepts and recent advances. Clin Orthop 204:76-85, 1986.
40. Errico T, Cooper PR. A new method of thoracic and lumbar body replacement for spinal tumors: technical note. Neurosurg 32:678-681, 1993.
41. Ibrahim A, Crockard A, Antoinietti P, et al. Does spinal surgery improve the quality of life for those with extradural (spinal) osseous metastases? An international multicenter prospective observational study of 223 patients. J Neurosurg Spine 8:271-278, 2008.
42. Mazel C, Balabaud L, Bennis S, et al. Cervical and thoracic spine tumor management: surgical indications, techniques, and outcomes. Orthop Clin North Am 40:75-92, 2009.
43. **Boriani S, Bandiera S, Biagini R, et al. Chordoma of the mobile spine: fifty years of experience. Spine 31:493-503, 2006.**
44. Ginsberg RJ, Martini N, Zaman M, et al. Influence of surgical resection and brachytherapy in the management of superior sulcus tumor. Ann Thorac Surg 57:1440-1445, 1994.
45. Komaki T, Mountain CF, Holbert JM, et al. Superior sulcus tumors: treatment selection and results for 85 patients without metastasis at presentation. Int J Radiat Oncol Biol Phys 19:31-36, 1990.
46. Maggi G, Casadio C, Pischedda F, et al. Combined radiosurgical treatment of Pancoast tumor. Ann Thorac Surg 57:198-202, 1994.
47. Wright CD, Moncure AC, Shepard JA, et al. Superior sulcus lung tumors. Results of combined treatment (irradiation and radical resection). J Thorac Cardiovasc Surg 94:69-74, 1987.

Chapter 38

Approaches and Techniques for C2 Tumors: Transpedicular Corpectomy and Spondylectomy

Justin K. Scheer, Azadeh Farin,
Frank Vrionis, Christopher P. Ames

Tumors of the upper cervical spine are associated with significant morbidity and mortality. Surgical management of C2 tumors remains very challenging, partly because of the close proximity of the vertebral arteries, the nerve roots, and the complex bony architecture, but it also requires complicated and technically demanding approaches. Because these tumors are rare, techniques for proper surgical resection have not been standardized. In this chapter we will provide an overview of the indications and contraindications for C2 tumor resection and a framework for preoperative evaluation, describe various techniques, and discuss outcomes of C2 tumor resection.

INDICATIONS AND CONTRAINDICATIONS

The indications for C2 body resection include primary and metastatic tumors. Functional recovery has been demonstrated to be superior when surgical decompression is performed in addition to radiation therapy, as compared with radiation alone.[1,2] However, surgical access from an anterior technique can be technically challenging and can result in high rates of swallowing and airway difficulties. For these reasons posterolateral transpedicular corpectomy, with piecemeal tumor resection and reconstruction of the axial vertebra, has been described. The posterolateral C2 transpedicular corpectomy has been influenced by the technique employed for thoracic metastatic disease, which evolved from transthoracic resection and reconstruction to a single-stage posterolateral approach that enables transpedicular tumor resection and reconstruction.[3] The posterolateral approach can be less invasive and is associated with less morbidity than other direct approaches but still facilitates radical resection and circumferential reconstruction in a single-stage procedure. The main advantage of the transpedicular approach at C2 is the ability to perform single-stage radical tumor resection and instrumented reconstruction without mandibular or pharyngeal splitting.[3] A single posterolateral surgical approach can be advantageous in cancer patients, because the dysphagia and aspiration associated with the transoral approach can be avoided. A single-stage approach further minimizes complications from wound healing, which is an important consideration in patients undergoing radiation therapy. These quality-of-life issues are relevant in the cancer patient population because these patients may already have a diminished quality of life and limited life span. However, not all C2 tumors warrant such an approach, with its concomitant risk of vertebral artery injury. Acosta and Ames[4] have reported favorable results with posterior stabilization alone and postoperative radiation in patients with highly aggressive tumors, without significant spinal cord compression and low predictive survival scores. Nonetheless, aggressive local resection, in addition to posterior stabilization and radiation therapy, may be warranted for less-aggressive tumors in younger patients with low burdens of disease when en bloc resection is not required to prolong survival.

Although the transpedicular approach for tumor resection and vertebral body reconstruction has been used extensively in the thoracic spine, its application in the cervical region has been less commonly described because of neural and vascular anatomic considerations. Still, the approach can be advantageous for lesions involving the C2 vertebral body, because C2 nerve root sacrifice results in sensory rather than motor deficits. Furthermore, the vertebral artery projects laterally in this location from the C2 foramen transversarium to the C1 tubercle, generating additional working room. Some dural retraction is possible in this region, because the spinal cord occupies a proportionally smaller portion of the canal volume at this level than more distal levels. The transpedicular approach with vertebral artery mobilization has been described for resection of ventral intradural tumors in the cervical spine.[5,6]

For primary bone tumors en bloc resection is indicated, with the most common tumor being chordoma (Fig. 38-1), a malignant, locally aggressive tumor with a high propensity for local recurrence after resection and a high risk of systemic metastasis despite adjuvant therapy.[7-9] This natural behavior has led most investigators to conclude that en bloc resection provides the best chance for prolonged disease-free survival and possible cure by preventing tumor cell contamination of surrounding tissues during removal of the solid tumor.[8,10-16] Marginal resection separates the surrounding tissue from the neoplasm by dissecting along a pseudocapsule and is thought to be less than ideal for avoiding a recurrence, compared with wide resection, although both marginal and wide resections are believed to have lower recurrence rates than intralesional

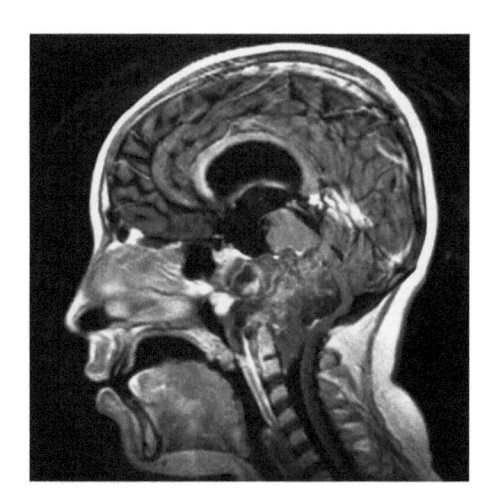

Fig. 38-1 Preoperative sagittal MRI scan showing clival chordoma.

resection.[9-11,14,17] Currently no randomized study has directly compared en bloc with piecemeal resection in the cervical spine. Still, the preponderance of evidence in the literature, scant as it may be, points to en bloc resection as the treatment of choice to prevent recurrence and to prolong survival. Standard treatment for clival chordoma is radical piecemeal resection to create safety zones around critical structures, with planned postoperative proton beam radiation therapy. For thoracolumbar and sacral tumors, the standard treatment is wide en bloc resection, when possible. The cervical spine represents a transitional area between these two alternative treatment strategies.

PREOPERATIVE EVALUATION

Careful study of the superior, inferior, and lateral extent of the tumor is critical to planning the surgical approach. Preoperative tracheostomy and gastrostomy tube feeding is favored for en bloc resection of lesions involving C1 or C2 and may be considered in sub axial lesions depending on tumor extent. Furthermore, preoperative angiography, test occlusion, and vertebral artery sacrifice via endovascular techniques should be considered when planning vertebral artery ligation at the time of surgery, or if the vertebral artery is at high risk for injury, such as in cases of prior surgery and irradiation. Points of fixation such as the thickness of the occipital keel and C2 pars and pedicle should be evaluated in the preoperative CT scan.

En bloc resection techniques have been well described for the appendicular musculoskeletal system and the lumbar and thoracic spine, with demonstrated beneficial effects on survival when lesions are removed en bloc with wide margins, compared to piecemeal resection.[18-25] When chordomas are of sacral origin, en bloc resection is also planned in accordance with evidence-based oncologic doctrines. In the cervical spine, en bloc resection involves the complete removal of one or more contiguous levels of the spinal column in two pieces from an anterior and posterior approach. En bloc removal of spine tumors does not always require en bloc spondylectomy. Histologic studies determine whether the specimen is intralesional or whether a marginal or wide excision should be performed (the latter is often not possible if the tumor is adjacent to dura). *Wide resection* indicates that a continuous zone of healthy tissue was demonstrated around the tumor; *marginal excision* indicates that the tumor was covered by a thin layer of reactive non-neoplastic tissue; and *intralesional* indicates that the tumor was found on the surface of the pathology specimen.

En bloc resection in the upper cervical spine is challenging because of critical anatomic considerations and the potential for morbidity, although it can optimize local control and possibly offer a cure.* Primary cervical tumors limited to osseous structures, sparing surrounding soft tissues, are more easily resected en bloc, but chordomas are not usually confined to the vertebral body by the time they are diagnosed. Complications from en bloc resection of cervical spine chordomas relate to the juxtaposition of the skull base, the intricate cervical pedicular architecture, the vasculature, the aerodigestive system, and the upper spinal cord and nerve roots. Patients must be aware that en bloc resection may be accompanied by deliberate nerve root sacrifice, excessive bleeding, injury to major vessels, the spinal cord, and nerve roots, contamination of tumor cells, severe dysphagia, aspiration, and spinal instability associated with the vertebrectomy. Bleeding may be reduced by preoperative embolization, the use of fibrin glue over the epidural venous plexus, or meticulous blunt resection.[24] The risk of tumor cell contamination may be reduced by using a T-saw for pediculotomy or anterior column osteotomy and rinsing with a combination of distilled water and concentrated cisplatin.[24,28,29] Analysis of the literature demonstrates that most patients will have at least one postoperative complication, with respiratory infections and distress being the most common. These anatomic constraints and complications explain why intralesional resection of cervical chordomas followed by radiation therapy appears to be the most common approach in the literature, rather than risking neurologic compromise, when the tumor abuts the dura or neural tissues.[17,30-36] Leitner et al[37] reported spondylectomy for chordoma at C4 with no epidural extension. Delgado et al[22] reported using a T-saw to perform a C5 spondylectomy for chordoma, with no evidence of recurrence after 9 years. Although not ideal, use of the dura mater as a margin is an option that is believed to result in a higher cure rate than piecemeal resection.[11,13,38-40] Boriani et al[14] described the first attempted en bloc parasagittal resection of a cervical (C5) chordoma, in which they also resected a segment of the vertebral artery but intentionally removed the tumor along the C6 nerve root intralesionally. Fourney et al[26] performed an en bloc C6 spondylectomy for osteosarcoma, with excision of intralesional margins around the remaining nerve roots and vertebral arteries. Recurrences resulting from intralesional resection can be challenging, but they can still be treated successfully with en bloc resection.

Multilevel chordomas pose even greater technical challenges because of the need to remove multiple segments of the spine in one piece without violating the tumor.[41,42] Despite this, an en bloc approach to multilevel primary cervical tumors should be considered as a potential cure, as compared with an intralesional procedure, with its concomitant recurrence rate and risk of metastatic disease.[11,14,16,21,43] Multilevel cervi-

---

*References 11, 14, 16, 21, 26, 27.

cal malignant tumor excision can be accomplished with wide margins and a planned marginal plane at the dura mater, albeit with some morbidity. The success of this type of procedure hinges on staging (Enneking and Weinstein-Boriani-Biagini staging systems), multidisciplinary discussions, setting appropriate expectations for patient recovery, possible functional outcomes, and quality of life, and meticulous preoperative and intraoperative planning, especially with regard to the vertebral arteries. Vertebral artery ligation for en bloc vertebrectomy, with the intent of maintaining a sound oncologic resection, has been legitimized by several reports in the literature, and successful en bloc marginal excision (negative surgical margins) of a multilevel C1-3 cervical chordoma has been described.[14,41,42] Talac et al[44] analyzed outcomes in 15 patients undergoing unilateral vertebral artery ligation to manage their cervical spine tumors and reported no adverse events resulting from brainstem, cerebellar, or spinal cord ischemia. The anatomy and the physiologic importance of the vertebral artery should be thoroughly investigated preoperatively, by means of angiography and balloon occlusion testing, in conjunction with cerebral blood flow studies, before contemplating its sacrifice during tumor resection.[45,46] Magnetic resonance angiography and intraoperative test occlusion of the artery, with monitoring of somatosensory and motor evoked potentials, can also be used.

Sciubba et al[42] reported the first en bloc resection of a multilevel cervical chordoma with C2-4 involvement, a large retropharyngeal component, vertebral artery encasement, and epidural extension in a 54-year-old man who presented with dysphagia, hoarseness, upper extremity numbness, and gait unsteadiness. A combined posterior-lateral/transmandibular circumglossal approach combined with right-sided neck dissection was used to generate wide anterior exposure from the C1 arch down to C5, enabling access to the upper portion of the tumor, which was necessary to achieve an extralesional resection. These investigators performed a total spondylectomy of C2-4, with sacrifice of the right C2-4 nerve roots and a segment of the right vertebral artery, which resulted in a marginal resection at the dura and paraspinous area, with dissection along the pseudocapsule in the latter.

For lateralized tumors, an alternative to performing multilevel spondylectomies is the use of parasagittal osteotomies for en bloc resection of chordomas, as reported by Tomita and Kawahara[47] This type of resection is not a complete spondylectomy; however, it does adhere to the oncologic principle of marginal en bloc excision. Boriani et al[14] described the en bloc removal of a chordoma at C5 by means of a similar technique, although they did not use the term *parasagittal osteotomy* to describe their single-level procedure. This technique is useful for multilevel lateralized chordomas, not only because it is technically easier to perform than multilevel spondylectomy, but also because it may pose less risk to the contralateral vertebral artery. Furthermore, this technique successfully maintains the oncologic principles of avoiding intralesional violation during chordoma resection. However, lack of data on long-term outcomes makes it difficult to judge its role versus that of the more technically demanding spondylectomy. A limitation of this technique is that it is primarily useful for lateralized tumors. There needs to be a clear margin of vertebral body through which the osteotomy can be performed.

TECHNIQUES

POSTEROLATERAL TRANSPEDICULAR C2 CORPECTOMY

The posterolateral transpedicular corpectomy begins with a wide C2 laminectomy.[3] The C2 pedicle is skeletonized with sacrifice of the C2 nerve roots. The foramen transversarium is entered with the use of a Kerrison rongeur at C2, and the vertebral artery is identified. While protecting the vertebral artery with a Penfield 4 dissector, the C2 pedicle and pars interarticularis are completely removed into the body of C2 with a high-speed drill (Fig. 38-2). The soft tumor in the vertebral body is removed through this transpedicular corridor. The C2 superior articular process and the C2-3 intervertebral disc are then removed. In cases where the tumor has caused severe narrowing of the vertebral artery on one side or where a nondominant or severely atretic vertebral artery is apparent, unilateral sacrifice and debulking from the affected side to enhance access may be preferable to bilateral vertebral artery manipulation, provided that the contralateral vertebral artery can deliver appropriate flow.

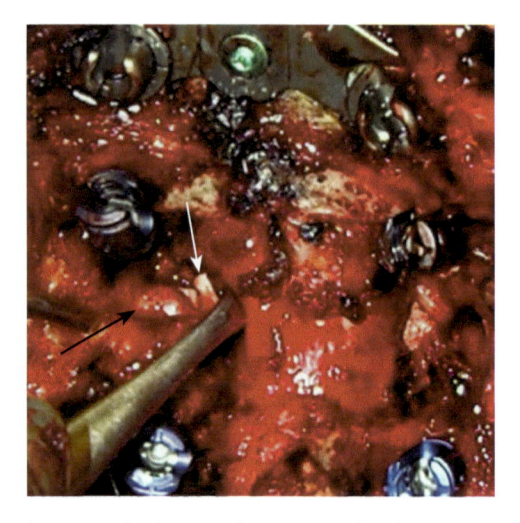

Fig. 38-2 Intraoperative photograph during the transpedicular corpectomy procedure shows the use of a Penfield 4 dissector to protect the skeletonized vertebral artery *(black arrow)* and pack methylmethacrylate into the resection cavity *(white arrow)*. (From Ames CP, Wang VY, Deviren V, et al. Posterior transpedicular corpectomy and reconstruction of the axial vertebra for metastatic tumor. Report of 3 cases. J Neurosurg Spine 10:111-116, 2009.)

C2 Spondylectomy

Total C2 spondylectomy, including the superior articular pillars, requires the placement of a load-bearing transfer mechanism from the C1 lateral mass to the C3 vertebrectomy or facet joints.[48] Cement or cage reconstruction of the thoracolumbar spine has been well established, but it can be impractical to fit a cage posteriorly from the C1 lateral mass to the C3 vertebrectomy. A less demanding option for reconstruction of the load-bearing construct is to place cages from the C1 lateral mass to the C3 lateral mass posteriorly with a long instrumented construct.[48] The integrity of the construct is critical, because many patients rely solely on the construct for stability, and they do not undergo fusion in the face of radiation and chemotherapy. Another construct option is Steinmann pins embedded in cement (Fig. 38-3). A drill is used to create pilot holes in the undersurface of the C1 lateral mass and the C3 endplate to fit a custom-cut Steinmann pin, which is placed into the vertebrectomy of C3, forced slightly deeper to allow the superior end to be placed under the C1 lateral mass, where it is then brought slightly out of the C3 vertebrectomy as it is brought up into the C1 lateral mass. This results in an angled trajectory from lateral to medial in the superoinferior direction. Methylmethacrylate is injected around the pins under direct vision and then sculpted with the use of a Woodson elevator to keep the cement away from the dura mater and to ensure complete embedding of the pins in the cement.

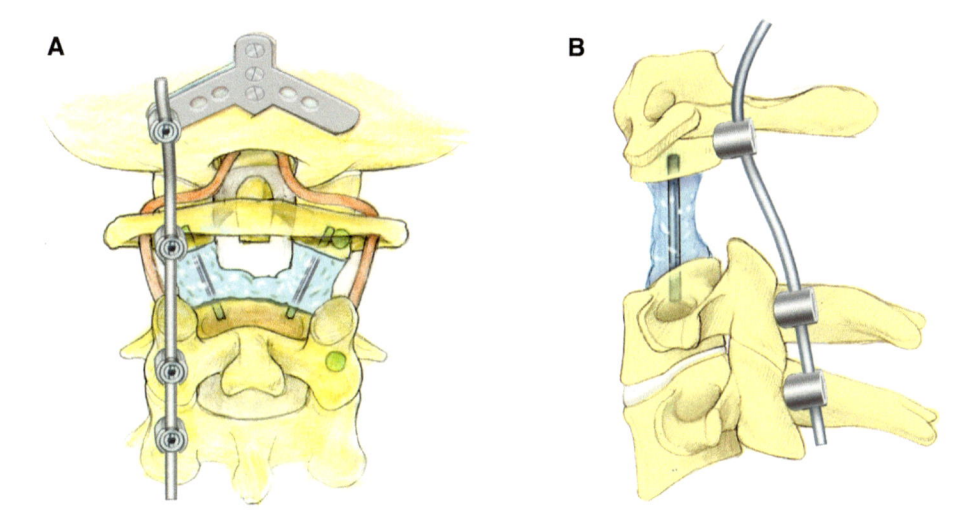

Fig. 38-3 **A,** Coronal and **B,** sagittal views for reconstruction of a C2 vertebrectomy with Steinmann pins and methylmethacrylate. (From Ames CP, Wang VY, Deviren V, et al. Posterior transpedicular corpectomy and reconstruction of the axial vertebra for metastatic tumor. Report of 3 cases. J Neurosurg Spine 10:111-116, 2009.)

En Bloc Resection

The standard transoral approach that is traditionally employed for rheumatoid arthritis and for en bloc resection of primary bone tumors of C2 can be limited, especially in lateral exposure, and can be complicated in the short term by dysphagia, aspiration, and pulmonary complications. Mandibular splitting and tracheostomy may be required for complete C2 vertebral body resection and reconstruction. This transglossal transmandibular approach (Fig. 38-4) permits access to the anterior aspect of the occipital condyles, C1 lateral mass, C2 body, and vertebral arteries at C2. The distinct disadvantage of the approach is the possibility of poor pharyngeal healing, especially when anterior instrumentation is placed and postoperative radiation therapy is planned. Supplementary posterior instrumentation is required to provide additional stability.

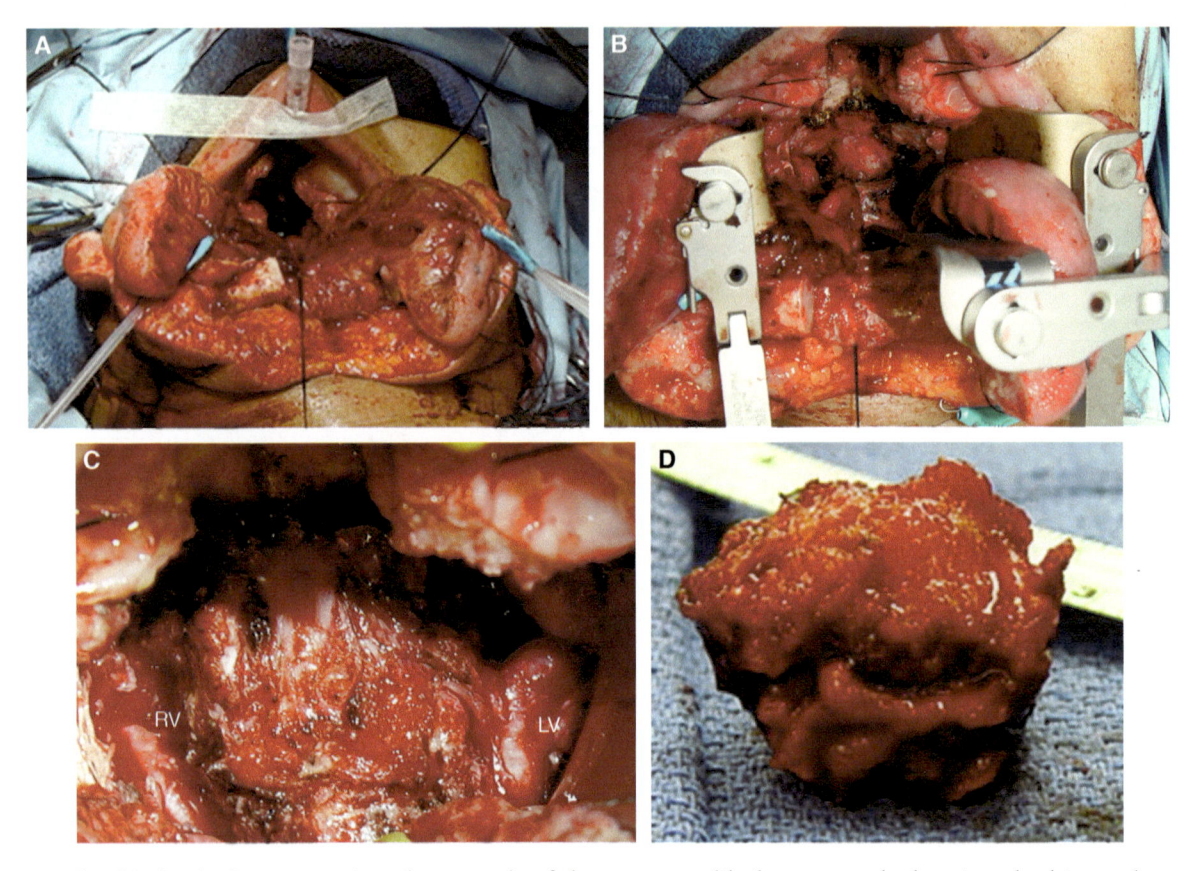

Fig. 38-4 **A,** Intraoperative photograph of the transmandibular approach showing the bisected tongue and mandible. **B,** The resection cavity after removal of the C2 body en bloc. **C,** The bilateral skeletonized vertebral arteries. (*LV,* Left vertebral artery; *RV,* right vertebral artery.) **D,** The specimen removed en bloc.

The transoral circumglossal retropharyngeal approach (Fig. 38-5) spares the tongue but provides difficult contralateral access, which becomes apparent with large tumors.

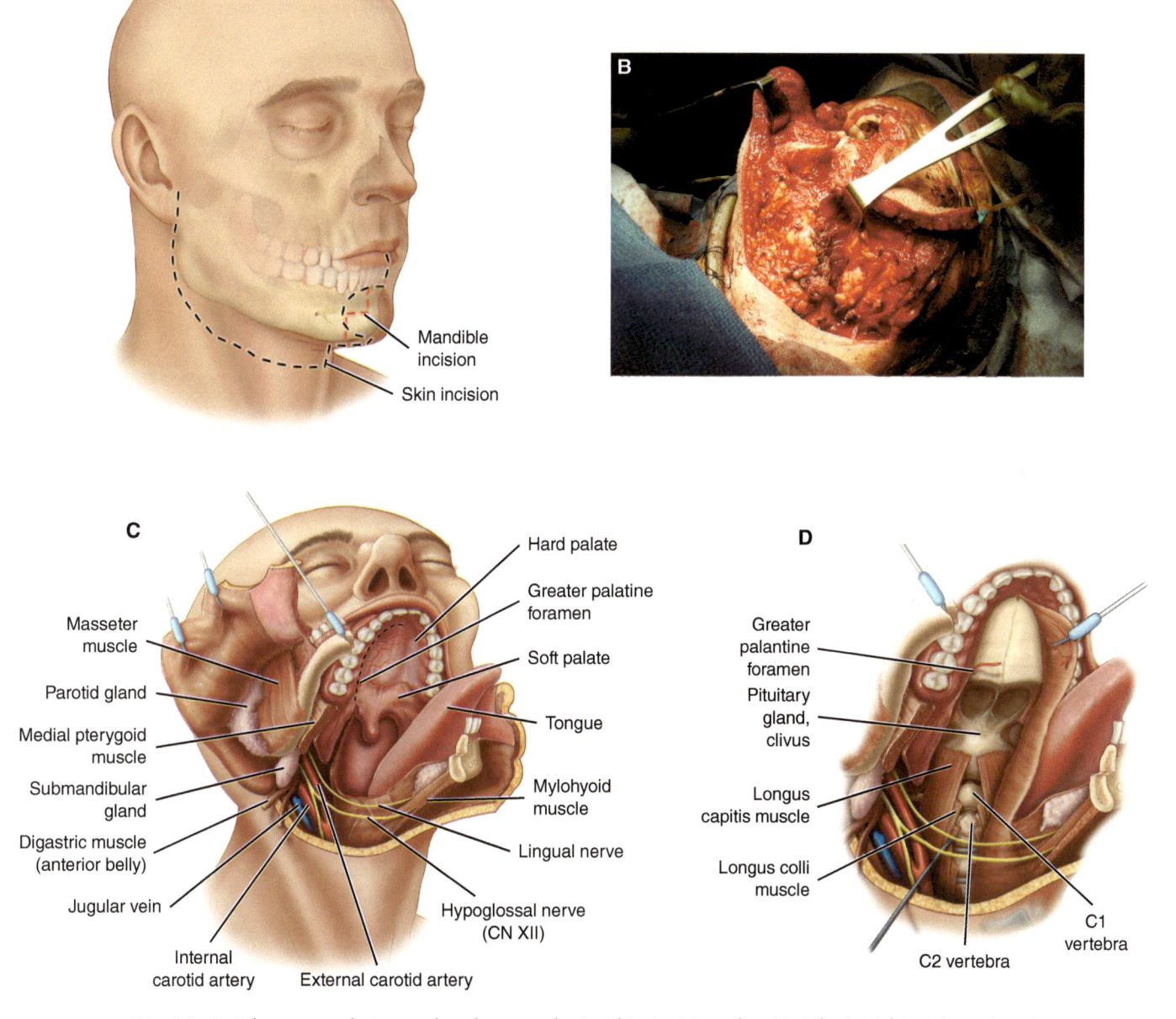

Fig. 38-5 The transoral circumglossal approach. **A,** Skin incision plan. **B,** The initial incision. **C** and **D,** Anatomic landmarks.

Continued

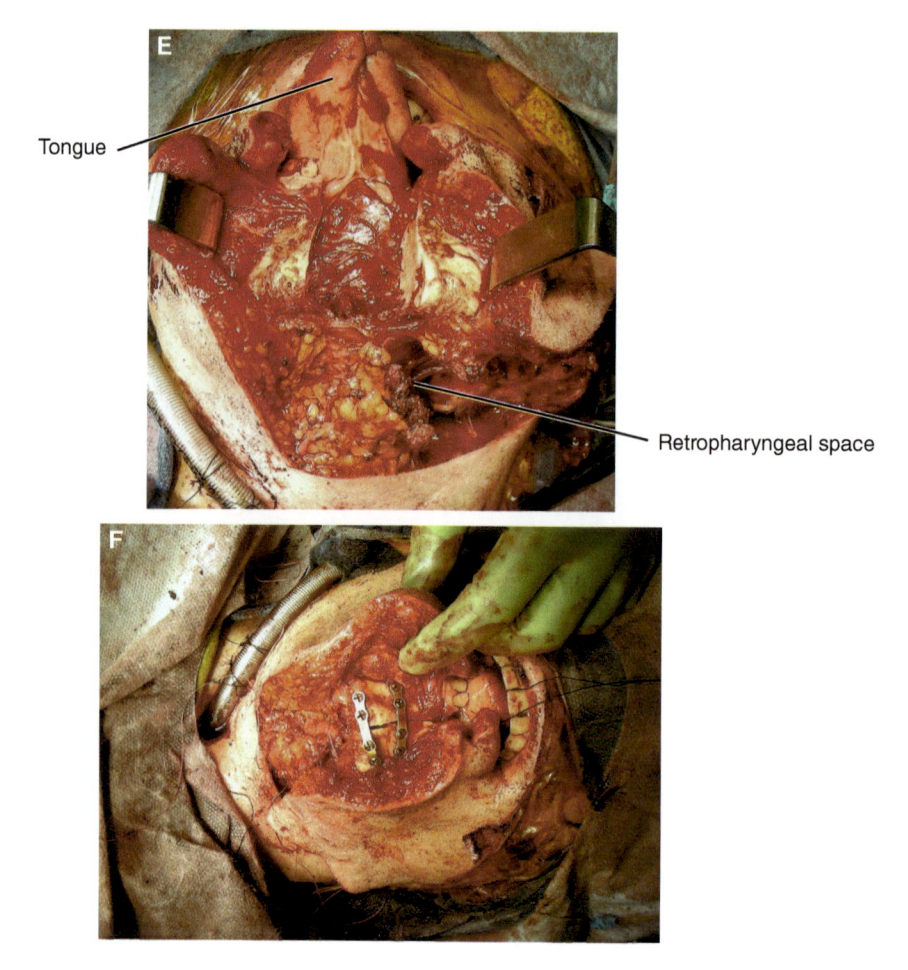

Fig. 38-5, cont'd **E,** Bisected mandible sparing the tongue. **F,** Closure of the mandible.

Parasagittal Osteotomy

A tumor-free region of the vertebral segment through which a parasagittal osteotomy is to be performed is identified on preoperative axial images; it must be sufficiently lateral from the tumor to avoid violation (Fig. 38-6). Note that in the absence of a lateralized tumor and with no good parasagittal tumor–free plane, spondylectomy remains the treatment of choice.

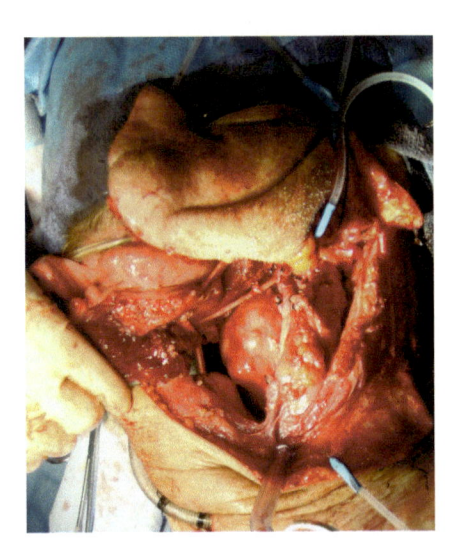

Fig. 38-6 Large parasagittal tumor.

Posterior stabilization and pedicle subtraction osteotomy with protective membrane placement is performed first. Fortunately, an easily dissectible plane is generally noted between the tumor and the dura, even in cases of severe compression. Placement of a silicone rubber sheet allows safe anterior osteotomy drilling, despite suboptimal visualization.

The posterior elements on the side of the planned anterior osteotomy are left intact for an arthrodesis surface, when possible. Selective nerve roots may be ligated if a true en bloc resection is mandated. When possible, the C5 nerve roots and below are preserved. Anteriorly, complete discectomies, with removal of the posterior longitudinal ligament, are performed at the rostral and caudal portions of the segment to be removed (see Fig. 38-6, and Chapter 39, p. 709).

OUTCOMES WITH EVALUATION OF RESULTS

Most published studies of cervical chordomas are hampered by poorly documented clinical outcomes. The frequency of surveillance to detect tumor recurrences varies among studies. Missing critical data points, such as Weinstein-Boriani-Biagini grade, Tomita score, follow-up data, a control group of patients who underwent piecemeal tumor resection for comparison, and information describing the anatomic location of the tumor, further limit the power of any analysis. Furthermore, because most descriptions of cervical spine tumors in the literature have been published as single case reports or small case series that limit analytic power, true survival data and rates of recurrence after en bloc resection are not known with scientific accuracy.

In Windle-Taylor's series[49] of 12 patients undergoing en bloc resection of cervical chordomas at two spine centers, the mean age at presentation was 60 years. The distribution of cases was almost evenly divided between those involving C1-2 and those involving the subaxial spine.

En bloc resection was attempted through an anterior approach in 33% of cases (29% C1-2; 40% subaxial), a posterior approach in 25% of cases (43% C1-2; 0% subaxial), and a combined approach in 42% of cases (29% C1-2; 60% subaxial).

Tumor margins were found to be wide in 2 of 12 cases (14% C1-2; 20% subaxial), marginal in 6 of 12 cases (29% C1-2; 80% subaxial), and contaminated in 3 of 12 cases (43% C1-2; 0% subaxial). No operative complications were reported.

Postoperative complications occurred in 5 of 12 patients (57% C1-2; 20% subaxial; $p < 0.05$) and included hoarseness, dysphagia, prolonged/permanent use of a feeding tube, and pneumonia. The average length of follow-up was 42 months.

Five of 12 patients had a recurrence (57% C1-2; 20% subaxial; $p < 0.05$). There was a higher incidence of postoperative complications and rates of recurrence for C1-2 tumors than for subaxial tumors.

Boriani et al[11] identified no recurrence of chordoma in the mobile spine in four patients who had undergone an en bloc resection, including marginal cases, whereas six of eight patients had a local recurrence after an intralesional excision. Wittig et al,[50] in their study of primary sarcomas of the mobile spine, reported recurrence rates of 11% in patients undergoing en bloc resection with negative margins, 33% in piecemeal resections with negative margins, and 50% to 70% in all resections with positive margins. Wright et al[51] reported on 16 patients with primary suboccipital and cervical chordomas undergoing piecemeal resection. With a mean 5-year follow-up (range 1 to 11 years), they reported a 40% recurrence rate and a 33% disease-related mortality rate.[51] York et al[52] published their series of 21 patients undergoing intralesional resection for giant cell tumors of the cervical spine. With a mean follow-up of 67.8 months (range 36 to 124 months), 7 patients (33.3%) had a recurrence, although only 1 of 13 underwent total piecemeal spondylectomy.[52] Zacay et al[53] reported their series of 7 patients with cervical chordomas who were treated with piecemeal resection; the recurrence rate was 28.6% with a follow-up of 23 months (range 7 to 169 months).

An analysis completed by the senior author (C.P.A), based on a complete Medline search for all articles reporting survival data for en bloc resections of primary tumors of the cervical spine in adults, yielded 18 cases with a mean follow-up of 47 months (range 1 to 149 months).[54] The mean age was 47 years, and of the 15 patients whose sex was reported, 9 were men. The mean operative time, estimated blood loss, and length of hospitalization were 18.6 hours, 2.9 L, and 34.6 days, respectively. In one case it reportedly took 56 hours to remove the mass en bloc.

There were 3 cases of local recurrences at 12, 44, and 113 months, respectively, and 1 case of distant metastasis at 12 months postoperatively. It was noted that although the recurrence rates may be lower than those reported for piecemeal resections, this has not been demonstrated with sufficient scientific validity.[51-53] No factors, including age, sex, tumor type, levels involved, or margin status, were found to be significantly associated with recurrence.

Based on this review, 1- and 5-year disease-free survival rates were 88.2% and 73.5%, respectively (Fig. 38-7). There were 12 cases of chordoma, 2 chondrosarcomas, 2 giant cell tumors, 1 malignant peripheral nerve sheath tumor, and 1 mesenchymal hamartoma. The mean number of levels involved was two.

All patients were managed by means of en bloc resection, with margins classified as wide in 5 patients, marginal in 6, intralesional in 6, and unreported in 1. Postoperative

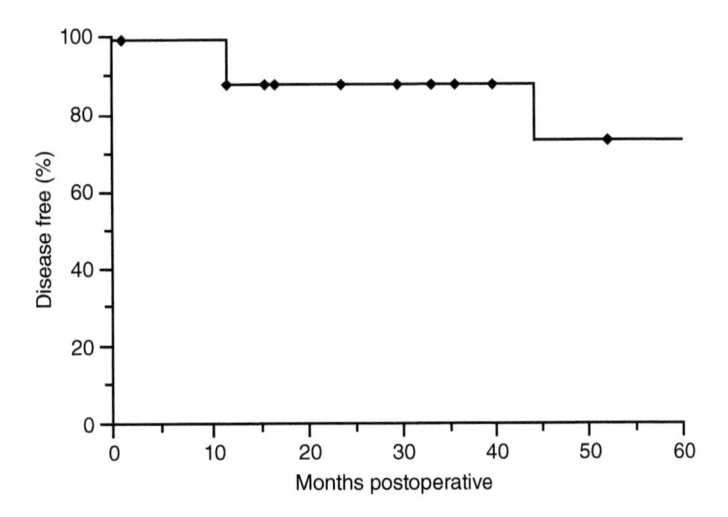

Fig. 38-7 Kaplan-Meier analysis of 18 patients who underwent en bloc resection. (From Cloyd JM, Chou D, Deviren V, et al. En bloc resection of primary tumors of the cervical spine: report of two cases and systematic review of the literature. Spine J 9:928-935, 2009.)

complications occurred in 8 of the 9 patients for whom these data were presented. The most common complications were dysphagia (55.6%) and pneumonia (44.4%). One patient, an 81-year-old woman who underwent excision of a C3 chordoma, died during the perioperative period from aspiration pneumonia 1 month after the initial operation. Only two groups have published outcomes data that used standardized measurements. For 8 patients at a mean of 35.8 months, the mean short-form 36 physical component score was 38. Local recurrence was defined as a recurrence of the original tumor within one spine level of the resection site. Total recurrence was defined as any recurrence (both local and distant) of the original tumor. In his review of all published en bloc resections for cervical spine tumors, the senior author (C.P.A.) calculated a total recurrence rate of 22.2%.

A separate analysis was performed exclusively for cases of chordoma. Among these 12 cases, the mean age was 54 years, 58% were men, the mean number of levels resected was 2.1, and most of the cases involved sacrifice of the vertebral artery and cervical nerve root. Wide margins were obtained in only 2 cases, and adjuvant radiation was used in 5 of the 8 cases in which this information was reported. With a median follow-up of 27 months, there was a 16.7% recurrence rate.

SIGNATURE CASES
POSTEROLATERAL TRANSPEDICULAR APPROACH

The following two patients both presented with metastatic disease involving the C2 vertebral body, cord compression, and C1-2 instability. These patients underwent piecemeal intralesional resection through a posterior transpedicular trajectory. These case reports demonstrate that tumors of the axis can be successfully resected from a transpedicular approach and that load-bearing transfer function can be effectively recreated from a solely posterior approach. Long-term follow-up is needed.

A 63-year-old woman with a history of breast and renal cell carcinoma presented with severe neck pain, especially when she turned her head. CT scans revealed destruction of the C2 vertebrectomy, and an angiogram revealed a vascular tumor fed by the left vertebral artery that could not be embolized (Fig. 38-8). She underwent a C1-3 laminectomy and C2 vertebrectomy through a left transpedicular approach, after ligation of the left C2 nerve root. Reconstruction was performed anteriorly with methyl methacrylate and posteriorly with C1-6 instrumentation. Pathologic findings were consistent with renal cell carcinoma. At 6 months postoperatively, she remained neurologically intact, and there was no instrumentation failure.

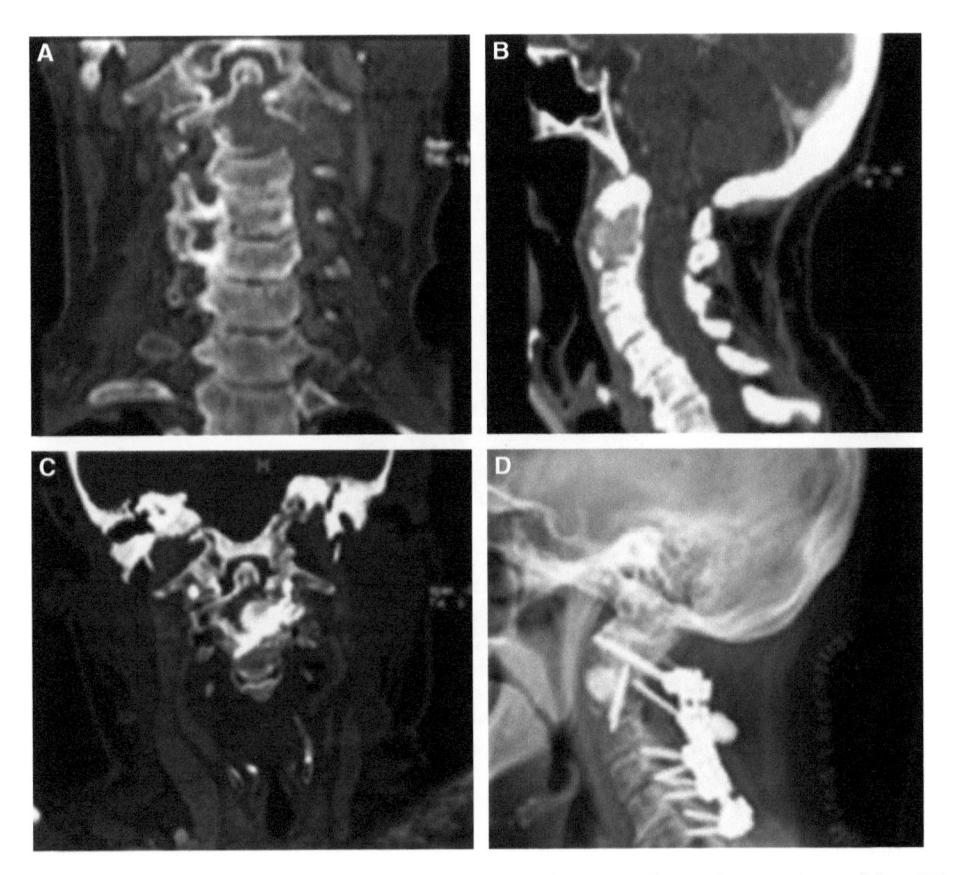

Fig. 38-8 **A,** Coronal and **B,** sagittal CT images revealing significant destruction of the C2 vertebrectomy. The patient underwent a C1-3 laminectomy and left transpedicular approach to the vertebrectomy for tumor resection. **C,** Methylmethacrylate was used to reconstruct the C2 vertebrectomy. **D,** This was supplemented with a C1-6 posterior fusion. (From Ames CP, Wang VY, Deviren V, et al. Posterior transpedicular corpectomy and reconstruction of the axial vertebra for metastatic tumor. J Neurosurg Spine 10:111-116, 2009.)

A 43-year-old woman, status post prior mastectomy, presented with severe neck pain and normal neurologic findings. MRI demonstrated a C2 lesion with cord compression and C1-2 subluxation (Fig. 38-9, *A*). A PET scan demonstrated no other area of metastatic disease. The patient underwent bilateral transpedicular corpectomy with vertebral artery preservation. The C2 region was reconstructed with methylmethacrylate and Steinmann pins bilaterally to restore the load-bearing column from the C1 lateral mass to the C3 vertebrectomy (Fig. 38-9, *B* through *E*). Supplementary occiput–C5 posterior fusion was also performed. The patient was discharged on postoperative day 5 and remained neurologically intact, with a 6-month 36-item short-form health survey physical health score of 43.4. There was no instrumentation failure or instability at 6 months.

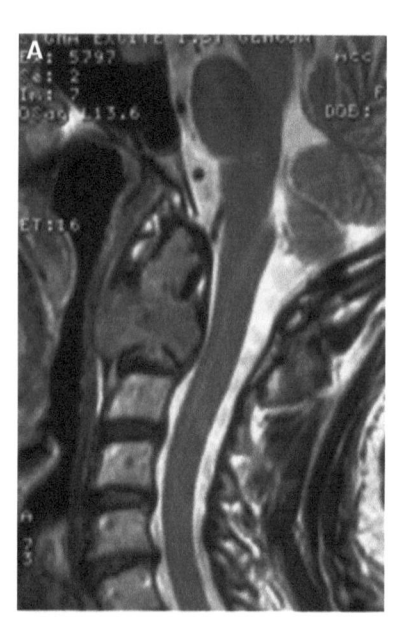

Fig. 38-9 **A,** Sagittal T2-weighted MRI scan demonstrating a lesion in the C2 vertebral body with spinal cord compression. (**B** and **D** from Ames CP, Wang VY, Deviren V, et al. Posterior transpedicular corpectomy and reconstruction of the axial vertebra for metastatic tumor. J Neurosurg Spine 10:111-116, 2009.)

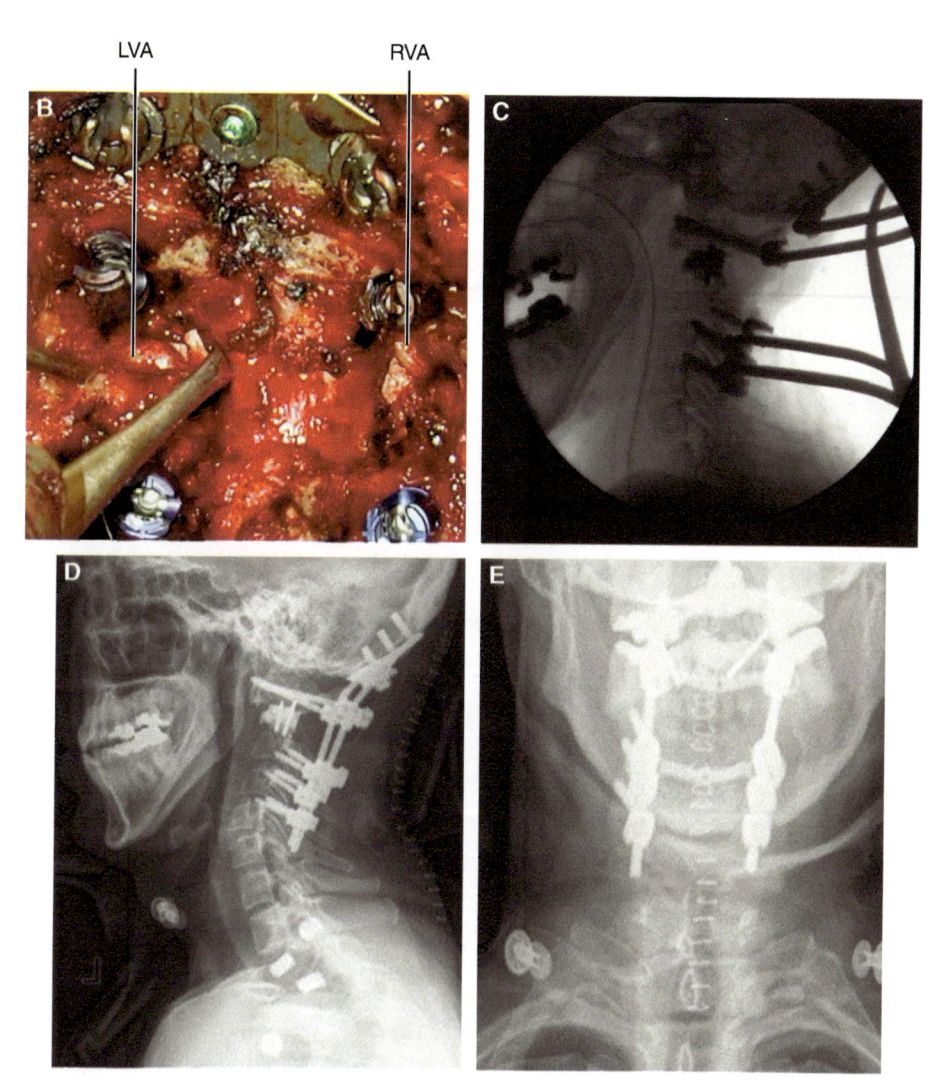

Fig. 38-9, cont'd **B,** Intraoperative photograph showing preservation of the left *(LVA)* and right *(RVA)* vertebral arteries. **C,** Intraoperative lateral radiograph demonstrating reconstruction with Steinmann pins and methylmethacrylate after transpedicular corpectomy of the axis. Further stabilization was achieved with a posterior occiput–C5 fusion, as shown in **D** and **E,** postoperative lateral and anteroposterior radiographs.

C2 Corpectomy With En Bloc Resection

A 76-year-old man, who initially presented with severe neck pain, underwent a C2-3 laminectomy and lateral mass fixation; the biopsy revealed chordoma (Fig. 38-10, *A* through *P*). He returned to the outside hospital several days later with bilateral foot paresthesia. Repeat imaging demonstrated collapse of the C2 vertebra with tumor progression. He was transferred to the senior author's institution (C.P.A.), where en bloc removal of C2 was planned. He first underwent posterior instrumented fusion from occiput to T2, C2 pedicle osteotomy, sacrifice of the C2 nerve root, and vertebral artery mobilization, with resection of the previous incision and scar. Several days later he underwent en bloc resection through a transmandibular transglossal approach.

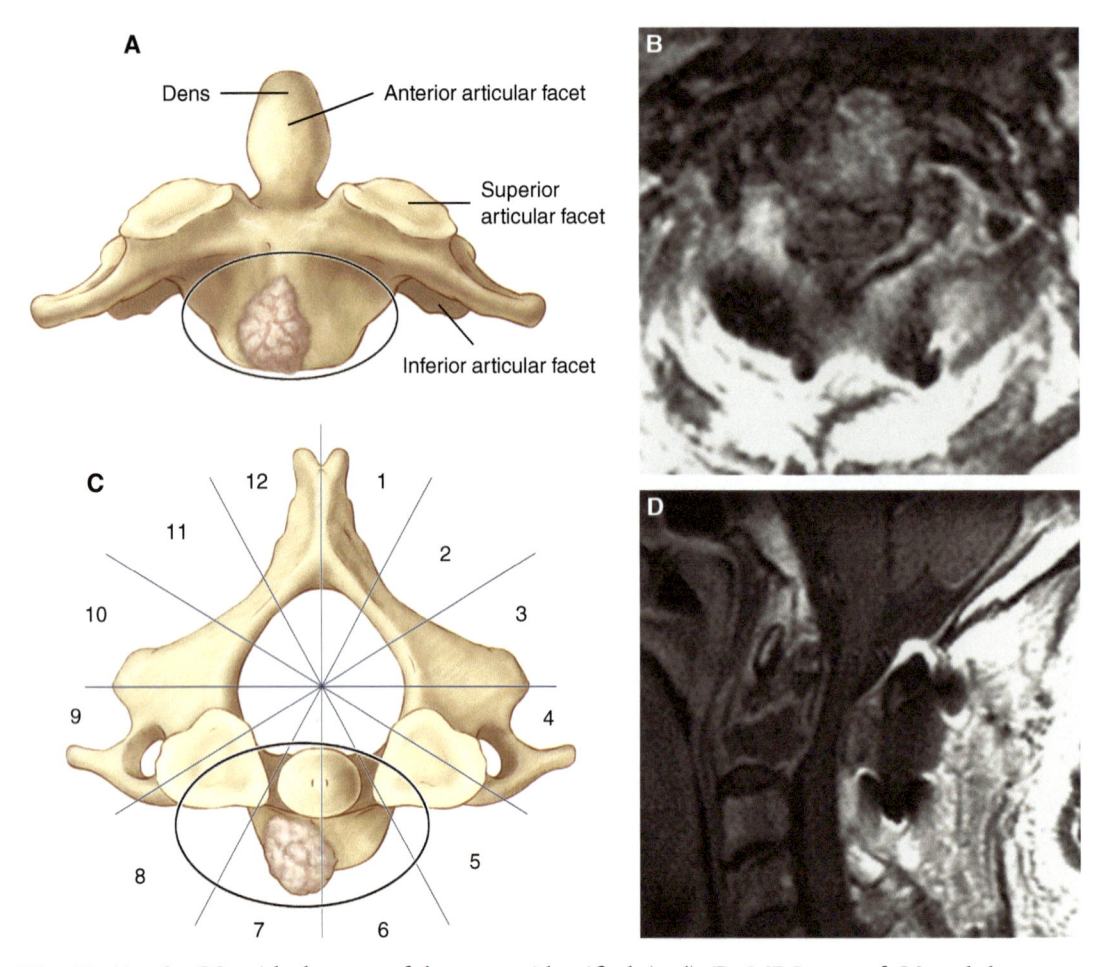

Fig. 38-10 **A,** C2, with the area of the tumor identified *(oval)*. **B,** MRI scan of C2 and the tumor. **C,** Axial view of C2 with the area of the tumor identified *(oval)*. **D,** Sagittal MRI showing the C2 tumor. (**K-P** from Journal of Neurosurgery: Spine, May 2010, vol 12, issue 5. Permission from AANS.)

A C2-3 discectomy was first performed, followed by a C2 corpectomy and removal of the tumor as a whole. Stabilization was achieved through a C1-3 anterior cervical fusion, with custom cages and iliac crest bone graft. Final pathologic findings revealed a marginal margin at the vertebral artery. Postoperatively he had dysphagia. After adjuvant proton beam therapy, he developed palatal wound dehiscence that required reoperation 9 months after the initial resection. At 17 months postoperatively, he was found to have further posterior pharyngeal wall breakdown and resultant hardware exposure, which was repaired with a radial forearm skin graft. At 30-month follow-up there was no evidence of disease on CT scans.

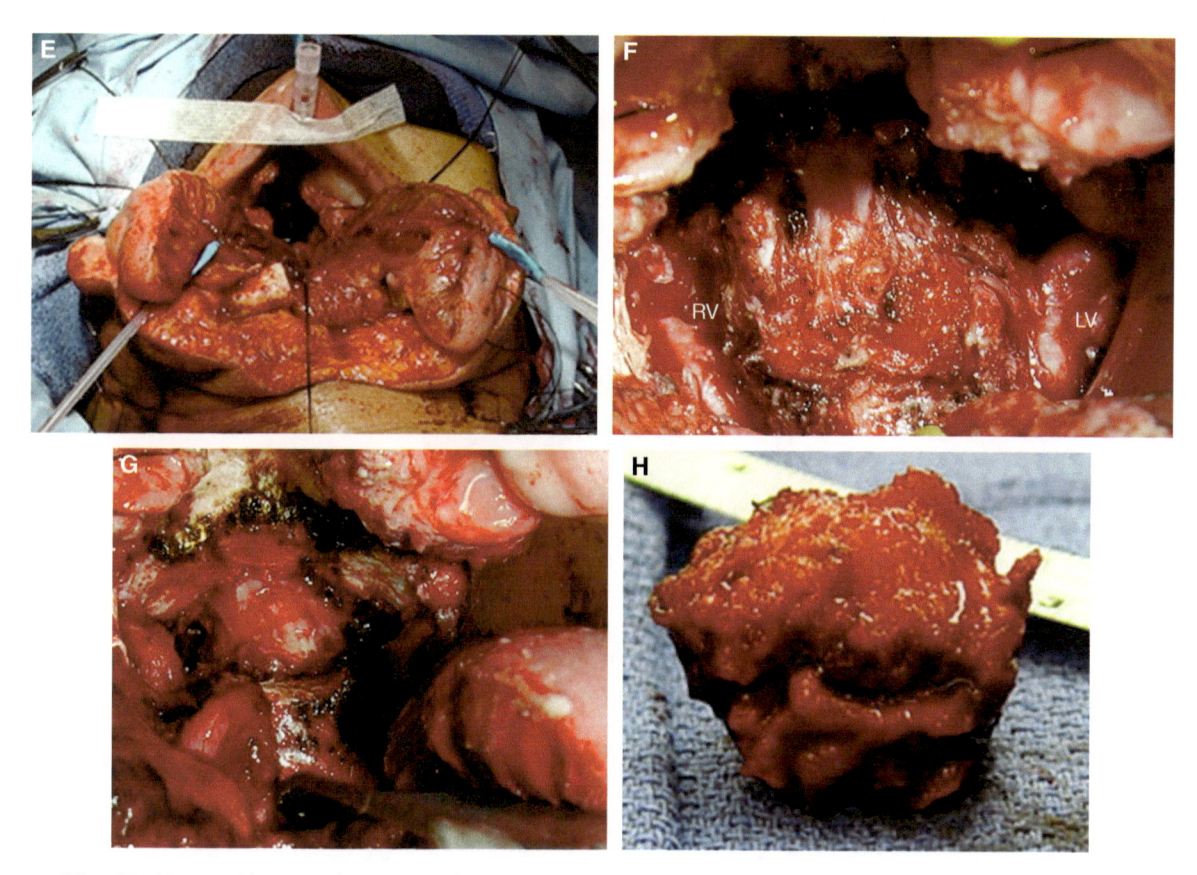

Fig. 38-10, cont'd **E,** The transoral transglossal approach. **F,** C2 tumor and the right *(RV)* and left *(LV)* vertebral arteries. **G,** Another view of the C2 tumor. **H,** The resected tumor.

Continued

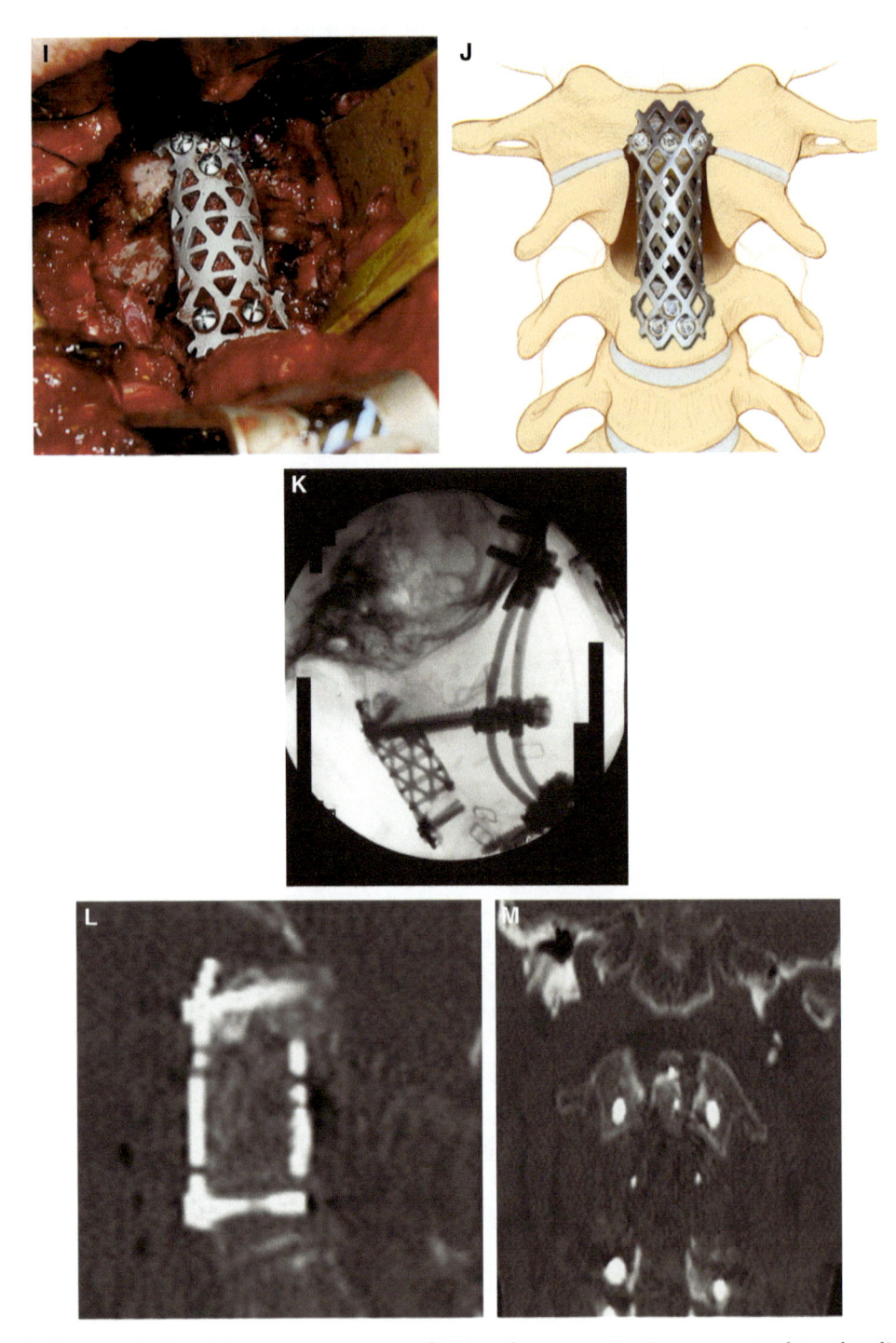

Fig. 38-10, cont'd **I** and **J**, Reconstruction of C2 with a cage. **K,** Postoperative lateral radiograph showing reconstruction with a cage and posterior instrumentation. **L,** Sagittal and **M,** anteroposterior CT scans showing the reconstruction.

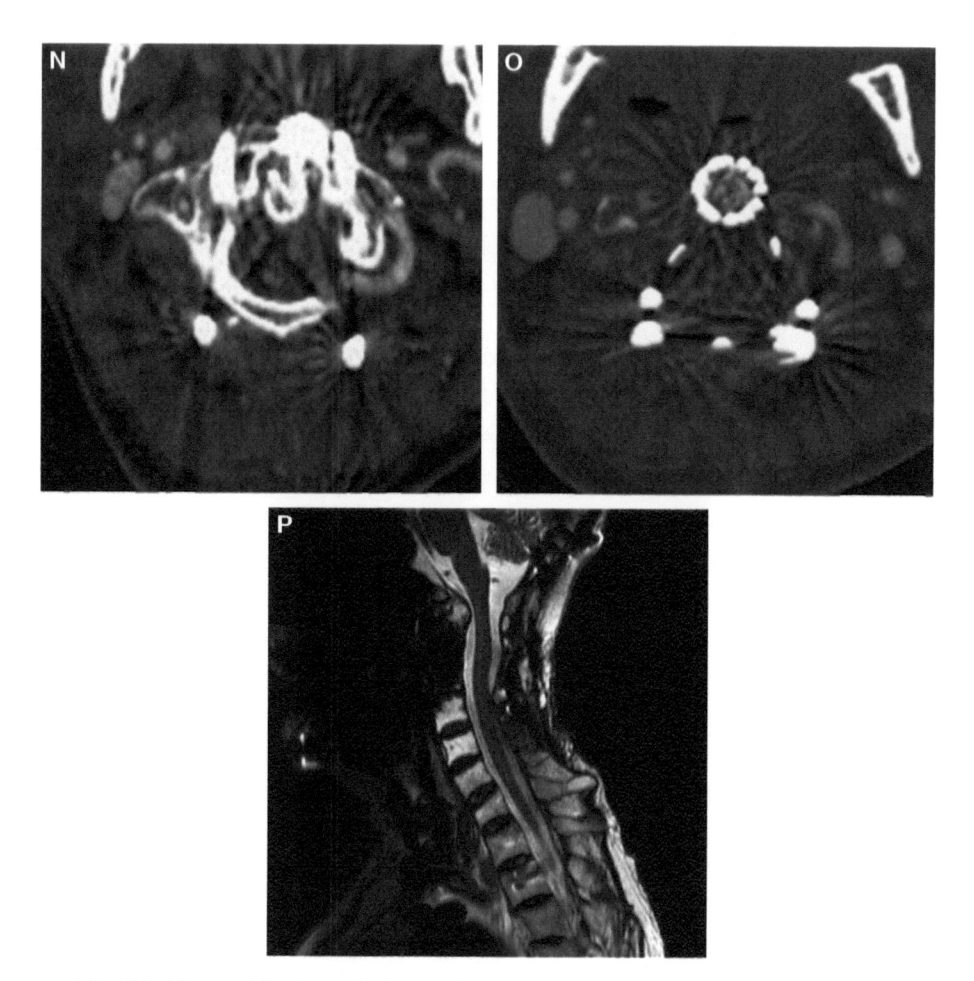

Fig. 38-10, cont'd **N** and **O,** Axial and **P,** sagittal postoperative MRI scans.

CONCLUSION

Transpedicular corpectomy with en bloc resection is possible for lesions involving C2. The risk of postoperative swallowing difficulties with anterior approaches at C2 remains very high. These risks and complications can have a significant impact on quality of life postoperatively. The C2 area represents a transition point between clival lesions in which radical intralesional debulking and postoperative radiation remain the treatments of choice and the subaxial cervical spine in which complete spondylectomy, even up to four levels, is possible. We currently favor en bloc resection for lesions below C2 and intralesional spondylectomy for lesions located between the clivus and the midpoint of C2.

BAILOUT TECHNIQUES

- Vertebral artery bleeding in soft tissue can be controlled with pressure over surgicel and a cottonoid. It is important to wait at least 5-10 minutes prior to removal to allow clot to form. Clips can be placed once better exposure is obtained and bleeding has slowed.
- Suture of a muscle graft around the area of bleeding can also be used if the artery cannot be sacrificed.
- Mesh cages can be secured to bone using maxillofacial screws as needed.
- In cases in which the angle of the defect is impossible to graft, Steinman pins and cement can be used.
- CSF leakage should be treated aggressively in this location with muscle or fat grafts, fibrin sealant, and lumbar drainage.

TIPS FROM THE MASTERS

- The most critical goal is radical and complete resection. In this deep and narrow corridor, if en bloc resection proves impossible (such as with condylar involvement) then radical and complete intralesional resection should be performed as a bailout. Postoperative adjuvant treatment is critical.
- Grafts and cages should be secured with screws or buttress plates to adjacent bone if possible as there is significant motion and loading at the cranial cervical junction.
- Coils should not be placed in the vertebral artery directly in the area of planned surgical ligation due to risk of coil dislodgement and bleeding.
- The transglossal technique provides the best bilateral lateral exposure.
- Postoperative positive pressure ventilation via mask or CPAP should be avoided especially in cases of CSF leak.

References (With Key References in Boldface)

1. Abdel-Wanis Mel-S, Tsuchiya H, Kawahara N, et al. Tumor growth potential after tumoral and instrumental contamination: an in-vivo comparative study of T-saw, Gigli saw, and scalpel. J Orthop Sci 6:424-429, 2001.
2. Abe E, Kobayashi T, Murai H, et al. Total spondylectomy for primary malignant, aggressive benign, and solitary metastatic bone tumors of the thoracolumbar spine. J Spinal Disord 14:237-246, 2001.
3. **Acosta FL Jr, Ames CP. Artificial pedicle screw reconstruction of the cervical spine after lateral paramedian transpedicular approach for lesions of the ventral cervical spinal canal. Neurosurgery 57:281-285; discussion 285, 2005.**
4. **Acosta FL Jr, Aryan HE, Chi J, et al. Modified paramedian transpedicular approach and spinal reconstruction for intradural tumors of the cervical and cervicothoracic spine: clinical experience. Spine 32:E203-E210, 2007.**

5. **Ames CP, Wang VY, Deviren V, et al. Posterior transpedicular corpectomy and reconstruction of the axial vertebra for metastatic tumor. J Neurosurg Spine 10:111-116, 2009.**
6. Arnautovic KI, Al-Mefty O. Surgical seeding of chordomas. J Neurosurg 95:798-803, 2001.
7. **Bailey CS, Fisher CG, Boyd MC, et al. En bloc marginal excision of a multilevel cervical chordoma. Case report. J Neurosurg Spine 4:409-414, 2006.**
8. Barrenechea IJ, Perin NI, Triana A, et al. Surgical management of chordomas of the cervical spine. J Neurosurg Spine 6:398-406, 2007.
9. Bergh P, Kindblom LG, Gunterberg B, et al. Prognostic factors in chordoma of the sacrum and mobile spine: a study of 39 patients. Cancer 88:2122-2134, 2000.
10. Bilsky MH, Shannon FJ, Sheppard S, et al. Diagnosis and management of a metastatic tumor in the atlantoaxial spine. Spine 27:1062-1069, 2002.
11. Boriani S, Chevalley F, Weinstein JN, et al. Chordoma of the spine above the sacrum. Treatment and outcome in 21 cases. Spine 21:1569-1577, 1996.
12. Boriani S, Weinstein JN, Biagini R. Primary bone tumors of the spine. Terminology and surgical staging. Spine 22:1036-1044, 1997.
13. Boriani S, Bandiera S, Biagini R, et al. Chordoma of the mobile spine: fifty years of experience. Spine 31:493-503, 2006.
14. Boriani S, Biagini R, De Iure F, et al. En bloc resections of bone tumors of the thoracolumbar spine. A preliminary report on 29 patients. Spine 21:1927-1931, 1996.
15. Bosma JJ, Pigott TJ, Pennie BH, et al. En bloc removal of the lower lumbar vertebral body for chordoma. Report of two cases. J Neurosurg 94:284-291, 2001.
16. Carpentier A, Blanquet A, George B. Suboccipital and cervical chordomas: radical resection with vertebral artery control. Neurosurg Focus 10:E4, 2001.
17. Chou D, Acosta F Jr, Cloyd JM, et al. Parasagittal osteotomy for en bloc resection of multilevel cervical chordomas. J Neurosurg Spine 10:397-403, 2009.
18. **Cloyd JM, Chou D, Deviren V, et al. En bloc resection of primary tumors of the cervical spine: report of two cases and systematic review of the literature. Spine J 9:928-935, 2009.**
19. Cohen ZR, Fourney DR, Marco RA, et al. Total cervical spondylectomy for primary osteogenic sarcoma. Case report and description of operative technique. J Neurosurg 97:386-392, 2002.
20. Currier BL, Papagelopoulos PJ, Krauss WE, et al. Total en bloc spondylectomy of C5 vertebra for chordoma. Spine 32:E294-E299, 2007.
21. D'Haen B, De Jaegere T, Goffin J, et al. Chordoma of the lower cervical spine. Clin Neurol Neurosurg 97:245-248, 1995.
22. Delgado TE, Garrido E, Harwick RD. Labiomandibular, transoral approach to chordomas in the clivus and upper cervical spine. Neurosurgery 8:675-679, 1981.
23. Enneking WF, Spanier SS, Goodman MA. Current concepts review. The surgical staging of musculoskeletal sarcoma. J Bone Joint Surg Am 62:1027-1030, 1980.
24. Enneking WF, Spanier SS, Goodman MA. A system for the surgical staging of musculoskeletal sarcoma. 1980. Clin Orthop Relat Res 415:4-18, 2003.
25. Fisher CG, Keynan O, Boyd MC, et al. The surgical management of primary tumors of the spine: initial results of an ongoing prospective cohort study. Spine 30:1899-1908, 2005.
26. Fourney DR, Abi-Said D, Rhines LD, et al. Simultaneous anterior-posterior approach to the thoracic and lumbar spine for the radical resection of tumors followed by reconstruction and stabilization. J Neurosurg 94:232-244, 2001.
27. Fujita T, Kawahara N, Matsumoto T, et al. Chordoma in the cervical spine managed with en bloc excision. Spine 24:1848-1851, 1999.
28. Graves VB, Perl J II, Strother CM, et al. Endovascular occlusion of the carotid or vertebral artery with temporary proximal flow arrest and microcoils: clinical results. AJNR Am J Neuroradiol 18:1201-1206, 1997.
29. Heary RF, Vaccaro AR, Benevenia J, et al. "En-bloc" vertebrectomy in the mobile lumbar spine. Surg Neurol 50:548-556, 1998.

30. Hoshino Y, Kurokawa T, Nakamura K, et al. A report on the safety of unilateral vertebral artery ligation during cervical spine surgery. Spine 21:1454-1457, 1996.
31. Hsu KY, Zucherman JF, Mortensen N, et al. Follow-up evaluation of resected lumbar vertebral chordoma over 11 years: a case report. Spine 25:2537-2540, 2000.
32. Ibrahim A, Crockard A, Antonietti P, et al. Does spinal surgery improve the quality of life for those with extradural (spinal) osseous metastases? An international multicenter prospective observational study of 223 patients. Invited submission from the Joint Section Meeting on Disorders of the Spine and Peripheral Nerves, March 2007. J Neurosurg Spine 8:271-278, 2008.
33. Junming M, Cheng Y, Dong C, et al. Giant cell tumor of the cervical spine: a series of 22 cases and outcomes. Spine 33:280-288, 2008.
34. Keynan O, Fisher CG, Boyd MC, et al. Ligation and partial excision of the cauda equina as part of a wide resection of vertebral osteosarcoma: a case report and description of surgical technique. Spine 30:E97-E102, 2005.
35. Kratimenos GP, Crockard HA. The far lateral approach for ventrally placed foramen magnum and upper cervical spine tumours. Br J Neurosurg 7:129-140, 1993.
36. Larsson SE, Lorentzon R, Boquist L. Giant-cell tumor of bone. A demographic, clinical, and histopathological study of all cases recorded in the Swedish Cancer Registry for the years 1958 through 1968. J Bone Joint Surg Am 57:167-173, 1975.
37. Leitner Y, Shabat S, Boriani L, et al. En bloc resection of a C4 chordoma: surgical technique. Eur Spine J 16:2238-2242, 2007.
38. Muhlbauer M, Knosp E. The lateral transfacetal retrovascular approach for an anteriorly located chordoma originating from the second cervical vertebra. Acta Neurochir (Wien) 143:369-376, 2001.
39. Nina P, Franco A, Barbato R, et al. Extradural low cervical chordoma. Case report. J Neurosurg Sci 43:305-309, 1999.
40. Patchell RA, Tibbs PA, Regine WF, et al. Direct decompressive surgical resection in the treatment of spinal cord compression caused by metastatic cancer: a randomised trial. Lancet 366:643-648, 2005.
41. **Rhines LD, Fourney DR, Siadati A, et al. En bloc resection of multilevel cervical chordoma with C-2 involvement. Case report and description of operative technique. J Neurosurg Spine 2:199-205, 2005.**
42. **Sciubba D, Molina C, Gokaslan Z, et al. En bloc resection of cervical chordomas: series of 12 patients and clinical outcomes. Presented at the Twenty-seventh Annual Meeting of the American Association of Neurological Surgeons/Congress of Neurological Surgeons Joint Section on Disorders of the Spine and Peripheral Nerves. Phoenix, AZ, 2011.**
43. **Suchomel P, Buchvald P, Barsa P, et al. Single-stage total C-2 intralesional spondylectomy for chordoma with three-column reconstruction. Technical note. J Neurosurg Spine 6:611-618, 2007.**
44. Talac R, Yaszemski MJ, Currier BL, et al. Relationship between surgical margins and local recurrence in sarcomas of the spine. Clin Orthop Relat Res 397:127-132, 2002.
45. Tomita K, Kawahara N, Murakami H, et al. Total en bloc spondylectomy for spinal tumors: improvement of the technique and its associated basic background. J Orthop Sci 11:3-12, 2006.
46. Tomita K, Kawahara N, Baba H, et al. Total en bloc spondylectomy for solitary spinal metastases. Int Orthop 18:291-298, 1994.
47. Tomita K, Kawahara N. The threadwire saw: a new device for cutting bone. J Bone Joint Surg Am 78:1915-1917, 1996.
48. Tomita K, Kawahara N, Baba H, et al. Total en bloc spondylectomy. A new surgical technique for primary malignant vertebral tumors. Spine 22:324-333, 1997.
49. Windle-Taylor PC. Cervical chordoma: report of a case and the technique of transoral removal. Br J Surg 64:438-441, 1977.

50. Wittig JC, Bickels J, Kellar-Graney KL, et al. Osteosarcoma of the proximal humerus: long-term results with limb-sparing surgery. Clin Orthop Relat Res 397:156-176, 2002.
51. Wright NM, Kaufman BA, Haughey BH, et al. Complex cervical spine neoplastic disease: reconstruction after surgery by using a vascularized fibular strut graft. Case report. J Neurosurg 90:133-137, 1999.
52. York JE, Kaczaraj A, Abi-Said D, et al. Sacral chordoma: 40-year experience at a major cancer center. Neurosurgery 44:74-79; discussion 79-80, 1999.
53. Zacay G, Eyal A, Shacked I, et al. Chordoma of the cervical spine. Ann Otol Rhinol Laryngol 109:438-440, 2000.
54. Zambelli PY, Lechevallier J, Bracq H, et al. Osteoid osteoma or osteoblastoma of the cervical spine in relation to the vertebral artery. J Pediatr Orthop 14:788-792, 1994.

Chapter 39

En Bloc Resection of Primary Tumors of the Cervical Spine

Frank L. Acosta, Jr., Doniel Drazin, Christopher P. Ames

Most primary malignant tumors of the cervical spine, including chordoma and chondrosarcoma, are relatively resistant to radiation therapy and chemotherapy. To achieve long-term disease control, en bloc resection with the absolute minimal marginal violation is recommended.[1-4] After gross and histologic examinations of the specimen, en bloc resection is further delineated as intralesional, marginal, or wide.[1] En bloc resection has been shown to reduce local recurrence rates and improve long-term survival in patients with cervical spine chordomas.[1] A recent review in the literature, by Cloyd et al,[5] of 18 cases of en bloc resection of cervical tumors, found that 88.2% and 73.5% of patients were disease free at 1 and 5 years, respectively.

Because of the constraints imposed by regional cervical anatomy, the standard unidirectional approaches (anterior and posterior) must frequently be combined to allow for an adequate tumor resection. Unilateral vertebral artery involvement is common, and often vertebral artery sacrifice, after preoperative test occlusion, is necessary to achieve adequate margins. Bilateral vertebral artery involvement usually mandates intentional marginal transgression at the dominant vessel or on the less involved side. Bypass is usually reserved for recurrent disease. In addition, after en bloc resection, anterior and posterior reconstruction is typically necessary to restore spinal stability. Different en bloc resection techniques, including multilevel spondylectomy and parasagittal osteotomy, have been described, with long-term disease-free survival.[6,7]

Nerve root sacrifice must also be carefully considered to achieve adequate marginal resections and should be weighed against other factors, such as patient age and the likelihood of clean margins in other areas. The functional consequences, including long-term dysphagia and permanent weakness resulting from nerve sacrifice, should be carefully discussed with the patient preoperatively. Recently we have begun using the CyberKnife Robotic Radiosurgery System for preoperative treatment in areas of planned transgression, such as critical nerve root margins, and in cases of bilateral vertebral artery involvement.

INDICATIONS AND CONTRAINDICATIONS

En bloc resection is indicated for patients with aggressive benign tumors (osteochondromas and giant cell tumors) or primary malignant tumors (chordomas and chondrosarcomas) that have high local recurrence rates and are resistant to radiation therapy and chemotherapy. Contraindications include multiple comorbid conditions and advanced age that would increase the risk of postoperative morbidity and mortality.

PREOPERATIVE EVALUATION
Diagnostic Studies

It is important to determine the degree of vertebral artery involvement by the tumor. The diagnostic studies include high-resolution computed tomographic (CT) angiography, magnetic resonance angiography, and/or intraarterial digital subtraction angiography. If the tumor encases the vertebral artery unilaterally, balloon test occlusion can help assess the risk of ligation.

Radiologic Studies

Preoperative plain cervical and three-foot standing radiographs and CT scans are obtained to evaluate general sagittal and coronal balance and bone quality, and to assess osseous involvement and possible erosion into multiple levels. Magnetic resonance imaging (MRI), with and without gadolinium, is used to assess the soft tissue component and determine the size, location, and boundaries of the tumor. Evidence of the tumor encasing the vertebral artery and any potential adherence of the tumor to cervical nerve roots can also be determined.

An adaptation of the Weinstein-Boriani-Biagini (WBB) staging system has been developed for use in the cervical spine (Fig. 39-1). Although small case numbers prevent the use of this system for outcome conclusions, it is useful as a preoperative planning exercise to determine the en bloc strategy and areas of planned marginal transgressions.

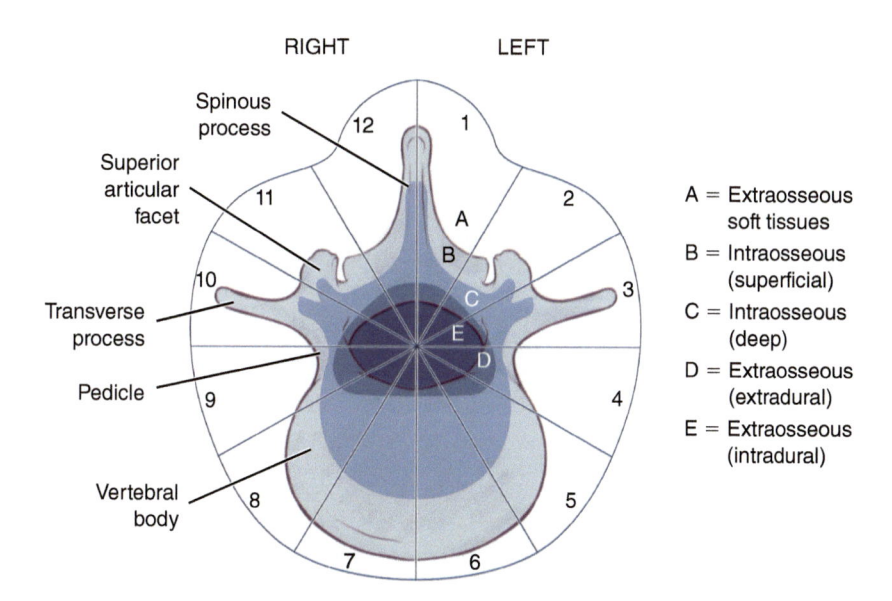

Fig. 39-1 Weinstein-Boriani-Biagini (WBB) surgical staging system. Concentric layers *A* through *E* are arranged from extraosseous to intradural, respectively. (Modified from Boriani S, Weinstein JN, Biagini R. Primary bone tumors of the spine. Terminology and surgical staging. Spine (Phila Pa 1976) 22:1036-1044, 1997.)

TECHNIQUE

En bloc resection of primary tumors of the cervical spine is performed in two stages. The first stage involves resection of the posterior elements of the cervical spine and osteotomies through one or both pedicles. The second stage is an anterior approach, with a parasagittal osteotomy through the involved vertebral bodies or transverse foramina.

ANTERIOR APPROACHES

There is no substitute for a wide exposure and excellent visualization for en bloc resection. A standard transoral approach is simply not adequate. For lesions primarily based at C2, we prefer a mandibulotomy approach with midline glossotomy, as needed. For lesions with significant C2 involvement but based in the subaxial spine, we use the transmandibular retropharyngeal circumglossal approach. For smaller subaxial lesions we use a standard transcervical. For large subaxial lesions we use a bilateral transcervical approach, working alternately through both exposures. Recurrent laryngeal nerve function must be assessed postoperatively before the tracheostomy tube is removed.

RESECTION OF POSTERIOR ELEMENTS

Preoperative antibiotics and steroids are administered, and general endotracheal anesthesia is induced. Somatosensory evoked potentials, transcranial motor evoked potentials, and electromyographs are monitored throughout the procedure. The patient's head is secured in a Mayfield frame. The patient is then positioned prone on chest bolsters, and the Mayfield frame is secured. Although in the thoracolumbar spine and sacrum, we prefer to excise the biopsy tract with a wide margin from the skin with the specimen, this is not possible in the cervical spine because most of these lesions are ventrally located and immediately adjacent to the trachea, pharynx, and esophagus and to the carotid sheath.

Wide exposure of the bilateral lamina and lateral masses is then accomplished, and posterior fixation is performed at three levels above and below the planned osteotomy. In the upper cervical spine, fixation is in the form of C1 lateral mass screws and C2 pedicle screws. (If required, fixation is extended to the occiput.) After fixation of the uninvolved segments, a wide laminectomy is performed through uninvolved bone. Both the inferior and superior articular process are removed, and a pediculectomy is then performed through uninvolved pedicles. For lateralized tumors the pediculectomy is performed on the side of ventral tumor involvement (Fig. 39-2, *A*). For large, midline tumors a bilateral pediculectomy is performed (Fig. 39-2, *B*) The vertebral artery is then identified at the top and bottom of the planned resection, just lateral to the pedicle. Weck clips are used to sacrifice the vessel, and the vessel is then transected. Next, in the upper cervical spine, the nerve roots may be sacrificed to improve exposure before pediculectomy. Predetermined nerve roots are then tied off and sacrificed unilaterally. The vertebral artery on the affected side may also be sacrificed, depending on the results of preoperative vertebral artery test occlusion. After nerve root and vertebral artery ligation, a pediculectomy is performed with an osteotome at the base of the vertebral body to completely release the posterior elements on the affected side or sides. For lateralized tumors the pediculectomy is performed on the side of tumor involvement (see Fig. 39-2, *A*). For large, midline tumors a bilateral pediculectomy is performed (see Fig. 39-2, *B*) for removal of the bilateral posterior elements. Once pediculectomy has been completed and the posterior elements removed, posterior fixation is completed. A silicone rubber sheet is then placed between the ventral tumor and the dura.

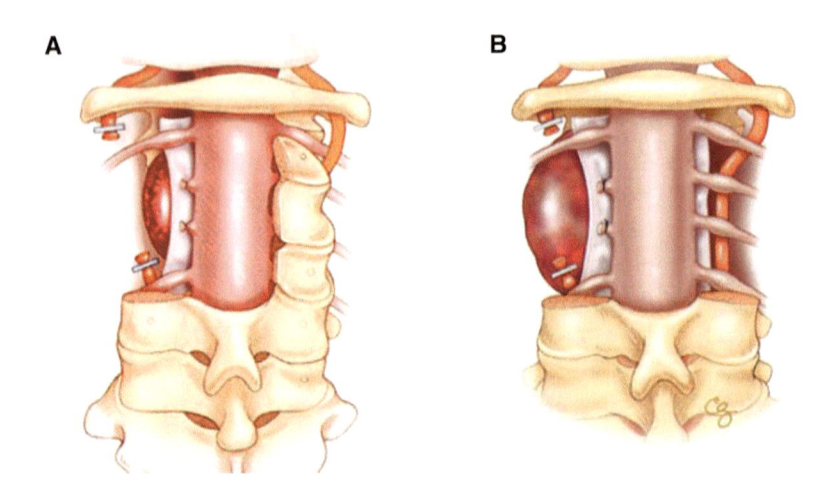

Fig. 39-2 **A,** Unilateral posterior element removal followed by vertebral artery and nerve root ligation, either retaining some unilateral posterior elements or **B,** completely removing all posterior elements. (From Chou D, Acosta F Jr, Cloyd JM, Ames CP. Parasagittal osteotomy for en bloc resection of multilevel cervical chordomas. J Neurosurg Spine 10:397-403, 2009.)

ANTERIOR COLUMN RESECTION

Parasagittal Osteotomy

After posterior column resection and instrumentation, attention is turned to en bloc anterior column resection. This is usually performed on a different day in a staged fashion. This takes the form of a parasagittal osteotomy for removal of various amounts of the anterior column (Fig. 39-3). First, discectomies at the levels above and below are performed, with posterior longitudinal ligament resection. A parasagittal osteotomy is performed through the involved vertebral bodies down to the membrane. For lesions involving more than 75% of the vertebral body, the osteotomy is carried out to the transverse foramen to allow for a complete en bloc vertebrectomy. This involves mobilization of the contralateral uninvolved vertebral artery out of the foramen transversarium, which is readily accomplished after removal of the anterior transverse process. The involved vertebral bodies are then removed en bloc. A Caspar pin inserted into the specimen can help to control it during removal and final manipulation. The spine is reconstructed with an appropriate-sized expandable cage with anterior plating.

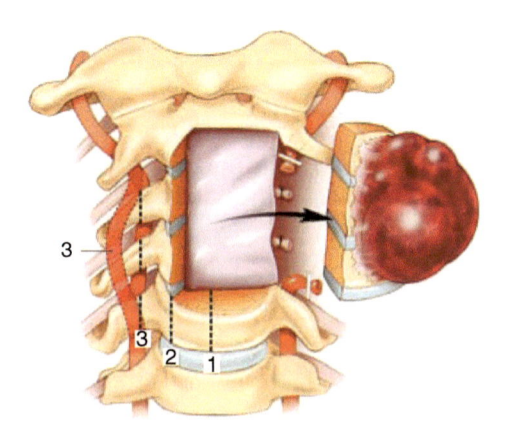

Fig. 39-3 Parasagittal osteotomy procedure performed to maintain oncologic margins while removing multiple levels of chordoma en bloc. Examples of parasagittal osteotomy locations are given for lateralized tumors involving less than 50% *(1)* and less than 75% *(2)* of the vertebral body. For tumors involving more than 75% *(3)* of the vertebral body, the osteotomy cuts lie at the very edge of the vertebral body or, in case of complete spondylectomy, the cuts lie on the transverse process of the transverse foramen with requisite vertebral artery mobilization.

OUTCOMES WITH EVALUATION OF RESULTS

In a systematic review of the literature, Cloyd et al[5] analyzed 18 patients with cervical spine tumors treated with en bloc resection: 12 with chordomas, two with chondrosarcomas, two with giant cell tumors, along with a malignant peripheral nerve sheath tumor, and one with a mesenchymal hamartoma. All patients were managed with en bloc resection with margins classified as follows: wide in five, marginal in six, intralesional in six, and not reported in one. The average number of levels involved was 2.1 ± 1.1 (range 1 to 4).

With an average follow-up of 47.4 ± 41.5 months, Cloyd et al[5] found 1- and 5-year disease-free survival rates of 88.2% and 73.5%, respectively, after en bloc resection of cervical spine tumors. Three patients had local recurrences, at 12, 44, and 113 months, respectively, and one patient had distant metastasis 12 months postoperatively. See Chapter 38, pp. 689-692 for additional information on outcomes with evaluation of results.

SIGNATURE CASES

A 59-year-old woman presented with right arm numbness. MRI showed a large mass involving the C3 and C4 vertebral bodies, with the mass affecting the spinal cord (Fig. 39-4, *A* and *B*). A subsequent angiogram demonstrated a dominant right vertebral artery. A biopsy specimen showed a chordoma. The patient was taken to the operating room for a posterior laminectomy with instrumented fixation from C2 to C6, with left C3-C4 nerve root ligations. The pedicles at C3 and C4 were amputated by means of an osteotomy at the base of the vertebral body to completely release the left-sided

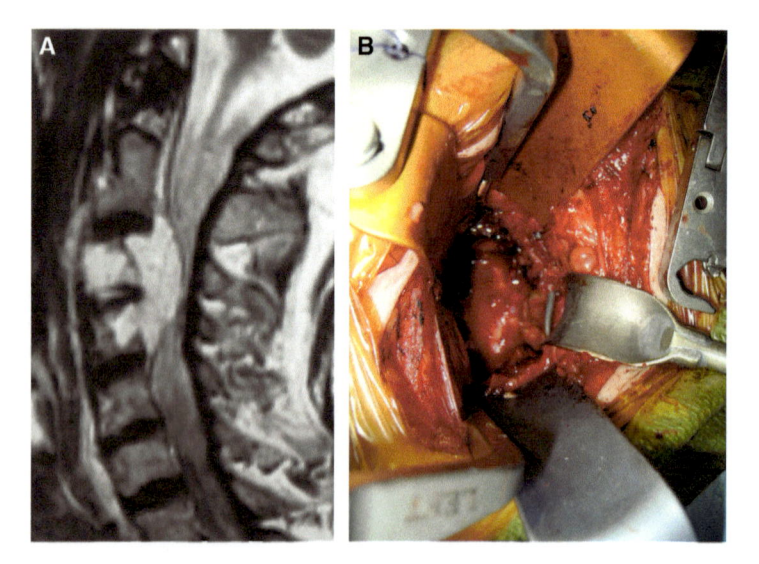

Fig. 39-4 **A,** Sagittal T2-weighted MRI scan demonstrating the extent of multilevel chordoma and epidural extension. **B,** Intraoperative view of the tumor. (**A-F** from Chou D, Acosta F Jr, Cloyd JM, et al. Parasagittal osteotomy for en bloc resection of multilevel cervical chordomas. J Neurosurg Spine 10:397-403, 2009.)

posterior elements from the anterior spine. The left vertebral artery was ligated, and the left posterior elements of C3 and C4 were removed en bloc. A silicone elastomer sheath was placed between the dura and the tumor.

Two days later, the patient underwent a discectomy through a standard anterior transcervical approach, with posterior longitudinal ligament resection at C2-3 and C4-5. A right-sided parasagittal osteotomy through the vertebral bodies of C3 and C4 was performed, using a high-speed burr to drill down to the dura, and the tumor involving C3 and C4 was removed en bloc. The spine was reconstructed with an expandable cage and anterior plating. The patient's postoperative course was complicated by posterior wound dehiscence at 1 month, which was treated by delayed primary closure. Follow-up MRI at 30 months showed the patient to be disease free, and postoperative radiographs verified that the construct was in a good position (Fig. 39-4, *C* through *F*).

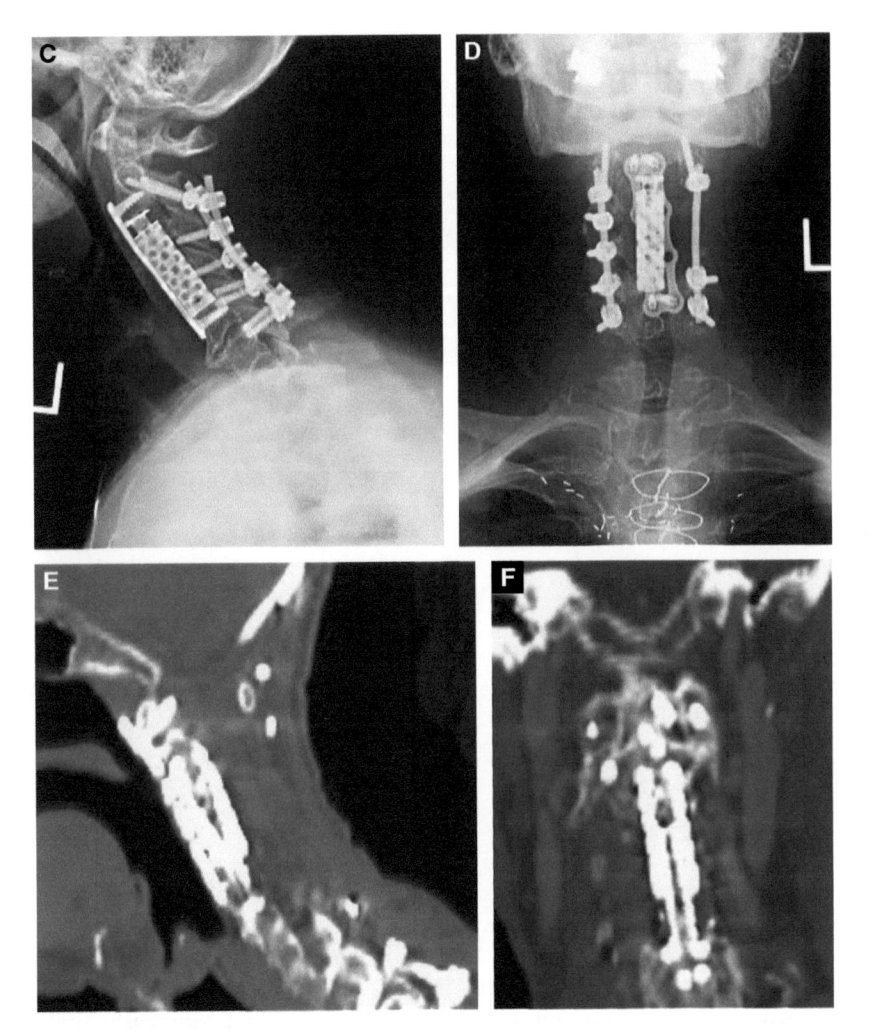

Fig. 39-4, cont'd **C,** Postoperative lateral and **D,** anteroposterior plain radiographs. **E,** Sagittal and **F,** coronal CT reconstructions.

A 61-year-old man had a 1-year history of throat discomfort. A CT scan demonstrated a mass in the vertebral body of C3 with extension from C2 to C4 (Fig. 39-5, *A*). The patient subsequently underwent a transoral biopsy procedure, and the diagnosis was a chordoma. An en bloc resection from the inferior aspect of C2 to the C4-5 disc space was planned. The patient first underwent a posterior instrumented fusion from the occiput to T2, followed by an osteotomy of the posterior elements from C2 to C4, with sacrifice of the left vertebral artery. The nerve roots of C3 to C5 were ligated.

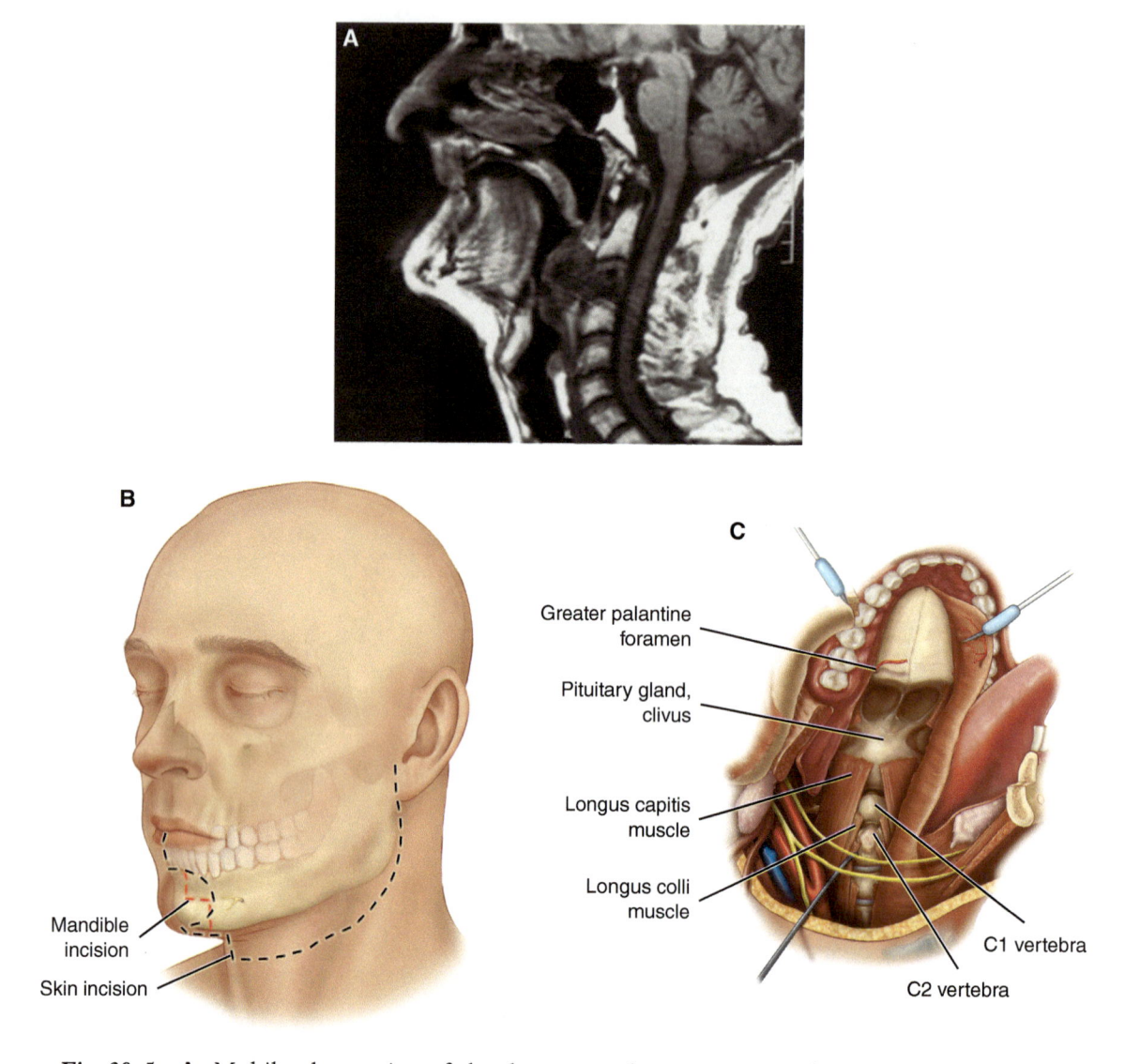

Fig. 39-5 **A,** Multilevel extension of chordoma mass shown on a sagittal T1-weighted MRI scan. **B,** Planned skin and mandible incisions for a transmandibular retropharyngeal circumglossal approach. **C,** Anatomic landmarks. (**A, E, F,** and **G** from Chou D, Acosta F Jr, Cloyd JM, Ames CP. Parasagittal osteotomy for en bloc resection of multilevel cervical chordomas. J Neurosurg Spine 10:397-403, 2009.)

The following day a transmandibular retropharyngeal circumglossal approach was used to perform a right parasagittal osteotomy through the bodies of C3 and C4 (Fig. 39-5, *B* and *C*). A complete discectomy was performed at C4-5. The inferior aspect of C2 was amputated with the use of a high-speed burr, and this cut was connected on the right side to the parasagittal osteotomy at C3-4. An en bloc resection of the tumor was performed, which involved the inferior aspect of C2 to the body of C4 (Fig. 39-5, *D* and *E*). The spine was reconstructed with the use of an expandable cage and a modified anterior cervical plate from C1 to C5 (Fig. 39-5, *F* through *I*).

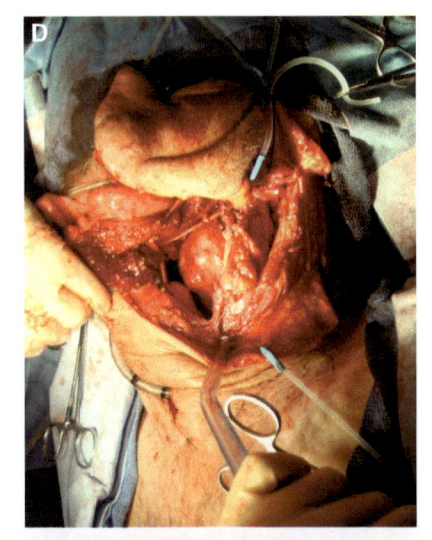

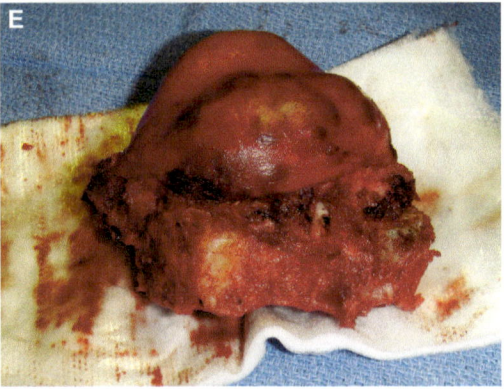

Fig. 39-5, cont'd Photograph of en bloc specimen of multilevel chordoma **D,** during and **E,** after removal.

Continued

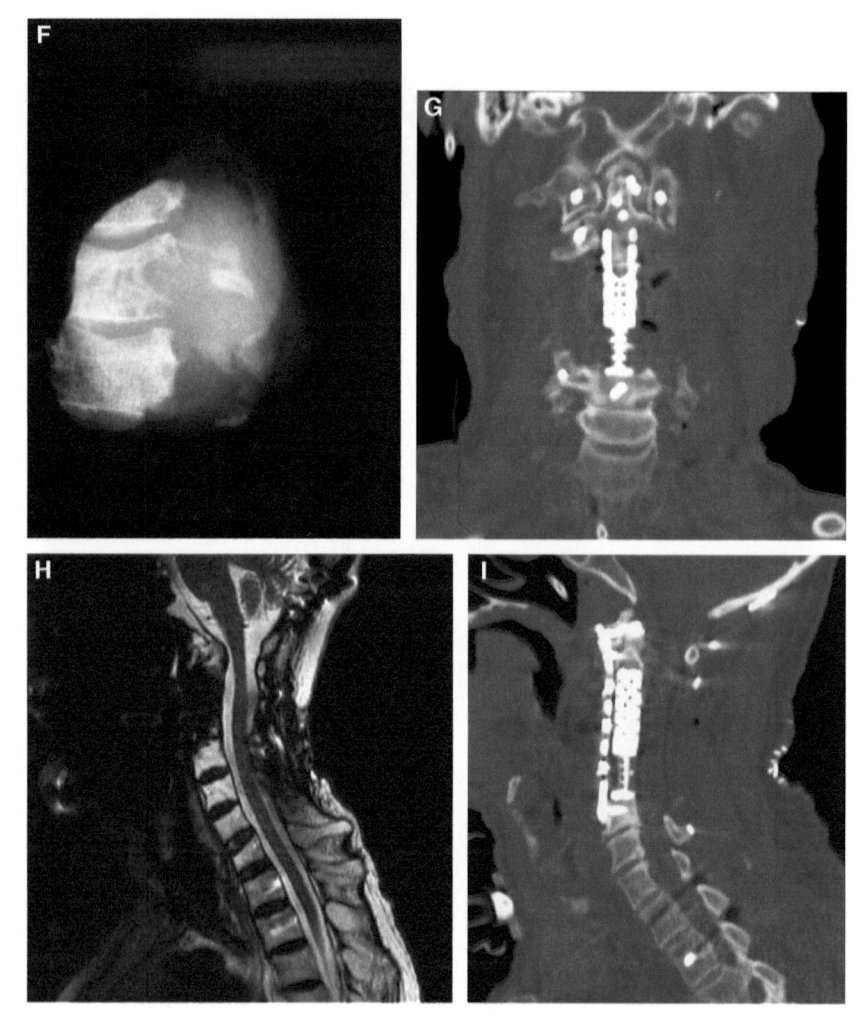

Fig. 39-5, cont'd Comparison of **F,** preoperative and **G,** 2-year postoperative MRI scans. **H,** Postoperative lateral MRI scans. **I,** Postoperative radiograph.

A 60-year-old woman with a history of neck pain was referred after a chiropractor palpated a large neck mass. MRI and CT scans demonstrated a giant tumor centered on the C4 vertebra, extending into the posterior elements of C4 and the anterior aspects of C3 and C5, and encasing the right vertebral artery (Fig. 39-6, A and B). Angiography showed the left vertebral artery to be patent, and so the right vertebral artery was occluded preoperatively. The patient was subsequently taken to the operating room where she underwent a C2-T1 laminectomy, transpedicular posterior osteotomies from C3 to C7, bilateral C4 and right C5 nerve root sacrifice, and occipital T3 posterior spine fusion with instrumentation. On postoperative day 7, the patient underwent en bloc resection of the four-level mass through a bilateral transcervical approach (Fig. 39-6, C and D). Stabilization was achieved with the use of expandable cages and synthetic bone graft material (Fig. 39-6, G through I). Results of pathologic examination demonstrated clean margins, with the exception of the planned transgression intralesional resection at the left vertebral artery.

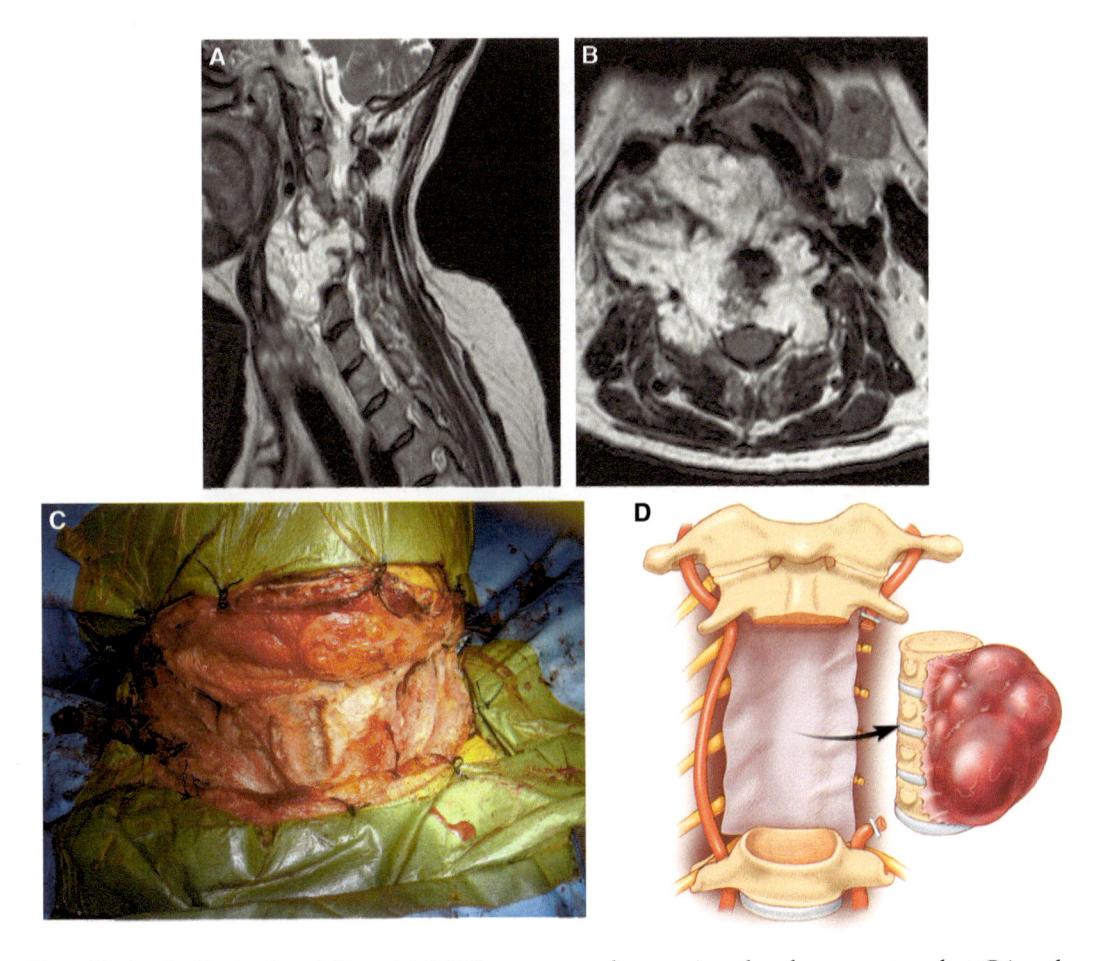

Fig. 39-6 **A,** Sagittal and **B,** axial MRI scans reveal a massive chordoma centered at C4 and extending to anterior aspects of C3-6. **C** and **D,** Patient underwent four-level en bloc resection with right-sided vertebral artery and C4 and C5 nerve root ligations. (From Cloyd JM, Chou D, Deviren V, Ames CP. En bloc resection of primary tumors of the cervical spine: report of two cases and systematic review of the literature. Spine J 9:928-935, 2009.)

Continued

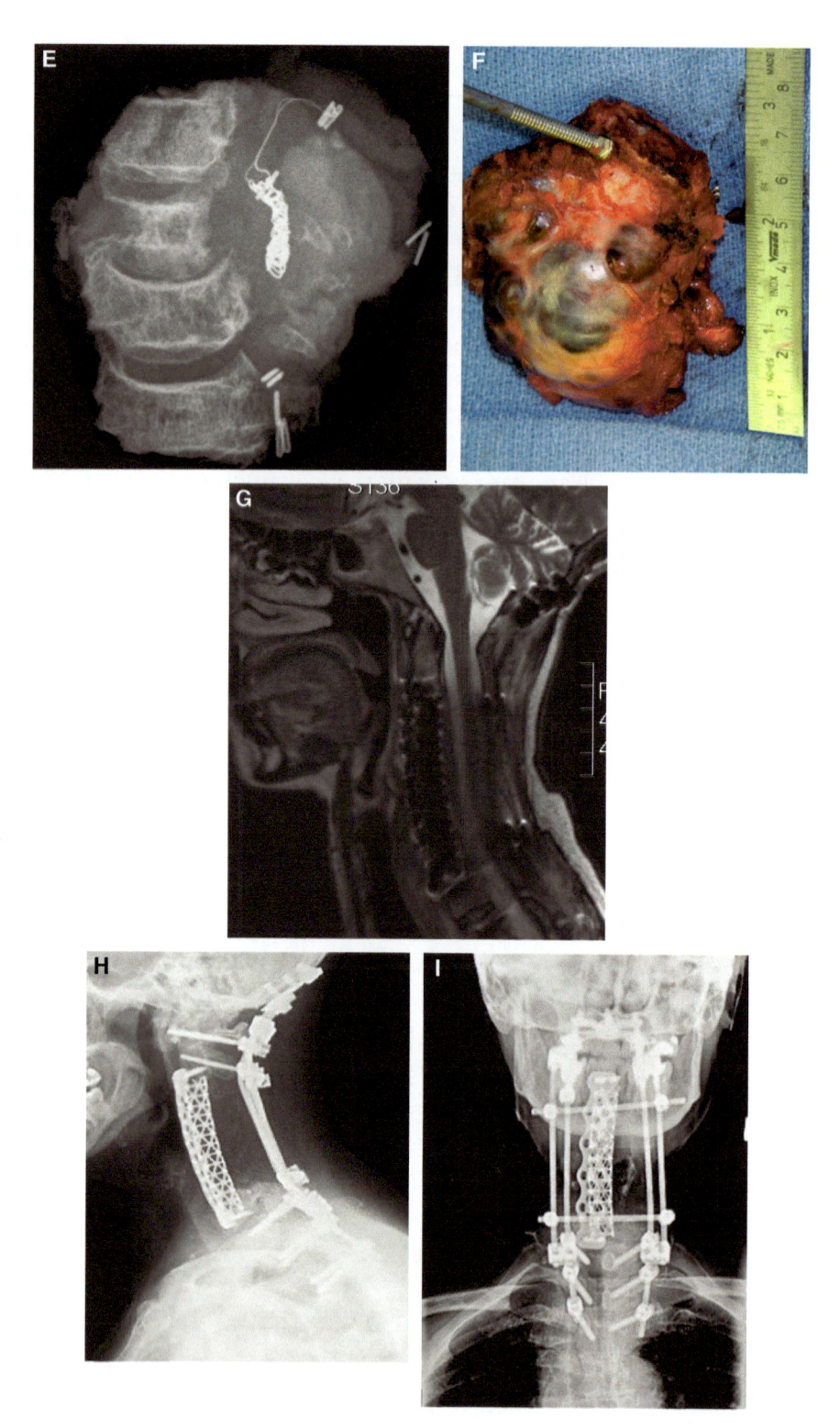

Fig. 39-6, cont'd **E** and **F,** Radiograph and postoperative photograph displaying the resected tumor and four levels of the cervical spine. **G-I,** Stabilization was achieved with an occipital–T3 posterior spine fusion and C3-6 anterior fusion with cage and synthetic bone graft.

CONCLUSION

Although challenging, en bloc resection of primary cervical spine tumors is possible. Borderline margins are typically obtained at the dura and anterior vital structures, such as the trachea, esophagus, and pharynx. Pediculectomy and resection of posterior elements are performed first. A parasagittal osteotomy is then performed for en bloc removal of the involved vertebral bodies and tumor. Reconstruction is performed with a posterior pedicle/lateral mass screw-rod construct and anterior cage-plate fixation. In a systematic review of the literature on en bloc resection of primary cervical spine tumors, 1- and 5-year disease-free survival rates were 88.2% and 73.5%, respectively.

BAILOUT TECHNIQUES

- In cases of obvious tumor trangression dural sealant or bone wax can be used to seal the area of unintentional contamination.
- Maxillofacial screws will fit through titanium mesh cages and can be used to stabilize the cage directly to the bone.
- Vascularized autograft fibula can be considered for cases of pseudarthrosis or challenging fusion environments, such as cases of prior irradiation with recurrence.

TIPS FROM THE MASTERS

- En bloc resection is the treatment of choice for lesions below C2. Dysphagia and other approach-related complications are increased with en bloc resections of lesions involving the greater portions of C2 and C1, but en bloc resections are not reasonable for lower clival-based lesions.
- Radical approaches, nerve sacrifice, and vertebral artery sacrifice should be approached with greater caution in older patients, and greater consideration should be given to planned transgressions and intralesional resections and preoperative and postoperative adjuvant treatments.
- Preoperative tracheostomy and insertion of a gastrostomy tube are strongly recommended.

References (With Key References in Boldface)

1. **Boriani S, Weinstein J, Biagini R. Primary bone tumors of the spine. Terminology and surgical staging. Spine 22:1036-1044, 1997.**
2. Fisher C, Keynan O, Boyd M, et al. The surgical management of primary tumors of the spine. Spine 30:1899-1908, 2005.
3. Talac R, Yaszemski M, Currier B, et al. Relationship between surgical margins and local recurrence in sarcomas of the spine. Clin Orthop 397:127-132, 2002.

4. **Tomita K, Kawahara N, Baba H, et al. Total en bloc spondylectomy. Spine 22:324-333, 1997.**
5. Cloyd JM, Chou D, Deviren V, et al. En bloc resection of primary tumors of the cervical spine: report of two cases and systematic review of the literature. Spine J 9:928-935, 2009.
6. Rhines LD, Fourney DR, Siadati A, et al. En bloc resection of multilevel cervical chordoma with C-2 involvement. Case report and description of operative technique. J Neurosurg Spine 2:199-205, 2005.
7. **Chou D, Acosta F Jr, Cloyd JM, et al. Parasagittal osteotomy for en bloc resection of multilevel cervical chordomas. J Neurosurg Spine 10:397-403, 2009.**

Chapter 40

En Bloc Spondylectomy: Single-Stage Thoracic Spine

Hideki Murakami, Katsuro Tomita,
Norio Kawahara, Satoru Demura

Spinal malignancies have historically been treated with curettage (piecemeal excision) of vertebral tumors in an effort to minimize the risk of injury to the neural elements and because of a lack of sophisticated surgical techniques and instrumentation. However, the clear disadvantages of this type of palliative surgery include the high risk of tumor cell contamination of surrounding structures and residual tumor tissue at the surgical site because it is difficult to distinguish between tumor and healthy tissue. In combination, these factors contribute to the high rate of local recurrence of spine tumors.

A number of surgeons have reported excellent clinical results with the use of total corpectomy or spondylectomy for reducing local recurrences of vertebral tumors.[1-9] We have developed a new surgical technique for spondylectomy (vertebrectomy), which we call *total en bloc spondylectomy* (TES), to avoid local recurrences.[10-16] Our technique is different from the aforementioned corpectomy in that it involves en bloc removal of the lesion—that is, removal of the entire vertebra, both the body and lamina, as a single compartment, with either wide or minimal margins.[17] The TES procedure was designed to achieve oncologic complete tumor resection en bloc, including the main lesion and satellite microlesions, in a vertebral compartment.

The surgical techniques of TES have improved remarkably on the basis of the knowledge acquired and in consideration of surgical anatomy, physiology, and biomechanics of both the spine and spinal cord.[18,19] This chapter presents a detailed description of the surgical techniques of TES at the thoracic spine.

INDICATIONS

Candidates for TES are primarily patients with the following pathologic conditions: primary malignant tumors, aggressive benign tumors, and isolated metastases in patients who have a long life expectancy.[18-20]

PREOPERATIVE EVALUATION

GENERAL CONDITIONS

When considering patients for surgery, especially those with spinal metastases, our prerequisite is a minimum score of three or less on the Eastern Cooperative Oncology Group (ECOG) performance status test[21] or 30% or more on the Karnofsky Performance Scale,[22] which are the same requirements for administrating chemotherapy.

RADIOLOGIC STUDIES

Computed tomography (CT) is required to assess the extent of bone involvement, whereas magnetic resonance imaging (MRI) demonstrates extraosseous extensions. Vertebral tumors most commonly extend farthest at the lateral part of the posterior longitudinal ligament vertically. We carefully check the vertical extension to adjacent vertebrae on MRI. The vertical extension of the spine tumor is important in the determining the craniocaudal surgical margins for TES.

Patients with malignant spine tumors should also undergo a systematic examination that included the following: bone scintigraphy to detect other bony lesions, MRI of the entire spine from C1 to the sacrum to search for other vertebral metastases, and CT scans of the chest, abdomen, and brain to detect distant metastases.

CLINICAL DECISION-MAKING

For primary malignant tumors, radical surgery with minimal or wide margins, such as TES, in addition to chemotherapy, is necessary. Aggressive benign tumors must be managed with thorough excision.

Scoring systems are used as a guideline in determining surgical strategy for patients with spinal metastases to determine the most technically appropriate and feasible surgery, for example, en bloc spondylectomy, debulking (piecemeal thorough excision), curettage, or palliative decompression.[20] From the standpoint of tumor growth, according to our surgical classification of spine tumors (Fig. 40-1), by which the extent of a spine tumor is stratified, TES is recommended only for patients with type 3, 4, 5, and 6 lesions. Patients with type 1 or type 2 lesions can be managed with radiation therapy, chemotherapy, corpectomy, or hemivertebrectomy. For patients with type 6 lesions, TES is recommended only when fewer than four vertebral bodies are involved. TES is not recommended for type 7 lesions. Systemic treatment or hospice care may be the treatment choice for patients with type 7 lesions.[18,19]

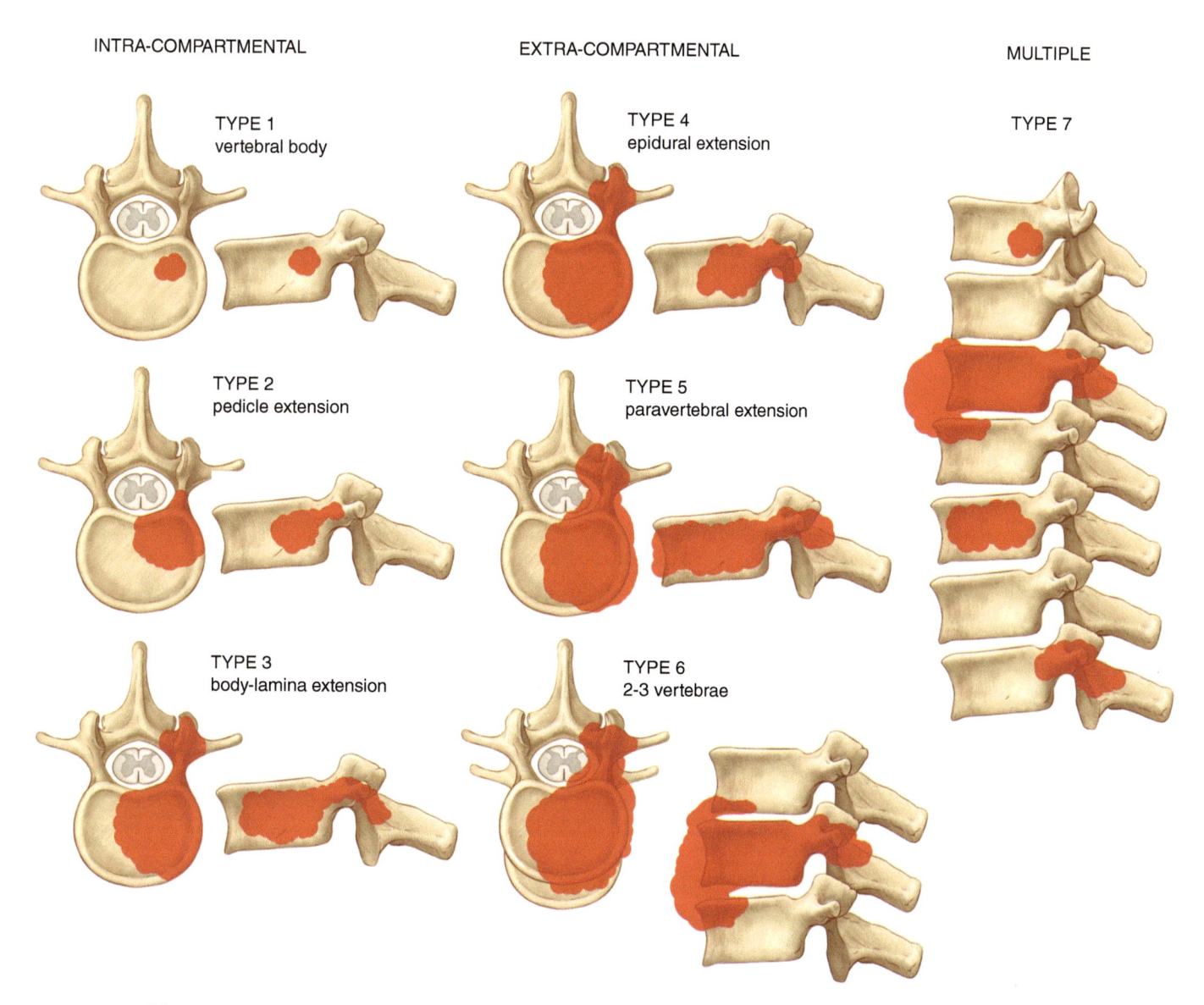

Fig. 40-1 Surgical classification of spine tumors. (Adapted from Tomita K, Kawahara N, Kobayashi T, et al. Surgical strategy for spinal metastases. Spine 26:298-306, 2001.)

TECHNIQUE

PREOPERATIVE EMBOLIZATION

Preoperative embolization of bilateral segmental arteries at three levels (i.e., embolization of bilateral segmental arteries of the tumors and two adjacent vertebrae, one cephalad and caudad) should be attempted 72 hours before the operation.[18,19] Embolization is carried out under local anesthesia by a radiologist. Following the aortic runoff, selective angiograms of segmental arteries supplying the targeted tumor and adjacent vertebrae (typically one level above and one level below the lesion) are obtained. Embolization coils or pieces of gelatin sponge are used for proximal embolization of the segmental arteries lateral to the vertebral bodies, and polyvinyl alcohol particles are used for peripheral embolization of the posterior branches of the segmental arteries to block the backward flow. The segmental artery or arteries that supply the anterior spinal artery (artery of Adamkiewicz) are not embolized to ensure that emboli are not delivered to the anterior spinal artery. This original embolization method has resulted in a dramatic decrease in intraoperative blood loss without compromising the spinal cord, as comparison with the method previously used at our hospital.[23-25] Of course a segmental artery does not exist at the upper thoracic spine (T1 to T4). Therefore, at these levels, embolization of feeding arteries to the tumor should only be carried out before TES.[26]

Approach

The single posterior approach is the method most commonly used at thoracic spine. Its principal advantage is the spinal cord can be carefully observed throughout the procedure, particularly during anterior spinal column osteotomy, corpectomy, and spinal reconstruction by posterior instrumentation. However, an anterior dissection through a thoracoscopic mini-open approach, followed by posterior TES, is safer than TES performed as a single posterior procedure in a patient whose segmental artery or arteries have tumor involvement as demonstrated on preoperative MRI.

Patients are placed prone over a Relton-Hall four-poster frame to avoid compression of the vena cava. A straight vertical midline incision is made over the spinous processes and is extended to three vertebrae above and three below the involved segment or segments.

Exposure

The paraspinal muscles are dissected from the spinous processes, the laminae, the facet joints, and the transverse processes, and they are then retracted laterally. A large articulated spinal retractor, especially designed for TES, is used. This retractor has a uniaxial joint in each of its limbs, and a wider exposure can then be achieved by spreading it. The ribs on the affected level, and one level below, are transected 3 to 4 cm lateral to the costotransverse joint after the pleura is bluntly separated from the ribs (Fig. 40-2). Then the superior articular processes of the vertebra affected by the tumor are achieved by osteotomizing the spinous and inferior articular processes of the upper neighboring vertebra and removing them by dissecting attached soft tissues, including the ligamentum flavum.

Introduction of the T-Saw Guide

To create a port for eliciting the tip of the T-saw guide through the nerve root canal, the soft tissue attached to the inferior aspect of the pars interarticularis is dissected and removed. A C-curved malleable T-saw guide is then introduced through the intervertebral foramen in a cephalocaudal direction. The tip of the T-saw guide should be introduced along the medial cortex of the lamina and the pedicle to avoid injuring the spinal cord (Fig. 40-3). After the T-saw guide is inserted, the tip of the guide at the exit

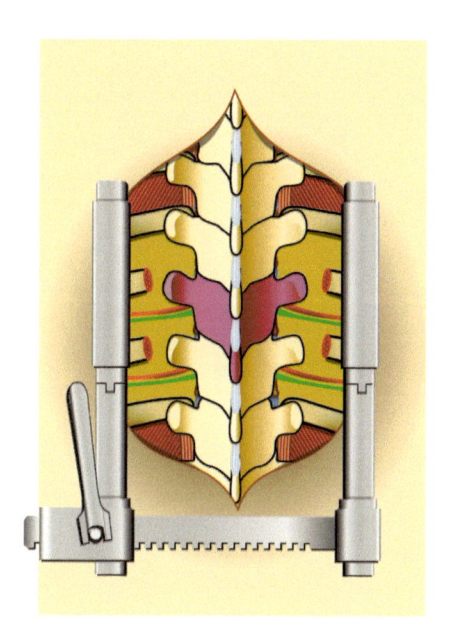

Fig. 40-2 Exposure. A large retractor is applied. Bilateral ribs on the affected level and one level below it are transected.

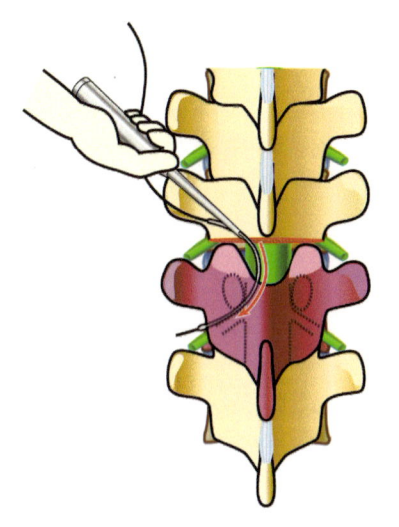

Fig. 40-3 Introducing the T-saw guide and T-saw. A C-curved malleable T-saw guide is introduced through the left intervertebral foramen in a cephalocaudal direction. The tip of the T-saw guide and the T-saw are found at the exit of the foramen. (Promedical Co. Ltd., Kanazawa, Japan.)

of the nerve root canal is located beneath the inferior border of the pars interarticularis. A T-saw (0.54 mm in diameter)[27] is passed through the hole in the T-saw guide, and the T-saw guide is removed. The T-saw is clamped with a T-saw holder at each end.

CUTTING THE PEDICLES AND EN BLOC LAMINECTOMY

Under steady tension, the T-saw is placed beneath the superior articular process with a specially designed T-saw manipulator. In this procedure the T-saw around the lamina is wrapped around the pedicle. With a reciprocating motion of the T-saw that uses two pulleys, the pedicles are cut, after which the entire posterior structure of the spine (the spinous process, the superior and inferior articular processes, and the pedicle) is removed in one piece (Fig. 40-4). The cut surfaces of the pedicle and the rib head are sealed with bone wax to reduce bleeding and minimize contamination by tumor

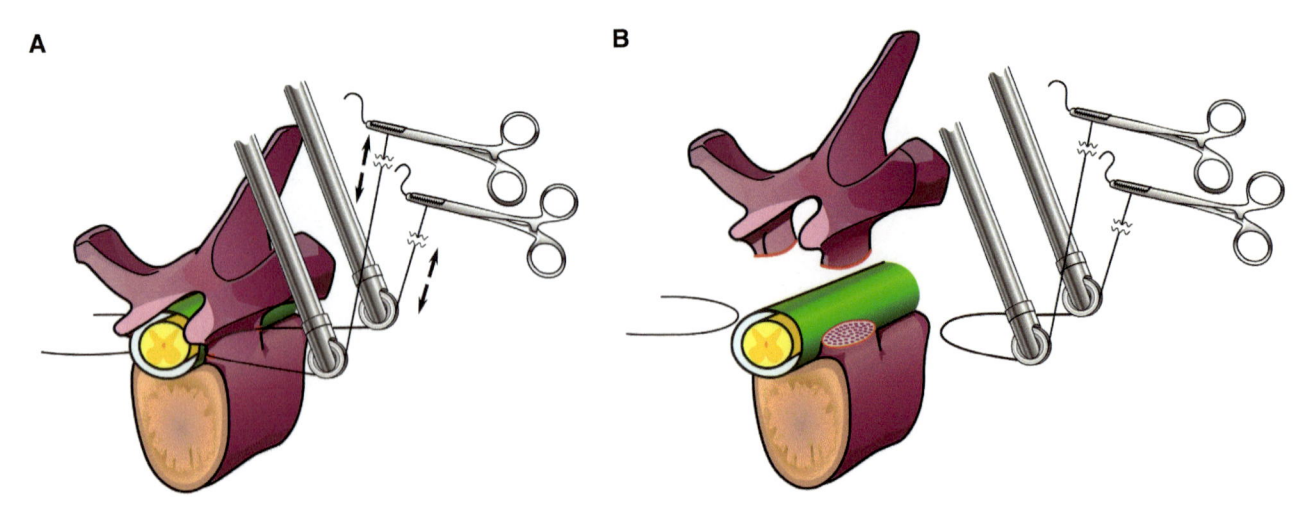

Fig. 40-4 **A,** Pediculectomy. Bilateral pedicles are cut by means of a reciprocating motion of the T-saw and the use of pulleys. **B,** En bloc laminectomy.

cells.[28] Double rinsing with distilled water and highly concentrated cisplatinum is recommended to eradicate contaminated cancer cells.[18] Fibrin glue (3 ml), injected manually into the epidural space in cranial and caudal directions of the involved vertebrae, helps to reduce oozing from the epidural venous plexus after en bloc laminectomy.[18]

BLUNT DISSECTION AROUND THE VERTEBRAL BODY

At the beginning of this step, the corresponding bilateral nerve roots are ligated and cut, so that the spinal branch of the segmental artery, which runs along the nerve root, is ligated and divided. Even if the spinal branch is the artery of Adamkiewicz, it is ligated and cut. Ligation of segmental arteries up to three vertebral levels, even including the artery of Adamkiewicz, may not affect the spinal cord evoked potentials or spinal cord function.[29] However, bilateral T1 nerve roots should be preserved if these nerve roots are not involved by the tumor (see case 2 in Signature Cases section, p. 730). The remaining rib heads are then dissected and resected. The blunt dissection is carried out on both sides through the plane between the pleura and the vertebral body. The segmental arteries are identified and dissected bilaterally from the vertebral body (Fig. 40-5). Usually the lateral aspect of the body is easily dissected with a "peanut" (cotton ball) and a curved vertebral spatula. By continuing dissection of both lateral sides of the vertebral body anteriorly, the aorta and azygos vein are carefully dissected anteriorly from the anterior aspect of the vertebral body with a spatula and the surgeon's fingers. When the surgeon's fingertips meet, anterior to the vertebral body (Fig. 40-6), a series of spatulas, starting with the smallest, is inserted sequentially to extend the dissection. Careful step-by-step dissection with anatomic consideration is fundamental. A pair of the largest spatulas is kept at the dissection site to prevent any iatrogenic injury to the surrounding tissues and organs and to extend the surgical field so that it is sufficiently wide to manipulate the anterior column. At this point, a cord spatula is used to mobilize the dural tube from the surrounding venous plexus and the ligamentous tissue at the proximal and distal cutting levels of the anterior column.

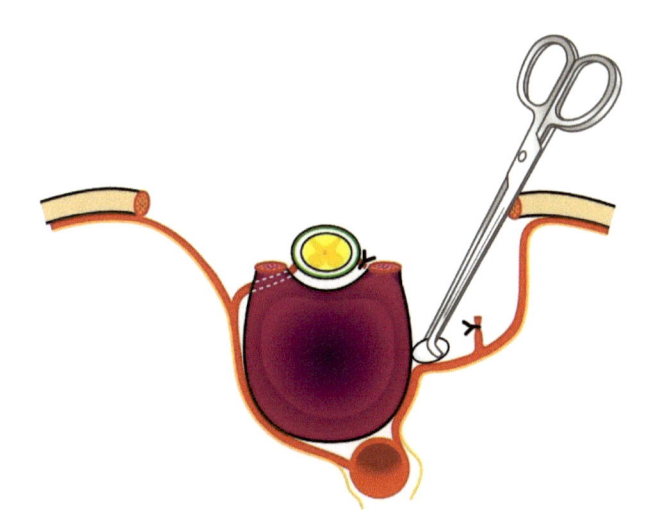

Fig. 40-5 Anterior dissection around the vertebral body. Bilateral segmental arteries are dissected by a peanut.

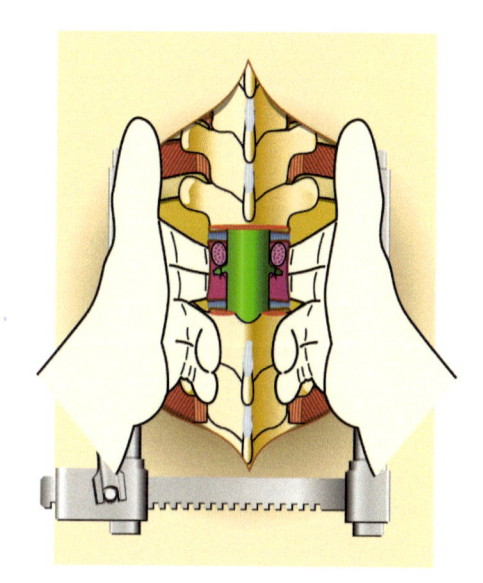

Fig. 40-6 Anterior finger dissection around the vertebral body.

EN BLOC CORPECTOMY

Posterior instrumentation (two above and two below the segmental fixation) must be performed to maintain stability after segmental resection of the anterior column (Fig. 40-7). For spinal shortening, we should use monoaxial screws in cranial side or the other to translate the vertebral body with parallel shift. Diamond T-saws are inserted at the proximal and distal cutting levels of the vertebral bodies after confirmation of the disc levels. The teeth-cord protector, which has teeth on both edges to prevent the T-saw from slipping, is then applied between the dural tube and the vertebral body. The anterior column of the vertebra is cut by the T-saw, together with the anterior and posterior longitudinal ligaments (Fig. 40-8). After the anterior column is cut, the mobility of the vertebra or vertebrae is again checked to ensure a complete corpectomy. In cases where the spinal cord is severely compressed by the epidural tumor extension, the tumorous vertebral body is pushed down in a ventral direction from the dural tube, which results in spinal cord decompression. An adhesion between the epidural tumor and the anterior aspect of the dura is safely dissected with a Penfield dissector

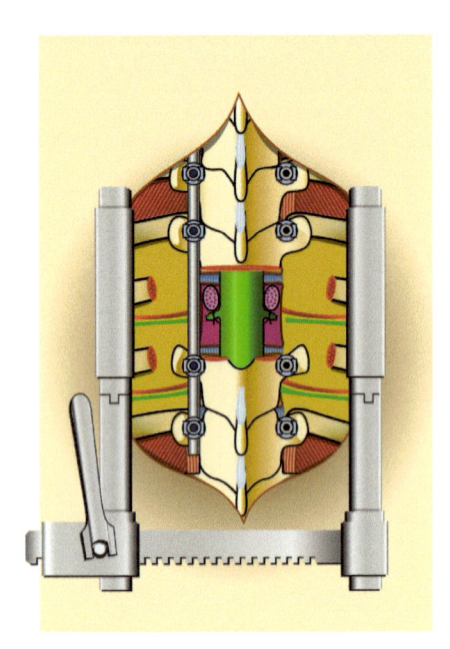

Fig. 40-7 Exposure before en bloc corpectomy. Posterior instrumentation is performed to maintain stability for segmental resection of the anterior column.

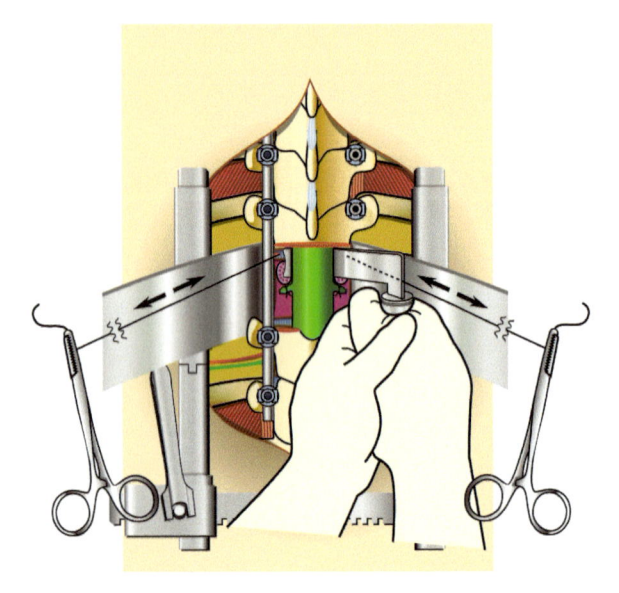

Fig. 40-8 Cutting the anterior column. The anterior column of the vertebra is cut by a diamond T-saw, together with the anterior and posterior longitudinal ligaments. The teeth–cord protector, which has teeth on both edges to prevent the T-saw from slipping, is applied between the dural tube and the vertebral body.

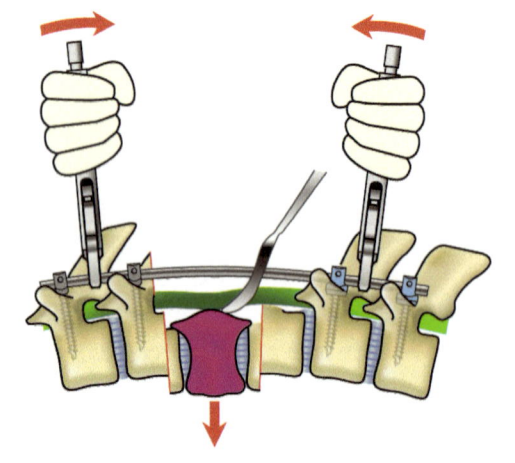

Fig. 40-9 Removal of the tumor with epidural extension. The vertebral bodies are pushed down for dissection to protect the spinal cord.

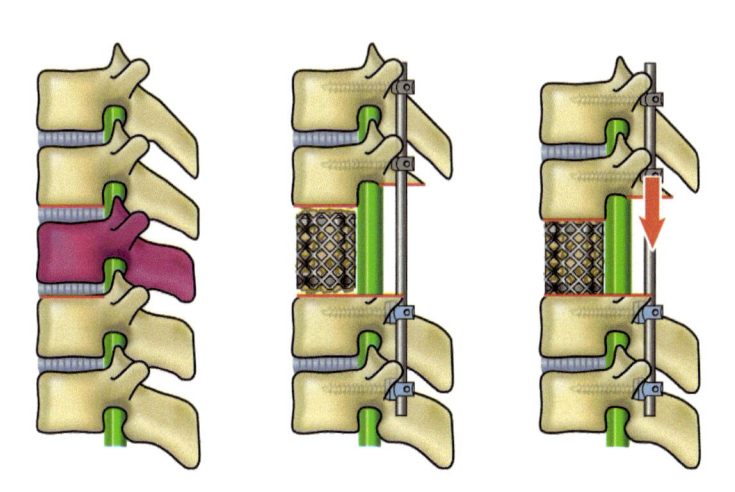

Fig. 40-10 Reconstruction (lateral view). The posterior instrumentation is adjusted to slightly compress the inserted vertebral spacer.

(Fig. 40-9). The freed anterior column is rotated around the spinal cord and carefully removed to avoid injury to the spinal cord. This procedure achieves complete anterior and posterior decompression of the spinal cord (circumferential decompression) and total en bloc resection of the vertebral tumor.

RECONSTRUCTION

A vertebral spacer, such as a titanium mesh cylinder cage with autograft or cement, is inserted precisely between the remaining healthy vertebrae.[30] After checking the appropriate position of the vertebral spacer by means of radiography, the posterior instrumentation is adjusted for slight (5 to 10 mm) compression of the inserted vertebral spacer (Fig. 40-10). Compression force should be applied to monoaxial screw heads for parallel shifting of the spinal column. This process offers three important advantages:
1. Enhanced stability of the anterior and posterior spinal column.
2. Anticipated earlier biological bony fusion.
3. Increased spinal cord blood flow, which is desirable for improving spinal cord function.[31]

If two or three vertebrae are resected, it is recommended that a connector device (artificial pedicle) be applied between the posterior rods and the anterior spacer (see case 2 in Signature Cases section, p. 730). Finally, the entire anterior and posterior reconstructed areas are covered with Marlex mesh to establish the compartment.

POSTOPERATIVE CARE AND REHABILITATION

Continuous suction is required for approximately 5 days, and perioperative intravenous antibiotics are continued until the drainage tubes are removed. Weight-bearing is allowed immediately after surgery. The patient wears an orthosis for 3 to 6 months until bony union has been established.

OUTCOMES WITH EVALUATION OF RESULTS

TES was performed in 182 patients between 1989 and 2009. Of these 182 patients, 129 had a metastatic tumor, 27 had a primary malignant tumor, and 26 had an aggressive benign tumor. The level of TES was thoracic in 118 patients and lumbar in 64. There were only two cases of neurologic deterioration after TES surgery. One patient had hyperesthesia immediately after the operation, which was attributed to distraction of the spinal cord due to a vertebral prosthesis that was too large. This patient recovered completely after immediate revision surgery to replace the vertebral prosthesis with a smaller one. In the other patient, paralysis occurred as a result of postoperative hematoma. After revision surgery, the paralysis improved to the same neurologic status as before TES. Five of the 118 patients undergoing thoracic TES had local recurrences, and the mean length of time to recurrence was 33 months. In all five patients, local recurrence was attributed to residual tumor tissue. In three patients the tumor extended further than expected into the adjacent level, and in the other two patients the tumor recurrence was from the dural area and was attributed to the epidural tumor extension.

SIGNATURE CASES

A 77-year-old woman with metastasis of renal cell carcinoma at T1 invading into the adjacent vertebrae above and below T1 (C7 and T2) was referred to our hospital (Fig. 40-11, *A*). She had undergone a nephrectomy for clear cell carcinoma of the left kidney 6 years earlier. She had mild neck pain and bilateral progressive muscle weakness of the lower extremities (grade C according to the Frankel classification of spinal cord

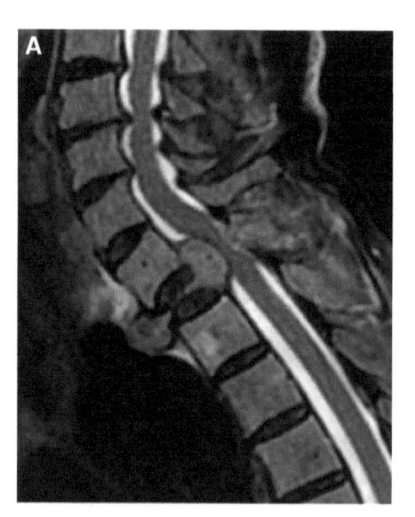

Fig. 40-11 **A,** Sagittal MRI scan at the cervicothoracic spine showing expansion of the epidural tumor in a craniocaudal direction from the T1 level.

injury). Embolization of feeding arteries to the tumor was undertaken 2 days before the surgery. TES of T1, including the lower half of C7 and the upper half of T2, was performed. During TES the left T1 nerve root was sacrificed because that nerve root was involved by the tumor (Figs. 40-11, *B* through *F*). Total operative time was 9 hours and 10 minutes, and the amount of bleeding was 1940 g. Muscle weakness of the bilateral lower extremities improved after TES. At follow-up (12 months after TES), she was classified as Frankel grade D.

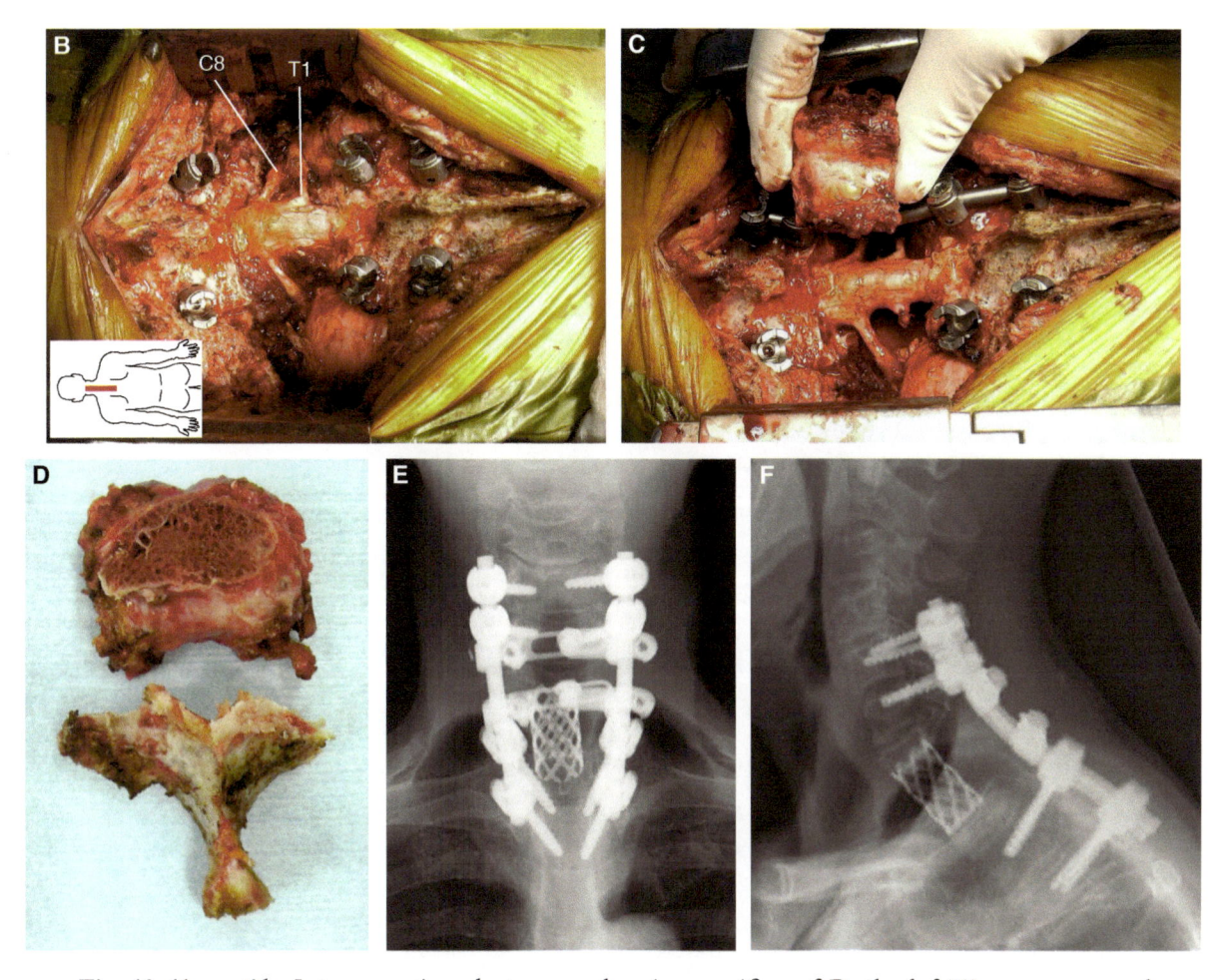

Fig. 40-11, cont'd Intraoperative photogram showing sacrifice of **B,** the left T1 nerve root and **C,** en bloc corpectomy. (*Inset* shows right C8 nerve root and T1 nerve root.) **D,** Axial view of resected T1 vertebral tumor. **E** and **F,** Postoperative radiographs after total en bloc spondylectomy.

A 47-year-old woman with metastasis of renal cell carcinoma at T10, invading into adjacent vertebrae above and below (T9 and T11), was referred to our hospital (Fig. 40-12, *A* and *B*). She had undergone a left nephrectomy 2½ years earlier. She had severe back pain without any paresis of the lower limbs (Frankel grade E). At angiography before TES, triple-level embolization (T9, T10, and T11) was performed. On the next day TES of T9, T10, and T11 was performed (Figs. 40-12, *C* through *J*). Total operative time was 9 hours and 20 minutes, and the amount of bleeding was 1340 g. She had no muscle weakness of the bilateral lower extremities after TES. Her Frankel grade remained E at follow-up (6 months after TES).

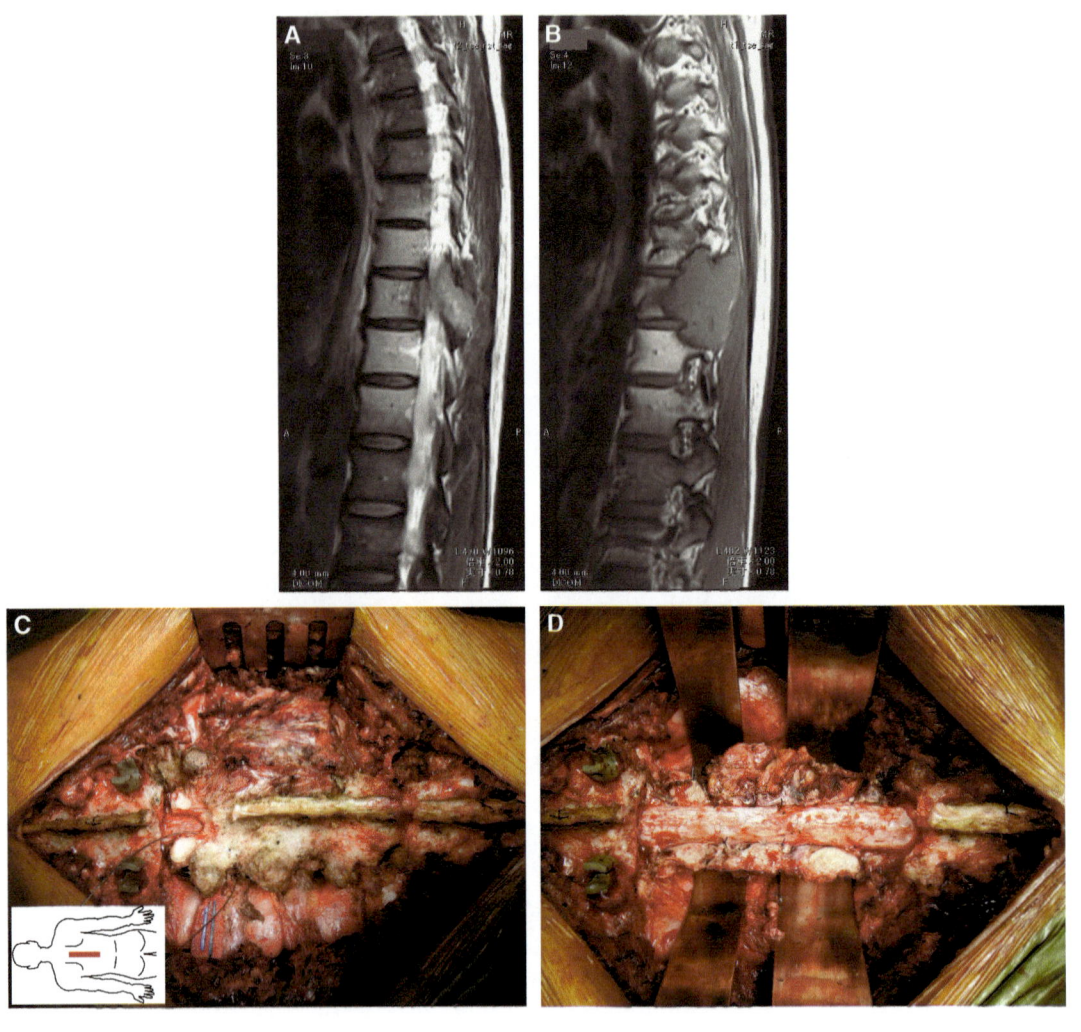

Fig. 40-12 **A** and **B,** Sagittal MRI scans of the thoracic spine. The T10 tumor has invaded in a craniocaudal direction adjacent to the vertebrae on the right side. Intraoperative photographs: **C,** T-saw was passed through the left intervertebral foramen at T9 for en bloc laminectomy. **D,** Spatulas were set for en bloc corpectomy after en bloc laminectomy of T9, 10, and 11.

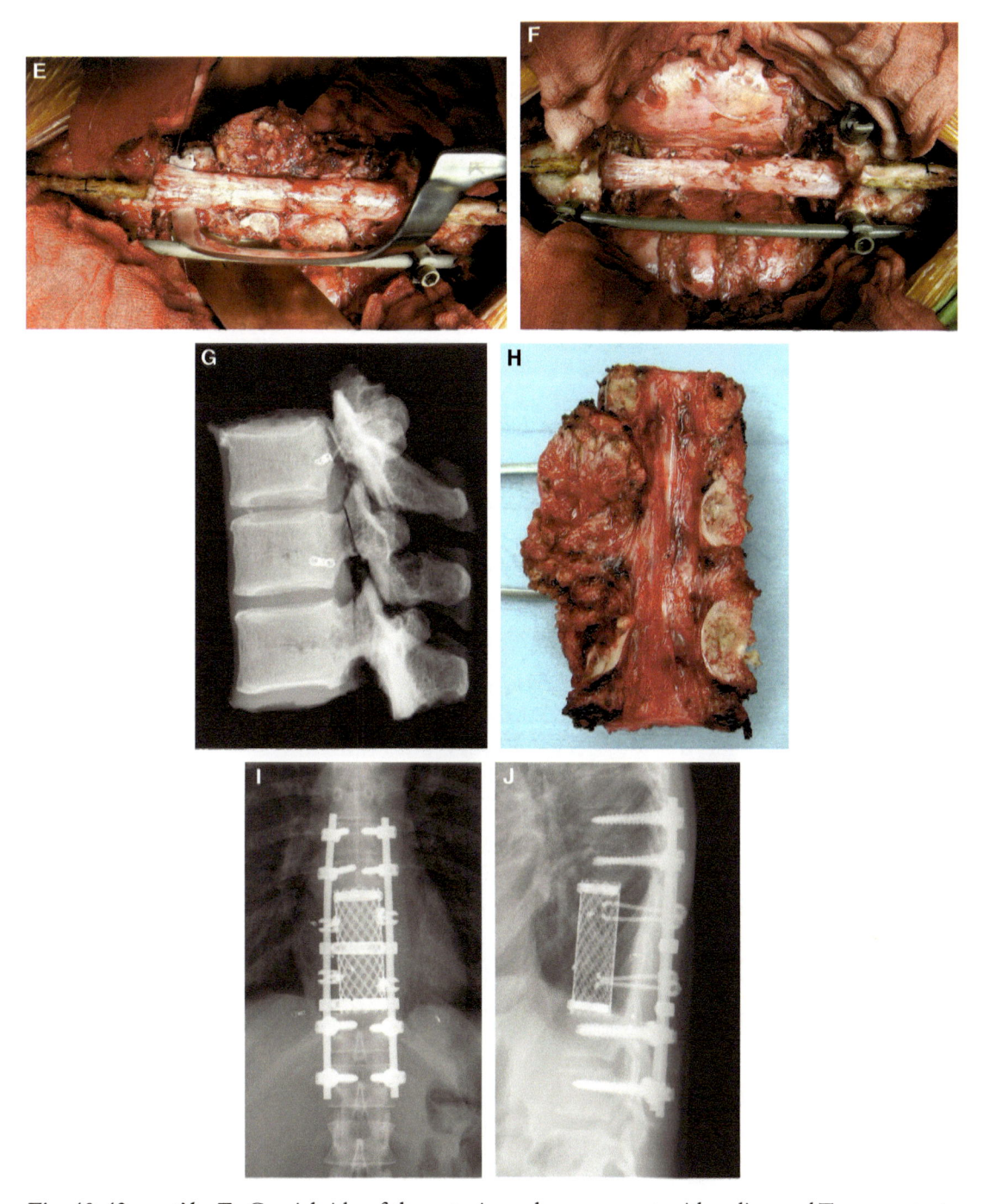

Fig. 40-12, cont'd **E,** Cranial side of the anterior column was cut with a diamond T-saw, protecting the spinal cord with a teeth-cord protector. **F,** En bloc corpectomy including three vertebrae. **G,** Lateral view radiograph of the resected specimens. **H,** Resected specimen of the T9, T10, and T11 vertebrae. **I,** Front and **J,** lateral postoperative radiographs after total en bloc spondylectomy. Two connector devices were placed.

CONCLUSION

The TES technique consists of two steps, including en bloc laminectomy and en bloc corpectomy, to salvage the spinal cord. In some cases the small part (the pedicle in most cases) becomes intralesional deliberately, but this must be confirmed to salvage the spinal cord. We believe that TES is the most radical method for treating malignant spine tumors, but offers the greatest potential for oncologic remission or curability in properly selected patients.

BAILOUT TECHNIQUE

If TES is not completed because of a serious problem such as massive bleeding or difficulty in dissecting around a tumor, the surgeon should perform decompression around the dura mater and stabilize the region to reduce a neurologic deficit and intractable pain. Radiation therapy to the remaining spine tumor can be initiated.

TIPS FROM THE MASTERS

- Preoperative embolization of bilateral segmental arteries at three levels should be attempted 72 hours before the operation.
- Ligation of segmental arteries up to three vertebral levels, even including the artery of Adamkiewicz, do not affect the spinal cord function.
- Usually the lateral aspect of the vertebral body is easily dissected with a "peanut" (cotton ball) and the surgeon's fingers.
- In cases where the spinal cord is severely compressed by the epidural tumor extension, the tumorous vertebral body is pushed down in a ventral direction from the dural tube after the anterior column is cut.
- Spinal shortening offers three important advantages: 1) enhanced stability, 2) earlier bony fusion, and 3) increased spinal cord blood flow.

References (With Key References in Boldface)

1. Roy-Camille R, Mazel CH, Saillant G, et al. Treatment of malignant tumor of the spine with posterior instrumentation. In Sundaresan N, Schmidek HH, Schiller AL, et al, eds. Tumor of the Spine. Philadelphia: WB Saunders, 1990, pp 473-487.
2. Roy-Camille R, Saillant G, Bisserie M, et al. Resection vertebrale totale dans la chirurgie tumorale au niveau du rachis dorsal par voie posterieure pure. Rev Chir Orthop 67:421-430, 1981.
3. Stener B. Total spondylectomy in chondrosarcoma arising from the seventh thoracic vertebra. J Bone Joint Surg Br 53:288-295, 1971.
4. Stener B. Complete removal of vertebrae for extirpation of tumors. Clin Orthop 245:72-82, 1989.

5. Stener B. Technique of complete spondylectomy in the thoracic and lumbar spine. In Sundaresan N, Schmidek HH, Schiller AL, et al, eds. Tumor of the Spine. Philadelphia: WB Saunders, 1990, pp 432-437.
6. Stener B, Johnsen OE. Complete removal of three vertebrae for giant cell tumour. J Bone Joint Surg Br 53:278-287, 1971.
7. Sundaresan N, Rosen G, Huvos AG, et al. Combined treatment of osteosarcoma of the spine. Neurosurgery 23:714-719, 1988.
8. Boriani S, Biagini R, De Iure F, et al. Vertebrectomia lombare per neoplasia ossea: tecnica chirurgica. Chir Organi Mov 79:163-173, 1994.
9. Boriani S, Chevalley F, Weinstein JN, et al. Chordoma of the spine above the sacrum. Treatment and outcome in 21 cases. Spine 21:1569-1577, 1996.
10. **Tomita K, Kawahara N, Baba H, et al. Total en bloc spondylectomy for solitary spinal metastasis. Int Orthop 18:291-298, 1994.**
11. Tomita K, Kawahara N, Baba H, et al. Total en bloc spondylectomy. A new surgical technique for primary malignant vertebral tumors. Spine 22:324-333, 1997.
12. Kawahara N, Tomita K, Fujita T, et al. Osteosarcoma of the thoracolumbar spine. Total en bloc spondylectomy. A case report. J Bone Joint Surg Am 79:453-458, 1997.
13. Kawahara N, Tomita K, Murakami H, et al. Total en bloc spondylectomy for spinal metastases. In Jasmin C, Coleman RE, Coia LR, et al, eds. The Textbook of Bone Metastases. Chichester, West Sussex, England: John Wiley & Sons, 2005, pp 215-223.
14. Kawahara N, Tomita K, Tsuchiya H. Total en bloc spondylectomy: a new surgical technique for malignant vertebral tumors. In Watkins RG, ed. Surgical Approach to the Spine, 2nd ed. New York, Springer-Verlag, 2003, pp 309-325.
15. Murakami H, Kawahara N, Abdel-Wanis ME, et al. Total en bloc spondylectomy. Semin Musculoskelet Radiol 5:189-194, 2001.
16. Tomita K, Toribatake Y, Kawahara N, et al. Total en bloc spondylectomy and circumspinal decompression for solitary spinal metastasis. Paraplegia 32:36-46, 1994.
17. Fujita T, Ueda Y, Kawahara N, et al. Local spread of metastatic vertebral tumors. A histologic study. Spine 22:1905-1912, 1997.
18. **Tomita K, Kawahara N, Murakami H, et al. Total en bloc spondylectomy for spinal tumors: improvement of the technique and its associated basic background. J Orthop Sci 11:3-12, 2006.**
19. **Kawahara N, Tomita K, Murakami H, et al. Total en bloc spondylectomy for spinal tumors: surgical techniques and related basic background. Orthop Clin North Am 40:47-63, 2009.**
20. Tomita K, Kawahara K, Kobayashi T, et al. Surgical strategy for spinal metastases. Spine 26:298-306, 2001.
21. Oken MM, Creech RH, Tormey DC, et al. Toxicity and response criteria of the Eastern Cooperative Oncology Group. Am J Clin Oncol 5:649-655, 1982.
22. Karnofsky DA, Burchenal JH. The clinical evaluation of chemotherapeutic agents in cancer. In MacLeod CM, ed. Evaluation of Chemotherapeutic Agents. New York: Columbia University Press, 1949, p 19.
23. Fujimaki Y, Kawahara N, Tomita K, et al. How many ligations of bilateral segmental arteries cause ischemic spinal cord dysfunction? An experimental study using a dog model. Spine (Phila Pa 1976) 31:E781-E789, 2006.
24. Numbu K, Kawahara N, Murakami H, et al. Interruption of bilateral segmental arteries at several levels. Influence on vertebral blood flow. Spine 29:1530-1534, 2004.
25. Ueda Y, Kawahara N, Tomita K, et al. Influence on spinal cord blood flow and spinal cord function by interruption of bilateral segmental arteries at up to three levels: experimental study in dogs. Spine 30:2239-2243, 2005.
26. Kawahara N, Tomita K, Baba H, et al. Cadaveric vascular anatomy for total en bloc spondylectomy in malignant vertebral tumors. Spine (Phila Pa 1976) 21:1401-1407, 1996.

27. Tomita K, Kawahara N. The threadwire saw: a new device for cutting bone. J Bone Joint Surg Am 78:1915-1917, 1996.
28. Abdel-Wanis ME, Tsuchiya H, Kawahara N, et al. Tumor growth potential after tumoral and instrumental contamination: an in-vivo comparative study of T-saw, Gigli saw, and scalpel. J Orthop Sci 6:424-429, 2001.
29. Kato S, Kawahara N, Tomita K, et al. Effects on spinal cord blood flow and neurologic function secondary to interruption of bilateral segmental arteries which supply the artery of Adamkiewicz: an experimental study using a dog model. Spine 33:1533-1541, 2008.
30. Akamaru T, Kawahara N, Sakamoto J, et al. The transmission of stress to grafted bone inside a titanium mesh cage used in anterior column reconstruction after total spondylectomy: a finite element analysis. Spine 30:2783-2787, 2005.
31. Kawahara N, Tomita K, Kobayashi T, et al. Influence of acute shortening on the spinal cord: an experimental study. Spine (Phila Pa 1976) 30:613-620, 2005.

Chapter 41

En Bloc Spondylectomy: Two-Stage Thoracic/Lumbar Spine

Dean Chou, Wali E. Danish

The treatment of cancers affecting the spine continues to evolve, with total en bloc spondylectomy being used more frequently. Historically laminectomies were performed for metastatic disease in an attempt to excise the tumor. It is now known that this method led to poor outcomes, resulting in a decreased role for this surgical technique.[1] Piecemeal excision of tumors also produced better results than laminectomies, but local recurrences remained a problem. Adjuvant therapy remains a critical component of management after piecemeal resection of tumors.[2]

Numerous studies reported that total en bloc spondylectomy subsequently improved results by reducing local recurrences.[1-3] Total en bloc spondylectomy differs from piecemeal spondylectomy in that the whole vertebra, body, and lamina are removed in two large pieces instead of many small pieces.[2] In total en bloc spondylectomy there is no communication between the remaining parts of the vertebral column because the entire affected vertebra is removed. Although the procedure is challenging, it is also versatile in that it allows en bloc resections of multiple levels, even at junctional levels.[4]

INDICATIONS AND CONTRAINDICATIONS

The oncologic value of this procedure is strongly evidenced by studies that show improvements in survival for both metastatic and primary malignant tumors.[1] Aggressive surgical resection has been found to be safe and effective, with good functional outcomes and improved quality of life.[1] In slow-growing malignant tumors, such as chordoma of the mobile spine (C2-L5), local control is better with en bloc resection at 5 years after surgery.[5] En bloc resection is also useful for other types of tumors. In cases of aggressive osteoblastoma (>4 cm), the high recurrence rate (>50%) warrants a more aggressive approach than the standard curettage previously used for conventional osteoblastomas.[6] En bloc resection may be useful in these cases.

The main indication for en bloc spondylectomy is resection of primary malignant tumors. Another relative indication for en bloc spondylectomy is isolated metastatic disease in patients who are otherwise healthy. Although the findings are not conclusive, there is some evidence to suggest that spondylectomy in such patients improves local control over piecemeal resection.[1] Because of the significant blood loss and lengthy operative time associated with en bloc spondylectomy, one contraindication is a patient's ability to tolerate this procedure. Total en bloc spondylectomy should not be performed in patients who are frail, elderly, or extremely ill.

Although en bloc spondylectomy can be performed in a single stage, it is technically formidable to accomplish. This procedure can also be done in two stages, which we describe herein.

PREOPERATIVE EVALUATION

Physical examination should include a thorough neurologic examination and documentation. The spine should also be evaluated for protuberances indicating kyphosis or paraspinal muscle invasion of the tumor.

Diagnostic studies should include magnetic resonance imaging (MRI) with contrast enhancement to identify tumor invasion, computed tomography (CT) to evaluate bone destruction, and standing anteroposterior and lateral radiographs to assess spinal alignment with gravity.

CLINICAL DECISION-MAKING

Treatment decisions should be carefully weighed, depending on pathologic findings (Table 41-1). For instance, biopsies of primary tumors should first be performed to confirm the diagnosis. If the diagnosis is primary malignant tumor, such as a chordoma, then detailed planning for a spondylectomy should be undertaken. Wide margins and no tumor violation should be the goals of the surgery, and an en bloc spondylectomy, if feasible, would be appropriate.

Table 41-1 **Treatment Decisions**

Primary malignant tumor	En bloc spondylectomy
Single isolated metastatic disease in a healthy patient	Consider en bloc spondylectomy
Diffuse metastatic disease, poor health, poor prognosis, invasive tumor with soft tissue and facet invasion	No spondylectomy

If the patient has an isolated metastasis, is healthy, and opts for aggressive management of the cancer, a spondylectomy can be considered. Some data suggest that spondylectomy may be more beneficial than piecemeal resection under these circumstances, but these data are far from conclusive.[1] However, for patients who have diffuse metastatic disease, a poor prognosis, or other major medical comorbidity, a spondylectomy would serve no purpose. In addition, the metastatic lesion should be relatively contained within the bony elements. If there is diffuse destruction, significant bone and soft tissue invasion to the point where a good margin cannot be obtained and tumor spillage would be inevitable, spondylectomy is not likely not have any advantage over piecemeal resection.

TECHNIQUE

The patient is positioned prone on a standard Jackson table, and the level of interest is identified with fluoroscopy. This is correlated with the results of MRI, and the level is checked and rechecked several times. A standard posterior spinal exposure is employed and, depending on bone quality, either two or three levels are exposed above and below the lesion. If the patient's bone quality is questionable, we instrument three levels above and below the lesion. If the bone quality is good, we instrument only two levels above and below. After a standard exposure is achieved, an intraoperative radiograph is obtained to confirm the level of interest. We routinely obtain two intraoperative radiographs for confirmation, and we place a marker on the pedicle or transverse process rather than on the interspinous space or spinous process. Pedicle screws are placed above and below the level of interest, except at the level just caudal to the spondylectomy site (Fig. 41-1, *A*). The screw hole is cannulated at this level, but the screw is not placed until later, because the screw head will interfere with the spondylectomy.

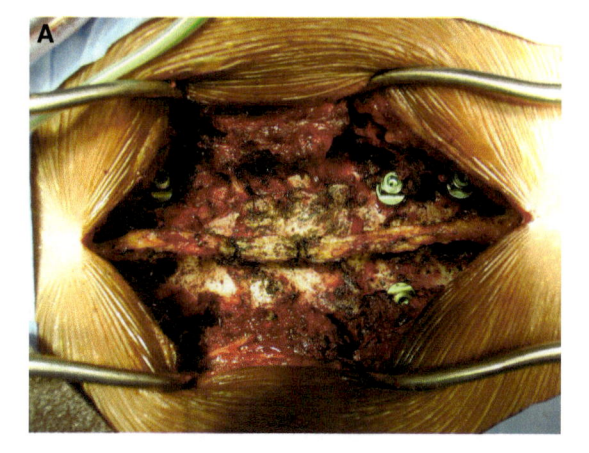

Fig. 41-1 **A,** Pedicle screws are placed above and below the level of interest, except at the level just caudal to the spondylectomy site.

The dissection is carried out all the way lateral to the transverse processes. Partial laminectomies are performed above and below the level of interest. Extreme care is taken not to violate any of the posterior elements of the level of interest. The facet joints are destroyed by means of electrocautery. The inferior articular process of the level above and the superior articular process of the level below are removed (Fig. 41-1, *B*). Again extreme care is taken not to violate any of the articular processes of the level of interest.

The pedicle screws in the immediate caudal vertebral body can now be placed once the facetectomies have been carried out. With the use of either a small osteotome or a wire saw, the pedicles on both sides are amputated (Fig. 41-1 *C*). This permits the entire posterior portion of the vertebra to be removed en bloc (Fig. 41-1, *D*), allowing direct visualization of the posterior aspect of the vertebral body, thecal sac, and nerve roots (note the incidental dural repair sutures placed by the senior author [D.C.]) (Fig. 41-1, *E*).

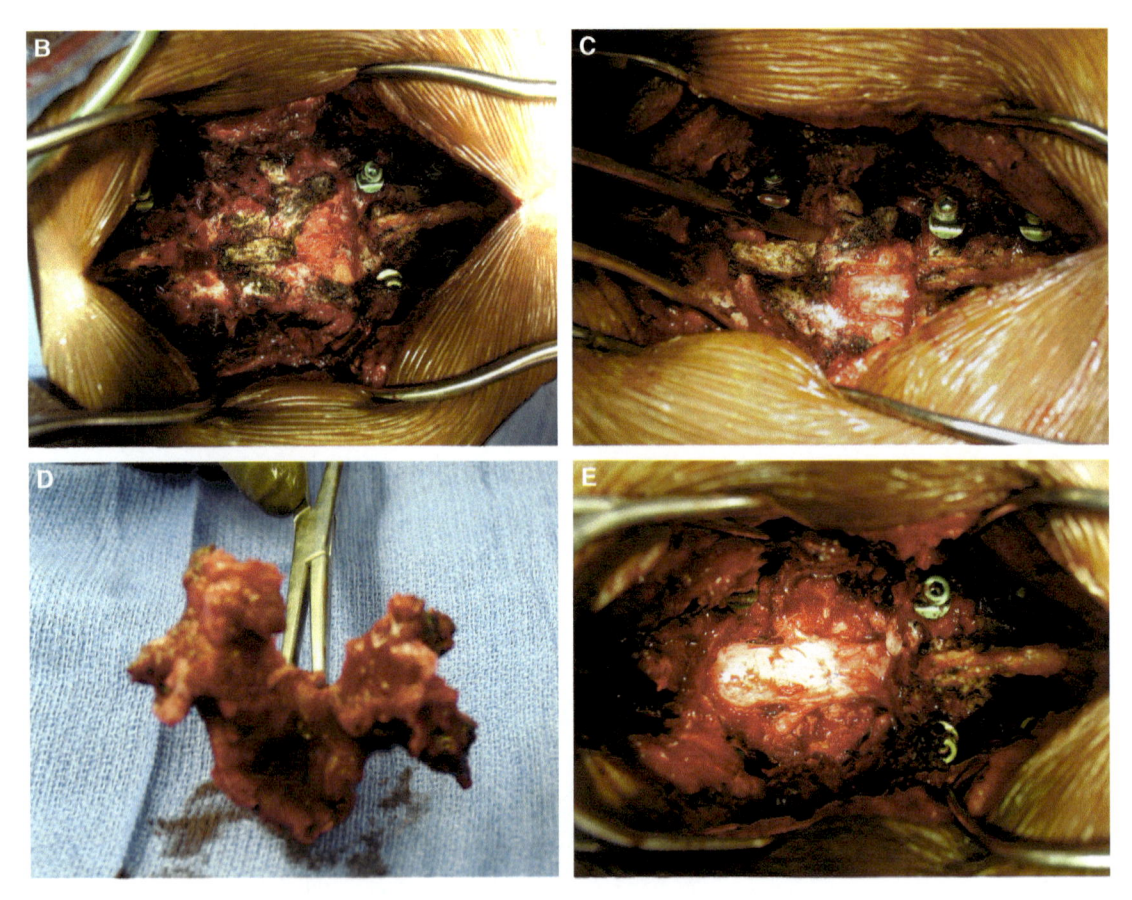

Fig. 41-1, cont'd **B,** The inferior articular process of the level above and the superior articular process of the level below are removed. With the use of either a small osteotome or a wire saw, the pedicles on both sides are **C,** amputated to allow the entire posterior portion of the vertebra to be **D,** removed en bloc and provides **E,** a view of the posterior aspect of the vertebral body, thecal sac, and nerve roots.

Because anterior resection of the vertebral body would be a left-sided approach, it is critical to release the contralateral side as much as possible from the posterior approach. Thus in this case we first ligated the right T12 nerve root. This allowed us access into the right lateral aspect of the vertebral body, which permitted us to disarticulate the rib, ligate the right segmental vessel (using bipolar cautery), dissect soft tissue, such as the crus of the diaphragm, off the vertebral body, and remove the discs. Because there is no view of the right side from a left-sided anterior approach, it is critical to perform as much dissection as possible of the right side during the posterior approach (Fig. 41-1, *F*). The posterior rods and cross-links are then placed (Fig. 41-1, *G*). A silicone rubber sheet is placed between the neural elements and the vertebral body, both for identification of the neural elements and to prevent scarring between the vertebral body and the dura (see Fig. 41-1, *G*).

After the posterior stage is completed, the standard anterior-retroperitoneal approach is performed. A confirmatory radiograph is obtained to identify the proper level. The psoas and crus muscles are dissected off laterally, and the segmental arteries are ligated. The discs above and below are completely removed, and the anterior longitudinal ligament is divided at both levels of the discs (Fig. 41-1, *H*). Extreme care is taken to protect the aorta and vena cava. Blunt dissection is performed to push these ventrally, and a saline-soaked sponge can be placed over them to protect them against inadvertent maneuvers of the spine tools. Once the vertebral body is free, it is gently rotated ventrally. It can then be lifted out of the body en bloc (Fig. 41-1, *I*). Posterior and anterior spinal elements placed together, demonstrating en bloc removal of spinal segments, are shown in Fig. 41-1, *J*. The anterior spinal column is then reconstructed, and the patient is mobilized as soon as possible.

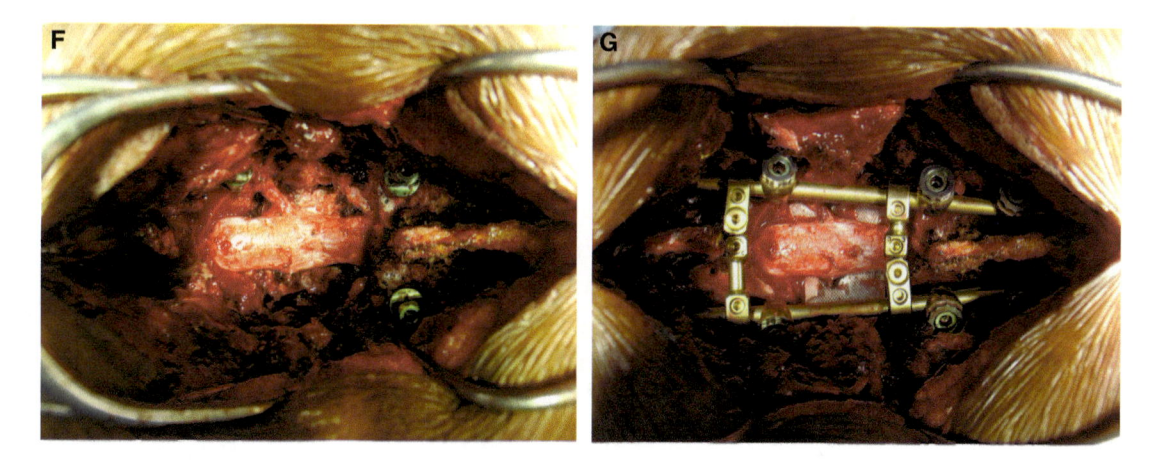

Fig. 41-1, cont'd **F,** It is critical to perform as much dissection as possible of the right side during the posterior approach. **G,** The posterior rods and crosslinks are then placed, and a silicone rubber sheet is placed between the neural elements and the vertebral body, both for identification of the neural elements and to prevent scarring between the vertebral body and the dura.

Continued

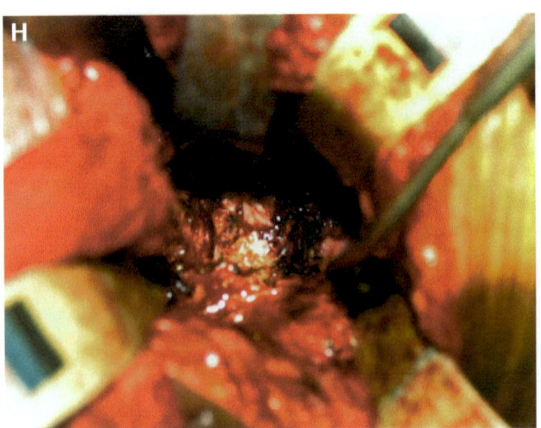

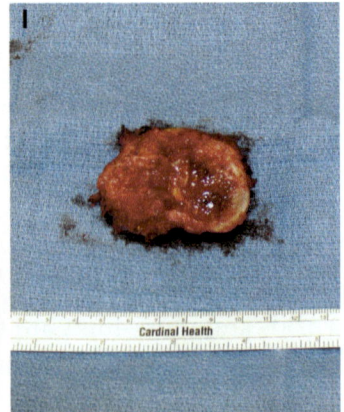

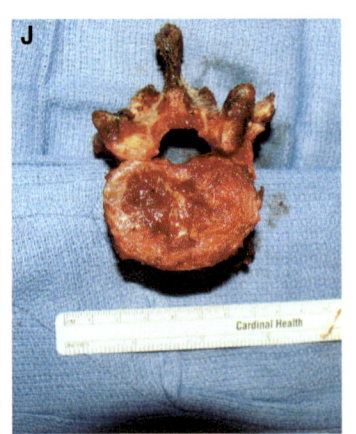

Fig. 41-1, cont'd **H,** The discs above and below are completely removed, and the anterior longitudinal ligament is divided at both levels of the discs. **I,** Once the vertebral body is free, it can then be lifted out of the body en bloc. **J,** Posterior and anterior spinal elements are placed together to demonstrate en bloc removal of the spinal segment.

OUTCOMES WITH EVALUATION OF RESULTS

En bloc spondylectomy with wide margins has proved to be a mainstay of increasing disease-free survival in malignant primary tumors of the mobile spine. In a combined retrospective and prospective evaluation of the treatments used to manage chordomas, en bloc resection has a considerably longer duration of disease-free survival compared with piecemeal resection.[5] The techniques used historically include radiation therapy with or without palliative surgery and intralesional excision with or without adjuvant therapy. A total of 100% of patients had a recurrence 18 to 20 months after radiation alone, palliative treatment, or intralesional intracapsular excision.[5] Seventy-five percent of patients had a recurrence 30 months, on average, after extracapsular excision and radiation, 50% had a recurrence 51 months after en bloc resection with inadequate margins and radiation, and only 20% had a recurrence 56 to 94 months after en bloc resection with appropriate margins.[5]

In addition to the improved chance of disease-free survival, preservation of functionality after en bloc resection further demonstrates the advantages of this technique, because patients undergoing en bloc resection have a better quality of life and are general free of spinal pain.[5] En bloc resection is not always indicated; for example, in recurrent or contaminated tumors, operations that only allow intralesional margins, and in some operations of the cervical spine where margins are mostly intralesional.[5] In these cases a careful risk-benefit analysis must be made. Complications of this surgical technique include problems with the instrumentation used in reconstruction and stabilization of the spine, as well as complications associated with surgery and anesthesia, which are always risks in such invasive procedures.

SIGNATURE CASE

A 55-year-old man with a known history of renal cell carcinoma, who had undergone a left nephrectomy, was seen by his urologist with evidence of a recurrence in the tumor resection bed. MRI indicated that he also had a lesion at T12 (Fig. 41-2, *A* through *C*).

Given that these were his only sites of disease and he was highly functional, he chose an aggressive approach to treatment. Thus a T12 spondylectomy was planned during resection of the lymph mode metastases. This was planned in two stages. The first stage would be a posterior stabilization: en bloc removal of the posterior elements and then dissection of the thecal sac and removal of the discs. The second stage would be an anterior approach, with en bloc removal of the vertebral body.

One year after surgery, the patient remains neurologically intact and working. He has had brain metastases during the intervening year, and these have been treated. The 1-year postoperative radiographs shown in Fig. 41-2, *D* and *E*, show the final construct.

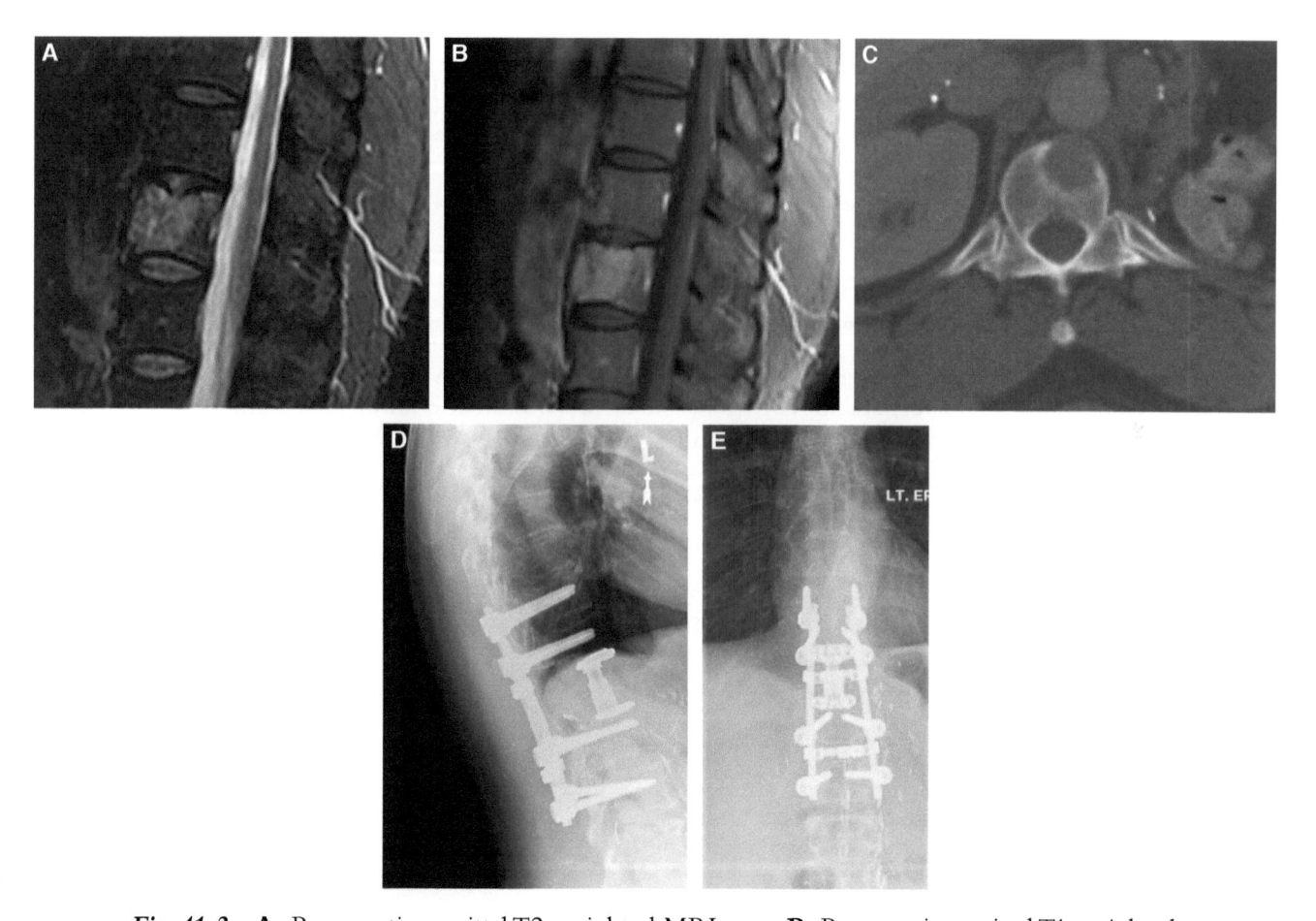

Fig. 41-2 **A,** Preoperative sagittal T2-weighted MRI scan. **B,** Preoperative sagittal T1-weighted MRI scan with gadolinium enhancement. **C,** Axial CT scan demonstrating bony destruction from the tumor. **D** and **E,** One-year postoperative radiographs.

CONCLUSION

En bloc spondylectomy should be performed for primary malignant tumors if a margin can be obtained. Meticulous preoperative planning should be performed. In selected cases spondylectomy can be performed for isolated metastatic lesions, but these must be considered very carefully because of the morbidity associated with spondylectomy.

BAILOUT TECHNIQUES

- When performing an osteotomy posteriorly, we find a ¼ inch curved osteotome to be most useful. If available, a T-saw (Medtronic, Memphis, TN) can also be used to remove the pedicle. Many times, when the osteotome is used, cuts must be made from cephalad, caudad, lateral to medial, and medial to lateral. It is important to make sure that a sharp osteotome is used and the dura is protected with a Penfield retractor.
- One problem that may arise is when the vertebral body cannot be easily removed en bloc. Usually it is the contralateral corners of the discs and annulus that hold it in place. A small Kerrison rongeur inserted into the disc space can be used to release the contralateral corner. If the posterior longitudinal ligament has not been completely cut, this can also be removed with a small Kerrison rongeur. The anterior longitudinal ligament must be fully released, and once this can be accomplished with a Kerrison rongeur.

TIPS FROM THE MASTERS

- Dissect as much as possible from the posterior approach before performing the anterior approach, especially contralateral to the side of the anterior approach.
- Remove as much of the corners of the discs and the ligamentous structures as possible; that is where the biggest anchor points will be.
- Consider the two-staged approach in the lumbar spine where the nerve roots cannot be sacrificed, but consider the single-staged approach in the thoracic spine if possible.
- Remove as much of the discs and posterior longitudinal ligament as possible from the posterior approach.
- When performing the posterior approach, consider the anterior view that you will have; use the posterior approach to dissect contralateral to your view.

References (With Key References in Boldface)

1. **Boriani S, Bandiera S, Biagini R, et al. Chordoma of the mobile spine: fifty years of experience. Spine (Phila Pa 1976) 31:493-503, 2006.**
2. Chou D, Wang V. Two-level en bloc spondylectomy for osteosarcoma at the cervicothoracic junction. J Clin Neurosci 16:698-700, 2009.
3. **Ibrahim A, Crockard A, Antonietti P, et al. Does spinal surgery improve the quality of life for those with extradural (spinal) osseous metastases? An international multicenter prospective observational study of 223 patients. Invited submission from the Joint Section Meeting on Disorders of the Spine and Peripheral Nerves, March 2007. J Neurosurg Spine 8:271-278, 2008.**
4. **Kawahara N, Tomita K, Murakami H, et al. Total en bloc spondylectomy for spinal tumors: surgical techniques and related basic background. Orthop Clin North Am 40:47-63, vi, 2009.**
5. Nishida K, Doita M, Kawahara N, et al. Total en bloc spondylectomy in the treatment of aggressive osteoblastoma of the thoracic spine. Orthopedics 31:403, 2008.
6. Tomita K, Kawahara N, Baba H, et al. Total en bloc spondylectomy. A new surgical technique for primary malignant vertebral tumors. Spine (Phila Pa 1976) 22:324-333, 1997.

Chapter 42

Transpedicular Approach for Anterior Decompression and Reconstruction

Sassan Keshavarzi, Dzenan Lulic, Henry E. Aryan

The spine is an extremely common site for metastasis, occuring in nearly 40% of cancer patients; with 5% to 10% of all cancer patients diagnosed with spinal metastasis.[1-7] In a series of 832 autopsies from patients who died of cancer, presented by Wong et al,[8] 36% had some evidence of spinal metastases. Currently 5% to 10% of cancer patients and 40% of patients with previous nonspinal bone metastases have spinal cord compression from epidural metastases.[4,8-12] Of patients with metastatic disease to the boney spine, 10% to 20% become symptomatic as a result of spinal cord compression.[11,13,14] Metastases from the prostate, breast, and lung make up 50% of all metastases to the spine and commonly cause spinal metastases in 90.5%, 74.3%, and 44.9%, respectively.[3-5,8,10,15-17] With advances in modern systemic therapy, more patients with spinal metastasis will present with symptomatic disease that warrants surgical intervention.

In the past, data did not always corroborate the need for surgical intervention. However, over the past decade our thinking has changed dramatically. Patchell et al[18] demonstrated that patients with spinal metastases presenting with neurologic deficits performed better (with respect to preservation and improvement of neurologic function) after undergoing surgery and radiation, as opposed to radiation alone. In large part this has come about because of advances in surgical techniques and technology, which has allowed improved decompression and stabilization. Surgeons attempting to resect spine tumors have a variety of options in terms of approaches that can be used.[3-5,19] The choice of approach will be dictated by the location of the tumor, the number of levels involved, the need for total excision, desired methods of resection and reconstruction, and the medical condition of each patient.[3,4,20] Anterior, posterior, anterolateral, posterolateral (including lateral extracavitary), combined anterior and posterior, staged anterior and posterior, and minimally invasive approaches have all been described.[3,16,21-23]

Corpectomy is one popular technique that provides exposure of the anterior spinal column, to facilitate treatment of disease spanning multiple levels or extending behind the posterior vertebral body, or treatment of vertebral body deformities.[22,24-26] Multilevel corpectomy can provide exposure of multiple levels of the spine to aid in resection of large tumors, but the morbidity associated with anterior approaches traditionally employed to achieve corpectomy is a concern.[19-21,24,27] Alternatively, the lateral extracavitary approach with corpectomy allows exquisite spinal exposure while avoiding the morbidity of anterior approaches, but few operations that use multilevel lateral extracavitary corpectomy have been described.[19,20,27]

Surgical techniques have markedly improved over the past couple of years, particularly with improvements in instrumentation and the introduction of expandable vertebral body cages, and have reduced the morbidity associated with surgical resection and stabilization. The upper limit of what can be done, from a technical standpoint, has expanded. This poses the dilemma of not whether certain surgery can be done but whether certain types of surgery *should* be performed, and whether such extensive surgery does, in fact, improve quality of life.

INDICATIONS AND CONTRAINDICATIONS

Although many factors influence our surgical planning, the management strategy for metastatic disease has three components: chemotherapy, surgery, and radiation. How we employ and combine these modalities has significantly changed over the past two decades. A number of previous studies proposed that laminectomy with adjuvant radiation therapy was no more effective than radiation alone in restoring or maintaining neurologic function.[28-35] Instead, such surgery was associated with infection and worsening of preexisting spinal instability. Based on these data, radiation was the initial treatment strategy employed by most physicians. However, spine surgery has come a long way over the past two decades, and this approach certainly no longer holds, especially for radiation-resistant tumors. Surgical intervention is directed at local disease control, decompression of neural elements, mechanical stabilization, and pain control. Common sites of metastases to the spine are the vertebral column (85%), the paravertebral region (10% to 15%), and rarely the epidural or subarachnoid/intramedullary space (<5%).[10,11,33] In 70% of spinal metastases the metastatic emboli seed the vertebral body, causing ventral spinal cord compression, thereby making significant decompression by means of laminectomy alone very unlikely. Laminectomy and posterior decompression without fusion often further destabilizes the spine in patients with an anterior column that is prone to instability and compression fractures. Thus it comes as no surprise that surgical intervention limited to a laminectomy does not contribute significantly to patient outcome. Surgical intervention has come to play a significant role because we have the ability to perform 360-degree decompression and stabilization, and to address the anterior column, which is most commonly affected by disease.

For those patients whose prognosis from a systemic standpoint is greater than 3 months, with a neurologic deficit (or impending neurologic deficit) caused by spinal metastasis, and whose medical condition would allow them to tolerate surgery, surgical stabilization may offer the best chance at preserving neurologic function. In selecting a treatment strategy, life expectancy is a significant factor, but other considerations include tumor radiosensitivity, previous failure of radiation therapy, stabilization, deformity, intractable pain, patient wishes, and status of systemic disease. Surgical planning is multifactorial and caters to each patient individually. Many surgeons use the scoring system of Tokuhashi et al[36] to determine patient survival, and also in an effort to standardize management strategy. This scoring system takes into consideration the Karnofsky score, number of extraspinal bone metastases, number of metastases in the spine, metastases to major internal organs, primary site of cancer, and myelopathy. Those patients with scores ≥5 generally die within 3 months, and those with scores ≥9 live for 12 months or more, on average.

PREOPERATIVE EVALUATION

- A history should be obtained to denote any signs of weakness, difficulty with ambulation, back pain, changes and difficulty with bowel or bladder habits, and an accurate time line of the patient's signs and symptoms.
- Standing plain radiographs should be obtained to evaluate sagittal balance and any deformity, especially acute kyphosis from compression fractures at the level with metastatic invasion.
- CT imaging to evaluate the integrity of the bony elements and their destruction by the tumor.
- MRI to evaluate the extent of spinal cord compression and signal changes in the spinal cord.
- MRI with contrast enhancement to define the location of the tumor dorsal/ventral and its circumferential compression of the spinal cord.
- Staging of primary disease should be performed. This should include imaging for distant systemic disease, generally by PET scan.
- In those patients who do not have a diagnosis of a primary lesion, a biopsy should be considered, because knowledge of the diagnosis and the radiosensitivity and chemosensitivity of tumors will influence surgical planning and the need for en bloc resection.
- Once the mass has been diagnosed, depending on the tumor, embolization should be considered to minimize intraoperative bleeding.

CLINICAL DECISION-MAKING
Treatment Decisions

Although surgical intervention is one of a number of options for treating metastatic disease, the following indications mandate surgical intervention:
- Acute neurologic deterioration secondary to compression of neural elements by the tumor or by advancing deformity
- Significant pain secondary to advancing deformity and the need for stabilization
- Extensive bone involvement and impending fracture
- Tumors resistant to chemotherapy and radiation

Choice of Technique

Surgical options include one of the following options:
- Dorsal decompression only, such as a laminectomy (because of poor results, this is not recommended/has been abandoned)
- Dorsal decompression and posterior instrumented stabilization, such as laminectomy and pedicle screw fixation
- Ventral decompression along with a purely ventral reconstruction:
  - Transthoracic corpectomy
  - Retroperitoneal corpectomy
  - Extreme lateral corpectomy
  - Dorsal decompression and 360-degree reconstruction through a completely posterior transpedicular approach

TECHNIQUE

The nature of these surgeries (extensive blood loss, risk of injury to neurovascular structures, and need for the patient to be in the prone position for 3 to 8 hours) make good and early communication between the surgical team and the anesthesia team paramount. Even before the operating room briefing or the induction of anesthesia, there should be a discussion regarding the need for antibiotics, the anesthetic needs to allow for neurophysiologic monitoring, the patient's risk of developing intraoperative coagulopathy, the possible need for transfusion, and the need to have the patient typed and crossmatched for blood.

After the patient has been placed under general anesthesia, arterial and central lines are often placed, antibiotics administered, and neuromonitoring electrodes placed. A set of somatosensory evoked potentials (SSEP) and motor evoked potentials (MEP) should be obtained both before and after positioning the patient. The patient should be positioned prone on an open-frame operating table. The open frame often takes pressure off of the abdomen, allowing better venous drainage and minimizing bleeding from epidural venous congestion. The open frame also allows the spine to reduce to its natural sagittal balance and lumbar lordosis, which is the ideal position for instrumentation and fixation of the spine. Because many times there is a need for multiple intraoperative radiographs, the use of a radiolucent operating table is very helpful.

The patient is prepared and draped, an incision is made, and the tissue dissection is performed exposing the appropriate levels. Exposure includes lateral masses in the cervical spine and the transverse processes in the lumbar spine, in addition to spinous processes and lamina. If the involved level is at the thoracic spine, the rib heads also need to be exposed at the level of the transpedicular resection. All of the appropriate levels should be instrumented with lateral mass screws or pedicle screws before tumor resection, because resection often further destabilizes the spine. A temporary stabilizing rod placed on the side contralateral to the surgical resection is very helpful and prevents intraoperative instability. It also prevents any translation that may injure neural elements.

Placement of the instrumentation before exposure of the neural elements with a laminectomy prevents inadvertent injury to the spinal cord during screw instrumentation. Screw stimulation electromyography (EMG) can be used to assess for pedicle wall breach and any nerve root injury in the lumbar spine. At the level of the vertebrectomy, begin by removing the spinous process and lamina (Fig. 42-1, *A* and *B*). Then proceed to remove the rib head and the transverse process that articulates at these levels (Fig. 42-1, *C* through *F*). The next step is to perform bilateral complete facetectomies by removing both the superior and inferior articulating facets at each level (Fig. 42-1, *G*). The nerve roots and pedicles should be easily visualized. Often nerve roots can be sacrificed in the thoracic spine, which makes the remaining portion of the osteotomy and reconstruction simpler. The pedicles can be drilled down to their junction with the vertebral body (Fig. 42-1, *H* and *I*).

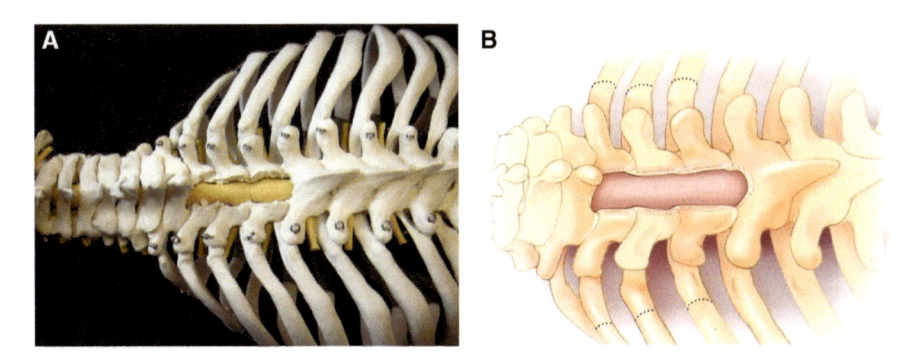

Fig. 42-1   **A** and **B,** At the level of the vertebrectomy, the spinous process and lamina are removed.

Continued

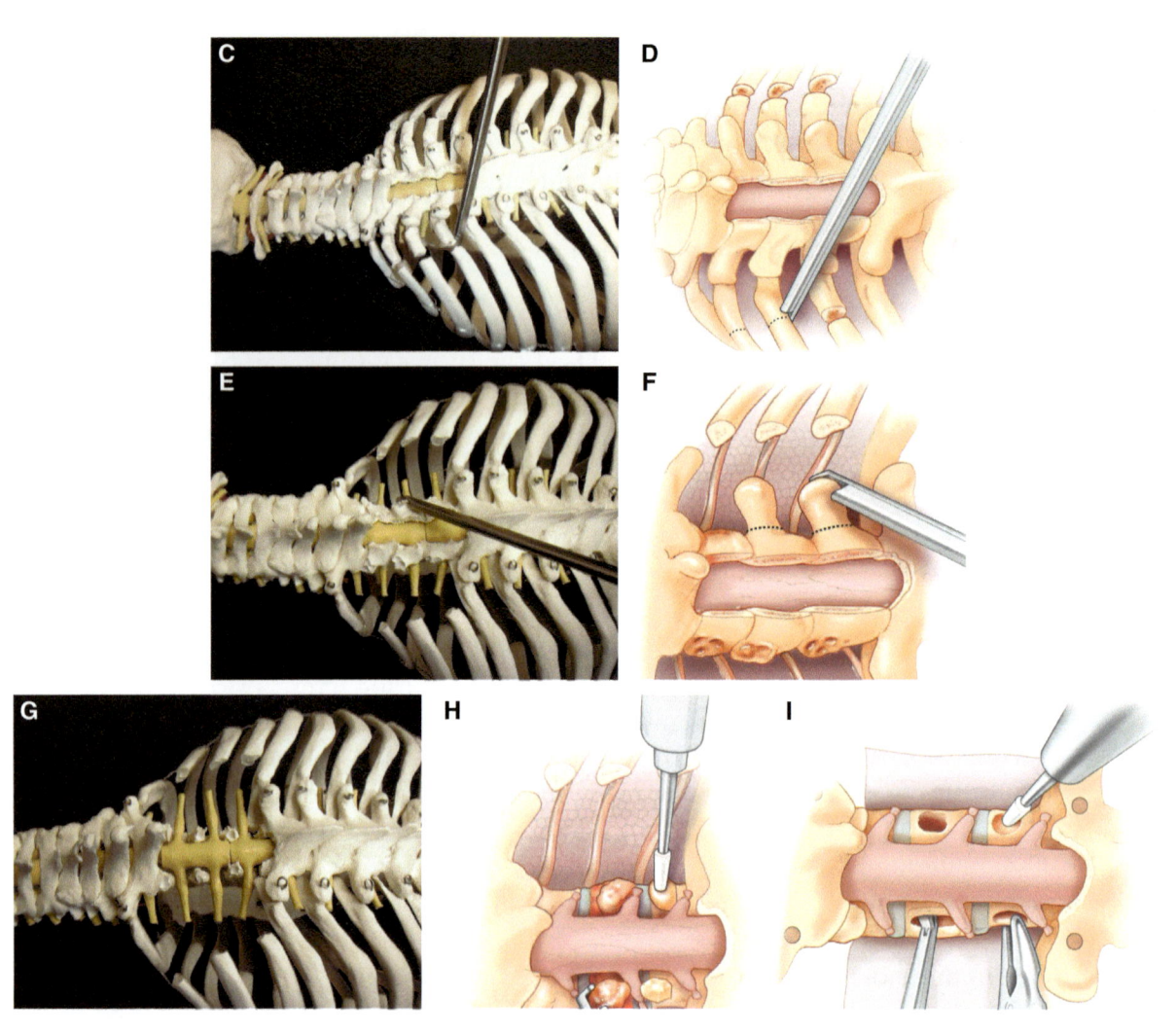

Fig. 42-1, cont'd **C-F,** The rib head and the transverse process, and finally, both the **G,** superior and inferior articulating facets at each level are removed. **H** and **I,** Next the pedicles can be drilled down to their junction with the vertebral body.

Once this is done, there is a safe access corridor to the vertebral body, and it can be resected by means of multiple instruments including a high-power hand drill, pituitary rongeurs, and curettes (Fig. 42-1, *J* through *M*). Once a substantial portion of the body has been removed by means of a decancellation osteotomy (eggshell procedure), the remaining portion under the posterior longitudinal ligament can be removed with an upgoing curette (see Fig. 42-1, *L*). An expandable cage, cement, or a static cage can be used to reconstruct and provide mechanical support anteriorly. The second rod may be placed and the sagittal alignment established with compression on the pedicle screws. If the goal is to correct the patient's alignment, further laminectomy is usually required above and below the resection, if there is a substantial amount of scar tissue from a previous surgery. The scar tissue should be resected to prevent any compression on the spinal cord resulting from closure of the osteotomy.

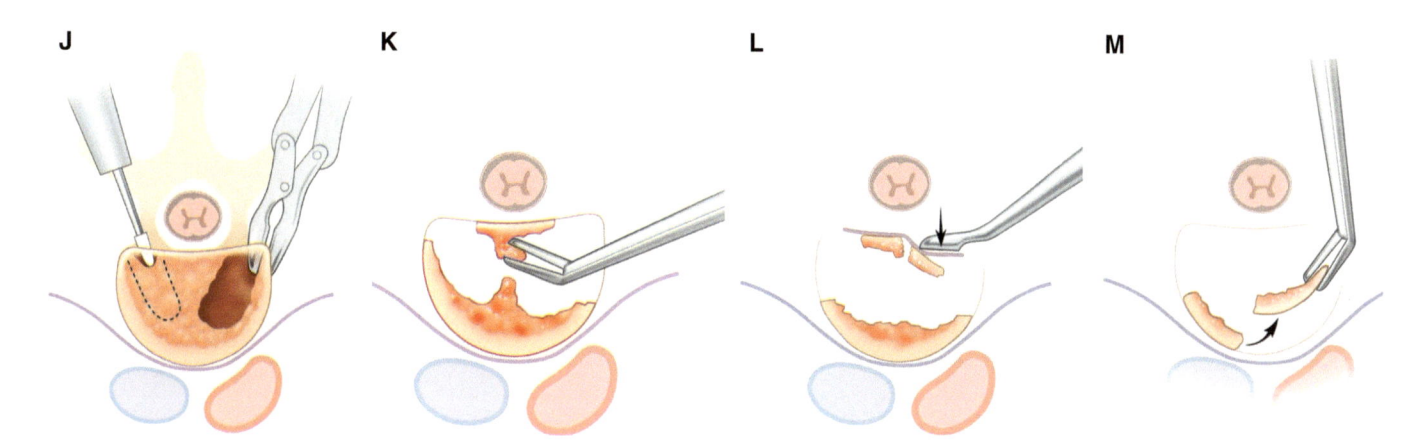

Fig. 42-1, cont'd **J** and **K,** With a safe access corridor to the vertebral body, it can be resected by means of multiple instruments including a high-power hand drill, pituitary rongeurs, and curettes. **L** and **M,** Once a substantial portion of the body has been removed by means of a decancellation osteotomy (eggshell procedure), the remaining portion under the posterior longitudinal ligament can be removed by means of an upgoing curette.

OUTCOMES WITH EVALUATION OF RESULTS

In a recently large multicenter study in which the senior author (H.E.A.) participated, 67 patients underwent a single-stage thoracolumbar vertebrectomy with circumferential reconstruction and arthrodesis.[37] The study cohort comprised 35 females and 32 males, with an average age of 54 years (range 14 to 86 years). Deformity of the vertebral column was caused by pathologic fractures in 37 patients (55%). Breast cancer was the most common malignancy in nine patients, followed by multiple myeloma in seven, lung cancer and prostate cancer in four each, and adenocarcinoma in three. Pathologic fractures treated in the current series were evenly distributed across the thoracic and upper lumbar spine. The majority of pathologic fractures were treated with single-level corpectomies (78%); only 22% required two-level corpectomies. Traumatic compression and burst fractures were encountered in 17 patients (25%). More than half of these fractures were located at the thoracolumbar junction at T12-L1. Traumatic fractures were exclusively treated with single-level corpectomies. Osteomyelitis was the cause of fractures of the anterior spinal column in 13 patients (20%). The majority of fractures with an infectious cause (69%) required multilevel corpectomies. Of note, 10% of the patients in the series had a history of previous spine surgery. The operative time for single-stage corpectomies with placement of a cage and posterior instrumentation was 324 minutes on average and did not differ significantly among pathologic, traumatic, and infectious fractures (range 157 to 692 minutes). The estimated average blood loss per case was 1511 ml (range 250 to 7800 ml). The estimated blood loss for pathologic and infectious fractures tended to be higher than for the repair of traumatic fractures. Vertebrectomies were most commonly performed at T12 (nine patients), L1 (eight patients), and T3 (seven patients). Fifty patients (75%) underwent a one-level corpectomy, 16 patients (24%) underwent two-level procedures, and one patient underwent a three-level procedure.

In the majority of cases involving the thoracic spine (88%), one or more nerve roots were sacrificed to facilitate cage placement. Only in a small percentage of operations involving the lumbar spine were nerve roots sacrificed (18%). Thus unilateral resections of nerve roots were performed at the level of L1 in two patients and L2 in one patient. The construct was stabilized using a posterolateral instrumented fusion in all patients. In eight patients (12%; three patients with pathologic fractures and five with traumatic fractures), a short-segment fixation was performed with one segment of stabilization cephalad and one caudal to the corpectomy. The majority of patients (53 patients; 79%) received long-segment fixation with two or three levels of stabilization cephalad and caudal to the corpectomy.

The postoperative hospital stay lasted a mean of 10 ± 5 days. Neurologic status was assessed using the ASIA outcome scale. Preoperatively, a third of patients were neurologically intact. Long-term follow-up data (20.5 months after the procedure) were available for 61 patients; six patients were lost to long-term follow-up. Of these six patients, five had osteomyelitic fractures.

Approximately half of the patients with long-term follow-up data had neurologic examinations unchanged from the preoperative examinations (31 patients), and 23 patients showed improvement in their neurologic function. However, 7 patients showed a decrease in lower extremity motor function, resulting from disease progression in 5 patients with pathologic fractures. A decrease in function was also seen in 1 patient with a traumatic L2 fracture and 1 patient with osteomyelitis. Radiographic evaluation before surgery revealed an average sagittal deformity of 17.1 degrees (range 2 to 33 degrees).

Posterior corpectomies and the placement of expandable titanium cages significantly reduced the sagittal deformity to 10.0 degrees (range 0 to 47 degrees; $p < 0.001$). An improvement in sagittal alignment was not significantly correlated with the type of pathology (traumatic, pathologic, or infectious fractures), number of corpectomies, or length of posterolateral fusion.

At the last follow-up 20.5 months after the procedure, Cobb angles were assessed on 29 CT scans and 38 radiographs. The average sagittal deformity was 10.9 degrees (range 0 to 47 degrees) and remained significantly different from preoperative values ($p < 0.001$); thus a mean sagittal deformity correction of 6.2 degrees (range 0 to 29.8 degrees) was achieved. During the follow-up period, Cobb angles were reduced by 0.9 degrees on average.

SIGNATURE CASES

A 64-year-old man with a history of prostate cancer had previously undergone kyphoplasty for pain and kyphotic deformity. However, the deformity continued to progress causing weakness, myelopathy, and severe back pain (Fig. 42-2, *A* and *B*). The patient was being treated with hormone therapy and had a low prostate-specific antigen level. He was taken to the operating room for posterior instrumented fusion, lateral extracavitary resection of the tumor, and placement of an expandable cage. Three months after surgery, the patient had significant resolution of the kyphosis (Fig. 42-2, *C* and *D*) and back pain, and improvement in lower extremity strength (to 5/5).

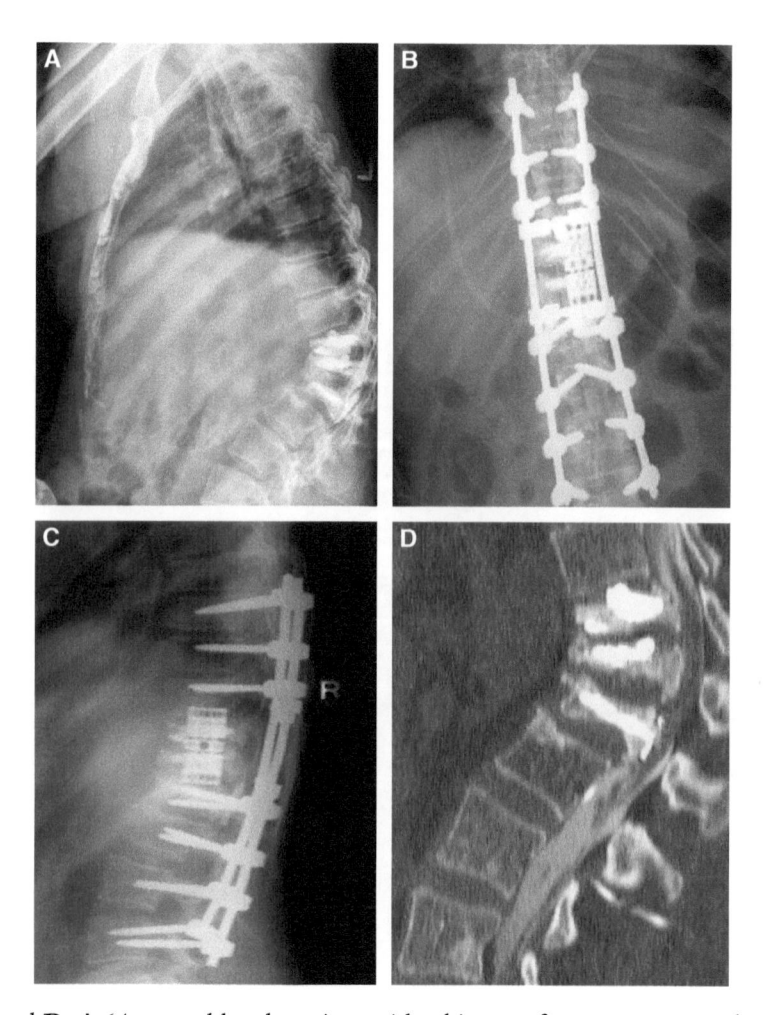

Fig. 42-2 **A** and **B,** A 64-year-old male patient with a history of prostate cancer, who had previously undergone kyphoplasty, had a progressive kyphotic deformity resulting in weakness. **C** and **D,** He was taken to the operating room for posterior instrumented fusion, lateral extracavitary resection of the tumor, and placement of an expandable cage that was stable at 3-month follow-up.

A 62-year-old woman with breast cancer presented with rapid neurologic deterioration 4 months after T2-T3 laminectomy and tumor debulking. Five days before she was seen, she had felt a "pop" in her head, and the deterioration progressed to an inability to ambulate. MRI showed that she had developed a complete collapse at the T3 vertebra with severe slippage of T2 over the T3/T4 vertebrae (Fig. 42-3, *A* and *B*). With severe stenosis/compression, the radiographic findings were consistent with the following physical examination findings: weakness, myelopathy, and loss of ambulation. There are many options for surgical management, but all of these options should include anterior decompression/reconstruction and realignment with posterior instrumentation/stabilization. The senior author (H.E.A.) elected to take the patient to the operating room for a T2-4 corpectomy and anterior reconstruction with an expandable cage (Fig. 42-3, *C* through *H*). The posterior instrumentation included lateral mass screws in C3-7 and pedicle screws in T1 and T5-8. Postoperatively, after reestablishment of her sagittal alignment, she improved to the point of ambulation (Fig. 42-3, *I*).

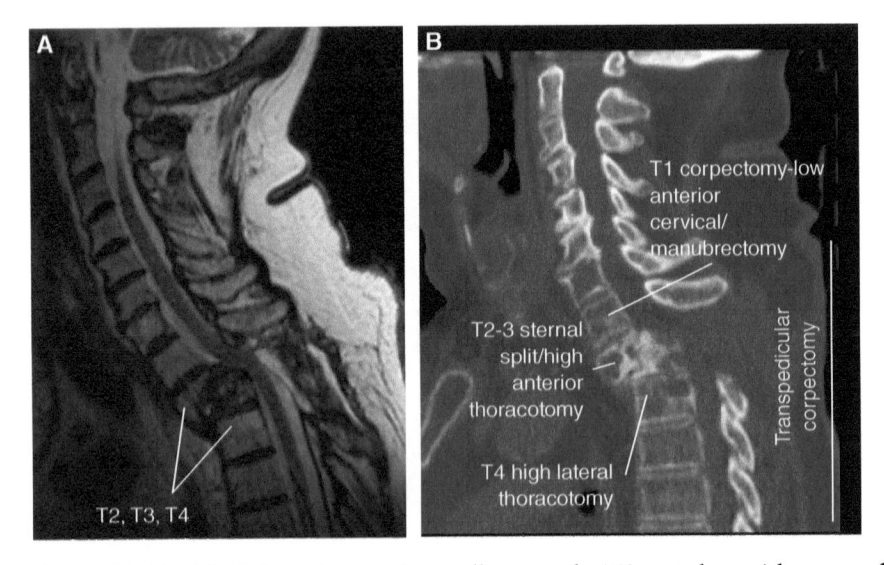

Fig. 42-3 **A** and **B,** On MRI there is complete collapse at the T3 vertebra with severe slippage of T2 over the T3/T4 vertebrae. Many surgical options are available, all of which include anterior decompression/reconstruction and realignment with posterior instrumentation/stabilization.

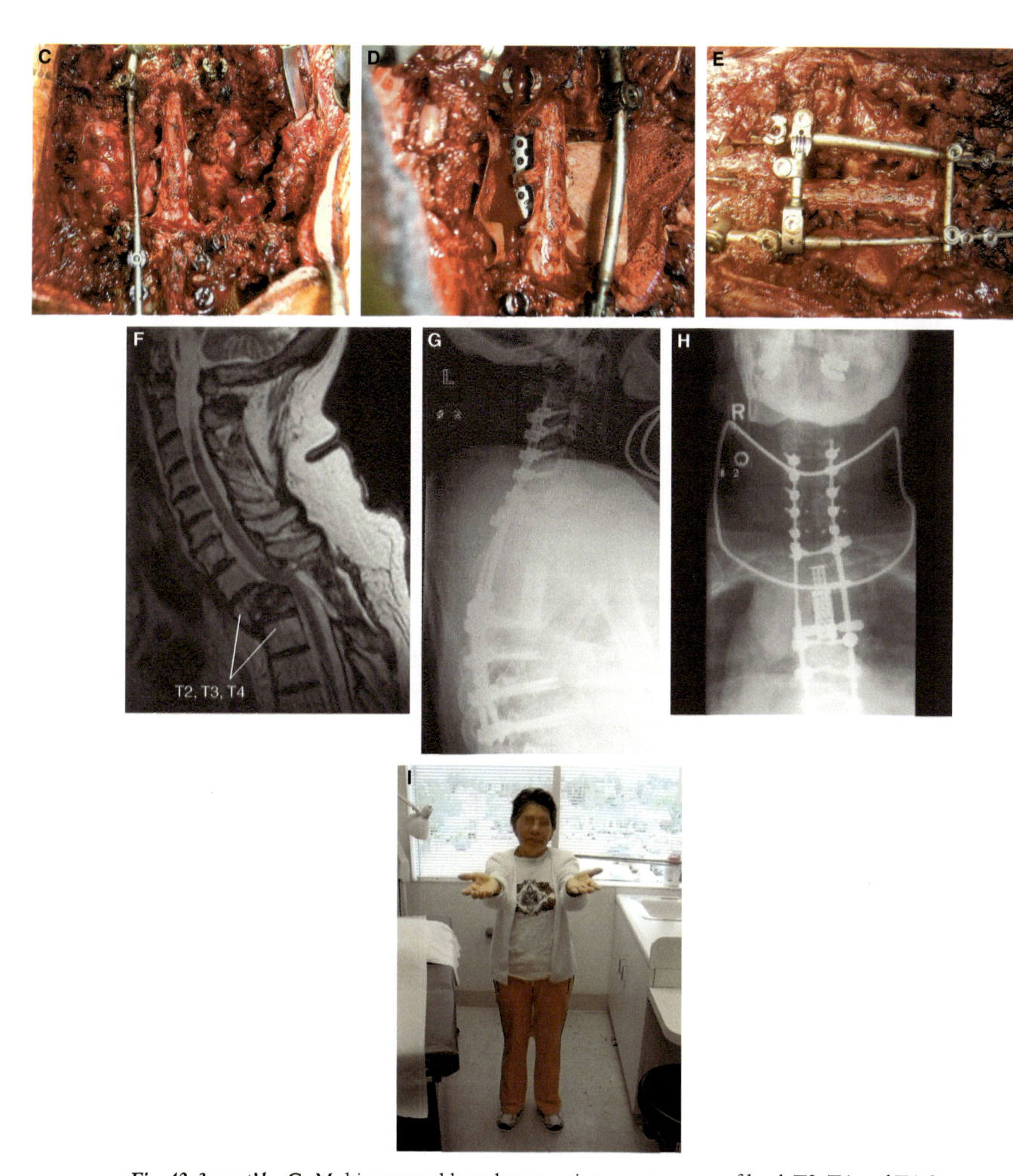

Fig. 42-3, cont'd **C,** Multisegmental lateral extracavitary corpectomy of levels T2, T4, and T6-8. **D,** An expandable cage was placed, with expansion of the cage to the appropriate height. **E,** Posterior instrumentation included lateral mass screws in C3-7 and pedicle screws in T1 and T5-8. **F-H,** Follow-up radiographs at 3 months demonstrate that the correction has been maintained. **I,** Patient has reestablishment of sagittal alignment and postoperative improvement to the point of ambulation.

CONCLUSION

The posterior transpedicular technique is an extremely powerful and versatile strategy for all areas of the thoracic and lumbar spine. An approach surgeon is not required, and complete circumferential canal decompression and stabilization can be achieved without violation of the pleural space. However, pulmonary complications, such as pleural effusion and pneumothorax, can still occur; therefore; chest radiographs should still be obtained in the postoperative period.

BAILOUT TECHNIQUES

- In the event of an intraoperative complication, it may be necessary to modify the procedure to reduce patient risk.
- The most common modification would be to stabilize the spine posteriorly but not decompress anteriorly. This provides an opportunity for some decompression, some stability, and for a later anterior-only approach.
- Alternatively a unilateral anterior decompression can be performed rather than bilateral, or an anterior decompression with reconstruction of the anterior column with cement rather than a cage.

TIPS FROM THE MASTERS

- A contralateral stabilizing rod should be positioned before decompression circumferential to provide some stability to the spine.
- Good anterior decompression can often be achieved through a unilateral approach. This reduces operative time and associated morbidity.
- Unilateral sacrifice of the thoracic nerve root is associated with minimal risk. The dorsal root ganglion (DRG) should be transected proximal to dorsal.

References (With Key References in Boldface)

1. Boriani S, Weinstein JN, Biagini R. Primary bone tumors of the spine: terminology and surgical staging. Spine 22:1036-1044, 1997.
2. **Tomita K, Kawahara N, Kobayashi T, et al. Surgical strategy for spinal metastases. Spine 26:298-306, 2001.**
3. Fourney DR, Gokaslan ZL. Use of "MAPs" for determining the optimal surgical approach to metastatic disease of the thoracolumbar spine: anterior, posterior, or combined. J Neurosurg Spine 2:40-49, 2005.
4. **Bilsky MH, Lis E, Raizer J, et al. The diagnosis and treatment of metastatic spinal tumor. Oncologist 4:459-469, 1999.**
5. Klimo P Jr, Schmidt MH. Surgical management of spinal metastases. Oncologist 9:188-196, 2004.
6. Yao KC, Boriani S, Gokaslan ZL, et al. En bloc spondylectomy for spinal metastases: a review of techniques. Neurosurg Focus 15:E6, 2003.

7. **Gokaslan ZL. Spine surgery for cancer. Curr Opin Oncol 8:178-181, 1996.**
8. Wong DA, Fornasier VL, MacNab I. Spinal metastases: the obvious, the occult, and the impostors. Spine 15:1-4, 1990.
9. Healey JH, Brown HK. Complications of bone metastases: surgical management. Cancer 88(Suppl 12):2940-2951, 2000.
10. Byrne TN. Spinal cord compression from epidural metastases. N Engl J Med 327:614-619, 1992.
11. Gerszten PC, Welch WC. Current surgical management of metastatic spinal disease. Oncology 14:1013-1024; discussion 1024, 1029-1030, 2000.
12. Barron KD, Hirano A, Araki S, et al. Experiences with metastatic neoplasms involving the spinal cord. Neurology 9:91-106, 1959.
13. Schaberg J, Gainor BJ. A profile of metastatic carcinoma of the spine. Spine 10:19-20, 1985.
14. Lada R, Kaminski HJ, Ruff R. Metastatic spinal cord compression. In Vecht C, ed. Neuro-oncology, Part III. Neurological Disorders in Systemic Cancer. Amsterdam: Elsevier Biomedical Publishers, 1997, pp 167-189.
15. **Sciubba DM, Gokaslan ZL, Suk I, et al. Positive and negative prognostic variables for patients undergoing spine surgery for metastatic breast disease. Eur Spine J 16:1659-1667, 2007.**
16. Shehadi JA, Sciubba DM, Suk I, et al. Surgical treatment strategies and outcome in patients with breast cancer metastatic to the spine: a review of 87 patients. Eur Spine J 16:1179-1192, 2007.
17. Tatsui H, Onomura T, Morishita S, et al. Survival rates of patients with metastatic spinal cancer after scintigraphic detection of abnormal radioactive accumulation. Spine 21:2143-2148, 1996.
18. Patchell RA, Tibbs PA, Regine WF, et al. Direct decompressive surgical resection in the treatment of spinal cord compression caused by metastatic cancer: a randomised trial. Lancet 366:643-648, 2005.
19. Senel A, Kaya AH, Kuruoglu E, et al. Circumferential stabilization with ghost screwing after posterior resection of spinal metastases via transpedicular route. Neurosurg Rev 30:131-137, 2007.
20. Acosta FL Jr, Aryan HE, Chi J, et al. Modified paramedian transpedicular approach and spinal reconstruction for intradural tumors of the cervical and cervicothoracic spine: clinical experience. Spine 32:E203-E210, 2007.
21. Muhlbauer M, Pfisterer W, Eyb R, et al. Noncontiguous spinal metastases and plasmacytomas should be operated on through a single posterior midline approach, and circumferential decompression should be performed with individualized reconstruction. Acta Neurochir (Wien) 142:1219-1230, 2000.
22. Visocchi M, Masferrer R, Sonntag VK, et al. Thoracoscopic approaches to the thoracic spine. Acta Neurochir (Wien) 140:737-743, 1998.
23. Keshavarzi S, Park MS, Aryan HE, et al. Minimally invasive thoracic corpectomy and anterior fusion in a patient with metastatic disease: case report and review of the literature. Minim Invasive Neurosurg 52:141-143, 2009.
24. Akeyson EW, McCutcheon IE. Single-stage posterior vertebrectomy and replacement combined with posterior instrumentation for spinal metastasis. J Neurosurg 85:211-220, 1996.
25. Douglas AF, Cooper PR. Cervical corpectomy and strut grafting. Neurosurgery 60(1 Suppl 1):S137-S142, 2007.
26. Medow J, Trost G, Sandin J. Surgical management of cervical myelopathy: indications and techniques for surgical corpectomy. Spine J 6(6 Suppl):S233-S241, 2006.
27. **Bilsky MH, Boland P, Lis E, et al. Single-stage posterolateral transpedicle approach for spondylectomy, epidural decompression, and circumferential fusion of spinal metastases. Spine 25:2240-2249, 2000.**
28. Stark RJ, Henson RA, Evans SJ. Spinal metastases: a retrospective survey from a general hospital. Brain 105:189-213, 1982.
29. Black P. Spinal metastasis: current status and recommended guidelines for management. Neurosurgery 5:726-746, 1979.
30. Young RF, Post EM, King GA. Treatment of spinal epidural metastases. Randomized prospective comparison of laminectomy and radiotherapy. J Neurosurg 53:741-748, 1980.

31. Findlay GF. Adverse effects of the management of malignant spinal cord compression. J Neurol Neurosurg Psychiatry 47:761-768, 1984.
32. Sørensen S, Børgesen SE, Rohde K, et al. Metastatic epidural spinal cord compression. Results of treatment and survival. Cancer 65:1502-1508, 1990.
33. Gilbert RW, Kim JH, Posner JB. Epidural spinal cord compression from metastatic tumor: diagnosis and treatment. Ann Neurol 3:40-51, 1978.
34. Constans JP, de Divitiis E, Donzelli R, et al. Spinal metastases with neurological manifestations. Review of 600 cases. J Neurosurg 59:111-118, 1983.
35. Martenson JA Jr, Evans RG, Lie MR, et al. Treatment outcome and complications in patients treated for malignant epidural spinal cord compression (SCC). J Neurooncol 3:77-84, 1985.
36. Tokuhashi Y, Matsuzaki H, Toriyama S, et al. Scoring system for the preoperative evaluation of metastatic spine tumor prognosis. Spine 15:1110-1113, 1990.
37. Hofstetter CP, Chou D, Newman CB, et al. Posterior approach for thoracolumbar corpectomies with expandable cage placement and circumferential arthrodesis: a multicenter case series of 67 patients. J Neurosurg Spine 14: 388-397, 2011.

Chapter 43

Hemipelvectomy and Hemicorporectomy: Hindquarter Amputation

Richard J. O'Donnell, Shane Burch

*A*mputation proximal to the shoulder or hip joint is sometimes necessitated by dire oncologic or infectious conditions. Especially when combined with resection of the chest wall and lung, a forequarter amputation is a quite extensive procedure, but hindquarter amputations (hemipelvectomy and hemicorporectomy) remain the most formidable ablative procedures that can be undertaken. In fact, hemicorporectomy is thought to be so aggressive that it is often challenged on ethical grounds. Although appropriately a part of discussions regarding treatment options for large lumbosacral and pelvic tumors, hemipelvectomy and hemicorporectomy are infrequently performed, principally because of the attendant expectation of grave complications, including death, as well as unacceptable oncologic and functional outcomes. Because any given center will perform few of these procedures, and given the poor prognosis often associated with the underlying medical problem, the literature contains little information in terms of longitudinal studies of patients undergoing hemipelvectomy or hemicorporectomy. This chapter seeks to highlight the indications, contraindications, preoperative decision-making, technique, outcomes, and literature review with respect to these rare but occasionally necessary operations.

INDICATIONS AND CONTRAINDICATIONS

The indications for hemipelvectomy and hemicorporectomy procedures are predicated on the assumption that these are procedures of last resort. Oncologic, infectious, and occasionally posttraumatic conditions are the most common categories for which these amputations are considered; congenital, developmental, metabolic, inflammatory, and degenerative diagnoses rarely require this type of intervention. In the simplest terms, hindquarter amputation would potentially be indicated when other less invasive forms of treatment would not be successful in providing acceptable palliative/curative control of tumors or suppression/cure of infections. All forms of medical (chemotherapy, antibiotics, analgesics), surgical (limb salvage, debridement, plastic surgical coverage), and radiation treatments should be attempted or ruled out before hindquarter amputations are discussed. The most common indication for hemipelvectomy is local control of sarcomas involving the sacrum, innominate bone, proximal femur, or soft tissues of the pelvis or buttock. A less frequent indication for hemipelvectomy would be intractable infections involving these tissues, particularly in patients with lower extremity paresis. The most common indication for hemicorporectomy is control of connective tissue malignancy or recalcitrant infections of the same structures, with extension to the lumbar spine.

Contraindications to hemipelvectomy and hemicorporectomy should be understood to be relative in the sense that even the most heroic amputation procedures are sometimes made appropriate by mutually agreed-on palliative goals. The most basic contraindication to hindquarter amputation would be medical or surgical reasons that would render the patient unable to survive the operation itself. Another contraindication would be a poor overall prognosis, without respect to hemipelvectomy or hemicorporectomy. Thus patients with a primary pelvic sarcoma and distant metastasis are generally not considered to be optimal candidates for hindquarter amputation. Similarly, patients with a secondary pelvic malignancy (e.g., metastatic carcinoma, melanoma, or bone marrow neoplasms) would not ordinarily be considered for these ablative operations.

Assuming a reasonably good short- to intermediate-term survival profile, hemipelvectomy and hemicorporectomy would still be contraindicated in the absence of an expectation of a reasonable likelihood of durable local control of the tumor or infection and maintenance of an acceptable quality of life. Some patients may be excluded from

---

Box 43-1 Relative Contraindications to Hemipelvectomy or Hemicorporectomy

Expectation of Poor Overall Survival
- Primary pelvic/lumbosacral malignancy with distant metastatic disease
- Secondary malignancy with pelvic/lumbosacral spread

Poor Probability of Local Control
- Likelihood of positive surgical margins in oncologic cases
- Difficulty of eradicating infection through amputation, flap coverage, and antibiotic treatment

Inability to Maintain an Acceptable Quality of Life
- Patient reluctance to undergo preparatory gastrointestinal/genitourinary diversion procedures
- Patient unwillingness to accept cosmetic and/or functional consequences

consideration because they are unwilling or unable to undergo extensive preparatory (intestinal and urinary diversion) or ancillary (plastic surgery) procedures or because they have unrealistic expectations regarding the rehabilitative consequences of these procedures (Box 43-1).

PREOPERATIVE EVALUATION
HISTORY

As is true for all areas of medicine, a complete history is crucial to better estimate a patient's suitability for surgery. For oncologic conditions, the nature and characteristics of the mass must be assessed in terms of palpability, growth rate, tenderness, and side effects, such as pain, swelling, and the neurologic sequelae of paresthesia, weakness, and bowel/bladder dysfunction. For patients with infections, local (erythema, warmth, tenderness, drainage), regional (lymphedema), and systemic (fever, sweats, chills, weight loss, fatigue) complications need to be documented. For all patients, a complete understanding of the patient's prior and planned diagnostic and therapeutic interventions must be achieved.

PHYSICAL EXAMINATION

A systematic approach to evaluation of a patient's mass or infection is paramount as a prerequisite for decision-making with respect to resectability and choice of technique for hemipelvectomy and hemicorporectomy. In addition to documentation of the neurologic side effects of axial diseases, physical examination of the local area of involvement is important for estimating the size, location, and mobility of tumors and the soft tissues surrounding infectious defects. In particular, indurations resulting from prior surgery, radiation therapy, or chronic infection may significantly alter a patient's candidacy for surgery or the choice of procedure. Depending on the location of the process, genitourinary and rectal examinations are an essential adjunct in preoperative planning.

DIAGNOSTIC STUDIES

Because of the magnitude of hindquarter amputation procedures, all pertinent radiologic and pathologic studies should be completed before the final decision to proceed is made. For the local process, necessary diagnostic studies include plain radiographs, nuclear medicine tests (technetium-99m total body bone scans for skeletal lesions, positron emission tomography [PET] for all oncologic conditions, and indium-labeled white blood cell scans for infections), computed tomography (CT), and magnetic resonance imaging (MRI). To rule out distant oncologic disease, a whole-body PET-CT scan is absolutely essential before a hemipelvectomy or hemicorporectomy is undertaken (Box 43-2). Identification of occult lesions should prompt consideration of a biopsy, because confirmation of distant disease is perhaps the most common rationale for avoiding a hindquarter procedure. Similarly, if any doubt exists with respect to the nature of the primary mass or infection, a temporally separate operative procedure should be scheduled so that sufficient tissue can be obtained for all necessary patho-

> **Box 43-2 Preparatory Diagnostic Studies for Hindquarter Amputations**
>
> **Laboratory Studies**
> - Serum
> - Urine
> - Microbiologic studies
>   - Wound cultures and stains
>
> **Radiologic Studies**
> - Plain radiographs
>   - Anteroposterior pelvis and obturator oblique pelvic studies
>   - Anteroposterior and lateral lumbar studies
> - Nuclear medicine
>   - Technetium-99m total body bone scan
>   - Indium-111–labeled white blood cell scan
> - Cross-sectional imaging
>   - Primary site
>   - Computed axial tomography with reconstruction images (CT)
>   - Magnetic resonance imaging (MR)
>   - Whole body
>   - 18-fluorodeoxyglucose positron emission tomography–computed axial tomography (PET-CT)
>
> **Pathologic Studies**
> - Percutaneous
>   - Fine-needle aspirate
>   - Core needle
>   - Image-guided
>   - Ultrasound
>   - CT
> - Open

logic and microbiological studies. Establishing a precise diagnosis under such circumstances can radically affect the decision to undertake surgery. In the case of suspected primary lumbosacral or pelvic malignancy, great care must be taken with respect to the manner in which the biopsy is performed. Percutaneous, especially image-guided, procedures are often best for tumors in these deep anatomic locations, so that biopsy tract contamination can be minimized.[1] Since sufficient material must be obtained to render an accurate diagnosis, open (incisional) biopsies are sometimes warranted, provided that attention is paid to incisional length and placement (in line with the definitive resection procedure), dissection through (rather than between) muscular planes, and avoidance of neurovascular exposure, bleeding, and infection.[2-4] Because an inappropriately performed biopsy can preclude a limb salvage effort or even an amputation, referral to a tertiary center skilled in the multidisciplinary management of musculoskeletal malignancies *before* a biopsy procedure is advisable.[5,6]

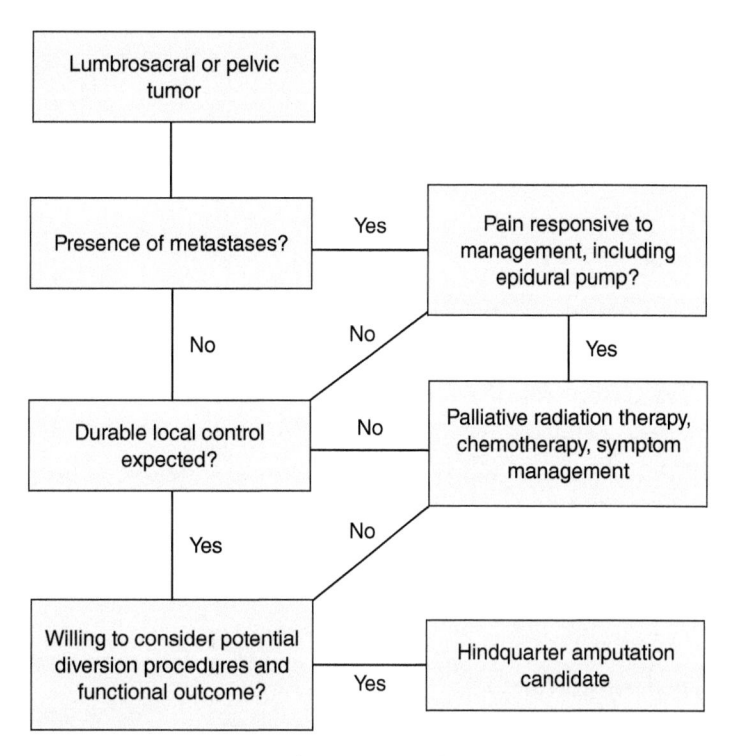

Fig. 43-1 Treatment algorithm for hindquarter amputation.

STAGING

As with all oncologic conditions, formal clinical and pathologic staging concludes the preoperative evaluation process. Staging should be done according to guidelines set forth by the American Joint Committee on Cancer.[7] For bone and soft tissue neoplasms, staging correlates directly with prognosis, which is of paramount importance when discussing expectations regarding hindquarter surgery with patients.

CLINICAL DECISION-MAKING

TREATMENT DECISIONS

As previously discussed, the decision as to whether to treat a patient with hemipelvectomy or hemicorporectomy rests on an estimation of whether the necessary surgical indications exist, based on a thorough preoperative evaluation and extensive discussions with the patient, the family, and caregivers to better understand their desires and goals. It is only then that a suitable technique can be chosen and a genuine shared decision-making process be concluded (Fig. 43-1).

CHOICE OF TECHNIQUE

Although hemicorporectomy, by definition, involves a translumbar amputation with the only variable essentially being the vertebral level, there are many variations of hemipelvectomy. Broadly speaking, choices in hemipelvectomy surgery include the following: (1) *extent:* partial, complete, or extended; (2) *lower extremity amputation:* internal or external; (3) *reconstruction:* presence or absence; and (4) *coverage:* none, anterior flap, posterior flap, or free flap. Selection of a technique largely depends on the location and extent of the oncologic or infectious process and the available options for soft tissue coverage.

Extent
The level of hemicorporectomy is quite simply determined by the most distal transection point that will allow for attainment of satisfactory surgical margins. For hemipelvectomy procedures, extent refers to the relative amounts of sacral and/or innominate bones that are resected. A partial (or "modified") hemipelvectomy involves only a portion of the innominate bone, which is roughly divided into the ischiopubic, acetabular, and iliac regions. A complete (or "standard") hemipelvectomy refers to resection of the entire innominate bone from the pubic symphysis to the sacroiliac joint. Finally, an extended hemipelvectomy includes removal of a portion (generally ≤50%) of the sacrum.

Lower Extremity Amputation
If the lower extremity is not amputated, the hemipelvectomy is referred to as internal. Otherwise, amputation of the pelvis and lower extremity results in the hemipelvectomy being classified as external.

Reconstruction
For internal hemipelvectomies, continuity between the lower extremity and the remainder of the body can be reestablished through the presence of reconstructive techniques, including endoprosthetic implants, alloprosthetic composites, allografts, autoclaved autografts, or arthrodeses.[8-12] In the absence of reconstruction, the lower extremity is said to be *flail*.[13]

Coverage
Hindquarter amputation wounds may be closed primarily or by use of a flap.[14-19] Options for locoregional rotational coverage include anterior (quadriceps) and posterior (gluteal) flaps. In rare circumstances, a free flap can be used to cover a hemipelvectomy defect.

Decision-Making Paths
Many permutations are the result of combining the various types of hemipelvectomy options outlined earlier in this chapter. The exact type of operation chosen depends on the location of the tumor or infectious process, the patient's desires, and the intraoperative findings. Options range from partial internal hemipelvectomy without reconstruction or a flap to extended external hemipelvectomy with free flap coverage.

TECHNIQUE
Assuming that appropriate surgical indications exist and that the patient fully understands the alternatives, benefits, and risks of surgery, several preoperative considerations

must be taken into account before proceeding with hemipelvectomy or hemicorporectomy.

In many cases, avoiding postoperative wound contamination by fecal material is of paramount importance. For instance, paraplegic patients, who may already lack sphincter control, often benefit from a diverting colostomy to minimize the chances of recurrent infection in the posterior wound bed, which, even under the best of circumstances, will remain subject to pressure effects from recumbency. At times urinary diversion is also beneficial, especially when loss of continence is an expected consequence of surgery. Patients are often understandably reluctant to accept such gastrointestinal and genitourinary interventions, but satisfactory performance of and recovery from such procedures is sometimes a necessary prerequisite for proceeding with hindquarter amputation.

In addition to optimization of the patient's overall cardiopulmonary and general medical health before such massive surgical procedures are undertaken, the use of neoadjuvant measures to alleviate the burden of local disease certainly plays a significant role in preparing for hindquarter amputation. In the case of infectious indications, preoperative cultures and maximal intravenous antibiotic coverage are essential. In the case of tumors, preoperative chemotherapy serves not only to limit the likelihood of progression of presumed systemic micrometastatic disease, but also may decrease the size of tumors to render a resection easier, safer, and more likely to yield negative surgical margins. Needless to say, bone marrow recovery from chemotherapy must be assured before proceeding with extensive surgery.

Since it is frequent for a substantial amount of time to elapse from when a patient is deemed to be a hindquarter amputation candidate until the proposed surgical date, it is important to repeat all relevant radiographic imaging studies just prior to the operation. In practical terms this would include plain radiographs (anteroposterior and lateral views of the lumbosacral spine; anteroposterior and oblique views of the pelvis) and MRI studies. In addition, a repeat whole-body fused PET-CT scan provides crucial information, including the metabolic response of the tumor to neoadjuvant chemotherapy and evaluation of potential interval development of occult metastatic disease that would preclude proceeding with extensive ablative surgery. Finally, in many cases of large lumbosacral and pelvic tumors, arrangements should be made for the patient to undergo arteriography and embolization just before surgery. This study provides optimal information regarding the correlation between the iliofemoral vasculature and the tumor process, and offers the opportunity to limit intraoperative hemorrhaging.

A final preparatory step before proceeding with surgery would be to ensure that all necessary surgical colleagues are available to render intraoperative assistance. Consultants who are customarily of assistance to the orthopedic and neurosurgical oncology team include general, vascular, urologic, and plastic surgeons. Some consideration should be given to enlisting the expertise of radiation oncologists to add intraoperative radiation therapy[20] or brachytherapy catheters to the operative bed. Time permitting, such techniques offer the opportunity to deliver adjuvant treatment directly to the tumor bed region most susceptible to local recurrence.

A combined epidural and general anesthesia technique is preferred; given the long operative time and often high blood loss, attention should be paid to establishment of central venous access and arterial monitoring.[21] In some cases cystoscopic placement of a ureteral stent is helpful in the identification of this important intraoperative landmark. Prevention of deep venous thrombosis is facilitated by the use of an intermittent pneumatic compression device on the contralateral lower leg. The patient is usually placed in the "lazy lateral" position, which is held with a well-padded beanbag, taking care to avoid putting pressure on bony prominences and the contralateral axilla. The goal of this form of decubitus positioning is to allow access and draping, if necessary, from the contralateral sacroiliac joint to the contralateral pubis. The entire ipsilateral extremity down to the toes is prepared and draped in a sterile fashion. The patient can then be shifted into a semiprone or semisupine position as required intraoperatively.

Specific details of the operative technique are difficult to catalog because of the wide variety of hemipelvectomies[22-25] and the rarity of hemicorporectomies[26-31]; each procedure must be individualized according to the differing requirements based on the precise oncologic or infectious indications for surgery. In general, an ilioinguinal or iliofemoral incision is chosen anteriorly to allow exposure of vital structures from the sacral promontory to the groin. For external procedures, exposure continues at a variable distance from the groin crease, across the buttock, ending along the posterolateral ilium. Proximal control of the major vessels is the first order of business, followed by identification of other important anatomic landmarks, including the nerves, ureters, and bowels.

Once a preliminary exploration of the tumor bed and surrounding relevant structures has been accomplished, the proper sequencing and tempo of the remaining portions of the operation must be kept in mind. In general, the order of subsequent steps is as follows: (1) creation of anterior or posterior plastic surgical flaps; (2) dissection of the tumor with a cuff of normal tissue; (3) anterior division of the pelvis through or lateral to the pubic symphysis; (4) posterior division of the pelvis through or medial to the sacroiliac joint; (5) transection of the lumbosacral nerve roots or sciatic nerve; (6) division and ligation of iliofemoral vessels; (7) division of the remaining soft tissue structures, such as the sacrotuberous and sacrospinous ligaments; (8) removal of the specimen; and (9) hemostasis and closure over drains. In this systematic approach, chronologic priority is given to aspects of the operation that are less bloody and challenging (flap creation), followed by the part that is often the most precise, demanding, and crucial (tumor dissection), with speed reserved for later steps that are most hemorrhagic (sacroiliac separation).

OUTCOMES WITH EVALUATION OF RESULTS

Because of the rarity of hindquarter amputation procedures, and given the often-poor patient survivorship, little medical literature exists with respect to longitudinal outcome studies for such procedures. Although more has been published with respect to internal hemipelvectomies, as compared with external hemipelvectomies and hemicorporectomies, the level of evidence for even most papers is generally grade IV or V. Nonetheless, over the past 75 years, several reasonably large case series of external hemipelvectomy patients have been published.[32-41] Two large series from the United Kingdom have shown that the peri-operative mortality rate has decreased from 22% in the first half of the twentieth century[32] to 1.3% in 2013 for 137 oncologic patients.[38] By contrast, a 2003 series of 56 United States Veterans Administration spinal cord injury patients still reported a 25% mortality rate with a hemipelvectomy procedure.[42] For oncologic patients, Grimer et al reported that major wound healing complications or infection arise in 45% of patients.[38] For patients treated with intent to cure, the overall 5-year survival and local recurrence rates were 45% and 15%, respectively.[38] Functional outcomes are, at best, fair,[43-46] with only 20% of patients using their prosthesis regularly.[38]

Most hemicorporectomy publications are case reports or very small case series. In 2009, Janis et al reported one of the largest experiences with nine paraplegic patients who underwent hemicorporectomy for terminal pelvic osteomyelitis.[47] The average survival after hemicorporectomy in this non-oncologic study was 11.0 years (range, 1.7 to 22.0 years). For the 66 hemicorporectomy cases that had been reported in the world literature until 2009, more than 50% of patients were alive at long-term follow-up.[47] As expected, prosthetic management and functional rehabilitation present enormous challenges.[48]

All conceivable intraoperative and perioperative complications can occur with hindquarter amputation procedures. Bleeding and the need for sometimes massive transfusions of blood and blood products is a given. Some form of infection, including superficial wound abscesses, deep pelvic infection, urinary tract infection, decubitus ulceration, and pneumonia, is a virtual certainty. Phantom pain and phantom sensation resulting from transection of major nerves and nerve roots is likely. Deep venous thrombosis and pulmonary embolism are distinct possibilities. All patients and their families need to accept the possibility of intraoperative or perioperative death. Most patients experience some, if not all, of these major and minor complications. After a successful recovery, all patients can expect to be subject to major lifelong functional impairment and disabilities.

SIGNATURE CASES
Partial Internal Hemipelvectomy With Reconstruction

A 54-year-old woman with a history of breast cancer presented with severe hip pain and inability to ambulate. Plain radiographs showed a very large lytic lesion destroying the acetabulum, extending from the ischiopubic region to the iliac wing (Fig. 43-2, *A*). A CT scan documented the extent of the bone and soft tissue neoplasm, while providing the opportunity to obtain tissue for histologic confirmation of metastatic breast carcinoma (Fig. 43-2, *B*). Arteriography and embolization immediately before surgical resection served to minimize intraoperative blood loss (Fig. 43-2, *C*). A partial internal hemipelvic resection was undertaken, followed by reconstruction with the use of a complex endoprosthetic "cup-cage-cup" acetabular device and a cemented total hip replacement (Fig. 43-2, *D* and *E*). Adjuvant radiation therapy and chemotherapy were administered, allowing the patient to remain disease free and productively employed 2 years after surgery.

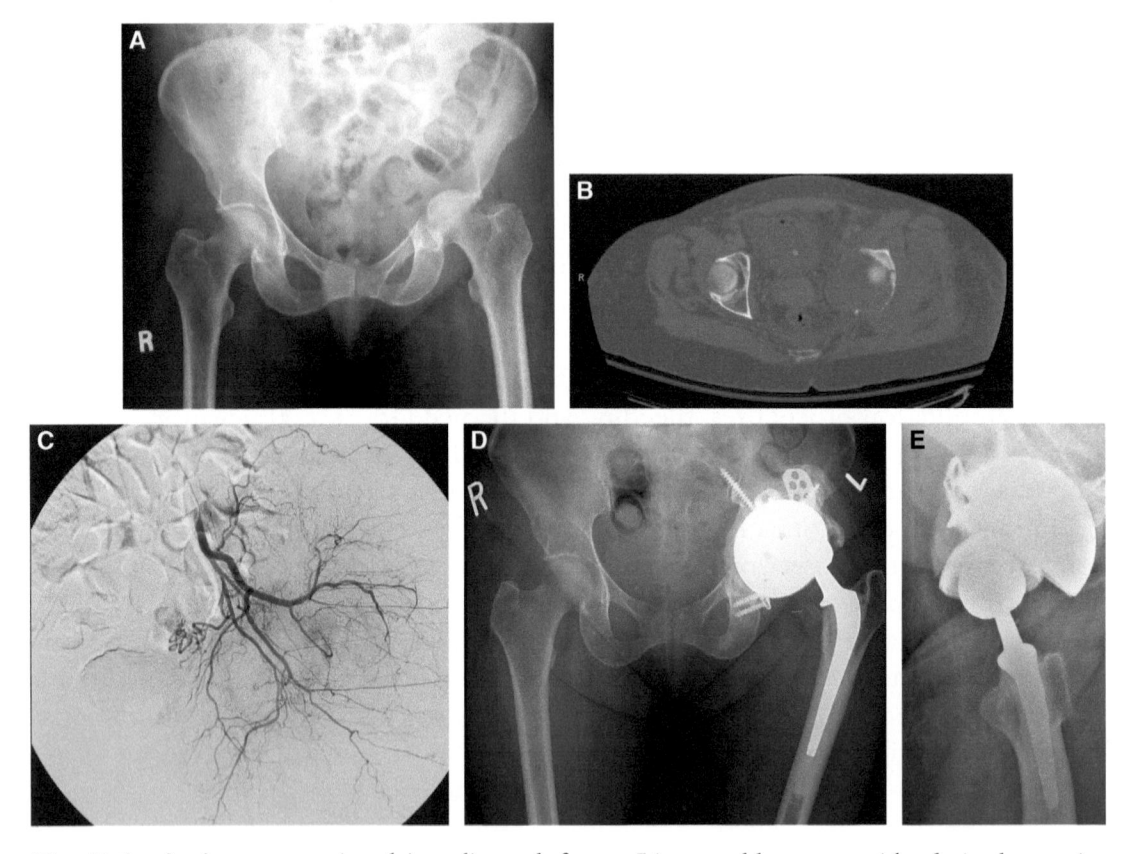

Fig. 43-2 **A,** Anteroposterior plain radiograph from a 54-year-old woman with a lytic, destructive left acetabular lesion and protrusion of the femoral head. **B,** Coronal CT scan reconstruction image showing the extent of hemipelvic destruction from the metastatic breast cancer, which extends from the iliac wing to the ischium. **C,** Digital subtraction angiogram showing preoperative embolization of a left acetabular tumor, performed to decrease intraoperative hemorrhage. **D,** Anteroposterior radiograph of the pelvis showing internal hemipelvic resection with total hip prosthetic reconstruction. **E,** Lateral hip radiograph showing "cup-cage-cup" hemipelvic reconstruction with a cemented femoral component.

Partial External Hemipelvectomy With Anterior Flap Coverage

A 70-year-old previously healthy woman was seen 3 months after she sustained a femoral pathologic fracture, treated with intramedullary rod fixation in a developing country (Fig. 43-3, *A*). The patient's technetium-99m total-body bone (Fig. 43-3, *B*) and PET (Fig. 43-3, *C*) scans demonstrated intense hypermetabolism throughout the thigh. MRI showed a massive tumor surrounding the femoral shaft circumferentially (Fig. 43-3, *D*). A subsequent incisional biopsy confirmed the diagnosis of osteosarcoma. Despite a large metastatic lung lesion (Fig. 43-3, *E*), the patient's hindquarter pain was so intractable that she requested palliative surgery. Because of contamination of the gluteal structures during rod insertion, the patient was judged not to be a candidate for limb salvage surgery. She consented to a partial external hemipelvectomy with anterior quadriceps flap coverage (Fig. 43-3, *F*). Within 6 months of surgery, she died of progressive pulmonary disease.

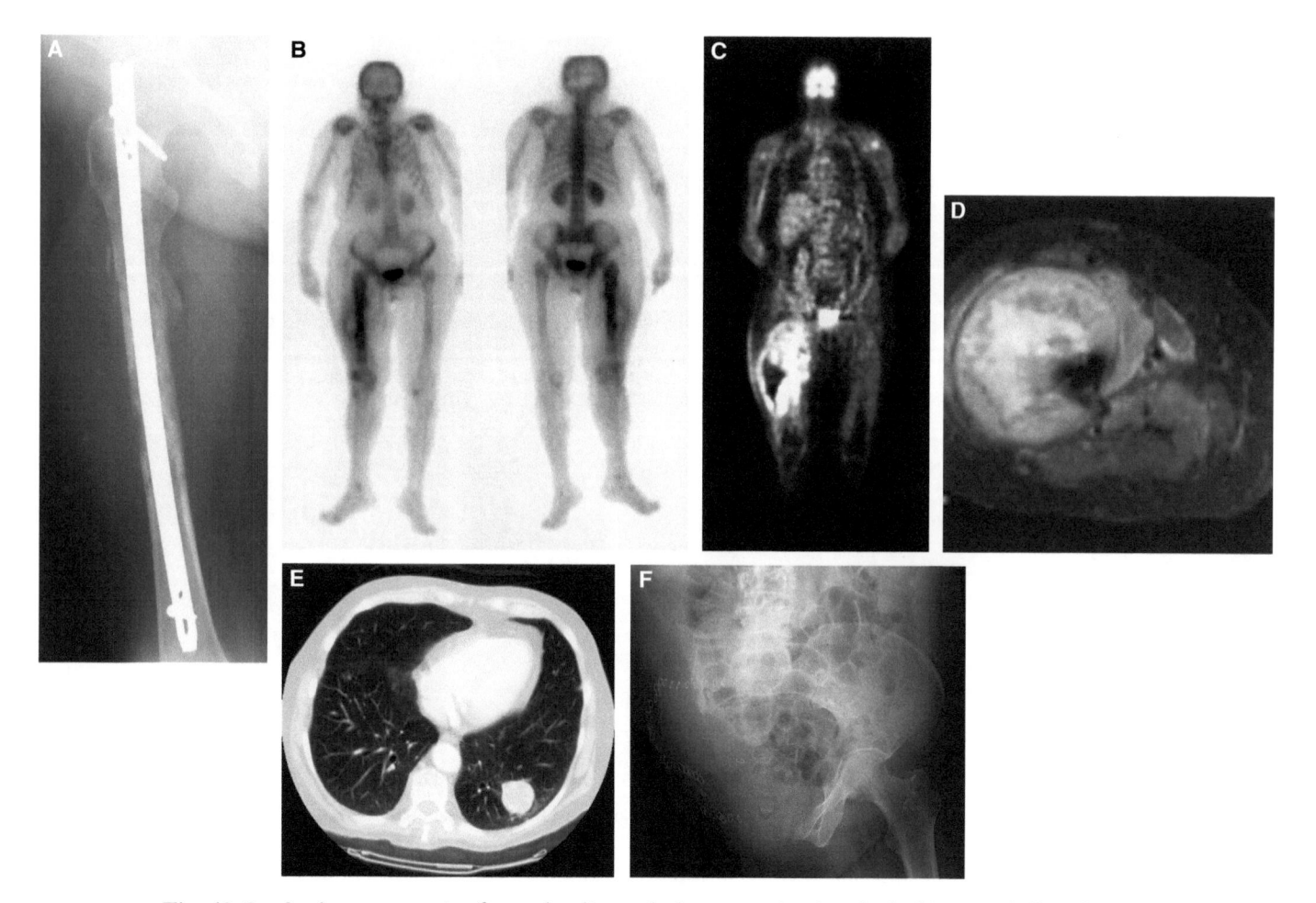

Fig. 43-3 **A,** Anteroposterior femoral radiograph demonstrating interlocked intramedullary femoral rod fixation of a diaphyseal pathologic fracture in a 70-year-old woman. **B,** Technetium-99m total-body bone scan demonstrating intense radiotracer uptake in the right femoral shaft. **C,** Coronal total-body PET scan showing marked metabolic activity in a thigh neoplasm. **D,** Axial T2-weighted MRI scan showing a massive osteosarcoma soft tissue mass surrounding the femoral shaft. **E,** Axial CT scan confirming the presence of a large left pulmonary metastatic osteosarcoma. **F,** Anteroposterior pelvic film showing partial external hemipelvectomy with small pubic and posterior iliac remnants.

PARTIAL EXTERNAL HEMIPELVECTOMY WITH ANTERIOR FLAP COVERAGE

A 20-year-old male patient was seen at an outside institution with progressive hip pain and disability (Fig. 43-4, A through C). He was treated with a cemented unipolar hemiarthroplasty hip replacement (Fig. 43-4, D). Subsequent review of the histologic material retrieved intraoperatively confirmed the presence of a high-grade telangiectatic osteosarcoma. After the patient was referred to a tertiary center, he was given standard multiagent chemotherapy, but extensive extracompartmental gluteal contamination from the prior procedure precluded any attempts at limb salvage. The patient then underwent an external hemipelvectomy with anterior flap coverage to obtain local control of the tumor (Fig. 43-4, E). Despite additional chemotherapy, the patient developed massive pulmonary metastatic disease within 10 months of the hindquarter amputation (Fig. 43-4, F).

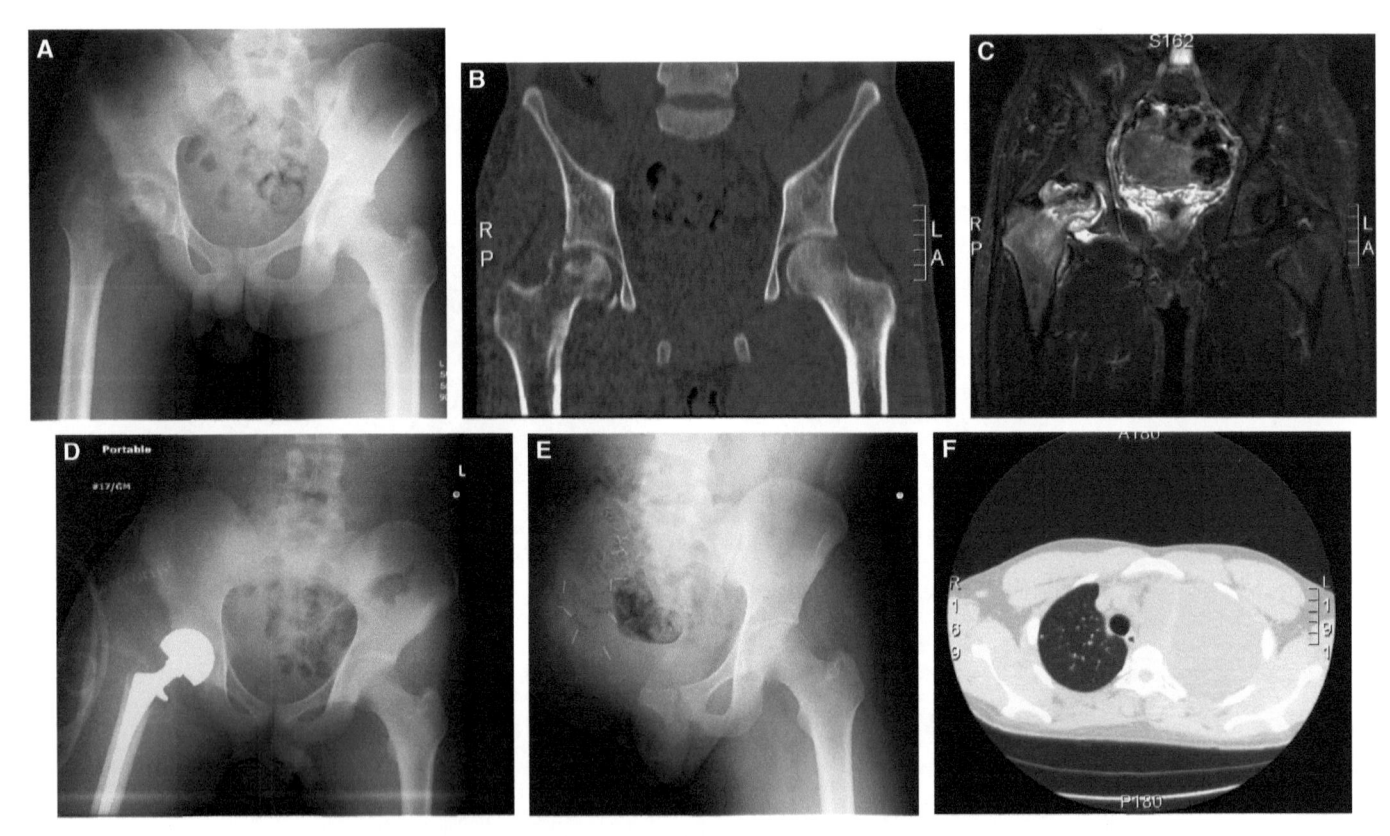

Fig. 43-4 **A,** Anteroposterior radiograph of the pelvis showing a displaced femoral neck fracture in a 20-year-old male patient. **B,** Coronal CT scan reconstruction image demonstrating lateral femoral head collapse. **C,** Coronal T2-weighted MRI scan demonstrating extensive bone and soft tissue process involving and surrounding the femoral head. **D,** Anteroposterior radiograph of the pelvis showing an uncemented unipolar hemiarthroplasty procedure performed before the discovery of a high-grade telangiectatic osteosarcoma. **E,** Anteroposterior radiograph of the pelvis demonstrating an external hemipelvectomy with a small pubic remnant. **F,** Axial CT scan confirming the presence of a massive left pulmonary metastatic osteosarcoma 10 months after hemipelvectomy.

PARTIAL EXTERNAL HEMIPELVECTOMY WITH POSTERIOR FLAP COVERAGE

A 43-year-old man presented with recurrent nonmetastatic right thigh synovial sarcoma, extending to the pelvis, that was not responsive to prior chemotherapy, surgery, and radiation therapy (Fig. 43-5, *A* and *B*). The patient proceeded with partial external hemipelvectomy through the sciatic notch and iliac wing with posterior flap coverage to obtain local control of the tumor (Fig. 43-5, *C*). He subsequently developed pulmonary metastatic disease.

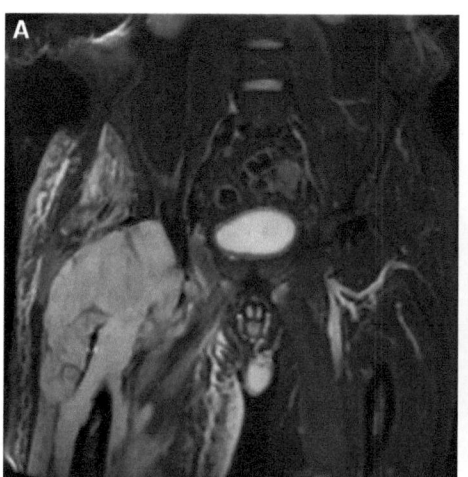

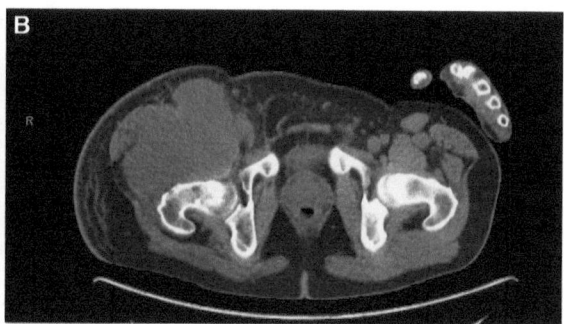

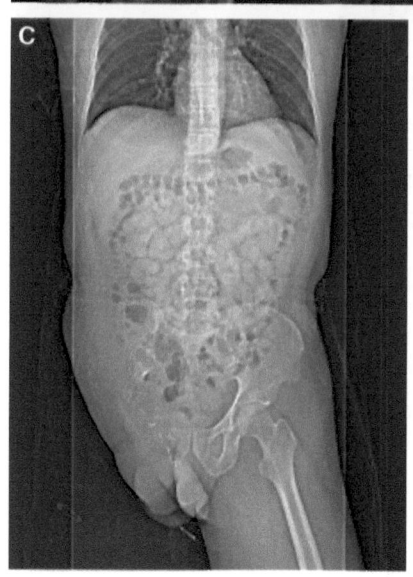

Fig. 43-5 **A,** Coronal T2-weighted MRI image demonstrating a recurrent synovial sarcoma mass extending to the pelvis. **B,** Axial CT scan images confirm neurovascular involvement not amenable to hip disarticulation. **C,** Anteroposterior radiograph showing a partial external hemipelvectomy through the sciatic notch.

Extended External Hemipelvectomy With Posterior Flap Coverage

A 56-year-old male patient presented with progressive nonmetastatic left acetabular dedifferentiated chondrosarcoma (Fig. 43-6, *A* and *B*). The patient underwent an extended external hemipelvectomy through the sacrum with posterior flap coverage to obtain local control of the tumor (Fig. 43-6, *C*). He subsequently developed pulmonary and hepatic metastases.

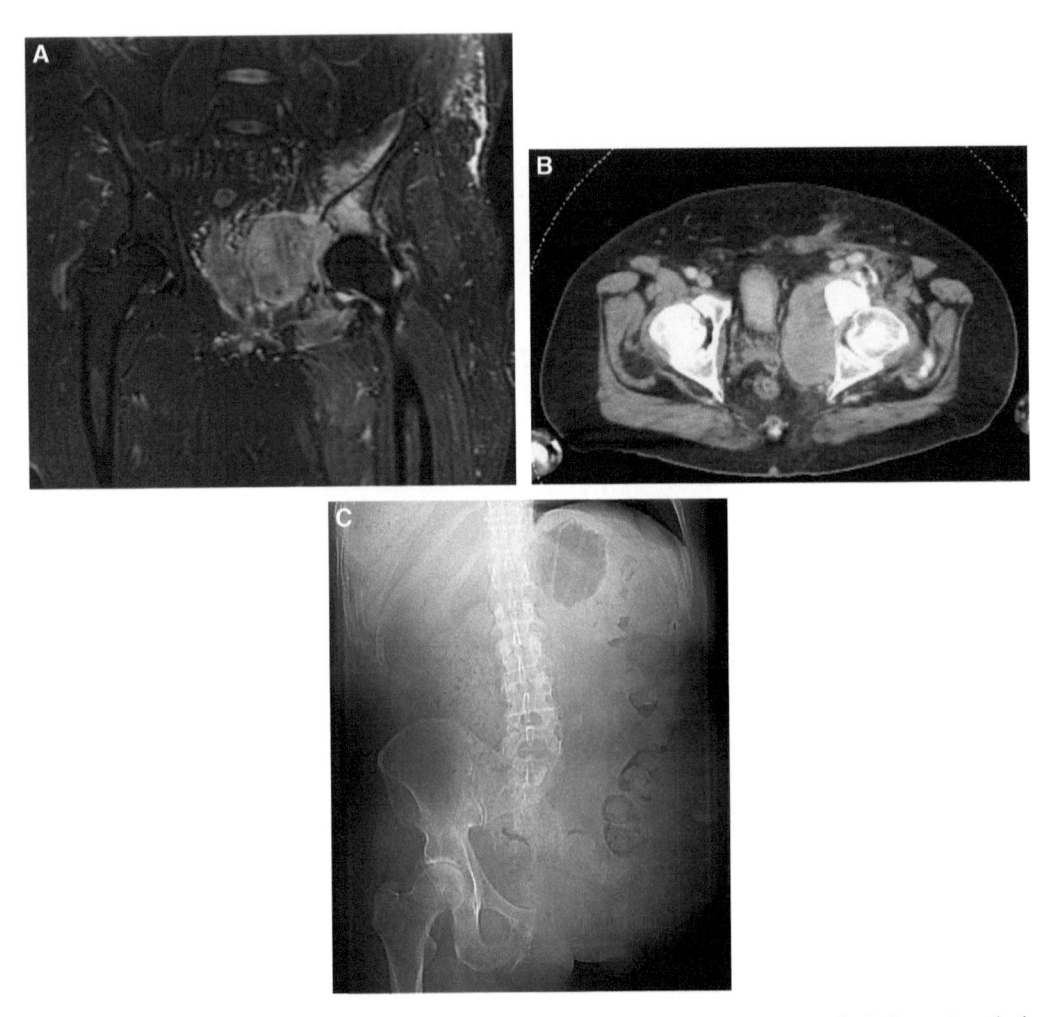

Fig. 43-6 **A,** Coronal T2-weighted MRI scan image showing a progressive dedifferentiated chondrosarcoma in the left acetabular region of a 56-year-old male patient. **B,** Axial CT scan images reveal a massive tumor not amenable to internal hemipelvectomy and reconstruction. **C,** Anteroposterior radiograph showing an extended external hemipelvectomy through the sacrum.

CONCLUSION

Hemipelvectomy and hemicorporectomy remain among the most massive, challenging, and formidable operations in the armamentarium of oncologic surgeons. Relatively few surgeons have the opportunity to become sufficiently experienced in these techniques so that they feel comfortable discussing the alternatives, benefits, and risks of the procedure and believe they can successfully undertake this operation. After extensive preoperative discussion and evaluation, and with careful intraoperative decision-making and perioperative care, these hindquarter amputations nonetheless offer the hope of significant palliative, and sometimes curative, outcomes.

BAILOUT TECHNIQUE

Needless to say, hemipelvectomy and hemicorporectomy procedures should not be undertaken lightly. Once preliminary exploration of the operative field has been completed and the tumor has been deemed resectable, a point of no return is very rapidly reached. In the face of intractable hemorrhage, abandonment of attempts to achieve negative surgical margins might be considered to be an acceptable "bailout technique" to save the life of the patient. Otherwise, with knowledge of the grave consequences that are at stake, the surgeon should strive to carry all hindquarter amputations, once begun, to safe and expeditious completion.

TIPS FROM THE MASTERS

- All forms of hemipelvectomy are extensive procedures that are considered with palliative and perhaps curative intent for massive, intractable pelvic neoplasms and infections.
- Hemicorporectomy is seldom performed, and generally only for the gravest of lumbosacral indications.
- Hindquarter amputations must be approached with careful preoperative radiologic planning, including a whole body PET-CT scan, as ruling out occult metastatic disease is generally considered to be a prerequisite before surgery.
- The shared decision-making process for hindquarter amputation procedures must include review of the alternatives, benefits, and risks of surgery, including the potential need for intestinal and urinary diversion, the possibility of perioperative profound morbidity and mortality, and the likelihood of profound alteration in functional status.
- The type of hindquarter amputation selected is based on the necessity of obtaining negative surgical margins and the soft tissues that remain available for defect coverage.
- Hemipelvectomies must proceed in a deliberate, expeditious fashion, from easier (generally anterior) to more difficult and hemorrhagic (generally posterior, sacroiliac).

References (With Key References in Boldface)

1. Virayavanich W, Ringler MD, Chin CT, Baum T, Giaconi JC, O'Donnell RJ, Horvai AE, Jones KD, Link TM. CT-guided biopsy of bone and soft-tissue lesions: role of on-site immediate cytologic evaluation. J Vasc Interv Radiol 22:1024-1030, 2011.
2. Mankin HJ, Lange TA, Spanier SS. The hazards of biopsy in patients with malignant primary bone and soft tissue tumors. J Bone Joint Surg Am 64:1121-1127, 1982.
3. Mankin HJ, Mankin CJ, Simon MA. The hazards of biopsy, revisited. J Bone Joint Surg Am 78:656-663, 1996.
4. Frassica FJ, McCarthy EF, Bluemke DA. Soft-tissue masses: when and how to biopsy. In Price CT, ed. Instructional Course Lectures. Rosemont, IL: American Academy of Orthopaedic Surgeons, 2000.
5. **von Mehren M, Benjamin RS, Bui MM, et al. Soft tissue sarcoma, version 2.2012: featured updates to the NCCN guidelines. J Natl Compr Canc Netw 10:951-960, 2012.**
6. **Biermann JS, Adkins DR, Benjamin RS, et al; National Comprehensive Cancer Network Bone Cancer Panel. NCCN clinical practice guidelines in oncology. Bone cancer. J Natl Compr Canc Netw 8:688-712, 2010.**
7. Edge SB, Byrd DR, Compton CC, Fritz AG, eds. AJCC Cancer Staging Manual, 7th ed. Philadelphia: Lippincott-Raven, 2009.
8. Dominkus M, Darwish E, Funovics P. Reconstruction of the pelvis after resection of malignant bone tumours in children and adolescents. In Tunn PU, ed. Treatment of Bone and Soft Tissue Sarcomas: Recent Results in Cancer Research. Berlin: Springer-Verlag, 2009.
9. Sherman CE, O'Connor MI, Sim FH. Survival, local recurrence, and function after pelvic limb salvage at 23 to 38 years of follow-up. Clin Orthop Relat Res 470:712-727, 2012.
10. Dai KR, Yan MN, Zhu ZA, et al. Computer-aided custom-made hemipelvic prosthesis used in extensive pelvic lesions. J Arthroplasty 22:981-986, 2007.
11. Hubert DM, Low DW, Serletti JM, et al. Fibula free flap reconstruction of the pelvis in children after limb-sparing internal hemipelvectomy for bone sarcoma. Plast Reconstr Surg 125:195-200, 2010.
12. Chang DW, Fortin AJ, Oates SD, et al. Reconstruction of the pelvic ring with vascularized double-strut fibular flap following internal hemipelvectomy. Plast Reconstr Surg 121:1993-2000, 2008.
13. Schwartz AJ, Kiatisevi P, Eilber FC, Eilber FR, Eckardt JJ. The Friedman-Eilber resection arthroplasty of the pelvis. Clin Orthop Relat Res 467:2825-2830, 2009.
14. Senchenkov A, Moran SL, Petty PM, et al. Soft-tissue reconstruction of external hemipelvectomy defects. Plast Reconstr Surg 124:144-155, 2009.
15. **Mat Saad AZ, Halim AS, Faisham WI, et al. Soft tissue reconstruction following hemipelvectomy: eight-year experience and literature review. Sci World J 2012:702904, 2012.**
16. Mavrogenis AF, Soultanis K, Patapis P, et al. Anterior thigh flap extended hemipelvectomy and spinoiliac arthrodesis. Surg Oncol 20:e215-e221, 2011.
17. Ross DA, Lohman RF, Kroll SS, et al. Soft tissue reconstruction following hemipelvectomy. Am J Surg 176:25-29, 1998.
18. Samant M, Chang EI, Petrungaro J, et al. Reconstruction of massive oncologic defects following extremity amputation. Ann Plast Surg 68:467-471, 2012.
19. Kong GX, Rudiger HA, Ek ET, et al. Reconstruction after external hemipelvectomy using tibia-hindfoot rotationplasty with calcaneo-sacral fixation. Int Semin Surg Oncol 5:1-4, 2008.
20. Tran QN, Kim AC, Gottschalk AR, Wara WM, Phillips TL, O'Donnell RJ, Weinberg V, Haas-Kogan DA. Clinical outcomes of intraoperative radiation therapy for extremity sarcomas. Sarcoma 10:1-6, 2006.

21. Molnar R, Emery G, Choong PF. Anaesthesia for hemipelvectomy—a series of 49 cases. Anaesth Intensive Care 35:536-543, 2007.
22. **Malawer MM, Wittig JC. Anterior flap hemipelvectomy. In Malawer MM, Wittig JC, Bickels J, eds. Operative Techniques in Orthopaedic Surgical Oncology. Philadelphia: Wolters Kluwer, 2012.**
23. **Malawer MM, Wittig JC. Posterior flap hemipelvectomy. In Malawer MM, Wittig JC, Bickels J, eds. Operative Techniques in Orthopaedic Surgical Oncology. Philadelphia: Wolters Kluwer, 2012.**
24. Chansky HA. Hip disarticulation and transpelvic amputation: surgical management. In Smith DG, Michael JW, Bowker JH, eds. Atlas of Amputations and Limb Deficiencies. Rosemont, IL: American Academy of Orthopaedic Surgeons, 2004.
25. Lackman RD, Crawford EA, Hosalkar HS, et al. Internal hemipelvectomy for pelvic sarcomas using a T-incision surgical approach. Clin Orthop Relat Res 467:2677-2684, 2009.
26. Wagman LD, Terz JJ. Hemipelvectomy and translumbar amputation. In Moore WS, Malone JM, eds. Lower Extremity Amputation. Philadelphia: WB Saunders, 1989.
27. **Wagman LD, Terz JJ. Translumbar amputation: surgical management. In Smith DG, Michael JW, Bowker JH, eds. Atlas of Amputations and Limb Deficiencies. Rosemont, IL: American Academy of Orthopaedic Surgeons, 2004.**
28. Barnett CC Jr, Ahmad J, Janis JE, et al. Hemicorporectomy: back to front. Am J Surg 196:1000-1002, 2008.
29. Weaver JM, Flynn MB. Hemicorporectomy. J Surg Oncol 73:117-124, 2000.
30. Ferrara BE. Hemicorporectomy: a collective review. J Surg Oncol 45:270-278, 1990.
31. Chang DW, Lee JE, Gokaslan ZL, Robb GL. Closure of hemicorporectomy with bilateral subtotal thigh flaps. Plast Reconstr Surg 105:1742-1746, 2000.
32. Gordon-Taylor G, Wiles P, Patey DH, et al. The interinnomino-abdominal operation: observations on a series of fifty cases. J Bone Joint Surg Br 34:14-21, 1952.
33. Pack GT, Miller TR. Exarticulation of the innominate bone and corresponding lower extremity (hemipelvectomy) for primary and metastatic cancer. A report of one hundred one cases with analysis of the end results. J Bone Joint Surg Am 46:91-95, 1964.
34. Senchenkov A, Moran SL, Petty PM, et al. Predictors of complications and outcomes of external hemipelvectomy wounds: account of 160 consecutive cases. Ann Surg Oncol 15:355-363, 2008.
35. Wirbel RJ, Schulte M, Mutschler WE. Surgical treatment of pelvic sarcomas: oncologic and functional outcomes. Clin Orthop Relat Res 390:190-205, 2001.
36. Baliski CR, Schachar NS, McKinnon JG, et al. Hemipelvectomy: a changing perspective for a rare procedure. Can J Surg 47:99-103, 2004.
37. Carter SR, Eastwood DM, Grimer RJ, et al. Hindquarter amputation for tumours of the musculoskeletal system. J Bone Joint Surg Br 72:490-493, 1990.
38. **Grimer RJ, Chandrasekar CR, Carter SR, et al. Hindquarter amputation: is it still needed and what are the outcomes? J Bone Joint Surg Br 95:127-131, 2013.**
39. Masterson EL, Davis AM, Wunder JS, et al. Hindquarter amputation for pelvic tumors. The importance of patient selection. Clin Orthop Relat Res 350:187-194, 1998.
40. Ziran BH, Smith WR, Rao N. Hemipelvic amputations for recalcitrant pelvic osteomyelitis. Injury 39:411-418, 2008.
41. Ham SJ, Schraffordt Koops H, Veth RP, et al. External and internal hemipelvectomy for sarcomas of the pelvic girdle: consequences of limb-salvage treatment. Eur J Surg Oncol 23:540-546, 1997.
42. Chan JW, Virgo KS, Johnso FE. Hemipelvectomy for severe decubitus ulcers in patients with previous spinal cord injury. Am J Surg 185:69-73, 2003.
43. Beck LA, Einertson MJ, Winemiller MH, et al. Functional outcomes and quality of life after tumor-related hemipelvectomy. Phys Ther 88:916-927, 2008.
44. Griesser MJ, Gillette B, Crist M, et al. Internal and external hemipelvectomy or flail hip in patients with sarcomas: quality-of-life and functional outcomes. Am J Phys Med Rehabil 91:24-32, 2012.

45. Carroll KM. Hip disarticulation and transpelvic amputation: prosthetic management. In Smith DG, Michael JW, Bowker JH, eds. Atlas of Amputations and Limb Deficiencies. Rosemont, IL: American Academy of Orthopaedic Surgeons, 2004.
46. Yari P, Dijkstra PU, Geertzen JHB. Functional outcome of hip disarticulation and hemipelvectomy: a cross-sectional national descriptive study in the Netherlands. Clin Rehabil 22:1127-1133, 2008.
47. **Janis JE, Ahmad J, Lemmon JA, et al. A 25-year experience with hemicorporectomy for terminal pelvic osteomyelitis. Plast Reconstr Surg 124:1165-1176, 2009.**
48. Gruman G, Michael JW. Translumbar amputation: prosthetic management. In Smith DG, Michael JW, Bowker JH, eds. Atlas of Amputations and Limb Deficiencies. Rosemont, IL: American Academy of Orthopaedic Surgeons, 2004.

Chapter 44

Reconstruction of the Sacroiliac Joint and Pelvis

Murat Pekmezci, Christopher P. Ames, Vedat Deviren

*T*umors of the sacrum are rare entities. However, they may incur significant morbidity and mortality. The diagnosis might be delayed for up to 6 years because of the increased accommodation of the pelvis.[1] Management of these tumors requires a multidisciplinary approach that includes a spine surgeon, plastic surgeon, vascular/colorectal surgeon, and oncologist. Therefore these patients should be treated at centers that specialize in treating musculoskeletal tumors. This chapter will focus on management of these lesions, with specific focus on reconstruction techniques.

ANATOMY AND BIOMECHANICS

Understanding the anatomy of the lumbosacral junction and pelvis is crucial for surgeons who manage sacral tumors. The sacrum is the keystone of the lumbosacral junction; it is a triangular bone that originates from five separate vertebrae fused along with the intervening intervertebral discs. The transverse lines that are observed at the ventral aspect of the sacrum represent these former disc spaces. The sacrum is triangular in shape with its apex aiming caudally. The base of the triangle forms the superior aspect of the sacrum. The dorsal surface of the sacrum is convex. The former spinous processes fuse and form the median crest. The facet joints also fuse and form intermediate crests. The laminae of the former vertebrae become the groove between the median and intermediate crests. There are four pairs of foramina posteriorly that allow passage of the dorsal sensory roots of the sacral nerves. Often the posterior elements of the fourth and fifth vertebrae are absent and form the sacral hiatus. The ventral surface of the sacrum is concave. There are four pairs of ventral sacral foramina that are located anterolaterally and at the level of the ventral ridges. The anterior divisions of the sacral nerves travel through these foramina. The vertebral bodies and the transverse processes then form the lateral masses of the sacrum.

The sacrum is attached to the iliac bones by means of sacroiliac joints. The stability of this articulation depends on the irregularity of the joint surfaces and mainly to the sacroiliac ligaments. The articulation spans the upper two sacral bodies. The ligaments that stabilize this joint involve anterior, posterior, and interosseous sacroiliac ligaments. The posterior ligaments are the strongest ligaments in the body and are primarily responsible for the stability of this junction. Sacrospinous and sacrotuberous ligaments are responsible for the rotational and vertical stability of the pelvis.

The lumbosacral junction is responsible for transfer of load from the spinal column to the lower extremities. The sacrum is a keystone of this equilibrium. Depending on the extent of the sacral resection, instrumentation of the lumbosacral junction might be necessary. Gunterberg et al[2] studied sacropelvic biomechanics in 1976. They sequentially increased the level of the transverse partial sacrectomy and loaded the specimens to failure. Partial sacrectomy at the level of the S1 foramen and mid–S1 body (1 cm below the promontory) resulted in 30% and 50% decreases in stability, respectively. These investigators concluded that patients could be allowed to bear weight, even after submaximal resection of the sacrum. On the other hand, Hugate et al[3] conducted a study where they loaded the specimens through the hip joints and used specimens from younger donors. These investigators showed that when the sacrum resection was performed above the S1 foramen (group I) and below the S1 foramen (group II), 75% and 84% of the sacroiliac joint was left intact, respectively. The load to failure was calculated as 2144N for group I and 1044N for group II. They reviewed the literature and calculated that the lumbosacral junction is subjected to a force of 2105N. They concluded that patients who had resections above the S1 foramen would require lumbopelvic reconstruction because the remaining pelvis could not carry normal loads. Recently Yu et al[4] studied the effects of transverse sacrectomy at different levels as U-S2 (S2-3 disc), U-1/2S2 (mid-S2 body), U-S1 (S1-2 disc), U-1/2S1 (above the S1 foramen), and right sacroiliac joint resection. The average sacroiliac joint area that remained intact was 75.2% after U-S1 and 27.7% after U-1/2S1. The rotational and compressive stiffness were similar to normal when the resection was made at mid-S2 body or lower, whereas the rotational stiffness was decreased without a change in compressive strength when the osteotomy was performed at U-S1. Both rotational and compressive stiffness decreased significantly when the osteotomy was carried out at the U-1/2S1 level. They recommended lumbopelvic reconstruction when the resection level was above the S1 foramen, because this resulted in a significant decrease in both rotational and compressive strength.

INDICATIONS AND CONTRAINDICATIONS
The common indications for partial or total sacrectomy include the following:
- Malignant tumors (primary or metastatic)
- Benign tumors (local aggressive)
- Osteomyelitis

The contraindications for sacrectomy include the following:
- Advanced-stage tumors with extensive local and systemic involvement
- Medically unstable patients who would not tolerate surgery

PREOPERATIVE EVALUATION
Physical Examination

Because there is a large potential space anterior to the sacrum, frequently the tumor reaches a considerable size by the time it causes symptoms. Therefore the delay in diagnosis ranges from 4 months to 6 years.[1] The most frequent presentation is low back pain caused by the mass effect of the lesion. As the tumor increases in size, radicular symptoms appear. Depending on the extent of involvement of the sacral nerve roots, patients may also complain of bowel and/or bladder symptoms, as well as sexual dysfunction. Extension of the tumor into the true pelvis may also interfere with rectal, bladder, and uterine function. Invasion of the piriformis and gluteus maximus muscles may cause pain and hip extension weakness. Finally, invasion of the sacroiliac joint results in severe pain with ambulation and even at rest.

Physical examination begins with an inspection to detect any skin involvement or visual mass effect in the posterior aspect of the sacrum. Palpation then follows to evaluate for tenderness over the sacrum or low back. Evaluation of the hip and sacroiliac joints is essential. Neurologic examination will help to determine whether a patient has weakness, reflex changes, or bowel/bladder dysfunction. The neurologic dysfunction is the result of either a pressure effect or direct invasion by the tumor. Depending on the region of the lumbosacral plexus that is involved, patients may have a variety of neurologic symptoms. The L5 nerve root is frequently involved at the extraforaminal region, and patients present with numbness on the outer aspect of the leg and foot and weakness on ankle dorsiflexion, big toe extension, knee flexion, and hip abduction. The S1 nerve root may be involved while it is coursing within the sacrum or in the presacral area. The manifestations include numbness on the bottom of the foot and weakness in ankle plantar flexion, knee flexion, and hip extension. A lesion of S2 would cause pain on the posterior aspect of the thigh, testicles, and labia and slight weakness in ankle plantar flexion. Pain in the outer thigh region, penis, and labia are typical of an S3 lesion, whereas pain in the inner perianal region and hyperesthesia reflects an S4-S5 lesion. Regarding bowel and bladder function, S3 is the key level. Unilateral lesions of S2 and S3 may cause mild bowel/bladder dysfunction. However, bilateral S2 or S3 lesions frequently cause significant bowel/bladder dysfunction.[5,6] Bilateral S4 or S5 lesions do not result in autonomic dysfunction. Several reflex changes can be seen, most commonly absence of ankle jerk, which is related to a disruption of afferent or efferent S1 root function. Pathology in afferent S1 or efferent S1 or S2 results in an absent plantar reflex. A lesion in the afferent or efferent S3 or S4 results in absence of a bulbocavernosus reflex. On the other hand, absence of anal reflex is related to a lesion in the S4 or S5 roots.

DIAGNOSTIC STUDIES

After a diagnosis of a sacral lesion, the next step is to obtain a histologic diagnosis, usually through a percutaneous biopsy. As is the case with all skeletal malignancies, biopsy of a lesion should ideally be planned and performed at the center where the definitive treatment will take place. Therefore it is important to refer these patients to a specialty center once the radiographic diagnosis has been made. Bergh et al[7] demonstrated that invasive diagnostic procedures or incomplete debulking surgery performed outside of major tumor centers were associated with an increased risk of local recurrence, as well as decreased survival. Because en bloc tumor resection with adequate margins is the only effective method for achieving long-term disease control or cure, management of these rare lesions should be performed at centers that have extensive experience with these lesions.

RADIOLOGIC STUDIES

Imaging of sacral pathologies usually requires computed tomography (CT) or magnetic resonance imaging (MRI). Conventional radiographs are insufficient for a variety of reasons. The sacrum is obscured because of the overlying bowel gas or stool, making interpretation of the images difficult. In addition, the sacrum does not have the distinctive trabecular pattern that can be assessed for disruption. Yet there are some landmarks that can be evaluated, such as the sacral foramina, which should be symmetrical. Sacroiliac joints should be visualized, as well as the iliac wings. Any irregularity or lucency in these regions should raise the question of a pathologic process. CT scans provide excellent resolution of the bony architecture and are frequently the next step in the evaluation of sacral pathologies. New multidetector CT scanners decrease the image acquisition time and radiation dose significantly. These scanners are very sensitive in determining the degree of destruction of the sacrum, and they are helpful in determining whether there is an impending fracture. On the other hand, MRI is the method of choice when there are associated neurologic symptoms. These images are helpful in determining the extent of a lesion, for example, whether it is extending beyond the presacral fascia or in association with nerve roots and other adjacent soft tissues. Bone scans are helpful in detecting distant metastases.

CLINICAL DECISION-MAKING
TREATMENT OPTIONS

The decision-making process depends on the location and extent of the lesion, and there are several questions that need to be answered. The first is the extent of resection. Although there is slight variation with regard to the nature of the individual tumor, the main goal is to achieve a wide resection with clean surgical margins. As has been discussed earlier in this chapter, local recurrence is directly correlated with surgical margins. *Wide resection* refers to excision of the tumor with normal tissue. Although resection of more normal soft tissue with the tumor will decrease the risk of local recurrence, the surgeon should balance the functional loss that is observed after this extensive resection with the intention to increase disease-free survival. Unfortunately, treatment of sacral tumors frequently results in significant morbidity. The sacral nerve roots distal to the level of resection should be ligated. Preservation of the L5 and S1 nerve roots, as well as the sciatic nerve, is a priority. However, if these structures pass through the tumor mass, they should also be sacrificed. At least 2 cm of normal bone should be resected to achieve wide resection margins. If there is invasion of the sacroiliac joint, then the adjacent portion of the ilium should also be resected. In addition, adjacent musculature should be included in the resection, particularly posterior structures, because it has been shown that the local recurrence rate is much higher in posterior than in anterior structures.[8] In cases of osteomyelitis, all of the infected sacrum should be resected, but the surgeon can be less aggressive in order to preserve function, and antibiotics can be used to treat residual infection.

The second question that should be answered is which approach to use. The options are a posterior-only approach versus an anteroposterior combined approach. Here the most important variable is the anterior extent of the tumor. Usually the presacral fascia is very strong and the tumor rarely invades past this natural barrier. If this fascia were invaded, then an anterior approach would become mandatory. Another indication for an anterior approach is the cephalad extent of the tumor. Usually, if the tumor is below S2, the surgeon can reach around both sides of the sacrum and dissect out the tumor from a posterior approach, as long as there is no invasion of the presacral fascia. If the tumor extends above S2, then anterior dissection through a posterior incision becomes more technically demanding, and a separate anterior dissection is strongly recommended. The anterior approach also allows preparation of a rectus flap to address the posterior soft tissue defect that remains after resection of the tumor.

The third question is whether pelvic stability would be lost and a lumbopelvic stabilization procedure would be necessary. Most of these tumors are below S2, and they can be treated by partial sacrectomy without destroying pelvic stability. As we discussed in the "Anatomy and Biomechanics" section, several biomechanical studies investigated the effects of sacrectomy at various levels, and the general consensus is when the resection is above the S1 foramen, reconstruction of the lumbosacral junction is recommended. The reconstruction techniques will be discussed in the following section.

CHOICE OF TECHNIQUE

There is no consensus on the optimal method of fixation after a total or subtotal sacrectomy that results in lumbopelvic instability. The first option is no instrumentation, which is favored by some investigators because of the high rate of infection that is observed with these lesions.[9,10] Patients remain recumbent for 2 to 3 months until sufficient scarring occurs to suspend the spinal column between the iliac wings. A lumbosacral orthosis has been to shown to decrease pain and improve mobility in these patients.[11] On the other hand, instrumentation allows earlier mobilization and enables the establishment of fusion between the pelvis and the lumbar spine. Parallel to advances in spinal implants, stronger constructs are now available to allow immediate weight-bearing after surgery. However, there is no gold standard, and it is recommended that surgeons use the construct with which they are most familiar.

Several techniques have been described for reconstructing the lumbosacral junction. Shikata et al[12] used two sacral bars that were attached to the lumbar spine by means of Harrington rods and massive autologous iliac crest and fibula grafts in two patients. Blatter et al[13] reported on the use of a construct in which two dynamic hip screws were inserted into the iliac wings and attached to an AO internal fixator in two patients. Both patients were ambulatory: one with assistive devices and one without.[13] Gokaslan et al[14] reported on the use of the Galveston technique in two patients after sacrectomy. Both patients had L3 ilium instrumentation with the Galveston L-rod technique, in addition to a threaded rod that connected the two iliac wings. One patient was ambulating unassisted, and the other was using a cane. Spiegel et al[15] modified this technique by exchanging the threaded rod for a pelvic reconstruction plate. Although the plate broke, the patient continued to have occasional back pain and was ambulatory with an ankle-foot orthosis. Santi et al[16] used Schanz pins that pass through the iliac wings and the L5 vertebral body and are later attached to the lumbar spine by means of rods and hooks. Their patient developed pseudarthrosis, and the hardware was removed. This patient later developed a stale painless pseudarthrosis between L5 and the ilium and was ambulating well with bilateral dynamic orthoses 2 years and 9 months after surgery. Tomita et al[17] used bars or AO plates to reconstruct the pelvis and then affixed it to the lumbar spine with Cotrel-Dubousset or Harrington rods. All three patient were ambulatory with the aid of a walker. Wuisman et al[18] used a custom-made prosthesis for a patient who had an extensive tumor that was invading bilateral iliac wings. The patient was ambulatory and pain free at 3 years' follow-up.[18]

A modified Galveston technique became popular over the past decade. This technique replaces the L-rod with one or two iliac screws that provide stronger fixation to the iliac crest.[19] McCord et al[20] compared 10 different lumbosacral fixation techniques and found that the strongest construct was medially directed iliac screws in combination with the Galveston-type iliac fixation. Kawahara et al[21] and Murakami et al[22] performed a finite element analysis on three different instrumentation systems. They compared the modified Galveston technique (two bilateral iliac screws), the triangular frame construct (two transiliac bars attached to spinal rods), and a new construct where L5 is translated distally and seated on the cephalad transiliac bar. They showed that there was excessive stress concentrated on the spinal rod between L5 and the iliac screws in the modified Galveston construct and at the iliac bar ileum junction in the triangular frame. They did not observe a particular stress concentration in the new construct where some load is transferred anteriorly. Kelly et al[23] recently tested a novel four-rod technique in an attempt to address the stress concentration observed at the rod between L5 and the iliac screws. They placed pedicle screws in a straight-ahead trajectory at L2 and L4, and a converging trajectory at L3 and L5, and placed separate rods into these different trajectories, which are connected to the ilium by one iliac screw. They reported one patient with no failure at 9 months.[23]

Mindea et al[24] reported on six patients in whom they used a titanium mesh cage, fixed by a transiliac bar underneath the L5 vertebral body, in addition to a modified Galveston instrumentation. All patients were ambulatory at discharge, which was, on average, 10 days after the procedure. Dickey et al[25] described another anterior column support in the form of fibular allografts that extend from the L5 body to the pelvic brim, as well as bilateral double iliac screws. They operated on nine patients, and seven of them were ambulating independently at the most recent follow-up. Newman et al[26] reported another modification of the triangular frame and used four iliac screws to attach the transiliac bars to the iliac wings. In addition, these investigators used carbon cages to achieve pelvic continuity. Based on the available biomechanical data, the most stable construct appears to be a modified Galveston instrumentation in association with an anterior column reconstruction would connect L5 to the ilium and participate in load transfer. This construct is also our preferred method of reconstruction.

TECHNIQUE

We prefer staged anterior release, osteotomy, if needed, and preparation of the vertical rectus abdominis myocutaneous (VRAM) flap, followed by posterior tumor resection and lumbopelvic reconstruction.

The first stage is performed in association with a vascular/colorectal surgeon and a plastic surgeon. The purpose of this stage is to dissect the anterior aspect of the tumor, ligate the vessels that supply the tumor, and prepare the VRAM flap.

The patient is positioned supine, and all of the bony landmarks are padded carefully. A midline laparotomy extending from the pubic symphysis to just above the umbilicus is performed. The dissection can be either retroperitoneal or transperitoneal. We prefer a transperitoneal approach because it provides the best exposure. The ureters and the iliac vessels are dissected bilaterally. The rectum is mobilized off of the tumor capsule. The tumor capsule is outlined taking special care not to violate it. Although every attempt is made to preserve the external iliac arteries, the internal iliac and middle sacral arteries are ligated if they are enclosed by the tumor. Encased iliac veins are mobilized to expose the osteotomy sites. The dissection should be carried down to the level of the greater sciatic notch, as well as laterally over the sacral ala, to expose the lumbosacral plexus. At this point an incomplete osteotomy can be performed at the intended level of the osteotomy to help the posterior-based osteotomy. If a total sacrectomy is planned, the L5-S1 disc should be removed. The anterior nerve roots are cut either as they exit the foramen or as they leave the tumor capsule. Bone wax is applied to the osteotomy sites to control the bleeding. A flexible, thin Silastic sheet be placed posterior to the vascular structures, the rectum, and anterior to the sacrum. This helps to prevent adhesions from forming and expedites the posterior stage. The prepared VRAM flap is placed in the pelvis. The abdominal wound is closed in layers, and a drain is placed.

Patients are positioned prone on a Jackson table with a four-poster frame. All of the bony prominences are carefully padded. A midline longitudinal incision is made from L2 down to the tip of the sacrum. The incision is modified so that any skin that is contaminated during the biopsy or involved by the tumor is resected along with the tumor. Based on preoperative MRI, the posterior musculature is left intact to enable en bloc resection of the tumor. Every attempt is made to avoid violating the tumor capsule. Posterior elements from the L3 to L5 vertebrae, posterior iliac spine, greater sciatic notch, and sciatic nerves are exposed. Depending on the intended level of resection, L5 or S1 laminectomy is performed. Sacral nerve roots are divided proximal to the intended level of resection, and the thecal sac is closed. The posterior sacroiliac ligaments and the sacrospinalis muscles are divided. The gluteus maximus is also partially divided through the tumor-free margin. Then the piriformis muscle and the superior gluteal and inferior gluteal vessels and nerves, along with the sciatic, pudendal, and posterior femoral cutaneous nerves, are identified. These neurovascular structures should be preserved whenever possible, whereas the piriformis muscle is divided at its musculotendinous junction. The sacrotuberous ligament is detached from the ischial tuberosity and the coccygeal muscles are cut, which is followed by resection of the sacrospinous ligaments. If the rectum is to be preserved, the anococcygeal ligament is released just proximal to the anal sphincter. If not, the anus is dissected circumferentially, and the levator muscle is also divided. Once the soft tissue dissection is completed, the osteotomies are finalized posteriorly, which circumferentially releases the sacrum. Finally, the entire sacrum is excised en bloc.

Depending on the extent of the resection and the surgeon's preference, one of the various spinopelvic reconstruction techniques is performed. Our preference is to uses double iliac screws posteriorly and titanium mesh cages anteriorly. After removal of the sacrum, bilateral pedicle screws are inserted from L3 to L5. Bilateral iliac screws are inserted into the posterior superior iliac spine. Then curved titanium mesh cages are inserted to serve as a buttress between the inferior endplate of L5 and the iliac wing. Small fragment screws are inserted through the cage into the iliac wing for supplemental fixation. The cages are filled with autograft/allograft. Then lumbar pedicle screw and iliac screws are connected by means of ¼-inch rods and transverse connectors.

Finally, the soft tissue coverage is addressed. Again various soft tissue coverage options have been described, but we prefer to use a VRAM flap. The flap that was prepared during the first stage is pulled through the defect. The skin is trimmed to fit the defect and sewn into the defect in layers.

OUTCOMES WITH EVALUATION OF RESULTS

Evaluation of the results of sacrectomy is difficult because most of the literature is dominated by patients with tumors where the outcome depends on tumor control and survival. Functional outcomes usually refer to bowel and bladder dysfunction, as well as ambulatory status. Sacrectomy affects ambulation depending on the extent of the neurologic deficit caused by the resection and reconstruction of the lumbopelvic junction. Bowel and bladder dysfunction is also dependent on the level of resection. Table 44-1 summarizes the selected articles in the literature that report on these outcomes.[27-32] Management of complications is discussed in the "Bailout Techniques" section.

Table 44-1 Sacrectomy Clinical Outcomes

Reference	No.	Follow-up	Survival	Ambulatory	Bowel and Bladder Dysfunction	Complications
Ramamurthy et al[32] (2009)	19	24 mo (range 2-240)	5-year survival 70%, 5-year disease-free survival 65%	All were ambulatory; no spinopelvic reconstruction	47%	58% had wound complications
Hulen et al[31] (2006)	16	5.5 yr	Four patients alive and disease free at 94.5 mo; six patients alive with disease at 55 mo	Only three ambulatory without assistive devices	15/16 dysfunctional	8 had wound complications
Fourney et al[30] (2005)	29	4.5 yr	Disease-free survival for chordoma 68 mo	All patients who underwent partial sacrectomy and unilateral sacroiliac joint resection were ambulatory	Seven patients who underwent low sacrectomy had normal function; one had stress incontinence; two patients with midsacrectomy had normal function and two had moderate dysfunction; 6-7 patients with high sacrectomy had severe dysfunction; 5-5 patients with total sacrectomy had complete dysfunction	Early complication rate 65%, late complication rate 10%
Guo et al[29] (2005)	50	N/A	N/A	One or more S1 sacrificed, 50% ambulatory; both S1 preserved, 76% ambulatory without assistance	25% bowel/bladder dysfunction if both S3 intact; 37.5% dysfunction if unilateral S3 intact; 75% dysfunction if both are not intact	
York et al[27] (1999)	27	3.6 yr (range 0.3-34)	Median overall survival time 7.4 yr	All patients remained ambulatory	20/27 bowel ± bladder dysfunction	
Bergh et al[28] (2000)	30	8.1 yr (range 0.2-23)	60% disease free at a mean of 8 yr	N/A	25/30 bladder/bowel problems	6/18 patients who had high sacral amputation had fractures

Many techniques have been discussed for reconstruction of the lumbopelvic junction. With the advances in instrumentation techniques, segmental spinal instrumentation is now the preferred technique. Biomechanical studies have shown that this type of reconstruction should include a posterior instrumentation augmented with an anterior column support. We prefer anterior titanium mesh cage reconstruction to restore the anterior column and posterior L3-ilium modified Galveston instrumentation with bilateral double iliac screws, because this is a more stable construct than the original Galveston technique that used a single rod or screw.

SIGNATURE CASES

A 56-year-old male who presented with a sacral cordoma that was involving S3-5 bodies (Fig. 44-1, *A*). He underwent anterior osteotomy of the sacrum, disection of the tumor and placement of a silastic sheet, followed by posterior partial sacrectomy below S2 without reconstruction (Fig. 44-1, *B* and *C*).

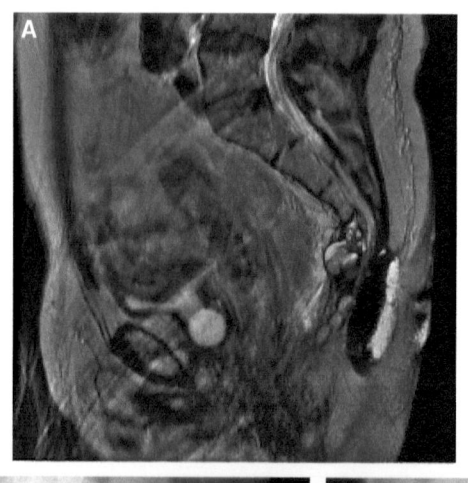

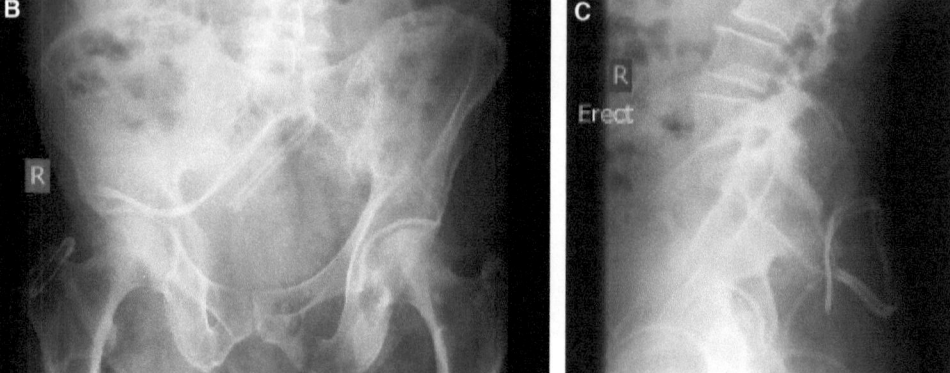

Fig. 44-1 Partial sacrectomy (ideally distal to S2). **A,** Preoperative MRI. **B,** Postoperative AP radiograph. **C,** Postoperative lateral radiograph.

A 77-year-old female presenting with a sacral cordoma originating from S2 body (Fig. 44-2, *A* and *B*). She had staged, anterior dissection, slastic sheet placement followed by posterior en-bloc resection and L3-ilium posterior instrumentation and cage reconstruction (Fig. 44-2, *C* and *D*).

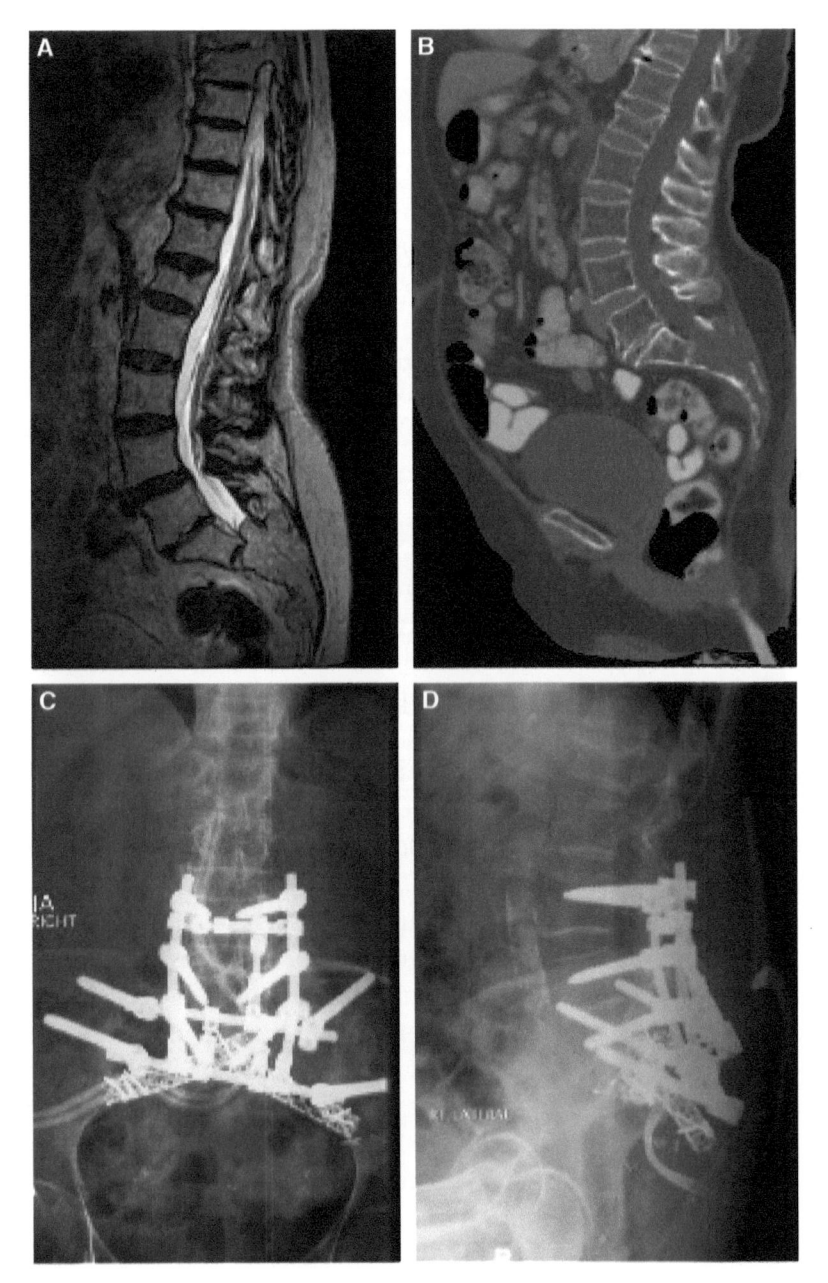

Fig. 44-2 Complete sacrectomy with reconstruction follow-up in 1 year. **A,** Preoperative pelvic MRI. **B,** Preoperative pelvic CT. **C,** Postoperative AP radiograph. **D,** Postoperative lateral radiograph.

CONCLUSION

Sacral tumors are rare but result in significant morbidity and mortality. The long-term outcome mandates wide resection, which frequently results in instability at the lumbopelvic junction. Reconstruction options range from no instrumentation to combined anterior and posterior reconstruction. There is no gold standard for the reconstruction technique, but current implant systems allow surgeons to create constructs that would allow early mobilization.

BAILOUT TECHNIQUES

INSTRUMENTATION

- Many techniques have been described for reconstruction of the lumbopelvic junction. Evaluation of preoperative imaging studies and detailed surgical planning would prevent surprises most of the time. Inadequate fixation can be balanced by delayed weight-bearing. Hardware failure, and the resulting pseudarthrosis, usually requires revision based on the individual characteristics of the reconstruction and bone stock, but in challenging cases instrumentation can be totally eliminated, as has been defined by several investigators.[9-11]

SOFT TISSUE COVERAGE

- Because wide resection is essential to reduce the risk of local recurrence, patients are left with a large defect after resection of sacral tumors. Several options exist for soft tissue coverage, such as bilateral gluteal advancement flaps, gluteal rotation flaps, gluteal/posterior thigh flaps, free flaps, and VRAM flaps. Disruption of local vasculature during resection of the tumor also affects the blood supply of the local flaps. Gluteal flaps have good potential, but they may not provide sufficient bulk to fill the large defect, and the addition of omentum to these flaps has been reported to overcome this problem.[33] In addition, mobilization of gluteal muscles to cover the defect may adversely affect gait. The problem is irradiation, which leads to thinning of the epidermis, loss of pliability, obliterative endarteritis, and fibroblast damage.[34] Therefore it is more reasonable to use nonirradiated tissue rather than local tissue. Some investigators recommend the use of local gluteal flaps in patients with no preoperative pelvic radiation therapy and intact gluteal vessels. In patients who have undergone preoperative pelvic radiation therapy or have damaged gluteal vessels, vertical rectus flaps should be used. In patients with a history of previous abdominal surgery, free flaps should be used. We prefer to use VRAM flaps, which provide ample skin and soft tissue for coverage and do not require microvascular techniques.[35] Although rare, if sacral herniation develops, a mesh repair can be performed.[36]

TIPS FROM THE MASTERS

- Management of these tumors requires a multidisciplinary approach that includes a spine surgeon, plastic surgeon, vascular/colorectal surgeon, and oncologist. Therefore these patients should be treated at centers that specialize in treating musculoskeletal tumors.
- Diagnostic procedures or incomplete debulking surgery performed outside of major tumor centers were associated with an increased risk of local recurrence, as well as decreased survival.
- Reconstruction of the lumbosacral junction is recommended when the resection is performed above the S1 foramen.
- Overall sacrectomy caries significant perioperative morbidity, detailed discussion should be done with the patient and family for shared decision.

References (With Key References in Boldface)

1. Murphy AS, Chandawarkar RY, Horattas M. Sacrococcygeal chordoma: a high index of suspicion in low backache. Contemp Surg 57:617-620, 2001.
2. Gunterberg B, Romanus B, Stener B. Pelvic strength after major amputation of the sacrum. An experimental study. Acta Orthop Scand 47:635-642, 1976.
3. **Hugate RR Jr, Dickey ID, Phimolsarnti R, et al. Mechanical effects of partial sacrectomy: when is reconstruction necessary? Clin Orthop Relat Res 450:82-88, 2006.**
4. **Yu B, Zheng Z, Zhuang X, et al. Biomechanical effects of transverse partial sacrectomy on the sacroiliac joints: an in vitro human cadaveric investigation of the borderline of sacroiliac joint instability. Spine (Phila Pa 1976) 34:1370-1375, 2009.**
5. Todd LT Jr, Yaszemski MJ, Currier BL, et al. Bowel and bladder function after major sacral resection. Clin Orthop Relat Res 397:36-39, 2002.
6. Nakai S, Yoshizawa H, Kobayashi S, et al. Anorectal and bladder function after sacrifice of the sacral nerves. Spine (Phila Pa 1976) 25(17):2234-2239, 2000.
7. Bergh P, Gunterberg B, Meis-Kindblom JM, et al. Prognostic factors and outcome of pelvic, sacral, and spinal chondrosarcomas: a center-based study of 69 cases. Cancer 91:1201-1212, 2001.
8. Hanna SA, Aston WJ, Briggs TW, et al. Sacral chordoma: can local recurrence after sacrectomy be predicted? Clin Orthop Relat Res 466:2217-2223, 2008.
9. Wuisman P, Lieshout O, Sugihara S, et al. Total sacrectomy and reconstruction: oncologic and functional outcome. Clin Orthop Relat Res 381:192-203, 2000.
10. Stener B, Gunterberg B. High amputation of the sacrum for extirpation of tumors. Principles and technique. Spine 3:351-366, 1978.
11. Guo Y, Yadav R. Improving function after total sacrectomy by using a lumbar-sacral corset. Am J Phys Med Rehabil 81:72-76, 2002.
12. Shikata J, Yamamuro T, Kotoura Y, et al. Total sacrectomy and reconstruction for primary tumors. Report of two cases. J Bone Joint Surg Am 70:122-125, 1988.
13. Blatter G, Halter Ward EG, Ruflin G, et al. The problem of stabilization after sacrectomy. Arch Orthop Trauma Surg 114:40-42, 1994.
14. Gokaslan ZL, Romsdahl MM, Kroll SS, et al. Total sacrectomy and Galveston L-rod reconstruction for malignant neoplasms. Technical note. J Neurosurg 87:781-787, 1997.
15. Spiegel DA, Richardson WJ, Scully SP, et al. Long-term survival following total sacrectomy with reconstruction for the treatment of primary osteosarcoma of the sacrum. A case report. J Bone Joint Surg Am 81:848-855, 1999.

16. Santi MD, Mitsunaga MM, Lockett JL. Total sacrectomy for a giant sacral schwannoma. A case report. Clin Orthop Relat Res 294:285-289, 1993.
17. Tomita K, Tsuchiya H. Total sacrectomy and reconstruction for huge sacral tumors. Spine (Phila Pa 1976) 15:1223-1227, 1990.
18. Wuisman P, Lieshout O, van Dijk M, et al. Reconstruction after total en bloc sacrectomy for osteosarcoma using a custom-made prosthesis: a technical note. Spine (Phila Pa 1976) 26:431-439, 2001.
19. Gallia GL, Haque R, Garonzik I, et al. Spinal pelvic reconstruction after total sacrectomy for en bloc resection of a giant sacral chordoma. Technical note. J Neurosurg Spine 3:501-506, 2005.
20. McCord DH, Cunningham BW, Shono Y, et al. Biomechanical analysis of lumbosacral fixation. Spine (Phila Pa 1976) 17(8 Suppl):S235-S243, 1992.
21. Kawahara N, Murakami H, Yoshida A, et al. Reconstruction after total sacrectomy using a new instrumentation technique: a biomechanical comparison. Spine (Phila Pa 1976) 28:1567-1572, 2003.
22. Murakami H, Kawahara N, Tomita K, et al. Biomechanical evaluation of reconstructed lumbosacral spine after total sacrectomy. J Orthop Sci 7:658-664, 2003.
23. Kelly BP, Shen FH, Schwab JS, et al. Biomechanical testing of a novel four-rod technique for lumbo-pelvic reconstruction. Spine (Phila Pa 1976) 33:E400-E406, 2008.
24. **Mindea SA, Salehi SA, Ganju A, et al. Lumbosacropelvic junction reconstruction resulting in early ambulation for patients with lumbosacral neoplasms or osteomyelitis. Neurosurg Focus 15:E6, 2003.**
25. Dickey ID, Hugate RR Jr, Fuchs B, et al. Reconstruction after total sacrectomy: early experience with a new surgical technique. Clin Orthop Relat Res 438:42-50, 2005.
26. Newman CB, Keshavarzi S, Aryan HE. En bloc sacrectomy and reconstruction: technique modification for pelvic fixation. Surg Neurol 72:752-756; discussion 756, 2009.
27. York JE, Kaczaraj A, Abi-Said D, et al. Sacral chordoma: 40-year experience at a major cancer center. Neurosurgery 44:74-79; discussion 79-80, 1999.
28. Bergh P, Kindblom LG, Gunterberg B, et al. Prognostic factors in chordoma of the sacrum and mobile spine: a study of 39 patients. Cancer 88:2122-2134, 2000.
29. **Guo Y, Palmer JL, Shen L, et al. Bowel and bladder continence, wound healing, and functional outcomes in patients who underwent sacrectomy. J Neurosurg Spine 3:106-110, 2005.**
30. **Fourney DR, Rhines LD, Hentschel SJ, et al. En bloc resection of primary sacral tumors: classification of surgical approaches and outcome. J Neurosurg Spine 3:111-122, 2005.**
31. Hulen CA, Temple HT, Fox WP, et al. Oncologic and functional outcome following sacrectomy for sacral chordoma. J Bone Joint Surg Am 88:1532-1539, 2006.
32. Ramamurthy R, Bose JC, Muthusamy V, et al. Staged sacrectomy—an adaptive approach. J Neurosurg Spine 11:285-294, 2009.
33. Diaz J, McDonald WS, Armstrong M, et al. Reconstruction after extirpation of sacral malignancies. Ann Plast Surg 51:126-129, 2003.
34. Yeh KA, Hoffman JP, Kusiak JE, et al. Reconstruction with myocutaneous flaps following resection of locally recurrent rectal cancer. Am Surg 61:581-589, 1995.
35. Glatt BS, Disa JJ, Mehrara BJ, et al. Reconstruction of extensive partial or total sacrectomy defects with a transabdominal vertical rectus abdominis myocutaneous flap. Ann Plast Surg 56:526-530; discussion 530-531, 2006.
36. Al-Haddad AA, Hellinger MD, Akerman SC. Surgisis mesh repair of a postsacrectomy perineal hernia along with posterior proctosigmoidectomy for concomitant stricture. Am Surg 73:1129-1132, 2007.

Chapter 45

Sacral Resection

Joyce Ho, Julio Garcia-Aguilar

*T*umors of the sacrum and the presacral region are relatively uncommon. Primary, benign, or malignant tumors of the sacrum account for less than 7% of all intraspinal primary tumors. Recurrent or metastatic tumors, multiple myeloma, and lymphoma are more common than primary sacral tumors. Many of the primary tumors are low grade, with a low tendency to metastasize, and are relatively resistant to radiation or chemotherapy. Most recurrent tumors have previously been treated with chemotherapy and radiation therapy before they invade the sacrum. Therefore, for most patients with tumors involving the sacrum, surgery is the primary, and often the only, form of treatment. Untreated sacral and presacral tumors tend to involve nerves and adjacent vascular, urologic, and gastrointestinal structures, causing significant morbidity. A cure for these locally invasive tumors of the sacrum would require complete resection under experienced hands. Because of the anatomic complexity of the region, a sacrectomy, with or without posterior or total pelvic exenteration, is a formidable operation that is best performed at a referral center by a specialized multidisciplinary team.

ANATOMY

The sacrum is composed of five fused vertebrae in adults. It is a large, triangular, wedge-shaped bone that is situated between the hip bones and forms the roof and posterosuperior wall of the posterior pelvic cavity. It articulates with the L5 vertebral body above (lumbosacral joint), the coccyx below (sacrococcygeal joint), and the ilium laterally (sacroiliac joint). The lumbosacral joint consists of articulation of the L5 and S1 vertebrae at the anterior intervertebral joint and at two posterior zygapophysial joints (facet joints) between the articular processes of these vertebrae. The sacrococcygeal joint is made up of fibrocartilage and ligaments that join the apex of the sacrum to the base of the coccyx. The sacroiliac joint is a strong weight-bearing synovial joint that connects the articular surfaces of the sacrum and ilium and ends at level S2 of the spinal cord. The sacroiliac joint plays the major role of anchoring the spine to the pelvis. Therefore resection of the S1 and S2 vertebrae destabilizes the pelvis.

The blood supply to the sacrum mainly derives from the median and lateral sacral arteries, which are branches of the internal iliac artery (Fig. 45-1). Presacral tumors often derive their major vascular supply from these arteries. The internal iliac arteries diverge from the common iliac arteries acutely and diverge caudally and dorsally into the pelvis. Their first major branches are the iliolumbar arteries. One or more lateral sacral arteries are the next branches of the internal iliac artery. They take a paramedian course on top of the piriformis muscle and in close relation to the anterior sacral foramina. The superior gluteal artery is the next and largest branch of the internal iliac artery. It courses posteriorly to penetrate the upper aspect of the sacral plexus at its exit from the pelvis through the greater sciatic foramen. The inferior gluteal artery intersects the lower sacral plexus in its path out of the greater sciatic foramen between the piriformis and coccygeal muscles. These arteries may need to be sacrificed during sacral resection.

Venous anatomy generally parallels arterial anatomy but is subject to a high degree of variability. Two common variations are the drainage of the middle sacral vein into the left common iliac vein rather than into the vena cava and the drainage of the iliolumbar veins into the common iliac veins rather than into the internal iliac vein.

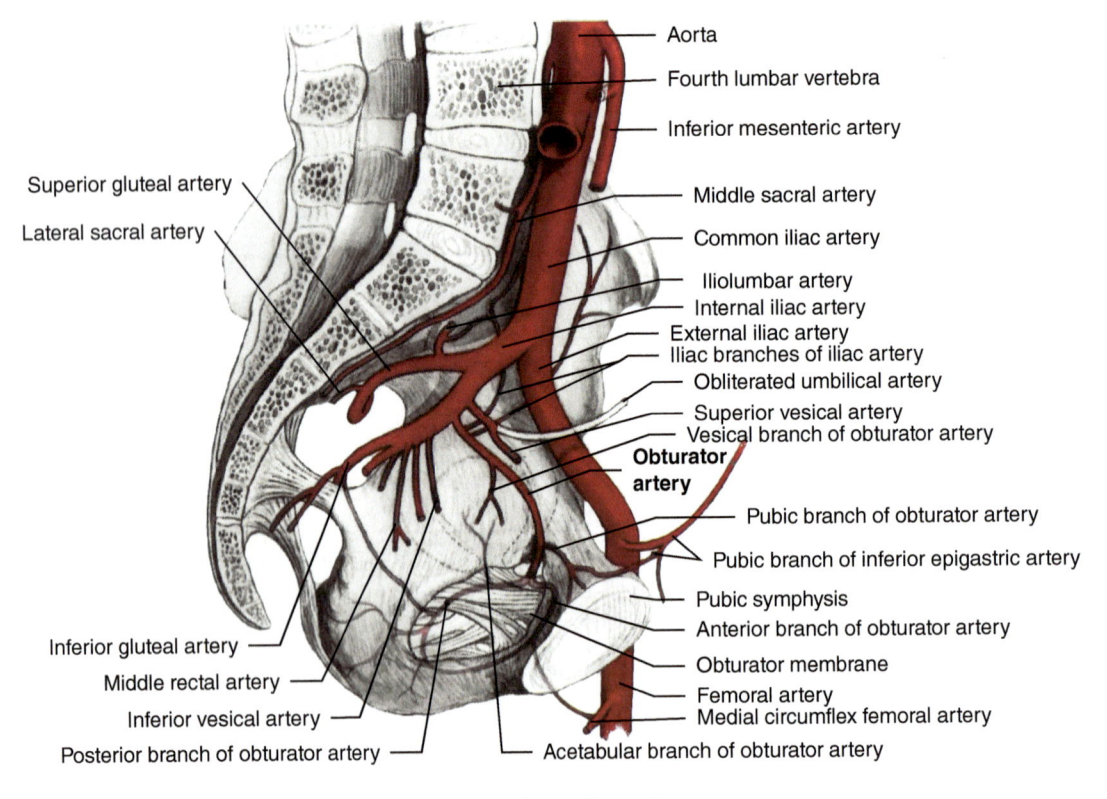

Fig. 45-1 Arterial supply to the sacrum.

The sacral plexus primarily derives from the lumbosacral trunk (the conjoined L4 and L5 roots), which courses caudally and laterally over the sacral alae (Fig. 45-2). The two most proximal branches of the sacral plexus are the superior and inferior gluteal nerves. The most important derivatives of the sacral plexus are the sciatic and pudendal nerves. The sciatic nerve is formed by the ventral rami of L4 to S3 that converge on the anterior surface of the piriformis. The articular branches of the sciatic nerve distribute to the hip joint, and its muscular branches innervate the flexors of the knee and thigh and all muscles in the leg and foot. Medial and caudal to the sacral plexus, branches of the anterior rami of S2 to S4 join to form the pudendal nerve. The pudendal nerve innervates the coccygeal and levator muscles of the pelvic floor, as well as the external anal sphincter. It is responsible for sensation to the genitals and innervates the muscular branches to the perineal muscles, external urethral sphincter, and external anal sphincter. The often ill-defined coccygeal plexus derives from the S4 and S5 nerve roots and the coccygeal roots and is responsible for perianal sensation.

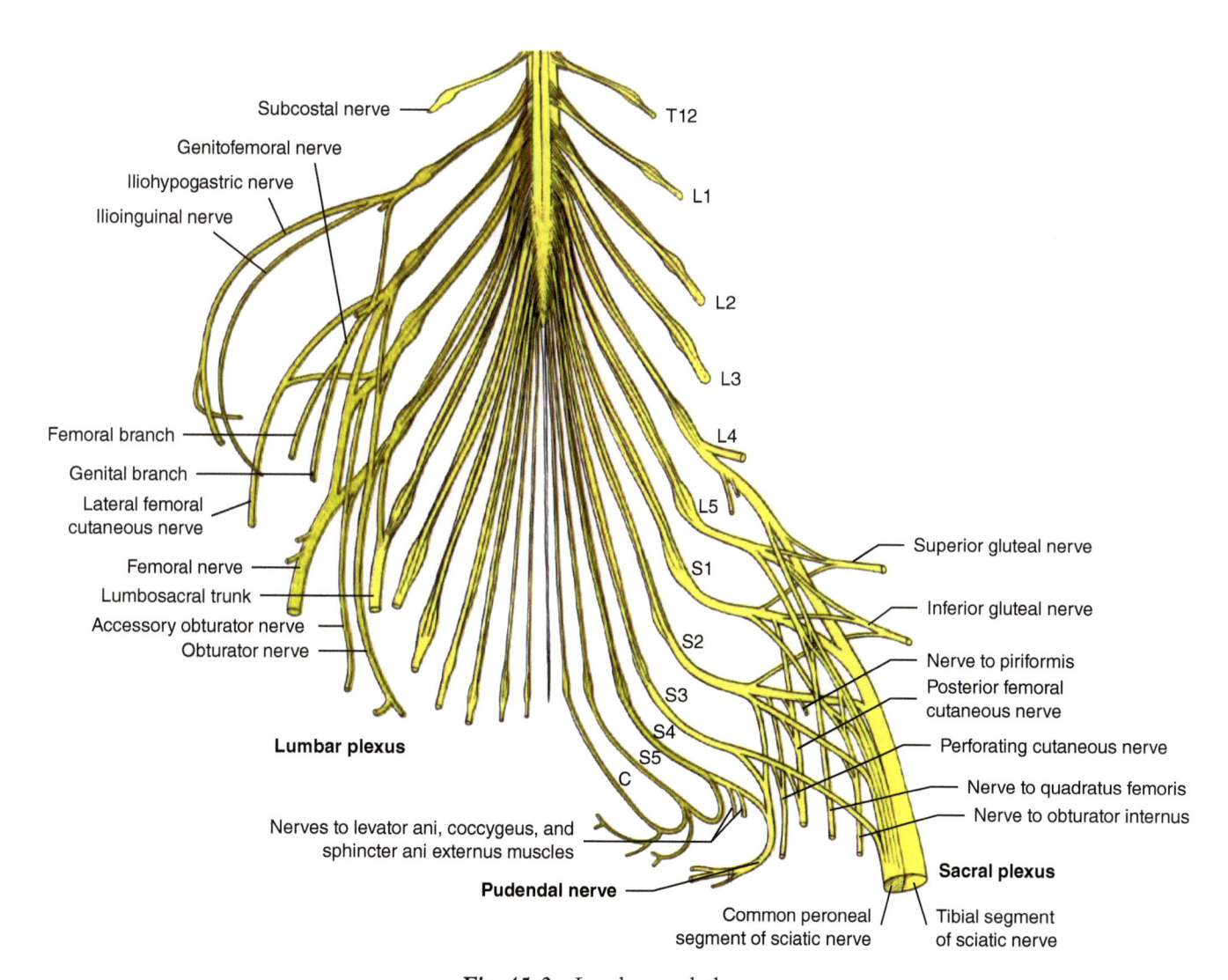

Fig. 45-2 Lumbosacral plexus.

The sympathetic system is important to male fertility because it coordinates reflexes for ejaculation. The parasympathetic system provides motor innervation to the detrusor muscle of the bladder and is primarily responsible for the vascular reflexes that sustain erectile function. The sympathetic and parasympathetic nerves have an intimate relationship with the sacrum. The superior epigastric plexus, also known as the presacral nerve, is situated in the midline from the bifurcation of the aorta to the promontory of the sacrum. In the area above, the plexus is formed by the condensation of the sympathetic lumbar nerves. Below, the plexus divides into the right and left hypogastric nerves that run from medial to lateral and distally to join the inferior hypogastric plexus. The hypogastric nerves contribute the sympathetic fiber to the inferior hypogastric plexus, while the parasympathetic fibers originate from the second, third, and fourth sacral segments of the spinal cord. The inferior hypogastric plexus is located laterally outside the rectum and the urogenital organs.

PATHOLOGY

The posterior pelvis includes the rectum, the retrorectal or presacral space, and the sacrum. It is an area where the neuroectoderm, the notochord, the hindgut, and the proctodeum undergo remodeling and regression in embryologic life. It can thus be the site of a heterogeneous group of benign and malignant tumors originating from vestigial tissue derived from the three germinal layers. These tumors are usually classified as congenital, inflammatory, neurogenic, osseous, or miscellaneous. According to the combined experience of seven different published series, 63% are congenital lesions, 10% are neurogenic, 8% are inflammatory, 7% are osseous, and 12% are miscellaneous. In all, 30% to 45% are malignant. The risk of malignancy is higher for solid tumors (60%) than for cystic lesions (10%). The relative frequencies of sacral and presacral tumors are different in children, in whom teratomas and myelomeningoceles are most common.

Primary pelvic malignancies involving the sacrum are rare, accounting for 1% to 7% of all spine tumors. These include chordoma, chondrosarcoma, some giant cell tumors, and Ewing's sarcoma. In addition, locally advanced rectal cancer has become one of the more common surgical indications for sacrectomy.

CONGENITAL TUMORS

The most common congenital tumor is a developmental cyst that often contains columnar or transitional epithelium (tailgut cysts or mucus-secreting cysts) or squamous epithelium with (dermoid cysts) or without (epidermoid cysts) skin appendages. These tumors are frequently asymptomatic; they are most commonly diagnosed in middle-aged women, and rarely undergo malignant transformation. Congenital tumors that can involve the sacrum are chordomas and teratomas.

CHORDOMAS

Chordomas are rare neoplasms that originate from notochordal remnants. They represent less than 3% of all primary bone tumors, but 50% are located in the retrorectal area. They affect individuals in the sixth and seventh decades of life and are more common in men. Men are affected twice as frequently as women. These tumors are slow growing and locally invasive into bone and surrounding soft tissues, and metastasize in 15% to 35% of patients. Chordomas are the most common primary malignant sacral neoplasms, accounting for 20% to 34% of neoplasms.

A dull pain in the buttock or lumbar area is usually the initial manifestation. Constipation, bladder dysfunction, and neurologic deficits in the lower extremities are late symptoms. Most chordomas are palpable by digital examination. Most patients have radiographic evidence of bone destruction, trabeculation, or calcification. Computed tomography (CT) and magnetic resonance imaging (MRI) provide an accurate assessment of the size and extent.

Chordomas are lobulated gelatinous tumors with areas of hemorrhage, cystic changes, or calcification. Histologically they contain cell aggregates separated by stromal tissue. In the center of the tumor, cords of cells with poorly defined boundaries appear to be floating in mucus. The physaliferous cells, which are large vacuolated cells, are pathognomonic.

TERATOMAS

Teratomas are true neoplasms originating in totipotent cells that are abnormally present in sequestered midline embryonic rests. Teratomas contain recognizable mature or immature elements representative of more than one germ layer. The sacrococcygeal area is the most frequent site of teratomas in infancy, occurring in 1 of 35,000 to 40,000 births. In adults sacrococcygeal teratomas are rare and are likely to be congenital. Teratomas in infancy are externally visible in most patients, but sacrococcygeal teratomas in adults are mostly confined to the retrorectal space. They are often cystic, although they may also be solid. Microscopically, teratomas contain a variety of tissues from more than one germ layer. Depending on the differentiation of their components, teratomas are classified as mature, immature, or malignant. Mature teratomas contain mature epithelial and mesenchymal tissues. Immature teratomas have areas of primitive endoderm, mesoderm, and ectoderm mixed with more mature elements. Malignant teratomas contain tissue of germ cell origin, such as embryonic tissue, germinoma, and choriocarcinoma. Teratomas that contain malignant non–germ cell elements, presumably derived from somatic tissue within the teratoma, are called teratomas with malignant transformation. Most teratomas in infancy and childhood are benign. In the pediatric population malignant teratomas tend to develop with increasing age. However, most teratomas in adults are benign.

Sacrococcygeal pain and perianal drainage are common symptoms, but some tumors are incidentally discovered during physical examination. Radiographic evidence of bone destruction is uncommon. Calcification inside the tumor is present in one fourth of the tumors. A pelvic CT or MRI scan helps confirm the diagnosis and extension inside the pelvis.

NEUROGENIC TUMORS

The most common neurologic tumors are schwannomas, neurofibromas, ependymomas, and ganglioneuromas. Two thirds of these tumors are benign. The most common neurogenic tumors in the sacrum are schwannomas. Sacral schwannomas and neurofibromas are intradural extramedullary masses that tend to grow within the sacral canal and only rarely expand through the anterior sacral foramina into the presacral space. Ependymomas arise from the ependymal cell clusters within the terminal filum and expand into the sacral canal. Ganglioneuromas are rare slow-growing tumors arising from sympathetic ganglion cells, and they can arise anywhere from the base of the skull to the pelvis. They are considered the benign counterpart of neuroblastomas. Neurogenic tumors developing in the retrorectal space can reach a large size before they become symptomatic. Local pain, with or without radicular lumbosacral radiation, is the most common presenting symptom. Sensorimotor and sphincter dysfunction usually follows. Tumors arising inside the spinal canal can cause devastating neurologic deficits. Complete resection is often curative.

OSSEOUS TUMORS

The variety and biological behavior of osseous tumors in the sacrum are similar to that of bone tumors elsewhere in the body. Giant cell tumors are the second most common tumors of the sacrum after chordomas. Although they are often found in long bones, typically in the distal femur, proximal tibia, and distal radius, up to 8% of giant cell tumors are located in the sacrum. Giant cell tumors are composed of osteoclastic giant cells within a spindle cell stroma. These tumors are generally benign; however, local malignant transformation has been reported in up to 16% of patients, and lung metastases have been found in 3% to 12% of patients. Giant cell tumors are commonly located in the proximal sacrum and are usually large, ranging from 5 to 11 cm at the time of diagnosis. They may also extend across the sacroiliac joint. Other osseous tumors, including osteomas, simple bone cysts, chondrosarcomas, osteosarcomas, Ewing's sarcomas, and aneurysmal bone cysts, can be found in the sacrum. Their clinical presentation is often characterized by progressive localized pain with radicular lumbosacral radiation, sensorimotor dysfunction, anal or urinary sphincter dysfunction, or constipation as a result of a direct effect of the mass on the rectum.

SECONDARY TUMORS

The sacrum can be secondarily involved either by hematogenous metastasis from distant tumors or by locally advanced or recurrent pelvic tumors, such as rectal, anal, or cervical cancer.

METASTATIC TUMORS

Metastatic tumors are the most common malignancies in the sacrum. Carcinomas that most frequently metastasize to the sacrum include breast, lung, prostate, renal cell, and gastrointestinal cancer, as well as multiple myeloma and thyroid cancer. Breast cancer is the most common cancer to metastasize to the sacrum. Presentation of metastatic disease in the sacrum typically involves an insidious onset of lower back pain and radiculopathy in the lower extremities. The onset of symptoms may be acute, compared with primary tumors, because of the aggressive invasive behavior of most metastatic lesions. Although most primary sacral tumors are treated by extensive surgical resection with curative intent, in cases of metastatic malignancies the chance for complete cure is often slim, and treatment is typically palliative. Combinations of surgical resection, debulking with adjuvant chemotherapy plus radiation therapy, or radiation alone, are reasonable treatment options.

RECURRENT OR LOCALLY ADVANCED PELVIC TUMORS

Although a primary locally advanced rectal cancer could potentially penetrate the presacral space and invade the sacrum, in most cases the sacrum is involved by recurrent disease or metastasis to the pelvic nodes. Most recurrences of rectal cancer are located within 1 cm of the previous anastomosis. They begin in the perirectal fat and are predominantly posterior, suggesting development from tumor deposits in lymph nodes left in portions of the mesorectum that were not removed during surgery. Consequently the posterior central pelvis is the most frequent place for a recurrence, surpassing the anterior central and lateral pelvis. The tendency for rectal cancer to recur in the posterior bony pelvis is associated with up to 30% sacral and coccyx involvement.

Pelvic recurrence of rectal cancer often presents with extensive local invasion, necessitating resection of adjacent structures or total pelvic exenteration and, in cases of posterior disease, requires resection of the sacrum. Although the sacrum is directly involved in less than 50% of cases, part of the sacrum may need to be resected en bloc to obtain negative margins.

DIAGNOSIS

The most common symptom of sacral and presacral tumors is a dull ache or pain located in the lower back or sacrococcygeal area. The pain may be the result of direct erosion of the bone or nerve compression. However, given the slow growth of some of these tumors and the capacity of the sacral canal and the pelvic cavity, tumors can reach a large size before becoming symptomatic. Some tumors, in particular some slow-growing teratomas, may be asymptomatic and are discovered incidentally during a routine physical examination.

Neurologic deficits arising from sacral tumors are caused by either compression of the sacral roots or direct involvement of the sacral plexus within the pelvis or the sciatic nerve near its exit from the pelvis. The most common neurologic deficits are loss of bowel and bladder control, as well as lower extremity weakness. Involvement of the S1 nerve root causes weakness in the gastrocnemius muscle and decreased plantar flexion at the ankle, whereas tumors sparing the S1 nerve root often present with perineal numbness, bowel and bladder incontinence, and sexual dysfunction.

A complete history and physical examination are mandatory. Many primary or secondary sacral and presacral tumors can be reached by digital rectal examination. They typically resemble a hard, fixed mass. Sexual function, bladder function, and bowel function should be clearly documented, because deficits may result after sacrectomy.

DIAGNOSTIC STUDIES

Sacral and presacral tumors may be indicated by radiographic evidence of bone destruction or ectopic calcification, but these findings are commonly overlooked on plain radiographs. CT and MRI are the imaging modalities of choice for diagnosing these tumors. CT scans with intravenous contrast enhancement provide excellent anatomic resolution, demonstrate bony details, and show areas of tumor calcification (Fig. 45-3, *A*). In addition to cross-sectional images, the new generation of CT scans also provides coronal and sagittal images that are particularly useful for detecting tumors located in the sacrum and for planning surgery. However, it is difficult to distinguish primary lesions from secondary lesions solely on the basis of CT findings. MRI scans have a higher resolution for assessing associated soft tissue masses, and the extent of bony destruction can also be better ascertained on MRI scans.

The various primary tumors of the sacrum have a particular appearance on CT and MRI scans. For example, giant cell tumors are frequently heterogeneous because of the presence of necrosis, hemorrhage, or cystic spaces. Low signal intensity on T2-weighted images is characteristic and is a result of the high hemorrhagic and fibrotic content of these tumors. Malignant tumors such as chordomas often show large lytic lesions, centered in the midline, with an associated soft tissue mass. Calcification is present in 30% to 70% of patients. Chordomas are isointense or hypointense on T1-weighted images and are typically hyperintense on T2-weighted images. These findings are characteristic of mucin accumulation within the tumor.

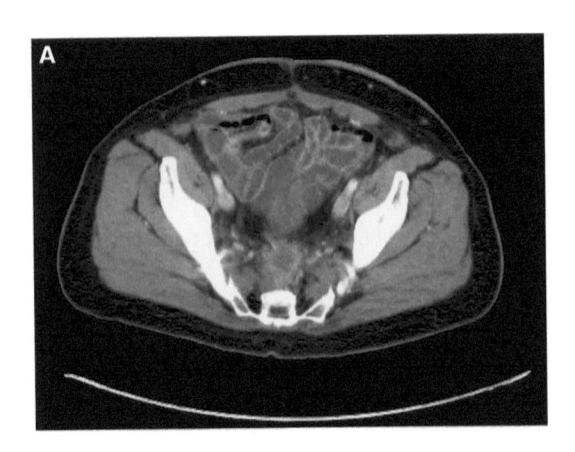

Fig. 45-3 **A,** CT scan from a patient with rectal cancer involving the sacrum above S2. This patient's disease was deemed unresectable.

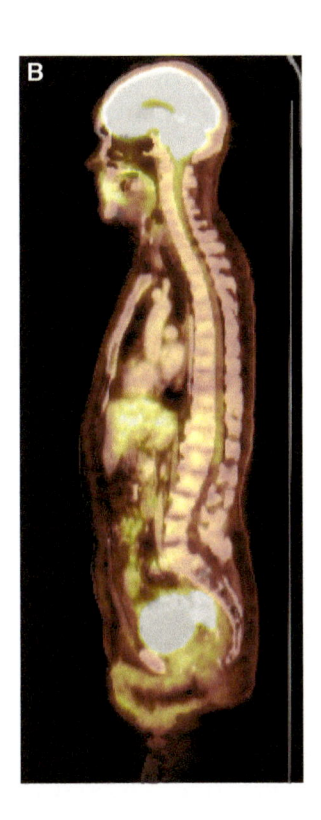

Fig. 45-3, cont'd **B,** Sagittal PET scan from the same patient showing high involvement of the sacrum.

Although CT and MRI are the mainstay diagnostic imaging modalities, other radiographic adjuncts may also be helpful. Positron emission tomography (PET) or PET-CT can be used for bone scans and is useful in evaluating distant disease and organ involvement (Fig. 45-3, *B*). Radionuclide bone scans may be useful for detecting bone destruction and assessing patients with metastatic lesions.

Flexible sigmoidoscopy or cystoscopy may help exclude rectal or bladder involvement. An intravenous pyelogram may also help define the relationship of the tumor to the ureters. In special situations an angiogram may be necessary to define the relationship between the tumor and the iliac vessels.

Biopsy

The differential diagnosis of solid tumors involving the sacrum or presacral space is extensive, and a precise histologic diagnosis may be useful in determining the treatment plan. Except for very superficial posterior tumors, the method of choice is a percutaneous biopsy performed under CT guidance. The skin entry should be located in the midline in an area that could be removed during the definitive operation. A tattoo mark at the entry site may help locate that site at the time of surgery. Transrectal biopsies should be avoided, except in rare cases where the tumor infiltrates the rectal wall.

INDICATIONS AND CONTRAINDICATIONS

Radical resection is often the only hope for cure of primary sacral malignancies. For most primary tumors of the sacrum, complete resection is advocated. In the case of chordomas, en bloc excision is the treatment of choice. The disease-free survival is largely determined by the extent of surgical resection. A radical wide margin, including the posterior margin of the gluteal muscle and at least one whole sacral segment beyond the area of gross disease, is recommended whenever possible. Schwannomas and neurofibromas are often confined to the sacral canal and can be resected completely using a posterior approach. For giant cell tumors, the most common osseous tumor of the sacrum, en bloc excision is the treatment of choice. However, complete resection is challenging because most giant cell tumors are large and involve the upper sacral segments, frequently abutting or extending beyond the sacroiliac joint. These tumors are large and hypervascular and usually involve necrosis, hemorrhage, and cystic spaces. Selective arterial embolization has been advocated to palliate symptoms or to downsize the tumor preoperatively. Total sacrectomy is also appropriate in some cases.

In the setting of metastatic disease, the prognosis is often far more dismal. For metastatic disease to the sacrum, including breast, lung, prostate, renal cell, and gastrointestinal cancers, multiple myeloma, and thyroid cancer, treatment is often palliative. Therefore surgical resection may only be indicated for palliative purposes, and patients may be treated with chemotherapy or radiation alone.

For local recurrences or locally advanced pelvic tumors involving the sacrum, most patients have already undergone chemotherapy or radiation, with or without a significant response. Therefore complete surgical resection is the only hope for a cure, provided there is absence of distant metastatic disease. Pelvic exenteration is often necessary, along with partial sacrectomy, to achieve negative resection margins.

In patients with metastatic or recurrent disease, sacrectomy may only be indicated in disease limited to the posterior bony pelvis and involving no higher than level S2 to S3 to preserve neurologic function (see Fig. 45-3). Lateral pelvic involvement, including the ureter, iliac vessels, and pelvic side wall, usually equate to unresectability. Involvement of the sciatic nerve is also a contraindication, because the morbidity resulting from resection of the nerve is too great. Distant metastasis must be ruled out, and candidates for sacrectomy should have a reasonable life expectancy, considering the significant morbidity associated with the operation.

CLINICAL DECISION-MAKING

Once an appropriate patient is selected, a multidisciplinary team approach to surgical planning is recommended. General oncologic surgeons, neurosurgeons, urologists, and plastic surgeons may all take part in the preoperative planning, execution, and reconstruction of an operation that is often technically challenging and requires extensive resources.

PREOPERATIVE PLANNING

A logical sequence of operative decision-making must be undertaken to optimize surgical success. Based on careful preoperative analysis of imaging studies and the level of sacral involvement, the level of clear margin resection should be determined. The level of division of the sacrum is also critically important because it has functional consequences.

The sacrectomy can be categorized as high or low according to the relationship between the level of the transection and the sacroiliac joint. High sacral resection involves removal of S1 and S2. High sacrectomies can be total, when both the S1 and S2 vertebrae are removed, or partial, when only a portion of the upper sacrum is removed. A high sacrectomy is a formidable operation because of the complexity of the surgical approach, the need to control large vessels with the potential for blood loss, the impact on the stability of the pelvis often requiring spinopelvic reconstruction, and the need to reconstruct a large soft tissue defect. Low sacrectomy involves the removal of S3 to S5 and has a minimal impact on the stability of the pelvis. A sacrectomy can be defined as simple when the sacrum is the only organ removed. In a complex sacrectomy the sacrum is resected en bloc with other pelvic organs. When tumor involvement of the rectum, ureter, bladder, or uterus is recognized preoperatively, the appropriate specialists should be consulted and involved in planning the resection and reconstruction.

SURGICAL TECHNIQUE

Selected small distal sacral tumors not involving the mesorectum can be fully mobilized and resected with a pure posterior approach. For most primary sacral tumors, even those that do not involve other pelvic structures, and for most recurrent tumors, a two-stage anterior and posterior approach is necessary. The abdominal approach, with the patient in a lithotomy position, is carried out first to mobilize and expose the anterior, lateral, and inferior margins of the tumor along with the involved organs. This is followed by a posterior approach, with the patient in the prone jackknife position, to perform the laminectomy and remove the sacrum in an en bloc fashion. The dual approach can often be performed on the same day, but in certain special circumstances it can be carried out as a staged procedure on two different days, 24 to 72 hours apart.

When indicated, ureteral stents should be placed at the beginning of the operation to facilitate intraoperative identification of the ureters. The patient is positioned in a modified low lithotomy position with legs in Allen stirrups. This position allows access to the rectum and vagina to help evaluate the relationship of the tumor to these structures. A midline incision is created and the abdominal cavity is entered. The presence of metastatic disease is excluded and the tumor is located by palpation.

For primary sacral tumors the location of the tumor should be assessed in relation to adjacent structures, such as the rectum, ureter, and hypogastric vessels. When the rectum or mesorectum is not involved, sacral tumors can be separated from the mesorectum by entering the areolar space behind the superior rectal vessels at the level of the promontory and following this plane along the presacral fascia. This approach requires opening the pelvic peritoneum on both sides of the rectum all the way to the anterior peritoneal reflection (cul-de-sac). For tumors that involve the distal portion of the sacrum, the dissection should be carried as far down as technically feasible. When the distal portion of the tumor cannot be reached from the pelvis, it is better to approach the distal dissection through the perineum.

When the rectum or mesorectum is involved, an en bloc resection is necessary. The space between the superior rectal vessels and the promontory is entered, and the areolar tissue is dissected until the tumor obliterates the space between the presacral fascia and the fascia propria of the rectum. At this point the mesentery and the bowel are divided at the level of the rectosigmoid junction. The peritoneum on both sides of the rectum is opened, and the dissection is kept lateral to the rectum. Anteriorly the peritoneum in the cul-de-sac is opened, and the dissection is carried out between the anterior rectal wall and the urogenital organs as far as necessary. For high tumors not involving the distal rectum, an en bloc resection may still be compatible with preservation of the sphincter, although sphincter function may be compromised if both S2 nerves have to be sacrificed. For lower sacral tumors involving the distal rectum, an en bloc excision often requires removal of the anal sphincter.

The ureter should be identified and kept safe during the operation. The internal iliac vessels should also be identified, but for most distal sacral tumors division of the main trunk is not necessary. However, the main trunk of the internal iliac vessels courses in front of the sacroiliac joint. For high tumors that require a complete sacrectomy or a high sacrectomy requiring division of the sacroiliac joints, the internal iliac vessels are ligated and divided. The primary trunk is then followed laterally, and its anterior and posterior branches are divided as they course toward the sciatic spine and the sciatic foramen.

Once the sacrum is mobilized, with or without adjacent organs, the pelvis is temporarily packed with a surgical sponge for hemostasis. A drain is placed in the pelvis with one end sutured onto the specimen so that it can be placed properly once the specimen is removed. In cases of rectal resection the proximal end of the colon is brought out as an end colostomy. In cases of pelvic exenteration, a urinary reconstruction may be required. If the rectus muscle is used for reconstruction, the flap is created and mobilized at this time and left in the pelvis. The midline incision is then closed in the usual fashion before the second stage of the procedure.

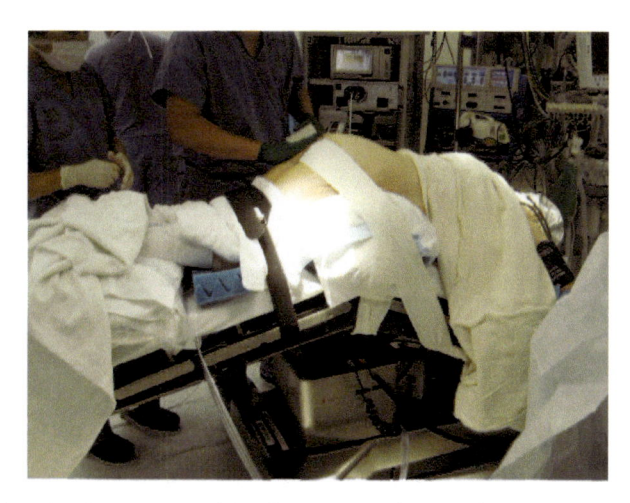

Fig. 45-4 Patient in the prone jackknife position during the second stage of sacrectomy.

The patient is repositioned in the prone jackknife position for the second stage of the operation. It is important to provide generous padding underneath the bony prominences of the pelvis to facilitate adequate exposure (Fig. 45-4). The surgical field should be prepared widely to encompass the lumbar region, bilateral thighs, and greater trochanters.

In cases of primary tumors sparing the rectum, a midline incision is made 2 to 3 cm above the anal verge and extended cephalad beyond the level of the tumor. The incision is carried down to the periosteum, and the gluteal muscle flaps are created from the periosteum of the sacrum, thereby exposing the part of the sacrum to be removed. The anococcygeal ligament is divided at the tip of the coccyx. The posterior aspect of the mesorectum is pushed down and separated from the anterior sacrum.

In patients requiring en bloc excision of the sacrum, other pelvic organs, and the anus, an elliptical incision is made on the perineum to encompass the anus and the vaginal introitus in female patients if the vagina is to be removed. The incision is then extended in the intergluteal crease as high as necessary to transect the sacrum above the level of the tumor. This incision is carried on both sides through the perirectal fat aiming toward the ischial tuberosities along the edge of the gluteal muscles on both sides. It is necessary to extend the incision at least one vertebral body above the level chosen for the transection of the sacrum. The insertion of the gluteus muscle should also be separated from the periosteum of the sacrum to expose the entire posterior cortex of the sacrum. In these patients it is preferable to enter the pelvis by incising the levator muscles laterally away from the area of the tumor. Once the attachment of the involved organs—rectum, vagina, and bladder—to the pelvic floor has been severed, the sacrectomy is begun.

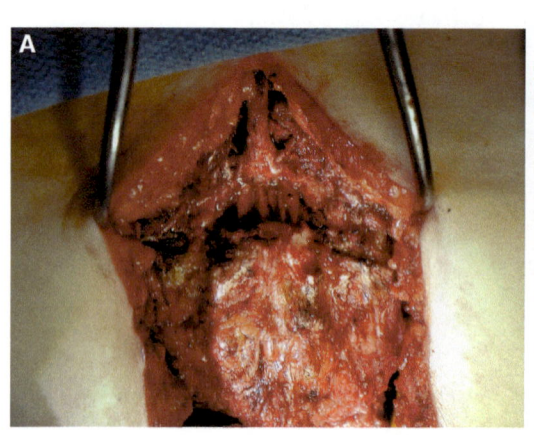

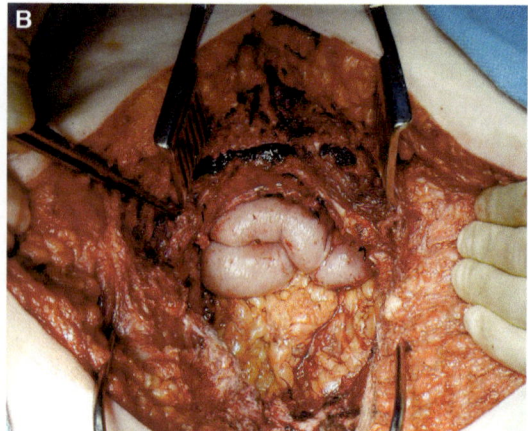

Fig. 45-5 **A,** Laminectomy at S2 in a patient with locally advanced rectal cancer showing clearing of the sacral roots. **B,** The resected rectum.

First the lateral attachments of the distal sacrum are severed by dividing the sacrotuberous and sacrospinous ligaments. If necessary, the piriformis muscle is divided to reach the apex of the sciatic notch. For high sacrectomies that require partial excision of the sacroiliac joint, the sciatic nerve has to be sacrificed. Laminectomy is then performed at the appropriate segment of the sacrum (Fig. 45-5, *A*). The dural sac of the filum terminale is ligated and divided; the sacral nerves are dissected and, when possible, preserved. Finally the anterior cortex of the sacrum is divided, and the specimen removed (Fig. 45-5, *B*).

Few cases of total sacrectomy have been reported because of the significant morbidity associated with the procedure. The technique of total sacrectomy involves bilateral ventral osteotomies along the entire length of the sacroiliac joints, and instead of a transverse osteotomy through the upper sacrum, an L5 to S1 discectomy is performed. The thecal sac is ligated below the L5 nerve roots. Lumboiliac fixation is required. Methods of reconstruction range from placement of transverse sacral bars to implantation of a custom-made prosthesis.

Frozen sections of the resection margins can be obtained to confirm negative margins before closure. Depending on the size of the perineal and gluteal defect, the wound can be closed primarily by local tissue rearrangement and mobilization of gluteal flaps or by reconstruction with a rectus abdominis myocutaneous transposition flap. For significant gluteal defects, bilateral gluteal fasciocutaneous V-Y advancement flaps may be used for reconstruction.

OUTCOMES WITH EVALUATION OF RESULTS

When considering the outcomes of sacrectomy for primary tumors or recurrent and metastatic tumors, it is necessary to take into consideration not only local tumor control and patient survival but also operative mortality and morbidity and long-term functional sequelae. Sacrectomies are long operations. High sacrectomies are often performed as staged procedures, with the posterior resection typically performed 26 to 48 hours after the initial transabdominal dissection. Even low sacrectomies can take more than 12 hours. Profuse bleeding requiring massive transfusion and intraoperative complications, including vascular injuries, dural tears, or bowel injury, are common during sacrectomies. The reported perioperative mortality rate ranges from 0% to 8.5%, but more than 50% of patients develop postoperative complications. The most common postoperative complications are wound separation, pelvic sepsis, hematoma, deep venous thrombosis, stress fractures, and cerebrospinal fluid leakage. Complications are more common in patients requiring high sacrectomy, those undergoing reoperative surgery, and those receiving preoperative radiotherapy. Patients without a colostomy who develop fecal incontinence have a higher risk of wound separation and sepsis. Postoperative complications prolong the hospital stay.

The margin status of the resection is paramount in determining outcomes for oncologic resection for primary or secondary tumors involving the sacrum. Local recurrence rates after surgical resection of sacral chordomas range from 14% to 84%, depending on the surgical margins. Resections with wide surgical margins have been associated with recurrences ranging from 5% to 17%. But resections with intralesional or marginal resection margins are associated with much higher local recurrence rates. Local recurrences can occur not only in the remaining portion of the sacrum but also in the surrounding soft tissue, such as the margins of the gluteus maximus or piriformis muscle. Therefore a wide excision of the surrounding soft tissue is also recommended. Approximately one third of patients treated for chordoma develop distant metastasis. Some series have reported overall 5-year survival rates of 84%, and even 95%, but in those same series only 42% to 56% of patients live without disease. Oncologic outcomes after sacrectomy for other less common primary sacral tumors, such as sarcomas, giant cell tumors, and nerve sheath tumors, depend on the biology of the tumors and the surgical margins achieved during surgery.

Most patients undergoing sacropelvic resection for recurrent rectal cancer have undergone preoperative radiation and chemotherapy; some receive additional intraoperative radiation. These patients often require a colostomy and urinary reconstruction, which increases the complexity of the operation and the risk of septic complications. In most series the mortality rate is lower than 5%, but between 50% and 59% of patients experience significant postoperative complications. Similar to patients undergoing surgery for primary sacral tumors, wound dehiscence and pelvic sepsis are the most common surgical complications, but urologic complications in patients undergoing urinary diversion are a common source of morbidity. Similar to patients with primary sacral tumors, a positive resection margin is a strong predictor of local recurrence and long-term survival. Despite strict selection criteria, only 62% to 84% of patients have a resection with negative margins. Positive resection margins are more often attributed to involvement of the pelvic side wall rather than the sacrum. Local tumor control is achieved in 36% to 57% of patients, but many develop distant metastasis and die of disseminated disease. The use of intraoperative radiation, either electron beam or brachytherapy, seems to improve local tumor control. The reported rate of 5-year disease-specific survival ranges from 20% to 45%, and the 5-year overall survival from 23% to 33%.

Functional preservation is also an important consideration in oncologic surgery, and the neurologic consequences of a sacrectomy are potentially very significant. Total sacrectomy compromises the stability of the pelvis, and although many variations of spinopelvic reconstruction have been devised, the benefit of reconstruction after sacrectomy remains debatable. Nonunion after sacropelvic reconstruction requiring removal of the instrumentation is not unusual, and assisted ambulation after sacrectomy without spinopelvic reconstruction is possible. The functional consequences of a partial sacrectomy depend on the preservation of the sacroiliac joints, the level of the osteotomy, and the sacral nerves resected. In general, sacroiliac stability will be preserved if the sacroiliac joint remains intact. From cadaveric studies of pelvic strength, it has been reported that if half of the sacroiliac joint, which corresponds to at least the upper half of the S1 segment, is left intact, then weight-bearing is safe after sacral resection. The sciatic nerve comprises L4 through the S3 nerve roots, the lumbosacral trunk courses over the sacral ala, and the S1 to S3 nerve roots course through the upper three anterior sacral foramina. Therefore a complete resection of the sacrum would result in denervation of both lower extremities in the distribution of the sciatic nerve, as well as bladder and bowel incontinence.

Most patients are able to ambulate with or without assistance after sacrectomy. Unilateral or bilateral severance of S1 results in leg weakness, and these patients require assistance, particularly when walking downstairs. Bilateral preservation of the S2 nerves is necessary for bowel, urinary, and sexual function. Severance of S2 and below results in a very mild decrease in strength in the legs, but severance of S3 has a minimal impact on muscle strength or ambulation. Severance of S3 or above is associated with fecal and urinary incontinence. The risk of incontinence is higher for patients who have bilateral S3 nerve resection (75%) compared with unilateral S3 nerve resection (37%). Fecal and urinary dysfunction is particularly relevant in patients undergoing sacrectomy for primary tumors, because in most of these patients the oncologic resection of the tumor does not require removal of the bladder or rectum. Therefore most patents undergoing a resection at S3 or above often require intermittent bladder catheterization and have liquid incontinence. Patients who undergo sacrectomies for recurrent rectal cancer often have the rectum and bladder removed before or after the sacrectomy.

SIGNATURE CASES

A 56-year-old man presented with persistent sacral pain. CT and MRI scans revealed a chordoma involving the sacrum invading S3 and S4 and extending along the bone and soft tissue (Fig. 45-6, *A* through *C*). The patient first underwent an anterior dissection to separate the mesorectum from the tumor, followed by a posterior laminectomy and partial sacrectomy at the S2 vertebral body (Fig. 45-6, *D*). The bilateral nerve roots at S2 were preserved, the rectum was dissected away from the anococcygeal ligament, and an en bloc sacrectomy with wide margins was completed (Fig. 45-6, *E*).

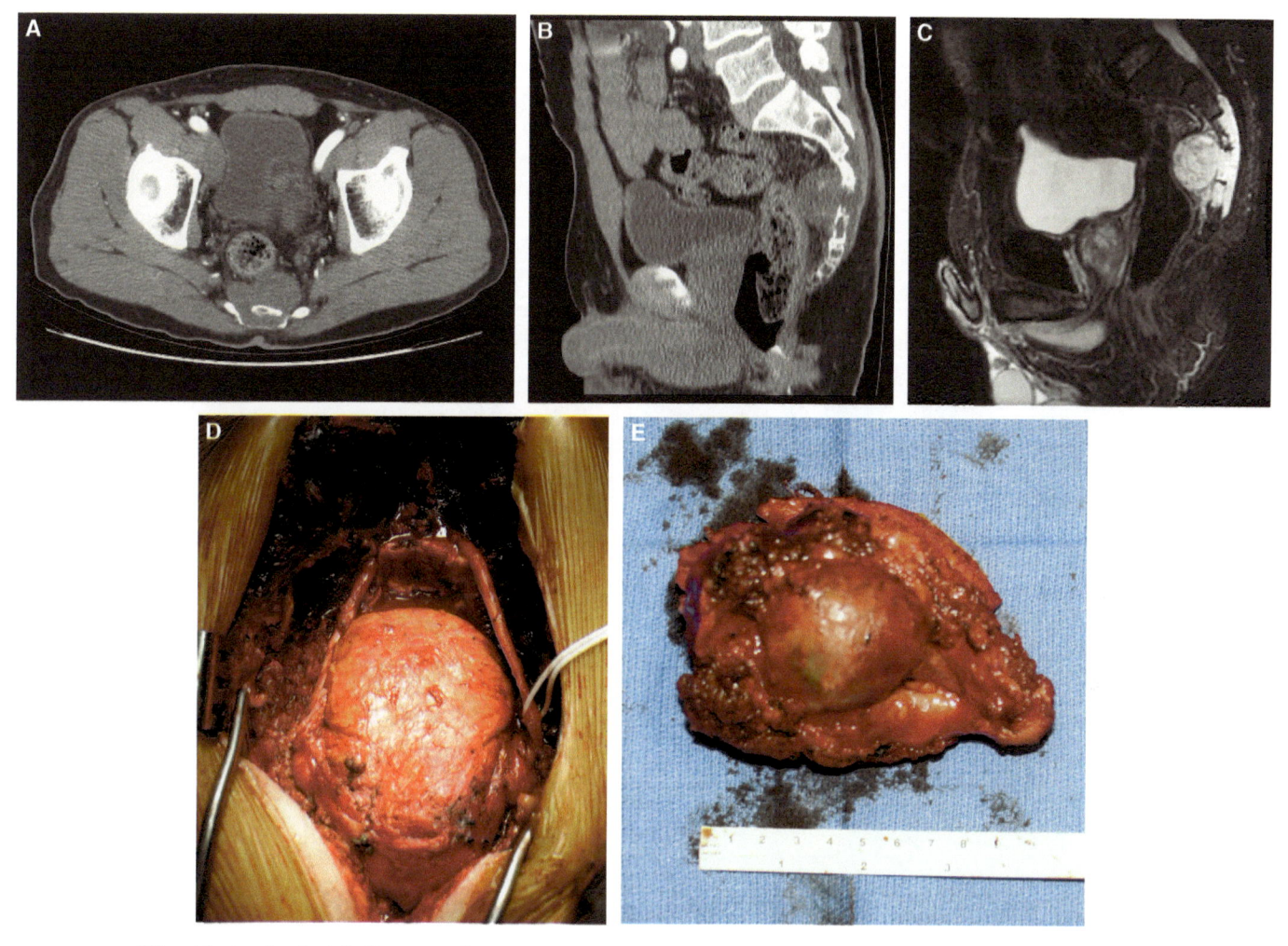

Fig. 45-6 **A,** Axial CT scan showing tumor invading the sacrum. **B,** Sagittal CT scan showing tumor invading the sacrum. **C,** Sagittal MRI scan of the tumor extending beyond the bone and soft tissue. **D,** View of the surgical field showing resection to the S2 vertebral body while preserving the S2 bilateral nerve roots. **E,** Surgical specimen showing successful completion of en bloc sacrectomy.

A 43-year-old man had a presacral recurrence after an abdominoperineal resection for locally advanced rectal cancer (Fig. 45-7, *A* and *B*). The patient had previously undergone neoadjuvant radiation and chemotherapy before abdominoperineal resection. He underwent an exploratory laparotomy with dissection of the pelvic content along the anterior surface of the sacrum to the level of the tumor (Fig. 45-7, *C*). The bladder attached to the tumor was mobilized, the urethra was transected, and the ileal conduit was created at this time. During the operation the patient received intraoperative electron beam radiation to the resection margin at the anterior aspect of S2 (Fig. 45-7, *D*). The abdomen was then closed, the patient was placed in the prone jackknife position, and pelvic exenteration with partial sacrectomy at the S2 level was performed (Fig. 45-7, *E*). The soft tissue defect (Fig. 45-7, *F*) was covered with a bilateral gluteal flap. The medial aspect of the flap was deepithelialized and pushed to fill the pelvic cavity (Fig. 45-7, *G* and *H*). The level of the sacral osteotomy is demonstrated in a plain radiograph that was obtained at the completion of the procedure (Fig. 45-7, *I*).

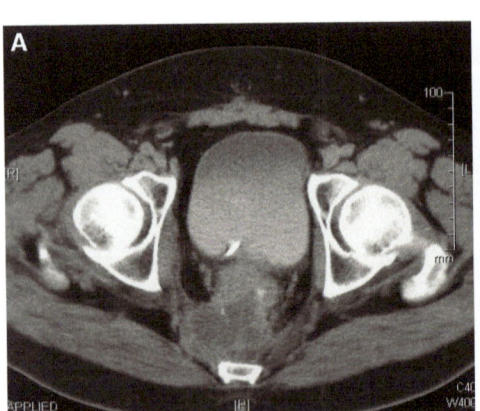

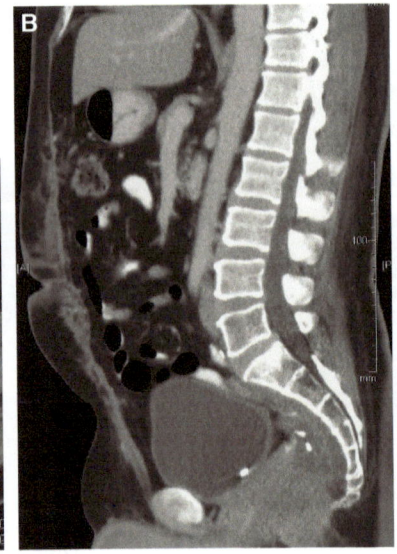

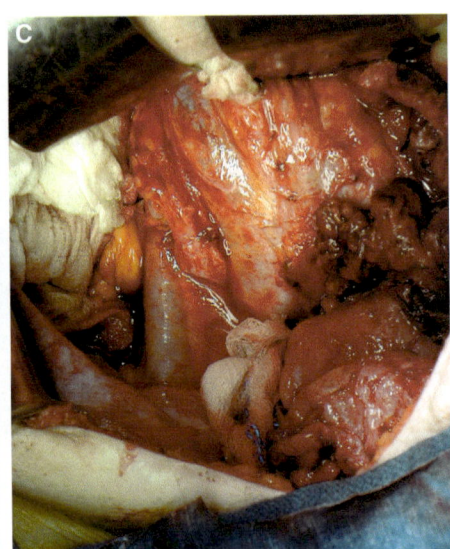

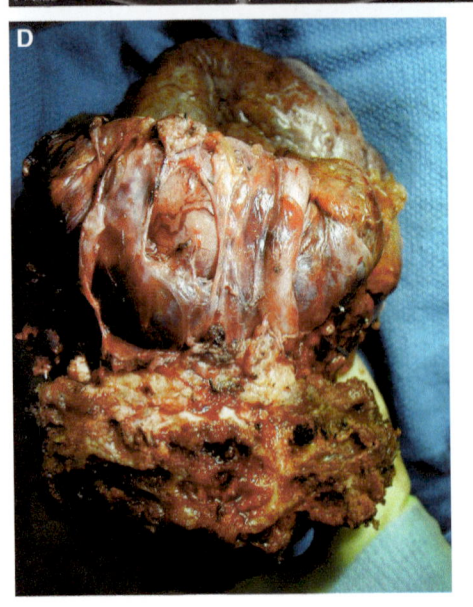

Fig. 45-7 **A,** CT scan showing presacral recurrence after abdominoperineal resection for locally advanced rectal cancer. **B,** Sagittal view showing presacral recurrence after abdominoperineal resection for locally advanced rectal cancer. **C,** Exploratory laparotomy with pelvic exenteration and sacrectomy involving a portion of the body of S2, S3, S4, and S5. **D,** Sacrum specimen.

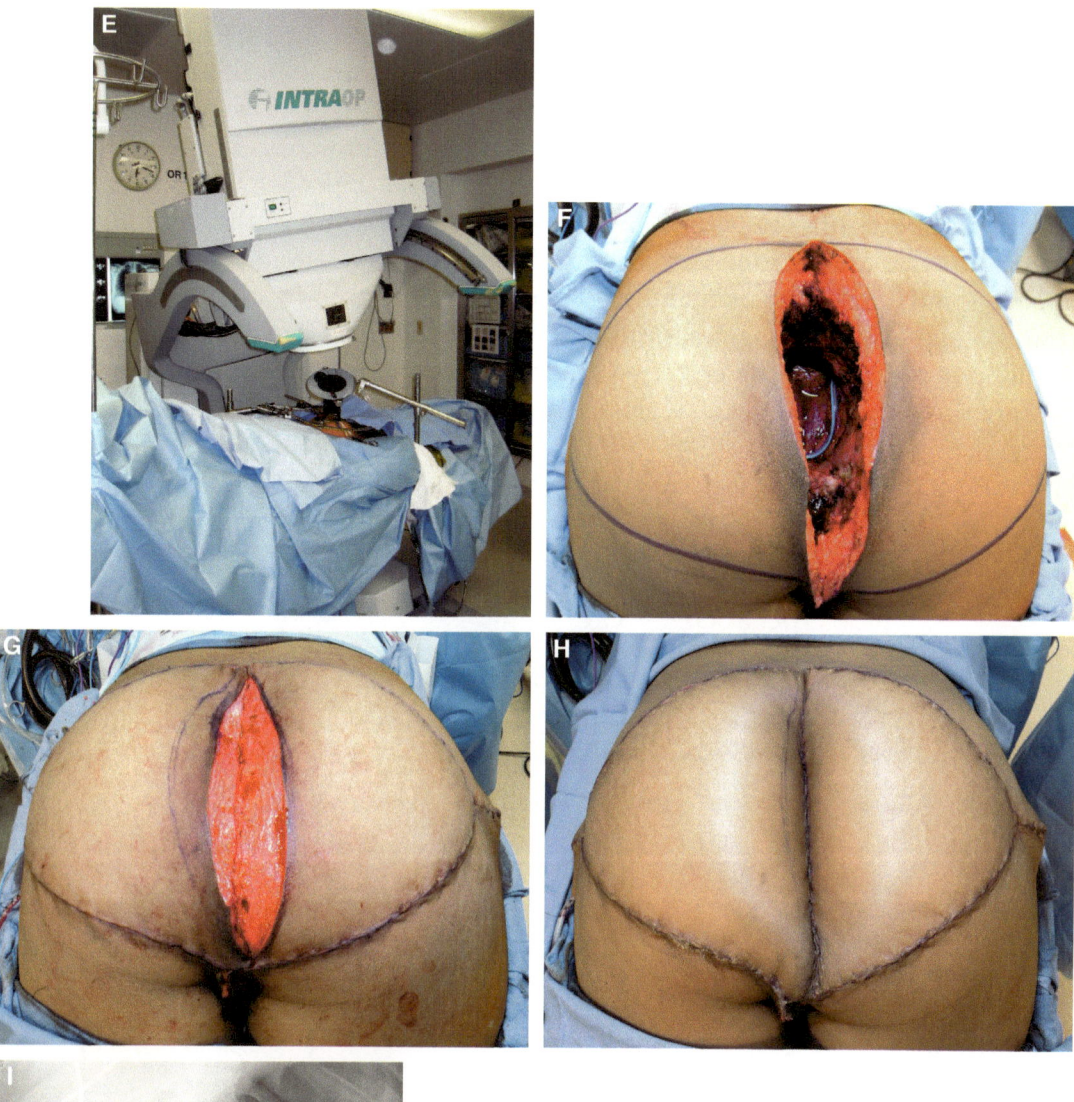

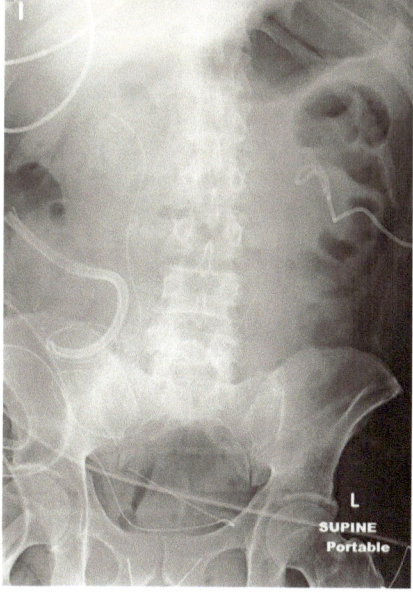

Fig. 45-7, cont'd **E,** Intraoperative electron beam radiation. **F,** Bilateral gluteal flap used to cover the soft tissue defect. **G,** The medial aspect of the flap was deepithelialized. **H,** The medial aspect of the flap was pushed to fill the pelvic cavity. **I,** Plain radiograph showing level of sacral osteotomy.

A 54-year-old woman with a history of rectal cancer was initially treated with abdominoperineal excision of the rectum. She remained in good health for 3 years until she was diagnosed with a perineal recurrence (Fig. 45-8, *A*) involving the sacrum (Fig. 45-8, *B*). She received 54 Gy of external beam radiation with concomitant sensitizing chemotherapy, with a good tumor response (Fig. 45-8, *C*). She eventually underwent an exploratory laparotomy for an en bloc resection of the small bowel, and posterior pelvic exenteration with a partial sacrectomy (including the vertebral bodies of S3, S4, and S5). This patient also underwent a hysterectomy, bilateral salpingoophorectomy, and posterior vaginectomy. A rectus muscle flap (Fig. 45-8, *D* through *G*) was used to reconstruct the posterior wall of the vagina and fill the pelvic cavity (Fig. 45-8, *H* through *J*), and bilateral gluteal flaps were used for soft tissue reconstruction of the sacroperineal defect (Fig. 45-8, *K* and *L*). The patient was without evidence of disease and had excellent performance status 2½ years after surgery (Fig. 45-8, *M*).

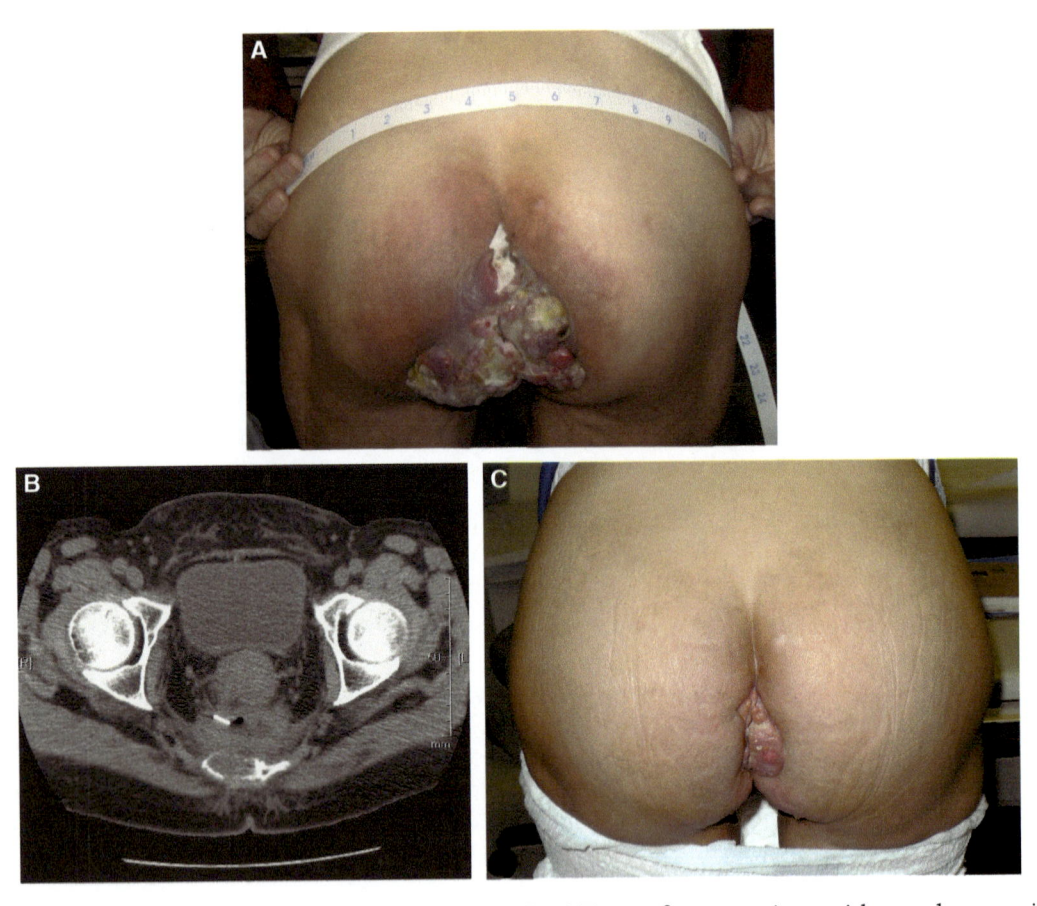

Fig. 45-8 **A,** Patient with perineal recurrence. **B,** CT scan from a patient with rectal cancer involving the sacrum. **C,** Tumor response after 54 Gy of external beam radiation with concomitant sensitizing chemotherapy.

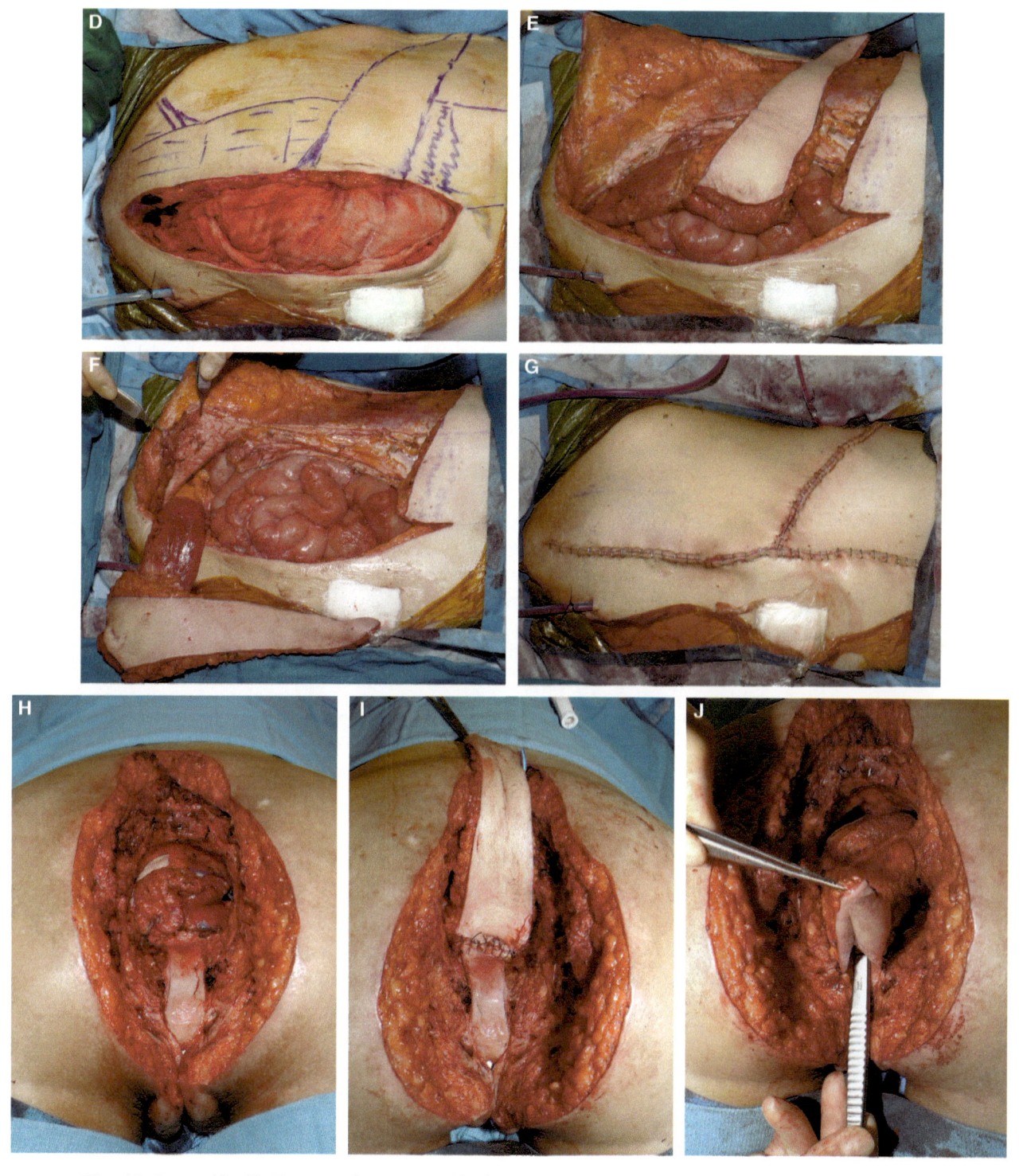

Fig. 45-8, cont'd **D,** Design of rectus muscle flap. **E,** Harvest of rectus muscle flap. **F,** Rectus muscle flap completely mobilized. **G,** Closure of abdominal donor site. **H,** Surgical field showing perineal defect after sacrectomy. **I,** Beginning of reconstruction with rectus muscle flap. **J,** Rectus muscle flap used to reconstruct the vagina.

Continued

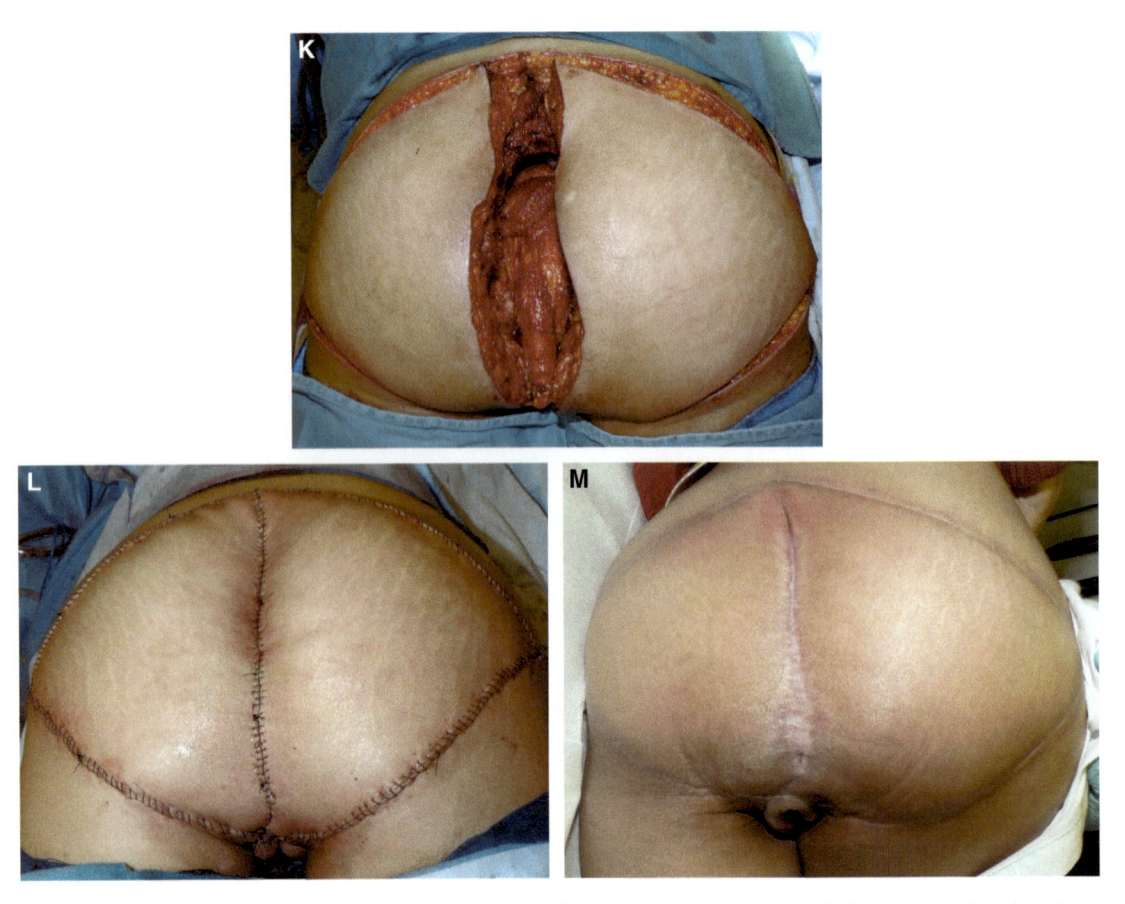

Fig. 45-8, cont'd K, Bilateral gluteal flaps for soft tissue reconstruction of the sacroperineal defect. **L,** Closure of gluteal flaps. **M,** Patient without evidence of disease and with excellent performance status 2½ years after surgery.

CONCLUSION

Primary tumors of the sacral and presacral region are uncommon but not exceptional. Untreated, these tumors are locally invasive, involving nerves and adjacent anatomic structures and resulting in significant gastrointestinal, urological, and vascular morbidity. Surgery is the primary treatment; cure requires complete resection. (In a nonprimary tumor metastatic to the sacrum, the possibility of cure is dim, and treatment is usually palliative.)

Resection of sacral malignancies often entails sacrectomy, with or without posterior or total pelvic exenteration. These difficult, lengthy procedures should only be undertaken after careful patient selection by highly experienced surgeons who have a perfect understanding of the complex anatomy involved. Surgical planning must be extensive and precise. Involvement of a multidisciplinary team is paramount: this includes colorectal, urologic, gynecologic, orthopedic, neurologic, vascular, radiologic, plastic, and reconstructive specialists. Operations of this magnitude are best performed at tertiary referral centers, where the necessary resources exist.

Acknowlegment

We thank Nicola Solomon, PhD, for assistance in writing and editing the manuscript.

Suggested Readings (With Key Suggested Readings in Boldface)

Bowers RF. Giant cell tumor of the sacrum: a case report. Ann Surg 128:1164-1172, 1948.

Fuchs B, Dickey ID, Yaszemski MJ, et al. Operative management of sacral chordoma. J Bone Joint Surg Am 87:2211-2216, 2005.

Fujimura Y, Maruiwa H, Takahata T, et al. Neurological evaluation after radical resection of sacral neoplasms. Paraplegia 32:396-406, 1994.

Garvey PB, Rhines LD, Feng L, et al. Reconstructive strategies for partial sacrectomy defects based on surgical outcomes. Plast Reconstr Surg 127:190-199, 2011.

Gokaslan ZL. Bowel and bladder continence, wound healing, and functional outcomes in patients who underwent sacrectomy. J Neurosurg Spine 3:106-110, 2005.

Gunterberg B, Romanus B, Stener B. Pelvic strength after major amputation of the sacrum. An experimental study. Acta Orthop Scand 47:635-642, 1976.

Guo Y, Palmer JL, Shen L, et al. Sites of local recurrence after surgery, with or without chemotherapy, for rectal cancer: implications for radiotherapy field design. Int J Radiat Oncol Biol Phys 55:138-143, 2003.

Hulen CA, Temple HT, Fox WP, et al. Oncologic and functional outcome following sacrectomy for sacral chordoma. J Bone Joint Surg Am 88:1532-1539, 2006.

Ishii K, Chiba K, Watanabe M, et al. Local recurrence after S2-3 sacrectomy in sacral chordoma. Report of four cases. J Neurosurg 97(1 Suppl):98-101, 2002.

Llauger J, Palmer J, Amores S, et al. Primary tumors of the sacrum: diagnostic imaging. AJR Am J Roentgenol 174:417-424, 2000.

Magrini S, Nelson H, Gunderson LL, et al. Sacropelvic resection and intraoperative electron irradiation in the management of recurrent anorectal cancer. Dis Colon Rectum 39:1-9, 1996.

Melton GB, Paty PB, Boland PJ, et al. Sacral resection for recurrent rectal cancer: analysis of morbidity and treatment results. Dis Colon Rectum 49:1099-1107, 2006.

Moriya Y, Akasu T, Fujita S, et al. Total pelvic exenteration with distal sacrectomy for fixed recurrent rectal cancer. Surg Oncol Clin N Am 14:225-238, 2005.

Murphey MD, Andrews CL, Flemming DJ, et al. From the archives of the AFIP. Primary tumors of the spine: radiologic pathologic correlation. Radiographics 16:1131-1158, 1996.

Nader R, Rhines LD, Mendel E. Metastatic sacral tumors. Neurosurg Clin N Am 15:453-457, 2004.

Ozdemir MH, Gürkan I, Yildiz Y, et al. Surgical treatment of malignant tumours of the sacrum. Eur J Surg Oncol 25:44-49, 1999.

Ruggieri P, Angelini A, Ussia G, et al. Surgical margins and local control in resection of sacral chordomas. Clin Orthop Relat Res 468:2939-2947, 2010.

Sahakitrungruang C, Chantra K, Dusitanond N, et al. Sacrectomy for primary sacral tumors. Dis Colon Rectum 52:913-918, 2009.

Sahakitrungruang C, Chantra K. One-staged subtotal sacrectomy for primary sacral tumor. Ann Surg Oncol 16:2594, 2009.

Schwab JH, Healey JH, Rose P, et al. The surgical management of sacral chordomas. Spine (Phila Pa 1976) 34:2700-2704, 2009.

Wanebo HJ, Koness RJ, Vezeridis MP, et al. Pelvic resection of recurrent rectal cancer. Ann Surg 220:586-595; discussion 595-597, 1994.

Wiig JN, Wolff PA, Tveit KM, et al. Location of pelvic recurrence after 'curative' low anterior resection for rectal cancer. Eur J Surg Oncol 25:590-594, 1999.

Yamada K, Ishizawa T, Niwa K, et al. Pelvic exenteration and sacral resection for locally advanced primary and recurrent rectal cancer. Dis Colon Rectum 45:1078-1084, 2002.

Chapter 46

Distal Sacrectomy

Dean Chou, Wali E. Danish

Tumors of the sacrum and related neurologic and pelvic structures are rare occurrences, accounting for only 1% to 7% of all clinically apparent tumors of the spine.[1] Proper evaluation of symptomatic sacral tumors is made difficult by their low occurrence rate and with the presentation of nonspecific symptoms. Sacral tumors often grow to a large size because of the long average delay between the onset of symptoms and diagnosis, which averages approximately 2 years. This is the result of the large capacity of the sacral canal and pelvis.[1] A correct diagnosis is further complicated by the nature of the pain associated with an early sacral tumor, which often mimics the pain experienced as a result of lumbar spondylosis.

Sacrectomy is indicated for primary malignant neoplasms of the sacrum. Sacrectomy is used for long-term disease-free survival, which is the reason for removal of the neoplasm in an en bloc fashion. Distal sacrectomy involves sparing S1 but removing the sacrum and coccyx below. At physiologic loads, S1 is sufficient for the pelvis to bear the load of the spine.[2] Thus amputation below S1 generally does not require reconstruction of the pelvis.

INDICATIONS AND CONTRAINDICATIONS

It has been shown that en bloc resection of such malignant primary neoplasms as chordomas or chondrosarcomas leads to improved long-term disease-free survival.[3-5] Accordingly, for tumors that are malignant for which en bloc resection improves survival, an en bloc sacrectomy should be planned. For those tumors responding to curettage, piecemeal resection, and radiation, an en bloc sacrectomy with nerve root sacrifice should not be performed. Such tumors would include metastatic lesions and benign primary lesions.

The patient's age and medical status should be considered. Careful consideration should be given to the advisability of performing surgery in elderly patients. The morbidity associated with sacrectomy is not negligible, and such patient factors as age, health status, expected survival, quality of life, and potential treatment with radiation only should all be considered.

PREOPERATIVE EVALUATION

The clinical presentation of a sacral tumor usually is pain. Oftentimes patients will complain of pain after sitting or with activity. Multiple evaluations for rectal or lumbar spine issues may have been initiated before the diagnosis of a sacral tumor. Physical examination may or may not show tenderness to palpation over the sacrococcygeal region. A mass may be palpated. Typically the physical examination findings will be unremarkable.

Appropriate diagnostic imaging includes MRI of the sacrum, with and without gadolinium, CT of the sacrum, and plain anteroposterior and lateral radiographs of the sacrum. On interpretation of these images, if a primary malignant neoplasm is suspected, a CT-guided biopsy is critical. It is imperative that the entry point for biopsy be indelibly marked with either a suture or tattoo ink, so that the biopsy tract can be widely resected during sacrectomy. En bloc resection of the biopsy tract is critical, because tumor cells can be seeded along this tract from the biopsy.

CLINICAL DECISION-MAKING

Subtotal resection or curettage of osteoid osteomas and osteoblastomas can lead to resolution of symptoms, but the probability of a recurrence is high with the use of these procedures for malignant neoplasms (such as chordoma or chondrosarcoma).[1] En bloc resection is the treatment of choice, with the degree of resection being a major determinant of the length of disease-free survival.[3] Classification of the sacral amputation is generally based on the level of nerve root sacrifice. Low sacral amputations involve sacrifice of at least one S4 nerve root or below, midsacral amputations involve sacrifice of at least one S3 nerve root, and high sacral amputations require sacrifice of at lease one S2 nerve root.[6] Total sacrectomy involves complete sacrifice of all sacral nerve roots.[7] These neurologic structures within or adjacent to the sacrum often must be sacrificed to ensure complete resection of malignant lesions, leading to loss of bowel or bladder control and sexual dysfunction.[1] Preservation of the S2 nerve root bilaterally is required for intact autonomic bowel, bladder, and sexual function, thus making distal sacrectomy (S3 or below) the preferred treatment when possible.[6] Treatment of sacral tumors traditionally involves radiation therapy, but the level of radiation necessary for effective treatment can cause radiation injury to surrounding structures, such as the rectum and pelvic organs.[1]

Sacroiliac stability is preserved if the tumor resection spares the sacroiliac joints, making reconstruction unnecessary, which leads to the patient's ameliorated functional status.[2] In contrast, in total sacrectomies, the axial spine is disconnected from the pelvis and usually necessitates reconstruction to provide support for such a biomechanically complex attribute of the region.

If the tumor is shown on biopsy to be a malignant primary neoplasm and the patient is a suitable candidate for surgery, en bloc sacrectomy should be carried out. The decision as to where to perform the sacral amputation depends on the appearance of the tumor on sagittal MRI. We find that T2-weighted sagittal images are the most useful for defining the extent of the tumor. Usually we prefer a margin of one sacral segment for amputation. For instance, if the tumor ends at the S3-4 interspace, we perform our amputation at the S2-3 interspace. This allows a wide margin of en bloc resection.

To determine the mediolateral extent of the tumor resection, we rely on axial T2-weighted images or T1-weighted images with gadolinium. These are measured from the midline to the right and to the left. The number of centimeters off the midline determines the mediolateral extent of the tumor. For wide resections we usually plan on 1 cm lateral to either side of the extent of the tumor.

At the level of the sacral amputation, the lowest nerves should be preserved. For instance, during an S1-2 sacral amputation, the S2 nerves should be preserved. This is to give the patient every chance of retaining bowel and bladder function. Ligation of nerves should be planned preoperatively, and extensive discussion with the patient regarding loss of bowel, bladder, and sexual function must take place. Patients must be made fully aware of the significant life changes that may ensue. A bowel preparation is performed the day before surgery to evacuate the rectum.

TECHNIQUE

The patient is placed on a Jackson table in the prone position. Plastic surgery is involved to reconstruct the gluteal attachments and skin closure, and colorectal surgery is involved to assist with dissection of the mesorectum and the anococcygeal ligament. A preoperative radiograph is obtained to confirm the level of sacral amputation. A mark is placed at this level. The anus is thoroughly cleansed, and gram-negative antibiotics, in addition to standard antibiotics, are administered. The skin resection is planned on the basis of the following two factors: (1) the biopsy insertion point and (2) the medial-lateral extent of the tumor.

It is important to include the biopsy tract in the excisional area. Also, the medial-lateral extent of the tumor must be taken into account. For very large tumors, further resection of muscle must be undertaken to avoid tumor violation. Although the skin resection does not have to be as wide as the tumor, it should be large enough to reach circumferentially around the sacrum for en bloc removal.

The elliptical incision is drawn and extended cephalad to a normal linear incision (Fig. 46-1, *A* and *B*). This allows for cephalad exposure of the sacrum in a normal fashion. An intraoperative radiograph is then obtained to confirm the level. Because there are no disc spaces in the sacrum, and it can be difficult to visualize the exact sacral level, we recommend counting the pedicles from S1 down. First, a confirmatory probe is placed under the S1 pedicle, and then each subsequent pedicle is noted to confirm the level.

The lateral aspects of the sacrum are then identified, and transaction of the gluteus maximus is performed. At all times, the tumor can be palpated (if large enough) to ensure that the excision is lateral to the tumor (Fig. 46-1, *C*). The muscle is bluntly dissected and then cut with a Bovie cautery to avoid inadvertent tumor violation. This dissection is taken all the way to the mesorectum, which is a soft, fatty layer that is clearly identifiable (Fig. 46-1, *D*). This is then carried out on both sides of the tumor until the coccyx begins to curve ventrally.

A laminectomy is performed at the level of the sacral amputation. For instance, if the level is at the S1-2 interspace, the laminectomy is performed at S2 (Fig. 46-1, *E*). Identification of the S2 pedicle is confirmed, and the S2 nerves are preserved (Fig. 46-1, *F*). The laminectomy is carried all the way laterally until no bone is present. The thecal sac and sacral nerves below S2 are tied off (Fig. 46-1, *G*). We obtain multiple radiographs and perform multiple identifications of the pedicles, with rechecking against the MRI scan to ensure that the proper level is identified before tying off the thecal sac.

The S2 pedicles are then amputated. A sagittal saw is used initially to start the osteotomy. This is done in the plane of the sacrum. To extend this laterally, a matchstick-type burr is used. Hemostasis is achieved with standard thrombin/Gelfoam products. The S2 nerves are then followed out until they are ventral to the sacrum (Fig. 46-1, *H*). Multiple dorsal branches of the S2 nerves must be ligated while preserving the ventral branches. The S2 can then be mobilized cephalad to the sacral amputation (now that the S2 pedicles are gone).

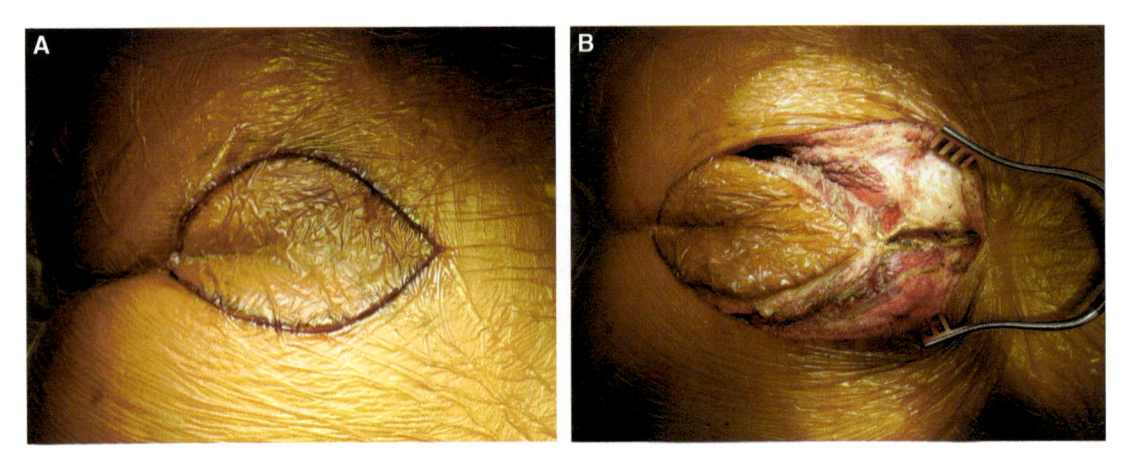

Fig. 46-1 **A,** The skin incision was first made according to the elipse, as shown. **B,** The midline skin incision was extended cephalad to find the normal S1 spinous process.

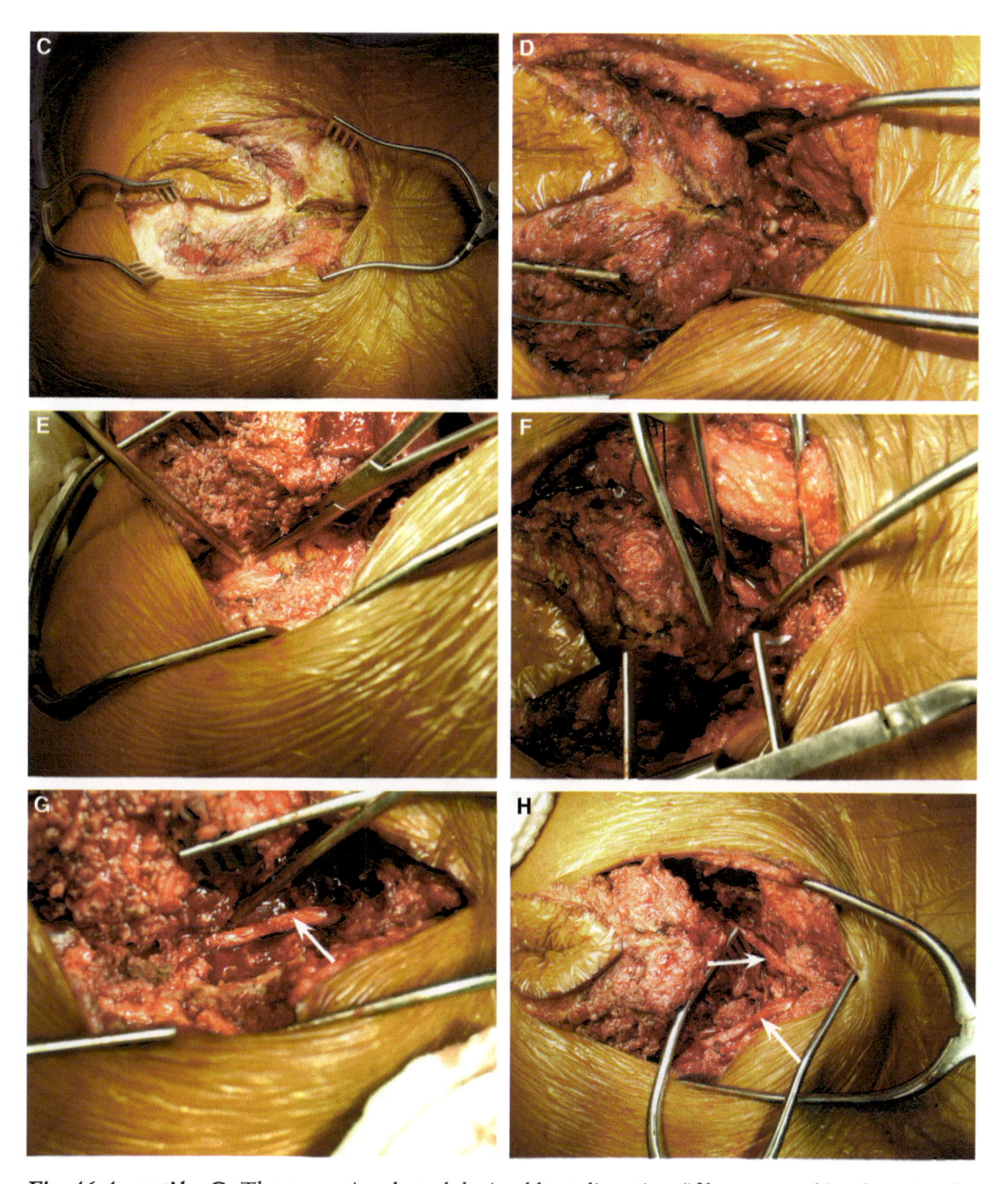

Fig. 46-1, cont'd **C,** The tumor is palpated during blunt dissection (if large enough); otherwise, the edge of the sacrum is palpated. **D,** The thecal sac is tied off, and **E,** blunt dissection of the mesorectum away from the ligament is performed. **F,** S1-2 osteotomy is performed, and **G,** the S2 nerves are identified, preserved, and their medial attachments released. **H,** The S2 nerves are freely mobilized away from the distal sacrum.

Continued

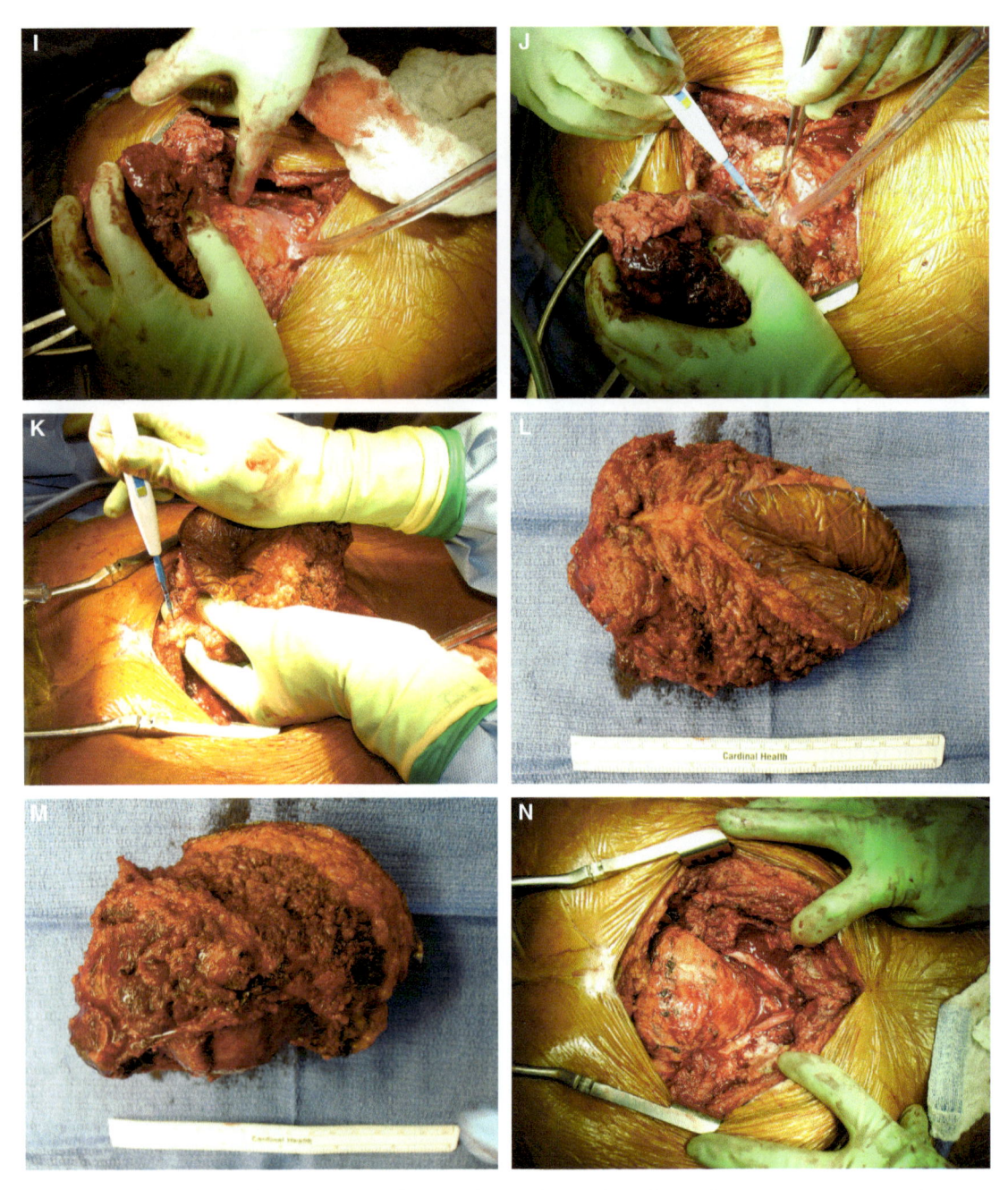

Fig. 46-1, cont'd **I,** The sacrum can be cantilevered up, identifying the mesorectum. **J,** The mesorectum is divided bluntly away from the distal sacrum, **K,** the anococcygeal ligament is divided, and **L** and **M,** the specimen is removed en bloc. **N,** The cavity now shows the mesorectum and the preserved S2 nerve roots.

The sacrum can then be gently cantilevered upward (Fig. 46-1, *I*), hinging on the anococcygeal ligament. Multiple fibrous attachments can be detached. As the sacrum is cantilevered upward, the mesorectum is identified. Blunt dissection techniques, with sponges held on instruments, are performed. The mesorectum is dissected away (Fig. 46-1, *J*) and, as caudad dissection is performed, the vascular supply of the sacrum is also encountered. These attachments are clipped, tied, or coagulated. The thick anococcygeal ligament is then manually palpated (Fig. 46-1, *K*). It is critical to dissect the mesorectum past the anococcygeal ligament to ensure that no damage to the rectum occurs. Once the anococcygeal ligament is cut, the sacrectomy is complete (Fig. 46-1, *L* through *N*).

Closure is then performed by plastic surgery. At our institution we tend to use Y flaps to mobilize the gluteal muscles medially for closure. In general, skin grafts are not needed. Patients are left on an airbed, lying on their sides or abdomens for 1 week, and then they are mobilized. They are not allowed to sit for 4 to 6 weeks, but they can stand and walk after the first week.

OUTCOME WITH EVALUATION OF RESULTS

We have found that en bloc sacrectomies give patients the best chance of disease-free survival. All patients are warned about bowel, bladder, and sexual dysfunction. For distal sacrectomies, preservation of S2 does not guarantee normal function. In fact, most patients have urinary and bowel dysfunction. Many patients with preservation of both S3 nerve roots will have normal function, but this is not universal. It is important to counsel patients preoperatively and explain that these are the long-term permanent sequelae of this operation. We also recommend proton beam radiation therapy, depending on the size of the tumor and the age of the patient. For instance, a 50-year-old male patient with a large tumor, with invasive characteristics on preoperative MRI, would be highly likely to receive proton beam therapy. But one could make the argument for serial imaging in a 70-year-old male patient with a small chordoma that was easily removed en bloc. It should be noted that any spillage of tumor during surgery would be an indication for proton beam therapy.

SIGNATURE CASE

A 61-year-old man had a 2-year history of pain in the buttocks and back. A complete workup demonstrated a sacral mass. Sagittal T2-weighted MRI demonstrated a sacral chordoma extending up into the S2 segment but not up to the S1-2 interspace (Fig. 46-2, *A*). Axial T1-weighted MRI with gadolinium demonstrated the extent of the tumor in the axial plane, as shown in Fig. 46-2, *B*.

The patient subsequently underwent a CT-guided biopsy of the lesion. The biopsy tract was indelibly marked. Pathologic findings confirmed that the patient had a chordoma. The patient was then scheduled for an en bloc sacrectomy, with an amputation at the S1-2 junction. It was explained to him that the S2 nerves would be preserved, but he would have permanent changes in bowel, bladder, and sexual function. A bowel preparation was given the night before to empty the rectum.

Surgery was coordinated with colorectal and plastic surgery. Six to 8 hours of surgery was planned. The specimen was removed en bloc (see Fig. 46-1, *L* and *M*). The patient did well after surgery, with a 9-day stay in the hospital. He did lose significant bowel and bladder function, as expected. He subsequently underwent postoperative proton beam therapy. The postoperative MRI scan shows resection of the chordoma (Fig. 46-2, *C*).

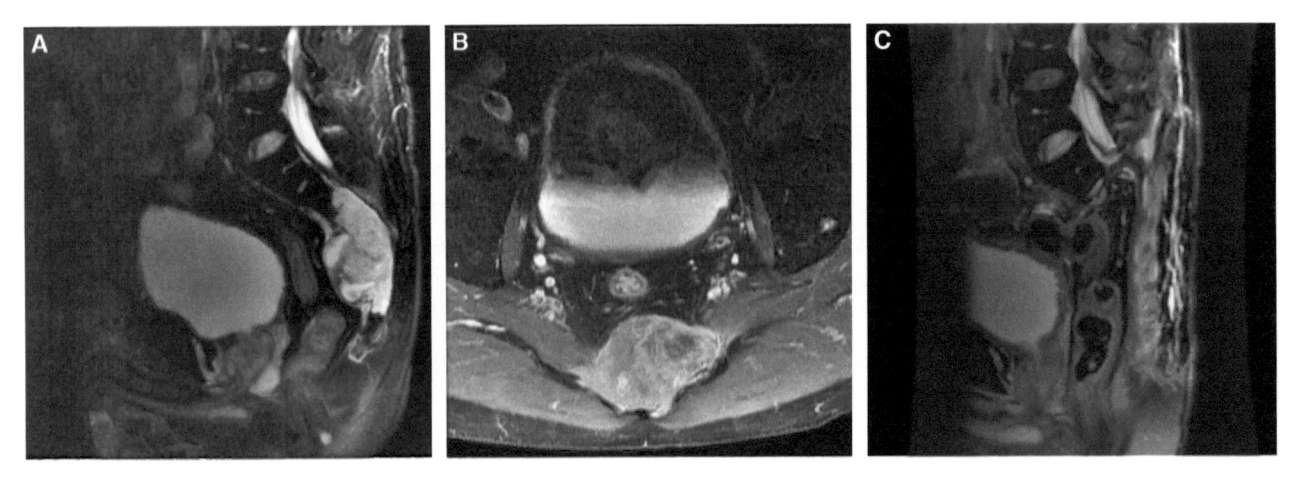

Fig. 46-2 **A,** Sagittal T2-weighted MRI demonstrating sacral chordoma extending up into the S2 segment, but not up to the S1-2 interspace. **B,** Axial T1-weighted MRI with gadolinium demonstrating the extent of tumor in the axial plane. **C,** Postoperative MRI scan showing resection of the chordoma.

CONCLUSION

Distal sacrectomy is a useful tool for managing malignant primary tumors of the sacrum. A biopsy to establish pathology is critical before undertaking any surgery of this magnitude. A detailed discussion with the patient regarding the significant morbidity associated with this operation is essential.

BAILOUT TECHNIQUE

If the tumor is violated during surgery, a figure-of-eight braided suture should be placed in an attempt to close the hole. A moist sponge should then be placed over that area to manipulate the tumor and potentially capture any tumor spillage. Any instruments that have come in contact with the violation should be removed from the field and disposed of, including sucker tips, needle drivers, gloves, and so forth.

TIPS FROM THE MASTERS

- Preoperative discussion with the patient regarding loss of bowel, bladder, and sexual function are paramount.
- Plan the osteotomy with wide margins to give the best chance of local control.
- Preservation of the most cephalad nerve root may improve the chances of increased control of bowel and bladder function.

References (With Key References in Boldface)

1. **Sciubba DM, Petteys RJ, Garces-Ambrossi GL, et al. Diagnosis and management of sacral tumors. J Neurosurg Spine 10:244-256, 2009.**
2. Yu B, Zheng Z, Zhuang X, et al. Biomechanical effects of transverse partial sacrectomy on the sacroiliac joints: an in vitro human cadaveric investigation of the borderline of sacroiliac joint instability. Spine (Phila Pa 1976) 34:1370-1375, 2009.
3. **Boriani S, Bandiera S, Biagini R, et al. Chordoma of the mobile spine: fifty years of experience. Spine (Phila Pa 1976) 31:493-503, 2006.**
4. York JE, Berk RH, Fuller GN, et al. Chondrosarcoma of the spine: 1954 to 1997. J Neurosurg 90:73-78, 1999.
5. York JE, Kaczaraj A, Abi-Said D, et al. Sacral chordoma: 40-year experience at a major cancer center. Neurosurgery 44:74-79; discussion 79-80, 1999.
6. **McLoughlin GS, Sciubba DM, Suk I, et al. En bloc total sacrectomy performed in a single stage through a posterior approach. Neurosurgery 63:ONS115-120; discussion ONS120, 2008.**
7. Fourney DR, Rhines LD, Hentschel SJ, et al. En bloc resection of primary sacral tumors: classification of surgical approaches and outcome. J Neurosurg Spine 3:111-122, 2005.

Chapter 47

Proximal Sacrectomy and Pelvic Reconstruction

Jamal McClendon, Jr., Tyler R. Koski, Stephen L. Ondra, Frank L. Acosta, Jr.

Sacral resections and osteotomies are performed for a variety of disease processes, including tumor, trauma, and osteomyelitis and for restoration of sagittal balance.[1] In most patients symptoms are the result of lumbopelvic junction instability that arises from the aforementioned pathologic conditions.[2] In the successful surgical management of proximal sacral resections and subsequent pelvic reconstructions, a clear understanding of this anatomic region is paramount. The sacrum is a large triangular bone that consists of five fused vertebrae, which articulates with the L5 vertebral body superiorly (lumbosacral joint), the coccyx below (sacrococcygeal joint), and the ilium bilaterally (sacroiliac joints).[3,4] In addition to the joints, the surrounding ligaments and joints connecting to the ilium are integral to the structural integrity of the spine and pelvis.[3]

The sacroiliac joint is a synovial structure formed between the articular surfaces of the sacrum and the ilium.[4,5] The sacral articular surface is covered by a thick hyaline cartilage, and a thin fibrocartilage overlies the articular surface of the ilium.[4] It also has an irregular lining and forms broad, interlocking surfaces with the ilium, which resist motion effectively.[1] The sacroiliac joint ends at the level of S2, and the posterior sacroiliac ligament also ends at the sacroiliac joint.

The strong sacroiliac, sacrotuberous, sacrospinous, and lumbosacral ligaments also play an important role in stabilization.[1] The interosseous, sacrospinous, and posterior sacroiliac ligaments are the strongest ligaments and function to resist movement of the sacroiliac joint and forward tilt of the upper end of the sacrum.[4,5] The sacrotuberous and sacrospinous ligaments resist the tendency of the lower end of the sacrum and coccyx to tilt backward.[4] The iliolumbar ligaments prevent the forward migration of L5 over the sacrum.[4] The combination of these ligamentous attachments renders the spinopelvic segment stable.[1]

In 1976 Gunterberg et al[6] conducted a detailed, biomechanical cadaveric study to evaluate sacropelvic mechanics and the effects of several transverse partial sacrectomies. Sacrectomies through the S1 foramina (between the S1 and S2 vertebral bodies) and through the S1 body (1 cm below the sacral promontory) were tested with regard to their compressive load to failure.[6] The results demonstrated weakening of the pelvis by 30% and 50%, respectively, as specimens were loaded vertically and tested to failure, but not enough to weaken the pelvis to the extent that they could no longer withstand normal standing forces imparted at the L5-S1 joint articulation.[6] The forces transmitted at the L5-S1 joint articulation are insufficient to withstand full weight-bearing after submaximal resection of the sacrum, as described earlier.[6] Controversy arose because the study created false loading and response conditions that were not entirely simulated by the in vivo loading environment, and this investigation largely evaluated the destruction strength of the pelvis rather than the stability of the sacroiliac joints under physiologic loading conditions.[5]

Yu et al[5] studied the pelvises of seven male human cadavers with normal bone mineral density to evaluate the biomechanical effects of transverse partial sacrectomy on the sacroiliac joints, and they investigated which level of transverse partial sacrectomy requires reconstruction. It was the first study to report the various effects of partial sacrectomy on sacroiliac joints of fresh cadavers. Statistically, significant differences in axial compressive forces and torsional stiffness were observed with osteotomy at a line passing through the superior border of the first sacral foramen (S1 vertebral body or sacral promontory), as compared with osteotomy at a line passing below the superior border of the second sacral foramen (S2 vertebral body) and osteotomy at a line passing below the inferior border of the second sacral foramen (S2-3 disc space). It was concluded that caudal sacrectomy to the level of the superior border of the second sacral foramen (S2 vertebral body) would not result in instability of the residual sacroiliac joints.[5] As such, lumboiliac reconstruction is not mandatory.[5] But a sacrectomy involving the superior border of the first sacral foramen requires consideration of reconstruction (Fig. 47-1).[5]

Tumors of the sacrum and related neural, retroperitoneal, and pelvic structures are rare, accounting for 1% to 7% of all clinically apparent spine tumors.[7] Diagnosis of these tumors is frequently delayed on the basis of late clinical symptoms, and the neoplasm may be very advanced at the time of presentation.[8] Symptoms may be mild, and these tumors are often large by the time they are diagnosed.[9] Thus because presentation is insidious and complicated by a deep location within the pelvis, these tumors often extend beyond the confines of the sacrum and into the adjacent soft tissues.[10] Approximately two thirds of all sacral tumors present at or below the level of S2.[1,11]

The sacrum not only contains important neurologic structures but also serves as the connection between the axial skeleton and the lower extremities by way of the sacro-

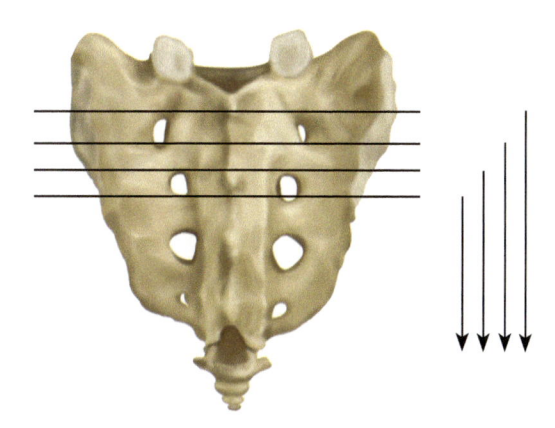

Fig. 47-1 Diagram illustrating sequential partial sacrectomies and percentage of axial compressive stiffness of residual sacroiliac joints, as compared with intact pelvis in human cadavers of normal bone mineral density (Adapted from Yu B, Zheng Z, Zhuang X, et al. Biomechanical effects of transverse partial sacrectomy on the sacroiliac joints: an in vitro human cadaveric investigation of the borderline of sacroiliac joint instability. Spine 34:1370-1375, 2009.)

iliac joints.[1] Based on the large volume at diagnosis, curative excision of sacral tumors often is technically demanding.[12-15] Sacrectomy provides an effective method of surgical treatment for aggressive benign and malignant sacral tumors, and radical treatment of malignant tumors of the sacrum may require en bloc resection that may violate the sacroiliac joint.[5,10] A radical surgical approach, such as partial or total sacrectomy, with sacrifice of sacral roots, is indicated when it is clinically advantageous to achieve total resection with wide margins.[9,16] The location of the tumor within the sacrum determines whether a partial or total sacrectomy will be necessary for radical resection.[17] The extent of sacral resection is influenced by the location and histopathologic findings of the tumor.[7,8,18-22] Radical resection has been demonstrated to prolong the progression-free survival period in patients harboring various primary sacral neoplasms that are not responsive to nonoperative therapy.[14,17,23-26]

Proximal sacrectomy can be used in patients with tumor extension present at the S1 endplate. Proximal sacrectomy cephalad to S1 is the key to determining clinically whether pelvic reconstruction is needed.[5] Various spinopelvic reconstruction techniques after sacrectomy have been reported, including iliac-sacral screw, posterior sacroiliac plating-screw, Galveston rod, and iliac screw fixations.[5,27-30]

INDICATIONS AND CONTRAINDICATIONS

The types of tumors that arise from or extend to the sacrum are diverse, and treatment options depend on the location, extent of the lesion, medical condition of the patient, and the biological aggressiveness of the lesion.[8] The complex anatomy of the sacral region and the advanced spine surgery techniques required to perform aggressive resections necessitate the expertise of a multidisciplinary surgical team to perform these demanding procedures.[8]

Chordoma is the most common primary bone tumor of the sacrum arising from the notochord remnant.[8,31,32] Local recurrence is the most important predictor of death in patients with chordoma and is related to the extent of the initial resection.* The surgical goal is gross total resection with negative margins for this type of tumor. Even after total en bloc resection for sacral chordoma, local recurrence is not unusual.[8,32,36] In patients whose lesions are successfully resected en bloc, with negative margins, the recurrence rate is approximately 25%.[31]

Giant cell tumors, osteosarcomas, and chondrosarcomas are other pathologic conditions that afflict the sacrum. Giant cell tumors are the second most frequent primary bone tumors of the sacrum.[8,38] Although histologically benign, these osteolytic expansive bone tumors are locally aggressive, often involving the vertebral body, and they have a high risk of recurrence after curettage alone.[8,31,38,39] Osteosarcoma is a malignant bone-forming tumor that occurs throughout the appendicular skeleton, involving the spine in 0.85% to 3% of cases.[31] These osteoblastic lesions, which have a bubble-like appearance on plain radiographs and CT scans, have a high rate of metastasis and exhibit locally aggressive behavior.[31] Most sacral chondrosarcomas are low-grade, slow-growing, locally aggressive tumors.[23,40] Significant factors associated with a worse prognosis, with respect to local control and/or survival, include a high histologic tumor grade, increasing patient age, primary surgery conducted outside a cancer center, incisional biopsy sampling compared with a noninvasive diagnostic procedure, and inadequate surgical margins.[23,41] These tumors are considered radioresistant, and chemotherapy with high-grade lesions appears to be of little benefit.[8,23] Primary malignant tumors of the sacrum respond best to multimodal treatment combining surgery, radiation, and chemotherapy.[31]

Radical resection may be the best available treatment for low-grade malignancies and aggressive, benign sacral tumors that are resistant to noninterventional therapies.[9] It can prolong the overall survival time.[9] Because of the limited life expectancy of patients with metastatic cancer, an approach that preserves and maintains quality of life is preferred.[31] Patients are typically treated with chemotherapy and/or radiation at first. Despite the potential neurologic and sexual dysfunction, total sacrectomy remains the best opportunity for reducing morbidity and mortality for both aggressive benign tumors, such as giant cell tumors, and low-grade malignant tumors, such as chordomas and chondrosarcomas.[16,30,42,43]

PREOPERATIVE EVALUATION

The preoperative evaluation includes a history and neurologic examination, and patients may present with low back pain, radicular pain, urinary incontinence, weakness, sphincter disturbances, saddle anesthesia, or paresthesias. For sacral tumors, pain generally increases with weight-bearing but can also occur at rest.[31] Pain at night is also not uncommon.[31]

Radiologic studies needed for complete evaluation include plain radiography, MRI, and in most cases CT scanning.[8] These studies determine the local extent of disease,

---

*References 8, 16, 25, 26, 32-37.

including the amount of sacral destruction, the presence of intrapelvic disease, and the presence of sacroiliac joint involvement.[8] Upright and sitting anteroposterior/lateral scoliosis plain radiographs are often required for deformity correction procedures involving osteotomies of the sacrum. Counseling is very important in discussing surgical resection of sacral lesions, because partial or complete sacrectomy involves the purposeful sacrifice of nerve roots with significant functional deficits.[8]

Diseases of the sacrum can be classified as infectious pathology, metastatic lesions, and primary bone tumors. Types of tumors of the sacral region include the following: chordoma, chondrosarcoma, giant cell tumor, osteosarcoma, osteochondroma, osteoblastoma, plasmacytoma, aneurysmal bone cyst, osteoid osteoma, myeloma, lymphoma, Ewing's sarcoma, neurofibrosarcoma, malignant fibrous histiosarcoma, metastasis, and malignant fibrous histiocytoma. Because the differential diagnosis of lesions in the sacral region is extensive, many investigators advocate preoperative biopsies.[8] Histologic diagnosis is often established by means of needle or open biopsy. With careful planning, the biopsy tract may be incorporated within the margins of the subsequent resection for sacral tumors.[8] A transrectal or transvaginal biopsy procedure should never be considered, because these otherwise uninvolved organs may become seeded with tumor cells, possibly necessitating subsequent radical surgery to remove the vagina or rectum.[8,36]

CLINICAL DECISION-MAKING

Metastatic disease is rare in the sacrum, in comparison with other sites, but metastatic disease in this region is still 40 times more frequent than primary bone tumors.[31] Tumors requiring en bloc resection with negative margins are metastatic, giant cell tumor, chordoma, chondrosarcoma, and Ewing's sarcoma.[4,44]

The initial evaluation of sacral tumors must take into account tumor vascularity, encroachment of the anterior pelvic fascia, and the tumor location relative to the S1 level.[2] Lesions below the S1 level are considered distal, and those at the S1 level are considered proximal.[2] In general, distal sacral lesions are structurally stable lesions, and the sacrum is often not reconstructed.[2,31] Proximal lesions may alter the biomechanics at the lumbosacral junction substantially, and a stabilization procedure is more frequently performed.[2,41,45-47]

Total sacrectomy for proximal sacral pathology involves removal of the entire sacrum, including all of S1 and below, creating a complete spinopelvic discontinuity.[10] Sacroiliac stability is not greatly affected by resection if 50% or more of the sacroiliac joint is intact (corresponding to at least the upper half of the S1 segment).[6,8,30,33] Resection involving more than 50% of the sacroiliac joint makes the pelvis unstable and requires reconstruction. After extensive sacral tumor resection that results in complete dissociation of the spine from the pelvis, it is necessary to restore continuity of the spine and the pelvic ring.*

---

*References 13, 15, 18, 27, 48, 49.

Assessing instability in the lumbosacropelvic region focuses on the anterior column, axial load transmission to the pelvis, posterior tension band, and pelvic ring competency.[2] Although all of these factors are essential for biomechanical stability, stability is predicated on a strong anterior column, which bears 80% of the axial load.[2] The absence of a strong anterior column causes increased stress to be placed on the posterior elements through cantilever forces, impairment of normal axial load transfer, and up to a 50% reduction in pelvic strength.* The integrity of the anterior column can be compromised because of tumor involvement, resection, degenerative process, or infection.[2]

Instability of the lumbosacral junction should be assessed in terms of the anterior column, axial load transfer to the pelvis from the anterior column, and posterior tension band competence.[31] The anterior column is rendered unstable when resection of the sacrum or erosion resulting from the primary disease process extends to 1 cm below the sacral promontory in more than two thirds of the sacral endplate surface.[6] If the sacrum is structurally competent, with more than 1 cm of bone preserved below the promontory over at least one third to one half the S1 endplate, no anterior column reconstruction is required after tumor resection.[31]

Total sacrectomy, with or without excision of adjacent parts of the ilium, produces a large osseous and soft tissue defect, causing vertical and rotational instability.[4] Some surgeons do not advocate reconstruction of the osseous defect after total sacrectomy because of potential major wound complications, especially deep wound infection.[30,54-57] It has been reported that the ambulatory status of patients does not improve with stabilization, because the lumbar spine migrates inferiorly and remains between the ilia after total sacrectomy, and the muscles and scar between the pelvis and spine form a biological sling and eventually stabilize the spine.[30,55,56]

Because of the risk of infection and hardware failure, some investigators have recommended that reconstruction be avoided.[8,12,54,57] Wuisman et al[12] reported successful mobilization in five patients more than 8 weeks after total sacrectomy, without any form of pelvic reconstruction. However, others advocate that reconstruction of the lumbosacral junction may facilitate early mobilization, with associated improvements in quality of life and reduction of comorbid conditions associated with immobilization.[8,30]

TECHNIQUE

A sequential anterior and posterior approach to facilitate high sacral amputation was described by Bowers,[58] in 1948. The treatment of primary tumors of the proximal sacrum requires en bloc resection through an anterior-posterior technique.[31] Indications for a combined anterior-posterior approach include extensive tumor vascularity, primary proximal sacral tumor encroaching on the lumbosacral junction in an ex-

---

*References 2, 6, 18, 27, 33, 45, 50-53.

tensive fashion (in particular, the S1 endplate), and disease that penetrates the anterior pelvic fascia.[2]

For an anterior approach the patient is positioned supine with the appropriate padding at all contact points. An access vascular surgeon may aid in meticulous dissection techniques in this region and help with handling of the vascular structures. Incision is created longitudinally in the midline, 2 to 3 cm above the umbilicus, to the symphysis pubis. Laparotomy is performed where a retroperitoneal dissection of the lower lumbar and pelvic area is accomplished. The rectosigmoid colon is dissected from the presacral fascia to the coccygeal region.[27] The internal and external iliac vessels are then released.[9,10,27] The common iliac vessels, distal vena cava, and aorta are then mobilized.[27] Colostomy is occasionally performed at this point, if indicated. If a proximal sacral tumor is encountered, the internal iliac and middle sacral arteries and veins are ligated, along with any tumor vessels, and both external arteries should be preserved. Control is gained of the hypogastric vessels to enable a safer posterior sacrectomy. If tumor is involved with the rectum, it is carefully dissected away without injury. Lateral dissection of the sacral ala allows identification of the lumbar trunk of the lumbosacral plexus.[27] The sacroiliac joint is identified laterally, and partial ventral osteotomies are performed, if needed, for en bloc tumor resection out laterally. Osteotomy cuts are performed for the resection lateral to the lesion or at the sacroiliac joints. An L5-S1 discectomy is performed at this point. The middle sacral, lower lumbar segmental, iliolumbar, and internal iliac vessels are ligated when necessary. A flexible thin Silastic sheath is placed dorsal to the vascular structures and the rectum, isolating them from the lumbar vertebrae and sacrum and inhibiting formation of adhesions.[27] The abdominal skin closure is conducted layer by layer, and a drain is often left in place.

For the posterior approach, this stage is begun with general endotracheal intubation and positioning of the patient on a Jackson table, where all contact points receive appropriate padding. Somatosensory evoked potentials and electromyography can be considered for routine monitoring during these operations. After the site is widely prepared and draped in the usual sterile fashion, a posterior midline incision from L3 to the sacrum would be made to expose the posterior elements. Subperiosteal dissection is performed with Bovie electrocautery. The posterior iliac crests, greater sciatic foramina, and sciatic nerves are exposed bilaterally, as well as the L3-5 spinous processes, facet joints, and transverse processes. Self-retaining retractors are positioned during the exposure. The lumbosacral flap is lifted from the sacrum and retracted rostrally, permitting wide lateral and caudal exposure without causing ischemic damage and the retractor-related muscular injury that can occur with straight lateral retraction of the posterior lumbosacral musculature.[4,59] The gluteus maximus and medius muscles are mobilized from the lateral aspects of the iliac crests. After dissecting and retracting the gluteal muscles, the sciatic notch should be identified. Pedicle screw segmental instrumentation is performed at the L3 through L5 levels using standard anatomic landmarks, described by Lenke. Depending on the needed distal reconstruction, bilateral iliac bolts are also placed at this time, ultimately to anchor the lumbar construct into the pelvis. An L5 laminectomy is performed, and the dural sac and L5 and S1 roots are identified. Bilateral L5 foraminotomies are often performed if the disease extends widely into the sacrum. If the tumor has significantly compromised the S1 endplate, a bilateral facetectomy would be performed. An L5-S1 discectomy is completed where the annulus and posterior longitudinal ligament have been removed with the use of a Leksell rongeur and Kerrison punches, and the anterior longitudinal ligament has been removed during the anterior portion. The sacral canal at the appropriate levels would be decompressed laterally to the border with the pedicles. This differs from a total sacrectomy, which would feature undoming the entire sacral canal and sacrificing sacral nerve roots. The lumbosacral nerve roots, thecal sac, and tumor are identified as part of the surgical dissection, and the tumor would be dissected free of the thecal sac by using an ultrasonic aspirator in conjunction with standard microscopic dissection techniques. After completion of the dissection, each nerve root that was decompressed is visualized and tracked as it enters the tumor or anterior wall of the sacrum. Additional exposure can be achieved by retracting the thecal sac and nerve roots, thus creating a corridor for the aspirator or microscopic instruments to function between nerve roots. Complete tumor resection and disease-infiltrated bone can be accomplished down to the anterior pelvic fascia. If a complete sacrectomy is being performed, the dural sac at L5-S1 (inferior to the takeoff of the L5 nerve roots) would be ligated and cut.[17] The nerves that transit the portion of the sacrum, S1-5, involved with tumor are double ligated with 2-0 silk ties and transected.[17,31] Posterior osteotomies are performed laterally and caudally to match the anterior cuts created during the anterior stage of the procedure for tumor resection; and posterior osteotomies of the pedicle subtraction type for sacral deformity are performed with the use of a Midas Rex drill and high-speed diamond AM8 drill bit and an osteotome with a mallet. The lateral resection of the sacrum may extend out but not through the sacroiliac joints, if reconstruction allowing mobilization is to be considered.[2,31] Care is taken to preserve the S2 nerve roots, because these function to principally control voluntary bowel and bladder sphincter function.[27,42]

The surgeon attempts to resect only the portion of the sacrum needed for local oncologic control, sparing much of the sacroiliac joint and as many of the lumbosacral nerve roots as possible.[1] After en bloc tumor resection with negative margins has been accomplished, reconstruction is completed. Rodding is performed next. There are different techniques involving distal rod instrumentation, including the modified Galveston technique, double iliac screw/bolt fixation, and the transiliac bar with interbody cage technique. In the modified Galveston technique (often used for total sacrectomy), distally the vertical Galveston L-rods are directed laterally into the ilium between the two cortices to establish a bilateral liaison between the lumbar spine and the ilia. Each Galveston rod forms a one-piece bridge between the lumbar spine and an ilium, and the transiliac rod (6 mm) completes the pelvic ring. This system provides stability around the horizontal axis of the spinal column while also preventing rotation around this axis.[27] A small osteotomy is made in the cortex of the medial posterior iliac crest to create a path for the Galveston rod into the ilia at approximately the S2-3 level. This allows placement of a pilot rod into the cancellous portion of the ilium to create a path for the contoured rod. The temporary rod is directed to a point 1.5 cm above the sciatic notch and between the two cortices of the ilium, and is tapped into place by a mallet to a depth of 2 cm or more. After the permanent rod is cut and appropriately contoured, it is tapped to a depth of approximately 4 to 5 cm into the ilium and proximally attached to the lumbar pedicle screws. Two to three cross-links are placed between the rods to provide added stability, especially for torsion. Sometimes a tibial or femoral shaft allograft strut is used to close the space between the two ilia and to augment the instrumentation, and a bone fusion promoter or demineralized bone matrix and allograft bone chips are added across the graft area to facilitate fusion of the entire defect after decortication.

The double iliac screw/bolt fixation technique is often performed before decompression and osteotomies. For the transiliac bar technique with interbody cage, a transverse threaded rod is placed to fix opposing iliac bones to each other and thereby prevent axial rotation of the lumboiliac union. The entire surgical field is then irrigated with copious amounts of saline and antibiotic solution. The transverse process, lamina, and facets of L3-5 are decorticated, and these areas are packed with allograft and demineralized bone matrix for arthrodesis. Abundant autogenous pelvic crest bone graft is used to facilitate fusion of the inferior lumbar vertebra to the allograft fixation and the iliac crests. Fusion is desired from the transverse processes and lamina of the distal lumbar spine to the medioposterior aspect of the ilium bilaterally. The paraspinous muscles are then reapproximated. Several drains are placed at this time. The fascial layers are closed, followed by the dermal layer and the skin. Rectus abdominis myocutaneous flap coverage is used, on occasion, to close large defects. This flap helps to eliminate the void created by high sacrectomy, and thereby assists with prolonged wound drainage and breakdown.[4] It involves transposition retroperitoneally to the sacral region of the patient, and the umbilicus is reconstructed anteriorly during that portion of the operation.[9] Local gluteal muscle flap can also be used before closure.

If a double iliac screw fixation is performed prior to decompression and osteotomies or tumor resection, the iliac screw entry points are identified by means of a curved osteotome to resect the appropriate portions of the posterior superior iliac spine. The iliac starter probe or Lenke probe is channeled for the inferior screw, where the two resected areas of the posterior superior iliac spine exist, between the two cortical plates of the ilium, and advanced just above the sciatic notch. A ball-tipped probe feeler confirms that no cortical breeches have been encountered. The inferior iliac screw path is tapped, and the screw is inserted into the inferior ilium. The inferior iliac screw must be long enough (70 to 80 mm in length) to endure weight-loading. The superior iliac screw is channeled parallel to the inferior screw, also above the sciatic notch. The superior iliac screw path is then tapped, and the iliac screw is inserted into the superior ilium (40 to 50 mm in length). This technique is performed on both sides. Before closure, two rods then connect the lumbar pedicle screws, and two offset short rods are used to connect the main rods and the superior iliac screws. In addition, two short rods connect the inferior iliac screws and the distal aspect of the main rod. Cross-links are placed between the main rods.

A Pyramesh titanium cage (Medtronic Sofamor-Danek, Memphis, TN) induces axial support, transferring the spinal axial load through a transiliac bar, and posterior segmental instrumentation in which pedicle screws and iliac bolts are used for reconstruction all provide immediate lumbosacropelvic stabilization.[2,31,60] This iliac bar traverses a mesh cage resting on the lower endplate of the L5 vertebral body.[60] This allows for immediate spinal-pelvic stability and early ambulation in patients with metastatic tumors who undergo subtotal resection.[60] Posterior column reconstruction alone does not allow transfer of the anterior column axial load to the pelvis. This can be accomplished by fitting a titanium mesh cage against the endplate of L5, where the cage is packed with bone graft material and has a passage that allows a 0.25 inch titanium rod to pass through.[31] A Kirschner wire is then passed through a stab incision in the skin on the lateral aspect of the hip. The Kirschner wire is passed under fluoroscopic guidance through the ipsilateral ilium, the cage, the contralateral ilium, and out through the contralateral hip.[31] A 0.25 inch cannulated reamer is passed over the Kirschner wire, and the ilium is perforated bilaterally.[31] A 0.25 inch titanium rod is passed through the ilium bilaterally and the cage.[31] Connectors are affixed to the rod to prevent movement.[31] The cage is immobile because of its placement flush up against the endplate of L5. Additional bone and graft material can be packed around the cage and rod to promote fusion or dense scarring to give added support to the construct.

OUTCOMES WITH EVALUATION OF RESULTS

Pelvic reconstruction techniques have evolved in parallel with improvements in spinal instrumentation, but presently the optimal reconstruction procedure has not been established after total sacrectomy.[61] The Galveston rod technique was first described for the treatment of neuromuscular scoliosis with pelvic obliquity.[4,62,63] It was proposed by Allen and Ferguson.[62] It was first used in conjunction with sublaminar wiring of the lumbar spine.[4,64] While originally not providing substantial torsional stability or significant resistance to extension, pedicle screws superseded these constructs.[4,64] Gokaslan et al[27] modified the original Galveston rod technique by placing lumbar pedicle screws for the sublaminar wiring and Harrington rods. Jackson and Gokaslan[59] found that the Galveston L-rod pelvic fixation was an effective way of achieving stabilization, providing significant pain relief, and maintaining ambulatory function.[4] The technique provides a long moment lever arm where an iliac rod extends anterior to the lumbosacral pivot point to withstand the forces exerted by the spine.[4,65] A threaded rod (transiliac bar) is placed anterior to the Galveston rods, and the ends outside the iliac cortical surfaces are secured with C-clamps.[17] The modified Galveston technique described by Jackson and Gokaslan[59] provides more rigidity than the wiring technique but has the disadvantage of requiring rod contouring, which can be time-consuming and difficult.[9]

The double iliac screw fixation with posterior lumbar fixation may be biomechanically stronger because it counteracts the rotational force of the spinopelvic axis more tightly than the modified Galveston technique.[4] Breakage of the spinal rod between the L5 pedicle screw and the iliac portion for modified Galveston reconstruction has been observed clinically because of the high stress transmitted to the pelvis by the spinal rods.[59,66,67] The L-shaped Galveston rods inserted into the ilia have shown signs of loosening. The system may have caudal migration because no connections between the transiliac rod and Galveston rods and the pelvic reconstruction plate have been noted to be broken bilaterally on routine follow-up radiographs.[30] The modified Galveston reconstruction technique does not optimally resist rotation around the horizontal axis.[17] Rotation around the horizontal axis is limited by the constrained position of the iliac portion of the Galveston rod and the position of the transiliac bar anterior to the Galveston rod.[33] This is clinically manifested as loosening noted of the Galveston rod within the ilium, resulting in radiolucencies (halo) around the iliac-based instrumentation.[17,59,68]

Another type of instrumented reconstruction consists of the triangular frame. It features the L5 vertebral body pulled distally and placed between the bilateral iliac crest. There is a risk of sacral rod loosening in the triangular frame reconstruction because of high stress of the cortical bone at the interface with the pelvis and L5 vertebral body. Rotation is limited by cross-connecting the lumbar rods to the rod connecting the iliac screws and to the transiliac bar.[17] Three-dimensional rod contouring is a challenge in the modified Galveston technique.[17] There has been no mechanical analysis of these reconstructions.[59,61,66,67]

Shikata et al[48] described the first lumbar-iliac fixation system for sacrectomy in which a combination of Harrington rods and hooks, sacral bars, and bone grafts were used. Iliac bones were jointed with the sacral bars, and the L5 vertebral body was lowered 2 cm and shifted anteriorly. This technique does not provide rotational stability around the horizontal axis of the spine, and the sacral bars connecting the soft posterior iliac wings do not provide firm fixation.[27,69]

In the treatment of sacral fracture, sacroiliac disruption, and partial sacrectomy, where 50% of the sacroiliac joint remains intact, the sacroiliac joint screw technique has been used.[4,70] The iliac-sacral screw fixation technique through the posterior approach is recommended after partial removal of the sacrum.[4,28,71] It has been shown to be associated with less failure than the Galveston technique.[4,28,71] It can be used with hooks or pedicle screws in the lumbar spine.[4,28,71] The posterior iliosacral plating and screw fixation technique through a posterior approach, after partial removal of the sacrum, is often used with sacroiliac joint screw placement.[4,29,71]

Functional outcomes have been evaluated by Guo et al,[72] who performed a retrospective analysis of 50 patients who underwent sacrectomy over a 9-year period and observed more wound infections in patients who had postoperative bowel incontinence, which led to wound infection, longer length of hospital stay, and delayed wound healing. They also appreciated a strong association between S3 nerve root integrity and bowel and bladder continence.[72] These complications can severely affect a patient's quality of life. Some surgeons often have their patients who require a sacrectomy undergo an elective colostomy for bowel diversion when there is likelihood that bowel function retraining may prove difficult on preoperative counseling.

There are several problems associated with sacral excision, such as bowel, bladder, and sexual dysfunction, infection, massive blood loss, and high incidence of local relapse.* Investigators including McDonnell et al[76] assigned early complications to major or minor categories. Major complications were defined as those that prolonged the length of hospital stay, and minor complications (including superficial wound infection and urinary tract infection) were defined as those that did not significantly alter the hospital course.[76] The risk of infection, loss of large amounts of blood, wound complications, and neurologic dysfunction are all problems associated with sacrectomy.[77-79] Gait abnormalities and lower extremity motor weakness are common complications as well. The extent of reconstruction and proximity of the incision to the rectum results in a high rate of wound complications that must be anticipated.† The risk of postoperative infection is high because of the large space vacated by the sacrum, the use of instrumentation, and the long duration of the surgery.[13] Serious wound complications after sacrectomy have been reported in as many as 25% to 46% of patients.[72,81-83] Chronic wound abscess and osteomyelitis of the sacroiliac joint can be observed. Other complications include pneumonia, urinary tract infection, and *Clostridium difficile* colitis.

Nonneurologic complications include internal iliac vein thrombosis, pulmonary embolus requiring an inferior vena cava filter, pneumonia, and disseminated intravascular coagulopathy.[2] Zileli et al[9] reported three deaths in their series, including stroke from fat embolus and septic shock from rectal perforation secondary to rectal wall ischemia. Foot drop is also seen from likely traction injury to the lumbosacral plexus or L5 nerve root.

Randall et al[10] reported significant bowel incontinence and bladder dysfunction in their series of total sacrectomies, requiring the need for a postoperative regimen of intermittent catheterization and suppository management. The status of bowel and bladder function is particularly relevant to the surgical management of sacral tumors.[19] En bloc sacrectomies sacrifice sacral roots, and it is critical that the function of these roots be preserved when possible.[9,12,19] Preservation of the S2 nerve roots bilaterally is required for intact autonomic bowel, bladder, and sexual function.‡ Sacrifice of the S3 nerve root causes sexual dysfunction, and loss of the bilateral S2 nerve roots causes loss

---

*References 13, 15, 33, 45, 48, 73-75.
†References 7, 50, 51, 54, 80, 81.
‡References 7, 8, 11, 19, 21, 84.

of normal urogenital and rectal function.[13,75] Patients undergoing amputations distal to S3 generally experience limited deficits, with preservation of sphincter function in the most of them and reduced perineal sensation in some.[8]

The morbidity associated with total sacrectomy is profound. The results of total sacrectomy reported by Fourney et al[8] showed that all five patients who underwent total sacrectomy suffered complete loss of bowel and bladder function and managed with intermittent urinary self-catheterization, laxatives for regular bowel evacuation, and manual emptying of the rectum on one occasion. These patients also experienced complete saddle anesthesia and sexual inability.[8]

Transverse partial sacrectomy is a surgical option for treating tumors of the caudal sacrum because it provides adequate surgical margins while maintaining pelvic ring and spinal column stability.[1] The mechanical consequences of transverse partial sacrectomy are poorly understood, and disarticulation of the spinopelvic segment may require bony stabilization and reconstruction using complex methods that involve lumbosacral-iliac arthrodesis.[1] This type of reconstruction can add surgical complexity and morbidity, but a transverse partial sacrectomy below the S2 foramina typically would not involve resection of the sacroiliac joints and would have little effect on stability.[1] Unfortunately the mechanical consequences of high partial-transverse sacrectomy are also not well understood by surgeons.[1] In a study of nine patients undergoing partial sacrectomies involving a portion of the S1 body for chordoma, three of them developed postoperative fractures, resulting in subsequent need for complex pelvic reconstruction by means of iliolumbar arthrodesis and spinal instrumentation.[11]

Hugate et al[1] performed a cadaveric study that examined the effects of transverse osteotomies involving the S1 and S2 sacral bodies. As seen in the cadaveric studies by Gunterberg et al[6] and Hugate et al,[1] examining the strength of the pelvis after specific osteotomy techniques, there were no failures at the sacroiliac joint. Hugate et al[1] found that the weak mechanical link was the inability of the base of the sacral ala to resist sagittal plane rotation.

Surgical management of patients needing proximal sacrectomies is quite complicated, and a perfect algorithm that would be applicable in all cases does not exist.[2] The goals of surgery should include restoration of the pelvic ring to facilitate axial load transfer from the spinal column to the pelvis.[2] In addition to stabilization and reconstruction, surgical objectives with regard to the treatment of the primary disease process include maximal decompression and tumor debulking for metastatic sacral tumors and maximal debridement of infected bone in osteomyelitis.[2] The goal for primary sacral tumors involves en bloc resection with sacrifice of neural elements to ensure maximal tumor debulking.[2,41,46,47,59] Pelvic ring competency must be ensured for a stable lumbopelvic construct.[2] The pelvic ring may be restored by a transiliac bar in cases where the sacrum is removed.[2] Pelvic ring competency is vital to the transfer of axial load onto the pelvis and then onto the femurs. Immediate spine stability is necessary to achieve early ambulation in patients requiring lumbosacropelvic reconstruction.[2]

SIGNATURE CASE

47-year-old woman with prior L3-S1 decompression and fusion who developed a sacral fracture and kyphosis. The patient underwent removal of implants and extension of fusion with bilateral dual iliac fixation. She then underwent stage II sacral (S2) subtraction osteotomy with osteotomy of bilateral sacral ala to complete sacral-pelvic dissociation and realignment. She underwent transiliac bar placement with plastics clo-

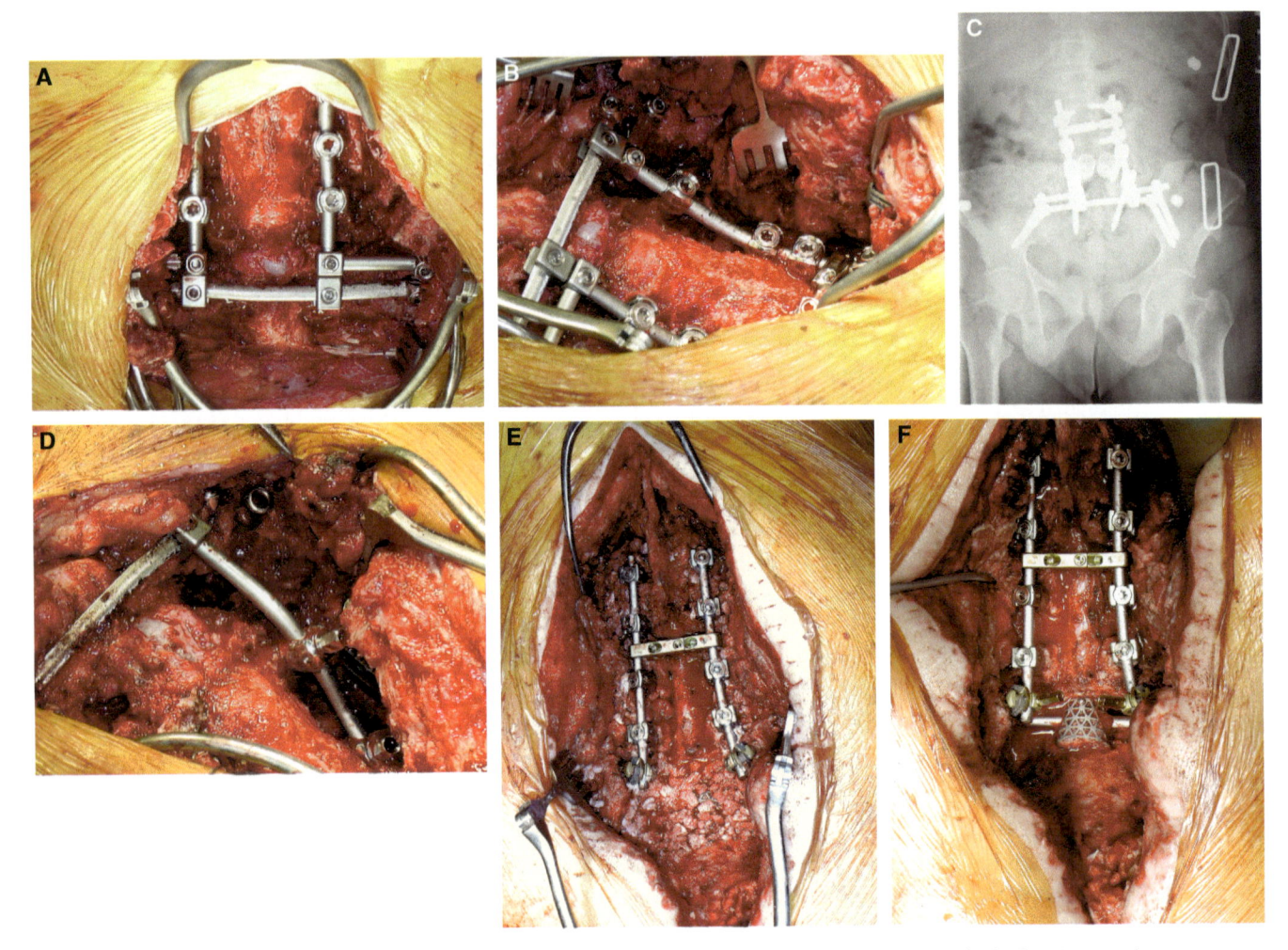

Fig. 47-2 **A** and **B,** Intraoperative photographs showing double iliac screw/bolt fixation technique with lumbar segmental instrumentation. Decompression of the thecal sac is also illustrated. **C,** Postoperative plain radiograph demonstrating lumbosacral pelvic reconstruction consisting of lumbar pedicle screws, sacral screws, bilateral iliac bolts, two interbody cages, and rodding system with cross-connector. **D,** Intraoperative photograph showing decompressed lumbar spine, sacrectomy, and instrumented pelvic reconstruction. **E,** Intraoperative photograph demonstrating lumbosacral pelvic segmental instrumentation after lumbar decompression and sacrectomy. **F,** Intraoperative photograph showing lumbar pedicle screw system with segmental instrumentation and bilateral rods, bilateral sacral bolts, and Pyramesh titanium cage with transiliac bar.

sure. The patient did well postoperatively but developed proximal junctional kyphosis and required L2 pedicle subtraction osteotomy and T10-S1/ilium posterior spinal fusion with removal of transiliac bar. The patient did well after surgery. She developed junctional kyphosis and required extension to T4 with a T10 vertebral column resection. The patient died from psychiatric complications several years later.

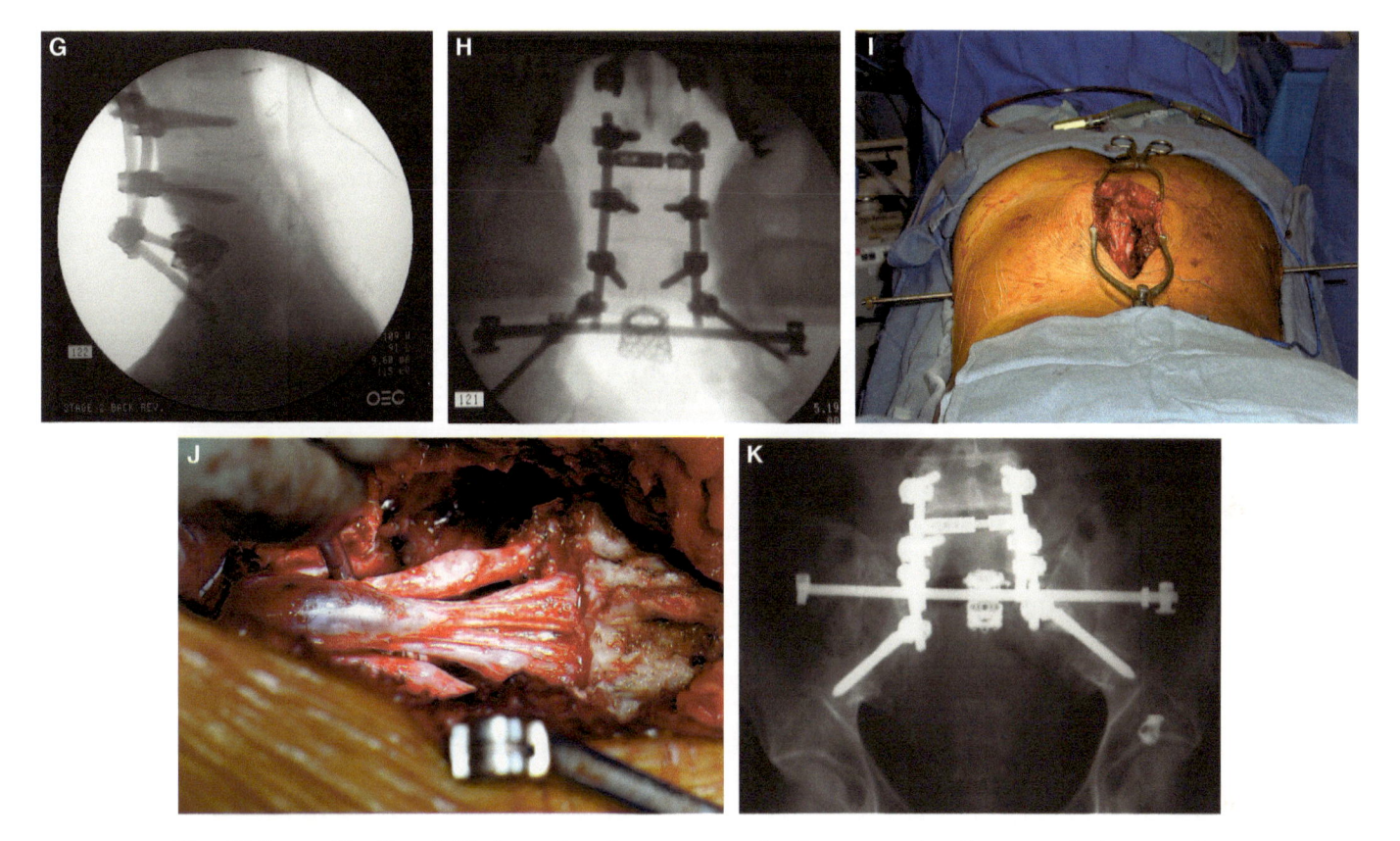

Fig. 47-2, cont'd **G** and **H,** Lateral and anteroposterior intraoperative fluoroscopic images after placement of Pyramesh titanium cage with transiliac bar and C-clamps for reconstruction of the pelvic ring. This technique also uses segmental lumbar pedicle screws, bilateral rods, and bilateral iliac bolts. **I,** Photograph showing the patient positioned in the operating room where the transiliac bar is placed. **J,** Intraoperative photograph showing decompressed thecal sac and sacral roots after proximal sacrectomy. **K,** Postoperative anteroposterior plain radiograph highlighting lumbosacral pelvic reconstruction featuring a Pyramesh cage with transiliac bar and C-clamps for the anterior column, and pedicle screws of the lumbar spine and bilateral bolts anchored in the ilium with bilateral rods connecting the construct. A cross-link is also featured.

CONCLUSION

Proximal sacrectomy with pelvic reconstruction has been demonstrated to be a safe and effective procedure for postinfectious process, deformity correction featuring osteotomy techniques, and tumor resection of the proximal sacrum. The medical fitness of the patient, the anatomic extent of the disease, and the appraisal of the biological behavior of the tumor are the major factors in determining candidacy for en bloc sacral resection.[8] The goal of en bloc surgical resection is to provide optimal long-term tumor control in appropriately selected patients.[8,10]

BAILOUT TECHNIQUES

- A combined surgical team consisting of neurosurgeons, vascular surgeons, and plastic surgeons is very useful for proximal sacrectomy.
- A multidisciplinary approach can make a proximal sacretomy a safe prodecure.

TIPS FROM THE MASTERS

- Proximal sacrectomy can be effective in treating sacropelvic deformity and tumor resection.
- Proper patient selection is important to ensure optimal outcomes.
- Biomechanically stable sacropelvic fixation is of utmost importance in reconstruction after sacrectomy.

References (With Key References in Boldface)

1. Hugate RR Jr, Dickey ID, Phimolsarnti R, et al. Mechanical effects of partial sacrectomy: when is reconstruction necessary? Clin Orthop Relat Res 450: 82-88, 2006.
2. Mindea SA, Salehi SA, Ganju A, et al. Lumbosacropelvic junction reconstruction resulting in early ambulation for patients with lumbosacral neoplasms or osteomyelitis. Neurosurg Focus 15:E6, 2003.
3. Hsieh PC, Ondra SL, Wienecke RJ, et al. A novel approach to sagittal balance restoration following iatrogenic sacral fracture and resulting sacral kyphotic deformity: technical note. J Neurosurg Spine 6:368-372, 2007.
4. Zhang HY, Thongtrangan I, Balabhadra RSV, et al. Surgical techniques for total sacrectomy and spinopelvic reconstruction. Neurosurg Focus 15:E5, 2003.
5. Yu B, Zheng Z, Zhuang X, et al. Biomechanical effects of transverse partial sacrectomy on the sacroiliac joints: an in vitro human cadaveric investigation of the borderline of sacroiliac joint instability. Spine 34:1370-1375, 2009.
6. Gunterberg B, Romanus B, Stener B. Pelvic strength after major amputation of the sacrum. An experimental study. Acta Orthop Scand 47:635-642, 1976.
7. Feldenzer JA, McGauley JL, McGillicuddy JE. Sacral and pre-sacral tumors: problems in diagnosis and management. Neurosurgery 25:884-891, 1989.

8. **Fourney DR, Rhines LD, Hentschel SJ, et al. En bloc resection of primary sacral tumors: classification of surgical approaches and outcome. J Neurosurg Spine 3:111-122, 2005.**
9. Zileli M, Hoscoskun C, Brastianos P, et al. Surgical treatment of primary sacral tumors: complications associated with sacrectomy. Neurosurg Focus 15:E9, 2003.
10. Randall RL, Bruckner J, Lloyd C, et al. Sacral resection and reconstruction for tumors and tumor-like conditions. Orthopedics 28:307-313, 2005.
11. Todd LT Jr, Yaszemski MJ, Currier BL, et al. Bowel and bladder function after major sacral resection. Clin Orthop Relat Res 397:36-39, 2002.
12. Wuisman P, Lieshout O, Sugihara S, et al. Total sacrectomy and reconstruction: oncologic and functional outcome. Clin Orthop Relat Res 381:192-203, 2000.
13. Ohata N, Ozaki T, Kunisada T, et al. Extended total sacrectomy and reconstruction for sacral tumor. Spine 29:E123-E126, 2004.
14. Ozaki T, Flege S, Liljenqvist U, et al. Osteosarcoma of the spine: experience of the Cooperative Osteosarcoma Study Group. Cancer 94:1069-1077, 2002.
15. Wuisman P, Lieshout O, van Dijk M, et al. Reconstruction after total en bloc sacrectomy for osteosarcoma using a custom-made prosthesis: a technical note. Spine 26:431-439, 2001.
16. Cheng EY, Ozerdemoglu RA, Transfeldt EE, et al. Lumbosacral chordoma: prognostic factors and treatment. Spine 24:1639-1645, 1999.
17. Gallia GL, Haque R, Garonzik I, et al. Spinal pelvic reconstruction after total sacrectomy for en bloc resection of a giant sacral chordoma: technical note. J Neurosurg Spine 3:501-506, 2005.
18. **Tomita K, Tsuchiya H. Total sacrectomy and reconstruction for huge sacral tumors. Spine 15:1223-1227, 1990.**
19. McLoughlin GS, Sciubba DM, Suk I, et al. En bloc total sacrectomy performed in a single stage through a posterior approach. Neurosurgery 63 (1 Suppl 1):ONS115-120; discussion ONS120, 2008.
20. Anson KM, Byrne PO, Robertson ID, et al. Radical excision of sacrococcygeal tumors. Br J Surg 81:460-461, 1994.
21. Fourney DR, Gokaslan ZL. Surgical approaches for the resection of sacral tumors. In Dickman CA, Fehlings MG, Gokaslan ZL, eds. Spinal Cord and Spinal Column Tumors: Principles and Practice. New York: Thieme Medical, 2006.
22. Sung HW, Shu WP, Wang HM, et al. Surgical treatment of primary tumors of the sacrum. Clin Orthop Relat Res 215:91-98, 1987.
23. Bergh P, Gunterberg B, Meis-Kindblom JM, et al. Prognostic factors and outcome of pelvic, sacral, and spinal chondrosarcomas: a center-based study of 69 cases. Cancer 91:1201-1212, 2001.
24. Bethke KP, Neifeld JP, Lawrence W Jr. Diagnosis and management of sacrococcygeal chordoma. J Surg Oncol 48:232-238, 1991.
25. Kaiser TE, Pritchard DJ, Unni KK. Clinicopathologic study of sacrococcygeal chordoma. Cancer 53:2574-2578, 1984.
26. York JE, Kaczaraj A, Abi-Said D, et al. Sacral chordoma: 40-year experience at a major cancer center. Neurosurgery 44:74-80, 1999.
27. **Gokaslan ZL, Romsdahl MM, Kroll SS, et al. Total sacrectomy and Galveston L-rod reconstruction for malignant neoplasms. Technical note. J Neurosurg 87:781-787, 1997.**
28. Freeman BL III. Scoliosis and kyphosis. In Canale ST, ed. Campbell's Operative Orthopedics, vol 3, 9th ed. St Louis: CV Mosby, 1998.
29. Fuchs B, Yaszemski MJ, Sim FH. Combined posterior pelvis and lumbar spine resection for sarcoma. Clin Orthop 397:12-18, 2002.
30. Doita M, Harada T, Iguchi T, et al. Total sacrectomy and reconstruction for sacral tumors. Spine 28:E296-E301, 2003.
31. Ondra SL, Salehi SA, Ganju A. Primary and metastatic disease of the sacrum and lumbar-sacral junction. In Batjer HH, Loftus CM, eds. Textbook of Neurological Surgery: Principles and Practice, vol 2. Philadelphia: Lippincott Williams & Wilkins, 2003.
32. Ishii K, Chiba K, Watanabe M, et al. Local recurrence after S2-3 sacrectomy in sacral chordoma. Report of four cases. J Neurosurg 97:98-101, 2002.

33. Stener B, Gunterberg B. High amputation of the sacrum for extirpation of tumors. Principles and technique. Spine 3:351-366, 1978.
34. Azzarelli A, Quagliuolo V, Cerasoli S, et al. Chordoma: natural history and treatment results in 33 cases. J Surg Oncol 37:185-191, 1988.
35. Bergh P, Kindblom LG, Gunterberg B, et al. Prognostic factors in chordoma of the sacrum and mobile spine: a study of 39 patients. Cancer 88:2122-2134, 2000.
36. Fourney DR, Gokaslan ZL. Current management of sacral chordoma. Neurosurg Focus 15:E9, 2003.
37. Yonemoto T, Tatezaki S, Takenouchi T, et al. The surgical management of sacrococcygeal chordoma. Cancer 85:878-883, 1999.
38. Turcotte RE, Sim FH, Unni KK. Giant cell tumor of the sacrum. Clin Orthop Relat Res 291:215-221, 1993.
39. Althausen PL, Schneider PD, Bold RJ, et al. Multimodality management of a giant cell tumor arising in the proximal sacrum: case report. Spine 27:E361-E365, 2002.
40. York JE, Berk RH, Fuller GN, et al. Chondrosarcoma of the spine: 1954 to 1997. J Neurosurg 90:73-38, 1999.
41. Rosen G, Caparros B, Nirenberg A, et al. Ewing's sarcoma: ten-year experience with adjuvant chemotherapy. Cancer 47:2204-2213, 1981.
42. Fujimura Y, Maruiwa H, Takahata T, et al. Neurological evaluation after radical resection of sacral neoplasms. Paraplegia 32:396-406, 1994.
43. Nakai S, Yoshizawa H, Kobayashi S, et al. Anorectal and bladder function after sacrifice of the sacral nerves. Spine 25:2234-2239, 2000.
44. Bridwell KH. Management of tumors at the lumbosacral junction. In Margulies JY, Floman Y, Farcy JPC, et al, eds. Lumbosacral and Spinopelvic Fixation. Philadelphia: Lippincott-Raven, 1996.
45. Samson IR, Springfield DS, Suit HD, et al. Operative treatment of sacrococcygeal chordoma. A review of twenty-one cases. J Bone Joint Surg Am 75:1476-1484, 1993.
46. Barwick KW, Huvos AG, Smith J. Primary osteogenic sarcoma of the vertebral column: a clinicopathologic correlation of ten patients. Cancer 46:595-604, 1980.
47. Weinstein JN, McLain RF. Primary tumors of the spine. Spine 12:843-851, 1987.
48. Shikata J, Yamamuro T, Kotoura Y, et al. Total sacrectomy and reconstruction for primary tumors: report of two cases. J Bone Joint Surg Am 70:122-125, 1988.
49. Clark J, Rocques PJ, Crew AJ, et al. Identification of novel genes, SYT and SSX, involved in the t (X;18) (p11.2;q11.2) translocation found in human synovial sarcoma. Nat Genet 7:502-508, 1994.
50. Gennari L, Azzarelli A, Quagliuolo V. A posterior approach for the excision of sacral chordoma. J Bone Joint Surg Br 69:565-568, 1987.
51. Localio SA, Eng K, Ranson JH. Abdominosacral approach for retrorectal tumors. Ann Surg 191:555-560, 1980.
52. Ozdemir MH, Gurkan I, Yildiz Y, et al. Surgical treatment of malignant tumours of the sacrum. Eur J Surg Oncol 25:44-49, 1999.
53. Wuisman P, Harle A, Matthiass HH, et al. Two-stage therapy in the treatment of sacral tumors. Arch Orthop Trauma Surg 108:255-260, 1989.
54. Michel A. Total sacrectomy and lower spine resection for giant cell tumor: one case report. Chir Organi Mov 75(Suppl):117-118, 1990.
55. Edwards CC. Spinal reconstruction in tumor management. In Uhthoff HK, ed. Current Concepts of Diagnosis and Treatment of Bone and Soft Tissue Tumors. New York: Springer-Verlag, 1984.
56. Cappanna R, Bricolli A, Campanacci LC, et al. Benign and malignant tumors of the sacrum. In Frymore JW, ed. The Adult Spine: Principles and Practice. Philadelphia: Lippincott-Raven, 1997.
57. Simpson AH, Porter A, Davis A, et al. Cephalad screw resection with a combined extended ilioinguinal and posterior approach. J Bone Joint Surg Am 77A:405-411, 1995.
58. Bowers RF. Giant cell tumor of the sacrum: a case report. Ann Surg 128:1164-1172, 1948.
59. **Jackson RJ, Gokaslan ZL. Spinal-pelvic fixation in patients with lumbosacral neoplasms. J Neurosurg 92:61-70, 2000.**

60. Salehi SA, McCafferty RR, Karahalios D, et al. Neural function preservation and early mobilization after resection of metastatic sacral tumors and lumbosacropelvic junction reconstruction. J Neurosurg 97:88-93, 2002.
61. Murakami H, Kawahara N, Tomita K, et al. Biomechanical evaluation of reconstructed lumbosacral spine after total sacrectomy. J Orthop Sci 7:658-664, 2002.
62. Allen BL Jr, Ferguson RL. The Galveston technique for L rod instrumentation of the scoliotic spine. Spine 7:276-284, 1982.
63. Allen BL Jr, Ferguson RL. The Galveston technique of pelvic fixation with L-rod instrumentation of the spine. Spine 9:388-394, 1984.
64. Ogilvie JW, Bradford DS. Sublaminar fixation in lumbosacral fusions. Clin Orthop 269:157-161, 1991.
65. Benzel EC. Biomechanics of Spine Stabilization. Rolling Meadows, IL: AANS Press, 2001.
66. Kawahara N, Murakami H, Yoskida A, et al. Reconstruction after total sacrectomy using a new instrumentation technique: a biomechanical comparison. Spine (Phila Pa 1976) 28:14, 1567-1572, 2003.
67. Kuroki H, Tajima N, Kubo S, et al. [Instrument failure after total sacrectomy and reconstruction of the sacrum] Nishinihonsekituikenkyukaisi 24:209-212, 1998.
68. Spiegel DA, Richardson WJ, Scully SP, et al. Long-term survival following total sacrectomy with reconstruction for the treatment of primary osteosarcoma of the sacrum. J Bone Joint Surgery Am 81:848-855, 1999.
69. Thomson J, Doty JR. Sacral biomechanics and reconstruction. In Doty JR, Rengachary SS, eds. Surgical Disorders of the Sacrum. New York: Thieme Medical, 1994.
70. Guyton JL. Fractures of hip, acetabulum, and pelvis. In Canale ST, ed. Campbell's Operative Orthopedics, vol 2, 9th ed. St Louis: Mosby, 1998.
71. Norris BL, Bosse MJ, Kellam JF, et al. Pelvic fractures: sacral fixation. In Wiss DA, ed. Fractures. Philadelphia: Lippincott-Raven, 1998.
72. Guo Y, Palmer JL, Shen L, et al. Bowel and bladder continence, wound healing, and functional outcomes in patients who underwent sacrectomy. J Neurosurg Spine 3:106-110, 2005.
73. Sundaresan N, Huvos AG, Krol G, et al. Postradiation sarcoma involving the spine. Neurosurgery 18:721-724, 1986.
74. Sundaresan N, Huvos AG, Krol G, et al. Surgical treatment of spinal chordomas. Arch Surg 122:1479-1482, 1987.
75. Ozaki T, Hillman A, Windelmann W. Surgical treatment of sacrococcygeal chordoma. J Surg Oncol 64:274-279, 1997.
76. McDonnell MF, Glassman SD, Dimar JR II, et al. Perioperative complications of anterior procedures on the spine. J Bone Joint Surg Am 78:839-847, 1996.
77. Gunterberg B. Effects of major resection of the sacrum. Clinical studies on urogenital and anorectal function and a biomechanical study on pelvic strength. Acta Orthop Scand Suppl 162:1-38, 1976.
78. Gunterberg B, Kewenter J, Petersen I, et al. Anorectal function after major resections of the sacrum with bilateral or unilateral sacrifice of sacral nerves. Br J Surg 63:546-554, 1976.
79. Gunterberg B, Norlen L, Stener B, et al. Neurologic evaluation after resection of the sacrum. Invest Urol 13:183-188, 1975.
80. Husmann OA, Cain MP. Fecal and urinary continence after ileal cecal cystoplasty for the neurogenic bladder. J Urol 165:922-925, 2001.
81. Magrini S, Nelson H, Gunderson LL, et al. Sacropelvic resection and intra-operative electron irradiation in the management of recurrent anorectal cancer. Dis Colon Rectum 39:1-9, 1996.
82. Touran T, Frost DB, O'Connell TX. Sacral resection. Operative technique and outcome. Arch Surg 125:911-913, 1990.
83. Wanebo HJ, Gaker DL, Whitehill R, et al. Pelvic recurrence of rectal cancer. Options for curative resection. Ann Surg 205:482-495, 1987.
84. Harrison SJ, McDonnell DE. Sacrectomy. In Doty JR, Rengacharry SS, eds. Surgical Disorders of the Sacrum. New York: Thieme Medical, 1994.

Chapter 48

Pediatric Spine and Spinal Cord Tumors

Andrew Jea, Nalin Gupta,
Peter P. Sun, Kurtis Ian Auguste

Tumors involving the spine and spinal cord in children are unique clinical entities that are distinct from their adult counterparts. Diagnosis of these lesions often requires careful attention to subtle clinical findings and an array of radiologic findings. Surgical options are designed with the specific characteristics of the immature spine in mind. Surgical techniques for the pediatric spine continue to evolve in their complexity, and, as a result, ever more challenging pediatric spinal pathology can be treated with success.

Pediatric spine tumors are categorized according to their location, and the differential diagnosis is broad. Spine tumors are classified as extradural (30%), intradural-extramedullary (45%), and intramedullary (25%).[1-4] The list of potential underlying pathologic findings includes tumors types of that appear much more frequently and at times exclusively in the pediatric population (Table 48-1). Ewing's sarcoma is the most common primary malignant spinal bone tumor in children.[5-7] Neuroblastoma is both the most common extracranial solid malignancy in infancy and childhood and the most common cause of spinal cord compression in the pediatric population.[8-10] Most intradural-extramedullary tumors arise from the leptomeningeal spread of primary brain tumors.[3]

The management of spinal column tumors has evolved significantly over the past 10 years. Advances in spinal instrumentation, surgical approaches, and techniques in children have enabled surgeons to treat these lesions more radically and to reconstruct the spinal column more effectively. The use of spinal stabilization in conjunction with the surgical treatment of these neoplasms has resulted in significant improvement in outcomes.[11] Fusion techniques derived from the adult spinal instrumentation tech-

Table 48-1 Summary of Pediatric Spine and Spinal Cord Tumors

Extradural	Intradural-Extramedullary	Intramedullary
Bone tumors	Neurofibroma	Astrocytoma
Ewing's sarcoma	Schwannoma	Ganglioglioma
Langerhan's cell histiocytosis/eosinophilic granuloma	Meningioma	Ependymoma
Osteoid osteoma/osteoblastoma	Ependymoma (myxopapillary)	Hemangioblastoma
Osteochondroma	Dermoid/epidermoid cyst	
Osteosarcoma	Atypical teratoid rhabdoid tumor	
Osteoclastoma/giant cell tumors	Primitive neuroectodermal tumor	
Aneurysmal bone cyst	Neurenteric cyst	
Chordoma	Arachnoid cyst	
Sacrococcygeal teratoma		
Hemangioma		
Neurofibroma		
Schwannoma		
Leukemia/lymphoma		
Extraspinal sarcoma		
Neuroblastoma		
Ganglioneuroma		
Germ cell tumor		
Metastases		

niques are applicable, with the exception of the youngest patients (<1 year old). Occipitocervical screw fixation has been used in children as young as 1.5 years of age,[12] obviating the need for external fixation devices, such halo-vest or cast immobilization, which may be poorly tolerated by children. Pedicle screw fixation is feasible in children as young as 4 years of age.[13] For children 8 years of age and older, the anatomy and configuration of the spine do not differ from the adult spine in terms of sensitivity or response to instrumentation.[14,15]

Preoperative thin-cut computed tomography (CT) through the area of interest should help the surgeon decide whether the bony anatomy is suitable for instrumentation. Screw length and screw trajectory should be estimated on the basis of preoperative CT scans. This is especially true for pediatric patients, given the wide variety of bone thicknesses in children of different ages.

Titanium alloy implants should be used in cases of neoplasms where frequent magnetic resonance imaging (MRI) is anticipated to monitor for evidence of local recurrence. The decreased ferromagnetic properties of titanium alloy, as compared with stainless steel, result in less scatter distortion of the image, permitting better follow-up of patients with tumors.[16] Segmental implants, such as cross-link members, should be omitted directly over or opposite the site of the tumor, as this may cause an unnecessary degradation in postoperative imaging.

Children past the infancy period can be successfully instrumented for spinal stability without increased risk or complications in the immediate postoperative period. However, follow-up studies are needed to determine the long-term effects, in terms of spinal alignment and growth, in the immature pediatric spine. Some reports studying the upper cervical spine after instrumented fusion have found minimal effects on alignment and growth[12]; however, effects on the pediatric spine below the C2 level have yet to be determined.

Anterior spinal instrumentation is used far less commonly than posterior spinal instrumentation in children. Still, surgical management of congenital deformities, such as kyphosis or scoliosis, often involves anterior instrumentation. Acquired deformities, such as those that arise as a result of trauma, inflammatory disorders, and especially tumors of the spine, may also occasionally require anterior instrumentation in children or adolescents.

INDICATIONS AND CONTRAINDICATIONS

Spine surgery in pediatric patients carries with it particular risks and complications, and patient selection is crucial. A recommendation of spine surgery should be based on a neurologic deficit, rapid progression of disease, or spinal destabilization. Patients with a fragile overall medical condition, immaturity, or a poor prognosis given the pathologic diagnosis should rarely undergo surgery. As a general rule, older pediatric patients tolerate open spine procedures better than younger patients. The potential for blood loss is proportionally less per body mass as children mature and grow. Underlying diagnoses should also be taken into consideration when spine surgery is being proposed, especially if multiple levels are planned or if the patient requires both anterior and posterior fusions, because these children risk greater blood loss.[17]

PREOPERATIVE EVALUATION

A full clinical history should be conducted before considering any surgical procedure, with a focus on symptoms that correspond to the underlying pathology. A history of persistent pain, especially pain that wakes the child from sleep, warrants further questioning. Details such as timing, quality, radiation, inciting events/activities, and methods of relief are particularly helpful. Children may also report abnormal sensations or weakness, often described as arm or leg heaviness. For patients too young to elaborate on their symptoms, a history of guarding with certain positioning or localized tenderness to palpation will often suffice. Other findings can include a history of stridor or dysphagia, neck or back stiffness, asymmetry noted with walking or crawling, and certainly alterations in bowel or bladder habits. Still, evolving neurologic deficits in children can be subtle, and the practitioner is not infrequently left with nonspecific findings, such as general malaise, irritability, and failure to achieve developmental milestones.

A review of comorbid conditions that would increase the risk of spine surgery should certainly be conducted before surgery. If necessary, an additional workup should be performed to ensure that the patient's cardiac, pulmonary, and renal status will tolerate a potentially lengthy surgical procedure. Standard laboratory testing should include complete blood counts, chemistry panels, and coagulation studies, and the results of these studies should be optimized.

Physical examination of children is often challenging, but it is a critical step in preoperative evaluation. Simple observation is often the most valuable and of highest yield when examining a child. Any differences in muscle bulk and tone should be documented. Asymmetrical extremity movements, with and without resistance, should be evaluated. Accurate sensory examinations are often only possible in older children, but asymmetric extremity withdrawal to tactile stimulation is informative in neonates and infants. The presence of deep tendon reflex abnormalities is helpful, but their absence is not uncommon in young children. Asymmetry, however, is pertinent spinal pathology that affects the craniocervical junction and will often produce the following bulbar findings on examination: stridor, weak or hoarse cry, and subtle head tilt with sternocleidomastoid weakness. Rectal tone and reflexes, such as the bulbocavernosus and anal wink, are sometimes notably diminished with spinal cord compression, although the psychological effects of attempting such examinations makes their yield questionable.

Careful review of the preoperative imaging results should be conducted to understand tumor size, location, and its involvement with or distortion of the surrounding spinal anatomy. Attention to the tumor's relationship to structures such as the neural foramina and its contents, as well as vascular anatomy such as the vertebral artery, is essential. To visualize this anatomy sufficiently, CT and MRI have become standard. CT scans are most useful in assessing bone thickness for instrumentation planning, characterizing bone tumors, and detecting calcifications in nonbone tumors. MRI scans should include phased-array surface coils and should be processed in all three planes of space. Standing, full-length, upright films are important for evaluating sagittal and coronal alignment. Preoperative review can also assist in planning the number of levels necessary for exposure, and/or the number of levels instrumented, should structural integrity be threatened. These images will also serve as baseline studies to detect postoperative changes in spinal alignment and the development of postoperative deformity. For bone tumors and highly vascular lesions, preoperative radionuclide bone scans and preoperative angiography should be considered. Radionuclide studies can assist in determining the extent of any multifocal disease. Lesions that are highly vascular could lead to substantial blood loss once a procedure is begun and thus preoperative angiography would provide an opportunity to embolize major feeding vessels prior to surgery.

CLINICAL DECISION-MAKING

The decision to operate is not always clearly defined, especially in a patient whose spine is in the process of maturing and is at risk for deformity as a result of surgery. The first priority in pediatric spine surgery should be to disturb as little anatomy as possible. The next priority is to restore as many tissue planes and structures to their natural states as possible. Finally, when preservation or restoration of anatomy is limited or if spinal stability is compromised, fusion techniques or instrumentation should be used.

In the surgical correction of spinal deformities, the addition of internal fixation serves the dual function of improving solid arthrodesis by rigid immobilization of the instrumented segments and correcting preexisting deformities by facilitated application of the corrective forces. Since the introduction of spinal pedicle screws by Boucher,[18] in the late 1950s, and the Harrington instrument,[19] in the early 1960s, internal pedicle screw fixation of the spine has gained widespread use in the correction of spinal deformities.[20-23]

Some advantages of anterior instrumentation compared with posterior instrumentation include preservation of motion segments and decreased blood loss with less muscle dissection.[24,25] Improved fusion rates and decreased operative times have also been proposed by some investigators.[24,26] Anterior instrumentation also provides a reduced rate of infection compared with posterior procedures. For patients who are skeletally immature, circumferential fusion incorporating anterior instrumentation serves to arrest further anterior and posterior column growth and prevents the occurrence of crankshaft deformity.[27]

The principle disadvantage of anterior approaches to the pediatric spine for placement of anterior hardware is that these approaches frequently require a second procedure for decompression of posterior pathology or placement of posterior spinal instrumentation. Currently many pediatric spine surgeons feel comfortable placing anterior spinal instrumentation through a posterior or posterolateral approach, gaining both anterior and posterior exposure of the spinal column through a single approach. A costotransversectomy or lateral extracavitary approach for the thoracic and lumbar spine allows simultaneous placement of anterior and posterior spinal instrumentation (Fig. 48-1).

As with posterior instrumentation, standard spinal instrumentation such as titanium or polyetheretherketone (PEEK) cages may have too large a profile for general pediatric use; careful study of preoperative CT scans is mandatory to determine whether the anatomy of the patient will be able to accept anterior instrumentation. Other potential complications include the risk of nerve root injury; implant loosening and migration; injury to critical vascular structures, such as the carotid artery, aorta, or inferior vena cava; injury to the spinal cord or its covering; visceral injury; adjacent level disease[28]; stenosis; and possible instability resulting from rigidity of the construct.[29]

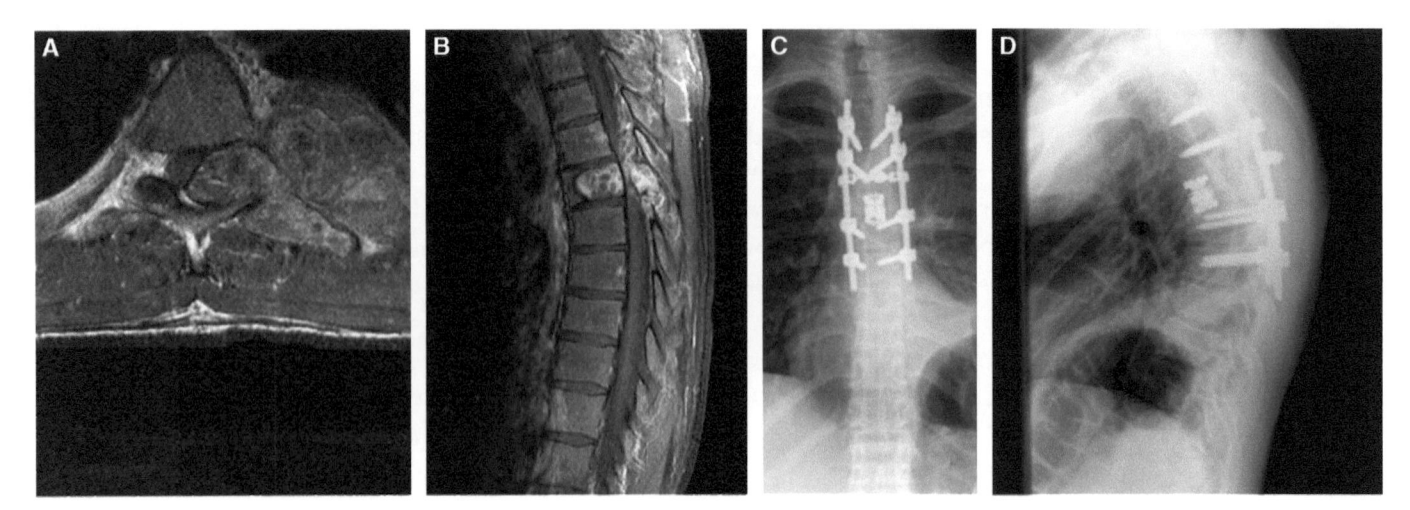

Fig. 48-1 Anterior instrumentation supplementing posterior fusion in the thoracic spine. An 18-year-old boy presented with a 1-year history of left-sided chest pain and 1 month of difficulty with balance and walking. On examination, the patient was found to have myelopathy. T1-weighted MRI scans **A,** without and **B,** with gadolinium showed a mass lesion centered at the T6 vertebral body, with extension into the left chest cavity, and spinal cord compression. The patient was taken to the operating room for a posterior-only approach and T6 vertebrectomy with spinal column reconstruction. Reconstruction was performed with **C** and **D,** an expandable titanium cage and pedicle screw fixation from T4 to T8. Pathologic examination revealed an aneurysmal bone cyst.

TECHNIQUE
PATIENT POSITIONING AND PREPARATION

The initial focus of each surgery should be proper positioning of the patient and preparation of the skin to avoid ischemia or infection. The vast majority of tumors in children can be addressed with the patient in the prone position. Pediatric patients rarely warrant the use of adult positioning devices, such as the Wilson frame or Jackson table, for prone positioning. Most commonly, gel or prefashioned padded bolsters suffice, for example, vertical placement of bolsters along the anterior axillary lines in larger children and horizontal placement above the xiphoid process and below the anterior superior iliac spine in smaller children (Fig. 48-2). At the conclusion of positioning, a final inspection is performed to free the abdomen, genitals, and nipples from direct compression, and all wires, intravenous lines, and other objects are separated from the skin with foam padding. Sterile preparation and draping is mandatory.

Tumors that impinge upon spinal cord or spinal nerves should have intraoperative neuromonitoring arranged as part of the surgical planning. Neuromonitoring can be used for patients with tumors involving the spinal cord or for patients requiring correction of deformities.[30,31] Changes in intraoperative somatosensory or motor-evoked potentials may represent early spinal cord injury. Corrective measures can be performed intraoperatively, which may prevent permanent injury to the spinal cord.

Vertical midline incisions are adequate for most posterior exposures and instrumentation. When lateral access to the retropleural (thoracic spine) or retroperitoneal (lumbar spine) spaces is necessary, the vertical incision can be continued in a right-angle,

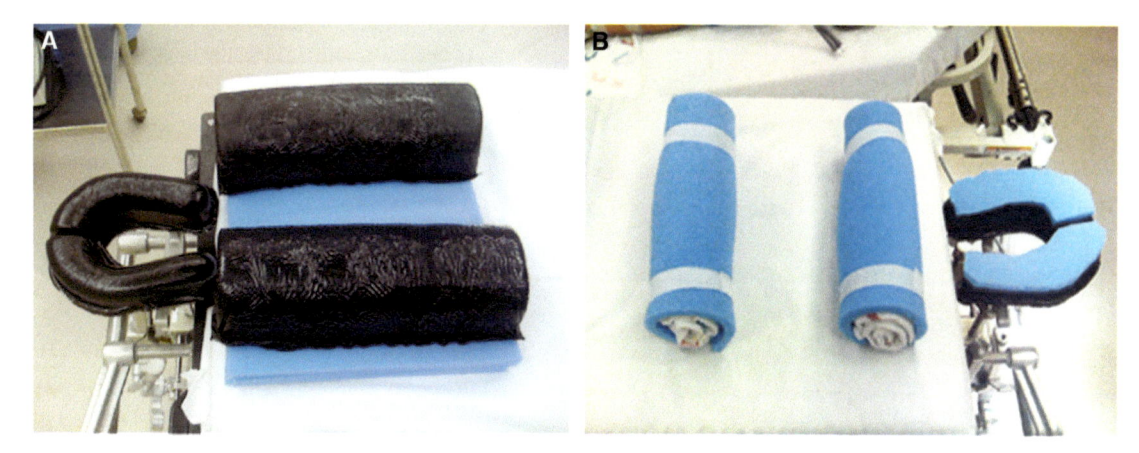

Fig. 48-2 Positioning bolsters for pediatric spine surgery patients. The use of Wilson frames and Jackson tables is rare in the pediatric population. More commonly used are **A,** gel and **B,** prefabricated blanket/padding bolsters arranged either vertically or horizontally, depending on the patient's size and weight.

horizontal fashion for further exposure (hockey-stick incision). Incisions are typically demarcated one level above and one level below a planned surgical exposure (for example, T1 to T5 for a T2 to T4 laminoplasty). Application of local anesthetic is invaluable, both for limiting postoperative discomfort and for hemostasis, when small amounts of epinephrine are included. Before the infusion of any local anesthetic, patient weight should be reviewed, and a safe, weight-based total dosage should be calculated.

TUMOR DISSECTION AND REMOVAL

Most pediatric spine tumors have well-defined borders and can be isolated from surrounding anatomy with meticulous dissection. An operating microscope is preferred over viewing with operating loupes and headlights. Softer tumors can be removed with some combination of suction, blunt and sharp microdissection, intermittent cauterization, and perhaps the use of an ultrasonic aspirator. For firmer tumors or bony tumors, high-powered ultrasonic aspiration or even low-powered drilling is necessary, although greater care must be exercised in protecting neighboring anatomy. To this end, the general strategy of internal debulking followed by "collapsing-in" of the tumor walls is often the most successful. Tumor margins that are in close approximation to spinal nerves can be tested with nerve stimulators to confirm the presence or absence of functional tissue. Also, as is the case with all pediatric patients, attention to hemostasis should be prioritized throughout tumor resection.

STANDARD LAMINOTOMY

The most common technique employed for posterior exposure of spine tumors and subsequent stabilization of the pediatric spine remains the osteoplastic laminotomy (Fig. 48-3). This method is preferable to laminectomy, which has been shown to result in scoliosis and kyphosis in children, especially with multilevel surgeries. With

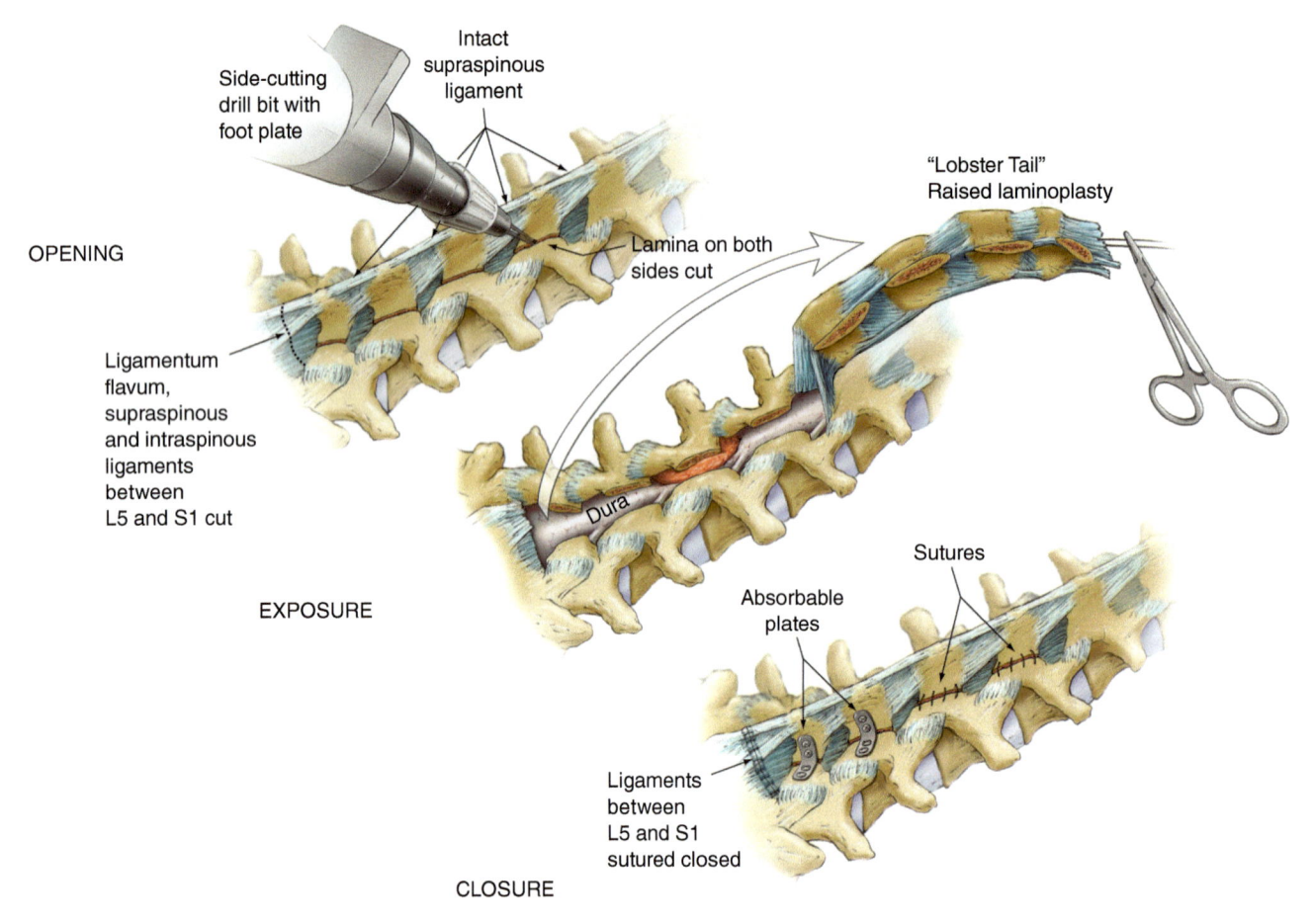

Fig. 48-3 Osteoplastic laminotomy. This bone-sparing technique is intended to restore the patient's anatomy as close to its original state as possible, in hopes of avoiding progressive postoperative deformities resulting from violation or removal of the posterior elements. A side-cutting drill is used to create parallel laminar cuts along the desired area of exposure. The rostral end of the laminotomy is preserved as an attachment point and wrapped with a moistened sponge. After the tumor is removed, the laminoplasty is fastened in place with either absorbable plates or heavy sutures. The interspinous and supraspinous ligaments are also secured with sutures.

the skin incised, the underlying subcutaneous tissues are dissected with a monopolar electrocautery device down to the level of the supraspinous ligament. At this point, self-retaining retractors are placed, and great care is taken to preserve the midline bony and ligamentous structures, the so-called *posterior tension band*, as the remainder of the dissection proceeds. We recommend creating two separate incisions lateral to the supraspinous ligament down to the superior, lateral surface of the spinous process. A lateral, subperiosteal dissection is then swept along the surfaces of the spinous processes and lamina, without disturbing either the neighboring joints or joint capsules.

Once the soft tissue dissection is completed, the laminotomy flap is raised in several steps. First, the supraspinous and interspinous ligaments are cut sharply below the lowest spinal level of the planned laminoplasty (between L4 and L5 for an L1-4 laminoplasty). As a precaution, a blunt dissecting instrument should be used to traverse interspinous ligament above the dura for protection, and then performing a sharp dissection down to the instrument secondarily. It is useful to cut an equidistant measure of ligament between the spinous processes to facilitate suture placement during closure. The inferior edge of the most caudal laminotomy level is dissected with a curette in preparation for drilling. A side-cutting drill bit with a footplate attachment is a safe and time-efficient means of creating the necessary laminar cuts. Drilling is initiated caudally and continued rostrally through the lateral margin of each shingled level. The underlying ligamentum flavum is dissected and cut sharply at each level. The laminotomy flap is then hinged rostrally, reminiscent of a "lobster tail," and covered with an antibiotic-soaked sponge. Where appropriate, epidural bleeding is controlled with electrocautery or the application of thrombin-soaked hemostatic agents.

This technique can be modified depending on the needs of exposure, patient anatomy and pathology, or surgeon preference. If bone preservation is not feasible or risk for residual bone tumor involvement is high, then complete bone removal by means of a laminectomy is preferable. Should difficulties arise in passing the side-cutting drill, the laminotomy cuts can be facilitated by or performed completely with rongeurs. In the event that the raised laminotomy flap obscures visualization, the flap can be completely released by severing the interspinous and supraspinous ligaments at the "hinge" of the flap rostrally, and the flap should be soaked in antibiotic irrigant. However, full flap removal is seldom necessary. Additional hinging is often attainable by releasing the rostral interspinous ligaments until the desired exposure is achieved.

Closure of the raised laminotomy flap is aimed at restoring the original anatomy without the need for permanent instrumentation. With the hinged flap uncovered and released, multiple sutures are placed in the caudal supraspinous and interspinous ligaments. Each lamina is then reapproximated to its original location and secured with absorbable plates or sutures, depending on the surface area of bone available. The paraspinous musculature is sutured to the interspinous ligament, the original paramedian cuts in the supraspinous ligament are sutured individually, and the subcutaneous tissue and skin are closed.

ONLAY SPINE FUSION

In the event that spine tumor resection results in significant spinal instability, the first and least invasive means of stabilization in children is the onlay fusion. This technique is reserved for the very immature spine, primarily neonates and young infants, whose anatomy cannot accommodate instrumentation of any form. The levels planned for postresection fusion should be cleaned of all soft tissue, which includes periosteum and facet joint cartilage. The bone surfaces should be decorticated until bleeding cancellous bone is exposed. Local autograft from spinous processes or autograft harvested from rib or iliac crest should be placed along the fusion bed. This can be supplemented with allograft in cases where the amount of autograft is insufficient.

Children who receive this form of autograft are best managed with external immobilization. This is achieved most commonly with halo immobilization devices. For children too small for halo devices, full- or half-body casts may need to be fashioned. Fusion progress would then be assessed with serial imaging of the spine.

OCCIPITAL SCREWS

Tumors that arise in or near the craniocervical junction may require stabilization after resection in the form of occcipitocervical stabilization. Numerous methods for obtaining occipitocervical stabilization have been described, including the use of methyl methacrylate, onlay bone graft with wires, contoured rods with wires, and metal plates with wires or screws.[32-37] Internal fixation is advised to guarantee postoperative stability and enhance the rate of arthrodesis. Occipital screws are most commonly employed in this setting.[35,38] When considering occipital screw placement for occipitocervical fusion, careful preoperative study of a thin-cut CT scan, including the occiput, is mandatory to confirm sufficient midline bone thickness to accommodate the shortest 6 mm occipital screw inserted obliquely.

Although bicortical screw placement may result in superior holding strength secondary to greater cortical purchase,[39] caution is needed to avoid overpenetration and potential neurologic injury.[40] Bicortical occipital screw insertion risks dural laceration, cerebrospinal fluid leakage, dural venous sinus injury/thrombosis, and subepidural/epidural hematoma formation.[41] Cerebrospinal fluid leakage and sinus bleeding can be stopped with placement of the occipital screws. If a screw cannot be placed, bone wax may be used to plug the drill hole in the bone.

Bicortical screw failure is directly related to screw length, and screw length is dictated by bone thickness.[42] Because the occiput is thickest in the region of the midline keel, multiple bicortical fixation points directed toward the midline have been advocated. The basiocciput below the external occipital protuberance and posterior to the foramen magnum represents the squamous portion and is the site of occipitocervical fusion.[43] Screw fixation is more secure in the bone above the inferior nuchal line, because bone below this landmark is thin. Screw purchase is improved closer to the superior nuchal line and external occipital protuberance. However, the superior nuchal line does not accurately reflect the location of the transverse sinus, ranging from 15 mm below the superior nuchal line to 17 mm above.[42] Unicortical screw purchase at and above the superior nuchal line may be warranted to decrease risk of dural venous sinus penetration.

Careful drilling with triangulation toward the midline should be performed millimeter by millimeter until the inner table of the occiput is breached. The dura should be palpable with a ball-tipped probe. This "stop-drill" technique is routinely used. With left-sided and right-sided screws directed toward the midline, screw paths may intersect, causing even more unwanted difficulty with screw placement. It is useful to stagger the screws on each side of midline, being conscientious to direct the next screw trajectories slightly more cephalad or caudad away from the previous trajectory (Fig. 48-4).

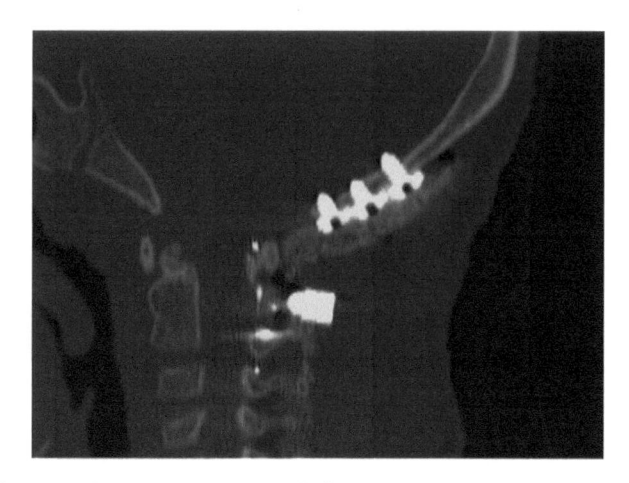

Fig. 48-4 Occipital screw placement. Prior to drilling, anatomic landmarks are identified. Four bony landmarks on the outer occipital cortex should be visible: the posterior rim of the foramen magnum, the superior nuchal line, the inferior nuchal line, and the external occipital protuberance. Safe placement of occipital instrumentation is placed between the inferior and superior nuchal line; 4.0 to 4.5 mm diameter occipital screws may be placed in a bicortical fashion using the stop-drill, or step-wise drill, technique in 2 mm increments. Drill and screw trajectories should be angled medially toward the thick midline keel. Left and right occipital screws are staggered to avoid intersection of screw paths.

C1 LATERAL MASS SCREWS AND C1-2 TRANSARTICULAR SCREWS

If screw fixation becomes necessary at C1, it is imperative that the entry point for the C1 lateral mass screw in the pediatric spine be placed at the confluence of the C1 lamina and the C1 lateral mass (Fig. 48-5). The pediatric spine is unsuitable to accept a C1 lateral mass screw at alternative entry sites, such as the C1 lamina itself, because of the high risk of violating the superior wall the lamina and injuring the vertebral artery in the sulcus arteriosus.[44,45]

It is also important to note how the pediatric atlas differs from the adult atlas. In the adult atlas, the medial side of the C1 lamina is typically flush with the medial C1 lateral mass. However, in the pediatric atlas, the medial aspect of the C1 lamina is typically 2 to 3 mm laterally stepped-off from the medial surface of the C1 lateral mass. An entry point based on the medial aspect of the C1 lamina will place the entry of the C1 lateral mass screw dangerously lateral in extreme proximity to the vertebral artery. Instead, the medial surface of the C1 lateral mass itself must be used as a landmark for starting the C1 lateral mass screw.

Bleeding from the venous plexus around the C2 nerve root can be substantial as dissection down to the junction of the C1 lamina and C1 lateral mass is carried out. This blood loss can be life-threatening in small children without a large blood volume to begin with and may lead to unwanted blood transfusions. Bipolar coagulation of the venous plexus and division of the C2 nerve root may obviate much of this venous hemorrhaging while improving exposure without incurring any significant neurologic sequelae.

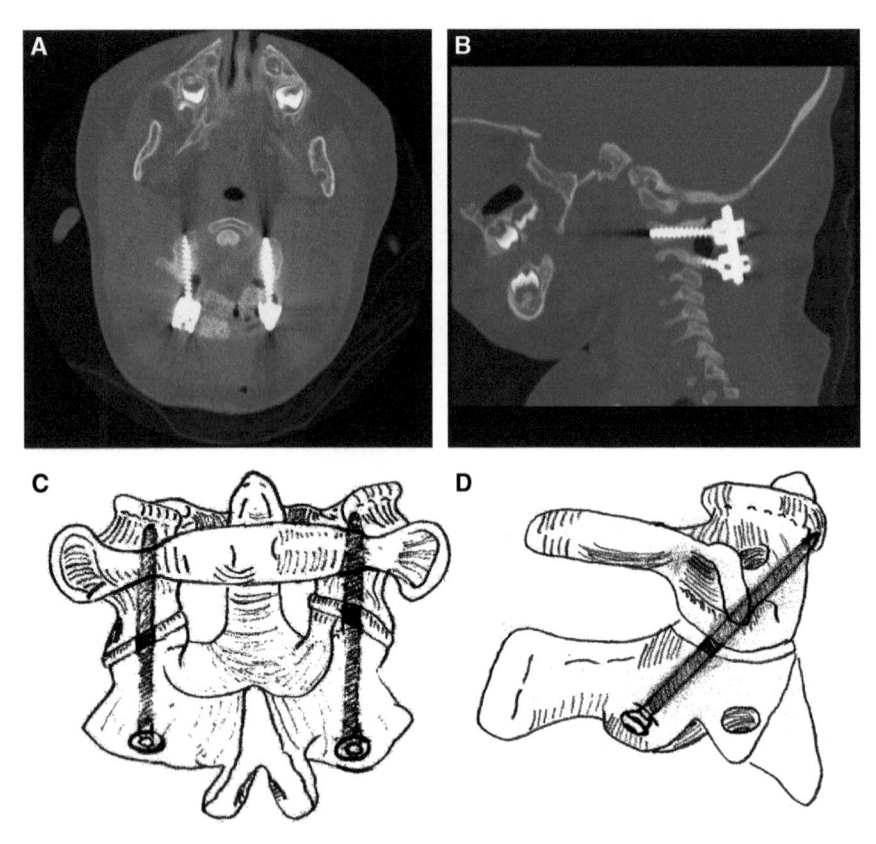

Fig. 48-5 C1 lateral mass and transarticular screws. For proper placement of **A** and **B**, C1 lateral mass screws, the posterior arch of C1 is identified and followed laterally to visualize the lateral masses. Notably, there is a step-off between the medial aspect of the C1 lamina and the medial surface of the C1 lateral mass; this anatomic feature is different than in adults where the medial C1 lamina is flush with the medial C1 lateral mass. Subperiosteal dissection of the C2 nerve roots and associated venous plexi from the junction between the posterior arch of C1 and lateral masses was performed to minimize bleeding. Alternatively, the C2 nerve roots and venous plexi can be coagulated with bipolar electrocautery and divided with little clinical significance. After palpating the medial and lateral surfaces of the lateral mass, a pilot hole may be drilled in the center of the lateral mass, usually no more than 2 to 3 mm from the medial surface. The rest of the placement of the C1 lateral mass screws proceeds using the technique described by Harms and Melcher, using either 3.5 mm or 4.0 mm diameter polyaxial screws. The drill and screw trajectory is angled 0 to 5 degrees **A**, medial and is aimed at the superior half of **B**, the anterior arch of C1 on fluoroscopy. Bicortical purchase is usually achieved about 4 mm from the anterior cortex of the anterior arch. **C** and **D**, C1 transarticular screw placement, a midline incision is made to expose the posterior elements from C1 to C3 with particular attention paid to C2-3 facet joints. The superior and medial aspects of the C2 pars are exposed. There is no reason to expose the lateral aspect of the C2 pars; in fact, this may be a dangerous maneuver because of the proximity of the vertebral artery. The roof of the C2 pedicle is followed to the C1-2 facet joint. The C2 entry point may be identified by first locating the medial edge of the C2-3 facet joint. The C2 entry site is just lateral and rostral to this point, and may be estimated by visualizing the course of the medial pars (approximately 3 mm up and 3 mm out). The drill or K-wire, either through a stab incision lateral to the T1 spinous process or through an extended incision, is typically directed 15 degrees medial, with the superior angle visualized by fluoroscopy. The drill or K-wire is directed down the C2 pedicle and across **C**, the C1-2 joint aiming at **D**, the anterior tubercle of C1. The tip of the drill or K-wire is advanced to a point 4 mm short of the anterior C1 tubercle, attaining purchase of the anterior cortex of C1. After tapping, a fully threaded 3.5- or 4.0-mm-diameter cortical screw is used. The necessary screw length can be measured directly from the drill or the K-wire. Screws are typically 34 to 44 mm in length. The technique is repeated on the contralateral side.

In the event that C1 lateral mass screw fixation is not feasible, C1-2 transarticular screw fixation is a suitable alternative. A midline incision is made to expose the posterior elements from C1 to C3 with particular attention paid to C2-3 facet joints. The superior and medial aspects of the C2 pars are exposed. There is no reason to expose the lateral aspect of the C2 pars; in fact, this may be dangerous a maneuver because of the proximity of the vertebral artery. The roof of the C2 pedicle is followed to the C1-2 facet joint.

The C2 entry point may be identified by first locating the medial edge of the C2-3 facet joint. The C2 entry site is just lateral and rostral to this point, and may be estimated by visualizing the course of the medial pars (approximately 3 mm up and 3 mm out). The drill or K-wire, either through a stab incision lateral to the T1 spinous process or through an extended incision, is typically directed 15 degrees medial, with the superior angle visualized by fluoroscopy. The drill or K-wire is directed down the C2 pedicle and across the C1-2 joint, aiming at the anterior tubercle of C1. The tip of the drill or K-wire is advanced to a point 4 mm short of the anterior C1 tubercle, attaining purchase of the anterior cortex of C1. After tapping, a fully threaded 3.5- or 4.0-mm-diameter cortical screw is used. The necessary screw length can be measured directly from the drill or the K-wire. Screws are typically 34 to 44 mm in length. The technique is repeated on the contralateral side.

C2 Pars/Pedicle and Translaminar Screws

The primary goal during C2 pars/pedicle screw placement is to avoid injury to the vertebral artery during placement. The isthmus of C2 is cleared of all soft tissue, and the subperiosteal plane is identified. The medial border of the C2 isthmus and thus the medial limits of proposed screw trajectory are palpated with an instrument. Screws inserted into the lateral mass of C2 begin between the upper and lower articular surfaces of C2 at a vertical line bisecting the articular mass. The screw is then oriented 25 degrees upward and 15 to 25 degrees medially (Fig. 48-6).

Wright[46,47] described a new technique for rigid screw fixation of the axis involving the insertion of polyaxial screws into the laminae of C2 in a bilateral crossing fashion and their feasibility for placement in the general adult population. Because the C2 translaminar screws are not in proximity to the vertebral artery, this technique allows rigid fixation of C2 through a safer technique. Recently teams of investigators have reported their experience with this technique of crossing and noncrossing screws in small series of children (Fig. 48-7).[48,49]

Lateral Mass Screws (C3-7)

The lateral mass should be adequately dissected of soft tissue and periosteum and can be considered square in shape. The entry point of lateral mass screws should be approximately 1 mm inferior and medial to the midpoint of the square. A 2.5 mm drill is then angled 20 to 25 degrees laterally and 30 to 40 degrees rostrally (or approximately parallel to the surface of the intervertebral joints). Drilling is performed

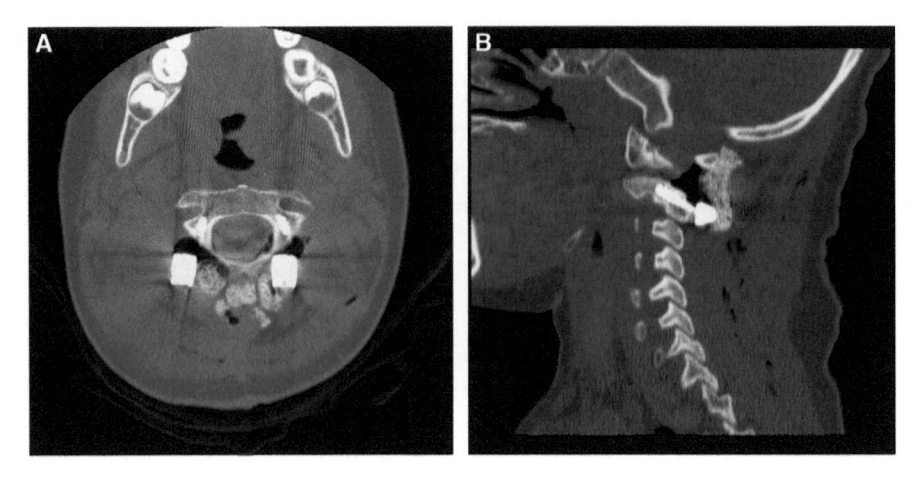

Fig. 48-6 C2 pars/pedicle screw placement. The entry point of a C2 pars/pedicle screw is similar to that of C1-2 transarticular screw placement. The medial, superior, and roof of the C2 pars/pedicle should be exposed, dividing the C2 nerve root and venous plexus, if necessary. The medial trajectory of the C2 pars/pedicle screw parallels **A,** the medial border of the C2 pars/pedicle, and the superior trajectory guided by fluoroscopy aiming for the anterior tubercle of C1; however, the C2 pars/pedicle screw stops short of **B,** the C1-2 joint. Screw length is typically half of the screw length for a C1-2 transarticular screw, measuring 16 to 22 mm in length.

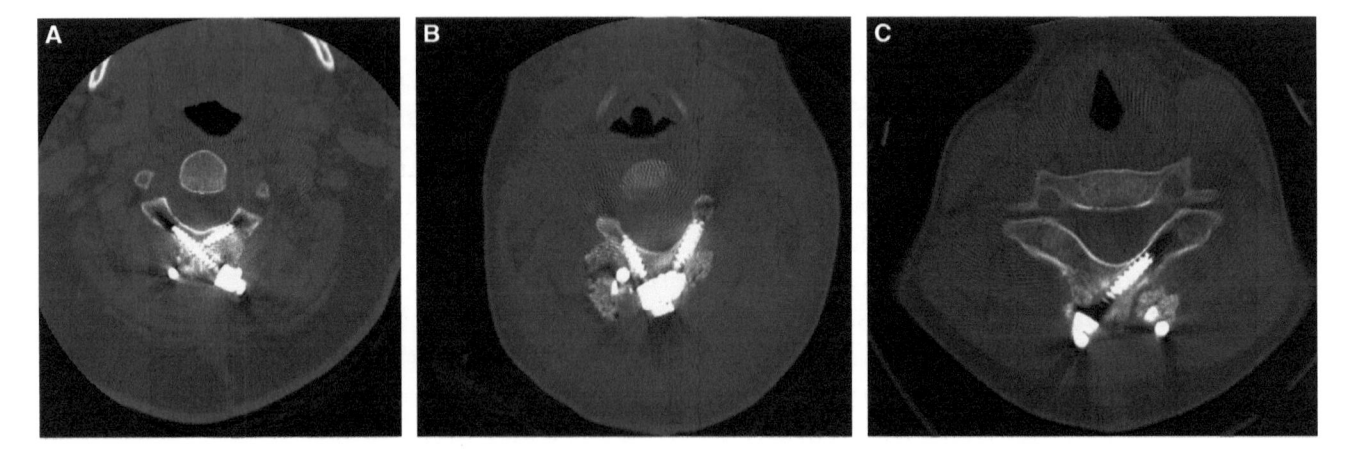

Fig. 48-7 Translaminar screw placement. **A-C,** Screws are crisscrossed along the lamina, providing a supplement or an alternative to lateral mass screws. This technique avoids any injury to the vertebral artery, and the hardware can be incorporated into neighboring lateral mass or pedicle screw constructs. A high-speed drill is used to open a small "entry" cortical window at the junction of the spinous process and lamina, close to the rostral margin of the lamina. Similarly, a high-speed drill is used to open a small "exit" cortical window at the junction of the facet and lamina, close to the rostral margin of the lamina. Using a hand drill as described by Wright, the contralateral lamina is carefully drilled along its length, with the drill visually aligned along the angle of the exposed contralateral laminar surface, aiming for the "exit" point. The drill tip should then be observed at the "exit" window. This gives confirmation that the drill did not violate the inner cortex of the lamina, allows bi-cortical screw purchase, and enables accurate measure of the appropriate screw length. Typically, a screw, 20 to 30 mm in length and 3.5 or 4.0 mm in diameter, could be placed. A small "entry" cortical window is then made at the junction of the spinous process and lamina, close to the caudal aspect of the lamina on the opposite side. The above technique is then repeated for this crossing translaminar screw. Fluoroscopy is not used during this technique. It neither guides screw trajectory nor confirms screw placement, as it is difficult to interpret on AP and lateral views where the screw lay in relation to the spinal canal.

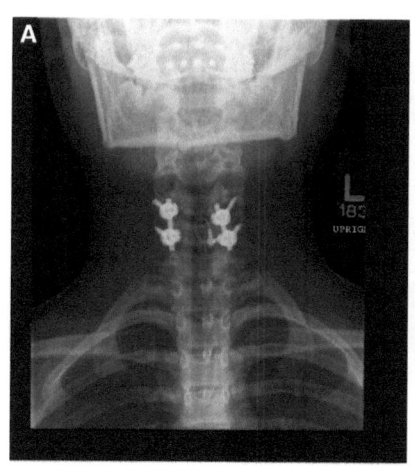

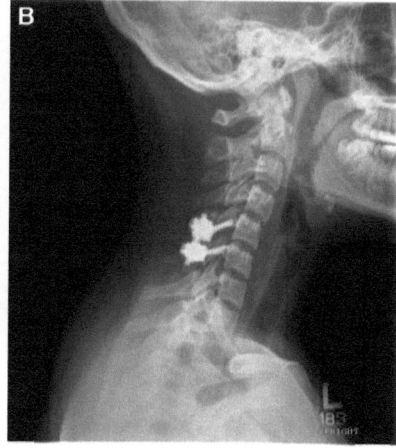

Fig. 48-8 Subaxial lateral mass screw placement. **A,** Anterior-posterior and **B,** lateral radiograph of the spine illustrating proper placement of lateral mass screws. The entire lateral mass of the subaxial cervical spine is exposed from its medial junction with the lamina to the lateral step-off. The entry point is identified approximately 1 mm inferior and 1 mm medial to the center of the 2D "square" posterior surface of the lateral mass. The drill and screw trajectory is directed superior and lateral (approximately 20 degrees up and 20 degrees out) to avoid the nerve root and vertebral artery, respectively, aiming for the superolateral "deep" corner of the 3D "cube" of the lateral mass in the mind's eye of the surgeon. Unicortical purchase is safe, but bicortical purchase may afford a biomechanical advantage. Fluoroscopy may be used, but is unnecessary. Boys usually tolerate 12 to 16 mm × 3.5 mm screws, and girls tolerate 10 to 14 mm × 3.5 mm screws.

in 2 mm increments and depth checked with a probe or gauge until the far cortex is penetrated. The holes can then be tapped and instrumented with screws (Fig. 48-8).

PEDICLE SCREWS

Pedicle screw placement at any spine level consists of proper selection of screw entry site, drilling, probing, tapping, and securing of the screw. The screw entry point in thoracic pedicles is below the upper facet joint, 1 to 3 mm lateral to the center of the joint. The screws are oriented 7 to 10 degrees toward the midline; increased medial angulation is necessary in the upper thoracic spine and decreased angulation is necessary for lower thoracic pedicle screws. Sagittal pedicle angulation is typically 10 to 20 degrees in a caudal direction. Lumbar pedicle screw entry sites occur at the intersection between a horizontal line bisecting the transverse processes and a vertical line along the lateral border of the superior articular process. Lumbar screws are oriented approximately 5 degrees near the thoracolumbar junction to approximately 15 degrees at the lumbosacral junction (Fig. 48-9).

TRANSLAMINAR SCREWS

Translaminar screw placement in the subaxial pediatric cervical spine has numerous potential advantages compared with current instrumentation techniques. The entire length of the subaxial cervical lamina can be readily visualized. Important neurovascular structures can be avoided. A screw can be placed of much longer length than

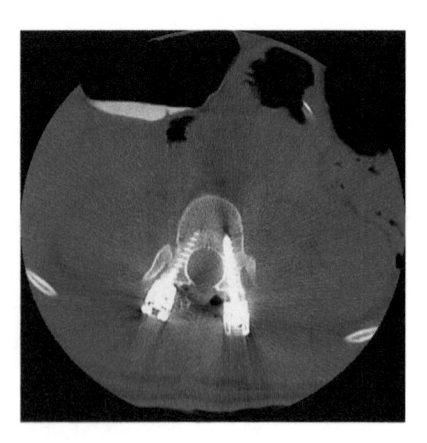

Fig. 48-9 Thoracic and lumbar pedicle screw placement. The entry point for pedicle screw placement may be consistently found at the confluence between the pars interarticularis and transverse process. A thorough knowledge of pedicle anatomy and the sagittal and axial angulation of the individual pedicles is mandatory for safe screw placement. Angles for the pedicle finder, tap, and screw are best judged using preoperative CT or MRI of the thoracic or lumbar region. Intraoperative real-time guidance with fluoroscopy or direct palpation of the pedicle through a laminotomy may aid in screw placement, as an alternative to free-hand placement.

a lateral mass screw at the same level to confer a greater degree of biomechanical advantage.

Potential drawbacks of this technique must also be noted. Although the dorsal laminar surface is exposed during surgery, the surgeon must be careful to avoid penetration of the nonvisualized ventral laminar wall, because penetration could lead to damage to the thecal sac or spinal cord. A modification of Wright's method of translaminar screw placement with an "exit" window in the dorsal lamina at the laminofacet line can help the surgeon avoid intracanalicular violation of the translaminar screw.[50] Preoperative fine-cut CT scans, with axial, sagittal, and coronal views, should be used to estimate the screw length and to determine whether the subaxial lamina can accept a minimum 3.5 mm diameter screw. We suggest that the acceptable width of the lamina should be at least 4.0 mm. Clearly, translaminar screws should not be used without intact posterior elements.

WIRING

A solid construct can be achieved in the lower cervical spine with adequate placement of interspinous wiring. Interconnecting holes are made on either side of the spinous process with a drill or perforating towel clamp. These holes should be made at the junction between the spinous process and the lamina. A flexible wire (1.2 mm) can then be threaded carefully through these holes and then wrapped around the caudal end of the spinous process inferior to the wired process. Once around, the ends of the wire are twisted and trimmed. An added measure of security can be achieved by decorticating the neighboring lamina and applying bone graft.

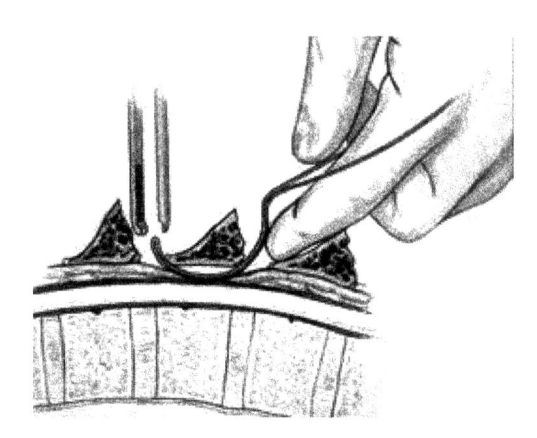

Fig. 48-10 Sublaminar wiring technique. Passing a metal wire or polyester band under the lamina does require a learning curve. The malleable metal end of the wire or polyester band is shaped into a gentle curve for passage around the lamina. The wire or band is always passed in a caudal-to-rostral direction. The tip of the wire or band is gripped with hemostats or forceps, and the rest of the passage follows a push-pull technique being mindful to keep tension so that a loop of band does not compress the thecal sac. After all of the sublaminar wires or bands have been passed, each of the wires or clamps is closed over the rods. The loop around the lamina is tightened with a tensioner. The final tension is primarily evaluated by the surgeon, taking into account the strength of the bone of the patient. Important points to consider when using this technique include: (1) the radius of curvature of the malleable metal tip should be at least equal to the length of the lamina; (2) the bend of the tip should not be greater than 45 degrees; (3) lateral passage of sublaminar metal wires or polyester bands should be avoided; (4) removal of additional bony lamina is not necessary because it does not significantly decrease the depth of band penetration but potentially weakens the lamina and increases the risk of instrumentation failure; (5) removal of the spinous process is recommended before direct midline passage of the sublaminar band; and (6) maintaining tension on the band throughout passage by using a push-pull technique to prevent bowing of the band into the spinal canal.

Sublaminar wiring is an additional option in children whose bones are too small for screw placement. The passage of sublaminar wires carries with it some risk to the underlying dura and spinal cord, however. Before insertion, the undersurface of the lamina should be probed with a thin dissector to free any ligamentous or soft tissue that would interfere with smooth passage of the wire. A soft bend in the wire will assist it along the undersurface of the lamina and facilitate visualization and accessibility of the wire tip when it has cleared the entire lamina (Fig. 48-10). The frailty of pediatric bone mandates that the wires be fastened tightly at the conclusion of placement, but excessive tightness risks laminar fracture and loss of the entire fusion construct.

POLYESTER BANDS

Recently polyester bands with a locking mechanism to provide rod coupling (Universal Clamp; Zimmer Spine, Warsaw, IN) were developed as an alternative to traditional anchors—wires, hooks, and screws (see Fig. 48-2). The material properties of polyester are characterized by its high tensile strength, high resistance to stretch, wet or dry, and resistance to degradation.[51] Polyester is biocompatible, without an excessive inflammatory reaction in surrounding tissue, including the dura. Polyester has been in use for more than 18 years in spinal implants in Europe (personal communication, 2007).

Its woven fabric makes it gentle, and its flexibility makes it an excellent alternative to implantation into the pediatric spine. This is most applicable when the anatomy is extraordinarily small to accept hooks or screws, or when the anatomy is marked by significant congenital structural abnormalities where free-hand or fluoroscopic-guided hook or screw placement may lead to an unacceptably high risk of neurologic injury. The polyester bands and locking mechanism to the rod may be placed at multiple levels, similar to wires, hooks, and screws, to effect segmental control, reduction, and fusion.

With the passage of any sublaminar instrumentation into the spinal canal, there is a risk of neurologic injury. Theoretically a polyester band, compared with a metal cable, should conform safely to the undersurface of the lamina, which may decrease the likelihood of neurologic injury. However, as illustrated in the above-mentioned case, neurologic injury is still a risk with passage of sublaminar polyester bands.

Similar to sublaminar wires, sublaminar polyester bands can directly traumatize the spinal cord.[52-58] Meticulous technique can reduce the risk of injury, particularly in the thoracic and thoracolumbar spine.[59] Because the metal tip is not visible during the sublaminar passage of the polyester band, the surgeon is unable to appreciate the depth of tip penetration into the spinal canal. Important points to consider when using this technique include the following:
1. The radius of curvature of the malleable metal tip should be at least equal to the length of the lamina.
2. The bend of the tip should not be greater than 45 degrees.
3. Lateral passage of sublaminar polyester bands should be avoided.
4. Removal of additional bony lamina is not necessary because it does not significantly decrease the depth of band penetration, but it potentially weakens the lamina and increases the risk of instrumentation failure.
5. Removal of the spinous process is recommended before direct midline passage of the sublaminar band.
6. Tension should be maintained on the band throughout passage, by using a push-pull technique, to prevent bowing of the band into the spinal canal.

Care must be taken not to overtighten the bands, which can cause the bands to pull through or fracture a weak or skeletally immature lamina, as occurred in one of our patients. Excessive laminotomy in preparing for band passage may weaken the lamina. Aggressive decortication in preparing the bony bed for arthrodesis may likewise decrease laminar strength and increase the risk of laminar fracture in the follow-up period.[60]

FUTURE TECHNIQUES

The future of pediatric spine surgery, as it pertains to stabilization after tumor resection, is sure to include more instrumentation as additional studies prove their safety, efficacy and durability. Product development will also likely cater to the dimensions and structural needs of pediatric patients. Furthermore, as minimally invasive techniques emerge and are refined, they will likely play a progressively larger role in pediatric spine surgeries. Access to the pediatric spine using minimally invasive tubular retraction systems are now well-described.[61] As these techniques develop, given their limited blood loss and reduction of postoperative pain, they will likely continue to increase in popularity.

OUTCOMES WITH EVALUATION OF RESULTS
LAMINECTOMY/LAMINOTOMY/LAMINOPLASTY

Spinal deformity after multilevel laminectomy has been well documented in children. The risk of deformity increases, with exposure spanning more than four levels, and is especially high in children undergoing laminectomy and radiation for malignant spine tumors.[62,63] Preoperative scoliotic deformity, an increasing number of resections, age less than 13 years, and surgery spanning the thoracolumbar junction have all been found to predict a greater risk of progressive spinal deformity after resection of intramedullary spinal cord tumors in children, as well as the presence of a tumor-associated syrinx.[64,65] Specifically, with respect to cervical intramedullary spine tumors, decompression spanning both the axial cervical spine (C1-2) and the cervicothoracic junction (C7-T1) increased the risk of progressive spinal deformity fourfold.[66] McGirt et al[67] report a 5% incidence of spinal deformity in children undergoing an osteoplastic laminotomy for intramedullary spinal cord tumor versus a 30% incidence in children undergoing laminectomy. If the spinal pathology spans multiple levels, anatomy-sparing techniques, such as multiple short-segment laminoplasties, have been proposed.[68] Spinal instrumentation after removal of pediatric intramedullary spinal cord tumors has been shown to be efficacious in preventing postlaminectomy deformities.[62] Postlaminoplasty kyphotic deformity has been described in the pediatric thoracic spine.[69]

OCCIPITAL SCREWS

Most of the limitations of occipitocervical fixation systems reside in the cranial part of the construct.[43,45] The occiput does not easily accommodate instrumentation.[42,43,70] The slope of the occipital bone and the angle it makes with the cervical spine impose unique geometric constraints. These limitations may lead to poor occipital screw purchase, screw loosening, pullout, breakage, and difficulties with screw insertion, culminating in catastrophic hardware failure.[71]

In a biomechanical investigation of occipital screw pullout strength, the bicortical pullout strength was found to be 50% greater than unicortical strength. Wire pullout strength was not significantly different from that of unicortical screws, although some investigators find a posteriorly wired contoured rod less likely to provide a good fusion environment because there is less stabilizing potential and greater potential and greater likelihood of loosening with fatigue.[44,72]

C1 Lateral Mass Screws and C1-2 Transarticular Screws

Transarticular C1-2 screws, as described by Jeanneret and Magerl,[73] provide a very rigid and biomechanically sound construct with the incorporation of four cortical surfaces, but the insertion procedure is technically demanding because of the danger of vertebral artery injury, especially in cases where atlantoaxial subluxation remains irreducible preoperatively. Although successful transarticular screw fixation of the atlantoaxial complex has been extensively reported in adult series, there have been only a handful of reports in the pediatric population. Analysis of clinical experience in the largest series of pediatric patients suggested a 4% rate of vertebral artery injury during screw placement.[36] None of these injuries resulted in any long-term morbidity or mortality. Although C1 lateral mass screw placement is still technically challenging and the potential risk of vertebral artery injury persists, our initial experience is that it is a feasible and efficacious part of an occipitocervical or atlantoaxial screw-rod construct in young patients.[74]

C2 Pars/Pedicle and Translaminar Screws

C1-2 transarticular screw placement is technically demanding because of the close proximity of the vertebral artery to the screw path. Vertebral artery injury has been reported to occur in 2% to 8% in several large series.[75-77] Pars/pedicle screws may have a lower incidence of arterial injury, but these screws still place the vertebral artery and spinal cord at risk.[78,79]

Lateral Mass Screws (C3-7)

Although lateral mass screw fixation in the cervical spine has been shown to provide excellent stability and high rates of fusion in adult patients,[80-82] little has been published about the use of subaxial lateral mass screws in the pediatric age group. Unlike the adult age group, there are limited cadaveric biomechanical analyses of these types of constructs. In addition, based on comparative biomechanical studies of the cervical fixation procedures, there is not much difference in stability between lateral mass screw fixation and conventional nonscrew fixation methods, such as sublaminar wiring.[83-87]

The two most popular techniques for lateral mass screws are the Roy-Camille and Magerl techniques. However, nerve roots, vertebral arteries, facet joints, and the dura and spinal cord are at risk during the placement of lateral mass screws. A recent review of the literature indicated that the youngest patient in whom subaxial lateral mass screws were successfully used was 8.2 years old.[88] This correlates with the age at which most authorities agree that the developing spine takes on an "adult" configuration.[89,90] Despite this, these investigators were only able to place 3.5 × 10 mm screws—the shortest screw length that is manufactured. Although a solid fusion was achieved in this case, after 3 months of rigid immobilization, another study of predominantly adult patients has suggested that a minimum subaxial lateral mass screw length of 14 mm is needed to confer any degree of biomechanical stability.[82]

PEDICLE SCREWS

Pedicle screw fixation systems have been widely used for reconstruction of the thoracic and lumbar spine because of their biomechanical superiority. Abumi et al[91,92] reported clinical results of pedicle screw fixation for reconstruction of traumatic and nontraumatic lesions of the middle and lower cervical spine. However, the procedure in the upper cervical spine has been criticized because of the potentially high risk to neurovascular structures, except at the C2 level.[93-95]

TRANSLAMINAR SCREWS

Recently translaminar screws have been promoted as a safe alternative to pedicle screws in the axis and in the upper thoracic spine, as they decrease the risk of violation of the transverse foramen and vertebral artery injury in the cervical spine and the risk of damage to the spinal cord and exiting nerve roots in the upper thoracic spine, without the need for image guidance.[46,96] We now propose that translaminar screw fixation in the subaxial cervical spine is a consideration, in highly selected cases, as an alternative to subaxial lateral mass screws in children with small lateral masses.

Although the biomechanics of lateral mass screw fixation of the subaxial cervical spine are well described, there is no report comparing construct stability or screw pullout strength of translaminar and lateral mass screws in this region. CT morphometric analysis for axial and subaxial translaminar screw placement in the pediatric cervical spine shows that the anatomy in 30.4% of patients younger than 16 years of age could accept bilateral C2 translaminar screws. However, the anatomy of the subaxial cervical spine only rarely could accept translaminar screws.[97] Nonetheless, the feasibility of translaminar screw placement in the subaxial cervical spine should be assessed on a case-by-case basis by careful study of preoperative thin-cut CT scans and sagittal and coronal reconstructions.

THORACOLUMBAR SPINE: WIRES, HOOKS, AND PEDICLE SCREWS

Noted advantages of pedicle screw fixation include three-column fixation, improved coronal, sagittal, and rotational correction, lower pseudarthrosis rates, lower implant failure rates, and few postoperative external orthosis requirements, when compared with hook and wire constructs.[98-101]

Despite their established role at the thoracolumbar, lumbar, and lumbosacral spine, the use of pedicle screws in the thoracic spine (T1 through T10) has had limited acceptance among spine surgeons.[100,102-105] This is because of concerns related to the small pedicle size and the tight proximity of vascular, nervous, and visceral structures in the thoracic cavity and the thoracic spine itself.[106-112] However, since the early 1990s, spine surgeons have been using pedicle screws for the management of thoracic deformities and serious vascular or visceral complications are, fortunately, rare.[101,105,113-118]

SIGNATURE CASES
OSTEOPLASTIC LAMINOPLASTY

The patient was a 6-year-old girl with a prior history of neurocutaneous melanosis diagnosed when she was 3 weeks of age. She presented with 3 weeks of progressive right lower extremity weakness and numbness. On initial examination, muscle strength testing yielded the following scores: right lower extremity at the iliopsoas 4/5, at the quadriceps 3/5, and strength in the remaining muscle groups 4/5. The left lower extremity demonstrated 4/5 strength. She had decreased proprioception in the right lower extremity.

MRI of the thoracic spine revealed a large intradural-extramedullary contrast-enhancing lesion, centered at T7, causing significant cord compression (Fig. 48-11, *A* and *B*). The patient was brought to the operating room where a T6-8 osteoplastic laminoplasty was performed (see Fig. 48-5). The intraoperative pathologic findings were consistent with a diagnosis of metastatic melanoma. Postoperative imaging revealed a gross total resection of the lesion and no spinal deformity (Fig. 48-11, *C* and *D)*. The patient returned to full strength, and her preoperative proprioceptive difficulties resolved.

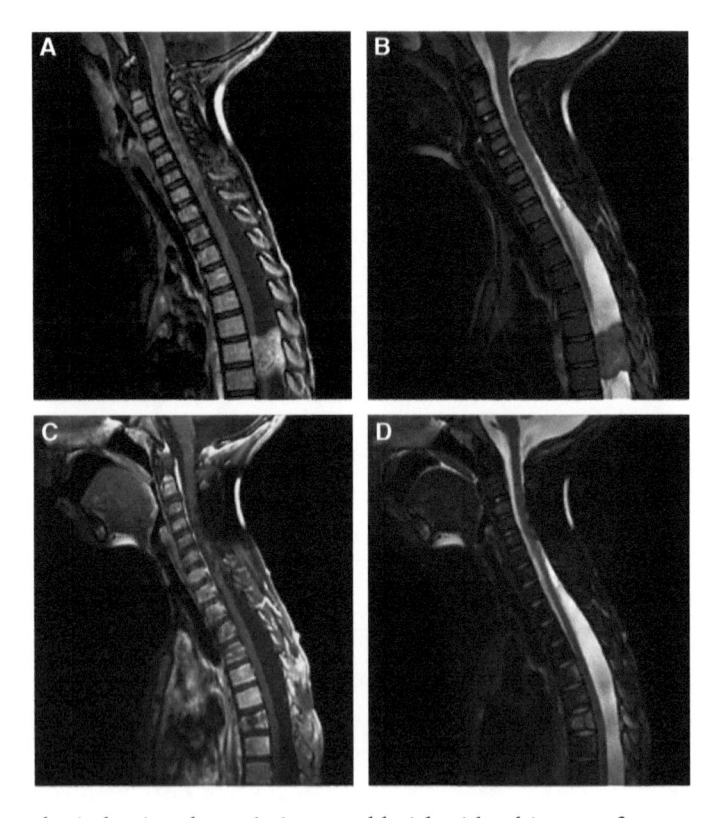

Fig. 48-11 Osteoplastic laminoplasty. A 6-year-old girl with a history of neurocutaneous melanosis presented with progressive right lower extremity weakness and numbness. **A,** Sagittal contrast-enhanced T1-weighted and **B,** T2-weighted MRI showed a T7 extradural mass displacing the spinal cord anteriorly. A T6-8 osteoplastic laminoplasty was performed for tumor resection. The intraoperative pathology was consistent with metastatic melanoma. The laminoplasty was secured with sutures at the conclusion of tumor removal. Sagittal contrast-enhanced **C,** T1-weighted and **D,** T2-weighted MRI showed a gross total resection of her lesion. Serial images over 3 years postoperative have shown no evidence of tumor recurrence or spinal deformity.

PEDICLE SCREW FIXATION

The patient was a 13-year-old female who presented with a 2-month history of left lower extremity dysesthesia and numbness. One week prior to presentation, she developed left leg weakness. Her motor exam at the time was 2/5 strength at the left iliopsoas muscle, 3/5 at the right iliopsoas, 4/5 in both hamstrings, 4/5 at the right extensor hallucis longus (EHL), 2/5 at the left EHL, and 3/5 plantarflexion bilaterally. Her neurologic exam was otherwise intact and she had no bowel or bladder dysfunction.

MRI of the spine revealed a lytic lesion involving the right posterior half of the T5 vertebral body extending into T5 posterior elements (Fig. 48-12, *A* and *B*) with spinal canal narrowing and cord compression at that level (Fig. 48-12, *C* and *D*). She underwent a T4-6 laminectomy for tumor resection that included a partial transpedicular corpectomy and a gross total resection was achieved. The intraoperative pathology was consistent with an aneurysmal bone cyst. She then underwent a posterior spinal fusion with pedicle screw fixation from T3 to T7, supplemented with iliac crest bone graft. Her preoperative dysesthesias resolved within weeks and her motor exam improved to full strength within 6 months. Serial postoperative images have shown stable hardware fixation and no progressive deformities (Fig. 48-12, *E* and *F*).

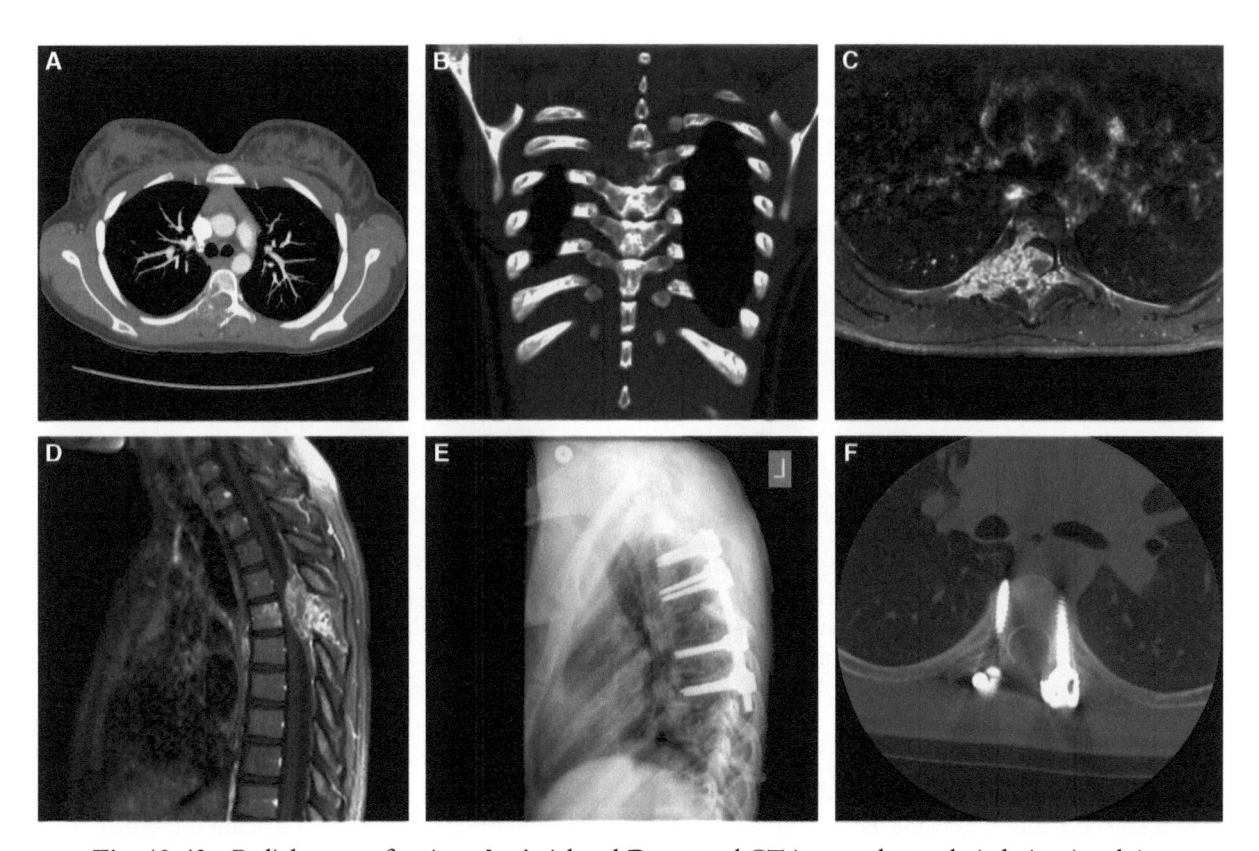

Fig. 48-12 Pedicle screw fixation. **A,** Axial and **B,** coronal CT images show a lytic lesion involving the right posterior aspect of the T5 vertebral body and posterior elements. **C,** Axial and **D,** sagittal T1-weighted MRI showed spinal canal compromise and cord compression. Following tumor removal, spinal stabilization was achieved with pedicle screw fixation from T3 to T7 as demonstrated on postoperative **E,** lateral radiograph and **F,** axial CT imaging.

VERTEBRECTOMY WITH ANTERIOR/POSTERIOR FUSION

The patient was a 6-year-old boy with a several history of a slowly enlarging right neck mass and progressive dysphagia. Evaluation with an MRI (Fig. 48-13, *A* and *B*) showed a mass lesion centered off the right aspect of the C5 and C6 vertebral bodies. The patient was taken to the operating room for staged anterior and posterior approaches. Through the anterior approach, C5 and C6 spondylectomies were performed with skeletonization of the right vertebral artery; a titanium cage and anterior plate were used to reconstruct the spinal column. The patient was taken back to the OR 2 days later for a posterior instrumented fusion from C3 to T2 to supplement the fusion (Fig. 48-13, *C* and *D*). Pathology revealed a chondroma.

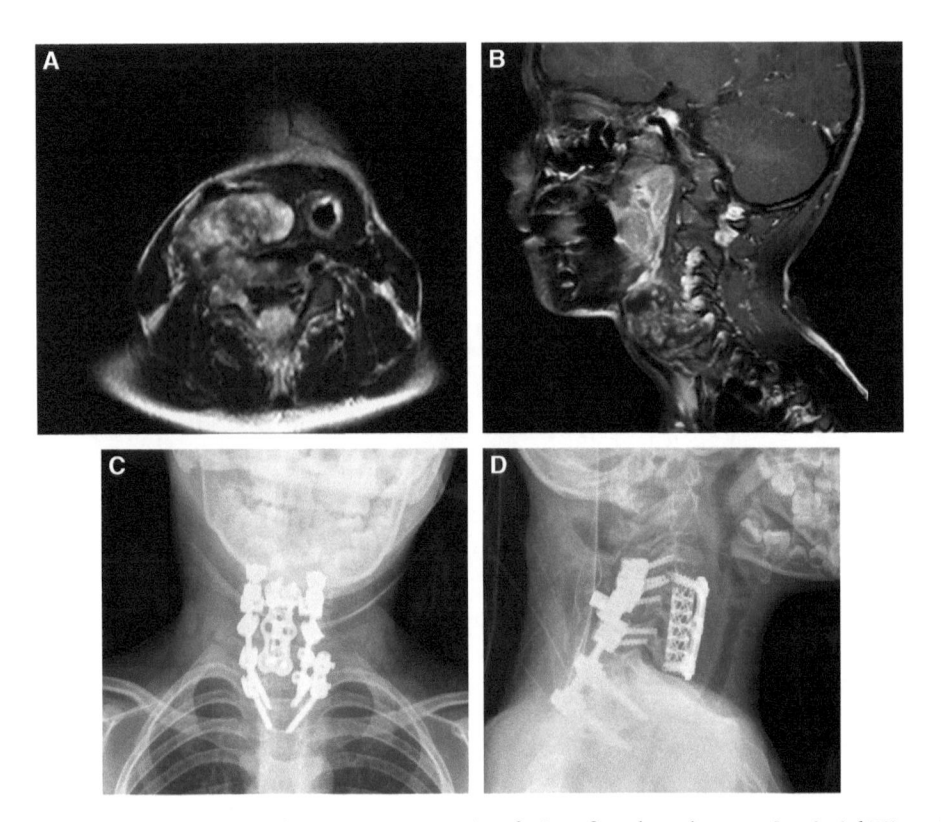

Fig. 48-13 Vertebrectomy with anterior/posterior fusion for chondroma. **A,** Axial T1-weighted MRI with gadolinium reveals a contrast-enhancing lesion of the C5 and C6 vertebra with involvement of the paraspinal soft tissue. **B,** The full extent of the paraspinal soft tissue involvement is seen on sagittal T1-weighted images with extension of the mass into retropharyngeal space. **C,** Anteriorposterior and **D,** lateral radiographs show a C5-6 titanium cage placed after spondylectomies from an anterior approach and a C3 to T2 posterior spinal fusion.

CONCLUSION

Instrumentation in the pediatric spine is increasingly more commonplace, and time has shown that these techniques, previously reserved for adults, can be performed safely and effectively in children. Nevertheless, pediatric neurosurgeons should be highly aware that interventions performed on the spinal column in the midst of its development carry some risk of deformity and the need for later stabilization procedures. Whenever possible, bone-sparing surgeries with preservation of anatomy are preferred.

BAILOUT TECHNIQUES

Not infrequently, the paucity of bone in the pediatric spine will eliminate the option of placing instrumentation due to lack of screw purchase. When this circumstance arises other methods of immobilization and spinal stabilization must be explored. This dilemma is especially frequent with neonates and infants. In these instances halo placement is commonly used. Children often have a propensity for autofusion with adequate immobilization, and halo placement alone can often result in sufficient fusion. For those patients who are too small for such a device, a full-body cast is sometimes the only option. Recent studies have advocated the use of bone morphogenetic protein in children, to assist with fusion in particularly challenging cases or in patients where bone formation is absolutely critical.[119]

Resecuring long-segment osteoplastic laminotomies or laminoplasties in children can often be challenging. The small flap laminae are often "floating" adjacent to native laminae once the supraspinous and intraspinous ligaments are reattached. Furthermore, the laminae are often too small to affix current plating systems. In these instances, small holes should be created with a 1 mm drill or a perforating towel clamp to secure the laminae with sutures. In these patients meticulous closure of muscle and fascia is paramount. Without the benefit of instrumentation to prevent kyphosis or scoliosis, surgeons must rely on the paraspinous muscles sutured to the neighboring interspinous ligaments to restore spinal stability.

Because of the anatomic limitations complicating transarticular screw placement in adults, and even more so in children, variations of C1-2 screw fixation have been reported in adult patients in whom independent C1 lateral mass screws and C2 pars/pedicle screws were connected with either a plate or a rod.[35,38] Atlantoaxial screw-rod fixation has been suggested as a safer procedure and perhaps, as we have found, the technique is applicable in more patients, despite anatomic variations, even in the smallest of pediatric patients.[74] It is an ideal technique to fix and reduce occipitoatlantoaxial deformities that remain irreducible with closed reduction.

TIPS FROM THE MASTERS

- For children 8 years of age and older, the anatomy and configuration of the spine do not differ significantly from the adult spine in terms of sensitivity or response to instrumentation.
- Preoperative thin-cut CT through the area of interest should help the surgeon decide whether the bony anatomy is suitable for instrumentation.
- Titanium alloy implants due to less metal artifact should be used in cases of neoplasms where frequent MRI is anticipated to monitor for evidence of local recurrence.
- Neuromonitoring can be used for patients with tumors involving the spinal cord or for patients requiring correction of associated spinal deformities.
- Placement of anterior spinal instrumentation or resection of tumor in the vertebral body through a posterior or posterolateral approach, gaining both anterior and posterior exposure of the spinal column through a single approach, is possible and preferred in children.
- While children may be successfully instrumented for spinal stability without increased risk or complications in the immediate postoperative period, continued follow-up with radiographic studies are needed to determine the long-term effects, in terms of spinal alignment and growth, in the immature (growing) pediatric spine.

References (With Key References in Boldface)

1. **Auguste KI, Gupta N. Pediatric intramedullary spinal cord tumors. Neurosurg Clin N Am 17:51-61, 2006.**
2. Binning M, Klimo P Jr, Gluf W, et al. Spinal tumors in children. Neurosurg Clin N Am 18:631-658, 2007.
3. Rossi A, Gandolfo C, Morana G, et al. Tumors of the spine in children. Neuroimaging Clin N Am 17:17-35, 2007.
4. Yamamoto Y, Raffel C. Spinal extradural neoplasms and intradural extramedullary neoplasms, in Albright AL, Pollack IF, Adelson PD, eds. Principles and Practice of Pediatric Neurosurgery. New York: Thieme, 1999, pp 685-696.
5. Hadfield MG, Quezado MM, Williams RL, et al. Ewing's family of tumors involving structures related to the central nervous system: a review. Pediatr Dev Pathol 3:203-210, 2000.
6. Weinstein JN, McLain RF. Primary tumors of the spine. Spine (Phila Pa 1976) 12:843-851, 1987.
7. Whitehouse GH, Griffiths GJ. Roentgenologic aspects of spinal involvement by primary and metastatic Ewing's tumor. J Can Assoc Radiol 27:290-297, 1976.
8. De Bernardi B, Pianca C, Pistamiglio P, et al. Neuroblastoma with symptomatic spinal cord compression at diagnosis: treatment and results with 76 cases. J Clin Oncol 19:183-190, 2001.
9. Plantaz D, Hartmann O, Kalifa C, et al. Localized dumbbell neuroblastoma: a study of 25 cases treated between 1982 and 1987 using the same protocol. Med Pediatr Oncol 21:249-253, 1993.
10. Plantaz D, Rubie H, Michon J, et al. The treatment of neuroblastoma with intraspinal extension with chemotherapy followed by surgical removal of residual disease. A prospective study of 42 patients—results of the NBL 90 Study of the French Society of Pediatric Oncology. Cancer 78:311-319, 1996.

11. Patchell RA, Tibbs PA, Regine WF, et al. Direct decompressive surgical resection in the treatment of spinal cord compression caused by metastatic cancer: a randomised trial. Lancet 366:643-648, 2005.
12. **Anderson RC, Kan P, Gluf WM, et al. Long-term maintenance of cervical alignment after occipitocervical and atlantoaxial screw fixation in young children. J Neurosurg 105:55-61, 2006.**
13. Rekate HL, Theodore N, Sonntag VK, et al. Pediatric spine and spinal cord trauma. State of the art for the third millennium. Childs Nerv Syst 15:743-750, 1999.
14. Givens TG, Polley KA, Smith GF, et al. Pediatric cervical spine injury: a three-year experience. J Trauma 41:310-314, 1996.
15. Kokoska ER, Keller MS, Rallo MC, et al. Characteristics of pediatric cervical spine injuries. J Pediatr Surg 36:100-105, 2001.
16. Torpey BM, Dormans JP, Drummond DS. The use of MRI-compatible titanium segmental spinal instrumentation in pediatric patients with intraspinal tumor. J Spinal Disord 8:76-81, 1995.
17. Shapiro F, Sethna N. Blood loss in pediatric spine surgery. Eur Spine J 13(Suppl 1):S6-S17, 2004.
18. Boucher HH. A method of spinal fusion. J Bone Joint Surg Br 41B:248-259, 1959.
19. Harrington PR. Treatment of scoliosis. Correction and internal fixation by spine instrumentation. J Bone Joint Surg Am 44A:591-610, 1962.
20. Boos N, Webb JK. Pedicle screw fixation in spinal disorders: a European view. Eur Spine J 6:2-18, 1997.
21. Krag MH, Beynnon BD, Pope MH, et al. An internal fixator for posterior application to short segments of the thoracic, lumbar, or lumbosacral spine. Design and testing. Clin Orthop Relat Res(203):75-98, 1986.
22. Roy-Camille R, Saillant G, Mazel C. Internal fixation of the lumbar spine with pedicle screw plating. Clin Orthop Relat Res (203):7-17, 1986.
23. Roy-Camille R, Saillant G, Mazel C. Plating of thoracic, thoracolumbar, and lumbar injuries with pedicle screw plates. Orthop Clin North Am 17:147-159, 1986.
24. Bernstein RM, Hall JE. Solid rod short segment anterior fusion in thoracolumbar scoliosis. J Pediatr Orthop B 7:124-131, 1998.
25. Majid ME, Castro FP Jr, Holt RT. Anterior fusion for idiopathic scoliosis. Spine (Phila Pa 1976) 25:696-702, 2000.
26. Turi M, Johnston CE II, Richards BS. Anterior correction of idiopathic scoliosis using TSRH instrumentation. Spine (Phila Pa 1976) 18:417-422, 1993.
27. Herring JA. Anterior spinal surgery. In Weinstein SL, ed. Pediatric Spine Surgery, 2nd ed. Philadelphia: Lippincott Williams & Wilkins, 2001, pp 239-246.
28. **Hilibrand AS, Carlson GD, Palumbo MA, et al. Radiculopathy and myelopathy at segments adjacent to the site of a previous anterior cervical arthrodesis. J Bone Joint Surg Am 81:519-528, 1999.**
29. Vaccaro AR, Balderston RA. Anterior plate instrumentation for disorders of the subaxial cervical spine. Clin Orthop Relat Res (335):112-121, 1997.
30. Sankar WN, Skaggs DL, Emans JB, et al. Neurologic risk in growing rod spine surgery in early onset scoliosis: is neuromonitoring necessary for all cases? Spine (Phila Pa 1976) 34:1952-1955, 2009.
31. Pelosi L, Lamb J, Grevitt M, et al. Combined monitoring of motor and somatosensory evoked potentials in orthopaedic spinal surgery. Clin Neurophysiol 113:1082-1091, 2002.
32. Rea GL, Mullin BB, Mervis LJ, et al. Occipitocervical fixation in nontraumatic upper cervical spine instability. Surg Neurol 40:255-261, 1993.
33. Elia M, Mazzara JT, Fielding JW. Onlay technique for occipitocervical fusion. Clin Orthop Relat Res (280):170-174, 1992.
34. Fehlings MG, Errico T, Cooper P, et al. Occipitocervical fusion with a five-millimeter malleable rod and segmental fixation. Neurosurgery 32:198-207; discussion 207-198, 1993.
35. Grob D, Dvorak J, Panjabi MM, et al. The role of plate and screw fixation in occipitocervical fusion in rheumatoid arthritis. Spine (Phila Pa 1976) 19:2545-2551, 1994.
36. Sasso RC, Jeanneret B, Fischer K, et al. Occipitocervical fusion with posterior plate and screw instrumentation. A long-term follow-up study. Spine (Phila Pa 1976) 19:2364-2368, 1994.

37. Smith MD, Anderson P, Grady MS. Occipitocervical arthrodesis using contoured plate fixation. An early report on a versatile fixation technique. Spine (Phila Pa 1976) 18:1984-1990, 1993.
38. Grob D, Schmotzer H. Posterior occipitocervical fusion. Spine State Art Rev 10:275-280, 1996.
39. Wittenberg RH, Shea M, Swartz DE, et al. Importance of bone mineral density in instrumented spine fusions. Spine (Phila Pa 1976) 16:647-652, 1991.
40. Ryken TC, Goel VK, Clausen JD, et al. Assessment of unicortical and bicortical fixation in a quasistatic cadaveric model. Role of bone mineral density and screw torque. Spine (Phila Pa 1976) 20:1861-1867, 1995.
41. Heywood AW, Learmonth ID, Thomas M. Internal fixation for occipito-cervical fusion. J Bone Joint Surg Br 70:708-711, 1988.
42. Roberts DA, Doherty BJ, Heggeness MH. Quantitative anatomy of the occiput and the biomechanics of occipital screw fixation. Spine (Phila Pa 1976) 23:1100-1107; discussion 1107-1108, 1998.
43. Nadim Y, Lu J, Sabry FF, et al. Occipital screws in occipitocervical fusion and their relation to the venous sinuses: an anatomic and radiographic study. Orthopedics 23:717-719, 2000.
44. Bambakidis NC, Feiz-Erfan I, Horn EM, et al. Biomechanical comparison of occipitoatlantal screw fixation techniques. J Neurosurg Spine 8:143-152, 2008.
45. Vale FL, Oliver M, Cahill DW. Rigid occipitocervical fusion. J Neurosurg 91:144-150, 1999.
46. Wright NM. Posterior C2 fixation using bilateral, crossing C2 laminar screws: case series and technical note. J Spinal Disord Tech 17:158-162, 2004.
47. Wright NM. Translaminar rigid screw fixation of the axis. Technical note. J Neurosurg Spine 3:409-414, 2005.
48. Chamoun RB, Relyea KM, Johnson KK, et al. Use of axial and subaxial translaminar screw fixation in the management of upper cervical spinal instability in a series of 7 children. Neurosurgery 64:734-739; discussion 739, 2009.
49. **Leonard JR, Wright NM. Pediatric atlantoaxial fixation with bilateral, crossing C-2 translaminar screws. Technical note. J Neurosurg 104:59-63, 2006.**
50. Jea A, Sheth RN, Vanni S, et al. Modification of Wright's technique for placement of bilateral crossing C2 translaminar screws: technical note. Spine J 8:656-660, 2008.
51. Seitz H, Marlovits S, Schwendenwein I, et al. Biocompatibility of polyethylene terephthalate (Trevira hochfest) augmentation device in repair of the anterior cruciate ligament. Biomaterials 19:189-196, 1998.
52. Ben-David B. Spinal cord monitoring. Orthop Clin North Am 19:427-448, 1988.
53. Burke SD, Matiko J. Segmental spinal instrumentation in neuromuscular spinal deformity. Orthop Trans 7:25-26, 1983.
54. Carlioz H, Ouaknine M. [Neurologic complications of surgery of the spine in children] Chirurgie 120:26-30, 1994.
55. Girardi FP, Boachie-Adjei O, Rawlins BA. Safety of sublaminar wires with Isola instrumentation for the treatment of idiopathic scoliosis. Spine (Phila Pa 1976) 25:691-695, 2000.
56. Herring JA, Wenger DR. Segmental spinal instrumentation: a preliminary report of 40 consecutive cases. Spine (Phila Pa 1976) 7:285-298, 1982.
57. Johnston CE II, Happel LT Jr, Norris R, et al. Delayed paraplegia complicating sublaminar segmental spinal instrumentation. J Bone Joint Surg Am 68:556-563, 1986.
58. Lonstein JE, Winter RB, Moe JH, et al. Neurologic deficits secondary to spinal deformity. A review of the literature and report of 43 cases. Spine (Phila Pa 1976) 5:331-355, 1980.
59. Lowe T. Morbidity and Mortality Committee Report. Presented at the Annual Meeting of the Scoliosis Research Society, Vancouver, BC, Canada 1987.
60. Aydingoz O, Bilsel N, Botanlioglu H, et al. Effect of decortication on laminar strength during sublaminar wiring: an experimental study. J Spinal Disord Tech 17:498-504, 2004.
61. Lu DC, Gupta N, Mummaneni PV. Minimally invasive decompression of a suboccipital osseous prominence causing rotational vertebral artery occlusion. Case report. J Neurosurg Pediatr 4:191-195, 2009.
62. Simon SL, Auerbach JD, Garg S, et al. Efficacy of spinal instrumentation and fusion in the prevention of postlaminectomy spinal deformity in children with intramedullary spinal cord tumors. J Pediatr Orthop 28:244-249, 2008.

63. de Jonge T, Slullitel H, Dubousset J, et al. Late-onset spinal deformities in children treated by laminectomy and radiation therapy for malignant tumours. Eur Spine J 14:765-771, 2005.
64. **McGirt MJ, Constantini S, Jallo GI. Correlation of a preoperative grading scale with progressive spinal deformity following surgery for intramedullary spinal cord tumors in children. J Neurosurg Pediatr 2:277-281, 2008.**
65. Yao KC, McGirt MJ, Chaichana KL, et al. Risk factors for progressive spinal deformity following resection of intramedullary spinal cord tumors in children: an analysis of 161 consecutive cases. J Neurosurg 107:463-468, 2007.
66. McGirt MJ, Chaichana KL, Attenello F, et al. Spinal deformity after resection of cervical intramedullary spinal cord tumors in children. Childs Nerv Syst 24:735-739, 2008.
67. **McGirt MJ, Chaichana KL, Atiba A, et al. Incidence of spinal deformity after resection of intramedullary spinal cord tumors in children who underwent laminectomy compared with laminoplasty. J Neurosurg Pediatr 1:57-62, 2008.**
68. Steinbok P. Multiple short-segment laminoplasties in children: a novel technique to avoid postoperative spinal deformity. Childs Nerv Syst 24:369-372, 2008.
69. Amhaz HH, Fox BD, Johnson KK, et al. Postlaminoplasty kyphotic deformity in the thoracic spine: case report and review of the literature. Pediatr Neurosurg 45:151-154, 2009.
70. Papagelopoulos PJ, Currier BL, Stone J, et al. Biomechanical evaluation of occipital fixation. J Spinal Disord 13:336-344, 2000.
71. Fehlings MG, Cooper PR, Errico TJ. Posterior plates in the management of cervical instability: long-term results in 44 patients. J Neurosurg 81:341-349, 1994.
72. Haher TR, Yeung AW, Caruso SA, et al. Occipital screw pullout strength. A biomechanical investigation of occipital morphology. Spine (Phila Pa 1976) 24:5-9, 1999.
73. Jeanneret B, Magerl F. Primary posterior fusion C1/2 in odontoid fractures: indications, technique, and results of transarticular screw fixation. J Spinal Disord 5:464-475, 1992.
74. Jea A, Taylor MD, Dirks PB, et al. Incorporation of C-1 lateral mass screws in occipitocervical and atlantoaxial fusions for children 8 years of age or younger. Technical note. J Neurosurg 107:178-183, 2007.
75. Dickman CA, Sonntag VK. Posterior C1-C2 transarticular screw fixation for atlantoaxial arthrodesis. Neurosurgery 43:275-280; discussion 280-271, 1998.
76. Farey ID, Nadkarni S, Smith N. Modified Gallie technique versus transarticular screw fixation in C1-C2 fusion. Clin Orthop Relat Res (359):126-135, 1999.
77. Madawi AA, Casey AT, Solanki GA, et al. Radiological and anatomical evaluation of the atlantoaxial transarticular screw fixation technique. J Neurosurg 86:961-968, 1997.
78. Howington JU, Kruse JJ, Awasthi D. Surgical anatomy of the C-2 pedicle. J Neurosurg 95:88-92, 2001.
79. Resnick DK, Lapsiwala S, Trost GR. Anatomic suitability of the C1-C2 complex for pedicle screw fixation. Spine (Phila Pa 1976) 27:1494-1498, 2002.
80. Deen HG, Birch BD, Wharen RE, et al. Lateral mass screw-rod fixation of the cervical spine: a prospective clinical series with 1-year follow-up. Spine J 3:489-495, 2003.
81. Roy-Camille R, Saillant G, Laville C, et al. Treatment of lower cervical spinal injuries—C3 to C7. Spine (Phila Pa 1976) 17(Suppl):S442-446, 1992.
82. Sekhon LH. Posterior cervical lateral mass screw fixation: analysis of 1026 consecutive screws in 143 patients. J Spinal Disord Tech 18:297-303, 2005.
83. Coe JD, Warden KE, Sutterlin CE III, et al. Biomechanical evaluation of cervical spinal stabilization methods in a human cadaveric model. Spine (Phila Pa 1976) 14:1122-1131, 1989.
84. Gill K, Paschal S, Corin J, et al. Posterior plating of the cervical spine. A biomechanical comparison of different posterior fusion techniques. Spine (Phila Pa 1976) 13:813-816, 1988.
85. Montesano PX, Jauch E, Jonsson H Jr. Anatomic and biomechanical study of posterior cervical spine plate arthrodesis: an evaluation of two different techniques of screw placement. J Spinal Disord 5:301-305, 1992.
86. Sutterlin CE III, McAfee PC, Warden KE, et al. A biomechanical evaluation of cervical spinal stabilization methods in a bovine model. Static and cyclical loading. Spine (Phila Pa 1976) 13:795-802, 1988.

87. Ulrich C, Woersdoerfer O, Kalff R, et al. Biomechanics of fixation systems to the cervical spine. Spine (Phila Pa 1976) 16(Suppl):S4-S9, 1991.
88. **Anderson RC, Ragel BT, Mocco J, et al. Selection of a rigid internal fixation construct for stabilization at the craniovertebral junction in pediatric patients. J Neurosurg 107:36-42, 2007.**
89. **Bailey DK. The normal cervical spine in infants and children. Radiology 59:712-719, 1952.**
90. **Brockmeyer DL, York JE, Apfelbaum RI. Anatomical suitability of C1-2 transarticular screw placement in pediatric patients. J Neurosurg 92:7-11, 2000.**
91. Abumi K, Itoh H, Taneichi H, et al. Transpedicular screw fixation for traumatic lesions of the middle and lower cervical spine: description of the techniques and preliminary report. J Spinal Disord 7:19-28, 1994.
92. Abumi K, Kaneda K. Pedicle screw fixation for nontraumatic lesions of the cervical spine. Spine (Phila Pa 1976) 22:1853-1863, 1997.
93. Borne GM, Bedou GL, Pinaudeau M. Treatment of pedicular fractures of the axis. A clinical study and screw fixation technique. J Neurosurg 60:88-93, 1984.
94. Roy-Camille R, Mazel C, Saillant G, et al. Rationale and techniques of internal fixation in trauma of the cervical spine. In Errico T, Bauer RD, Waugh T, eds. Spinal Trauma. Philadelphia: JB Lippincott, 1991, pp 163-191.
95. Roy-Camille R, Saillant G, Mazel C. Internal fixation of the unstable cervical spine by a posterior osteosynthesis with plates and screws. In Study TCSR, ed. The Cervical Spine, 2nd ed. Philadelphia: JB Lippincott, 1989, pp 390-403.
96. Kretzer RM, Sciubba DM, Bagley CA, et al. Translaminar screw fixation in the upper thoracic spine. J Neurosurg Spine 5:527-533, 2006.
97. Chern JJ, Chamoun RB, Whitehead WE, et al. Computed tomography morphometric analysis for axial and subaxial translaminar screw placement in the pediatric cervical spine. J Neurosurg Pediatr 3:121-128, 2009.
98. Belmont PJ Jr, Klemme WR, Dhawan A, et al. In vivo accuracy of thoracic pedicle screws. Spine (Phila Pa 1976) 26:2340-2346, 2001.
99. Liljenqvist U, Lepsien U, Hackenberg L, et al. Comparative analysis of pedicle screw and hook instrumentation in posterior correction and fusion of idiopathic thoracic scoliosis. Eur Spine J 11:336-343, 2002.
100. Liljenqvist UR, Halm HF, Link TM. Pedicle screw instrumentation of the thoracic spine in idiopathic scoliosis. Spine (Phila Pa 1976) 22:2239-2245, 1997.
101. Suk SI, Kim WJ, Lee SM, et al. Thoracic pedicle screw fixation in spinal deformities: are they really safe? Spine (Phila Pa 1976) 26:2049-2057, 2001.
102. Amiot LP, Lang K, Putzier M, et al. Comparative results between conventional and computer-assisted pedicle screw installation in the thoracic, lumbar, and sacral spine. Spine (Phila Pa 1976) 25:606-614, 2000.
103. Delorme S, Labelle H, Aubin CE, et al. A three-dimensional radiographic comparison of Cotrel-Dubousset and Colorado instrumentations for the correction of idiopathic scoliosis. Spine (Phila Pa 1976) 25:205-210, 2000.
104. Jonsson B, Sjostrom L, Olerud C, et al. Outcome after limited posterior surgery for thoracic and lumbar spine metastases. Eur Spine J 5:36-44, 1996.
105. Suk SI, Lee CK, Kim WJ, et al. Segmental pedicle screw fixation in the treatment of thoracic idiopathic scoliosis. Spine (Phila Pa 1976) 20:1399-1405, 1995.
106. Cinotti G, Gumina S, Ripani M, et al. Pedicle instrumentation in the thoracic spine. A morphometric and cadaveric study for placement of screws. Spine (Phila Pa 1976) 24:114-119, 1999.
107. Ebraheim NA, Jabaly G, Xu R, et al. Anatomic relations of the thoracic pedicle to the adjacent neural structures. Spine (Phila Pa 1976) 22:1553-1556; discussion 1557, 1997.
108. Kothe R, O'Holleran JD, Liu W, et al. Internal architecture of the thoracic pedicle. An anatomic study. Spine (Phila Pa 1976) 21:264-270, 1996.

109. Krag MH, Weaver DL, Beynnon BD, et al. Morphometry of the thoracic and lumbar spine related to transpedicular screw placement for surgical spinal fixation. Spine (Phila Pa 1976) 13:27-32, 1988.
110. Papin P, Arlet V, Marchesi D, et al. Unusual presentation of spinal cord compression related to misplaced pedicle screws in thoracic scoliosis. Eur Spine J 8:156-159, 1999.
111. **Vaccaro AR, Rizzolo SJ, Allardyce TJ, et al. Placement of pedicle screws in the thoracic spine. Part I: Morphometric analysis of the thoracic vertebrae. J Bone Joint Surg Am 77:1193-1199, 1995.**
112. **Vaccaro AR, Rizzolo SJ, Balderston RA, et al. Placement of pedicle screws in the thoracic spine. Part II: An anatomical and radiographic assessment. J Bone Joint Surg Am 77:1200-1206, 1995.**
113. Bransford R, Bellabarba C, Thompson JH, et al. The safety of fluoroscopically-assisted thoracic pedicle screw instrumentation for spine trauma. J Trauma 60:1047-1052, 2006.
114. Di Silvestre M, Parisini P, Lolli F, et al. Complications of thoracic pedicle screws in scoliosis treatment. Spine (Phila Pa 1976) 32:1655-1661, 2007.
115. Kim YJ, Lenke LG, Bridwell KH, et al. Free hand pedicle screw placement in the thoracic spine: is it safe? Spine (Phila Pa 1976) 29:333-342; discussion 342, 2004.
116. Kuklo TR, Lenke LG, O'Brien MF, et al. Accuracy and efficacy of thoracic pedicle screws in curves more than 90 degrees. Spine (Phila Pa 1976) 30:222-226, 2005.
117. Suk SI, Lee CK, Chung SS. Comparison of Zielke ventral derotation system and Cotrel-Dubousset instrumentation in the treatment of idiopathic lumbar and thoracolumbar scoliosis. Spine (Phila Pa 1976) 19:419-429, 1994.
118. Winter RB, Hall JE. Kyphosis in childhood and adolescence. Spine (Phila Pa 1976) 3:285-308, 1978.
119. Lu DC, Sun PP. Bone morphogenetic protein for salvage fusion in an infant with Down syndrome and craniovertebral instability. Case report. J Neurosurg 106:480-483, 2007.

SECTION IV

Complications and Outcomes

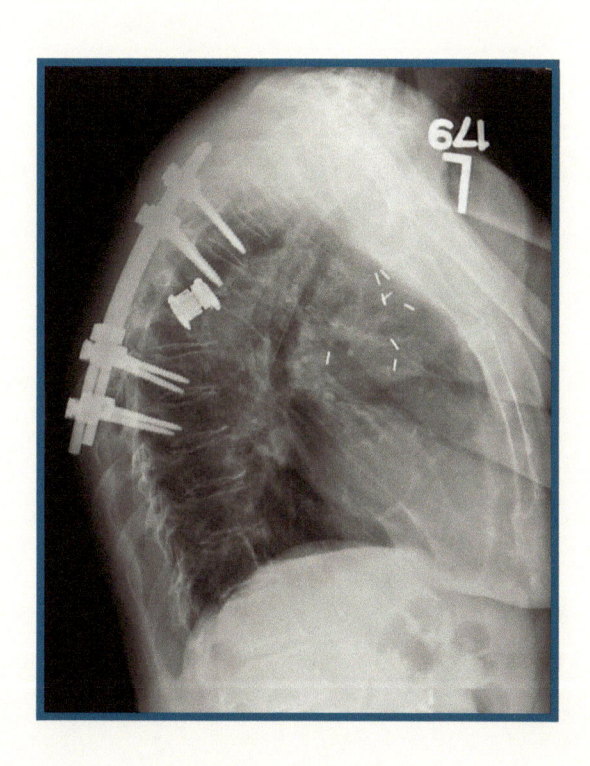

Chapter 49

Complications in Spine Tumor Surgery

Jean-Paul Wolinsky, Daniel M. Sciubba

Complications that are encountered during surgery for spinal column tumors are not all unique, but the frequency of complications may be greater than that found in nononcologic patients, and the consequences can be grave. The spine segment to be surgically treated and the type of surgery contemplated (intralesional versus en bloc) dictate the potential complication profile. There are certain complications that are not unique to any portion of spine surgery, but others occur more frequently with certain procedures.

BLOOD LOSS

Complications associated with bleeding are directly related to the type of tumor being treated. Certain malignancies are highly vascular, for example, renal cell carcinoma, hepatocellular carcinoma, follicular cell thyroid carcinoma, pheochromocytoma, and hemangiopericytoma (Box 49-1). Knowledge of the tumor type preoperatively can be useful for predicting the potential vascularity of a tumor. If a particularly vascular

---

Box 49-1 Vascular Tumors of the Spine

- Renal cell carcinoma
- Thyroid cancer (follicular)
- Hepatocellular cancer
- Pheochromocytoma
- Melanoma
- Sarcoma
- Hemangiopericytoma
- Myeloma
- Giant cell tumor
- Aneurysmal bone cysts

tumor is anticipated, then preoperative embolization of the tumor can be useful to minimize intraoperative blood loss (Fig. 49-1). In addition, during the operation, a clear understanding of the normal anatomy surrounding the tumor can help predict the margins of the tumor and can help predict where displaced structures, such as the spinal cord and nerve roots, might be encountered. By clearly defining the normal anatomy surrounding a tumor during surgery, before proceeding with tumor resection, the chances of minimizing the injury to vital structures can be improved. As tumor resection proceeds, and as a tumor hemorrhages, the surgical field can be obscured. Hemorrhaging might not be controllable until the entire tumor has been resected, and therefore rapid resection of the tumor may be required to avoid exsanguination. Such expedient operating, combined with aggressive resuscitation of the patient with blood products (packed red blood cells, fresh-frozen plasma, platelets, and cryoprecipitate), may be needed to achieve surgical resection and the avoid complications associated with massive blood loss.

Primary tumors of the spinal column necessitating en bloc resection to achieve control can be associated with large blood losses during surgery. These operations usually require massive and unique exposures that pose challenges to obtaining complete vascular control. Although the tumor itself may not be vascular, because an en bloc resection is designed to avoid violation of a vascular tumor, the dissection can be slow and continued blood loss from normal tissues can be expected. For instance, osteotomies through normal bone can bleed until delivery of the specimen has been completed. For this reason, a wide selection of hemostatic agents should be available at all times in the operating room. Specifically, Gelfoam, Gelfoam powder mixed with thrombin, Surgicel, and bone wax can all be used to control focal areas of hemorrhage, and cottonoids, sponges, and towels can be used to pack larger cavities.

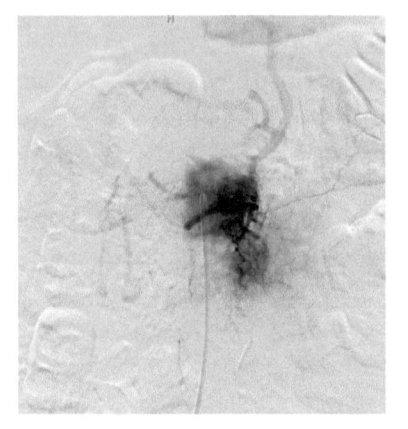

Fig. 49-1   Angiogram of renal cell carcinoma metastasis to the spine showing extensive tumor blush after infusion of contrast material.

Large vascular structures (aorta, inferior vena cava, vertebral arteries, carotid arteries, segmental vessels, iliac arteries, and veins) can all be injured during the dissection, and exposure for primary repair may not be possible until the specimen has been delivered. Hemorrhaging from these structures can be rapid, and therefore the amount of vascular reserve that a patient may have can be rapidly depleted. To increase this reserve, and allow more time to achieve vascular control or repair, the patient's blood volume and hemodynamic status need to be maintained at a higher level than would normally be tolerated during other operations. Discussions with the anesthesiologist before and during surgery should thus be directed at maintaining a higher intraoperative hemoglobin level to be prepared for rapid, unexpected blood loss.

INFECTION

Chemotherapy, radiation therapy, steroids, length of surgery, blood loss, and tumor location are all potential risk factors for developing wound infections.[1,2] The rate of wound infections in oncologic spine surgery compared with degenerative spine surgery, can be 10 times greater, 3% to 4% in degenerative cases versus up to 38% in sacral tumor surgeries.[3,4] The various chemotherapeutic agents used to treat different spine tumors are quite numerous and beyond the scope of this chapter, but the effects of these agents can be deleterious and prevent the body from mounting an appropriate immune response to combat infection. The absolute neutrophil count can be depressed, the function of the white blood cells can be altered, and the ability to form normal scar tissue can be hampered. Compounding these difficulties is the frequent need for high-dose steroids with spinal column tumors and neurologic dysfunction, which further increases the challenges of proper wound healing.

It is well known that preoperative radiation therapy also decreases the wound-healing capacity of the body.[1] If possible, surgery should precede radiation therapy. If this is not possible, then surgery should be delayed for at least 3 to 4 weeks to lessen the chances of wound complications. Postoperative radiation therapy can also delay wound healing and increase the chances of wound dehiscence and infection and, if possible, radiation therapy should be delayed for at least 2 weeks postoperatively. Advances in radiation delivery, in the form of stereotactic and fractionated stereotactic radiation, appear to be promising in their ability to limit toxicity to normal tissues and decrease the chances of radiation-associated complications, but currently the experience with these modalities is limited.[5,6]

Length of surgery and the degree of blood loss are also factors that may also increase the risk of infection.[2,4] These factors directly correlate with the complexity of the tumor resection and also most likely with the size and extent of the tumor. There has been speculation that increased blood transfusion correlates with a higher risk of infection, but this must be balanced with the deleterious effects of profound anemia from withholding transfusion.

The location of a tumor to be resected also plays a significant role in the risk for perioperative infections. Sacral tumor resections have a significantly higher rate of infection (up to 38%) when compared with infections for resections of tumors of the mobile spine.[1,3] The proximity of the incision with the anus and subsequent postoperative wound contamination can increase the potential for infection. In addition, these operations tend to be longer, are associated with greater blood losses, and will tend to have more soft tissue resection and larger tissue defects to close. Because of the regional anatomy, the complex myocutaneous flaps available for closure are quite limited in this region. The plastic surgery flaps commonly used for closure of these large defects include gluteal rotational flaps, myocutaneous rectus abdominis flaps, and omental flaps. Compounding the tissue closure issues, these wounds are in a very dependent portion of the body, and it is very difficult to limit pressure on the postoperative wound as the patient recovers. Also, when a patient who has undergone a sacral tumor resection is ambulating postoperatively, there may be significant amount of stress placed on the wound.

NERVE INJURY OR NERVE SACRIFICE

Nerve roots exiting the spinal cord can be injured during resection of the tumor. In certain instances, particularly with en bloc resections, sacrifice of a nerve root can be intentional. The potential complications of nerve root injury or sacrifice must be understood (Table 49-1).

The C1-4 nerve roots in isolation can be sacrificed without clinically significant motor consequences. Sacrifice of C3 and C4 unilaterally can result in weakness of the diaphragm. Transection of C3 through C5 will result in paralysis of the diaphragm and could have devastating consequences. Injury to C5, C6, C8, or T1, in isolation or in combination, can produce significant disability in a patient. Of the motor roots of the brachial plexus, C7 injury or sacrifice is usually well tolerated.

Ligation of the thoracic nerve roots below T1 is well tolerated. The result will be a bandlike numbness along the nerve root and usually inconsequential loss of intercostal muscle function. If a nerve root is to be sacrificed, ligation and transection proximal to the dorsal root ganglion can limit postoperative dysesthetic pain syndrome. A watertight ligation of the nerve root in this location is critical to avoid leakage of spinal fluid from the nerve root sleeve. Such closure is especially relevant close to the pleural space, because the negative intrathoracic pressures that are transmitted can create a substantial cerebrospinal fluid (CSF) fistula and persistent CSF pleural effusion.[7] It has been suggested that spinal cord ischemia is a potential complication of multiple thoracic nerve root or segmental vessel ligation, but this has not been the experience of the senior author (J.P.W.).

In the lumbar spine, sacrifice of the L3 and L4 nerve roots is not well tolerated. This results in disability from weakness of the quadriceps muscles. Transection of L1 or L2 in isolation may initially cause iliopsoas weakness, but over time the remaining root usually is able to compensate. Isolated L5 nerve root sacrifice can result in weakness as

Table 49-1 Expected Deficits After Intentional Sacrifice of a Spinal Root

Spinal Root	Expected Deficit
C1-4 (isolated)	No significant motor deficit
C3 and C4 (unilateral)	Unilateral diaphragm weakness
C3, C4, and C5 (unilateral)	Unilateral diaphragm paralysis
C5	Deltoid paralysis and biceps weakness
C6	Biceps weakness
C7	Triceps and wrist extension weakness (usually well tolerated)
C8 or T1	Intrinsic hand weakness
T2-12	No significant motor deficit
L1 or L2	Iliopsoas weakness (usually well tolerated)
L3 or L4	Quadriceps weakness, potential foot drop with L4
L5	Foot drop and/or weakness of extensor hallucis longus
S1	Weakness of plantar flexion
S2, S3, S4, and S5	Bowel, bladder, and sexual dysfunction
S3, S4, and S5	Abnormal but present bowel, bladder, and sexual function
S4 and S5 only	Normal bowel, bladder, and sexual function

minimal as extensor hallucis longus weakness but can also be more profound, manifesting as a complete foot drop.

The sympathetic nerves controlling sexual function lie ventral to the lumbar spine. Manipulation of these nerves or sacrifice of these nerves can result in retrograde and/or painful ejaculation in men. The incidence of this complication from anterior surgery is variable, but if an en bloc resection is being contemplated at L4 or L5, discussion of this possible outcome with male patients is advisable.

The distal sacral nerve roots (S4 and S5) can be sacrificed with minimal consequence. Unilateral sacrifice of S3 (with bilateral S4 and S5) can result in fairly normal bowel, bladder, and sexual function. Bilateral S3 to S5 nerve root loss will result in a change in bowel, bladder, and sexual function, but patients still might have acceptable function. Loss of S2-5 will result in complete loss of bowel, bladder, and sexual function. A patient with unilateral loss of S2-5 can also have bowel, bladder, and sexual function. S1 nerve root loss will result in weakness of the gastrocnemius muscle but is well tolerated. Conversely, loss of L5 and the sacral nerve roots will result in the inability for a patient to ambulate.[8]

SPINAL FLUID LEAK

A CSF leak that occurs during resection of a spine tumor can be as challenging to deal with as with degenerative disorders. Persistent fluid leaks can result in headaches, meningitis, and epidural hematomas.[9,10] Strategies for dealing with such leaks are highly varied, and no one strategy can be used for all types of leaks. It is of paramount importance when dealing with these leaks to determine from where the leak is emanating and then achieve the most watertight dural closure possible during the initial surgery.

In situations when the dura has been resected or is lacking sufficient substance, a dural patch will need to be employed. Patches can be obtained locally from fascia or muscle, or they can be harvested from another site, such as tensor fascia lata grafts, which can be a common source. Exogenous graft material is also widely available, and all have varying handling characteristics. These substances are usually collagen-based grafts or Gore-Tex–based grafts.

Tissue glues are often commonly used to reinforce a dural closure. These can be made from the patient's serum in the form of fibrin glue. Commercially available fibrin glues are another source. Some are from pooled serum and some are from synthetic sources. All types of fibrin glue appear to work well, and the type used is usually at the discretion of the surgeon. An ample amount of sealant should be used to reinforce the closure, but is limited to avoid creating a complication stemming from an iatrogenic epidural mass.

Certain regions of the body are particularly troublesome if a dural laceration is encountered. Sealing of ventral spinal fluid leaks in the thoracic spine can be challenging. The negative pressure in the chest during inspiration can promote a spinal fluid fistula. Various strategies have been employed to try to control such leaks. After a watertight dural closure has been achieved, and the suture line has been reinforced with fibrin glue, a pleural flap can be elevated and rotated over the leak. If this is not suitable, an intercostal muscle flap with an intercostal vascular pedicle can be mobilized and placed over the dural closure. The negative inspiratory pressure can be minimized by using bilevel positive airway pressure postoperatively.[11] In addition, if a visceral pleural leak was not encountered during the thoracotomy, and a pneumothorax is not present postoperatively, the thoracostomy tube can be placed on water seal to minimize propagation of the CSF fistula. Finally, a lumbar drain can be placed to decrease the intradural pressure and promote closure of the leak.

SPINAL CORD INJURY

Spinal column tumor resections can be massive operations that put the spinal cord at risk during surgery. Blood loss can result in hypotension, and the patient must be properly resuscitated to avoid ischemic injury to the cord. Traumatic injury can occur during resection of the tumor or with manipulation of a large specimen during an en bloc resection. Accidental avulsion of a nerve root can result in tension on the spinal cord, and an injury can occur as a result.

Identification of the injury at the time of insult may be useful to try to minimize the injury. The use of somatosensory evoked potentials (SSEPs) and motor evoked potentials (MEPs) can be useful to determine whether a potential spinal cord injury has occurred. The interpretation and explanation of SSEPs and MEPs is beyond the scope of this chapter. If a change is suggestive of an injury, and the change is considered to be a real change by the neuromonitoring team, the anesthesia team, and the surgeon, then measures can be instituted to try to minimize the injury. The blood pressure should be increased to keep the mean arterial pressure above 80 to 90 mm Hg. Steroids can be administered. Increasing the blood pressure and administering steroids are adjuncts that are thought to be helpful in preventing an injury, but this has never been proved to be effective, and the dosage is not certain in spine tumor surgery.

During large spinal exposure and resection, multiple segmental arteries may need to be sacrificed. Concern exists over the total number of vessels taken, if bilateral vessels are sacrificed, and if the artery of Adamkiewicz is taken. Results of experimental studies in dog models suggest that spinal cord damage occurs after bilateral sacrifice of four or more vessels, including the artery of Adamkiewicz.[12] Intraoperatively, all efforts should be made to save as many vessels as possible. In addition, maintaining high mean arterial pressure (>80 mm Hg) should be a goal during spinal cord monitoring while such vessels are being taken.

Of note, during large spinal column resections, including vertebrectomy, spondylectomy, or any large osteotomy procedure, there can be substantial destabilization of the spine that puts the spinal cord and its vascular supply at risk. Such procedures may shorten, lengthen, or twist the spinal cord transiently during tumor resection or manipulation of instrumentation. For this reason, it is highly recommended that temporary or permanent stabilizing instrumentation be used sparingly during the operation to avoid iatrogenic and unexpected destabilization of the spine during tumor manipulation or specimen removal.

THORACIC DUCT INJURY

Injury to the thoracic duct can lead to a persistent chyle leak. This is most often encountered during transthoracic approaches to the spine on the left side of the chest. The thoracic duct can also be injured during en bloc vertebral body resections with the use of the Roy-Camille or the Tomita technique, in which manipulation of soft tissues ventral to the spine is conducted from a posterior approach with more limited visibiliy.[9,13] In fact, with the use of either of these techniques, a thoracic duct injury must be universal but is not universally symptomatic or recognized. Persistent chyle leaks manifest themselves as continued high-volume fluid output through a thoracostomy or as an accumulation or progression of a pleural effusion, the latter of which can be diagnosed as a chylothorax through percutaneous aspiration. Ultimately such leaks can result in malnutrition, because absorption of fats into the venous system is hindered. If recognized at the time of surgery, the treatment option is direct ligation of the thoracic duct. High-fat solutions, such as cream, can be placed through a nasogastric tube to stimulate chyle production and thus aid in identifying the leak intraoperatively. If a leak is suspected and confirmed postoperatively, conservative treatment is usually successful in controlling the injury. Maintaining the patient on a low-fat, low-triglyceride diet, nothing by mouth, and on total parenteral nutrition will decrease the production of chyle and hopefully allow the leak to spontaneously close. Thoracostomy drainage is maintained during this time period. If a chyle leak persists despite conservative management, surgical exploration and closure may be indicated. Before surgery, a lymph node angiogram may be useful in identifying the leak. The procedure itself may actually lead to sclerosis of the chyle leak.[14] Caution must be exercised when proceeding with lymphangiography, because an idiosyncratic reaction may occur with the contrast medium being used, resulting in encephalitis.

INSTRUMENTATION FAILURE/PSEUDARTHROSIS

The degree of bony resection during removal of tumors of the spinal column usually results in instability, necessitating reconstruction of the spine with instrumentation and arthrodesis. The environment in which this needs to be accomplished is usually fairly hostile. Chemotherapy, malnutrition, chronic disease, and radiation therapy all make achieving a solid arthrodesis difficult. The bone quality in patients with certain types of tumors (i.e., multiple myeloma) or in patients who have already received some type of treatment for their tumors (chemotherapy or radiation therapy) is usually poor. Tumors requiring en bloc resection usually will necessitate an operative plan that results in complete disassociation of the spine and complete spinal instability. Establishing a solid instrumentation base in such an environment can be challenging, and if arthrodesis is not achieved, and if the patient's survival is long enough, instrumentation will ultimately fail.

Instrumentation constructs that are designed for reconstruction after resection of spine tumors tend to be significantly more robust compared with degenerative disorders. When planning reconstruction options for degenerative disorders, maintaining motion and sacrificing as few motion segments as possible are usually the goals. In designing constructs for oncologic resections, more is less. More instrumentation tends to be needed to stabilize the spine, and sacrifice of motion to achieve this goal is usually beneficial as a tradeoff to instrumentation failure and complications. Complications of spinal instability in conjunction with a tumor may require additional repeat operations and lengthen the recovery time. This lengthened recovery time can significantly impede the ability to deliver needed chemotherapy and radiation therapy, and missing a window of opportunity could result in recurrence of tumors and ultimately complete failure of the initial goal of surgery.

Bone quality plays a significant role in achieving a solid construct (Fig. 49-2). The degree of osteopenia and osteoporosis may be increased as a result of exposure to chemotherapy. Radiation therapy will also change the bone quality. Irradiated bone tends to undergo changes in cancellous bone and results in replacement of the cancellous

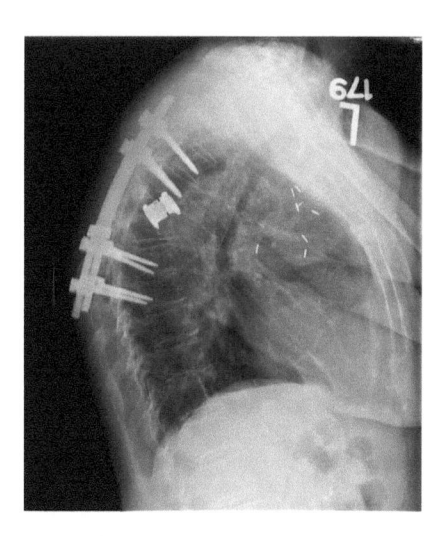

Fig. 49-2 Lateral radiograph of the thoracic spine after vertebrectomy for breast cancer metastasis and reconstruction with pedicle screws, rods, and distractible vertebral cage. Significant subsidence of the cage into the osteoporotic bone has occurred.

architecture with fatty marrow. Certain tumors also tend to result in worsening bone quality. Patients with multiple myeloma are considered high risk for surgery, because their bone quality is usually quite poor, and instrumentation tends to easily fail. Strategies have been devised to try to navigate these hazards in bone quality. One option is to increase the anchor points of the instrumentation, which often results in instrumentation of more spine segments. Another strategy is to incorporate laminar hooks and pedicle hooks at the ends of the construct to supply additional anchor points at the stronger cortical bone to resist screw pullout. In addition, augmenting the holes made in the bone with polymethylmethacrylate (PMMA) cement can increase the pullout strength of pedicle screws in weakened bone.[15]

Arthrodesis in the face of tumor resection can be difficult to achieve and is unpredictable. The life expectancy of the patient plays a role in determining whether there will be suitable time to achieve a bony fusion. The extent of bony resection can also hinder the ability to achieve a bony fusion; in addition, large gaps in the spine will need to grow bone in order to achieve an arthrodesis. This is particularly difficult after an en bloc resection. In such cases vascularized structural autografts have been used, and some investigators have suggested that they increase the chance of arthrodesis.[16] Furthermore, there are specific areas in which arthrodesis may be difficult, regardless of the presence of a spine tumor, including the craniocervical junction and the lumbopelvic junction. In such biomechanically high-stress environments, extra care should be taken to provide as much stability to the construct as possible, to avoid catastrophic instrumentation failures. Such strategies will increase the complexity of the operation, increase operative site exposure, and may increase the overall risk of an operation; however, such maneuvers may still be more beneficial to the patient in the long term.

CONCLUSION

Complications occur with all types of spine surgery, but spine tumor surgery places patients at increased risk. First, because of the tumor burden, these patients are at higher risk for wound complications, blood loss, and bone healing before any surgery. Intraoperatively the tumor anatomy may place local structures (neural and vascular) at greater risk. In addition, soft tissues may be more severely damaged in an attempt to isolate and remove the lesion. Finally, instrumentation can be challenging, given the altered bony anatomy from tumor growth or removal, and bone purchase may be weakened by osteoporosis, cachexia, and/or radiation. For these reasons, extra care should be taken when approaching any patient with a suspected spine tumor.

References (With Key References in Boldface)

1. Demura S, Kawahara N, Murakami H, et al. Surgical site infection in spinal metastasis: risk factors and countermeasures. Spine (Phila Pa 1976) 34:635-639, 2009.
2. Pull ter Gunne AF, Cohen DB. Incidence, prevalence, and analysis of risk factors for surgical site infection following adult spinal surgery. Spine (Phila Pa 1976) 34:1422-1428, 2009.
3. Sciubba DM, Nelson C, Gok B, et al. Evaluation of factors associated with postoperative infection following sacral tumor resection. J Neurosurg Spine 9:593-599, 2008.
4. **Olsen MA, Nepple JJ, Riew KD, et al. Risk factors for surgical site infection following orthopaedic spinal operations. J Bone Joint Surg Am 90:62-69, 2008.**
5. **Gibbs IC, Patil C, Gerszten PC, et al. Delayed radiation-induced myelopathy after spinal radiosurgery. Neurosurgery 64(2 Suppl):A67-A72, 2009.**
6. Gerszten PC, Burton SA, Ozhasoglu C. CyberKnife radiosurgery for spinal neoplasms. Prog Neurol Surg 20:340-358, 2007.
7. Hentschel SJ, Rhines LD, Wong FC, et al. Subarachnoid-pleural fistula after resection of thoracic tumors. J Neurosurg 100(4 Suppl Spine):332-336, 2004.
8. Fourney DR, Rhines LD, Hentschel SJ, et al. En bloc resection of primary sacral tumors: classification of surgical approaches and outcome. J Neurosurg Spine 3:111-122, 2005.
9. **Tomita K, Kawahara N, Murakami H, et al. Total en bloc spondylectomy for spinal tumors: improvement of the technique and its associated basic background. J Orthop Sci 11:3-12, 2006.**
10. Sciubba DM, Kretzer RM, Wang PP. Acute intracranial subdural hematoma following a lumbar CSF leak caused by spine surgery. Spine 30:E730-E732, 2005.
11. Yoshor D, Gentry JB, Lemaire SA, et al. Subarachnoid-pleural fistula treated with noninvasive positive-pressure ventilation. Case report. J Neurosurg 94(2 Suppl):319-322, 2001.
12. **Kato S, Kawahara N, Tomita K, et al. Effects on spinal cord blood flow and neurologic function secondary to interruption of bilateral segmental arteries which supply the artery of Adamkiewicz: an experimental study using a dog model. Spine 33:1533-1541, 2008.**
13. Kawahara N, Tomita K, Murakami H, et al. Total en bloc spondylectomy for spinal tumors: surgical techniques and related basic background. Orthop Clin North Am 40:47-63, 2009, vi.
14. Matsumoto T, Yamagami T, Kato T, et al. The effectiveness of lymphangiography as a treatment method for various chyle leakages. Br J Radiol 82:286-290, 2009.
15. Chang MC, Liu CL, Chen TH. Polymethacrylate augmentation of pedicle screw for osteoporotic spinal surgery: a novel technique. Spine 33:E317-E324, 2008.
16. Wright NM, Kaufman BA, Haughey BH, et al. Complex cervical spine neoplastic disease: reconstruction after surgery by using a vascularized fibular strut graft. Case report. J Neurosurg 90(1 Suppl):133-137, 1999.

Chapter 50

Outcomes Reporting in Tumor Surgery

John Street, Charles G. Fisher

Patients with tumors of the spine, whether primary or metastatic, are burdened by their disease in a manner that is distinct from patients with disorders of the spine that are degenerative, developmental, or traumatic. Similarly, these patients will experience significant impairment in quality-of-life domains distinct from those with malignant disease elsewhere. Patients with tumors of the spine often present with progressive neural compromise, functional limitations, pain, deformity, and important considerations regarding mental health and social function. Without exception, established outcome instruments for oncology and for spinal disorders are not designed for patients with tumors of the spine and may be less sensitive and specific to changes in health status that result from nonoperative and operative care.

According to the American Cancer Society, approximately 2500 new cases of primary bone cancer and 10,500 cases of soft tissue sarcomas are diagnosed in the United States each year. Of these, approximately 5% to 7% involve the spine. The incidence of primary spinal neoplasms has been estimated to be 2.5 to 8.5 per 100,000 per year. The most common primary lesions include osteosarcoma (35%), chondrosarcoma (25%), Ewing's sarcoma (15%), chordoma (10%), and malignant fibrous histiocytoma including fibrosarcoma (5%). According to the National Cancer Data Base of the American College of Surgeons, for cases with a minimum 5-year follow-up from 1985 to 1998, the relative 5-year survival rate was 54% for osteosarcoma, 75% for chondrosarcoma, and 50% for Ewing's sarcoma.[1,2]

The spinal column is the most frequent site of bone metastasis, and between 30% and 70% of patients with cancer will have evidence of spine metastasis at autopsy. It is estimated that there are approximately 25,000 cases of spinal cord compression resulting from metastases annually in the United States, most of which are the result of prostate, breast, and lung cancer.[3] The morbidity associated with spinal metastases includes not only pain, fractures, spinal instability, cord compression, and immobility, but also the specific symptoms associated with the primary tumor and the myriad physical and psychosocial aspects of metastatic disease. This is particularly important because the presence of bony metastases in the spine often signals an incurable disease.

Nevertheless, patients with spinal metastases are living significantly longer with their disease. With the recent trend of improved survival and advances in medical treatment (e.g., bisphosphonates and antiangiogenic tumor modulation), in stereotactic radiotherapy, and in surgical technique, there has been an interest in reviewing and refining the contribution of Health-Related Quality of Life (HRQOL) outcome measures of treatment in metastatic disease of the spine.[4-8]

In recent times there have also been dramatic changes in the management of primary tumors of the spine. Advances in staging, radiology, and surgical technique and adjuvant therapies have all brought promise, but despite these advances, treatment of spine tumors is still largely not standardized. Most clinical studies remain retrospective reviews of heterogeneous tumor types and varied treatment modalities spanning many years. A critical component of this shortcoming is the lack of uniform outcome measurements in this unique patient group.

Tumors of the spine have a distinct, important, and measurable impact on HRQOL. Patients with malignant disease of the spine have significant impairment of physical function, neural function, pain, mental health, and social roles. The literature on this complex group of patients is generally of poor quality. The use of standardized clinical outcomes is limited and characterized by outcome measures that are process variables, including survival, local recurrence, complications, and gross measures of function (ambulatory status, Frankel score), with more limited use of direct patient self-assessments of their health status. The reporting of these process variables does not reflect patients' overall experience with their health care and the impact of their care on changing the quality of their lives. The use of patient self-assessment instruments would permit a direct measure of the value of care as perceived by the recipient. Any disease-specific self-assessment instrument is intended to maximize the specificity of the instrument for a disorder and the sensitivity of the instrument to detect change in the condition. Although there are distinct differences between primary and metastatic tumors of the spine, with respect to their presentations, treatment options, and prognoses, probably just one outcome tool would likely suffice for both disease processes. The relative rarity of primary tumors of the spine may make a unique outcome tool impractical; however, distinct outcomes related to primary disease, such as "disease-free survival," must be considered when choosing domains for an outcome tool.[9]

This chapter is designed to examine the concepts of outcome, particularly quality-of-life outcome assessment, in spine tumor surgery. We will review the currently available literature for both primary and metastatic disease, explore some of the conceptual and methodologic issues in HRQOL assessment in this specific patient population, and finally review some recent efforts to establish and validate an outcomes tool that is specific to malignant disease of the spine.

GENERAL CONCEPTS OF OUTCOMES REPORTING IN TUMOR SURGERY

Measuring and understanding the outcome of treatment from the patient's perspective captures the essence of patient-centered care, and incorporating this information into clinical decision-making is essential. To date, much of our reporting on either primary or metastatic diseases of the spine has focused on process variables and complications of our surgical interventions. This is a direct consequence of the low prevalence of primary spine tumors and the inherent heterogeneity of metastatic disease.

Quality of life is a concept that is easy to grasp intuitively but difficult to define. In medicine and surgery what we wish to measure is "health-related" quality of life—that is, the extent of the impact of the disease process and/or our treatment on physical, psychological, and social aspects of a person's life and feeling of well-being. These different aspects of quality of life are called *domains*. Quality-of-life "instruments" or "tools" can measure different domains. Depending on their purpose, domains can be measured in two "dimensions": (1) objective assessment of functioning or health status (e.g., process variables) and (2) subjective assessment by the patient of his or her own perceived health. Objective measures or process variables are attractive to clinicians and researchers because they are more easily quantifiable and reproducible. However, it is the change in the patient's perception of his or her own health and function that is the truest measure of the appropriateness of our intervention. This has been highlighted in a number of previous publications related specifically to the care of patients with a wide variety of spinal pathologies.

In oncology, in general, patient-based outcomes include survival time, disease-free survival time, and outcomes reported by the patients themselves, such as HRQOL and satisfaction with care. Clearly, survival as an endpoint of care is appropriate for primary tumors of the spine and, in general, the morbidity of the surgery and its complications and, in particular, of planned neurologic, visceral, or vascular sacrifices, is considered in the light of a potential for cure, or at least a lengthy disease-free survival. In the context of primary tumors of the spine, secondary outcomes including HRQOL, while they are also critically important, are potentially of secondary importance. It is interesting, of itself, that we must assume the relative importance of these primary (disease-free survival) and secondary (HRQOL) outcomes because of the lack of appropriate literature.

In the palliative surgical setting of metastatic disease of the spine, however, disease-free survival time is not a consideration, and survival time, invariably, is more a function of the primary disease and total body metastatic burden. In this setting, unique HRQOL domains are more relevant and so would be more appropriate as the main treatment endpoints. Thus incorporating HRQOL into outcomes reporting in spine tumor surgery is complex and requires additional methodologic design to ensure that outcomes are sufficiently robust to inform clinical practice and that the unique differences between primary and metastatic disease are considered.

There is a wide range of critical elements that have an impact on patients with metastatic disease, as well as on their caregivers. Preventing and treating pain and other symptoms related to either primary or metastatic lesions, supporting families and caregivers, ensuring the continuity of care, ensuring respect for persons and informed decision-making, attending to well-being, including existential and spiritual concerns, and supporting function and survival duration are general issues that are common to most patients with metastatic disease. Studies, not specifically of metastatic disease of the spine, have shown that among the factors that improve utilization outcomes and patient-centered outcomes are multidisciplinary teams involving nurses and social services, continuity of care and service coordination, and facilitated communication.

The low prevalence of primary spine tumors and the inherent heterogeneity of metastatic disease of the spine oblige us to rely on the lower end of the evidence-based pyramid (e.g., small case series) in interpreting outcomes and determining optimal care for these complex and challenging patients. The solution to this problem is found, undoubtedly, in merging data from different centers, so that sample size becomes significant enough to produce meaningful analyses. The prerequisite for such multicenter pooling of information is the standardization of terminology and treatment algorithms, and the universal adoption of standardized outcome tools, to create a universal language shared by all practitioners in the field.

Over the past three decades, there has been an explosion of quality-of-life (QOL) studies in the medical literature. A Medline search using *quality of life* as a key word reveals a significant increase in the number of articles related to the topic over a period of 30 years, from 32 in 1973 to 5444 in 2004. In a systematic review of the quality of QOL publications in the spine literature,[10] we reported that the total number of articles published increased by 36%, whereas the number of QOL articles increased by 102% over the study period from 2000 to 2004. In 2000, 18% of the articles published dealt with QOL issues, whereas this figure rose to 30% for 2004. In 2004, when a QOL instrument was used, it was more often disease specific, validated, and appropriate to the stated hypothesis of the paper than in 2000. Our analysis confirmed that the overall "quality" of the published QOL articles had improved, at least as assessed by the lesser criteria set down by Velanovich.[11] No such "quality" improvement, however, was observed for the more demanding criteria of Gill and Feinstein.[12] These 10 criteria involve much more complex methodologic challenges than the criteria of Velanovich.[11] These criteria will be enumerated and discussed in greater detail later in this chapter.

HRQOL measures in cancer may be classified as either generic, general cancer, or primary or secondary site specific or cancer problem/symptom specific. A generic HRQOL measure can be applied to a range of diseases and conditions that may be, but need not be, cancer related. Examples include the Medical Outcomes Study Short

Form (SF-36) and a number of other psychometrically based measures, as well as the Sickness Impact Profile (SIP), Nottingham Health Profile (NHP), EuroQol Group (EQ-5D), Health Utility Index (HUI), and indeed, most preference-based measures. A general cancer measure is intended for application across the full range of cancer-related events, regardless of the patient's tumor type. Among the many examples are the following:

- European Organization for Research and Treatment of Cancer QLQ-C30 (EORTC)
- Eastern Cooperative Oncology Group Performance Status (ECOG-PS), Health Utility Index (HUI)
- Functional Assessment of Cancer Therapy Scale (FACT-G)
- Functional Living Index Cancer questionnaire (FLIC)
- Karnofsky Index of Quality of Life

A cancer site–specific or cancer problem–specific HRQOL measure is tailored, respectively, to a particular type of primary tumor (EORTC-QLQ-BR2331 for breast cancer or the Musculoskeletal Tumor Society score), problem area (FACT N32 for febrile neutropenia associated with adjuvant chemotherapy), or treatment modality (FACT BRM33 for treatment with biological response modifiers, such as interferon). No such site-specific or disease-specific HRQOL instrument exists for either primary or metastatic tumors affecting the spine.

The validity of measures of HRQOL can be established by use of the International Classification of Functioning, Disability and Health (ICF). The ICF consists of two major parts, each containing two separate components. Part 1 covers functioning and disability and includes the components *body functions (b), structure (s),* and *activities and participation (d)*. Part 2 covers contextual factors and includes the components *environmental factors (e)* and *personal factors (pf)*. The conceptual connection between HRQOL and the ICF has been previously studied for many primary cancers, and the ICF has been validated as a benchmark tool for the comparison of different HRQOL instruments. The correlation of established HRQOL measures and ICF is measured to validate existing outcomes instruments. This tool does not consider etiology of illness and thus has the capacity to include all aspects of disease burden, as experienced by a patient with a tumor affecting the spine.[13-19]

SPECIFIC CONSIDERATIONS IN REPORTING SURGICAL OUTCOMES

Deciding on a suitable outcome tool to study HRQOL in patients with malignant disease of the spine involves the consideration of a number of important factors related to the context and aims of the study itself. In this way the specific domains within the questionnaire would be matched to the objectives of the study. The particular HRQOL domains relevant to a given study will be unique to the study objectives (long-term disease-free survival or immediate perioperative morbidity), the type and goals of the interventions being studied (en bloc resection or intralesional surgery), the disease type (primary or metastatic tumor), and the patient group. A thorough understanding of the natural history of the disease, the anticipated progression without treatment, and the expected effects of the intervention are required to ensure that the most appropriate outcome tool is selected.

With regard to surgical intervention for malignant disease of the spine, the specific nature of the anticipated effects of intervention and the expected timeline for them to be exerted will influence the type of HRQOL measure selected and the timing and frequency of its administration. A measure should be selected that is sensitive to capture both the positive and negative effects of the intervention, because the side effects of treatments (combined anterior and posterior approaches for metastatic disease) may outweigh the potential benefits to HRQOL (such as symptom alleviation) perceived by patients. An understanding of whether these effects are transient or long lasting will further influence the timing of the HRQL assessments and how assessments from different time points should be interpreted. These distinctions are particularly relevant when one considers the inherent differences between primary and metastatic tumors of the spine. With primary tumors of the spine, the potential for cure or for significant disease-free survival allows consideration of significant morbidity that would not be contemplated in the palliative setting of diffuse metastatic disease. These differences must be incorporated into any outcome tool for malignant disease of the spine and, ultimately, may mandate the use of different outcome tools for both primary and metastatic disease. That said, at this time, with the relatively poor quality of literature that is available and the rarity of primary tumors, it is probably more important that we establish one outcome tool (however limited) that would be used in all centers. Further refining of the tools and incorporation of other domains of HRQOL can be performed subsequently.

Generic cancer HRQOL measures are designed to assess multiple general HRQOL issues. They assess physical, social, and emotional function, as well as common symptoms that occur, such as fatigue, pain, and nausea and vomiting. However, their generic nature means that they are often rather lengthy and may be less sensitive to changes in the condition-specific symptoms and aspects of HRQOL relevant to a given disease. In contrast, condition-specific HRQOL instruments address the complex and unique areas of function known to be impaired in specific cancers. They are typically more sensitive to changes in clinical status but at the expense of being less useful in comparing different populations and patient groups.

As we outlined earlier, patients with tumors of the spine often present with progressive neural compromise, functional limitations, pain, deformity, and important considerations regarding mental health and social function. It is, therefore, essential to pick or design a condition-specific questionnaire that adequately covers these domains. There are many disease-specific questionnaire modules published by the EORTC Quality of Life and the FACT groups that contain scales and single items covering a whole range of symptoms and functional issues associated with different types and treatments of cancer. However, none are specific to the progressive neural compromise, functional limitations, pain, and deformity that are commonplace with tumors of the spine. Although it is uncommon to assess a single domain of HRQOL in a clinical trial, dimension-specific measures may be used in conjunction with other generic measures, if further detailed analysis of a specific issue is required. Generic aspects of HRQOL may also be secondary endpoints, and they will provide information that can be used to understand whether relief of symptoms also leads to improvement in other aspects of HRQOL. For the study of primary and metastatic disease of the spine, therefore, we would recommend that both a generic and a disease-specific measure be used.

Respondent item burden is an important consideration in selecting an instrument or combining instruments or tools, especially when studying patients who must contend with complex treatment regimens, progressive disease, and, as is the case with metastatic disease of the spine, the end of life. Little research has been done to address item burden, but some factors that contribute are relevance of measurement domains and items to respondents, length of a questionnaire and time for completion, sequence and timing of administration, and overall impact on the respondent, such as time commitment, physical exhaustion, and emotional distress from answering questions that may be upsetting. It is equally important to determine the optimal point during the course of the disease trajectory, the individual readiness of patients, and their cognitive capacity for completing questionnaires.[20,21]

Consideration of the complexity and nature of a questionnaire's scoring system is also critical. Overall summary scores may be obtained with some HRQOL instruments, particularly the generic ones, and they have the attraction of producing a single score that can be used to compare different populations and patient groups. For instance, patients with primary tumors of the spine could be compared with those who have primary tumors of the extremities. Overall scores, however, may fail to identify where interventions lead to improvement in one aspect of HRQOL but deterioration in another. Surgery for patients with primary tumors of the spine, for instance, may result in significant disease-free survival but at the cost of loss of neurologic function. It is, therefore, recommended that multidimensional questionnaires with relevant symptoms and functional scales be used to provide HRQOL data to inform treatment decisions.

Obviously, interpretation of results from quality-of-life studies becomes complicated when investigators do not use a consistent conceptual basis to define quality of life or if they fail to even define quality of life. This uneven, inappropriate usage, for instance, sometimes leads researchers to conclude that patients have a good quality of life just because they are employed, do not report symptoms or require medication, or are not in need of reoperation. To address some of these difficulties, both Velanovich[11] and Gill and Feinstein,[12] in different publications, proposed criteria to determine the conceptual and methodologic rigors of the methods used in studies purporting to measure HRQOL. We would propose that criteria such as these would be used when considering the development of an outcomes tool specific to malignant disease of the spine (Boxes 50-1 and 50-2).

> **Box 50-1** Velanovich Criteria for Assessment of a "Quality-of-Life" Publication*
>
> 1. Was a Quality-of-Life instrument used?
> 2. What was the type of instrument (generic, disease specific, or ad hoc)?
> 3. Was the instrument validated and reliable?
> 4. Was it appropriate for the stated study hypothesis?
> 5. Was statistical analysis performed appropriately?
>
> *According to the publication by Velanovich.[11] From Street J, Lenehan B, Fisher C. The quality of quality of life publications in the spinal literature: are we getting any better? J Neurosurg Spine 11:512-517, 2009.

> **Box 50-2** Gill and Feinstein Criteria for Assessment of a "Quality-of-Life" Publication*
>
> **Investigator Specific Criteria**
>
> 1. Did the investigators conceptually identify what they meant by Quality of Life?
> 2. Did they state the domains they wanted to measure as components of Quality of Life?
> 3. Did investigators give reasons for choosing the instruments used?
> 4. Did investigators aggregate the results from multiple items, domains, or instruments into a single Composite Score for Quality of Life?
>
> **Instrument Specific Criteria**
>
> 5. Were patients asked to give their own Global Rating for Quality of Life?
> 6. Was overall quality of life distinguished from Health-Related Quality of Life?
> 7. Were patients invited to supplement the items listed in the instruments offered by investigators?
> 8. If so, were these supplemental items incorporated into the final rating?
> 9. Were patients asked to indicate which items (either specified by the investigator or added by the patients) were personally important to them?
> 10. If so, were these importance ratings incorporated into the final rating?
>
> $$\text{Summary score} = \frac{\text{Sum of No. of criteria fulfilled} \times 100}{\text{No. of criteria by which an article is eligible to be judged*}}$$
>
> *Criteria according to Gill and Feinstein.[12] From Street J, Lenehan B, Fisher C. The quality of quality of life publications in the spinal literature: are we getting any better? J Neurosurg Spine 11:512-517, 2009.

It is clear that the selection of appropriate domains within a questionnaire for a particular objective is essential in planning any data collection. A thorough examination and evaluation of the most appropriate domains along various criteria is necessary. Psychometric properties (e.g., reliability, validity, and sensitivity) and application-related features (e.g., administration mode, scales used, time needed for completion, and so forth), as well as translation into relevant languages, need to be accounted for. Thus it is of particular interest to examine the content covered by any newly proposed questionnaire. A content comparison based on a universally accepted, well-defined, and standardized reference system that allows for a detailed exploration and comparison of all contents of the questionnaire would, therefore, be valuable. The newly available International Classification of Functioning, Disability and Health (ICF) serves as such a universal framework. The ICF belongs to the World Health Organization family of international health classifications. Although the well-known International Classification of Diseases (ICD) classifies diagnoses, the ICF classifies functioning. The ICF is based on the biopsychosocial model of functioning, disability, and health and offers a detailed and etiologically neutral classification. Several investigators have dealt with the conceptual connections between the HRQOL and the ICF. The ICF is a useful tool to encourage multicenter-multinational assessment of functioning. It is crucial to understand that the ICF is a reference to facilitate measurement of functioning, but it is not a QOL instrument itself.[13-19,22-24]

REVIEW OF THE CURRENT LITERATURE

To explore the current literature, we have considered the following two primary questions:
1. What currently available generic and cancer-specific outcome tools should be used to develop domains in a disease-specific instrument for tumors of the spine?
2. What outcome instruments have been used in the published literature to measure HRQOL in patients with cancer and, more specifically, tumors of the spine?

We reported a systematic review of the HRQOL outcome measures used in the published literature on metastatic disease of the spine. We reviewed English-language biomedical journals from 1966 to December 2008.[3] Two separate literature searches were carried out, as outlined in the preceding primary questions. Only those original studies analyzing the outcomes or results of surgical management of metastatic disease of the spine were retained. The outcome tools used were enumerated, and the individual studies were graded by means of the classification of evidence, according to the criteria described by Guyatt. The content validity of the six most frequently used measures of cancer-related HRQOL was then established using the International Classification of Functioning, Disability and Health.[25] In the review of the cancer literature, in general, the most commonly used cancer-specific tools were the ECOG, EORTC QLQ-C30, and EuroQol-5D. The most commonly used generic tools were the SF-36, SIP-5, and activities of daily living. These cancer-specific HRQOL tools had excellent content validity when directly compared with the universal World Health Organization ICF tool. Thus it would be appropriate to include domains from any of these outcome tools in the non–disease-specific component of the assessment of HRQOL as it relates to patients with metastatic disease of the spine. Based on frequency of citation and on correlation with ICF, both ECOG as a cancer-specific tool and SF-36 as a generic HRQOL outcome tool could be used while a disease-specific tool for metastatic disease of the spine is being developed.

The value of disease-specific measures in disorders of the spine is that the instrument may be more specific to impairment caused by the condition and may be more sensitive to change. None of these instruments, however, specifically address the concerns and impairments of patients with tumors affecting the spine, and we understand that the choice of an appropriate instrument for the population studied has a significant effect on patient responsiveness and instrument performance. On review of the literature on spinal metastases, in particular, only 34 of 141 studies used a patient self-assessment instrument to assess health status. These included ECOG, Oswestry Disability Index (ODI), SF-36, and Functional Independence Measure (FIM). None of these instruments have been validated for patients with tumors affecting the spine. None of the 141 studies selected for review provided a definition for HRQOL, and none attempted to justify the use of their chosen instrument. No study presented a case for choice based on the specific needs and concerns of persons with metastatic disease of the spine. Analysis of the results depicted also reflects the importance of pain and neurologic function in patients with metastatic disease of the spine. We found that among 141 studies, 73 measured pain by means of a visual analog scale, 53 assessed ambulatory status, and 36 used the Frankel grading system for neurologic deficits, followed by the more recently developed and more comprehensive American Spinal Injury Association (ASIA) score in 11. There was no consensus on the use of a uniform HRQOL instrument in the literature and significant disparity in the choice of instruments.

In their review of the morbidity of en bloc resections, Boriani et al[26] discuss death, recurrence, surgical complications, and event-free survival as outcome variables. Although this study clearly puts the feasibility and burden of this treatment into perspective, it does not offer a validated HRQOL outcome measure. The only validated HRQOL outcome used in reports of primary tumors of the spine has been the SF-36. Liljenqvist et al[27] concluded that HRQOL analysis (SF-36) revealed only slightly decreased physical component and normal mental component scores compared with normal scores in those patients with no evidence of residual or recurrent disease. These investigators proposed that en bloc spondylectomy enables wide or marginal resection of malignant lesions of the spine, in most cases, with acceptable morbidity. They concluded that intralesional resection, poor histologic response, and solitary spinal metastases of Ewing's sarcoma and osteosarcoma are associated with a poor prognosis. Fisher et al[28] reported that the HRQOL, using the SF-36, shows acceptable morbidity with these procedures (physical component summary = 37.73 ± 11.52, mental health component summary = 51.69 ± 9.54). They concluded that the principles of wide surgical resection, commonly applied in appendicular oncology, can and should be used for the treatment of primary bone tumors of the spine, with anticipated acceptable morbidity and satisfactory survival.

The remainder of the literature on primary tumors has reported on process variables, such as recurrence, event-free survival, neurologic status, and surgical and postoperative complications. The complications enumerated have included hardware failures, wound infection and dehiscence, and residual neurologic deficits (e.g., bowel and bladder dysfunction). Although the reporting of these process variables is an essential component of gathering and assimilating data from multiple centers, it does not provide a tangible measure of patient perspective on "outcome" from treatment.[26-38]

This synthesis of the literature on outcomes in patients with tumors affecting the spine demonstrates that there is no disease-specific questionnaire that is widely accepted and used to measure HRQOL. The most commonly used measures were process variables rather than measures of HRQOL. Survival, pain, ambulation, neurologic deficit, and sphincter control are each indirect measures of health status and utility, and they are often misleading measures of "quality of life." The studies that included patient self-assessment instruments did not justify their use of the chosen instrument, and none of the instruments chosen were validated for patients with either primary or metastatic tumors affecting the spine. Although no consistency could be found in the studies, the variability and disparity of these data indicate the need for disease-specific domains in a future outcome tool for use in patients with tumors affecting the spine.

A SPECIFIC TOOL FOR OUTCOMES REPORTING IN TUMOR SURGERY

The Spine Oncology Study Group has developed an Outcome Questionnaire (SOSGOQ) specific for patients with malignant disease of the spine (see Boxes 50-1 and 50-2). It was developed by a consensus of an international expert working group after direct consultation with patients and patient advocacy groups, in order to determine the most appropriate domains to be included. When developing a new outcomes tool, investigators are often faced with a wide, sometimes confusing, array of options in terms of domains to be included. Also, metastatic disease of the spine summarizes a selection of different primary cancer sites, tumor stages, and treatment modalities.

When we examined the content of the Spine Oncology Outcomes Questionnaire, based on the ICF as the frame of reference, we identified the HRQOL questionnaires routinely used in studies of spinal malignancy.[39] These were the *Edmonton Symptom Assessment System* (ESAS), Karnofsky Performance Scale, and ODI. We then examined the contents of these questionnaires based on their translation ("linkage") to the ICF, and finally we compared the contents of the SOSG Outcomes Questionnaire with these other tools, based on the ICF as a reference. We found that the SOSGOQ includes all of the domains considered relevant for the measurement of function and disability (body structures-*s*, body functions-*b*, activity and participation-*d,* and environmental factors-*e*), and that the SOSGOQ has far superior content capacity to measure the disease burden, as experienced by a patient with malignant disease of the spine, than do any of the patient self-assessment instruments previously identified from a systematic review of the literature.

The conceptual connection between HRQOL and the ICF has been previously studied for many primary cancers, and the ICF has been validated as a benchmark tool for the comparison of different HRQOL instruments. The correlation of established HRQOL outcome tools and ICF is a measure of content validity. The content validity of a number of cancer-specific outcome tools of HRQOL has been established using the International Classification of Functioning, Disability and Health (ICF). This validation has been performed for outcome tools such as the European Organization for Research and Treatment of Cancer (EORTC) Quality of Life Questionnaire, Functional Assessment of Cancer Therapy quality-of-life instrument (FACT), Breast Cancer Chemotherapy Questionnaire (BCQ), Cancer Rehabilitation Evaluation System-Short Form (CARES-SF), and the Functional Living Index-Cancer (FLIC).

These tools have all been found to have good-to-excellent ICF linkage reliability. In comparison, the SOSGOQ has superior content validity, more comprehensive concept inclusion, and more specific ICF linkage than any patient self-assessment instrument previously identified in the literature on primary or metastatic disease of the spine. The SOSGOQ also compares very favorably with the ICF linkage reliability reported for the cancer-specific outcome tools EORTC, FACT, BCQ, CARES-SF, and FLIC.

CONCLUSION

In this chapter we examined the concepts of outcome assessment in spine tumor surgery. We reviewed the current available literature for both primary and metastatic disease and explored some of the conceptual and methodologic issues in HRQOL assessment in this specific patient population.

Tumors of the spine have distinct, important, and measurable impacts on HRQOL. Patients with malignant disease of the spine have significant impairment of physical function, neural function, pain, mental health, and social roles. The literature on this complex patient group is generally of poor quality. The use of standardized clinical outcomes is limited and characterized by outcome measures that are process variables. The use of patient self-assessment instruments would permit a direct measure of the value of care, as perceived by the recipient. Given the distinct differences between primary and metastatic tumors of the spine, their presentations, and treatment options and prognoses, individual outcome tools would be ideal for both disease processes but are probably not practical at the present time.

An appropriate outcome tool for malignant disease of the spine would have to provide a coherent conceptual framework of interrelated quality-of-life concepts that will allow us to better understand health and well-being as experienced by patients with tumors of the spine.

Thus we conclude that there is little consensus or uniformity in the choice of outcome measures for patients with tumors affecting the spine. The lack of uniformity in outcome measures prevents effective combination of studies in meta-analysis and limits the value of published literature in demonstrating the impact of operative and nonoperative management in the treatment of spinal metastasis. The creation of a single valid and reliable spinal oncology–specific outcome measure for use in future studies would allow greater applicability and provide a more robust measure of HRQOL in this complex patient population. Until such time as this specific tool is available we recommend the use of ECOG and SF-36, perhaps in conjunction with the visual analog scale for pain, ambulatory status, and the Frankel grading system for all future studies. Recurrence, survival, and event-free and disease-free survival should specifically be reported for primary tumors.

References (With Key References in Boldface)

1. **Chi JH, Bydon A, Hsieh P, et al. Epidemiology and demographics for primary vertebral tumors. Neurosurg Clin N Am 19:1-4, 2008.**
2. Schellinger KA, Propp JM, Villano JL, et al. Descriptive epidemiology of primary spinal cord tumors. J Neurooncol 87:173-179, 2008.
3. **Street J, Berven S, Fisher C, et al. Health related quality of life assessment in metastatic disease of the spine: a systematic review spine. Spine (Phila Pa 1976) 34(22 Suppl):S128-S134, 2009.**
4. Berven S, Deviren V, Demir-Deviren S, et al. Studies in the modified Scoliosis Research Society Outcomes Instrument in adults: validation, reliability, and discriminatory capacity. Spine 28:2164-2169; discussion 2169, 2003.
5. Bombardier C. Outcome assessments in the evaluation of treatment of spinal disorders: summary and general recommendations. Spine 25:3100-3103, 2000.
6. Bridwell KH, Cats-Baril W, Harrast J, et al. The validity of the SRS-22 instrument in an adult spinal deformity population compared with the Oswestry and SF-12: a study of response distribution, concurrent validity, internal consistency, and reliability. Spine 30:455-461, 2005.
7. Skolasky RL, Riley LH III, Albert TJ. Psychometric properties of the Cervical Spine Outcomes Questionnaire and its relationship to standard assessment tools used in spine research. Spine J 7:174-179, 2007.
8. Stucki G, Liang MH, Fossel AH, et al. Relative responsiveness of condition-specific and generic health status measures in degenerative lumbar spinal stenosis. J Clin Epidemiol 48:1369-1378, 1995.
9. **Siddiqui F, Kachnic LA, Movsas B. Quality-of-life outcomes in oncology. Hematol Oncol Clin North Am 20:165-185, 2006.**
10. **Street J, Lenehan B, Fisher C. The quality of quality of life publications in the spinal literature: are we getting any better? J Neurosurg Spine 11:512-517, 2009.**
11. Velanovich V. Using quality-of-life measurements in clinical practice. Surgery 141:127-133, 2007.
12. Gill TM, Feinstein AR. A critical appraisal of the quality of quality-of-life measurements. JAMA 272:619-626, 1994.
13. Cieza A, Geyh S, Chatterjee S, et al. Identification of candidate categories of the International Classification of Functioning, Disability and Health (ICF) for a Pi-by-no ICF Core Set based on regression modelling. BMC Med Res Methodol 6:36, 2006.
14. Cieza A, Stucki G. Content comparison of health-related quality of life (HRQOL) instruments based on the International Classification of Functioning, Disability and Health (ICF). Qual Life Res 14:1225-1237, 2005.
15. Cieza A, Stucki G, Weigl M, et al. ICF core sets for low back pain. J Rehabil Med (44 Suppl):69-74, 2004.
16. Prodinger B, Cieza A, Williams DA, et al. Measuring health in patients with fibromyalgia: content comparison of questionnaires based on the International Classification of Functioning, Disability and Health. Arthritis Rheum 59:650-658, 2008.
17. Stucki G, Kostanjsek N, Ustun B, et al. ICF-based classification and measurement of functioning. Eur J Phys Rehabil Med 44:315-328, 2008.
18. Tschiesner U, Linseisen E, Baumann S, et al. Assessment of functioning in patients with head and neck cancer according to the International Classification of Functioning, Disability, and Health (ICF): a multicenter study. Laryngoscope 119:915-923, 2009.
19. Tschiesner U, Rogers SN, Harreus U, et al. Content comparison of quality of life questionnaires used in head and neck cancer based on the International Classification of Functioning, Disability and Health: a systematic review. Eur Arch Otorhinolaryngol 265:627-637, 2008.
20. Cella DF, Tulsky DS, Gray G, et al. The Functional Assessment of Cancer Therapy scale: development and validation of the general measure. J Clin Oncol 11:570-579, 1993.
21. Schipper H, Clinch J, McMurray A, et al. Measuring the quality of life of cancer patients: the Functional Living Index-Cancer: development and validation. J Clin Oncol 2:472-483, 1984.

22. Kuenstner S, Langelotz C, Budach V, et al. The comparability of quality of life scores. A multitrait multimethod analysis of the EORTC QLQ-C30, SF-36 and FLIC questionnaires. Eur J Cancer 38:339-348, 2002.
23. Grill E, Mansmann U, Cieza A, et al. Assessing observer agreement when describing and classifying functioning with the International Classification of Functioning, Disability and Health. J Rehabil Med 39:71-76, 2007.
24. Offenbächer M, Cieza A, Brockow T, et al. Are the contents of treatment outcomes in fibromyalgia trials represented in the International Classification of Functioning, Disability, and Health? Clin J Pain 23:691-701, 2007.
25. Guyatt G, Gutterman D, Baumann MH, et al. Grade strength of recommendations and quality of evidence in clinical guidelines: report from an american college of chest physicians task force. Chest 129:174-181, 2006.
26. Boriani S, Bandiera S, Donthineni R, et al. Morbidity of en bloc resections in the spine. Eur Spine J 19:231-241, 2010.
27. Liljenqvist U, Lerner T, Halm H, et al. En bloc spondylectomy in malignant tumors of the spine. Eur Spine J 17:600-609, 2008.
28. **Fisher CG, Keynan O, Boyd MC, et al. The surgical management of primary tumors of the spine: initial results of an ongoing prospective cohort study. Spine 30:1899-1908, 2005.**
29. Hsieh PC, Xu R, Sciubba DM, et al. Long-term clinical outcomes following en bloc resections for sacral chordomas and chondrosarcomas: a series of twenty consecutive patients. Spine 34:2233-2239, 2009.
30. Cloyd JM, Chou D, Deviren V, et al. En bloc resection of primary tumors of the cervical spine: report of two cases and systematic review of the literature. Spine J 9:928-935, 2009.
31. Bacci G, Boriani S, Balladelli A, et al. Treatment of nonmetastatic Ewing's sarcoma family tumors of the spine and sacrum: the experience from a single institution. Eur Spine J 18:1091-1095, 2009.
32. Henderson FC, McCool K, Seigle J, et al. Treatment of chordomas with CyberKnife: Georgetown University experience and treatment recommendations. Neurosurgery 64(2 Suppl):A44-A53, 2009.
33. Rao G, Suki D, Chakrabarti I, et al. Surgical management of primary and metastatic sarcoma of the mobile spine. Neurosurg Spine 9:120-128, 2008.
34. Bilsky MH, Gerszten P, Laufer I, et al. Radiation for primary spine tumors. Neurosurg Clin N Am 19:119-123, 2008.
35. Chi JH, Sciubba DM, Rhines LD, et al. Surgery for primary vertebral tumors: en bloc versus intralesional resection. Neurosurg Clin N Am 19:111-117, 2009.
36. Zileli M, Kilinçer C, Ersahin Y, et al. Primary tumors of the cervical spine: a retrospective review of 35 surgically managed cases. Spine J 7:165-173, 2007.
37. Melcher I, Disch AC, Khodadadyan-Klostermann C, et al. Primary malignant bone tumors and solitary metastases of the thoracolumbar spine: results by management with total en bloc spondylectomy. Eur Spine J 16:1193-1202, 2007.
38. Boriani S, Bandiera S, Biagini R, et al. Chordoma of the mobile spine: fifty years of experience. Spine 31:493-503, 2006.
39. **Street J, Lenehan B, Berven S, et al. Introducing a new health-related quality of life outcome tool for metastatic disease of the spine: content validation using the International Classification of Functioning, Disability, and Health; on behalf of the Spine Oncology Study Group. Spine (Phila Pa 1976) 35:1377-1386, 2010.**

Index

A

Abiraterone for prostate cancer
  after chemotherapy, 357-358
  before chemotherapy, 358-359
ABT-869 for advanced non–small cell lung cancer, 307
Acquired immune deficiency syndrome, 80
Activities of daily living, 131, 139-142; *see also* Occupational therapy
Activity demands, 142
Acute transverse myelopathy, 79
Adaptability in ambulation, 139
Adaptive performance skills, 142
ADLs, 131, 139-142; *see also* Occupational therapy
ADT
  preserving bone integrity with, 362-364
  for prostate cancer, 355-356
Advancement flap
  latissimus dorsi, 118, 119
  V-Y gluteal, 120, 121
AFO, 150, 151
AIDS, 80
Alar ligament, 6
Alar voids, 20
ALL, 6, 24
Ambulation, 138-139
American Joint Committee on Cancer (AJCC) staging system
  for breast cancer, 329, 330
  for Pancoast tumors, 566-568
  for renal cell carcinoma, 316-317
American Spinal Injury Association scale, 132, 133, 898
AMPS, 142
Amputation, hindquarter; *see* Hindquarter amputation
Anatomic localization of spine tumors, 36-37
Anatomic regions of back, 113, 114
Anatomy, 3-37
  cervical spine, 3-8
  intervertebral discs, 23-24
  lumbar spine, 14-18
  other critical structures, 33-35
  paraspinal muscles, 25-29
  sacrum, 19-22
  spine ligaments, 24-25
  thoracic spine, 9-14
  transitional vertebra, 22
  uncovertebral and facet joints, 22-23
  vascular supply
    of spinal cord, 31-33
    of vertebral column, 30-31
Androgen deprivation therapy
  preserving bone integrity with, 362-364
  for prostate cancer, 355-356
Aneurysmal bone cysts, 225-235
  bailout techniques and expert advice on, 233
  biopsy of, 226-227
  choice of treatment for, 228-229
  clinical features of, 225, 226
  diagnosis of, 225-226
  genetics of, 225
  histologic findings in, 225
  imaging of, 226
  outcomes for, 230
  pedicle screw fixation for, 867
  radiation therapy for, 227-228
  selective arterial embolization for
    choice of, 228-229
    outcomes for, 230
    signature cases on, 231-233
    technique for, 229
  staging of, 226
  surgical treatment of
    preoperative evaluation for, 226-227
    pros and cons of, 227
    technique for, 229-230
  tips from masters on, 233
  treatment options for, 227-228
  vertebra plana due to, 226
Angiogenesis in breast cancer, 343
Angiography, 37
  anesthesia and adjunctive measures for, 439
  bowel motion during, 439
  catheters for, 441-442
  equipment for, 438
  noninvasive imaging prior to, 437-438
  protocol for, 443-444
  provocative testing prior to, 439-441
Angiosarcoma, 282-283
  sagittal osteotomy for en bloc resection of, 640-641
Ankle-foot orthosis, 150, 151
Annulus fibrosus, 6, 24
Anterior arches of cervical vertebrae, 3
Anterior decompression and reconstruction, transpedicular approach for, 745-756
  bailout techniques on, 756
  clinical decision-making on, 748
  indications and contraindications for, 746-747
  outcomes of, 751-752
  preoperative evaluation for, 747
  signature cases on, 753-755
  technique for, 748-751
  tips from masters on, 756
Anterior longitudinal ligament, 6, 24
Anterior segmental medullary vein, 33
Anterior spinal artery, 31, 32
Anterior spinal vein, 32-33
Anterior sulcal vein, 32
Anterior transcervical approach for Pancoast tumor, 577
Anterior/lateral lesions, combined lateral/posterior approach for large, 647-675
  clinical decision-making on, 651-653
  hypervascular metastases with paraspinal extension as
    clinical decision-making on, 652
    signature case on, 670-671
    technique for, 658-661
  indications and contraindications for, 648-649
  outcomes for, 666-667
  Pancoast tumor with spinal involvement as
    clinical decision-making on, 651
    results of, 667

Anterior/lateral lesions, combined lateral/
  posterior approach for large—cont'd
 Pancoast tumor with spinal involvement
    as—cont'd
   signature case on, 668-669
   technique for, 654-658
  preoperative evaluation for, 649-651
  primary spinal tumor involving chest wall as
   clinical decision-making on, 652-653
   signature case on, 672-674
   technique for, 661-666
  signature cases on, 668-674
  technique for, 653-666
  tips from masters on, 675
Anterolateral thoracotomy with median
  sternotomy-trapdoor incision,
  598-599
Antiandrogens for prostate cancer, 355
Antoni A areas in schwannomas, 380, 381
Antoni B areas in schwannomas, 380, 381
Apoptosis, 87
Arachnoid, 7
Aromatase inhibitors for breast cancer, 339
Arterial embolization; see Embolization
Arterial supply
 of spinal cord, 32
 of vertebral column, 30
Arteriovenous fistula and subacute necrotiz-
  ing myelopathy, 80, 81
Artery of Adamkiewicz, 31, 32
Artery of cervical enlargement, 445
Artery of lumbar enlargement, 31, 32
Arthrodesis, 887
Articular facets, 23
Articular processes, 23
ASA, 31, 32
Ashworth Scale, Modified, 134
ASIA scale, 132, 133, 898
Aspen cervical collar, 144
Aspiration
 defined, 169
 silent, 164, 169
Assessment of Motor and Process Skills, 142
Assistive devices in physical therapy evaluation, 130-131
Astrocytomas, 68-72, 460
 anaplastic, 68
 diffuse, 68, 69
 vs. ependymomas, 70
 fibrillary, 68, 70
 gangliogliomas as, 71-72
 glioblastoma multiforme as, 68, 70
 grading of, 460
 imaging of, 69-70, 460
 pathology of, 68, 460
 pilocytic, 68, 69
 prevalence of, 68, 460
 treatment of, 460
Atlantoaxial joint, 3

Atlantooccipital joint, 3
Atlantooccipital membranes, 6
Atlas, 3
Avastin (bevacizumab)
 for advanced non–small cell lung cancer,
   306-307
 for breast cancer, 343
 for renal cell carcinoma, 318
AVF and subacute necrotizing myelopathy,
  80, 81
Axillary node staging, 336
Axillary thoracotomy, 600-601
Axis, 3
Axitinib for advanced non–small cell lung
  cancer, 307

B

Babinski test, 134
Balance in ambulation, 138-139
Balloon test occlusion, 447-449, 552, 556-557
Basiocciput, 6
Bathing
 lower body, 142
 upper body, 141
Bathroom, environmental modification of,
  143-144
BCQ, 899-900
Beam delivery for stereotactic radiosurgery,
  101-102
Beam-hardening artifact, 36
Bed mobility, 135, 137
Benadryl (diphenhydramine) for iodine con-
  trast allergy, 435, 436
Benign bone tumors, Enneking surgical clas-
  sification of, 217
Bevacizumab (Avastin)
 for advanced non–small cell lung cancer,
   306-307
 for breast cancer, 343
 for renal cell carcinoma, 318
BHD syndrome and renal cell carcinoma, 315
BIBF1120 for advanced non–small cell lung
  cancer, 307
Bicalutamide for prostate cancer, 355
Biological therapy for breast cancer, 340
Biomechanics and reconstruction, 39-50
 of cervicothoracic junction, 46-47
 key principles of, 39-40
 of lumbosacral-pelvic region, 49-50, 777-
   778, 791-794, 825-826
 of occipitocervical junction, 40-43
 of subaxial cervical spine, 43-45
 of thoracolumbar spine, 47-48
Biopsy
 core needle, 416
 fine-needle aspiration, 416
 percutaneous image-guided; see Percutaneous spine biopsy

Birt-Hogg-Dubé syndrome and renal cell
  carcinoma, 315
Bisphosphonates
 for advanced non–small cell lung cancer,
   309
 with androgen deprivation therapy, 362-
   363
 for breast cancer, 345
 for renal cell carcinoma, 319
Bladder incontinence, postoperative, 152-153
Bleeding during surgery, 879-881
Blood loss during surgery, 879-881
BMD with androgen deprivation therapy,
  362-364
BMS-690514 for advanced non–small cell
  lung cancer, 307
Bone cysts, aneurysmal; see Aneurysmal bone
  cysts
Bone metastases
 of breast cancer, 345
 of non–small cell lung cancer, 309
 of renal cell carcinoma, 319
Bone mineral density with androgen deprivation therapy, 362-364
Boots to prevent skin breakdown, 154
Bowel incontinence, postoperative, 152-153
Bowel motion during angiography and embolization, 439
Bracing, postoperative, 150-151
Bragg peak, 89
BRCA1 and *BRCA2*, 327-328, 346
Breast cancer, 325-347
 advanced
  management of, 342-343
  prognosis for, 333, 334-335
 characterization of, 330-333
 diagnosis of, 329
 early-stage
  locoregional treatment of, 335-337
   radiation therapy for, 336-337
   surgery for, 335-336
  prognosis for, 333-334
  systemic therapy for, 337-342
   biological, 340
   chemotherapy as, 339-340
   decision-making algorithm for, 341
   factors affecting, 337, 338
   hormonal, 338-339
   neoadjuvant, 342
 epidemiology of, 325
 estrogen and progesterone receptors in, 331
 future research on, 347
 gene expression in, 333
 grading of, 332-333
 hemipelvectomy for, 768
 HER2 in, 331-332, 340, 342-343, 344
 histology of, 331
 inflammatory, 331
 isolated tumor cell in, 329

in men, 346
metastatic
   to bone, 345
   to CNS, 343-345
   management of, 342-343
   micro-, 329, 337
   prognosis for, 333, 334-335
pathogenesis of, 325-326
prevention of, 346
prognosis for, 333-335
risk factors for, 326-328
staging of, 329-330
stereotactic radiosurgery for, 103-104
subtypes of, 331
transpedicular approach for anterior decompression and reconstruction for, 754-755
triple-negative, 332
Breast Cancer Chemotherapy Questionnaire, 899-900
Breast cancer susceptibility genes 1 and 2, 327-328, 346
Breast conservation surgery, 335, 336
Breast disease, benign, 328
Bremsstrahlung, 88
BTO, 447-449, 552, 556-557

C

C1, 3
C1 lateral mass screws for pediatric tumors, 855-857, 864
C1-2 transarticular screws for pediatric tumors, 857, 864
C1-C2 articulation, 6
C2, 3
C2 pars/pedicle screws for pediatric patients, 857, 858, 864
C2 translaminar screws for pediatric patients, 857, 858, 864
C2 tumors, 679-700
   C2 spondylectomy for, 685
   en bloc resection for
      indications and contraindications for, 680-681
      outcomes for, 690-692
      preoperative evaluation for, 681-683
      signature case on, 696-699
      technique of, 686-688
   indications and contraindications for surgical management of, 679-681
   outcomes for, 690-692
   parasagittal osteotomy for, 190-191, 683, 689
   posterolateral transpedicular C2 corpectomy for
      indications and contraindications for, 679

      signature case on, 692-695
      technique of, 684
   preoperative evaluation for, 681-683
   signature cases on, 692-699
   surgical techniques for, 684-689
C3-7 lateral mass screws for pediatric patients, 857-859, 864
CAB for prostate cancer, 355
Cancer Rehabilitation Evaluation System-Short Form (CARES-SF), 899-900
Carbon ion beams in heavy-particle radiation, 90-91
Caregiver support, evaluation of, 130, 141
Catheter(s) for angiography and embolization, 37, 441-442
Cauda equina syndrome, 398
cEBRT as initial treatment, 99-100, 102-103
Celiac artery, 34
Celiac ganglia, 34
Celiac plexus, 34
Celiac trunk, 34
Cell death and radiation dosage, 89
Cementable screws in thoracoscopic spine surgery, 626-627
Central nervous system metastases of breast cancer, 343-345
Cerebrospinal fluid leak, 884
Cervical chordoma, 679-700
   anterior approach for, 185
   C2 spondylectomy for, 685
   clinical presentation of, 179
   en bloc resection for
      indications and contraindications for, 680-681
      outcomes for, 690-692
      preoperative evaluation for, 681-683
      signature case on, 696-699, 710-716
      technique of, 686-688
   indications and contraindications for surgical management of, 679-681
   outcomes for, 690-692
   parasagittal osteotomy for, 190-191, 683, 689
   posterolateral transpedicular C2 corpectomy for
      indications and contraindications for, 679
      technique of, 684
   preoperative evaluation for, 681-683
   signature case on, 696-699
   surgical techniques for, 684-689
Cervical collar, 144
Cervical cord segments, 7
Cervical intervertebral discs, 6
Cervical nerves, 7
Cervical paraspinal muscles, 26
Cervical precautions, 144-145
Cervical region, critical structures to avoid in, 33

Cervical spinal cord, 7
Cervical spine anatomy, 3-8
Cervical spine biopsy, 417-420
   anterior transoral approach for, 419
   anterolateral approach for, 417-418
   new technique for, 420
   posterolateral approach for, 418
   prebiopsy evaluation for, 417
Cervical spine tumors
   en bloc resection of, 705-717
      anterior approaches for, 707
      anterior column resection in, 709
      indications and contraindications for, 706
      outcomes of, 710
      parasagittal osteotomy in, 709
      preoperative evaluation for, 706-707
      resection of posterior elements in, 707-708
      signature cases on, 710-716
      technique for, 707-709
      tips from masters on, 717
   occupational therapy after surgical management of, 144-145
   paramedian transpedicular approach for, 497-509
      bailout technique for, 509
      clinical decision-making on, 499
      indications and contraindications for, 498
      intraoperative monitoring during, 499
      outcomes of, 504-505
      positioning for, 499
      postoperative care after, 504
      preoperative evaluation for, 498
      signature cases on, 506-508
      technique for, 499-504
         contralateral spinal instrumentation placement in, 499
         exposure of ventral spinal canal in, 500, 501
         facetectomies in, 500, 501
         incision in, 499
         laminectomies in, 500
         pedicle resection in, 500, 501
         reconstruction in, 502, 503
         tumor resection in, 502, 503
         vertebral artery mobilization in, 500, 501
      tips from masters on, 509
   transoral and transcervical approaches for, 529-549
      bailout techniques with, 548
      clinical decision making on, 532-533
      indications and contraindications for, 530-531
      outcomes for, 542-543
      preoperative evaluation for, 531-532

Cervical spine tumors—cont'd
　transoral and transcervical approaches for—cont'd
　　signature cases on, 544-547
　　techniques for, 533-542
　　tips from master on, 548-549
　T-saw laminoplasty for dumbbell, 487-495
Cervical sympathetic chain, 34
Cervical vertebrae, 3, 7
Cervicothoracic ganglion, 34
Cervicothoracic junction
　access to, 593-598
　biomechanics and tumor reconstruction of, 46-47
Cervicothoracic spine tumors, paramedian transpedicular approach for, 497-509
　bailout technique for, 509
　clinical decision-making on, 499
　indications and contraindications for, 498
　intraoperative monitoring during, 499
　outcomes of, 504-505
　positioning for, 499
　postoperative care after, 504
　preoperative evaluation for, 498
　signature cases on, 506-508
　technique for, 499-504
　　contralateral spinal instrumentation placement in, 499
　　exposure of ventral spinal canal in, 500, 501
　　facetectomies in, 500, 501
　　incision in, 499
　　laminectomies in, 500
　　pedicle resection in, 500, 501
　　reconstruction in, 502, 503
　　tumor resection in, 502, 503
　　vertebral artery mobilization in, 500, 501
　tips from masters on, 509
Chair transfer, 136
Chemotherapy
　for breast cancer, 339-340
　for chordoma, 182, 188
　for non–small cell lung cancer, 302-305, 306
　for osteosarcoma, 263-264, 288-289
　for Pancoast tumors, 575-576
　for prostate cancer, 355-356
　for renal cell carcinoma, 317
　and wound healing, 881
Chest wall involvement, combined lateral/posterior approach for primary spinal tumor with
　clinical decision-making on, 652-653
　signature case on, 672-674
　technique for, 661-666
Children; see Pediatric tumors
Chondroma, 201-220
　clinical presentation of, 204-205
　epidemiology of, 201

imaging of, 205-206
pathology of, 202
treatment of, 207-209
vertebrectomy with anterior/posterior fusion for, 868
Chondrosarcoma, 201-210
　clear cell, 204
　clinical presentation of, 204-205
　conventional, 203
　cytogenetic abnormalities of, 204
　dedifferentiated, 203
　epidemiology of, 201
　grading of, 202-203
　hemipelvectomy for, 772
　imaging of, 205-206
　mesenchymal, 203-204
　pathology and staging of, 202-204
　sacral, 828
　stereotactic radiosurgery for, 108-109
　treatment of, 207-209
Chordoma, 175-194
　biology of, 177-179
　biopsy of, 181
　cervical; see Cervical chordoma
　chemotherapy for, 182, 188
　chondroid, 178
　clinical decision-making on, 180-181
　clinical presentation of, 179
　clival
　　far-lateral approach for, 526
　　imaging of, 681
　conventional, 178
　dedifferentiated (with sarcomatous transformation), 178, 188
　defined, 175
　epidemiology of, 175-176
　genetic studies of, 179
　gross appearance of, 175, 185-186
　heavy-particle radiation for, 93
　lumbar, 184-185
　metastasis of, 177-178
　microscopic appearance of, 186
　natural history of, 176
　pathogenesis of, 175
　radiation therapy for, 181, 187-188
　sacral; see Sacral chordoma
　and sarcomas, 176
　signature cases on, 190-193
　surgical treatment of, 181-189
　　anterior or lateral retroperitoneal approach for, 184
　　in cervical spine, 185
　　complications of, 185
　　with dural resection, 183-184
　　goal of, 181
　　indications and contraindications for, 177
　　local recurrence after, 176-177, 186

　　in lumbar spine, 184-185
　　outcomes of, 185-189
　　posterior approaches for, 183
　　postoperative care after, 185
　　preoperative evaluation for, 180
　　preoperative planning for, 182
　　for recurrent lesions, 181-182
　　rehabilitation after, 156-159
　　specimens and margins in, 185-187
　　supine or lateral decubitus position for, 184
　　technique for, 182-185
　　wound closure after, 185
　treatment of choice for, 182
　vertebral body, 188-189
Chyle leak, 885-886
Cimetidine (Tagamet) for iodine contrast allergy, 435, 436
C-ion beams in heavy-particle radiation, 90-91
Circumferential fixation of subaxial cervical spine, 44
Circumglossal approach, 538
Classification
　of ependymomas, 65
　of functioning, disability, and health, 893, 896-897, 899-900
　of giant cell tumors, 217
　of Pancoast tumors, 566-569
　of spinal metastases, 53-54
　surgical
　　of benign bone tumors, 217
　　of soft tissue sarcomas, 275-277
　　of spinal tumors, 58
Client-centered rehabilitation, 143
Clinical target volume in stereotactic radiosurgery, 101
Clival chordoma
　far-lateral approach for, 526
　imaging of, 681
Clonus test, 134
CNS metastases of breast cancer, 343-345
Combined androgen blockade for prostate cancer, 355
Combined lateral/posterior approach for large anterior/lateral lesions, 647-675
　clinical decision-making on, 651-653
　hypervascular metastases with paraspinal extension as
　　clinical decision-making on, 652
　　signature case on, 670-671
　　technique for, 658-661
　indications and contraindications for, 648-649
　outcomes for, 666-667
　Pancoast tumor with spinal involvement as
　　clinical decision-making on, 651
　　results of, 667

signature case on, 668-669
    technique for, 654-658
  preoperative evaluation for, 649-651
  primary spinal tumor involving chest
      wall as
    clinical decision-making on, 652-653
    signature case on, 672-674
    technique for, 661-666
  signature cases on, 668-674
  technique for, 653-666
  tips from masters on, 675
Complication(s), 879-888
  blood loss as, 879-881
  CSF leak as, 884
  infection as, 881-882
  instrumentation failure/pseudarthrosis as,
      886-887
  nerve injury or nerve sacrifice as, 882-883
  spinal cord injury as, 884-885
  thoracic duct injury as, 885-886
Compton, Arthur Holly, 87
Compton effect, 87
Compton scattering, 87
Computed tomographic angiography, 37
Computed tomographic myelography, 36
Computed tomography, 36, 37
  prior to heavy-particle radiation, 91
  for stereotactic radiosurgery, 101
Computed tomography-guided biopsy, 414-
    416
Congenital tumors of sacrum, 794
Contact guard assist level, 135
Continence disorders, postoperative, 152-153
Contrast-enhanced images, 64, 65
Conventional external-beam radiation
    therapy as initial treatment, 99-100,
    102-103
Conventional fraction radiation, 102
Conventional radiography, 37
Coordination
  evaluation of, 133-134
  postoperative deficits of, 152
Cord expansion on MRI, 65
Core needle biopsy, 416
Core strengthening, 137-138
Corpectomy
  C2 transpedicular
    indications and contraindications for,
        679
    signature case on, 692-695
    technique of, 684
  en bloc, 725-727
  for hemangiomas, 241, 244
Costal facets, 10
Costotransverse articulations, 11
Costotransverse ligaments, 11
Costotransversectomy for intradural extra-
    medullary tumors, 482-483

Costovertebral articulations, 11
Craniocervical junction tumors, combined
    far-lateral approaches and recon-
    struction for, 511-527
  bailout techniques and expert advice on,
      527
  bone removal and dural opening for, 518-
      521
  choice of technique for, 514
  for clival chordoma, 526
  closure for, 521, 527
  for foramen magnum meningioma, 512,
      522-524
  indications and contraindications for, 512
  for jugular foramen schwannoma, 525
  outcomes of, 521
  positioning and setup for, 515-516
  preoperative evaluation for, 513
  signature cases on, 522-526
  skin incision and bony exposure for, 516-
      518
  treatment decisions for, 514, 515
  vascular injuries during, 527
Critical structures, 33-35
CSF leak, 884
CT; see Computed tomography
CTJ
  access to, 593-598
  biomechanics and tumor reconstruction
      of, 46-47
CTV in stereotactic radiosurgery, 101
Curettage, defined, 651
CXCR4 in osteosarcoma, 264-265
CyberKnife radiosurgery, 101, 105
Cybertech brace, 146
Cyclotron, 89, 90
Cysts
  aneurysmal bone; see Aneurysmal bone
      cysts
  on MRI, 65
  of sacrum, 794

D

DCIS, 328
Deep venous thrombosis, postoperative, 155
Deglutition; see Swallow(s) and swallowing
Denosumab
  for advanced non–small cell lung cancer,
      309
  with androgen deprivation therapy, 363-
      364
Dens, 3
Dependent assistance level, 135
Dermoid cysts of sacrum, 794
Developmental cyst of sacrum, 794
Devic's syndrome, 79
Diaphragmatic crura, 34

Diffusion tensor imaging, 70
Dimethyl sulfoxide, ethylene vinyl alcohol
    dissolved in, for embolization, 451,
    452
Diphenhydramine (Benadryl) for iodine
    contrast allergy, 435, 436
Disease-free survival time, 891
Docetaxel
  for advanced non–small cell lung cancer,
      304, 306
  for prostate cancer, 355-356
Domains in quality of life assessment, 891
Dorsal sacroiliac ligament, 21
Dorsolateral spinal arteries, 31
Double iliac screw/bolt fixation technique
    for reconstruction after sacrectomy,
    833-834, 835, 838
Double swallows, 168
Dressing
  lower body, 142
  upper body, 141
Dressing stick, 146, 147
Drop metastases, 20
DSAs, 31
Ductal carcinoma, infiltrating, 331
Ductal carcinoma in situ, 328
Dumbbell tumor of cervical spine, T-saw
    laminoplasty for, 487-495
Dura, 7
Durable medical equipment in physical
    therapy evaluation, 130-131
Dural sac, 20
DVT, postoperative, 155
Dynamic sitting balance, 136, 137
Dynamic standing balance, 136, 137
Dysphagia, 161-171
  assessment of, 163-166
  causes of, 169
  defined, 161
  pharyngeal phase, 166-167
  signature cases on, 170-171
  with transoral and transcervical approaches,
      531, 532, 533, 542-543
  treatment and strategies for, 168

E

Eastern Cooperative Oncology Group per-
    formance status (ECOG-PS)
  for advanced non–small cell lung cancer,
      305
  in quality of life assessment, 893, 897, 898
  in surgical decision-making, 57
EBRT as initial treatment, 99-100, 102-103
Edmonton Symptom Assessment System, 899
Effortful swallow, 168
EGFR in advanced non–small cell lung can-
    cer, 308-309

Ejaculatory dysfunction, postoperative, 153
Embolization, 435-453
   anesthesia and adjunctive measures for, 439
   for aneurysmal bone cysts
      choice of, 228-229
      outcomes for, 230
      signature cases on, 231-233
      technique for, 229
   angiographic protocol for, 443-444
   bowel motion during, 439
   catheters for, 441-442
   complications of, 452
   equipment for, 438
   evaluation of cervical spine tumors for, 445-449
      balloon test occlusion for, 447-449
   evaluation of thoracic and lumbar spine tumors for, 449
   future directions for, 452-453
   for giant cell tumors, 219
   for hemangioblastomas, 450-451
   for hemangiomas, 241-242
   indications and contraindications for, 453
   with iodine contrast allergy, 453, 454
   material for, 451-452
   noninvasive imaging prior to, 437-438
   provocative testing prior to, 439-441
   renal function assessment prior to, 436-437
   technique for, 449-451
   prior to thoracic total en bloc spondylectomy, 721-722
   tips from masters on, 453
Embosphere Microspheres, 451
En bloc corpectomy, 725-727
En bloc laminectomy, 723-724
En bloc resection, 268
   of C2 tumors
      indications and contraindications for, 680-681
      outcomes for, 690-692
      preoperative evaluation for, 681-683
      signature case on, 696-699
      technique of, 686-688
   defined, 651
   of lateralized spine tumors, 629-644
      anterior approach in, 633-634
      bailout techniques for, 644
      clinical decision-making on, 632
      indications for, 631
      outcomes for, 639
      posterior approach in, 634-639
      preoperative evaluation for, 631-632
      signature cases on, 640-644
      technique for, 633-639
      tips from masters on, 644
   of primary cervical spine tumors, 705-717
      anterior approaches for, 707
      anterior column resection in, 709

      indications and contraindications for, 706
      outcomes of, 710
      parasagittal osteotomy in, 709
      preoperative evaluation for, 706-707
      resection of posterior elements in, 707-708
      signature cases on, 710-716
      technique for, 707-709
      tips from masters on, 717
En bloc spondylectomy
   single-stage thoracic spine, 719-732
      approach for, 722
      bailout technique for, 732
      blunt dissection around vertebral body in, 724-725
      clinical decision-making for, 720-721
      cutting of pedicles and en bloc laminectomy in, 723-724
      en bloc corpectomy in, 725-727
      exposure in, 722, 723
      indications for, 720
      introduction of T-saw guide in, 722-723
      outcomes of, 728
      postoperative care and rehabilitation after, 727
      preoperative embolization prior to, 721-722
      preoperative evaluation for, 720
      reconstruction in, 727
      signature cases on, 728-731
      technique of, 721-727
      tips from masters on, 732
   two-stage thoracic/lumbar, 735-742
      bailout techniques for, 742
      clinical decision-making on, 736-737
      indications and contraindications for, 735-736
      outcomes of, 740
      preoperative evaluation for, 736
      signature case on, 741
      technique of, 737-740
      tips from masters on, 742
Enchondromas, 202
Endonasal and transoral approach, 544
Endoscopic-assisted spine surgery; see Thoracoscopic spine surgery
Enhancement on MRI, 64, 65
Enneking surgical classification
   of benign bone tumors, 217
   of soft tissue sarcomas, 275-277
Environmental modifications, 143-144
EORTC, 893, 894, 897, 899-900
Ependymal tumors, 399-401
   definition/clinical presentation of, 399
   pathologic differential diagnosis of, 400
   practical points on, 401
   prognosis for, 401

   radiologic/pathologic correlation for, 400
   typical macroscopic and microscopic findings with, 399-400
Ependymomas, 65-68, 458-459
   anaplastic, 65
   vs. astrocytomas, 70
   classification of, 65
   epidemiology of, 458
   imaging of, 66-67
   myxopapillary, 65, 67, 399-401, 459
   pathology of, 65-66
   prevalence of, 65
   sacral, 400, 796
   sub-, 65, 68, 459-460
   surgical management of, 458-459
Epidermal growth factor receptor in advanced non–small cell lung cancer, 308-309
Epidermoid cysts of sacrum, 794
Epidural sinuses, 31
EQ-5D, 893, 897
erbB2 gene in breast cancer, 332
Erectile dysfunction, postoperative, 153
Erector spinae, 28
Erlotinib for advanced non–small cell lung cancer, 308
ESAS, 899
Esophageal phase of swallow, 163
Estrogen receptors in breast cancer, 331, 338
Ethylene vinyl alcohol dissolved in dimethyl sulfoxide (DMSO) for embolization, 451, 452
European Organization for Research and Treatment of Cancer QLQ-C30, 893, 894, 897, 899-900
EuroQol Group, 893, 897
Everolimus
   for breast cancer, 342
   for renal cell carcinoma, 318-319
External venous plexus, 31
External-beam radiation therapy as initial treatment, 99-100, 102-103
Extracompartmental lesions, 58
Extradural compartment, 36, 37
Extramedullary compartment, 36

F

Facet joint anatomy, 22-23
FACT-G, 893, 894, 899-900
Family support, evaluation of, 130, 141
Far-lateral approaches and reconstruction for craniocervical junction tumors, 511-527
   bailout techniques and expert advice on, 527
   bone removal and dural opening for, 518-521

choice of technique for, 514
for clival chordoma, 526
closure for, 521, 527
for foramen magnum meningioma, 512, 522-524
indications and contraindications for, 512
for jugular foramen schwannoma, 525
outcomes of, 521
positioning and setup for, 515-516
preoperative evaluation for, 513
signature cases on, 522-526
skin incision and bony exposure for, 516-518
treatment decisions for, 514, 515
vascular injuries during, 527
Fasciocutaneous flaps, 113, 115
Fast spin-echo sequences, 64
Fat-suppressed sequences, 35-36
Fecal incontinence, postoperative, 152-153
Female sexual dysfunction, postoperative, 154
Fiberoptic endoscopic evaluation of swallowing (FEES), 165-166
Fibrin glue, 884
Fibrosarcoma, 279-280
  nerve sheath, 290
Fibrous histiocytomas, malignant, 278-279
Fibrous tumors, solitary; see Solitary fibrous tumors
Fibrous xanthomas, malignant, 278-279
Fibular flap, vascularized, 124
FIM, 898
Fine-needle aspiration biopsy, 416
Finger-nose-finger test, 133-134
Flaps
  advancement, 118, 119
  fasciocutaneous, 113, 115
  free, 115, 123-124
  gluteus maximus, 120-121
  latissimus dorsi, 117-118, 119, 123
  local skin, 124
  muscle, 115
  musculocutaneous, 113, 115
  omental, 122
  paraspinous muscle, 115, 118-120
  rectus abdominis, 122, 123
  reverse, 118, 119
  selection of, 115
  transverse back, 122, 123
  trapezius, 116-117
  vascularized fibula, 124
FLIC, 893, 899-900
Floating ribs, 11
Fluoroscopic-guided biopsy, 413-414, 430-431
Flutamide for prostate cancer, 355
FNAB, 416
Foramen magnum meningioma, far-lateral approach for, 512, 522-524
Fractionation schedules, 102

Free flaps, 115, 123-124
Free tissue transfer, 115, 123-124
FSE sequences, 64
Fuhrman grading system for renal cell carcinoma, 314, 315
Functional ability, evaluation of, 130-131
Functional Assessment of Cancer Therapy Scale, 893, 894, 899-900
Functional assist level, 135
Functional Independence Measure, 898
Functional Living Index-Cancer questionnaire, 893, 899-900
Functional mobility, 135-136, 143

G

Gait, 136, 138
Gait assistive device, 139
Galveston technique, modified, for reconstruction after sacrectomy, 782-783, 832-833, 834-835
Gamma Knife units, 88
Gangliogliomas, 71-72, 461
Ganglion impar, 21
Ganglioneuromas of sacrum, 796
GCTs; see Giant cell tumors
Gefitinib for advanced non–small cell lung cancer, 308, 309
Gemcitabine for advanced non–small cell lung cancer, 304
Gesellschaft fur Schwerionenforschung, 90
Giant cell tumors, 213-224
  of cervical spine, 220
  classification of, 217
  clinical presentation of, 213
  defined, 213
  genetics of, 217
  gross pathology of, 216
  histologic findings in, 216
  imaging of, 214-215
  outcomes for, 218, 221-222
  radiographic differential diagnosis of, 215
  of sacrum, 220-221, 796, 828
  signature case on, 222-223
  staging of, 217
  of thoracolumbar spine, 220
  tips from masters on, 223
  treatment of, 217-221
    combined lateral/posterior approach for, 672-674
    cryotherapy for, 219-220
    embolization for, 219
    en bloc resection for, 220
    intralesional procedures for, 218
    radiation therapy for, 218-219
    surgical techniques for, 220-221
GivMohr sling, 158
GKUs, 88

Glioblastoma multiforme, 68, 70
Glossotomy, midline, 545
Glucagon for bowel motion during angiography and embolization, 439
Gluteal island flap, 120, 121
Gluteus maximus flap, 120-121
Goserelin for prostate cancer, 355
Grooming, 141
Gross tumor volume (GTV) in stereotactic radiosurgery, 101
G-VAX for prostate cancer, 359, 362

H

H_1 blocker for iodine contrast allergy, 435, 436
H_2 blocker for iodine contrast allergy, 435, 436
Hadrons, 88
Hand splint, resting, 150
Hare, Edwin, 565
Harmonic scalpel in thoracoscopic spine surgery, 614
Harvard cyclotron, 90
Health Utility Index, 893
Health-Related Quality of Life outcome measures
  cancer-related, 893, 894
  general concepts of, 891-893
  generic, 892-893, 894
  renewed interest in, 890
  review of current literature on, 897-899
  in SOSGOQ tool, 899
  specific considerations in reporting surgical outcomes with, 893-895
  validity of, 893
Heavy Ion Medical Accelerator group, 90
Heavy-particle radiation, 87-96
  advantages of, 90-91
  clinical decision-making for, 92
  history of, 90-91
  indications and contraindications for, 91
  mechanism of action of, 88, 89
  outcomes of, 93
  preoperative evaluation for, 91-92
  signature cases on, 93-95
  sources of, 88
  technique of, 92
Hemangioblastomas, 72-75, 401-404, 461
  vs. astrocytomas, 70
  definition/clinical presentation of, 401
  embolization for, 450-451
  genetics of, 403
  imaging of, 73-75
  pathogenesis of, 461
  pathologic differential diagnosis of, 403
  pathology of, 73
  practical points on, 404

Hemangioblastomas—cont'd
  prevalence of, 72-73
  prognosis for, 404
  radiologic/pathologic correlation for, 403
  surgical treatment of, 461
  typical macroscopic and microscopic findings with, 402
  in von Hippel-Lindau syndrome, 401, 403, 404, 461
Hemangioblastomatosis, 401, 404
Hemangiomas, 237-247
  asymptomatic or incidental, 240
  cavernous vs. capillary, 239
  clinical decision making for, 240-243
  clinical features of, 237, 240-241
  diagnosis of, 238-239
  epidemiology of, 237
  imaging of, 237, 238-239
  pain due to, 241
  percutaneous ethanol injections for, 243
  percutaneous vertebroplasty for, 242
  preoperative transarterial embolization for, 241-242
  radiation therapy for, 242-243
  signature cases of, 245-246
  spinal cord compression due to, 241
  surgical management of
    complications of, 245
    corpectomy or vertebrectomy for, 241, 244
    emergency decompression with laminectomy for, 241, 242-243
    indications and contraindications for, 237, 241
    outcomes for, 245
    preoperative evaluation for, 238-239
    technique for, 243-244
  tips from masters on, 247
Hemangiopericytoma, 395-397
  definition/clinical presentation of, 395
  genetics of, 396
  lipomatous, 396
  pathologic differential diagnosis of, 396
  practical points on, 397
  prognosis for, 397
  radiologic/pathologic correlation for, 397
  typical macroscopic and microscopic findings with, 395-396
Hemiclamshell incision, anterolateral thoracotomy with, 598-599
Hemicorporectomy, 759-773
  bailout technique for, 773
  clinical decision-making on, 763-764
  indications and contraindications for, 759-761
  outcomes of, 767
  preoperative evaluation for, 761-763

technique for, 764-766
tips from masters on, 773
Hemipelvectomy, 759-773
  bailout technique for, 773
  clinical decision-making on, 763-764
  extended external with posterior flap coverage, 772
  indications and contraindications for, 759-761
  outcomes of, 767
  partial external with anterior flap coverage, 769-770
  partial external with posterior flap coverage, 771
  partial internal with reconstruction, 768
  preoperative evaluation for, 761-763
  signature cases on, 768-772
  technique for, 764-766
  tips from masters on, 773
Hemorrhaging during surgery, 879-881
Hemostatic agents, 880
HER2 in breast cancer, 331-332, 340, 342-343, 344
Hereditary leiomyomatosis renal cell carcinoma, 315
Hereditary papillary renal cell carcinoma, 315
Hindquarter amputation, 759-773
  bailout technique for, 773
  clinical decision-making on, 763-764
  indications and contraindications for, 759-761
  outcomes of, 767
  preoperative evaluation for, 761-763
  signature cases on, 768-772
  technique for, 764-766
  tips from masters on, 773
Histiocytomas, malignant fibrous, 278-279
HLRCC, 315
Home setup, evaluation of, 129-130
Hormonal therapy for breast cancer, 338-339
Horner syndrome due to Pancoast tumor, 570-571
HPC; see Hemangiopericytoma
HPRCC, 315
HRQOL outcome measures; see Health-Related Quality of Life outcome measures
HUI, 893
Human epidermal growth factor receptor type 2 in breast cancer, 331-332, 340, 342-343, 344
Hyaline cartilage plate, 24
Hydrocortisone for iodine contrast allergy, 436
Hygiene, 141
Hyperreflexia, postoperative, 152
Hypertonia, evaluation of, 134

Hypertonicity, postoperative, 152
Hypervascular metastases, combined lateral/posterior approach for
  clinical decision-making on, 652
  signature case on, 670-671
  technique for, 658-661
Hypofractionated radiation, 102, 104
Hypogastric nerves, 794
Hyporeflexia, postoperative, 152
Hypotension, orthostatic postoperative, 155
Hypotonicity, postoperative, 152

I

IASLC staging system for Pancoast tumors, 567-568
ICF, 893, 896-897
  review of current literature on, 897
  and SOSGOQ tool, 899-900
IDEAL technique, 64
IDEM tumors; see Intradural extramedullary tumors
IFN-α for renal cell carcinoma, 317-318
IGRT, 102
IL-2 for renal cell carcinoma, 317-318
Iliac screw fixation, 49
Iliocostalis muscle, 28
Iliolumbar ligament, 17
Image-guided biopsy; see Percutaneous spine biopsy
Image-guided intensity-modulated radiation therapy, 102
Imaging, 63-82
  of astrocytomas, 68-72
  of ependymomas, 65-68
  of hemangioblastomas, 72-75
  of lymphoma, 75-76
  of metastases, 76-77
  modalities for, 35-36, 63-64
  of non–neoplastic lesions, 78-82
  of spine tumors, 36-37, 65-82
Immobilization for stereotactic radiosurgery, 101
IMRT, 102
Incontinence, postoperative, 152-153
Independent level, 135
Infection, postoperative, 881-882
Inferior hypogastric plexus, 794
Infiltrating ductal carcinoma, 331
Inflammatory breast cancer, 331
Instrumental ADLs, 141
Instrumentation failure, 886-887
Integument, postoperative care for, 154
Intensity-modulated radiation therapy, 102
Intercostal artery, 30
Interferon-α for renal cell carcinoma, 317-318

Interleukin-2 for renal cell carcinoma, 317-318
Internal carotid artery, balloon test occlusion of, 447
Internal venous plexus, 31
International Association for the Study of Lung Cancer staging system for Pancoast tumors, 567-568
International Classification of Functioning, Disability and Health, 893, 896-897
　review of current literature on, 897
　and SOSGOQ tool, 899-900
International Union Against Cancer staging system for Pancoast tumors, 567-568
Interosseous ligament, 21
Interspinalis muscle, 28
Interspinous wiring for pediatric patients, 860
Intertransversarii muscle, 28
Intervertebral discs
　anatomy, 23-24
　cervical, 6
Intervertebral veins, 31, 33
Intracompartmental lesions, 58
Intradural compartment, 36
Intradural extramedullary tumors, 379-404, 473-485
　clinical features of, 473-474
　ependymal tumors as, 399-401
　hemangioblastomas as, 401-404
　meningiomas as, 389-392
　mesenchymal nonmeningothelial neoplasms as, 392-399
　　hemangiopericytoma as, 395-397
　　paragangliomas as, 398-399
　　solitary fibrous tumors as, 392-394
　peripheral nerve sheath tumors as, 380
　　malignant, 388-389
　　neurofibromas as, 384-388
　　schwannomas as, 380-384
　surgical management of, 473-485
　　bailout techniques, 484-485
　　in cervical and upper thoracic spine, 475-481
　　　for C1-2 tumors, 477-478
　　　paramedian transpedicular approach for, 497-509
　　　posterior subscapular technique for, 480-481
　　　selection of surgical approach for, 475, 476
　　　vertebral artery in, 478-480
　　complications of, 475
　　indications for, 474
　　intraoperative monitoring during, 474-475

　　in lumbar spine, 483-484
　　　midline posterior approach for, 483
　　　paramedian approach for, 484
　　　retroperitoneal approach for, 483
　　in middle and lower thoracic spine, 481-483
　　　costotransversectomy and transpedicular approach for, 482-483
　　　thoracoscopic approach for, 481-482
　　　thoracotomy for, 481
　　signature case on, 484
　　surgical approaches for, 475, 476
　tips from masters on, 404
Intralesional specimen, defined, 681
Intramedullary compartment, 36-37
Intramedullary spinal cord tumors, 457-470
　astrocytomas as, 68-72, 460
　ependymomas as, 65-68, 458-459
　epidemiology of, 457
　ganglioglioma as, 461
　hemangioblastomas as, 72-75, 461
　imaging of, 63-82
　　modalities for, 63-64
　　vs. non-neoplastic lesions, 78-82
　lymphoma as, 75-76, 462
　melanoma as, 462
　metastases as, 76-77
　other rare, 462
　subependymoma as, 459-460
　surgical management of, 457-470
　　anatomy and neurophysiologic monitoring during, 462-463
　　for astrocytoma, 460
　　challenges of, 458
　　for ependymoma, 458-459
　　for ganglioglioma, 461
　　goals of, 457
　　for hemangioblastoma, 461
　　incision for, 464
　　laminectomy or laminotomy in, 464
　　for lymphoma, 462
　　for melanoma, 462
　　midline myelotomy in, 465-466
　　opening of dura in, 464-465
　　operative approach for, 463-464
　　for other rare tumors, 462
　　postoperative care after, 468
　　reapproximation and wound closure in, 468
　　for subependymoma, 459-460
　　techniques for, 463-469
　　tumor removal in, 466-468, 469
Iodine contrast allergy, 435, 436
Ionization density of heavy particles, 90
Irinotecan for advanced non–small cell lung cancer, 304

Isocenter verification for stereotactic radiosurgery, 101
Isolated tumor cell (ITC) in breast cancer, 329
Item burden, 895
Iterative decomposition of water and fat with echo asymmetry and least-squares estimation technique, 64

J

Jaffe-Lichtenstein disease, 225
Jugular foramen schwannoma, far-lateral approach for, 525

K

KAFO, 150
Kaplan-Meier curves with spinal metastases, 59-60
Karnofsky Index of Quality of Life, 893, 899
Karnofsky performance scale, 57
　for advanced non–small cell lung cancer, 305
KELS, 142
Ketoconazole for prostate cancer, 355
Key muscle level, 132
Ki-67 in breast cancer, 332
Kirschner wire (K-wire)
　for reconstruction after sacrectomy, 834
　in thoracoscopic spine surgery, 615-616
Knee-ankle-foot orthosis, 150
Kohlman Evaluation of Living Skills, 142
Kyphosis of thoracic spine, 9

L

Laminae of lumbar vertebrae, 16
Laminectomy
　and emergency decompression for hemangiomas, 241, 242-243
　en bloc, 723-724
　for intramedullary spinal cord tumors, 464
　for pediatric tumors, 851, 863
Laminoplasty
　for pediatric tumors
　　outcomes of, 863
　　signature case on, 866
　　technique of, 852-853
　T-saw; see T-saw laminoplasty
Laminotomy
　for intramedullary spinal cord tumors, 464
　for pediatric tumors
　　outcomes of, 863
　　signature case on, 866
　　technique of, 851-853
Lapatinib for breast cancer, 343

Laryngeal function examination, 164
Laryngeal penetration, 169
Lateral costotransverse ligament, 11
Lateral mass screws (C3-7) for pediatric patients, 857-859, 864
Lateral masses of cervical vertebrae, 3
Lateral thoracotomy, 600-601
Lateralized spine tumors, sagittal osteotomy for en bloc resection of, 629-644
   anterior approach in, 633-634
   bailout techniques for, 644
   clinical decision-making on, 632
   indications for, 631
   outcomes for, 639
   posterior approach in, 634-639
   preoperative evaluation for, 631-632
   signature cases on, 640-644
   technique for, 633-639
   tips from masters on, 644
Latissimus dorsi flap, 117-118, 119, 123
Lawrence Berkley Laboratory, heavy-particle radiation at, 90
LCIS, 328
Leg lifter, 146, 147
Leiomyosarcoma, 281
Leptomeningeal metastases of breast cancer, 344-345
LET, 90
Leuprolide for prostate cancer, 355
LHRH agonists for prostate cancer, 355
Li-Fraumeni syndrome and breast cancer, 328
Linear accelerators (linacs), 88
Linear energy transfer, 90
Linear-quadratic model for cell death and radiation dosage, 89
Liposarcoma, 281, 282
Lobular carcinoma, 331
Lobular carcinoma in situ, 328
Local skin flaps, 124
Locomotor training, 138-139
Log-rolling technique, 137
Loma Linda University Proton Beam Center, 90, 93
Longissimus muscle, 28
Lower extremity bracing after surgery, 150-151
Lower third of back, 113, 114
   reconstructive surgery of, 115, 118-123
Lumbar artery, 30
Lumbar nerve roots, 18
Lumbar plexus, 793
Lumbar precautions, 145-148
Lumbar region
   biomechanics and tumor reconstruction of, 49-50
   critical structures to avoid in, 34
Lumbar spine anatomy, 14-18
Lumbar spine biopsy, 424-427
   posterolateral approach for, 424
   transpedicular (bull's-eye, en face), 424, 425-427

Lumbar spine tumors
   occupational therapy after surgery for, 145-148
   sagittal osteotomy for en bloc resection of lateralized, 629-644
      anterior approach in, 633-634
      bailout techniques for, 644
      clinical decision-making on, 632
      indications for, 631
      outcomes for, 639
      posterior approach in, 634-639
      preoperative evaluation for, 631-632
      signature cases on, 640-644
      technique for, 633-639
      tips from masters on, 644
   two-stage en bloc spondylectomy for, 735-742
      bailout techniques for, 742
      clinical decision-making on, 736-737
      indications and contraindications for, 735-736
      outcomes of, 740
      preoperative evaluation for, 736
      signature case on, 741
      technique of, 737-740
      tips from masters on, 742
Lumbar vertebrae, 7, 14-17
Lumbar-iliac fixation system for sacrectomy, 835
Lumbopelvic junction instability, 825, 830
Lumbopelvic junction reconstruction
   bailout techniques for, 788
   clinical decision-making on, 780-783
   signature cases on, 787
   technique of, 783-784
   tips from masters on, 789
Lumbosacral angle, 19
Lumbosacral corset, 145
Lumbosacral joint anatomy and biomechanics, 777-778, 791, 825-826
Lumbosacral junction instability, 830
Lumbosacral junction reconstruction
   bailout techniques for, 788
   clinical decision-making on, 780-783
   signature cases on, 787
   technique of, 783-784
   tips from masters on, 789
Lumbosacral ligament, 825-826
Lumbosacral pivot point, 49
Lumbosacral plexus, 21, 793
Lumbosacral region, biomechanics and tumor reconstruction of, 49-50
Lumbosacral transition point, 50
Lumbosacral trunk, 21
Lung cancer, 301-310
   epidemiology of, 301
   non–small cell, 302-309
      cytotoxic chemotherapy for, 302-305
      preventing/neutralizing metastases of, 309

      second-line cytotoxic chemotherapy for, 306
      targeting EGFR pathway for, 308-309
      targeting VEGF pathway for, 306-308
   small cell, 302
   stereotactic radiosurgery for, 106-107
   thoracoscopic spine surgery for, 624-625
Luteinizing hormone-releasing hormone (LHRH) agonists for prostate cancer, 355
Lymphoma, 75-76, 462

M

MACS-TL anterolateral spinal implant, 611-612
MACS-TL screws, 615-616
Maffucci syndrome, chondromas in, 205
Magnetic resonance angiography, 37
Magnetic resonance imaging, 35-36, 37, 63-64, 65
   prior to heavy-particle radiation, 91
   for stereotactic radiosurgery, 101
Magnetic resonance imaging-guided biopsy, 414, 416
Magnetic susceptibility artifacts, 36, 64
Male sexual dysfunction, postoperative, 153
Malignant fibrous histiocytomas, 278-279
Malignant fibrous xanthomas, 278-279
Malignant neurofibromas, 290
Malignant peripheral nerve sheath tumors, 290-293, 294, 388-389
Malignant schwannomas, 290
Mammalian target of rapamycin
   in breast cancer, 342
   in renal cell carcinoma, 318
Mammography, 329, 346
Manual muscle testing, 132
Marginal excision, defined, 681
Masako maneuver, 168
Massachusetts General Hospital, heavy-particle radiation at, 90
Maxillotomy approach, 535-537
Maximum assistance level, 135
MBSS, 164-165
MDR1 gene in osteosarcoma, 264
MDV3100 for prostate cancer, 359
Median sacral crest, 20
Median sternotomy, anterolateral thoracotomy with, 598-599
Medical history in physical therapy evaluation, 129
Medical Outcomes Study Short Form, 892-893, 898
Medrol (methylprednisolone) for iodine contrast allergy, 436
Medullary feeder arteries, 31
Melanoma, 462
Mendelsohn maneuver, 168
Meninges, 7

Meningiomas, 389-392
  definition/clinical presentation of, 389
  fibrous (fibroblastic), 390
  of foramen magnum, far-lateral approach for, 512, 522-524
  genetics of, 391
  meningothelial, 390
  pathologic differential diagnosis of, 391
  practical points on, 392
  prognosis for, 392
  radiologic/pathologic correlation for, 391-392
  vs. schwannomas, 382-383
  transitional (mixed), 390
  typical macroscopic and microscopic findings with, 390-391
MEPs
  to minimize spinal cord injury, 885
  with Pancoast tumor, 581-582
  during provocative testing, 440
Mesenchymal nonmeningothelial neoplasms, 392-399
  hemangiopericytoma as, 395-397
  paragangliomas as, 398-399
  solitary fibrous tumors as, 392-394
Metabolic cell death, 87
Metallic magnetic susceptibility artifacts, 36, 64
Metastasis(es)
  bone
    of breast cancer, 345
    of non–small cell lung cancer, 309
    of renal cell carcinoma, 319
  of breast cancer
    to bone, 345
    to CNS, 343-345
    management of, 342-343
    micro-, 329, 337
    prognosis for, 333, 334-335
  of chordoma, 177-178
  combined lateral/posterior approach for hypervascular
    clinical decision-making on, 652
    signature case on, 670-671
    technique for, 658-661
  drop, 20
  imaging of, 76-77
  as intramedullary spinal cord tumors, 76-77
  preventing non–small cell lung cancer, 309
  skip, 265
  spinal, 76-77
    classification of, 53-54
    imaging of, 77
    outcomes with, 59-60
    pathology of, 77
    prevalence of, 76
    scoring systems for, 54-56
    surgical decision-making for, 57-59
Metastatic tumors, 76-77
  classification of, 53-54
  imaging of, 77
  outcomes with, 59-60
  pathology of, 77
  prevalence of, 76
  quality of life with, 891-892
  of sacrum, 797
  scoring systems for, 54-56
  stereotactic radiosurgery for; see Stereotactic radiosurgery (SRS)
  surgical decision-making for, 57-59
Methylprednisolone (Medrol) for iodine contrast allergy, 436
MFHs, 278-279
Miami J collar, 156, 157
Microcatheters for angiography and embolization, 441-442
Micrometastases of breast cancer, 329, 337
Middle third of back, 113, 114
  reconstructive surgery of, 115, 118, 119
Midline awareness, 137
Midline glossotomy, 545
Midline posterior approach for lumbar intradural extramedullary tumors, 483
Minimal assistance level, 135
Minimally invasive thoracoscopic spine surgery; see Thoracoscopic spine surgery
Mitosis-linked cell death, 87-88
Mobility, functional, 135-136, 143
Model of Human Occupation, 142
Moderate assistance level, 135
Modified Ashworth Scale, 134
Modified barium swallow study, 164-165
Modified Galveston technique for reconstruction after sacrectomy, 782-783, 832-833, 834-835
Modified independent level, 135
Moment arms, 40
  of lumbosacral region, 49, 50
  at occipitocervical junction, 41
  of subaxial cervical spine, 43, 44
  of thoracolumbar spine, 47, 48
Motesanib for advanced non–small cell lung cancer, 307
Motion artifacts, 36
Motor evoked potentials
  to minimize spinal cord injury, 885
  with Pancoast tumor, 581-582
  during provocative testing, 440
Motor function loss after surgery, 149-151
Movement disorders, postoperative, 152
MPNSTs, 290-293, 294, 388-389
MR angiography, 37

MRI; see Magnetic resonance imaging
MS, 78-79
mTOR
  in breast cancer, 342
  in renal cell carcinoma, 318
Mucomyst (N-acetylcysteine) for iodinated contrast with renal insufficiency, 436, 437
Mucus-secreting cysts of sacrum, 794
Multifidus muscle, 28
Multiple chondromatosis syndrome, 205
Multiple myeloma, 371-376
  clinical features of, 371
  defined, 371
  instrumentation failure with, 887
  medical management of, 371-372
  surgical management of
    bailout techniques and expert advice on, 376
    clinical decision-making in, 373
    indications and contraindications for, 372
    outcomes of, 374-375
    preoperative evaluation for, 372-373
    signature cases for, 375
    technique for, 374
    tips from masters on, 376
Multiple sclerosis, 78-79
Multiple-drug-resistant-1 gene in osteosarcoma, 264
Multipodus boot, 154
Muscle flaps, 115
Muscle tone disorders, postoperative, 152
Musculocutaneous flaps, 113, 115
Myelitis, radiation, 80, 81
Myelography, 64
  for stereotactic radiosurgery, 101
Myeloma
  multiple; see Multiple myeloma
  plasma cell, heavy-particle radiation for, 94
Myelopathy
  acute transverse, 79
  radiation, 80, 81-82
  after stereotactic radiosurgery, 105
  subacute necrotizing, 80, 81
Myxopapillary ependymoma, 65, 67, 399-401, 459

N

N-acetylcysteine (Mucomyst) for iodinated contrast with renal insufficiency, 436, 437
n-Butyl cyanoacrylate (n-BCA) for embolization, 451-452
Neoadjuvant chemotherapy
  for early-stage breast cancer, 342
  for osteosarcoma, 263-264, 288-289

Nerve injury, 882-883
Nerve plexuses, 34
Nerve sacrifice, 882-883
Nerve sheath fibrosarcomas, 290
Nerve sheath tumors
   clinical features of, 473-474
   epidemiology of, 473-474
   peripheral, 380
      malignant, 290-293, 294, 388-389
      neurofibromas as, 384-388
      schwannomas as, 380-384
   surgical management of, 473-485
      bailout techniques and expert advice on, 484-485
      in cervical and upper thoracic spine, 475-481
         for C1-2 tumors, 477-478
         paramedian transpedicular approach for ventral, 497-509
         posterior subscapular technique for, 480-481
         selection of surgical approach for, 475, 476
         vertebral artery in, 478-480
      complication of, 475
      indications for, 474
      intraoperative monitoring during, 474-475
      in lumbar spine, 483-484
         midline posterior approach for, 483
         paramedian approach for, 484
         retroperitoneal approach for, 483
      in middle and lower thoracic spine, 481-483
         costotransversectomy and transpedicular approach for, 482-483
         thoracoscopic approach for, 481-482
         thoracotomy for, 481
      signature case on, 484
      surgical approaches for, 475, 476
Neural foramina
   cervical, 7
   lumbar, 18
Neurofibromas, 384-388
   definition/clinical presentation of, 384-385
   diffuse, 385
   genetics of, 386
   localized intraneural, 385
   malignant, 290
   pathologic differential diagnosis of, 386
   plexiform, 385-386
   practical points on, 388
   prognosis for, 387
   radiologic/pathologic correlation for, 387
   of sacrum, 796
   vs. schwannomas, 382
   typical macroscopic and microscopic findings with, 385-386

Neurofibromatosis 1, 384, 386, 387
   malignant peripheral nerve sheath tumors in, 290, 292, 293, 388
Neurofibromatosis 2, schwannomas in, 380, 383
Neurofibrosarcomas, 290
Neurogenic tumors of sacrum, 796
Neurologic complications, postoperative, 149-154
Neuropathy, evaluation of, 131
Nexavar (sorafenib)
   for advanced non–small cell lung cancer, 307
   for renal cell carcinoma, 318, 319
NF1, 384, 386, 387
   malignant peripheral nerve sheath tumors in, 290, 292, 293, 388
NF2, schwannomas in, 380, 383
NHP, 893
Nilutamide for prostate cancer, 355
Nitrous oxide toxicity, 80
Non-neoplastic lesions, imaging of, 78-82
Non–small cell lung cancer, 302-309
   cytotoxic chemotherapy for, 302-305
   epidemiology of, 301
   Pancoast tumors in, 566
   preventing/neutralizing metastases of, 309
   second-line cytotoxic chemotherapy for, 306
   targeting EGFR pathway for, 308-309
   targeting VEGF pathway for, 306-308
Notochord, 175
Nottingham Health Profile, 893
NSCLC; see Non–small cell lung cancer
NSTs; see Nerve sheath tumors
Nuclear medicine bone scans, 36
Nucleus pulposus, 6, 24

O

Objective assessment of quality of life domains, 891
OC junction, biomechanics and tumor reconstruction of, 40-43
OC stabilization in pediatric patients, 854-855, 863
O-C1 transarticular screws, stability of, 42
Occipital condyles, 3, 6
Occipital keel screws, stability of, 42
Occipital screws for pediatric tumors, 854-855, 863
Occipitocervical junction, biomechanics and tumor reconstruction of, 40-43
Occipitocervical stabilization in pediatric patients, 854-855, 863
Occupational performance, 141-142
Occupational profile, 141

Occupational therapy, 139-156
   aims of, 139-141
   evaluation for, 141-142
   postoperative, 142-156
      after cervical surgery, 144-145
      of deep vein thrombosis, 155
      environmental modifications in, 143-144
      goals and expectations of, 142-143
      of integument, 154
      monitoring vital signs during, 143
      of neurologic complications, 149-154
      of orthostasis, 155
      of psychological factors, 155-156
      after sacral surgery, 148-149
      after thoracic and lumbar surgery, 145-148
   signature case on, 156-159
ODI, 898, 899
Odontoid process, 3
Odynophagia, 169
Ollier disease, chondromas in, 205
Omental flap, 122
Onlay spine fusion for pediatric tumors, 853-854
On-Q PainBuster postoperative analgesia system, 605
Onyx (ethylene vinyl alcohol dissolved in dimethyl sulfoxide) for embolization, 451, 452
Oral preparatory phase of swallow, 162
Oral transit phase of swallow, 162
Oral-motor examination, 164
Oropharyngeal swallow
   evaluation of, 163-166
   stages of, 161-163
Orthostatic hypotension, postoperative, 155
Orthotics, 150-151
Osseous tumors of sacrum, 796
Osteoblastoma(s), 251-257
   epidemiology of, 251
   histology findings for, 252
   imaging of, 254-255
   natural history and clinical presentation of, 253
   outcomes for, 256
   staging of, 252
   tips from masters on, 257
   treatment of, 255-256
Osteoblastoma-like osteosarcoma, 252
Osteogenic sarcoma; see Osteosarcoma
Osteoid osteomas, 251-257
   epidemiology of, 251
   histology findings for, 252
   imaging of, 254-255
   natural history and clinical presentation of, 253
   outcomes for, 256

tips from masters on, 257
treatment of, 255-256
Osteoplastic laminotomy for pediatric tumors
  outcomes of, 863
  signature case on, 866
  technique of, 851-853
Osteoporosis with androgen deprivation therapy, 362-364
Osteosarcoma, 259-272, 283-289
  biopsy of, 261-262, 288
  chondroblastic, 262, 263
  clinical presentation of, 260, 286
  epidemiology of, 259-260, 283, 284-285
  fibroblastic, 262, 263
  hemipelvectomy for, 769, 770
  imaging of, 261, 285-288
  immunohistochemical markers for, 285
  medical management of, 263-265
  microscopic features of, 284-285
  molecular biomarkers for, 264-265
  neoadjuvant chemotherapy for, 263-264, 288-289
  osteoblastic, 262, 263
  osteoblastoma-like, 252
  pathology of, 262-263, 283-285, 286-287
  prognosis for, 260
  radiation therapy for, 264, 288, 289
  risk factors for, 260
  of sacrum, 828
  secondary, 262
  staging and grading of, 265-266, 267, 268
  subtypes of, 259, 262, 263
  surgical approaches for, 268-271, 288
  surgical planning for, 266-268
  tips from masters on, 272
Outcomes reporting in tumor surgery, 889-900
  general concepts of, 891-893
  review of current literature on, 897-899
  specific considerations in, 893-897
  specific tool for, 899-900
Owestry Disability Index, 898, 899

P

Paclitaxel for advanced non–small cell lung cancer, 304
Pain evaluation, 131
Pain sensation loss, postoperative, 151
Palliative setting, quality of life in, 891-892
Pancoast, Henry Kunrath, 565
Pancoast syndrome, 565-566
Pancoast tumors, 565-585
  anesthetic considerations for, 576
  bailout techniques for, 585
  classification of, 566-569
    surgical, 568-569
    TNM system for, 566-568
  clinical features of, 570-571
  complications with, 583-584
  defined, 565
  diagnosis of, 574-575
  epidemiology of, 566
  imaging of, 572-573, 574
  intraoperative monitoring for, 581-582
  patient selection and decision-making on, 571-573
  postoperative management of, 582-583
  preoperative radiation therapy and chemotherapy for, 575-576
  preoperative staging evaluation of, 574
  surgical anatomy of, 569-570
  surgical approaches for, 576-579
    anterior transcervical, 577-578
    combined lateral/posterior
      clinical decision-making on, 651
      results of, 667
      signature case on, 668-669
      technique for, 654-658
    posterolateral, 576-577, 578-581
    trapdoor, 577-578
  surgical results with, 585
  surgical techniques for, 579-581
    en bloc resection with planned transgression as, 572
    posterior midline approach and second-stage posterolateral thoracotomy as, 580-581
    single-stage posterolateral thoracotomy as, 579-580
  therapeutic management of, 571-585
  type A, 568, 569
    single-stage posterolateral thoracotomy for, 579-580
    surgical approaches for, 578
  type B, 569
    posterior midline approach and second-stage posterolateral thoracotomy for, 580-581
    surgical approaches for, 579
  type C, 569
    imaging of, 572-573
    posterior midline approach and second-stage posterolateral thoracotomy for, 580-581
    type B, 579
Pancoast-Tobías syndrome, 565-566
Paragangliomas, 398-399
Paramedian approach for lumbar intradural extramedullary tumors, 484
Paramedian transpedicular approach for ventral intradural extramedullary tumors of cervical and cervicothoracic spine, 497-509
  bailout technique for, 509
  clinical decision-making on, 499
  indications and contraindications for, 498
  intraoperative monitoring during, 499
  outcomes of, 504-505
  positioning for, 499
  postoperative care after, 504
  preoperative evaluation for, 498
  signature cases on, 506-508
  technique for, 499-504
    contralateral spinal instrumentation placement in, 499
    exposure of ventral spinal canal in, 500, 501
    facetectomies in, 500, 501
    incision in, 499
    laminectomies in, 500
    pedicle resection in, 500, 501
    reconstruction in, 502, 503
    tumor resection in, 502, 503
    vertebral artery mobilization in, 500, 501
  tips from masters on, 509
Parasagittal osteotomy
  for C2 tumors, 190-191, 683, 689
  for primary cervical spine tumors, 709
Paraspinal muscles, anatomy, 25-29
Paraspinous muscle flap, 115, 118-120
Parathyroid hormone-related peptide in advanced non–small cell lung cancer, 309
Paravertebral muscles, 25-29
Patient-based outcomes, 891
Pazopanib for advanced non–small cell lung cancer, 307
Pediatric tumors, 845-870
  anterior vs. posterior instrumentation for, 849-850
  bailout techniques for, 869
  C1 lateral mass screws and C1-2 transarticular screws for
    outcomes of, 864
    technique of, 855-857
  C2 pars/pedicle and translaminar screws for
    outcomes of, 864
    technique of, 857, 858
  clinical decision-making on, 848
  dissection and removal of, 851
  future techniques for, 862-863
  indications and contraindications for surgical management of, 847
  laminectomy/laminotomy/laminoplasty for
    outcomes of, 863
    signature case on, 866
    technique of, 851-853
  lateral mass screws (C3-7) for
    outcomes of, 864
    technique of, 857-859

Pediatric tumors—cont'd
  occipital screws for
    outcomes of, 863
    technique of, 854-855
  outcomes for, 863-865
  patient positioning and preparation for, 850-851
  pedicle screws for
    outcomes of, 865
    signature case on, 867
    technique of, 859, 860
    in thoracic spine, 865
  polyester bands for, 861-862
  preoperative evaluation for, 847-848
  signature cases on, 866-868
  spine fusion for
    onlay, 853-854
    vertebrectomy with anterior/posterior, 868
  in thoracolumbar spine, 865
  tips from masters on, 870
  translaminar screws for
    outcomes of, 865
    technique of, 859-860
  types of, 845, 846
  wiring for
    outcomes of, 865
    technique of, 860-861
Pedicle(s)
  of lumbar vertebrae, 16
  of thoracic vertebrae, 12
Pedicle screw fixation for pediatric patients
  outcomes of, 865
  signature case on, 867
  technique of, 859, 860
  in thoracic spine, 865
Pelvic ligaments, 21
Pelvic reconstruction, 777-789
  bailout techniques for, 788
  biomechanics and, 49-50
  clinical decision-making on, 780-783, 829-830
  outcomes of, 834-837
  proximal sacrectomy and, 825-840
  signature cases on, 787, 838-839
  technique of, 783-784, 832-834
  tips from masters on, 789
Pelvic tumors, recurrent or locally advanced, 797
Pemetrexed for advanced non–small cell lung cancer, 304, 306
Percutaneous spine biopsy, 411-432
  approaches for, 413-414
  cervical, 417-420
    anterior transoral approach for, 419
    anterolateral approach for, 417-418
    new technique for, 420

posterolateral approach for, 418
prebiopsy evaluation for, 417
complications of, 429
core needle, 416
CT-guided, 414-416
fine-needle aspiration, 416
fluoroscopic-guided, 413-414, 430-431
indications and contraindications for, 412
lumbar, 424-427
  posterolateral approach for, 424
  transpedicular (bull's-eye, en face), 424, 425-427
of malignant tumors, 425, 426-427
MRI-guided, 414, 416
needle for, 416, 429
nondiagnostic, 429
positioning and patient preparation for, 413
preoperative evaluation for, 413
sacral, 427-428
of sclerotic lesions, 425
signature cases on, 430-431
for spine infections, 425, 426
technique of, 413-416
thoracic, 420-424
  intercostal approach for, 423
  paraspinal approach for, 421
  transcostovertebral approach for, 422-423
  transforaminal approach for, 421, 424
  transpedicular approach for, 420, 421
tips from masters on, 432
ultrasound-guided, 416
Peripheral nerve sheath tumors, 380
  malignant, 290-293, 294, 388-389
  neurofibromas as, 384-388
  schwannomas as, 380-384
Pertuzumab or breast cancer, 343
PET, 36
  prior to heavy-particle radiation, 91
Peutz-Jeghers syndrome and breast cancer, 328
P-glycoprotein (P-gp) in osteosarcoma, 264
Pharyngeal phase disorders, 166-167
Pharyngeal phase of swallow, 162-163
Philadelphia collar, 144
Photons, 88
Physical therapy, 128-139
  defined, 128
  functions and goals of, 128-129
  postoperative, 137-139
  signature case on, 156-159
Physical therapy evaluation, 129-136
  diagnosis in, 129
  objective measures in, 131-136
    of coordination, 133-134
    of functional mobility, 135-136
    of proprioception, 133

of range of motion, 131
of sensory impairment, 133
of skin integrity, 133
of spasticity, 134
of strength, 132
previous medical and surgical history in, 129
subjective measures in
  pain as, 131
  previous level of function/durable medical equipment owned as, 130-131
  social history as, 129-130
Pia, 7
Planning target volume in stereotactic radiosurgery, 101
Plasma cell myeloma, heavy-particle radiation for, 94
Plasmacytoma, 371-376
  clinical features of, 371
  defined, 371
  medical management of, 371-372
  surgical management of
    bailout techniques and expert advice on, 376
    clinical decision-making in, 373
    indications and contraindications for, 372
    outcomes of, 374-375
    preoperative evaluation for, 372-373
    signature cases for, 375
    technique for, 374
    tips from masters on, 376
Plastic surgery; see Reconstructive surgery
PLL, 6, 24-25
Polar caps, 66
Polar cysts, 65, 66
Polyester bands for pediatric patients, 861-862
Polyvinyl alcohol for embolization, 450, 451
Positron emission tomography, 36
  prior to heavy-particle radiation, 91
Posterior arches of cervical vertebrae, 3
Posterior longitudinal ligament, 6, 24-25
Posterior midline approach for Pancoast tumor, 579, 580-581
Posterior segmental medullary vein, 33
Posterior spinal vein, 33
Posterior sulcal vein, 33
Posterior tension band in pediatric osteoplastic laminotomy, 852
Posterolateral thoracotomy
  classic, 602-603
  for Pancoast tumor, 576-577
    second-stage, 579, 580-581
    single-stage, 578, 579-580
Posterolateral transpedicular corpectomy for C2 tumors
  indications and contraindications for, 679
  signature case on, 692-695
  technique of, 684

Prednisone for iodine contrast allergy, 435, 436
Preoperative transarterial embolization; see Embolization
Presacral nerve, 794
Presacral space, 19
Presbyphagia, 162, 169
Prevertebral anastomoses, 30
Progesterone receptors in breast cancer, 331
Prognostic scoring systems for spinal metastases, 54-56
Proprioception
  evaluation of, 133
  postoperative deficits in, 151-152
Prostate cancer, 353-366
  abiraterone for
    after chemotherapy, 357-358
    before chemotherapy, 358-359
  androgen deprivation therapy and chemotherapy for, 355-356
  beyond androgen deprivation therapy for, 356
  epidemiology of, 353-354
  MDV3100 for, 359
  nonmedical considerations for, 364
  novels therapies in clinical development for, 365
  preserving bone integrity with, 362-364
  radiation therapy for, 364
  surgical decompression for, 364
  thoracoscopic spine surgery for, 622-623
  tips from masters on, 366
  transpedicular approach for anterior decompression and reconstruction for, 753
  vaccine therapy for, 359-362
Prostate-specific antigen screening, 353
PROSTVAC-VF for prostate cancer, 359, 362
Proton(s), 89-90; see also Heavy-particle radiation
Proton beam radiation therapy for chordoma, 187-188
Provocative testing prior to embolization, 439-441
PSA screening, 353
Pseudarthrosis, 886-887
Pseudocapsule, 265
Psoas muscles, 28
Psychological factors, postoperative, 155-156
Psychosocial symptoms, postoperative, 155-156
PTH-rp in advanced non–small cell lung cancer, 309
PTV in stereotactic radiosurgery, 101
Pudendal nerve, 793
Pulmonary embolism, postoperative, 155

PVA for embolization, 450, 451
Pyramesh titanium cage for reconstruction after sacrectomy, 834, 838-839

Q

Quadratus lumborum muscles, 28
Quality of life (QOL), 891
  in medical literature, 892

R

Radiate ligament, 11
Radiation myelitis, 80, 81
Radiation myelopathy, 80, 81
Radiation therapy
  for aneurysmal bone cysts, 227-228
  for breast cancer, 336-337
  cell death and dosage in, 89
  for chordoma, 181, 187-188
  conventional external-beam, 99-100, 102-103
  current sources of, 88-90
  for giant cell tumors, 218-219
  for hemangiomas, 242-243
  image-guided intensity-modulated, 102
  mechanism of action of, 87-88
  for osteosarcoma, 264, 288, 289
  for Pancoast tumors, 575-576
  for prostate cancer, 364
  undesired effects of, 88
  and wound healing, 881
Radical resection, defined, 651
Radiculomedullary arteries, 31
Radiography, conventional, 37
Radiosensitivity, 89
Radiosurgery, stereotactic; see Stereotactic radiosurgery (SRS)
Range of motion evaluation, 131
RANK
  in advanced breast cancer, 345
  in advanced non–small cell lung cancer, 309
RANK-L inhibitor, with androgen deprivation therapy, 363-364
Rapid alternating movement evaluation, 133
Rate of perceived exertion journal, 158
RCC; see Renal cell carcinoma
Reacher, 146, 147
Reactive oxygen free radical species, 88
Recapping T-saw laminoplasty; see T-saw laminoplasty
Receptor activator of nuclear factor kB
  in advanced breast cancer, 345
  in advanced non–small cell lung cancer, 309

Receptor activator of nuclear factor kB ligand inhibitor, with androgen deprivation therapy, 363-364
Reconstructive surgery, 113-125
  anatomic regions for, 113, 114
  biomechanics and, 39-50
    of cervicothoracic junction, 46-47
    key principles of, 39-40
    of lumbosacral-pelvic region, 49-50, 777-778, 791-794, 825-826
    of occipitocervical junction, 40-43
    of subaxial cervical spine, 43-45
    of thoracolumbar spine, 47-48
  clinical decision-making for, 114-115
  free flaps for, 123-124
  general techniques of, 115
  indications and contraindications for, 113
  local skin flaps for, 124
  of lower third, 118-123
  of middle third, 118, 119
  postoperative care after, 124-125
  preoperative evaluation for, 114
  of upper third, 115-118
    caudal portion, 117-118
    cephalic portion, 116-117
Rectal cancer, pelvic recurrence of
  clinical features of, 797
  imaging of, 798-799
  sacrectomy for, 804, 805-806, 808-812
Rectus abdominis flaps, 122, 123
Recurrent laryngeal nerve in transoral and transcervical approaches, 533, 541, 542-543, 547, 548
Reflexive deficits, postoperative, 152
Rehabilitation, 127-159
  client-centered, 143
  defined, 127
  factors in success of, 128
  goals of, 128
  occupational therapy for, 139-156
  physical therapy for, 128-139
  signature case on, 156-159
  value of, 127
Renal cell carcinoma, 313-320
  diagnosis of, 314
  en bloc spondylectomy for
    single-stage, 728-731
    two-stage, 741
  epidemiology of, 313-314
  genetic syndromes of, 314-315
  grading of, 314, 315
  histopathology of, 314, 315
  prognosis for, 319-320
  risk factors for, 314
  staging of, 316-317
  stereotactic radiosurgery for, 103
  tips from masters on, 320

Renal cell carcinoma—cont'd
　treatment of, 317-319
　　for bone metastases, 319
　　chemotherapy for, 317
　　combined lateral/posterior approach for
　　　clinical decision-making on, 652
　　　signature case on, 670-671
　　　technique for, 658-661
　　immunotherapy for, 317-318
　　molecular agents for, 318-319
　　surgery for, 317
Renal function assessment prior to embolization, 436-437
Residue, 169
Respondent item burden, 895
Resting hand splint, 150
Retroperitoneal approach for lumbar intradural extramedullary tumors, 483
Reverse flap, latissimus dorsi flap as, 118, 119
Ribs
　floating, 11
　and thoracic spine, 10-11
Rolling, 135, 137
ROM evaluation, 131
RPE journal, 158

S

Sacral ala, 19-20
Sacral canal, 20
Sacral chordoma
　clinical features of, 795
　outcomes for, 189
　sacrectomy for
　　distal, 822
　　en bloc, 807
　　　and posterior reconstruction, 192-193, 787
　　indications and contraindications for, 827-828
　　posterior partial, 786
　　signature cases on, 192-193, 786-787, 807, 822
Sacral cornu, 20
Sacral ependymomas, 400
Sacral foramina, 20, 777
Sacral hiatus, 20, 777
Sacral ligaments, 20
Sacral nerves, 777
Sacral plexus, 21, 793
Sacral precautions, 148-149
Sacral promontory, 19
Sacral region
　biomechanics and tumor reconstruction of, 49-50
　critical structures to avoid in, 34
Sacral resection; see Sacrectomy
Sacral spine biopsy, 427-428

Sacral sympathetic plexus, 21
Sacral tumors
　biopsy of, 799
　diagnosis of, 797-798, 826
　epidemiology of, 826
　imaging of, 798-799
　pathology of, 794-797
Sacral vertebrae, 19
Sacrectomy, 791-812
　anatomy and biomechanics relevant to, 778, 791-794, 825-827
　for chordomas, 786-787, 795
　clinical decision-making on, 800
　for congenital tumors, 794
　distal, 815-823
　　bailout technique for, 823
　　clinical decision-making on, 816-817
　　indications for, 815-816
　　outcome for, 821
　　preoperative evaluation for, 816
　　signature case on, 822
　　technique for, 817-821
　　tips from masters on, 823
　high vs. low, 801
　indications and contraindications for, 778-779, 800
　for metastatic tumors, 797
　for neurogenic tumors, 796
　occupational therapy after, 148-149
　for osseous tumors, 796
　outcomes of, 784-786, 804-806, 836-837
　preoperative evaluation prior to, 779-780
　preoperative planning for, 801
　proximal, 825-840
　　bailout techniques for, 840
　　clinical decision-making on, 829-830
　　indications and contraindications for, 827-828
　　outcomes for, 834-837
　　preoperative evaluation for, 828-829
　　signature case on, 838-839
　　technique for, 830-834
　　tips from masters on, 840
　reconstruction after, 777-789
　　bailout techniques for, 788
　　clinical decision-making on, 780-783
　　outcomes of, 834-837
　　signature cases on, 787, 838-839
　　technique of, 783-784, 832-834
　　tips from masters on, 789
　for secondary tumors, 796
　signature cases on, 786-787, 807-812
　simple vs. complex, 801
　surgical technique for, 801-804
　for teratomas, 795-796
　transverse partial, 778, 826, 827, 837
Sacrococcygeal joint anatomy and biomechanics, 19, 791, 825-826

Sacroiliac joint anatomy and biomechanics, 19, 21, 778, 791-792, 825-826
Sacroiliac joint reconstruction, 777-789
　bailout techniques for, 788
　clinical decision-making on, 780-783
　signature cases on, 787
　technique of, 783-784
　tips from masters on, 789
Sacroiliac joint screw technique, 835
Sacroiliac ligaments, 21, 778, 825-826
Sacrospinous ligament, 21, 825-826
Sacrotuberous ligament, 21, 825-826
Sacrum, anatomy and biomechanics of, 19-22, 777-778, 791-794, 825-827
Sagittal balance, 40
　of cervicothoracic junction, 46
　in lumbosacral region, 49, 50
　of occipitocervical junction, 41-42
　of subaxial cervical spine, 43
　of thoracolumbar spine, 47
Sagittal osteotomy for en bloc resection of lateralized tumors of lumbar spine, 629-644
　anterior approach in, 633-634
　bailout techniques for, 644
　clinical decision-making on, 632
　indications for, 631
　outcomes for, 639
　posterior approach in, 634-639
　preoperative evaluation for, 631-632
　signature cases on, 640-644
　technique for, 633-639
　tips from masters on, 644
Sarcoma(s)
　chordomas and, 176
　hemipelvectomy for synovial, 771
　osteogenic; see Osteosarcoma
　soft tissue; see Soft tissue sarcomas
Satellite cysts on MRI, 65
SCD, 80, 81
Schwannomas, 380-384
　cellular, 382
　definition/clinical presentation of, 380
　genetics of, 383
　of jugular foramen, far-lateral approach for, 525
　malignant, 290, 384
　melanotic, 382, 384
　pathologic differential diagnosis of, 382-383
　practical points on, 384
　prognosis for, 384
　"psammomatous" variant of, 382
　radiologic/pathologic correlation for, 383-384
　sacral, 796
　　plasma cell, 95
　typical macroscopic and microscopic findings with, 380-382

Schwannomatosis, 380
Sciatic nerve, 793
SCLC, 301, 302
Sclerotic lesions, biopsy of, 425
Scoring systems for spinal metastases, 54-56
Screw placement in thoracoscopic spine surgery, 615-616
SDF-1 in osteosarcoma, 264
Secondary tumors of sacrum, 796
Segmental arteries, 30
Selective arterial embolization; *see* Embolization
Self-feeding, 141
Sensory considerations, postoperative, 151
Sensory impairment, evaluation of, 133
Sentinel node biopsy for breast cancer, 336
SEPs
    to minimize spinal cord injury, 885
    with Pancoast tumor, 581, 582
    during provocative testing, 440
Sexual dysfunction, postoperative, 153-154
SF-36, 892-893, 898
SFTs; *see* Solitary fibrous tumors
Sharpey's fibers, 24
Shoehorn, long-handled, 146, 147
Shoelaces, elastic, 146
Short-T1 inversion-recovery sequences, 64
Sickness Impact Profile, 893
Silent aspiration, 164, 169
Single-fraction radiation, 102
SIP, 893
Sipileucel-T for prostate cancer, 359-361
Sit to stand, 136, 138
Sitting balance, 136, 137-138
Skin breakdown, postoperative, 154
Skin care, postoperative, 154
Skin integrity, evaluation of, 133
Skin island, 115
    latissimus dorsi flap with, 117
    trapezius flap with, 117, 118
Skip metastases, 265
Small cell lung cancer, 301, 302
Social history in physical therapy evaluation, 129-130
Sock aid, 146, 147
Sodium bicarbonate for iodinated contrast with renal insufficiency, 436, 437
Soft tissue sarcomas, 275-289
    angiosarcoma as, 282-283
    epidemiology of, 275
    fibrosarcoma as, 279-280
    leiomyosarcoma as, 281
    liposarcoma as, 281
    malignant fibrous histiocytomas as, 278-279
    osteogenic sarcoma (osteosarcoma) as, 283-289
    risk factors for, 275
    sagittal osteotomy for en bloc resection of, 642-644
    staging of, 275-277
    survival rates for, 278
    tips from masters on, 294
Solitary fibrous tumors, 392-394
    definition/clinical presentation of, 392
    genetics of, 393
    pathologic differential diagnosis of, 393
    practical points on, 394
    prognosis for, 394
    radiologic/pathologic correlation for, 394
    typical macroscopic and microscopic findings with, 392-393
Somatosensory evoked potentials
    to minimize spinal cord injury, 885
    with Pancoast tumor, 581, 582
    during provocative testing, 440
Sorafenib (Nexavar)
    for advanced non–small cell lung cancer, 307
    for renal cell carcinoma, 318, 319
SOSGOQ, 899-900
Spasticity
    evaluation of, 134
    postoperative, 152
Speech therapy, signature case on, 170-171
Speech-language pathologist, assessment of dysphagia by, 163-166
Spinal catheter angiography, 37
Spinal compartments, 36-37
Spinal cord, vascular supply of, 31-33
Spinal cord decompression, stereotactic radiosurgery for, 104-105, 108-109
Spinal cord injury, 884-885
Spinal metastases, 76-77
    classification of, 53-54
    imaging of, 77
    outcomes with, 59-60
    pathology of, 77
    prevalence of, 76
    scoring systems for, 54-56
    surgical decision-making for, 57-59
Spinal nerve(s), 7
Spinal nerve root monitoring with Pancoast tumor, 582
Spinal Oncology Study Group Outcome Questionnaire, 899-900
Spinalis muscle, 28
Spine fusion for pediatric tumors
    onlay, 853-854
    vertebrectomy with anterior/posterior, 868
Spine ligaments, 24-25
Spinous processes
    of lumbar vertebrae, 17
    sacral, 20
    of thoracic vertebrae, 12
Splanchnic nerves, 34
Spondylectomy, 268
    for C2 tumors, 685
    en bloc single-stage thoracic, 719-732
        approach for, 722
        bailout technique for, 732
        blunt dissection around vertebral body in, 724-725
        clinical decision-making for, 720-721
        cutting of pedicles and en bloc laminectomy in, 723-724
        en bloc corpectomy in, 725-727
        exposure in, 722, 723
        indications for, 720
        introduction of T-saw guide in, 722-723
        outcomes of, 728
        postoperative care and rehabilitation after, 727
        preoperative embolization prior to, 721-722
        preoperative evaluation for, 720
        reconstruction in, 727
        signature cases on, 728-731
        technique of, 721-727
        tips from masters on, 732
    en bloc two-stage thoracic/lumbar, 735-742
        bailout techniques for, 742
        clinical decision-making on, 736-737
        indications and contraindications for, 735-736
        outcomes of, 740
        preoperative evaluation for, 736
        signature case on, 741
        technique of, 737-740
        tips from masters on, 742
Sponge, long-handled, 147
SRS; *see* Stereotactic radiosurgery
SSEPs
    to minimize spinal cord injury, 885
    with Pancoast tumor, 581, 582
    during provocative testing, 440
Stairs, 136
Standby assist, supervision level, 135
Standing balance, 136, 138
Standing exercises, 138
Static sitting balance, 136, 137
Static standing balance, 136
Stauffer's syndrome, 314
Stellate ganglion, 34
Stener, Bertil, 268
Stepping in ambulation, 138
Stereotactic radiosurgery, 99-110
    complications of, 105
    defined, 100
    image-guided techniques for, 101-102
    as initial treatment, 103-104, 106-107
    as postoperative adjuvant therapy, 104-105, 108-109

Stereotactic radiosurgery—cont'd
  principles of, 100-101
  signature cases on, 106-109
  target identification in, 100-101
  treatment planning for, 101
Steroids for iodine contrast allergy, 435, 436
STIR sequences, 64
Strength evaluation, 132
Stress shielding, 39-40
    of lumbosacral region, 50
    at occipitocervical junction, 41, 43
    of subaxial cervical spine, 43, 44
    of thoracolumbar spine, 47
Stromal cell-derived factor 1 in osteosarcoma, 264
Subacute combined degeneration, 80, 81
Subacute necrotizing myelopathy, 80, 81
Subaxial cervical spine, biomechanics and tumor reconstruction of, 43-45
Subependymoma, 65, 68, 459-460
Subjective assessment of quality of life domains, 891
Sublaminar wiring for pediatric patients, 861
Suboccipital/sublaminar wired contoured rod, stability of, 42
Sunitinib (Sutent)
  for advanced non–small cell lung cancer, 307
  for renal cell carcinoma, 318, 319
Superior articular facets of lumbar vertebrae, 17
Superior costotransverse ligament, 11
Superior epigastric plexus, 794
Superior pulmonary sulcus, 565
Superior sulcus tumors; see Pancoast tumors
Supine to sit edge of bed, 135, 137
Supraglottic swallow, 168
Surgical classification of spinal tumors, 58
Surgical decision-making for spinal metastases, 57-59
Surgical history in physical therapy evaluation, 129
Survival curves with spinal metastases, 59-60
Survival time, 891
Survivin in osteosarcoma, 265
Sutent (sunitinib)
  for advanced non–small cell lung cancer, 307
  for renal cell carcinoma, 318, 319
Swallow(s) and swallowing
  clinical evaluation of, 163-164
  double, 168
  effortful, 168
  fiberoptic endoscopic evaluation of, 165-166
  stages of, 161-163
  supraglottic, 168

Swallow management, 161-171
  signature cases on, 170-171
  treatment and strategies for, 168
Swallow study, modified barium, 164-165
Swallowing disorders, 161
  assessment of, 163-166
  causes of, 169
  pharyngeal phase, 166-167
  signature cases on, 170-171
  with transoral and transcervical approaches, 531, 532, 533, 542-543
  treatment and strategies for, 168
Sympathetic chain with cervical nerve sheath tumors, 480
Sympathetic trunk, 34
Synchrotron, 89
Synovial sarcoma, hemipelvectomy for, 771

T

T1-weighted images, 35, 64
T2-weighted images, 35, 64
Tagamet (cimetidine) for iodine contrast allergy, 435, 436
Tailgut cysts, 794
Tamoxifen for breast cancer, 338-339
Target identification in stereotactic radiosurgery, 100-101
Target localization for stereotactic radiosurgery, 101
Target volume
  in heavy-particle radiation, 92
  in stereotactic radiosurgery, 101
TDM-1 for breast cancer, 343
Temperature sensation loss, postoperative, 151
Temsirolimus for renal cell carcinoma, 318
Teratomas of sacrum, 795-796
Terminal growth inhibition, 87
TES; see Total en bloc spondylectomy
TEST for spinal metastases, 59-60
Testosterone in prostate cancer, 355
Therapeutic use of self, 141
Thoracic duct injury, 885-886
Thoracic nerve roots, 12
Thoracic precautions, 145-148
Thoracic region, critical structures to avoid in, 33-34
Thoracic spine
  anatomy, 9-14
  kyphosis of, 9
Thoracic spine biopsy, 420-424
  intercostal approach for, 423
  paraspinal approach for, 421
  transcostovertebral approach for, 422-423
  transforaminal approach for, 421, 424
  transpedicular approach for, 420, 421

Thoracic spine tumors
  occupational therapy after surgical treatment of, 145-148
  single-stage en bloc spondylectomy for, 719-732
    approach for, 722
    bailout technique for, 732
    blunt dissection around vertebral body in, 724-725
    clinical decision-making for, 720-721
    cutting of pedicles and en bloc laminectomy in, 723-724
    en bloc corpectomy in, 725-727
    exposure in, 722, 723
    indications for, 720
    introduction of T-saw guide in, 722-723
    outcomes of, 728
    postoperative care and rehabilitation after, 727
    preoperative embolization prior to, 721-722
    preoperative evaluation for, 720
    reconstruction in, 727
    signature cases on, 728-731
    technique of, 721-727
    tips from masters on, 732
  surgical approaches for, 591-606
    for access to cervicothoracic junction, 593-598
    anterolateral thoracotomy with median sternotomy–trapdoor incision as, 598-599
    axillary thoracotomy as, 600-601
    classic posterolateral thoracotomy as, 602-603
    indications and contraindications for, 592
    postoperative concerns with, 604-605
    preoperative evaluation for, 593
    tips from masters on, 606
    video-assisted thoracoscopic surgery as, 603-604
  two-stage en bloc spondylectomy for, 735-742
    bailout techniques for, 742
    clinical decision-making on, 736-737
    indications and contraindications for, 735-736
    outcomes of, 740
    preoperative evaluation for, 736
    signature case on, 741
    technique of, 737-740
    tips from masters on, 742
Thoracic vertebrae, 7, 9-10
Thoracolumbar paraspinal muscles, 28
Thoracolumbar spine, biomechanics and tumor reconstruction of, 47-48

Thoracolumbosacral orthosis, 145, 146
Thoracoscopic spine surgery, 603-604, 607-627
　advantages and disadvantages of, 610
　anesthesia and patient positioning for, 612, 625
　bailout techniques for, 625-627
　cementable screws in, 626-627
　chest tube placement and closure in, 619-620
　complications of, 621-622
　exposure in, 613-614, 626
　indications and contraindications for, 608
　for intradural extramedullary tumors, 481-482
　localization and access in, 612-613, 625-626
　placement of vertebral body screws in, 615-616
　preoperative evaluation for, 608-609
　preoperative planning for, 610-611
　results of, 620-621
　room layout and instruments for, 611-612
　signature cases on, 622-625
　tips from masters on, 627
　tumor and vertebral body resection in, 616-617, 626
　vertebral body reconstruction and stabilization in, 618-619, 626
Thoracotomy
　anterolateral with median sternotomy-trapdoor incision, 598-599
　axillary (lateral), 600-601
　for intradural extramedullary tumors, 481
　posterolateral, 602-603
　　for Pancoast tumor, 576-577
　　　second-stage, 579, 580-581
　　　single-stage, 578, 579-580
TLSO, 145, 146
TNM staging system; see Tumor-node-metastasis staging system
Tobías, J.W., 565
Toileting, 142
Total en bloc spondylectomy
　single-stage thoracic, 719-732
　　approach for, 722
　　bailout technique for, 732
　　blunt dissection around vertebral body in, 724-725
　　clinical decision-making for, 720-721
　　cutting of pedicles and en bloc laminectomy in, 723-724
　　en bloc corpectomy in, 725-727
　　exposure in, 722, 723
　　indications for, 720
　　introduction of T-saw guide in, 722-723
　　outcomes of, 728

　　postoperative care and rehabilitation after, 727
　　preoperative embolization prior to, 721-722
　　preoperative evaluation for, 720
　　reconstruction in, 727
　　signature cases on, 728-731
　　technique of, 721-727
　　tips from masters on, 732
　two-stage thoracic/lumbar, 735-742
　　bailout techniques for, 742
　　clinical decision-making on, 736-737
　　indications and contraindications for, 735-736
　　outcomes of, 740
　　preoperative evaluation for, 736
　　signature case on, 741
　　technique of, 737-740
　　tips from masters on, 742
Total excisional surgery for spinal metastases, 59-60
Transarterial embolization; see Embolization
Transcervical approaches, 529-549
　bailout techniques with, 548
　clinical decision making on, 532-533
　indications and contraindications for, 530-531
　outcomes for, 542-543
　preoperative evaluation for, 531-532
　signature cases on, 546-547
　special considerations with, 547
　techniques for, 539-542
　tips from master on, 548-549
Transcervical-transmandibular approach, 542, 546
Transfer from sit to stand, 136, 138
Transglossal approach, 537
　for C2 tumors, 686, 697
Transiliac bar technique for reconstruction after sacrectomy, 782-783, 833, 834, 835, 837, 838-839
Transitional vertebra, 22
Translaminar screws for pediatric patients, 859-860, 865
Transmandibular-transcervical approach, 542, 546
Transmandibular-transglossal approach, 537-538
　for C2 tumors, 686
Transnasal approach, 538-539
Transoral approaches, 529-549
　bailout techniques with, 548
　for C2 tumors, 686-688, 697
　clinical decision making on, 532-533
　indications and contraindications for, 530-531
　outcomes for, 542-543

　preoperative evaluation for, 531-532
　signature cases on, 544-545
　special considerations with, 547
　techniques for, 533-539
　tips from master on, 548-549
Transoral circumglossal retropharyngeal approach for C2 tumors, 687-688
Transoral-transpharyngeal approach, 533-534
Transpalatal approach, 534-535
Transpedicular approach
　for anterior decompression and reconstruction, 745-756
　　bailout techniques on, 756
　　clinical decision-making on, 748
　　indications and contraindications for, 746-747
　　outcomes of, 751-752
　　preoperative evaluation for, 747
　　signature cases on, 753-755
　　technique for, 748-751
　　tips from masters on, 756
　for intradural extramedullary tumors
　　cervical, 481
　　thoracic, 482-483
Transpedicular corpectomy for C2 tumors
　indications and contraindications for, 679
　signature case on, 692-695
　technique of, 684
Transverse back flap, 122, 123
Transverse ligament, 6
Transverse processes
　of cervical vertebrae, 3
　of thoracic vertebrae, 11
Trapdoor approach
　anterolateral thoracotomy with, 598-599
　for Pancoast tumor, 577
Trapezius flap, 116-117
Trastuzumab derivative of maytansine-1 for breast cancer, 343
Trastuzumab emtansine for breast cancer, 343
Trastuzumab for breast cancer, 340, 342-343
Triangular frame reconstruction after sacrectomy, 835
Triple-negative breast cancer, 332
Triptorelin for prostate cancer, 355
T-saw laminoplasty, 487-495
　equipment for, 487-488
　outcomes of, 491-494
　position and exposure for, 488-489
　posterior arch reconstruction with, 491
　signature cases for, 492-494
　surgical approach for, 488
　technique of, 489
　tips from masters on, 495
　tumor removal during, 490-491
　vertebral artery during, 488
Tumoral cysts on MRI, 65

Tumor-node-metastasis staging system
  for breast cancer, 329, 330
  for Pancoast tumors, 566-568
  for renal cell carcinoma, 316-317
  for soft tissue sarcomas, 275, 276-277
Tyrosine kinase inhibitors
  for advanced non–small cell lung cancer, 306-309
  for renal cell carcinoma, 318

U

Ultrasound-guided biopsy, 416
Uncinate processes, 23
Uncovertebral joints, 22-23
Upper extremity bracing after surgery, 150
Upper sternal split, 594, 595-598
Upper third of back, 113, 114
  reconstructive surgery of, 115-118
Urinary incontinence, postoperative, 152-153

V

Vaccine therapy for prostate cancer, 359-362
Vascular endothelial growth factor
  in advanced non–small cell lung cancer, 306-308
  in breast cancer, 343
  in renal cell carcinoma, 318
Vascular supply
  of spinal cord, 31-33
  of vertebral column, 30-31
Vascular tumors, preoperative embolization of; see Embolization
Vascularity of tumor, 879-880
Vascularized fibula flap, 124
VATS; see Thoracoscopic spine surgery
VEGF
  in advanced non–small cell lung cancer, 306-308
  in breast cancer, 343
  in renal cell carcinoma, 318
Venous drainage
  of spinal cord, 32-33
  of vertebral column, 31
Ventral sacroiliac ligament, 21
Verocay bodies in schwannomas, 380, 381
Vertebra(e)
  anomalous number of, 22
  cervical, 3
  lumbar, 14
  plana, 226
  sacral, 19
  thoracic, 9-10
  transitional, 22
Vertebral artery, 551-562
  anatomy of, 32, 34
  anomalies of, 555-556
  in anterior approaches, 554, 555
  in anterolateral approaches, 552, 554
  bailout techniques for, 562
  balloon test occlusion of, 447-449, 552, 556-557
    evaluation prior to, 445-446
  with cervical nerve sheath tumors, 478-480
  in clinical decision-making, 551-554
  exposure and mobilization of, 558-560
  factors increasing risk of injury to, 555-556
  in lateral approaches, 554
  in posterior approaches, 554, 555
  release of extrinsic intermittent compression of, 554
  sacrifice of, 556-558
  surgery without exposure of, 554-555
  tips from masters on, 562
  transposition of, 561
Vertebral bodies, thoracic, 9-10
Vertebral body fracture after stereotactic radiosurgery, 105
Vertebral body screw placement in thoracoscopic spine surgery, 615-616
Vertebral column, vascular supply of, 30-31
Vertebrectomy, 268
  with anterior/posterior spine fusion for pediatric tumors, 868
Vertical rectus abdominis myocutaneous flap for sacroiliac and pelvic reconstruction, 783-784, 788
VHL; see von Hippel-Lindau syndrome/disease
VHLD; see von Hippel-Lindau syndrome/disease
Video-assisted thoracoscopic surgery; see Thoracoscopic spine surgery
Vinorelbine for advanced non–small cell lung cancer, 304
Vitamin B_{12} deficiency, subacute combined degeneration due to, 80, 81
Vocal cord paresis, 169
von Hippel-Lindau syndrome/disease, 73
  hemangioblastomas in, 401, 403, 404, 461
  and renal cell carcinoma, 314-315
VRAM flap for sacroiliac and pelvic reconstruction, 783-784, 788
V-Y gluteal advancement flap, 120, 121

W

Weinstein-Boriani-Biagini (WBB) staging system, 630
  for aneurysmal bone cysts, 226
  for cervical spine tumors, 706-707
  for osteosarcoma, 267
  for soft tissue sarcomas, 277, 278
WHO Zubrod Scale for advanced non–small cell lung cancer, 305
Wide resection, defined, 681, 780
Wiring for pediatric patients
  outcomes of, 865
  technique of, 860-861
Wolff's law, 40
World Health Organization Zubrod Scale for advanced non–small cell lung cancer, 305
Wound closure, 115
Wound coverage, primary vs. secondary, 114
Wound dehiscence, 124
Wound infection, 124-125, 881-882

X

Xanthomas, malignant fibrous, 278-279
Xanthosarcomas, 278-279

Z

Zellballen in paragangliomas, 398
Zoledronic acid
  for advanced non–small cell lung cancer, 309
  with androgen deprivation therapy, 362-363
  for breast cancer, 345
  for renal cell carcinoma, 319
Zubrod Scale for advanced non–small cell lung cancer, 305